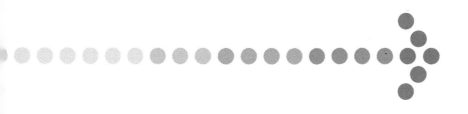

ACSM's
Resource Manual for
Guidelines
for Exercise Testing
and Prescription

FIFTH EDITION

SENIOR EDITOR

Leonard A. Kaminsky, PhD, FACSM
ACSM Program Director® Certified
ACSM Exercise Test Technologist® Certified
Human Performance Laboratory
Adult Fitness/Cardiac Rehabilitation Program
Ball State University
Muncie, Indiana

SECTION EDITORS

Kimberly A. Bonzheim, MS, FACSM
ACSM Program Director® Certified
Noninvasive Cardiology
William Beaumont Hospital
Royal Oak, Michigan

Carol Ewing Garber, PhD, RCEP®, FACSM
ACSM Program Director® Certified
ACSM Exercise Test Technologist® Certified
ACSM Health Fitness Instructor® Certified
Bouvé College of Health Sciences
Northeastern University
Boston, Massachusetts

Stephen C. Glass, PhD, FACSM
ACSM Exercise Specialist® Certified
Department of Movement Science
Grand Valley State University
Allendale, Michigan

Larry F. Hamm, PhD, FACSM
ACSM Program Director® Certified
ACSM Exercise Test Technologist® Certified
ACSM Exercise Specialist® Certified
Cardiac Rehabilitation Program
Neuroscience Center
National Rehabilitation Hospital
Washington, DC

Harold W. Kohl III, PhD, FACSM
Centers for Disease Control and Prevention
National Center for Chronic Disease Prevention and
Health Promotion
Division of Nutrition and Physical Activity
Physical Activity and Health Branch
Atlanta, Georgia

Alan Mikesky, PhD, FACSM
Department of Physical Education
Indiana University–Purdue University Indianapolis
Indianapolis, Indiana

ACSM's
RESOURCE MANUAL
FOR GUIDELINES
FOR EXERCISE
TESTING AND
PRESCRIPTION

FIFTH EDITION

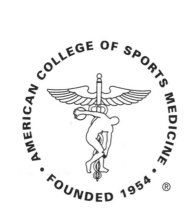

**AMERICAN COLLEGE
OF SPORTS MEDICINE**

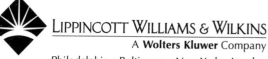

LIPPINCOTT WILLIAMS & WILKINS
A **Wolters Kluwer** Company

Philadelphia • Baltimore • New York • London
Buenos Aires • Hong Kong • Sydney • Tokyo

Acquisitions Editor: Peter Darcy
Managing Editor: Matthew J. Hauber
Marketing Manager: Christen D. Murphy
Production Editor: Jennifer Ajello/Sirkka E. H. Bertling
Designer: Risa Clow
Compositor: Seven Worldwide
Printer: Courier—Kendallville

ACSM's Publications Committee Chair: Jeffrey L. Roitman, EdD, FACSM
ACSM Group Publisher: D. Mark Robertson

351 West Camden Street
Baltimore, MD 21201

530 Walnut Street
Philadelphia, PA 19106

Printed in the United States of America

First Edition, 1988
Second Edition, 1993
Third Edition, 1998
Fourth Edition, 2001

Library of Congress Cataloging-in-Publication Data

American College of Sports Medicine.
   ACSM's resource manual for Guidelines for exercise testing and prescription / American College of Sports Medicine; [Leonard A. Kaminsky ... et al., editors].—5th ed. p. cm. Includes bibliographical references and index.
   ISBN 0-7817-4591-8

   1. Exercise therapy—Handbooks, manuals, etc. 2. Exercise tests—Handbooks, manuals, etc. I. Title: Resource manual for Guidelines for exercise testing and prescription. II. Kaminsky, Leonard A., 1955-III. American College of Sports Medicine. Guidelines for exercise testing and prescription. IC. Title.

RM725.R42 2005
615.8'2—dc22   2004063299

The publishers have made every effort to trace the copyright holders for borrowed material. If they have inadvertently overlooked any, they will be pleased to make the necessary arrangements at the first opportunity.

To purchase additional copies of this book, call our customer service department at **(800) 638-3030** or fax orders to **(301) 824-7390**. International customers should call **(301) 714-2324**.

Visit Lippincott Williams & Wilkins on the Internet: http://www.LWW.com. Lippincott Williams & Wilkins customer service representatives are available from 8:30 am to 6:00 pm, EST.

For more information concerning American College of Sports Medicine Certification and suggested preparatory materials, call **(800) 486-5643** or visit the American College of Sports Medicine web site **www.acsm.org**.

06 07 08 09
2 3 4 5 6 7 8 9 10

Foreword

It is with great pleasure that I introduce to you the fifth edition of the *American College of Sports Medicine's Resource Manual for Guidelines for Exercise Testing and Prescription*. For many years, this resource has served thousands of students and professionals as a valuable companion to the *ACSM Guidelines*. The editorial team members and individual chapter contributors have compiled a compendium of topics that not only extend the exercise and health related information provided in the *Guidelines*, but cover areas well beyond the scope of the *Guidelines*. Chapters are written by a prestigious group of scientists, clinicians, researchers and health/fitness practitioners. These pages contain the most current, science-based information regarding exercise and health.

There is no question that one of the greatest challenges facing our culture as we embark on the 21st century is the myriad of disorders associated with a sedentary lifestyle. While we have made substantial progress in understanding the risks associated with physical inactivity, we are far from the ultimate goal of having a society that is active at a level that promotes both health and longevity. We must continue to pursue effective strategies to mobilize the population to be more active. To achieve this goal, our society will likely benefit from a large cadre of clinical and health and fitness professionals who are thoroughly educated in the information and trained in the skills covered within this text.

As you will see, this revision of the *Resource Manual* has been reconfigured to provide a better link with content contained within the seventh edition of the *ACSM Guidelines*, enhancing its value within educational programs, and it is intended to expand upon the *Guidelines* by providing practical examples, and in most cases, offer a greater depth of coverage for each of the topics. This text has something for everyone, from serving as a primer for those in formal educational programs to serving as a science-based reference guide for the practicing professional. For this latter group, the content contained within this text can provide much needed continuing education on a wide range of topics.

So, I encourage you to venture into these pages and learn something new. No matter who your next patient or client may be, he or she will benefit from the insights you will gain from the authors of this text. Then share your new expertise and knowledge with colleagues. Together, you and other readers of the *ACSM's Resource Manual* can make a difference in the health of Americans—one step at a time!

Mitchell H. Whaley, Ph.D., FACSM

Preface

The American College of Sports Medicine (ACSM) first published *Guidelines for Exercise Testing and Prescription* in 1975. After the publication of the third edition of the *Guidelines*, ACSM issued the first edition of the *Resource Manual for Guidelines for Exercise Testing and Prescription* in 1988. The original purpose of the *Resource Manual* was to serve as a companion to the *Guidelines*, and this remains a fundamental purpose of the book. Additionally, it is recognized that the *Resource Manual* can and should serve as a valuable aide for professionals who provide exercise services for fitness, health, and clinical reasons and for those who teach courses that are preparatory for exercise-related careers.

Changes to the Fifth Edition

A number of significant changes have been made in this edition of the *Resource Manual*. First, the book was substantially reorganized with the number of sections reduced to seven (from 13) and the number of chapters reduced to 50 (from 80). Most of the content areas from the fourth edition were retained, however, material that was considered not to be "resourceful" for content included in the *Guidelines* was eliminated. The second change is the reduction of redundant presentation of material that already exists in the *Guidelines* or in other chapters within the *Resource Manual*. Readers will find many cross-references throughout this book, which direct them to relevant material presented elsewhere in the *Guidelines* or the *Resource Manual*. The third change is a significant reordering of the presentation of material to facilitate locating the relevant resource material for sections in the *Guidelines*. The introductory section (Section 0) presents the scientific foundations and bases for the principles of exercise testing and training. The following four sections (I. Lifestyle Factors Associated with Health and Disease; II. Physical Fitness and Clinical and Diagnostic Assessments; III. Exercise Prescription, Exercise Programming, and Adaptations to Exercise Training; and IV. Exercise Testing and Training for Individuals with Chronic Disease) correspond to the three sections in the *Guidelines* (Health Appraisal, Risk Assessment, and Safety of Exercise; Exercise Testing; and Exercise Prescription). The *Resource Manual* includes two additional sections of importance to exercise and allied health professionals: V. Human Behavioral Principles Applied to Physical Activity and VI. Exercise Program Administration. Additionally, new topics covered in the *Resource Manual* and those with increased emphasis are Chapter 8, Physical Activity Assessment; Chapter 17, Clinical Exercise Testing in Individuals with Disabilities Caused by Neuromuscular Disorders; Chapter 27, Applied Exercise Programming; Chapter 34, Exercise in Patients with End-Stage Renal Disease; Chapter 36, Arthritic Diseases and Conditions; Chapter 37, Neuromuscular Diseases and Exercise; Chapter 38, Immunological Conditions; Chapter 40, Channels for Delivering Behavioral Programs; and Chapter 45, Exercise Program Professionals and Related Staff.

New Features

In this edition, readers will find three new features in each chapter. A list of *Key Terms* and definitions is provided in each chapter, and these terms are highlighted in the text to assist readers in understanding key concepts. Each chapter also has a listing of *Selected Readings for Further Study*. Although the *Resource Manual* attempts to provide an in-depth overview of topics important to exercise testing and prescription, it is not possible to be completely comprehensive. Thus, we have provided recommendations for additional literature that will further readers' understanding of the material presented in the chapters. In some cases, the selected readings are textbooks or textbook chapters; however, we also have provided key references from journals. The third new feature is a list of recommended websites. We have identified websites with educational content related to the topics; however, some sites are more generally related to the topic area (e.g., professional organizations) where the reader may find multiple resources.

A major point of emphasis for the editorial team was to include the most current information available and to emphasize consensus reports when they are available. For example, the authors were encouraged to incorporate the main points from all position stands of the ACSM on topics related to the content of their chapters. Additionally, consensus scientific statements, reports from expert panels, and reports from other professional organizations were reviewed and referenced as appropriate. A listing of the reports referred to in this edition is provided at the end of the preface.

It was our intention that readers can derive a good understanding of the topic from the material presented in the *Resource Manual* and, when more in-depth knowledge is needed on a topic, readers are able to use the references to the consensus reports, selected readings, and websites.

Presentation of Knowledge, Skills, and Abilities

The past two editions of the *Resource Manual* provided a listing of specific knowledge, skills, and abilities (KSAs) at the beginning of each chapter. The ACSM Committee on Certification and Registry Boards (CCRB) performed a job task analysis survey in 2004 for all ACSM certifications and the registry. Results from this survey were used to supplement the review and revision of the KSAs. The CCRB determined that KSAs might need to be more dynamic to stay abreast with changes in knowledge and application of scientific and clinical information. Thus, this edition does not provide a direct link to specific KSAs because they may change from year to year. However, this edition of the *Resource Manual* does provide a listing of KSA content areas that are covered in each chapter to assist candidates in preparing for the ACSM Certification and Registry examinations.

Summary

We expect that the fifth edition of the *Resource Manual* will appeal to a broader audience than the previous editions because of its expanded content, reorganization, and new features. The fifth edition will certainly continue to be a valuable resource for ACSM certification and registry examination candidates and as a reference manual for those working in an occupation that uses exercise programming for health or clinical benefits. Many academic programs already use the *Guidelines* as a required text for the study of the effects of exercise and physical activity on health, fitness, and clinical outcomes, and we believe that the *Resource Manual* will be an excellent academic resource. With the simultaneous publication schedule, the reorganization of the *Resource Manual* to follow a similar topic order as the *Guidelines*, and the cross-linking of material between the *Guidelines* and the *Resource Manual*, this edition should appeal to instructors of a variety of classes in both undergraduate and graduate curricula as an excellent companion to the *Guidelines*.

Major Reports References in the Fifth Edition

CHAPTER 5

AHA/ACC guidelines for preventing heart attack and death in patients with atherosclerotic cardiovascular disease: 2001 update.

AHA Dietary Guidelines: Revision 2000: A statement for healthcare professionals from the Nutrition Committee of the American Heart Association.

AHA guidelines: Evidence-based guidelines for cardiovascular disease prevention in women.

AHA scientific statement: Exercise and physical activity in the prevention and treatment of atherosclerotic cardiovascular disease.

Summary of the scientific conference on dietary fatty acids and cardiovascular health. Conference summary from the Nutrition Committee of the American Heart Association.

Hormone replacement therapy and cardiovascular disease: a statement for healthcare professionals from the American Heart Association.

Implication of recent clinical trials for the National Cholesterol Education Program adult treatment panel III guidelines.

Third report of the National Cholesterol Education Program (NCEP) expert panel on detection, evaluation, and treatment of high blood cholesterol in adults. (Adult treatment panel III).

U.S. Department of Agriculture and U.S. Department of Health and Human Services: Nutrition and your health: dietary guidelines for Americans, 5th ed.

CHAPTER 6

ACCP/AACVPR Pulmonary Rehabilitation Guidelines Panel: Pulmonary rehabilitation: joint ACCP/AACVPR evidence-based guidelines.

AHA/ACSM: Recommendations for cardiovascular screening, staffing, and emergency policies at health/fitness facilities.

AHA: Resistance exercise in individuals with and without cardiovascular disease: benefits, rationale, safety and prescription.

American College of Sports Medicine: Position stand: Exercise and physical activity for older adults.

American College of Sports Medicine: Position stand: Exercise and type 2 diabetes.

American College of Sports Medicine: Position stand: Osteoporosis and exercise.

American College of Obstetricians and Gynecologists: Exercise during pregnancy and the postpartum period.

American Diabetes Association: Physical activity/exercise and diabetes mellitus.

Exercise standards for testing and training: A statement for healthcare professionals from the American Heart Association.

National High Blood Pressure Education Program: The seventh report of the Joint National Committee on Detection, Evaluation, and Treatment of High Blood Pressure (JNC VII).

CHAPTER 7

U.S. Department of Health and Human Services. Physical activity and health: a report of the Surgeon General.

AHA Guidelines for Primary Prevention of Cardiovascular Disease and Stroke: 2002 Update: Consensus panel guide to comprehensive risk reduction for adult patients without coronary or other atherosclerotic vascular diseases. American Heart Association Science Advisory and Coordinating Committee.

CHAPTER 8

Measurement of Physical Activity: The Cooper Institute Conference Series. Proceedings from the 9th Measurement and Evaluation Symposium.

Physical activity and public health: a recommendation from the Centers for Disease Control and Prevention and the American College of Sports Medicine.

CHAPTER 9

ACOG Practice Bulletin: Clinical management guidelines for obstetrician-gynecologists. Osteoporosis.

AHA Dietary Guidelines: Revision 2000: A statement for healthcare professionals from the Nutrition Committee of the American Heart Association.

American College of Endocrinology: Position statement of insulin resistance syndrome.

American Heart Association guide for improving cardiovascular health at the community level: A statement for public health practitioners, healthcare providers, and health policy makers from the American

Heart Association expert panel on population and prevention science.

The Expert Committee on the Diagnosis and Classification of Diabetes Mellitus. Report of the expert committee on the diagnosis and classification of diabetes mellitus.

Expert Panel on the Identification, Evaluation, and Treatment of Overweight and Obesity in Adults: Clinical guidelines on the identification, evaluation, and treatment of overweight and obesity in adults.

Institute of Medicine, National Academy of Sciences: Dietary reference intakes energy, carbohydrate, fiber, fat, fatty acids, cholesterol, protein and amino acids.

NIH Consensus Development Panel on Osteoporosis Prevention, Diagnosis, and Therapy: Osteoporosis prevention, diagnosis, and therapy.

Report of a Joint WHO/FAO Expert Consultation: Diet, nutrition and the prevention of chronic diseases.

Standing Committee on the Scientific Evaluation of Dietary Reference Intakes, Food and Nutrition Board, Institute of Medicine, National Academy of Sciences: Dietary reference intakes for calcium, phosphorus, magnesium, vitamin D, and fluoride.

Summary of the scientific conference on dietary fatty acids and cardiovascular health: Conference summary from the nutrition committee of the American Heart Association.

CHAPTER 10

Institute of Medicine: Dietary Reference Intakes [6 reports].

U.S. Departments of Agriculture and Health and Human Services. Nutrition and your health: Dietary guidelines for Americans, 5th edition.

CHAPTER 11

Cardiac rehabilitation: Clinical practice guidelines. Rockville, MD: Agency for Health Care Policy and Research and the National Heart, Lung and Blood Institute.

U.S. Department of Health and Human Services: Mental health: a report of the Surgeon General.

U.S. Department of Health and Human Services Office of Public Health and Science: Healthy people 2010 objectives.

CHAPTER 13

American College of Sports Medicine: Position stand: The recommended quantity and quality of exercise for developing and maintaining cardiorespiratory and muscular fitness, and flexibility in healthy adults.

CHAPTER 14

American College of Sports Medicine: Position stand: Exercise and hypertension.

CHAPTER 15

American Thoracic Society: Standards for the diagnosis and care of patients with chronic obstructive pulmonary disease.

American Thoracic Society/American College of Chest Physicians: ATS/ACCP statement on cardiopulmonary exercise testing.

CHAPTER 16

ACC/AHA Guidelines for the clinical application of echocardiography. A report of the American College of Cardiology/American Heart Association Task Force on Practice Guidelines (Committee on

Clinical Application of Echocardiography). Developed in collaboration with the American Society of Echocardiography.

ACC/AHA 2002 guideline update for exercise testing: Summary article. A report of the American College of Cardiology/American Heart Association Task Force on Practice Guidelines.

ACC/AHH guidelines for exercise testing: A report of the American College of Cardiology/American Heart Association Task Force on Practice Guidelines (Committee on Exercise Testing).

American College of Cardiology/American Heart Association clinical practice guidelines: Part II (evolutionary changes in a continuous quality improvement project).

American Diabetes Association: Consensus development conference on the diagnosis of coronary heart disease in people with diabetes.

Guidelines for clinical use of cardiac radionuclide imaging. Report of the American College of Cardiology/American Heart Association Task Force on Assessment of Diagnostic and Therapeutic Cardiovascular Procedures (Committee on Radionuclide Imaging). Developed in collaboration with the American Society of Nuclear Cardiology.

26th Bethesda conference: Recommendations for determining eligibility for competition in athletes with cardiovascular abnormalities. Task Force 5: Coronary artery disease.

CHAPTER 17

Paralyzed Veterans of America: Fatigue and multiple sclerosis: evidence-based management strategies for fatigue in multiple sclerosis.

Paralyzed Veterans of America: Multiple sclerosis clinical practice guidelines. Disease modifying therapies in multiple sclerosis: evidence-based management strategies for disease modifying therapies in multiple sclerosis.

CHAPTER 18

ACC/AHA Guidelines for the Management of Patients with Acute Myocardial Infarction: 1999 Update: a report of the American College of Cardiology/American Heart Association Task Force on Practice Guidelines (Committee on Management of Acute Myocardial Infarction).

Air pollution and cardiovascular disease. A statement for healthcare professionals from the Expert Panel on Population and Prevention Science of the American Heart Association.

American Association of Cardiovascular and Pulmonary Rehabilitation: Guidelines for cardiac rehabilitation and secondary prevention programs.

Cardiovascular advisory panel guidelines for the medical examination of commercial motor vehicle drivers.

Exercise standards: a statement for healthcare professionals from the American Heart Association.

CHAPTER 19

ACC/AHA/ASE 2003 guideline update for the clinical application of echocardiography: a report of the American College of Cardiology/American Heart Association Task Force on Practice Guidelines (ACC/AHA/ASE Committee to Update the 1997 Guidelines for the Clinical Application of Echocardiography).

ACC/AHA/ASNC guidelines for the clinical use of cardiac radionuclide imaging: a report of the American College of Cardiology/American Heart Association Task Force on Practice Guidelines (ACC/AHA/ASNC Committee to Revise the 1995 Guidelines for the Clinical Use of Radionuclide Imaging).

ACC/AHA 2002 guideline update for exercise testing: a report of the American College of Cardiology/American Heart Association Task Force on Practice Guidelines (Committee on Exercise Testing).

ACC/AHA 2002 guideline update for the management of patients with chronic stable angina: a report of the American College of Cardiology/American Heart Association Task Force on Practice

Guidelines (Committee to Update the 1999 Guidelines for the management of Patients with Chronic Stable Angina).

CHAPTER 22

Statement on exercise: benefits and recommendations for physical activity programs for all Americans. A statement for health professionals by the Committee on Exercise and Cardiac Rehabilitation of the Council on Clinical Cardiology, American Heart Association.

CHAPTER 25

American College of Sports Medicine: Position stand: Exercise and physical activity for older adults.

American College of Sports Medicine: Position stand: Progression models in resistance training for healthy adults.

Resistance exercise in individuals with and without cardiovascular disease: benefits, rationale, safety, and prescription: An advisory from the Committee on Exercise, Rehabilitation, and Prevention, Council on Clinical Cardiology, American Heart Association; Position paper endorsed by the American College of Sports Medicine.

CHAPTER 26

American College of Sports Medicine: Position stand: Appropriate intervention strategies for weight loss and prevention of weight regain for adults.

National Athletic Trainers' Association: Position statement: Exertional heat illnesses.

National Athletic Trainers' Association: Position statement: Fluid replacement for athletes.

CHAPTER 28

American College of Sports Medicine: Heat and cold illnesses during distance running.

American College of Sports Medicine/American Heart Association Joint Position Statement: Automated external defibrillators in health/fitness facilities.

American Diabetes Association: Diabetes mellitus and exercise.

American Heart Association/American College of Sports Medicine Joint Scientific Statement: Recommendations for cardiovascular screening, staffing, and emergency policies at health/fitness facilities.

OSHA: The OSHA Bloodborne Pathogens Standard.

CHAPTER 29

AHA/ACC guidelines for preventing heart attack and death in patients with atherosclerotic cardiovascular disease: 2001 update. A statement for healthcare professionals from the American Heart Association and the American College of Cardiology.

27th Bethesda conference: Matching the intensity of risk factor management with the hazard for coronary disease events.

Writing Group for the Women's Health Initiative Investigators: Risks and benefits of estrogen plus progestin in healthy postmenopausal women: principal results from the Women's Health Initiative controlled trial.

CHAPTER 30

ACC/AHA guidelines for ambulatory electrocardiography: Executive summary and recommendations. A report of the American College of Cardiology/American Heart Association Task Force on Practice Guidelines (Committee to Revise the Guidelines for Ambulatory Electrocardiography).

ACC/AHA guidelines for coronary artery bypass graft surgery: Executive summary and recommendations: A report of the American College of Cardiology/American Heart Association Task Force on Practice Guidelines (Committee to Revise the 1991 Guidelines for Coronary Artery Bypass Graft Surgery).

ACC/AHA guidelines for the evaluation and management of chronic heart failure in the adult.

ACC/AHA guidelines for percutaneous coronary intervention: Executive summary and recommendations: a report of the American College of Cardiology/American Heart Association Task Force on Practice Guidelines (Committee to Revise the 1993 Guidelines for Percutaneous Transluminal Coronary Angioplasty).

ACC/AHA guidelines for the management of patients with ST-elevation myocardial infarction—Executive summary: a report of the American College of Cardiology/American Heart Association Task Force on Practice Guidelines (Writing Committee to Revise the 1999 Guidelines for the Management of Patients With Acute Myocardial Infarction).

ACC/AHA guideline update for the management of patients with unstable angina and non-ST-segment elevation myocardial infarction.

American College of Cardiology/American Heart Association Task Force on Practice Guidelines; European Society of Cardiology Committee for Practice Guidelines and Policy Conferences (Committee to Develop Guidelines for the Management of Patients with Atrial Fibrillation); North American Society of Pacing and Electrophysiology. ACC/AHA/ESC Guidelines for the Management of Patients with Atrial Fibrillation: Executive summary: a report of the American College of Cardiology/American Heart Association Task Force on Practice Guidelines and the European Society of Cardiology Committee for Practice Guidelines and Policy Conferences (Committee to Develop Guidelines for the Management of Patients with Atrial Fibrillation). Developed in collaboration with the North American Society of Pacing and Electrophysiology.

American College of Cardiology/American Heart Association Task Force on Practice Guidelines/North American Society for Pacing and Electrophysiology Committee to Update the 1998 Pacemaker Guidelines. ACC/AHA/NASPE 2002 guideline update for implantation of cardiac pacemakers and antiarrhythmia devices. Summary article: a report of the American College of Cardiology/American Heart Association Task Force on Practice Guidelines (ACC/AHA/NASPE Committee to Update the 1998 Pacemaker Guidelines).

American College of Cardiology; American Heart Association Task Force on Practice Guidelines. Committee on the Management of Patients with Chronic Stable Angina: ACC/AHA 2002 guideline update for the management of patients with chronic stable angina—Summary article: a report of the American College of Cardiology/American Heart Association Task Force on Practice Guidelines (Committee on the Management of Patients with Chronic Stable Angina).

American College of Sports Medicine: Position stand: Exercise and hypertension.

American Heart Association. Evidence-based guidelines for cardiovascular disease prevention in women.

American Heart Association Council on Clinical Cardiology Subcommittee on Exercise, Rehabilitation, and Prevention, American Heart Association Council on Nutrition, Physical Activity, and Metabolism Subcommittee on Physical Activity: Exercise and physical activity in the prevention and treatment of atherosclerotic cardiovascular disease: a statement from the Council on Clinical Cardiology (Subcommittee on Exercise, Rehabilitation, and Prevention) and the Council on Nutrition, Physical Activity, and Metabolism (Subcommittee on Physical Activity).

Cigarette smoking, cardiovascular disease, and stroke: a statement for healthcare professionals from the American Heart Association. American Heart Association Task Force on Risk Reduction.

Exercise standards for testing and training: a statement for healthcare professionals from the American Heart Association.

Guidelines for carotid endarterectomy.

Guidelines for the management of patients with valvular heart disease: executive summary. A report of the American College of Cardiology/American Heart Association Task Force on Practice Guidelines (Committee on Management of Patients with Valvular Heart Disease).

National Heart, Lung and Blood Institute, American College of Cardiology Foundation. Women's Ischemic Syndrome Evaluation: Current status and future research directions: report of the National Heart, Lung and Blood Institute workshop.

Prevention Conference VI: Diabetes and cardiovascular disease.

Principles for national and regional guidelines on cardiovascular disease prevention: A scientific statement from the World Heart and Stroke Forum.

Safety and utility of exercise testing in emergency room chest pain centers: An advisory from the Committee on Exercise, Rehabilitation, and Prevention, Council on Clinical Cardiology, American Heart Association.

CHAPTER 31

Cardiac rehabilitation clinic practice guidelines no. 17. Rockville, MD; U.S. Department Of Health And Human Services, Public Health Service Agency For Health Care Policy And Research And The National Heart, Lung And Blood Institute, 1995.

Resistance exercise individuals with and without cardiovascular disease: benefits, rationale, safety, and prescription: an advisory from the Committee on Exercise, Rehabilitation, and Prevention, Council on Clinical Cardiology, American Heart Association. 2000.

American College of Sports Medicine: Position stand: Progression models in resistance training for healthy adults. 2002.

CHAPTER 32

American College of Cardiology/American Heart Association Task Force on Practice Guidelines (Committee to Revise the 1995 Guidelines for the Evaluation and Management of Heart Failure); International Society for Heart and Lung Transplantation; Heart Failure Society of America. ACC/AHA Guidelines for the Evaluation and Management of Chronic Heart Failure in the Adult: Executive Summary A Report of the American College of Cardiology/American Heart Association Task Force on Practice Guidelines.

American College of Chest Physicians. Medical therapy for pulmonary arterial hypertension: ACCP evidence-based clinical practice guidelines.

American College of Chest Physicians. Screening, early detection, and diagnosis of pulmonary arterial hypertension: ACCP evidence-based clinical practice guidelines.

American College of Chest Physicians. Surgical treatments/interventions for pulmonary arterial hypertension: ACCP evidence-based clinical practice guidelines.

American Thoracic Society: Dyspnea: mechanisms, assessment, and management. A consensus statement.

American Thoracic Society Statement: Lung function testing: selection of reference values and interpretative strategies.

ATS Committee on Proficiency Standards for Clinical Pulmonary Function Laboratories: ATS statement: guidelines for the six-minute walk test.

ATS/ACCP statement on cardiopulmonary exercise testing.

Expert Panel Report 2: Guidelines for the diagnosis and management of asthma.

Global strategy for the diagnosis, management, and prevention of chronic obstructive pulmonary disease. NHLBI and WHO Global Initiative for Chronic Obstructive Lung Disease.

Pulmonary rehabilitation: Joint ACCP/AACVPR evidence-based guidelines. ACCP/AACVPR Pulmonary Rehabilitation Guidelines Panel. American College of Chest Physicians. American Association of Cardiovascular and Pulmonary Rehabilitation.

Standards for the diagnosis and care of patients with chronic obstructive pulmonary disease. American Thoracic Society.

CHAPTER 33

American Diabetes Association: Gestational diabetes mellitus: Position statement.

American Diabetes Association: Implications of the Diabetes Control and Complications Trial: Position statement.

American Diabetes Association: Implications of the United Kingdom Prospective Diabetes Study: Position statement.

American Diabetes Association: Physical activity/exercise and diabetes: Position statement.

American Diabetes Association: Standards of medical care in diabetes: Position statement.

Diabetes and cardiovascular disease: A Statement for Healthcare Professionals From the American Heart Association.

Report of the Expert Committee on the Diagnosis and Classification of Diabetes Mellitus.

CHAPTER 34

National Kidney Foundation. National Kidney Foundation practice guidelines for chronic kidney disease: evaluation, classification, and stratification.

CHAPTER 35

American College of Sports Medicine: Position stand: The female athlete triad.

National Osteoporosis Foundation. Physician's guide to prevention and treatment of osteoporosis.

National Institutes of Health: Osteoporosis prevention, diagnosis, and therapy. NIH Consensus Statement.

An update on the diagnosis and assessment of osteoporosis with densitometry. Committee of Scientific Advisors, International Osteoporosis Foundation.

U.S. Preventive Services Task Force: Clinical guidelines: screening for osteoporosis in postmenopausal women: recommendations and rationale.

CHAPTER 36

American College of Rheumatology: Guidelines for the management of rheumatoid arthritis.

The orthopaedic forum: NIH consensus statement on total knee replacement.

CHAPTER 38

World Health Organization consensus statement. Consultation on AIDS and sports.

CHAPTER 40

U.S. Department of Health and Human Services: Healthy people 2010: understanding and improving health.

CHAPTER 43

Depression in Primary Care: Volume 1. Detection and diagnosis. Clinical practice guideline.

Depression in primary care: Volume 2. Treatment of major depression. Clinical practice guideline.

CHAPTER 47

American College of Cardiology/American Heart Association: Guidelines for the evaluation and management of chronic heart failure in the adult.

American College of Cardiology/American Heart Association: Guidelines for the management of patients with acute myocardial infarction.

American College of Cardiology/American Heart Association: 2002 guidelines for the management of patients with chronic stable angina.

American Diabetes Association: Clinical practice recommendations: summary of revisions for the 2001 clinical practice recommendations.

Core components of cardiac rehabilitation/secondary prevention program.

Guidelines for preventing heart attack and death in patients with atherosclerotic cardiovascular disease: 2001 update: a statement for healthcare professionals from the AHA/ACC.

U. S. Department of Health and Human Services, Public Health Services, Agency for Health Care Policy and Research, and the National Heart, Lung and Blood Institute: Guide for smoking cessation specialists.

CHAPTER 49

American College of Sports Medicine and American Heart Association: Automated external defibrillators in health/fitness facilities.

American College of Sports Medicine and American Heart Association: Joint statement: Recommendations for cardiovascular screening, staffing, and emergency policies at health/fitness facilities.

Joint Commission on Accreditation of Healthcare Organizations, 1996: Comprehensive Accreditation Manual for Hospitals.

CHAPTER 50

American Association for Cardiovascular and Pulmonary Rehabilitation: Core competencies for cardiac rehabilitation specialists.

American Heart Association: Guidelines for cardiopulmonary resuscitation and emergency cardiac care.

American Heart Association: The AHA medical/scientific statement on cardiac rehabilitation programs.

American Heart Association: The AHA medical/scientific statement on exercise.

National Strength and Conditioning Association: Strength and conditioning professional standards and guidelines.

Acknowledgments

This section is probably the most difficult to write as there have been so many people that deserve recognition and thanks for their support of this project. I will make an earnest attempt to recognize all those that played a significant role, however, my thanks go out to many more unnamed individuals for their assistance. Also, the order of presentation of those mentioned is not based on their level of support or importance, as all played a significant role.

This is the fifth edition of this Resource Manual. I certainly want to recognize all those that contributed to this book in the past. Having such excellent content to work with made the revision process much easier. I want to especially thank Jeff Roitman, the Senior Editor of the third and fourth editions. Jeff's assistance and guidance with learning the editorial process was invaluable.

Thanks to Mitch Whaley, senior editor of the seventh edition of the ACSM's Guidelines for Exercise Testing and Prescription. You recruited your Associate Editors, Pete Brubaker and Bob Otto, wisely. I have so much respect for all three of you and appreciate you involving me in the editorial review sessions for the Guidelines, it certainly helped the Resource Manual editorial group understand the changes being made in the Guidelines and allowed us to develop content that resources that material.

Thanks to an outstanding group or Section Editors – Alan Mikesky, Bill Kohl, Larry Hamm, Steve Glass, Carol Garber, and Kim Bonzheim. I truly enjoyed working with all of you and appreciate your willingness to volunteer your time to this project. You are all so knowledgeable, talented, and passionate about your work. You did a great job recruiting excellent authors and guiding them through the writing process. I look forward to continued professional involvement with each of you in the future.

Thanks to all of the authors for your important contributions to this Resource Manual. The readers of this book will benefit greatly from your wisdom. Your willingness to volunteer your time and expertise is very much appreciated. Thanks also to all the reviewers for their helpful comments.

Thanks to the staff of our publisher, Lippincott, Williams, and Wilkins. I received excellent support and advice from Matt Hauber, Senior Managing Editor. Matt's promptness and expertise in handling my many queries was much appreciated. Thanks also to Sirkka Bertling, Production Editor, for her excellent assistance in getting this manuscript into the published form.

Thanks to Jeff Roitman, ACSM Publications Committee Chair and D. Mark Robertson, ACSM Assistant Executive Vice President, Publications, Editorial Services, Advancement, Membership & Chapter Services, and Pete Darcy, Executive Editor, WK Health/Lippincott Williams & Wilkins. Your behind the scenes administrative support was helpful to all of us involved with this project.

Thanks to all the dedicated professionals who work in programs that utilize physical activity and exercise to improve peoples' health and quality of life. Your understanding and support of the need for rigorous academic training for individuals who work in physical activity and exercise programs will ultimately payoff in improved quality of care for our patients and clients.

To my colleagues, students, and friends at Ball State University, thank you for your support during this writing and editorial project.

To my wife, Mary, and daughters, Lauren and Bonnie, thanks for your continual love, for helping me keep things in perspective, and for being understanding of my involvement in this project.

Lenny Kaminsky

Contributors

Leonard A. Kaminsky, PhD, FACSM
ACSM Program Director® Certified
ACSM Exercise Test Technologist® Certified
Human Performance Laboratory
Adult Fitness/Cardiac Rehabilitation Program
Ball State University
Muncie, Indiana

Kent Adams, PhD, FACSM
Exercise Physiology Lab
University of Louisville
Louisville, Kentucky

Simon Bacon, PhD
Department of Psychiatry
Duke University Medical Center
Durham, North Carolina

Rafael E. Bahamonde, PhD, FACSM
Department of Physical Education
Indiana University–Purdue University Indianapolis
Indianapolis, Indiana

Susan G. Beckham, PhD, FACSM, RCEP®
ACSM Program Director® Certified
ACSM Exercise Test Technologist® Certified
Noninvasive Cardiology
Dallas VA Medical Center
Dallas, Texas

Valerie Bishop, PhD, RCEP®
ACSM Health Fitness Instructor® Certified
ACSM Exercise Specialist® Certified
Independent Consultant
Ojai, California

James A. Blumenthal, PhD
Department of Psychiatry
Duke University Medical Center
Durham, North Carolina

Clinton A. Brawner, CES
ACSM Exercise Specialist® Certified
Preventive Cardiology
Henry Ford Hospital
Detroit, Michigan

Suzanne Brodney-Folse, PhD, RD
Department of Community Health
Brown University
Providence, Rhode Island

Cedric X. Bryant, PhD, FACSM
Educational Services
American Council on Exercise
Redmond, Washington

Barbara N. Campaigne, PhD, FACSM
Diabetes and Endocrine Platform Team
Eli Lilly and Company
Indianapolis, Indiana

Brian Carlin, MD
Division of Pulmonary and Critical Care Medicine
Drexel University
Philadelphia, Pennsylvania

Ruth Ann Carpenter, MS, RD, LD
Cooper Institute
Dallas, Texas

Cynthia Castro, PhD
Stanford Prevention Research Center
Stanford University School of Medicine
Stanford, California

Heather O. Chambliss, PhD
The Cooper Institute
Southaven, Mississippi

Timothy Church, MD, MPH, PhD
Center for Medical & Laboratory Research
Cooper Institute
Dallas, Texas

Christopher B. Cooper, MD, FRCP, FACSM, FCCP
ACSM Health Fitness Director® Certified
Departments of Medicine and Physiology
UCLA—David Geffen School of Medicine
Los Angeles, California

Kerry S. Courneya, PhD
Faculty of Physical Education
University of Alberta
Edmonton, Alberta

Joel T. Cramer, PhD, HFI; CSCS,*D; NSCA-CPT, *D
ACSM Health Fitness Instructor® Certified
Department of Kinesiology
The University of Texas at Arlington
Arlington, Texas

Tim L.A. Doyle, MSc, CSCS
Exercise Biomechanics
University of Notre Dame Australia
Fremantle WA Australia

Eric L. Dugan, PhD
Biomechanics Laboratory
Ball State University
Muncie, Indiana

Andrea Dunn, PhD, FACSM
Klein Buendel, Inc.
Golden, Colorado

Gregory B. Dwyer, PhD, FACSM, RCEP®
ACSM Program Director® Certified
ACSM Exercise Specialist® Certified
ACSM Exercise Test Technologist® Certified
Movement Studies and Exercise Science Department
East Stroudsburg University
East Stroudsburg, Pennsylvania

Kyle Ebersole, PhD
Department of Human Movement Science
University of Wisconsin, Milwaukee
Milwaukee, Wisconsin

Jonathan K. Ehrman, PhD, FACSM
ACSM Program Director® Certified
ACSM Exercise Specialist® Certified
Department of Preventive Cardiology
Henry Ford Heart & Vascular Institute
Detroit, Michigan

Eve V. Essery, PhD
Department of Nutrition and Food Sciences
Texas Woman's University
Denton, Texas

Tammy K. Evetovich, PhD, FACSM
ACSM Health Fitness Instructor® Certified
Department of Health, Human Performance and Sport
Wayne State College
Wayne, Nebraska

Brian W. Findley, MEd
Health Sciences Department
Palm Beach Community College
Boca Raton, Florida

Shannon J. Fitzgerald, PhD
Department of Kinesiology, Health Promotion, &
Recreation
University of North Texas
Denton, Texas

Carl Foster, PhD, FACSM
ACSM Program Director® Certified
Department of Exercise and Sport Science
University of Wisconsin-LaCrosse
LaCrosse, Wisconsin

Barry A. Franklin, PhD, FACSM
ACSM Program Director® Certified
ACSM Exercise Specialist® Certified
Preventive Cardiology
Beaumont Health Center
Royal Oak, Michigan

Neil F. Gordon, MD, PhD, FACSM
Center for Heart Disease Prevention
St. Joseph's/Candler Health System
Savannah, Georgia

B. Sue Graves, EdD, FACSM
ACSM Health Fitness Instructor® Certified
Department of Exercise Science and Health Promotion
Florida Atlantic University
Davie, Florida

Suzanne L. Groah, MD, MSPH
Rehabilitation Research and Training Center on
Secondary Conditions after Spinal Cord Injury
National Rehabilitation Hospital
Washington, DC

Larry R. Gurchiek, PhD
Department of Health, Physical Education, & Leisure
Studies
University of South Alabama
Mobile, Alabama

Chad Harris, PhD
Department of Kinesiology
Boise State University
Boise, Idaho

David L. Herbert, JD
Herbert and Benson, Attorneys at Law
Canton, Ohio

William G. Herbert, PhD, FACSM
ACSM Program Director® Certified
Department of Human Nutrition, Foods, and Exercise
Virginia Polytechnic Institute and State University
Blacksburg, Virginia

Brendan Humphries, PhD
School of Science and Primary Industries
Charles Darwin University
Darwin, Northern Territory, Australia

Kurt Jackson, PhD, GCS
Kettering Medical Center
Kettering, Ohio

Anthony S. Kaleth, PhD, RCEP®
ACSM Program Director® Certified
ACSM Health Fitness Instructor® Certified
ACSM Exercise Specialist® Certified
Department of Physical Education
Indiana University–Purdue University Indianapolis
Indianapolis, Indiana

Peter T. Katzmarzyk, PhD, FACSM
School of Physical and Health Education
Queen's University
Kingston, Ontario

NiCole Keith, PhD
Department of Physical Education
Indiana University–Purdue University Indianapolis
Indianapolis, Indiana

Steven John Keteyian, PhD,FACSM, RCEP®
Henry Ford Heart & Vascular Institute
Detroit, Michigan

Abby King, PhD, FACSM
Training Program
Stanford University School of Medicine
Palo Alto, California

Duane V. Knudson, PhD, FACSM
Department of Kinesiology
California State University, Chico
Chico, California

John E. Kovaleski, PhD
Department of Health & Physical Education
University of South Alabama
Mobile, Alabama

Len Kravitz, PhD
ACSM Health Fitness Instructor® Certified
Department of Physical Performance & Development
University of New Mexico
Albuquerque, New Mexico

Jessica Krenkel, MS, RD, CNSD
Division of Medical Nutrition
University of Nevada School of Medicine
Reno, Nevada

Doina Kulick, MD
Division of Medical Nutrition
University of Nevada School of Medicine
Reno, Nevada

Richard Mearl Lampman, PhD, FACSM
Department of Surgery
St. Joseph Mercy Hospital
Ann Arbor, Michigan

John A. Larry, MD
Division of Cardiology
The Ohio State University Medical Center
Columbus, Ohio

Richard F. Leighton, MD
Medical College of Ohio
Toledo, Ohio

Beth Lewis, PhD
Health Partners Research Foundation
Minneapolis, Minnesota

Bess H. Marcus, PhD
Division of Behavioral Medicine
The Miriam Hospital
Providence, Rhode Island

John E. Martin, PhD
Department of Psychology
San Diego State University
San Diego, California

Sara McGlynn, MBA, CPA
Cardiology
William Beaumont Hospital
Royal Oak, Michigan

Stephen P. Messier, PhD, FACSM
Department of Health & Exercise Science
Wake Forest University
Winston-Salem, North Carolina

Aryan N. Mooss, MD
Division of Cardiology
Creighton University School of Medicine
Omaha, Nebraska

James R. Morrow, Jr., PhD, FACSM
Department of Kinesiology, Health
Promotion & Recreation
University of North Texas
Denton, Texas

Janet A. Mulcare, PhD, FACSM
Department of Physical Therapy
Andrews University
Berrien Springs, Michigan

Melissa A. Napolitano, PhD
Centers for Behavioral and Preventive Medicine
Brown Medical School and the Miriam Hospital
Providence, Rhode Island

David L. Nichols, PhD, FACSM
Department of Kinesiology
Texas Woman's University
Denton, Texas

David C. Nieman, DrPH, FACSM
Department of Health, Leisure and Exercise Science
Appalachian State University
Boone, North Carolina

Nancy E. O'Hare, ScD, FACSM
Cardiovascular Division
Beth Israel Deaconess Medical Center
Boston, Massachusetts

Patricia Painter, PhD, FACSM
Department of Physiological Nursing
University of California at San Francisco
San Francisco, California

Albert Washington Pearsall IV, MD
Department of Orthopaedic Surgery
University of South Alabama Medical Center
Mobile, Alabama

Laura Peno-Green, MD, FCCP
Marietta Pulmonary Medicine
Marietta, Georgia

James A. Peterson, PhD, FACSM
Healthy Learning
Monterey, California

John P. Porcari, PhD, FACSM, RCEP®
ACSM Program Director® Certified
Department of Exercise and Sport Science
University of Wisconsin-La Crosse
LaCrosse, Wisconsin

Judith J. Prochaska, PhD, MPH
Department of Psychiatry
University of California, San Francisco
San Francisco, California

Jeanne E. Ruff, MS
Cardiovascular Rehab and Health Promotion
Peninsula Regional Medical Center
Salisbury, Maryland

Khaleel Salahudeen, MD
Pulmonary Laboratory
Allegheny General Hospital
Pittsburgh, Pennsylvania

James F. Sallis, PhD, FACSM
Department of Psychology
San Diego State University
San Diego, California

Robert Scales, PhD
Albuquerque, New Mexico

Stephen F. Schaal, MD
Division of Cardiology
The Ohio State University Medical Center
Columbus, Ohio

John Schairer, DO
Advanced Cardiovascular Health Specialists
Livonia, Michigan
Henry Ford Heart & Vascular Institute
Detroit, Michigan

Lois Sheldahl, PhD
Veteran's Administration Medical Center
Milwaukee, Wisconsin

Ray W. Squires, PhD, FACSM
ACSM Program Director® Certified
ACSM Exercise Specialist® Certified
Division of Cardiovascular Diseases & Internal Medicine
Mayo Clinic and Foundation
Rochester, Minnesota

Satchiko St. Jeor, PhD
Division of Medical Nutrition
University of Nevada School of Medicine
Reno, Nevada

Stephen J. Tharrett, MS
Club Corps of America
Dallas, Texas

Larry S. Verity, PhD, FACSM
ACSM Exercise Specialist® Certified
Department of Exercise & Nutritional Sciences
San Diego State University
San Diego, California

Stella Lucia Volpe, PhD, RD, FACSM
ACSM Exercise Specialist® Certified
Department of Nutrition
University of Massachusetts
Amherst, Massachusetts

Janet P. Wallace, PhD, FACSM
ACSM Program Director® Certified
ACSM Exercise Specialist® Certified
Adult Fitness Program
Indiana University
Bloomington, Indiana

Joe P. Weir, PhD, FACSM
Department of Physical Therapy
Des Moines University
Des Moines, Iowa

Michael Whitehurst, EdD, FACSM
Department of Exercise Science & Health Promotion
Florida Atlantic University
Davie, Florida

Jessica Whiteley, PhD
The Centers for Behavioral and Preventative Medicine
Brown Medical School/The Miriam Hospital
Providence, Rhode Island

Reviewers

Committee on Certification and Registry Boards (CCRB) Reviewers

Dalynn Badenhop, PhD, FACSM
Medical College of Ohio
Toledo, Ohio

Madeline Paternostro-Bayles, PhD, FACSM
Indiana University of Pennsylvania
Indiana, Pennsylvania

Clinton Brawner, BS
ACSM Exercise Specialist® Certified
Henry Ford Hospital
Detroit, Michigan

Virginia Byers-Kraus, MD, PhD
Duke University Medical Center
Durham, North Carolina

Shala Davis, PhD, FACSM
ACSM Program Director® Certified
ACSM Exercise Specialist® Certified
East Stroudsburg University
East Stroudsburg, Pennsylvania

Adam De Jong, MA
ACSM Exercise Specialist® Certified
William Beaumont Hospital
Oxford, Michigan

Shawn Drake, PhD
ACSM Program Director® Certified
ACSM Exercise Specialist® Certified
Arkansas State University
State University, Arkansas

Greg Dwyer, PhD, FACSM
East Stroudsburg University
East Stroudsburg, Pennsylvania

Jon Ehrman, PhD, FACSM
ACSM Program Director® Certified
ACSM Exercise Specialist® Certified
Henry Ford Hospital
Detroit, Michigan

Tonya Goyal, PhD
Duke University
Durham, North Carolina

Bryan Haddock, PhD, RCEP®
ACSM Health Fitness Director® Certified
ACSM Health Fitness Instructor® Certified
California State University, San Bernardino
San Bernardino, California

Mark Ketterer, PhD
Henry Ford Hospital
Detroit, Michigan

Steven Keteyian, PhD, FACSM, RCEP®
Henry Ford Hospital
Detroit, Michigan

Matthew Vukovich, PhD, FACSM
South Dakota State University
Brookings, South Dakota

Chris Womack, PhD, FACSM
ACSM Exercise Specialist® Certified
Michigan State University
East Lansing, Michigan

External Reviewers

Rick Albrecht, PhD
Grand Valley State University
Allendale, Michigan

Bryan Blissmer, PhD
University of Rhode Island
Kingston, Rhode Island

David R. Brown, PhD, FACSM
Centers for Disease Control and Prevention
Atlanta, Georgia

Lee Brown, EdD, FACSM
ACSM Health Fitness Instructor® Certified
California State University, Fullerton
Fullerton, California

Marilyn A. Cairns, ScD
Northeastern University
Boston, Massachusetts

Bernard Clark, MD, FACC
St. Francis Hospital and Medical Center/
University of Connecticut Medical School
Hartford, Connecticut

Gerilynn Connors, BS, RRT
Inova Fairfax Hospital
Falls Church, Virginia

Dino G. Costanzo, MS, RCEP®
ACSM Exercise Test Technologist® Certified
ACSM Program Director® Certified
New Britain General Hospital
New Britain, Connecticut
Bradley Memorial Hospital
Southington, Connecticut

Ronald Davis, PhD
Ball State University
Muncie, Indiana

JoAnn Eickhoff-Shemek, PhD, FACSM, FAWHP
ACSM Exercise Test Technologist® Certified
ACSM Health Fitness Director® Certified
ACSM Health Fitness Instructor® Certified
University of South Florida
Tampa, Florida

Pamala K. Gandolfi, BS
ACSM Exercise Specialist® Certified
MidMichigan Medical Center
Houghton Lake, Michigan

Anne M. Gavic, MPA
ACSM Exercise Specialist® Certified
ACSM Exercise Test Technologist® Certified
Evanston Northwestern Healthcare
Evanston, Illinois

Ernest V. Gervino, PhD, FACSM
Beth Israel Deaconess Medical Center/
Harvard Medical School
Boston, Massachusetts

Fred Goss, PhD, FACSM
ACSM Program Director® Certified
University of Pittsburgh
Pittsburgh, Pennsylvania

Brian Hatzel, PhD
Grand Valley State University
Allendale, Michigan

Gregory W. Heath, DHSc, MPH, FACSM
ACSM Program Director® Certified
Centers for Disease Control and Prevention
Atlanta, Georgia

Laurie Hoffman-Goetz, PhD, MPH, FACSM
University of Waterloo
Waterloo, Ontario
Canada

Edward S. Horton, MD
Joslin Diabetes Center—Harvard Medical School
Boston, Massachusetts

Terry Housh, PhD, FACSM
University of Nebraska
Lincoln, Nebraska

Deborah A. Jones, PhD
Centers for Disease Control and Prevention
Atlanta, Georgia

Carol Kennedy, MS
ACSM Health Fitness Instructor® Certified
Indiana University
Bloomington, Indiana

C. Dexter Kimsey, PhD
Centers for Disease Control and Prevention
Atlanta, Georgia

Shel Levine, MS, MSA, CES
ACSM Exercise Specialist® Certified
ACSM Exercise Test Technologist® Certified
Eastern Michigan University
Ypsilanti, Michigan

Melinda Manore, PhD, RD, FACSM
Oregon State University
Corvallis, Oregon

Michelle Maynard, PhD
Centers for Disease Control and Prevention
Atlanta, Georgia

Timothy S. Maynard, MSS
ACSM Program Director® Certified
Providence Hospital
Mobile, Alabama

Kay N. Mikesky, MS, HFI
ACSM Health Fitness Instructor® Certified
Factual Fitness
Zionsville, Indiana

Wayne C. Miller, PhD, FACSM
George Washington University
Washington, DC

Mark S. Nash, PhD, FACSM
University of Miami School of Medicine
Miami, Florida

David Nieman, DrPh, FACSM
Appalachian State University
Boone, North Carolina

Donald Nicholas, PhD
Ball State University
Muncie, Indiana

Claudio Nigg, PhD
University of Hawai'i at Manoa
Honolulu, Hawai'i

Jeffrey Pauline, EdD
Ball State University
Muncie, Indiana

Timothy Quinn, PhD, FACSM
ACSM Exercise Specialist® Certified
University of New Hampshire
Durham, New Hampshire

Deborah Riebe, PhD, FACSM
ACSM Health Fitness Instructor® Certified
University of Rhode Island
Kingston, Rhode Island

Sanjeeb Sapkota, MD, MPH
Centers for Disease Control and Prevention
Atlanta, Georgia

Andrea J. Speight-Watson, RN, MSN
ACSM Exercise Specialist® Certified
William Beaumont Hospital
Royal Oak, Michigan

Thomas W. Storer, PhD
Division of Health Sciences, El Camino College
Torrance, California

Katherine W. Tauney, PhD, FACSM
University of North Carolina
Chapel Hill, North Carolina

Mark G. Urtel, EdD
Indiana University–Purdue University Indianapolis
Indianapolis, Indiana

Mitchell H. Whaley, PhD, FACSM
ACSM Program Director® Certified
Ball State University
Muncie, Indiana

Andrea T. White, PhD, FACSM
University of Utah Health Sciences Center
Salt Lake City, Utah

Mary Yoke, MA, MM
Adelphi University
Long Island, New York

Contents

Section 0 Scientific Foundations for Exercise Testing and Prescription

Section Editor: Alan Mikesky, PhD, FACSM

Section I Lifestyle Factors Associated with Health and Disease

Section Editor: Harold W. Kohl III, PhD, FACSM

Section II Physical Fitness and Clinical and Diagnostic Assessments

Section Editor: Larry F. Hamm, PhD, FACSM

Section III Exercise Prescription, Exercise Programming, and Adaptations to Exercise Training

Section Editor: Stephen C. Glass, PhD, FACSM

Scientific Foundations for Exercise Testing and Prescription

SECTION EDITOR: ALAN MIKESKY, PhD, FACSM

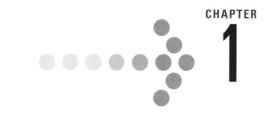

Functional Anatomy

RAFAEL BAHAMONDE AND ANTHONY S. KALETH

Anatomical Position and Definitions of Anatomical Locations and Planes

The **anatomical position** is the universally accepted reference position used to describe regions and spatial relationships of the human body and to make reference to body positions (e.g., joint motions). In the anatomical position, the body is erect with feet together and the upper limbs hanging at the sides, palms of the hands facing forward, thumbs facing away from the body, and fingers extended (Fig. 1-1). Other common anatomical terms and definitions are shown in Table 1-1.

Another useful tool used to describe anatomical motions are the body planes, or **planes of motion**. There are three basic imaginary planes that pass through the body. The *sagittal plane* divides the body or structure into the right and left sides. The *frontal* or *coronal plane* divides the body or structure into anterior and posterior portions. The *transverse plane* (also called the *cross-sectional* or *horizontal plane*) divides the body or structure into superior and inferior portions (Fig. 1-2). Table 1-1 lists some terms commonly used to reference anatomical spatial relationships.

Cardiovascular Anatomy

GENERAL COMPONENTS AND FUNCTIONS

The cardiovascular system is a continuous closed arrangement that includes a pump (the heart) and more than 60,000 miles of conduits (blood vessels)[1]. The primary function of the cardiovascular system is to provide an environment for the transport of nutrients and removal of waste products. The cardiovascular system assists with maintenance of homeostasis at rest and during exercise.

The cardiovascular system performs the following specific functions[2–4]:

1. Transports oxygenated blood from the lungs to tissues and deoxygenated blood from the tissues to the lungs
2. Distributes nutrients (e.g., glucose, free fatty acids, amino acids) to cells
3. Removes metabolic wastes (e.g., carbon dioxide, urea, lactate) from the periphery for elimination or reuse
4. Regulates pH to control acidosis and alkalosis
5. Transports hormones and enzymes to regulate physiological functions
6. Maintains fluid volume to prevent dehydration
7. Maintains body temperature by absorbing and redistributing heat

The following sections provide an overview of the basic structures and functions of the heart and blood vessels.

Heart

Location and General Landmarks

The adult heart is approximately the size of a fist and weighs between 250 and 350g[5]. The heart is positioned obliquely within the thoracic cavity in a space known as the *mediastinum* (Fig. 1-3). It is anterior to the vertebral column and posterior to the sternum. The lungs flank the heart bilaterally and slightly overlap it.

The heart has four chambers. The two superior chambers are the *atria*, and the two inferior chambers are the *ventricles*. The external deep grooves of the heart (called *sulci*) define the boundaries of the four chambers of the heart[4,6]. The coronary sulcus separates the atria from the ventricles; the interventricular sulcus separates the left

KEY TERMS

Agonist: Muscle or muscle group that is the prime mover of an exercise or activity

Anatomical position: The universally accepted reference position used to describe regions and spatial relationships of the human body and to make reference to body positions.

Antagonist: Muscle or muscle group that opposes the actions of the prime movers

Appendicular skeleton: All of the bones other than those of the axial skeleton that are found in the limbs of the body

Axial skeleton: The bones of the skeleton that form the central or supportive core, including the bones of the skull, vertebral column, ribs, and sternum

Contractile proteins: Specialized proteins found within muscle cells that interact with one another to cause muscle force production. The contractile proteins are actin and myosin.

Joints: The articulations between bones, typically classified according to structure as being fibrous, cartilaginous, or synovial (synovial joints are the most common in the body)

Muscle fiber architecture: The orientation of the muscle fibers (i.e., cells) to the longitudinal axis of the muscle. Terms commonly used to describe muscle fiber architecture include fusiform or longitudinal, pennate, unipennate, bipennate, and multipennate.

Planes of motion: Perpendicularly arranged planes that divide the human body and can be used to describe various body movements. The three planes of motion are commonly known as the sagittal, frontal, and transverse planes.

Regulatory proteins: Specialized proteins found within muscle cells that block the binding of the contractile proteins to one another and thus keep the muscle in a relaxed state. The regulatory proteins are troponin and tropomyosin.

Respiratory membrane: The membrane formed by the walls of alveoli and capillaries as they come in contact with one another in the lungs. The significance of the respiratory membrane is that this is where diffusion of oxygen and carbon dioxide occurs within the lungs.

Sliding-filament theory: The theory that describes how muscles shorten during contraction. In brief, specialized contractile proteins within the muscle cells interact such that they slide over one another rather than physically changing length during contractions.

Synergist: Muscle or muscle group that assists the agonist in performing an exercise or activity

Ventilation: The act of breathing in which air is moved into and out of the lungs. Inspiration and expiration are the processes that enable ventilation to occur.

---

and right ventricles (LV, RV). The sulci also contain the major arteries and veins that provide circulation to the heart.

The heart has a base and an apex. The base of the heart consists mainly of the left atrium (LA), part of the right atrium (RA), and parts of the proximal portion of the large veins that enter the heart posteriorly. The base is located superiorly and near the right sternal border at the level of second and third ribs. The apex of the heart is located inferiorly and to the left of the base at the level of the fifth intercostal space. Approximately two thirds of the mass of the heart is to the left of the midsternal border. As the heart is palpated at the apex (between the fifth and sixth ribs), the contraction can be easily felt. This is referred to as the *point of maximal intensity (PMI)*[3].

The heart also has borders. The superior border consists of both atria and the bases of the pulmonary trunk and the aorta. The right border is formed by the RA. The left border consists of the LV and a small part of the LA. The inferior border is formed primarily by the RV and a portion of the LV at the apex.

The heart is rotated to the left in the chest so that the anterior portion of the heart forms the sternocostal surface, which consists mainly of the RA and RV. The diaphragmatic surface consists mainly of the LV where it slopes and rests on the diaphragm.

Tissue Coverings and Layers of the Heart

The heart is covered by a double-walled, loose-fitting membranous sac called the *pericardium* (Fig. 1-4). The outer wall of the pericardium, the parietal pericardium, has both a fibrous (tough) layer and a serous (smooth) layer. The fibrous layer serves to strengthen the pericardium and anchor it within the mediastinum. The thin serous layer adheres to the fibrous layer of the parietal pericardium and forms a tight covering over the heart surface. This serous

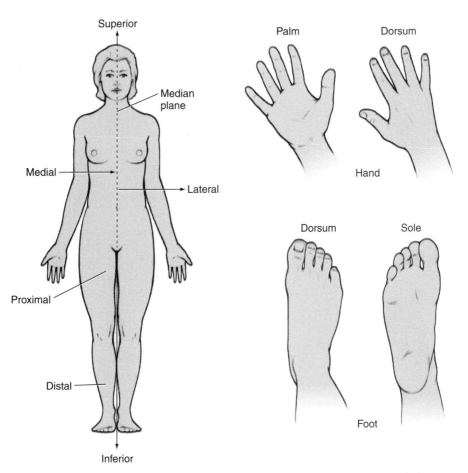

FIGURE 1-1. Anatomical position: the body is erect with the feet together, with the upper limbs hanging at the side, palms or the hands facing forward, thumbs facing away from the body, and fingers extended. Typically, all anatomical references to the body relate to this position.

covering is called the visceral pericardium, or *epicardium*. Between the parietal and visceral layers is the *pericardial cavity*. The pericardial cavity contains *pericardial fluid*, which acts as a lubricant, reducing friction between the membranes during contractions. If the pericardium becomes inflamed, *pericarditis*, a condition characterized by painful adhesions, can result.

The thickest layer of tissue in the heart is the *myocardium*. The myocardium is composed of cardiac

muscle. Within the myocardium is a network of criss-crossing dense connective tissue fibers called the *cardiac skeleton*. This cardiac skeleton provides insertion points for the fibers of the cardiac musculature, support for the valves of the heart, and some separation between the atria and the ventricles.

The inner layer of the myocardium is lined with a thin layer of endothelium called the *endocardium*. The endocardium forms the innermost lining of the walls of the various heart chambers as well as the heart valves. The endocardium joins with the endothelial linings of the blood vessels as they leave and enter the heart[7].

TABLE 1-1. Definitions of Anatomical Locations

Term	Definition
Anterior	The front of the body; ventral
Deep	Below the surface
Distal	Farthest away from any reference point
Inferior	Away from the head; lower
Lateral	Away from the midline of the body; to the side
Medial	Toward the midline of the body
Posterior	The back of the body; dorsal
Proximal	Closer to any reference point
Superficial	Located close to or on the body surface
Superior	Toward the head; higher

Heart Chambers, Valves, and Blood Flow

The heart is two pumps in a single unit with four chambers or cavities: the RA, LA, RV, and LV (Fig. 1-5). The right heart (RA and RV) and the left heart (LA and LV) make up the two pumps. The right side of the heart collects blood from the periphery and pumps it through the lungs (pulmonary circuit). The left side of the heart collects blood from the lungs and pumps it throughout the body (systemic circuit)[8–12].

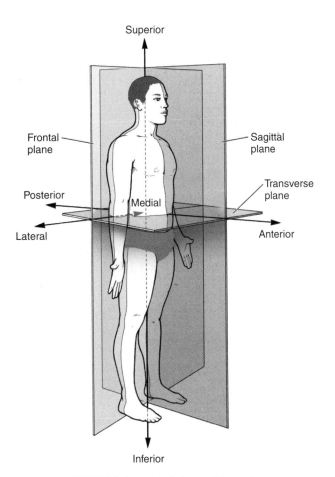

FIGURE 1-2. Anatomical planes of the body.

The atria of the heart are separated by the *interatrial septum* and the ventricles, by the *interventricular septum*. The atria are smaller and have thinner walls than the ventricles. The LV walls and interventricular septum are two to three times thicker than the RV walls. The thicker myocardium of the LV allows the left side of the heart to pump blood against the greater resistance offered by the large vascular tree that makes up the systemic circuit. Conversely, the RV only has to pump blood a relatively short distance through the pulmonary circuit.

The heart has four valves whose function is to maintain unidirectional blood flow. The *AV valves* separate the atria from the ventricles. The *semilunar valves* separate the ventricles from the aorta and pulmonary artery trunk. The AV valves are named for the number of leaflets, or *cusps*, formed by the endocardium (Fig. 1-6). Whereas the right AV valve has three cusps and is called the *tricuspid valve*, the left AV valve has only two cusps and is called the *bicuspid (or mitral) valve*. The tricuspid valve controls the flow of blood from the RA to the RV, and the mitral valve controls blood between the LA and LV. The cusps of the AV valves are attached to *chordae tendineae* (strong fibrous bands) that extend from the *papillary muscles*. The papillary muscles arise from folds and ridges of the myocardium that project into the ventricular chambers. During ventricular contraction, the papillary muscles shorten, thus pulling the chordae tendineae taut and preventing the AV valves from swing-

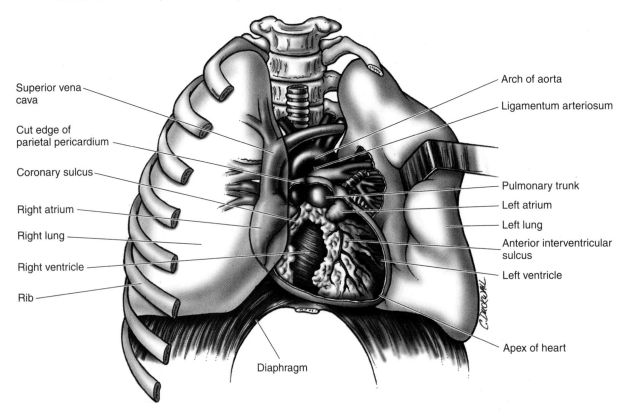

FIGURE 1-3. Anterior view of the thorax showing the position of the heart in the mediastinum.

ing back into the atria, thus preventing retrograde blood flow during ventricular contraction[13].

There are two semilunar valves in the heart, each with three cusps. The *pulmonary valve* lies between the RV and the pulmonary artery. The *aortic valve* is located between the LV and the aorta. The cusps of the semilunar valves prevent the backflow of blood from the arteries to the ventricles.

Blood flow through the heart is accomplished by the following sequence of events, beginning with the return of systemic blood to the RA:

1. Venous blood flows into the RA via the superior and inferior vena cava, coronary sinus, and anterior cardiac veins.
2. The RA free wall (contractile section of the RA heart wall) contracts, and blood moves through the tricuspid valve into the RV.
3. The RV free wall contracts, the tricuspid valve closes, and blood flows through the pulmonary valve into the pulmonary artery and the branches of that system.
4. Blood ultimately reaches the alveolar capillaries, where gas exchange occurs.
5. Blood flows back to the LA via the pulmonary veins.
6. The LA free wall contracts, and blood flows through the bicuspid valve and into the LV.

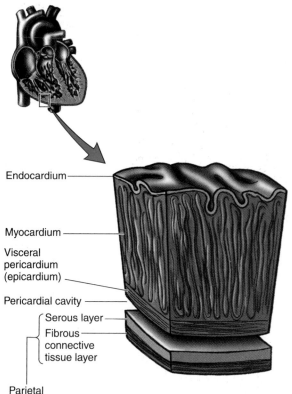

Endocardium

Myocardium

Visceral pericardium (epicardium)

Pericardial cavity

Serous layer

Fibrous connective tissue layer

Parietal pericardium

FIGURE 1-4. The endocardium, myocardium, and pericardium.

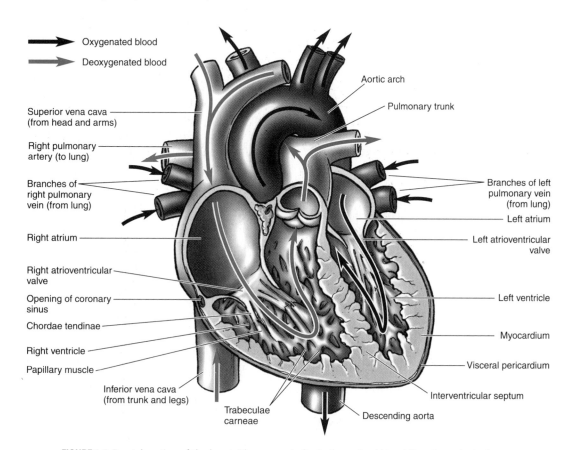

Oxygenated blood

Deoxygenated blood

Aortic arch

Pulmonary trunk

Superior vena cava (from head and arms)

Right pulmonary artery (to lung)

Branches of right pulmonary vein (from lung)

Branches of left pulmonary vein (from lung)

Left atrium

Right atrium

Left atrioventricular valve

Right atrioventricular valve

Opening of coronary sinus

Left ventricle

Chordae tendinae

Myocardium

Right ventricle

Visceral pericardium

Papillary muscle

Inferior vena cava (from trunk and legs)

Interventricular septum

Trabeculae carneae

Descending aorta

FIGURE 1-5. Frontal section of the heart. The *arrows* indicate the path of blood flow through the heart.

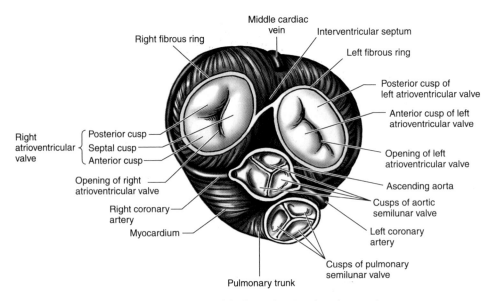

FIGURE 1-6. Superior view of the heart showing the valve openings.

7. The LV free wall contracts, the bicuspid valve closes, and blood flows through the aortic valve into the aorta and its branches, where it is distributed to the coronary circulation and the systemic circulation[13–16].

Heart Blood Supply

Although the interiors of the heart chambers are continuously bathed with blood, only the endocardium is nourished directly. The myocardium is too thick to permit adequate diffusion of nutrients and oxygen to the cardiac muscle cells and epicardium. The functional supply of blood for the heart is delivered via the *left* and *right coronary arteries (LCA, RCA)* (Figs. 1-7 and 1-8). The coronary arteries arise from the *aortic sinus* at the base of the aorta just superior to the semilunar valve cusps of the aortic valve (Fig. 1-9).

The LCA angles toward the left side of the heart for about 1 to 2 cm before branching into the *left anterior descending (LAD)* coronary artery and the *circumflex artery (CxA)*[17]. The LAD artery supplies blood to the interventricular septum and anterior walls of both ventricles. The CxA branches toward the left margin of the heart in the coronary sulcus and supplies blood to the laterodorsal walls of the LA and LV. Both the LAD artery and CxA curve around the left ventricular wall and supply small branches that interconnect (*anastomose*) with the RCA.

The RCA supplies blood to the right side of the heart as it follows the AV groove before curving to the back of the heart, giving off a *posterior interventricular artery* (*posterior descending artery*, or *PDA*). The RCA and PDA have numerous branches that supply blood to the anterior, posterior, and lateral surfaces of the RV and to the RA.

After blood circulates through the coronary artery system, which ends at the myocardial capillaries, it is collected by the cardiac veins. The blood then travels a path similar to that of the coronary arteries but in the opposite direction. On the posterior aspect of the heart, the cardiac veins form an enlarged vessel, the *coronary sinus*, which empties the blood into the RA. Some smaller anterior cardiac veins also empty directly into the RA.

Conduction System of the Heart

Cardiac muscle has intrinsic properties that allow it to depolarize and contract without neural stimulation. Cardiac cells interconnect end to end and form *intercalated discs*[2]. These intercalated discs allow electrical impulses to spread from cell to cell and cause the myocardium to act as a single unit or functional *syncytium*. The components of the heart's conduction system include the sinoatrial (SA) node, the AV node, AV bundle (bundle of His), right and left bundle branches, and the Purkinje fibers (Fig. 1-10).

The electrical impulse, which initiates cardiac contraction, begins at the *SA node*, or intrinsic pacemaker, of the heart. The cells of the SA node, which lie in the wall of the RA near the opening of the superior vena cava, depolarize spontaneously about 60 to 80 times per minute at rest[18]. From the SA node, the electrical impulse spreads via internodal gaps through both atria until it reaches the *AV node*, in the inferior part of the interatrial septum. The electrical impulse is delayed at the AV node for approximately 0.13 seconds to allow the atria to contract and fill the ventricles[18]. The impulse then moves rapidly through the *AV bundle of His*, through the *right and left bundle branches*, and through the network of *Purkinje fibers* in the myocardium of both ventricles. The Purkinje fibers

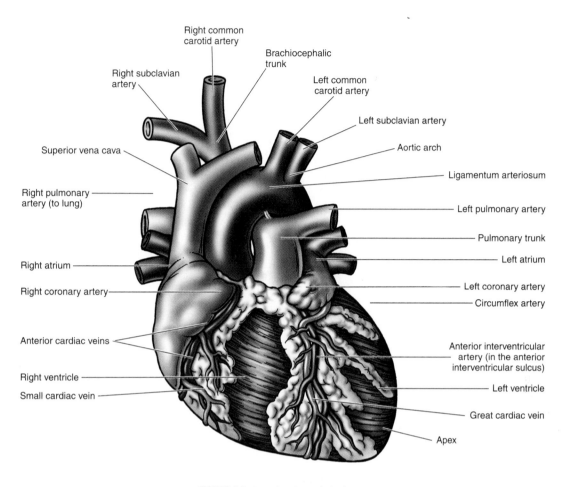

FIGURE 1-7. Anterior view of the heart.

are specialized fast-conducting cells that allow rapid conduction to the ventricles. This rapid conduction allows the ventricles to contract at approximately the same time.

The rate and forcefulness of heart contraction does not depend on intrinsic nerve stimulation but rather are influenced by extrinsic factors, such as autonomic nerve control and hormone activity. Sympathetic nerves and hormones (e.g., norepinephrine and epinephrine) stimulate the atria and ventricles of the heart to beat faster (*chronotropic effect*) and more forcefully (*inotropic effect*). Parasympathetic nerves (vagi) control the atria and slow the heart rate.

Blood Vessels

After blood flows from the heart, it enters the vascular system, which is composed of numerous blood vessels. The blood vessels form a closed system to deliver blood to the tissues; help promote the exchange of nutrients, metabolic wastes, hormones, and other substances with the cells; and ultimately return blood back to the heart.

Arteries carry blood away from the heart (Fig. 1-11). Large arteries branch into smaller arteries and eventually to smaller *arterioles*. Arterioles branch into capillaries,

which allow the exchange of blood with various tissues (e.g., digestive system, liver, kidneys). On the venous side of the circulation, capillaries converge into small *venules*, which converge to form larger vessels called *veins*. The large veins (e.g., superior and inferior vena cava, pulmonary veins) return blood to the heart.

The walls of the various blood vessels vary in thickness and size because of the presence or absence of one or more layers of tissues (Fig. 1-12). The *tunica intima* consists of the endothelium and a thin connective tissue basement membrane. The tunica intima is the only layer common to all of the blood vessels. The internal elastic lamina separates the tunica intima from the middle layer of smooth muscle fibers and elastic fibers known as the *tunica media*. The smooth muscle fibers of the tunica media can be influenced by neural control (parasympathetic and sympathetic nerves), hormones (e.g., acetylcholine, norepinephrine, epinephrine), or local factors (e.g., pH, oxygen levels, carbon dioxide levels), which can cause them to vasoconstrict or vasodilate. The external elastic lamina separates the tunica media from the outermost layer of connective tissue called the *tunica adventitia (externa).* The adventitia helps attach vessels to surrounding tissues[4].

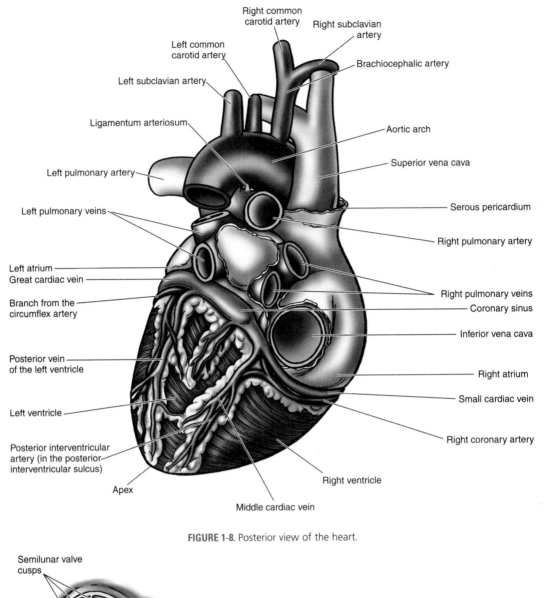

FIGURE 1-8. Posterior view of the heart.

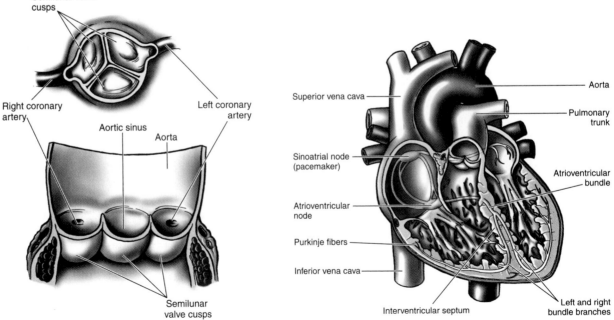

FIGURE 1-9. The origin of the coronary arteries.

FIGURE 1-10. The electrical conduction system of the heart.

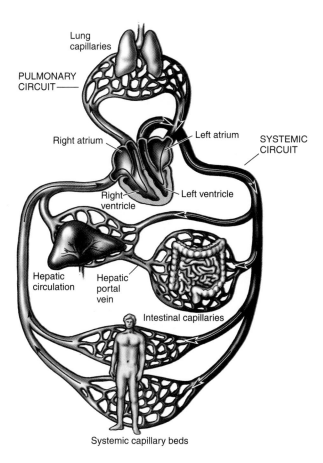

FIGURE 1-11. Schematic diagram of blood circulation.

Arteries

Arteries can be classified as *elastic* or *muscular* according to their size and function. Large arteries such as the aorta and those of the pulmonary trunk are called elastic arteries. The tunica media of these vessels is thick and contains many elastic fibers (see Fig. 1-12). The elastic nature of these arteries helps maintain pressure within the vessels. Other smaller arteries distribute blood throughout the body. These arteries are called muscular arteries, and their tunica media contains primarily smooth muscle fibers. Muscular arteries are less distensible than elastic arteries.

Arterioles

Arterioles are very small microscopic arteries that deliver blood to the capillaries. They have lumens smaller than 0.5 mm, and their tunica media is largely composed of smooth muscle with scattered elastic fibers[4]. Arterioles play a major role in regulating blood flow to the capillaries because of their ability to vasoconstrict or vasodilate. Also, changes in arteriole diameter can affect systemic blood pressure (BP).

Capillaries

Capillaries are also microscopic vessels that connect the arterioles with the venules. Capillaries form dense networks that branch throughout all tissues. The average capillary is 1 mm in length and 0.01 mm in diameter. This is just large enough for a single red blood cell to pass through[3] (Fig. 1-12). Capillaries have extremely thin walls made of a single layer of cells and a basement membrane. In contrast to the other blood vessels, capillaries do not have a tunica media or tunica adventitia. This unique characteristic of capillaries allows for the exchange of materials between blood and the tissue cells.

Venules and Veins

Venules, which form from capillaries, consist mainly of tunica intima and tunica adventitia. Venules collect blood from capillaries. *Veins* receive blood from the

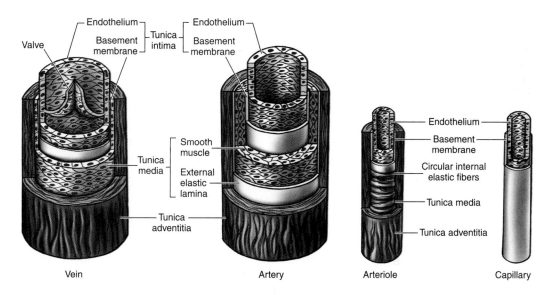

FIGURE 1-12. Comparison of the structure of blood vessels.

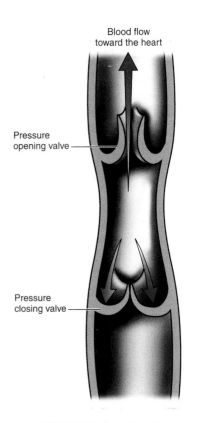

FIGURE 1-13. Valves of a vein.

ANATOMICAL SITES FOR BLOOD PRESSURE AND HEART RATE DETERMINATION

Measurement of arterial BP before, during, and after an exercise test or training session is routine. The systolic and diastolic BPs (SBP and DBP) are taken to ensure patient safety and to obtain important diagnostic and prognostic information. The most common method used for determination of BP is brachial artery auscultation. The brachial artery courses through a groove formed by the bifurcation of the triceps and biceps brachii muscles on the medial aspect (inside) of the arm. (Fig. 1-14).

Exercise professionals may measure peripheral pulses to obtain an index of resting heart rate, training bradycardia, or aerobic exercise intensity. Large, superficial arteries are preferable for pulse determination because they are easily palpable. Two conventional palpation sites are the common carotid and radial arteries. The right and left common carotid arteries are located on the anterior portion of the neck in the groove formed by the larynx (Adam's apple) and the sternocleidomastoid muscles (large muscles on the lateral sides of the neck) just below the mandible (lower jaw)[1]. The radial artery courses deep on the lateral (thumb side) aspect of the forearm and becomes superficial near the distal head of the radius[1]. Radial pulses may be difficult to obtain in individuals with large amounts of subcutaneous fat over the palpation site. Pulses may be taken at any arterial site. Other arterial palpation sites include temporal (temple region of skull), popliteal (behind the knee), femoral (inguinal fold of groin), and dorsal pedis (top of foot). Lower extremity pulses may provide information regarding the adequacy of peripheral blood flow.

venules and have the same three tissue layers as arteries. However, the tunica media of the veins is thinner than that found in the arteries. In general, the veins are thinner and more compliant than arteries and act as blood reservoirs. The walls of some veins, such as those in the legs, contain one-way valves that help maintain venous return to the heart by preventing retrograde blood flow even under relatively low pressures (Fig. 1-13). The valves in the veins are made up of folds of tunica intima (endothelium) and are similar in nature to the semilunar valves of the heart. A special type of vein formed by a thin layer of endothelial cells surrounded with dense connective tissue for support is called a *venous sinus* (e.g., coronary sinus of the heart).

At rest, most (60%) of the blood volume is in veins and venules, which is why they are called blood reservoirs. Capillaries hold only about 5% of the blood volume, and arteries and arterioles hold about 15%. Blood stored in the veins and venules can be quickly redistributed to the arterial side via vasoconstriction, which is caused by smooth muscle located in the venous walls. The muscle pump provided by increased skeletal muscle activity, such as during exercise, can also assist in redistribution of the venous blood, thereby providing greater blood volume to the active muscles.

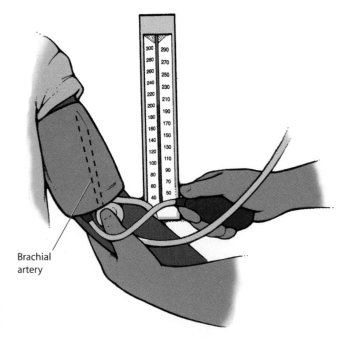

FIGURE 1-14. Positions of the stethoscope head and pressure cuff.

SUMMARY

In summary, the cardiovascular system is a closed system of pumps, valves, and conduits that coordinate to function both anatomically and physiologically to maintain a constant internal environment (see Chapter 3). The heart is a hollow, four-chambered organ that works with the circulatory system to pump blood through elastic blood vessels to the lungs and systemic circulation. The compliance and elasticity of these blood vessels helps maintain BP at rest and during exercise. In times of increased cardiovascular work, the cardiovascular system functions in an even more sophisticated manner to meet those demands while it continues to maintain BP and meet tissue demand requirements.

Respiratory Anatomy

GENERAL COMPONENTS AND FUNCTIONS

This section describes the basic anatomy of the respiratory system as it relates to function. The lungs of an average-sized person weigh about 1 kg. However, if spread out, the tissue would occupy an approximate surface area of 70 m^2 (750 ft^2), which is roughly the size of a handball court[1]. The anatomy of the respiratory system supports the basic function of exchanging carbon dioxide (CO_2), a byproduct of cellular metabolism, and oxygen (O_2), which is necessary for cellular activity[19]. Other important functions include production and metabolism of vasoactive substances and filtering systemic venous blood before entry into the LV. The structural components of the respiratory system (Fig. 1-15) are the framework for the corresponding functions of the system (Table 1-2)[20,21].

The respiratory system consists of two major divisions, the upper and lower respiratory tracts. Functionally, the respiratory system can be separated in two portions: the *conducting portion*, which is a system of interconnecting cavities and tubes (i.e., nose, mouth, pharynx, larynx, trachea, bronchi), and the *respiratory portion*, where the exchange of gases occurs (e.g., respiratory bronchioles, alveolar ducts, and alveoli) (Figs. 1-15, 1-16).

Upper Respiratory Tract

The upper respiratory tract, which includes the nose, paranasal sinuses, pharynx, and larynx (see Fig. 1-15), acts as a conduction pathway for the movement of air

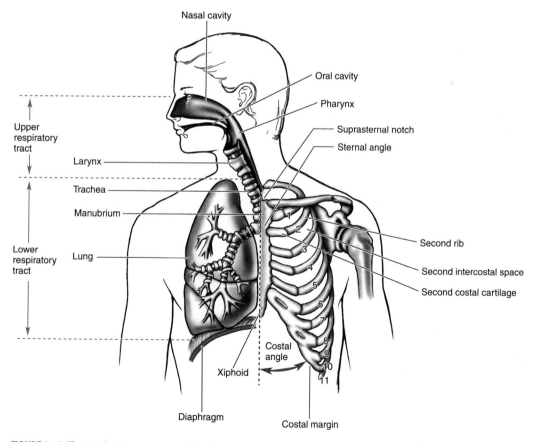

FIGURE 1-15. The respiratory system consists of an upper respiratory tract (nose, pharynx, and larynx) and a lower respiratory tract (tracheobronchial tree and lungs).

TABLE 1-2. Structural Components of the Respiratory System and Their Corresponding Function

Structural Components	Function
Respiratory center	Control of breathing
Peripheral chemoreceptors	
Afferent and efferent nerves	
Upper respiratory tract	Distribution of ventilation
Conducting airways	
Respiratory bronchioles	
Chest wall, respiratory muscles, and pleura	Ventilatory pump
Pulmonary arteries, capillaries, and veins	Distribution of blood flow
Functional respiratory unit	Gas exchange
Mucociliary escalator	Bronchial clearance
Alveolar macrophages	
Lymphatic drainage	Lung clearance and defense

into the lower respiratory tract. The function of these structures is to purify, warm, and humidify ambient air before it reaches the gas exchange units. During normal quiet breathing, inspired air is heated to body temperature and the relative humidity is increased to more than 90% during passage through the nose. Outside air goes into the nasal cavity via the nostrils. As air enters the nostrils, it passes through the vestibule, which is lined with skin that has coarse hairs that help filter out large dust

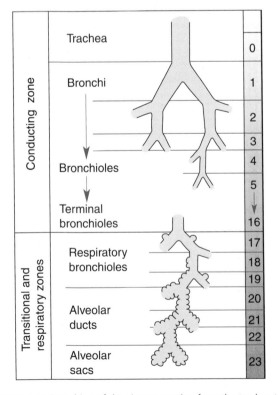

FIGURE 1-16. Branching of the airways starting from the trachea to the alveolar sacs. There are approximately 23 generations of branching in the tracheobronchial tree.

particles. Air is then moved to the upper nasal cavity. The upper nasal cavity is lined with a membrane rich in capillaries, which are responsible for warming the air. *Mucus* secreted by cells moistens the air and trap dust particles. Mucus is removed by the cilia in the pharynx, where it is eliminated from the respiratory tract via swallowing or spitting. The pharynx or throat is a funnel-shaped tube about 13 cm long that begins at the internal nares (internal nostrils), anterior to the cervical vertebrae and posterior to the nasal and oral cavities and larynx. The pharynx is made of skeletal muscles and lined with mucous membrane. It functions to serve as a passage for air and food and serves as a resonating chamber for speech. The pharynx is divided by the soft palate into the *nasopharynx* and the *oropharynx*. The *epiglottis*, located at the base of the tongue, protects the laryngeal opening during swallowing. The *larynx*, or voice box, contains the vocal cords, which contribute to speech and participate in coughing, and connects the pharynx with the next respiratory organ, the trachea, which is the first organ of the lower respiratory tract.

Lower Respiratory Tract

The lower respiratory tract begins in the *trachea* (windpipe) just below the larynx and includes the bronchi, bronchioles, and alveoli (see Figs. 1-15 and 1-16.). There are approximately 23 generations of airways; the first 16 are conducting airways, and the last seven are respiratory airways ending in approximately 300 million alveoli, which form the gas exchange surface. The structural components of the airways match their functional properties. For example, whereas the volume of the conducting zone is approximately 1 mL of air per pound of body weight and does not contribute to gas exchange, the areas where gas exchange occurs occupy a proportionately greater volume in the lungs.

Trachea

The trachea, or windpipe, begins at the base of the neck and extends approximately 10 to 12 cm to an internal ridge called the *carina* (see Fig. 1-15), where it divides into the right and left main bronchi. It is anterior to the esophagus, extending from the larynx to about the fifth thoracic vertebra. The trachea consists of a series of anteriorly located horseshoe-shaped cartilaginous rings, which are closed posteriorly by a longitudinal muscle bundle. The mucous membrane of the carina is highly sensitive and is associated with the cough reflex.

Bronchi and Bronchioles

At the sternal angle, the trachea divides into *right and left primary bronchi*, which branch into the right and left lung, respectively. The major bronchi contain cartilage that maintains the free passage of air as well as large numbers

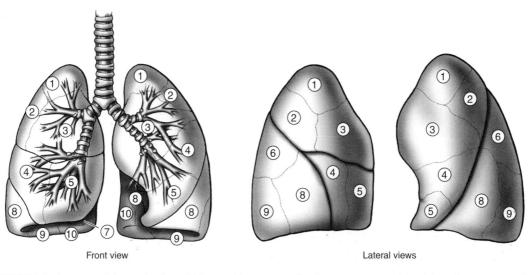

FIGURE 1-17. Structure of the tracheobronchial tree with corresponding lung segments, which originate from segmental bronchi. The right upper lobe contains segments 1 to 3, the right middle lobe contains segments 4 and 5, and the right lower lobe contains segments 6 to 10. The left upper lobe contains segments 1 to 5, and the left lower lobe contains segments 6 to 10.

of mucous glands that produce secretions in response to irritation, infection, or inflammation. Once in each lung, the primary bronchi divide into smaller bronchi called *secondary (lobar) bronchi* because they go to each of the lobes of the lungs (three lobes in the right lung and two on the left lung) (Figs. 1-16 and 1-17). The secondary bronchi continue to branch into *tertiary (segmental) bronchi* (10 on the right and 10 on the left), then *bronchioles*, and end in *terminal bronchioles*. Beyond the terminal bronchioles are respiratory bronchioles, alveolar ducts, and the alveoli (see Figs. 1-16 and 1-17). This branching is commonly referred as the *bronchial tree*. The structural makeup of the bronchial tree changes as it extends to its terminal branches. The C-shaped cartilage rings in the airway walls are gradually replaced by smaller plates of cartilage and then totally disappear in the bronchioles. Smooth muscles make up more of the airway wall as the cartilage decreases. In addition, the inside layer of epithelium experiences structural changes as there is a transition to squamous cells in the alveoli. This transition of the epithelium is important to facilitate gas exchange.

Alveoli

Respiratory bronchioles subdivide into *alveolar ducts*, which lead to *alveolar sacs* with alveoli. Alveolar sacs are air spaces or openings shared by two or more alveoli. *Alveoli* are cup-shaped pouches lined with type I and II epithelium surrounded by a thin elastic membrane for support. The *Respiratory (alveolar-capillary) Membrane* consists of the alveolar epithelium; the interstitium, containing the basement membrane, and the pulmonary capillary endothelial cells (Fig. 1-18). Type II epithelial cells, found primarily at the junctions of alveolar walls, produce *surfactant*. A thin layer of surfactant lines the

alveolus and functions to lower the surface tension in the alveolus. This helps to keep the alveolus open and to prevent collapse.

Respiratory Gas Exchange

Gas exchange occurs by way of two anatomical structures, the functional respiratory unit and the alveolus. As illustrated in Figure 1-19, a terminal bronchiole enters the center of the functional respiratory unit accompanied by

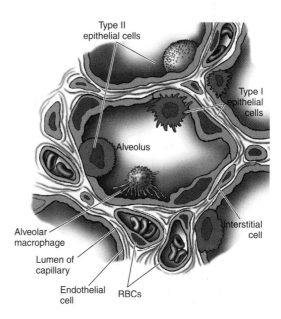

FIGURE 1-18. The major cells of the alveolus include epithelial cells (types I and II), endothelial cells of the pulmonary capillary, and alveolar macrophages. Also shown are lumen of capillary with red blood cells (RBCs).

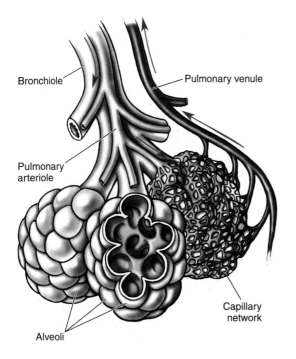

FIGURE 1-19. The functional respiratory unit. It consists of a bronchiole and corresponding blood supply; the pulmonary arteriole carries deoxygenated blood, and the pulmonary venule carries oxygenated blood. The rich capillary network supplies the alveoli for the purpose of gas exchange.

a pulmonary arteriole carrying deoxygenated blood from the body tissues and muscles. The arteriole divides into a rich network of pulmonary capillaries that lie adjacent to the alveolar walls and then drain into pulmonary venules and veins.

The exchange of respiratory gases takes place by passive diffusion across the respiratory membrane. The respiratory membrane wall is very thin, about 0.5 μm in thickness and 1/16 the diameter of a red blood cell (RBC). The combination of a large surface area and a thin respiratory membrane make for rapid diffusion of the respiratory gases into and out of the blood.

Blood Supply to the Lungs

The pulmonary circulation is a low-pressure system with a normal mean pressure of approximately 15 mm Hg at rest. The lungs receive blood from the pulmonary arteries, which contain systemic venous blood from the RV, and bronchial arteries, which contain oxygenated blood from the LV (Fig. 1-20). The pulmonary arteries deliver blood that is oxygenated within the alveoli, and the blood within the bronchial arteries provides nourishment for the rest of the lung tissue.

Deoxygenated blood coming from the systemic circulation via the right atrium and ventricle of the heart passes through the pulmonary trunk dividing into the right and left pulmonary arteries. The pulmonary arteries

divide into branches corresponding to the divisions of the bronchial tree and supply the pulmonary arterioles. In the lungs, blood releases CO_2 and gets replenished with O_2 (*respiratory gas exchange*). Oxygenated blood is then transported from the pulmonary capillaries to four pulmonary veins, which empty into the left atrium. The pulmonary veins also receive blood from the bronchial circulation, which accounts for a right-to-left shunt that normally occurs in the lungs and includes up to 5% of cardiac output. Oxygenated blood passes from the LA into the LV, where it is pumped into the coronary arteries of the heart and the systemic circulation via the aorta and its branches.

VENTILATORY PUMP AND MECHANICS OF BREATHING

The ventilatory pump consists of the chest wall, the respiratory muscles, and the pleural space (Figs. 1-21 and 1-22). These components of the ventilatory pump provide for the processes of *inspiration* (air moving into the lungs) and *expiration* (air moving out of the lungs). Breathing involves both inspiration and expiration so that **ventilation** (exchange of air) of the lungs is accomplished. Inspiration is initiated by activation of the respiratory muscles, particularly the diaphragm. The respiratory muscles increase the thoracic dimensions such that the pressure in the pleural space is lower than

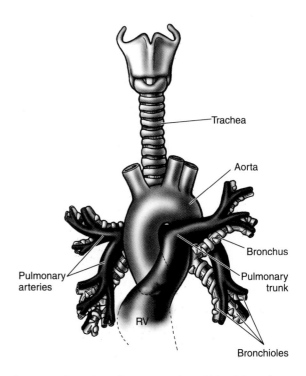

FIGURE 1-20. The major pulmonary arteries, which originate from the right ventricle (RV). Branches of the pulmonary artery are adjacent to the bronchi and bronchioles.

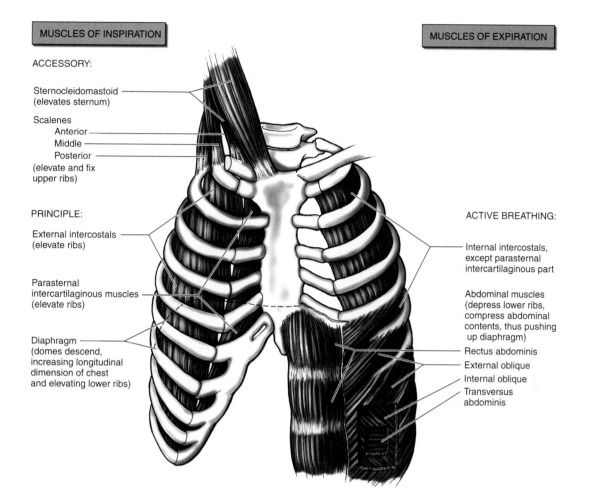

FIGURE 1-21. The major muscles of respiration. The principal inspiratory muscles, shown on the *left*, include the diaphragm, external intercostal muscles, and parasternal muscles. The principal expiratory muscles, shown on the *right*, include the internal intercostal muscles and the abdominal muscles (rectus, transversus, and internal and external oblique muscles).

the outside atmospheric pressure. Air enters the lung until the *intrapulmonary* (inside the lung) gas pressure equals atmospheric pressure. During expiration, the respiratory muscles relax and thoracic dimensions are decreased (e.g., the ribs fall back down and the diaphragm moves upward into the thorax), thus increasing intrapulmonary pressure relative to the outside atmospheric pressure. As a result, air flows from the lungs to outside the body, thus completing the process of breathing.

Chest Wall

The chest wall includes the intercostal muscles, which are considered respiratory muscles, (see Fig. 1-21) and bones (the spine, ribs, and sternum). The ribs articulate with the spine so that the ribs can move upward and outward during inspiration and downward and inward during expiration. This hinging movement contributes to the changes in thoracic volume that are critical for driving ventilation.

Respiratory Muscles

The muscles of respiration are the only skeletal muscles essential to life. The muscles of inspiration and expiration are illustrated in Figures 1-21 and 1-22. The *diaphragm*, the major muscle of inspiration, is innervated by the *phrenic nerve*, which originates from the third to fifth cervical spinal segments. Spinal cord transection caused by injury at or above this level compromises respiratory muscle function and, consequently, ventilation.

The diaphragm consists of a flat crural part (i.e., dome-like portion of the diaphragm) and vertical muscles called the *costal portion*. The diaphragm functions as a piston, with contraction and relaxation of the vertically oriented muscle fibers. With contraction, the crural portion moves downward and displaces the abdominal contents so that the abdomen and the chest wall move outward. Expiration is normally passive (i.e., it requires no muscular work) under quiet breathing because of the elastic recoil of the lung tissue and gravity, which causes the ribs

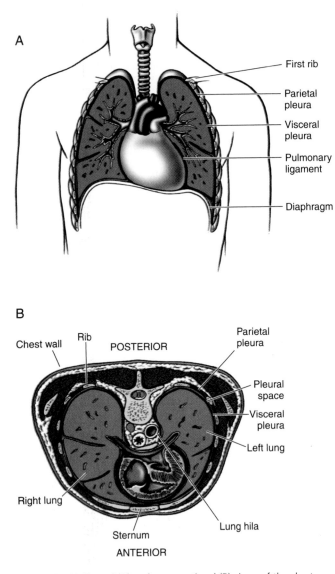

FIGURE 1-22. Frontal (**A**) and cross-sectional (**B**) views of the chest and lungs showing the pleural layers (visceral and parietal) and the pleural space. With inspiration, negative pressure develops in the pleural space. This allows air to move from the atmosphere into the tracheobronchial tree for gas exchange. The negative intrathoracic pressure also facilitates return of venous blood into the right atrium.

to fall back to their natural position. However, during active breathing, when ventilatory requirements are increased (e.g., during exercise), the muscles of expiration are recruited. The major muscles of expiration are the intercostal and the abdominal muscles (rectus abdominis, external and internal oblique, and transversus abdominis).

In patients with airflow obstruction (e.g., acute bronchoconstriction in asthma or emphysema), hyperinflation of the lungs stretches the lung tissue and leads to additional elastic recoil, forcing the crural portion of the diaphragm downward and shortening the vertical muscle fibers. This places the diaphragm at a mechanical disad-

vantage because of the altered length–tension relationship (see Chapter 3).

Pleura

The visceral pleura (i.e., inner layer intimately covering the lungs) and parietal pleura (i.e., layer lining the inside of the chest wall and diaphragm) are thin membranes between the lungs and the chest wall; they converge at the lung hila (Fig.1-22)[22]. The pleural space, which lies between the visceral and parietal pleura, contains a small amount of fluid (Fig.1-22). Because the pleural space is airtight and the chest wall and lung tissue pull against each other across the pleural space, negative pressure is produced at rest. During inspiration, both the visceral and parietal pleura expand outward and more negative pressure develops in the pleural space.

Air can enter the pleural space (i.e., *pneumothorax*) by spontaneous rupture of a subpleural cyst or by trauma to the chest wall (e.g., a fractured rib with penetration of the parietal pleura). With a pneumothorax, the lungs collapse while the chest wall expands because of its intrinsic elastic properties. The parietal pleura contain abundant pain fibers, and irritation of this membrane by a pneumothorax or inflammation produces local chest pain exacerbated by motion of the pleura (e.g., deep inspiration).

SUMMARY

The major function of the respiratory system is the exchange of carbon dioxide and oxygen, which is necessary for metabolism. The respiratory system is divided functionally into conducting zones, which filter, warm, and moisten incoming air, and respiratory zones, where gas exchange occurs. Other important functions include the production and metabolism of vasoactive substances and the filtering of particulate material before entry into the systemic circuit. The structural components of the respiratory system are the framework for these and other important functions at rest and with physical activity.

Musculoskeletal Anatomy

GENERAL COMPONENTS AND FUNCTIONS

A major objective of exercise training is improvement in musculoskeletal fitness. The physiological adaptation of muscle to exercise training may be manifested through improvements in muscle force production, muscular endurance, and resistance to injury. Inherent in designing effective training programs is a thorough understanding of muscle structure and function. This section provides a brief overview of the fundamentals of musculoskeletal anatomy. For in-depth study, the reader is referred to a variety of excellent sources[13,23–26].

Skeletal System (Axial Skeleton, Appendicular Skeleton, and Bone Tissue)

Beyond supporting soft tissue, protecting internal organs, and acting as an important source of nutrients and blood constituents, the bones of the skeletal system serve as rigid levers for locomotion. The skull, vertebral column, sternum, and ribs are considered the **axial skeleton**; the remaining bones, in particular those of the upper and lower limbs, are considered the **appendicular skeleton**. The major bones of the body are illustrated in Figure 1-23. The skeletal system consists of cartilage, periosteum, and bone (osseous) tissue. The structure of a bone can be explained using a typical long bone such as the humerus. The main portion of a long bone or shaft is called the *diaphysis* (Fig. 1-24). The ends of the bone are called the *epiphyses*. The epiphyses are covered by *articular cartilage*. Cartilage is a resilient, semirigid form of connective

tissue that reduces the friction and absorbs some of the shock in synovial joints. The region of mature bone where the diaphysis joins the epiphyses is called the *metaphysis*. In an immature bone, this region includes the *epiphyseal plate*, also called the *growth plate*. The *medullary cavity*, or marrow cavity, is the space inside the diaphysis. Lining the marrow cavity is the endosteum, which contains cells necessary for bone development. The *periosteum* is a membrane around the surface of bones that are not covered with articular cartilage. The periosteum is composed of two layers, an outer fibrous layer and an inner highly vascular layer that contains cells for the creation of new bone. The periosteum serves as point attachment for ligaments and tendons and is critical for bone growth, repair, and nutrition.

There are two types of bones: compact and spongy. The main difference is in the amount of matter and space they contain. *Compact bone* contains few spaces and

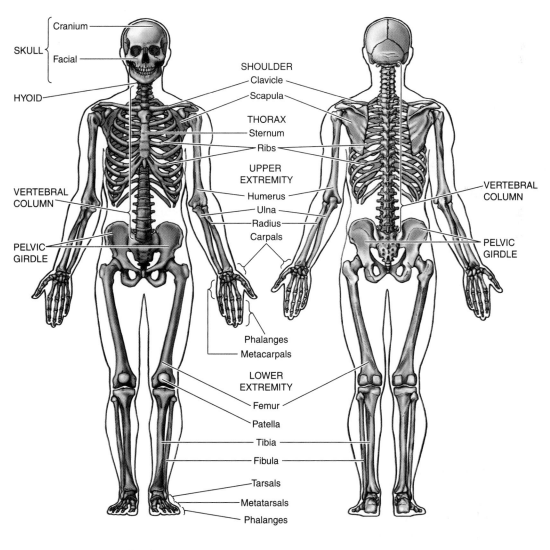

Anterior   Posterior

FIGURE 1-23. Divisions of the skeletal system.

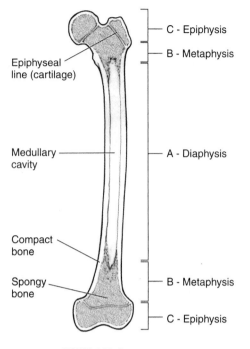

Epiphyseal line (cartilage)

C - Epiphysis

B - Metaphysis

Medullary cavity

A - Diaphysis

Compact bone

Spongy bone

B - Metaphysis

C - Epiphysis

FIGURE 1-24. Bone anatomy.

Structure and Function of Joints in Movement

Joints are the articulations between bones, and along with bones and ligaments, they constitute the articular system. *Ligaments* are tough, fibrous connective tissues anchoring bone to bone. Joints are typically classified as *fibrous,* in which bones are united by dense fibrous connective tissue; *cartilaginous,* in which the bones are united by cartilage; or *synovial,* in which a fibrous articular capsule and an inner synovial membrane enclose the joint cavity. Table 1-3 summarizes the joint classifications and examples in the human body.

Synovial (Diarthrodial) Joints

The most commonly occurring joint in the human body is the synovial joint. Figure 1-25 illustrates its unique capsular arrangement, which is a critical concern to exercise professionals. There are four distinct features of a synovial joint: it has a joint cavity, the articulating surfaces of the bones are covered with articular cartilage, it is enclosed by a fibrous joint capsule, and the capsule is lined with synovial membrane. The *synovial membrane* produces *synovial fluid,* which provides constant lubrication during movement to minimize the wearing effects of friction on the cartilaginous covering of the articulating bones. Synovial joints are sometimes reinforced by ligaments. These ligaments are either separate or are a thickening of the outer layer of the joint capsule. Some synovial joints have other structures such as articular discs (e.g., knee). There are six major types of synovial joints classified by the shape of the articulating surface or type of movement allowed (see Table 1-3). Table 1-4 summarizes commonly used joints, joint motions, and the plane in which they occur (Fig. 1-26).

Joints are typically well perfused by numerous arterial branches and are innervated by branches of the nerves

forms the external layer of all bones of the body and a large portion of the diaphysis of the long bones, where it provides support for bearing weight. In contrast, *spongy bone* is characterized as being much less dense. It consists of a three-dimensional lattice composed of beams or struts of bone called *trabeculae.* Open spaces are present between the trabeculae, unlike in compact bone. The trabeculae are oriented to provide strength against the stresses normally encountered by the bone. In some bones, the space within these trabeculae is filled with *red bone marrow,* which produces blood cells.

TABLE 1-3. Classification of Joints in the Human Body

Joint Classification	Features and Examples
Fibrous	
Suture	Tight union unique to the skull
Syndesmosis	Interosseous membrane between bone (e.g., the union along the shafts of the radius and ulna, tibia and fibula)
Gomphosis	Unique joint at the tooth socket
Cartilaginous	
Primary (synchondroses; hyaline cartilaginous)	Usually temporary to permit bone growth and typically fuse; some do not (e.g., at the sternum and rib [costal cartilage])
Secondary (symphyses; fibrocartilaginous)	Strong, slightly movable joints (e.g., intervertebral discs, pubic symphysis)
Synovial	
Plane (arthrodial)	Gliding and sliding movements (e.g., acromioclavicular joint)
Hinge (ginglymus)	Uniaxial movements (e.g., elbow, knee extension and flexion)
Ellipsoidal (condyloid)	Biaxial joint (e.g., wrist flexion and extension, radio-ulnar deviation)
Saddle (sellar)	Unique joint that permits movements in all planes, including opposition (e.g., the carpometacarpal joint of the thumb)
Ball and socket (enarthrodial)	Multiaxial joints that permit movements in all directions (e.g., hip and shoulder joints)
Pivot (trochoidal)	Uniaxial joints that permit rotation (e.g. humeroradial joint)

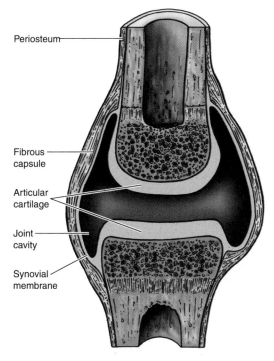

Periosteum

Fibrous
capsule

Articular
cartilage

Joint
cavity

Synovial
membrane

FIGURE 1-25. A synovial joint.

supplying the adjacent muscle and overlying skin. Proprioceptive feedback is an important joint sensation, as is pain, owing to the high density of sensory fibers in the joint capsule. This feedback has obvious importance in regulating human movement and in preventing injury.

Joint Movements and Range of Motion

The degree of movement within a joint is typically called the *range of motion (ROM)*. ROM can be *active (AROM)*, the range that can be reached by voluntary movement, or *passive (PROM)*, the ROM that can be achieved by external means (e.g., an examiner or device). Joints are typically limited in range by the articulations of bones (as in the limitation of elbow extension by the olecranon process of the ulna); ligamentous arrangement; and soft tissue limitations, as occurs in elbow and knee flexion.

Movement at one joint may influence the extent of movement at adjacent joints because a number of muscles and other soft tissue structures cross multiple joints. For example, finger flexion decreases in the presence of wrist flexion because muscles that flex both the wrist and fingers cross multiple joints. Tables 1-5 and 1-6 summarize major joint movements and the muscles that produce those movements, with example resistance exercises for the muscles.

Muscular System

Bones provide support and leverage to the body, but without muscles, we would not be able to move. There are three types of muscle tissue: skeletal, cardiac (see Heart—Location and General Landmarks: *myocardium*) and smooth muscle. Skeletal muscle is primarily attached to bones and is responsible for moving the skeletal

TABLE 1-4. Major Joint Motions and Planes of Motion

Major Joints	Type of Joints	Joint Movements	Planes
Scapulothoracic	Not a true joint	Elevation–depression	Frontal
		Upward–downward rotation	Frontal
		Protraction–retraction	Transverse
Glenohumeral	Synovial: ball and socket	Flexion–extension	Sagittal
		Abduction–adduction	Frontal
		Internal–external rotation	Transverse
		Horizontal abduction–adduction	Transverse
		Circumduction	
Elbow	Synovial: hinge	Flexion–extension	Sagittal
Proximal radioulnar	Synovial: pivot	Pronation–supination	Transverse
Wrist	Synovial: ellipsoidal	Flexion–extension	Sagittal
		Ulnar–radial deviation	Frontal
Metacarpophalangeal	Synovial: ellipsoidal	Flexion–extension	Sagittal
		Abduction–adduction	Frontal
Proximal interphalangeal	Synovial: hinge	Flexion–extension	Sagittal
Distal interphalangeal	Synovial: hinge	Flexion–extension	Sagittal
Interverterbral	Cartilagenous	Flexion–extension	Sagittal
		Lateral flexion	Frontal
		Rotation	Transverse
Hip	Synovial: ball and socket	Flexion–extension	Sagittal
		Abduction–adduction	Frontal
		Internal–external rotation	Transverse
		Horizontal abduction–adduction	Transverse
		Circumduction	
Knee	Synovial: hinge	Flexion–extension	Sagittal
Ankle: talocrural	Synovial: hinge	Dorsi flexion–plantarflexion	Sagittal
Ankle: subtalar	Synovial: gliding	Inversion–eversion	Frontal

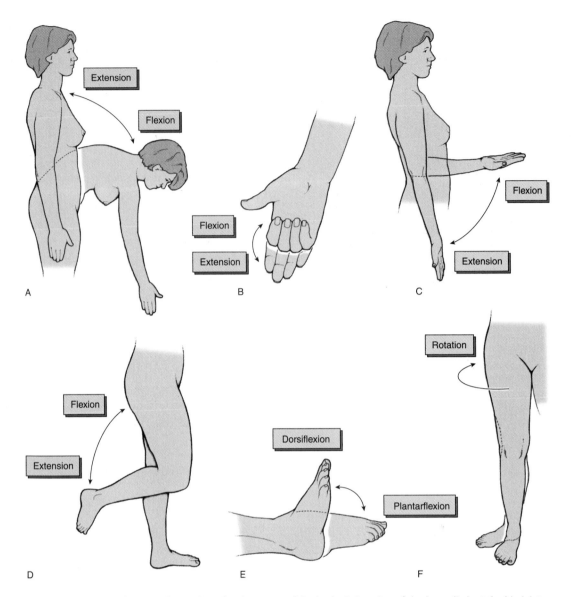

FIGURE 1-26. A–E. Flexion and extension of various parts of the body. **F.** Rotation of the lower limb at the hip joint.

system, stabilizing the body (posture), and generating heat. Skeletal muscle tissue is under voluntary control and is called *striated* because of the dark and light bands visible under a microscope. In general, all muscle tissue has four important characteristics: a) excitability (the ability to respond to stimuli by generating an electrical signal, or action potential), b) contractility (the ability to shorten and thicken), c) extensibility (the ability to stretch), and d) elasticity (the ability to return to its original shape after stretching or contracting).

Skeletal Muscle Structure

The individual *muscle fibers* (muscle cells) that make up skeletal muscles are held together by a hierarchical organization of several connective tissue membranes (Fig. 1-27).

The outermost layer surrounding the whole muscle is the *epimysium*. Skeletal muscles are composed of multiple bundles of muscle fibers, varying in size from 15 to 150 muscle fibers. These bundles of muscle fibers are known as *fasciculi* (an individual bundle is a fasciculus). Each fasciculus is covered and thus separated from other fasciculi by *perimysium*. A third connective tissue layer known as the *endomysium* envelops individual muscle fibers. Blood vessels, nerves, and lymphatic vessels pass into the muscle to reach the individual muscle fibers. An additional thin elastic membrane is found just beneath the endomysium and is called the *sarcolemma*. The sarcolemma is the true cell boundary and encloses the cellular contents of the muscle fiber, nuclei, local stores of fat, glucose (in the form of glycogen), enzymes, **contractile proteins**, and other specialized structures such as the mitochondria.

TABLE 1-5. Major Movements of the Upper Extremities

Joint	Movement	Major Agonist Muscles	Examples of Resistance Exercises
Scapulothoracic	Fixation	Serratus anterior	Push-ups
		Pectoralis minor	Parallel bar dips
		Trapezius	Upright rows
		Levator scapulae	Shoulder shrugs
		Rhomboids	Seated rows
Glenohumeral	Flexion	Anterior deltoid	Front raises
		Pectoralis major (clavicular head)	Incline bench press
	Extension	Latissimus dorsi	Dumbbell pullovers
		Teres major	Chin-ups
		Pectoralis major (sternocostal head)	Bench press
	Abduction	Middle deltoid	Lateral raises, Dumbbell press
		Supraspinatus	Low pulley lateral raises
	Adduction	Latissimus dorsi	Lats pulldown
		Teres major	Seated row
		Pectoralis major	Cable crossover fly
	Medial (internal) rotation	Latissimus dorsi	Back latissimus pulldowns,
		Teres major	bent rows
		Subscapularis	One-arm dumbbell
		Pectoralis major	rows
		Anterior deltoid	Rotator cuff exercises
			Dumbbell press, parallel bar dips
			Front raises
	Lateral (external) rotation	Infraspinatus	External rotation exercises
		Teres minor	
		Posterior deltoid	Back press, bent-over
			lateral raises
Elbow	Flexion	Biceps brachii	Curls
		Brachialis	Preacher curls
		Brachioradialis	Hammer curls
	Extension	Triceps brachii	Triceps dips, triceps extensions
		Anconeus	Pushdowns, triceps kickback
Radioulnar	Supination	Supinator	Dumbbell supination
		Biceps brachii	
	Pronation	Pronator teres, pronator quadratus	Dumbbell pronation
Wrist	Flexion	Flexor carpi radialis and ulnaris	Wrist curls
		Palmaris longus	
		Flexor digitorum superficialis	
	Extension	Extensor carpi radialis longus, brevis and ulnaris	Reverse wrist curls
		Extensor digitorum	
	Adduction (ulnar deviation)	Flexor and extensor carpi ulnaris	Wrist curls, reverse wrist curls
	Abduction (radial deviation)	Extensor carpi radialis longus and brevis	Wrist curls, reverse wrist curls
		Flexor carpi radialis	

Skeletal muscles are anchored to the skeleton by extensions of the epimysium, perimysium and endomysium. These connective tissues extend beyond the end of a muscle and converge to form *tendons*. In most cases, tendons are dense cords of connective tissue that attach a muscle to the periosteum of the bone. When the tendon is flat and broad, it is called an *aponeurosis*. Tendons and aponeuroses provide the mechanical link between skeletal muscle and bone.

Skeletal muscles have different **muscle fiber architecture** (arrangement of muscle fiber relative to the line of pull of the muscle). Muscles can have a *parallel or fusiform fiber arrangement* (i.e., the muscle fibers run in line with the pull of the muscle) or *pennate arrangement* (Fig. 1-28).

In pennate muscle, the fibers run obliquely or at an angle to the line of pull. Pennate muscles can be classified as *unipennate* (fibers only on one side of the tendon, e.g., vastus lateralis), *bipennate* (fibers on both sides of a centrally positioned tendon, e.g., rectus femoris), or *multipennate* (two or more fasciculi attaching obliquely and combined into one muscle, e.g., deltoid). The muscle fiber architecture of a muscle can affect muscle force generation, velocity of shortening, and ROM. For example, muscles composed of long muscle fibers tend to have parallel arrangements and demonstrate greater ROM and velocity of shortening than pennate muscles. In contrast, pennate muscles are composed of large numbers of short fibers, providing a larger cross-sectional area capable of generat-

TABLE 1-6. Major Movements of the Lower Extremities

Joint	Movement	Major Agonist Muscles	Examples of Resistance Exercises
Intervertebral	Trunk flexion	Rectus abdominis	Sit-ups, crunches, leg raises
		External obliques	Machine crunches
		Internal obliques	High pulley crunches
	Trunk extension	Erector spinae	Back extensions, dead lifts
	Lateral flexion	Rectus abdominis	Roman chair side bends
		External obliques	Dumbbell side bends
		Internal obliques	Hanging leg raises
	Rotation	External obliques	Broomstick twist
		Internal obliques	Machine trunk
			Rotations
Hip	Flexion	Iliacus	Leg raises
		Psoas major	Incline leg raises
		Rectus femoris	Machine crunches
		Sartorius	Leg raises
		Pectineus	Cable adductions
	Extension	Gluteus maximus	Squats, leg presses, lunges
		Hamstrings (semitendinosus, semimembranosus, long head of biceps femoris)	Leg curls (standing, seated, lying) Good mornings
	Abduction	Tensor fasciae latae	Cable hip abductions
		Sartorius	Standing machine abductions
		Gluteus medius	Floor hip abductions
		Gluteus minimus	Seated machine abductions
	Adduction	Adductor longus, brevis, and magnus	Power squats
		Gracilis	Cable adductions
		Pectineus	Machine adductions
	Medial rotation	Semitendinosus	Leg curls (standing, seated, lying)
		Semimembranosus	Floor hip adduction
		Gluteus medius	Machine abductions
		Tensor fascia latae	
		Gracilis	
	Lateral rotation	Biceps femoris	
		Adductor longus, brevis, magnus	
		Gluteus maximus	
Knee	Flexion	Hamstrings	Leg curls (standing, seated, lying)
		Gracilis	
		Sartorius	
	Extension	Quadriceps femoris (rectus femoris, vastus lateralis, medialis, and intermedius)	Lunges, squats, leg extensions
Ankle: talocrural	Dorsiflexion	Tibialis anterior	Ankle dorsiflexion against resistance
		Extensor digitorum longus	
		Extensor hallucis longus	
	Plantarflexion	Gastrocnemius, soleus, tibialis posterior	Standing calf raises, Donkey calf raises
		Flexor digitorum longus	Seated calf raises
		Flexor hallucis longus	
Ankle: subtalar	Eversion	Peroneus longus and brevis	Exercises against resistance
	Inversion	Tibialis anterior and posterior	Exercises against resistance

ing greater force production, but less ROM, than muscles with parallel fiber architecture.

Muscles can also be described by the number of joints they act upon. For example, a muscle that causes movement at one joint is *uniarticular* (e.g., brachialis) (Figs.1-29 and 1-30). Muscles that cross more than one joint are referred to as *biarticular* (having actions at two joints, e.g., the hamstring muscles, biceps brachii) or *multiarticular* muscles. The main advantage of bi- and multiarticular

muscles is that only one muscle is needed to generate tension in two or more joints. This is more efficient and conserves energy. In many instances, the length of the muscle stays within 100% to 130% of the resting length: as one side of the muscle shortens, the other side stretches, maintaining a near constant length. This property of bi- and multiarticular muscles enhances tension production (for further explanation, see length–tension relationship in Chapter 3).

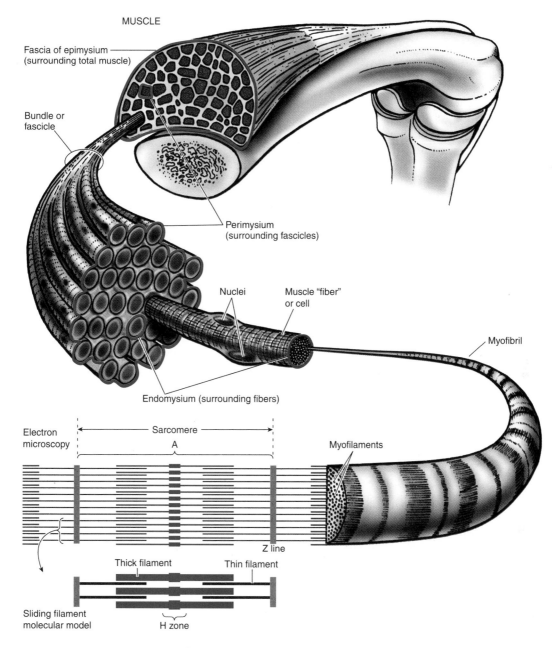

FIGURE 1-27. Cross-section of skeletal muscle and the arrangement of its connective tissue wrappings.

Skeletal Muscle Microanatomy

Skeletal muscle fibers are approximately 10 to 100 microns in diameter and frequently many centimeters long. Each muscle fiber contains several hundred to several thousand regularly ordered, threadlike *myofibrils*. These myofibrils extend lengthwise throughout the cell and are connected to the plasma membrane by intermediate filaments. Myofibrils contain the apparatus that contracts the muscle cell, which consists primarily of two types of myofilaments: thick filaments (*myosin*) and thin filaments (*actin*). The myosin and actin filaments are arranged longitudinally in the smallest contractile unit of

skeletal muscle, the *sarcomere*. Each myofibril is composed of numerous sarcomeres joined end to end at the Z *lines*. The dark *A band* represents the region that contains both thick myosin filaments and thin actin filaments. The *H zone* is the central portion of the A band that appears only when the sarcomere is in a resting state and it is occupied only by thick filaments (see Fig. 1-28). A thick filament contains approximately 200 myosin molecules with the heads of the molecules (called crossbridges) protruding outwards at regular intervals. They occur in the A band, where they overlap at either end with thin filaments. The thin filaments consist of the contractile protein *actin* and **regulatory proteins** *tropomyosin* and

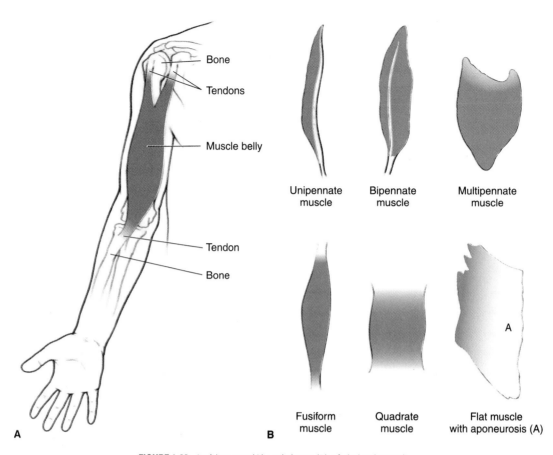

FIGURE 1-28. Architecture (**A**) and shape (**B**) of skeletal muscles.

troponin. Each actin filament has one end inserted in to a Z line, with the opposite end extending toward the center of the sarcomere, lying in the space between the myosin filaments. The actin protein has a binding site that, when exposed, serves as an attachment point for to the myosin crossbridge. It is this arrangement of the myosin and actin filaments that give skeletal muscle its striated appearance when viewed through a microscope.

Muscle Fiber Actions and Fiber Types

Approximately 5% of skeletal muscle weight is constituted of the high-energy phosphates, key minerals and energy sources needed for force production; another 20% of muscle composition is protein, principally the contractile elements *myosin*, *actin*, and *tropomyosin*. Water constitutes 75% of muscle composition[8]. Physical training results in a significant alteration of these constituents, depending on the specific training stimulus.

Given the wide shift in blood supply shunted to active skeletal muscle during vigorous exercise, a highly competent vascular bed must exist throughout muscles. Likewise, the body has the ability to enhance blood supply through formation of new capillary networks stimulated by physical training that involves endurance or aerobic training.

Skeletal muscles are controlled by the central nervous system (CNS), both at higher centers and in individual spinal segments, and by proprioceptive structures (e.g., muscle spindles, Golgi tendon organs) inherent to the muscle and tendon complex. The integration is complex yet remarkably efficient. Although it has never been conclusively proven, the preponderance of scientific evidence indicates that when stimulated to contract, muscle tissue shortens or lengthens because the myosin and actin myofilaments slide past each other without changing individual length. The contact between filaments is known as *crossbridging*, and it controls shortening and lengthening of muscles during contractile movements. Box 1-1 summarizes the **sliding-filament theory**[27]. This continual process of advancing and releasing crossbridges permits the generation of tension. Force production continues as long as the muscle is stimulated, but the ability of the muscle to perform may be limited by intrinsic factors such as diminished production of adenosine triphosphate (ATP), decreased pH, and accumulation of metabolic byproducts (see the discussion of fatigue in Chapter 3).

Three common terms describing muscle contraction are *twitch*, *summation*, and *tetanus*. *Twitch* refers to a single, brief muscle contraction caused by a single action potential traveling down a motor neuron. *Summation* is the adding together of individual twitch contractions to increase the intensity of the overall muscle contraction. Progressive stimulation frequencies increase the amount

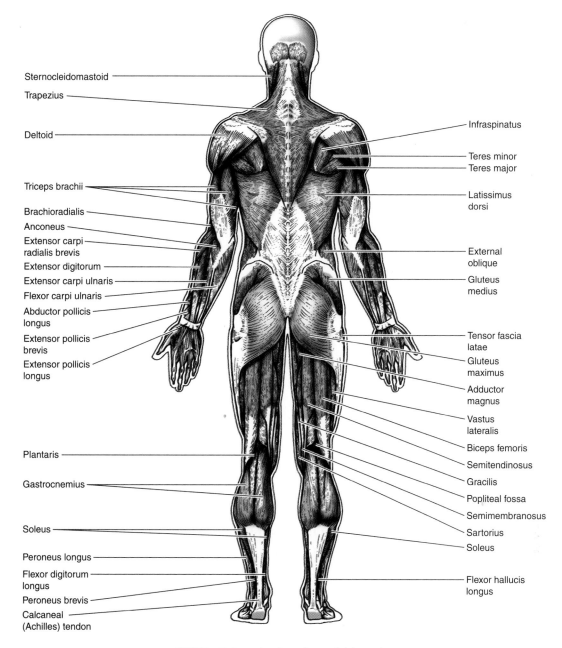

Sternocleidomastoid

Trapezius

Deltoid

Triceps brachii

Brachioradialis

Anconeus

Extensor carpi
radialis brevis

Extensor digitorum

Extensor carpi ulnaris

Flexor carpi ulnaris

Abductor pollicis
longus

Extensor pollicis
brevis

Extensor pollicis
longus

Plantaris

Gastrocnemius

Soleus

Peroneus longus

Flexor digitorum
longus

Peroneus brevis

Calcaneal
(Achilles) tendon

Infraspinatus

Teres minor
Teres major

Latissimus
dorsi

External
oblique

Gluteus
medius

Tensor fascia
latae

Gluteus
maximus

Adductor
magnus

Vastus
lateralis

Biceps femoris

Semitendinosus

Gracilis

Popliteal fossa

Semimembranosus

Sartorius

Soleus

Flexor hallucis
longus

FIGURE 1-29. Posterior view of superficial muscles.

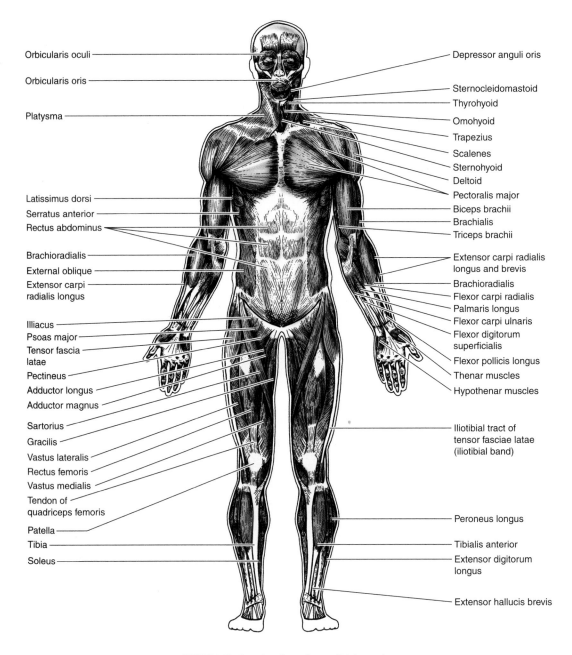

Orbicularis oculi

Orbicularis oris

Platysma

Latissimus dorsi
Serratus anterior
Rectus abdominus

Brachioradialis
External oblique
Extensor carpi
radialis longus

Illiacus
Psoas major
Tensor fascia
latae
Pectineus
Adductor longus
Adductor magnus

Sartorius
Gracilis
Vastus lateralis
Rectus femoris
Vastus medialis
Tendon of
quadriceps femoris

Patella
Tibia
Soleus

Depressor anguli oris

Sternocleidomastoid
Thyrohyoid
Omohyoid
Trapezius
Scalenes
Sternohyoid
Deltoid
Pectoralis major
Biceps brachii
Brachialis
Triceps brachii
Extensor carpi radialis
longus and brevis
Brachioradialis
Flexor carpi radialis
Palmaris longus
Flexor carpi ulnaris
Flexor digitorum
superficialis
Flexor pollicis longus
Thenar muscles
Hypothenar muscles

Iliotibial tract of
tensor fasciae latae
(iliotibial band)

Peroneus longus

Tibialis anterior
Extensor digitorum
longus

Extensor hallucis brevis

FIGURE 1-30. Anterior view of superficial muscles.

BOX 1-1	Sliding Filament Summary of Muscle Contraction and Relaxation

RESTING MUSCLE

Calcium ions are bound to the SR

Tropomyosin–troponin complex blocks attachment sites for myosin ATP is bound to myosin heads

MUSCLE CONTRACTION

Nerve impulse exceeding resting potential spreads across sarcolemma and down transverse tubules, causing release of calcium from the SR

Calcium binds with troponin, which permits actin and myosin to form cross bridges

Myosin ATPase is activated, splitting ATP; this transfer of energy causes movement of the myosin cross bridges, generating tension

Crossbridges uncouple when ATP binds to the myosin bridge

RELAXATION

Coupling and uncoupling continue until calcium concentration becomes insufficient

When the nerve impulse ceases, calcium is taken up the SR; actin and myosin return to a resting state

ATP = adenosine triphosphate; SR = sarcoplasmic reticulum.

of force developed because the muscle cannot completely relax from the previous stimulus before the next stimulus arrives. As soon as the frequency of stimulation is high enough, full summation is achieved. This is referred to as *tetanus* and is the maximal amount of force the motor unit can develop. At this point, muscle fiber stimulation is of such high frequency that it is unable to return to its resting length between contractions[8].

The human body has the ability to perform a wide range of physical tasks combining varying composites of speed, power, and endurance. No single type of muscle fiber possesses the characteristics that would allow optimal performance across this continuum of physical challenges. Rather, muscle fibers possess certain characteristics that result in relative specialization. For example, motor units of specific fiber types are selectively recruited by the body for speed and power tasks of short duration, and others are recruited for endurance tasks of long duration and relatively low intensity. When the challenge requires elements of speed or power but also has an endurance component, yet another type of muscle fiber is recruited.

These different fiber types, to be described more specifically later, should not be thought of as mutually exclusive. In fact, intricate recruitment and switching occurs in muscle over the performance of many tasks, and fibers designed to be optimal for one type of task can contribute to the performance of another. The net result is a functioning muscle that can respond to a wide variety of tasks, and although the composition of the muscle may lend itself to performing best in endurance activities, it still can accomplish speed and power tasks to a lesser degree.

Fortunately, the human body can respond adequately to most physical tasks encountered in everyday living. In the presence of muscle impairment, specific training regimens may restore performance to normal function. Likewise, normal function can be enhanced through exercise training to accomplish physical tasks that are in excess of the demands of daily living, such as athletics[28,29].

Over the years, there has been a fair amount of controversy about the classification of muscle fiber types[30]. In addition, questions remain about whether these types can change in response to an intervention such as endurance training[31–34]. In either case, there is general agreement that relative to exercise performance, two distinct fiber types—type I (slow twitch) and type II (fast twitch, with their proposed subdivisions)—have been identified and classified by contractile and metabolic characteristics[35,36]. To illustrate the variation in fiber types within the population, Table 1-7 lists fiber type distribution in elite athletes relative to the normal population.

TABLE 1-7. Muscle Fiber Composition in Selected Populations

Sport	% Type I (Slow Twitch)	% Type II (Fast Twitch)
Distance runners	60–90	10–40
Track sprinters	25–45	55–75
Weight lifters	45–55	45–55
Shot putters	25–40	60–75
Nonathletes	47–53	47–53

Reprinted with permission from Powers SK, Howley ET: Exercise Physiology. Dubuque, IA: WC Brown; 1990:160.

TABLE 1-8. Structural and Functional Characteristics of Slow Twitch (ST) and Fast Twitch (FT$_A$ and FT$_B$) Muscle Fibers

Characteristics	Fiber Type		
	ST	FT$_A$	FT$_B$
Neural aspects			
Motor neuron size	Small	Large	Large
Motor neuron recruitment threshold	Low	High	High
Motor nerve conduction velocity	Slow	Fast	Fast
Structural aspects			
Muscle fiber diameter	Small	Large	Large
Sarcoplasmic reticulum development	Less	More	More
Mitochondrial density	High	High	Low
Capillary density	High	Medium	Low
Myoglobin content	High	Medium	Low
Energy substrates			
Phosphocreatine stores	Low	High	High
Glycogen stores	Low	High	High
Triglyceride stores	High	Medium	Low
Enzymatic aspects			
Myosin-ATPase activity	Low	High	High
Glycolytic enzyme activity	Low	High	High
Oxidative enzyme activity	High	High	Low
Functional aspects			
Twitch (contraction) time	Slow	Fast	Fast
Relaxation time	Slow	Fast	Fast
Force production	Low	High	High
Energy efficiency, "economy"	High	Low	Low
Fatigue resistance	High	Low	Low
Elasticity	Low	High	High

Courtesy of Fox EL, Bowers RW, Foss ML: The Physiological Basis of Physical Education and Athletics, 4th ed. Dubuque, IA: WC Brown; 1989:110.

Type I Muscle Fibers. The characteristics of type I muscle fibers, listed in Table 1-8, are consistent with muscle fibers that resist fatigue. Thus, type I fibers are selected for activities of low intensity and long duration. Within whole muscle, type I motor units asynchronously contract; that is,

TABLE 1-9. Adaptation in Skeletal Muscle Relative to Specific Training Regimens

Muscle Factor	Training			
	Slow Twitch		Fast Twitch	
	ST	ET	ST	ET
Percent composition	0 or ?	0 or ?	0 or ?	0 or ?
Size	+	0 or +	+ +	0
Contractile property	0	0	0	0
Oxidative capacity	0	+ +	0	+
Anaerobic capacity	? or +	0	? or +	0
Glycogen content	0	+ +	0	+ +
Fat oxidation	0	+ +	0	+
Capillary density	?	+	?	? or +
Blood flow during work	?	? or +	?	?

ST = strength training; ET = endurance training

0 = no change; ? = unknown; 1 = moderate increase; 11 = large increase.

Adapted with permission from Gollnick PD, Sembrowich WI: Adaptations in human skeletal muscle as a result of training. In Amsterdam E, ed. Exercise and Cardiovascular Health and Disease. New York: Yorke Medical Books; 1977:90 and from McArdle W, Katch F, Katch V: Exercise Physiology, 4th ed. Baltimore: Williams & Wilkins; 1996:334.

in addition to their inherent fatigue resistance, endurance is prolonged by the constant switching that occurs to ensure freshly charged muscle as the exercise stimulus continues. Sedentary persons have approximately 50% type I fibers, and this distribution is generally equal throughout the major muscle groups of the body[37]. In endurance athletes, the percentage of type I fibers is greater, but this is thought to be largely a genetic predisposition, despite some evidence suggesting that prolonged exercise training can alter fiber type (Table 1-9)[38,39].

Essentially, those most successful at endurance activities generally have a high proportion of type I fibers, and this is most likely attribuable to genetic factors supplemented through appropriate exercise training. From a metabolic perspective, type I fibers are those frequently called aerobic because the generation of energy for continued muscle contraction is met through the ongoing oxidation of available foodstuffs (carbohydrates and fats). Thus, with minimal accumulation of anaerobically produced metabolites, continued muscle contraction is favored in type I fibers.

Type II Muscle Fibers. At the opposite end of the continuum, individuals who achieve the greatest success in power and high-intensity speed tasks usually have a greater proportion of type II muscle fibers distributed through the major muscle groups. Because force generation is so important, type II fibers shorten and develop tension considerably faster than type I fibers[40]. These fibers are typically thought of as type IIB fibers, the "classic" fast-twitch fiber. Metabolically, these fibers are the classic anaerobic fibers because they rely on energy sources intrinsic to the muscle, not the fuels used by type I fibers. When an endurance component is introduced, such as in events lasting upward of several minutes (800–1500 meter races, for example), a second type of fast-twitch fiber, type IIA, is recruited. As noted in Table 1-8, the type IIA fibers represent a transition of sorts between the needs met by the type I and type IIB fibers. Metabolically, although type IIA fibers have the ability to generate a moderately large amount of force, they also have some aerobic capacity, although not as much as type I fibers. This is a logical and necessary bridge between the types of muscle fibers and the ability to meet the variety of physical tasks imposed. Reference to the existence of the type IIC fiber is necessary in a complete description of human muscle fiber types. The IIC fiber has been described as a rare and undifferentiated muscle fiber type that is probably involved in reinnervation of impaired skeletal muscle[41].

How Muscles Produce Movement

Skeletal muscles produce force that is transferred to the tendons, which, in turn, pull on the bones and other structures (skin). Most muscles cross a joint, so when a muscle contracts, it pulls one of the articulating bones toward the other. Usually, both articulating bones do not move equally; one of the articulating bones stays more stationary. The attachment that is more stationary and usually more proximal (especially in the extremities) is called the *origin*. The muscle attachment that moves the most and is usually located more distally is called the *insertion*.

Levers.   Mechanically, to produce movement, the muscles, joints, and bones work as a system of levers. The bone acts as the lever, the joint functions as the center of rotation (COR), and the muscles produce the force or effort (F) to move the lever. The resistance (R), or the force that opposes the movement of the lever, could be the weight of the body part or, as in a case of lifting weights, the external resistance provided by the weights. Levers are classified into three types according to the position of the fulcrum and the forces of effort and resistance (Fig. 1-31). Third-class levers (Fig. 1-31C) are the most common type of levers in the human body and are designed for ROM and speed of movement (see Fig. 1-31).

Muscle Actions.   *Muscle action* is the neuromuscular activation that leads to the production of force and contributes to the movement or the stabilization of the musculoskeletal system[42]. Muscle can perform three basic actions: isometric, concentric, and eccentric. In an *isometric or static action*, the muscle generates force in the absence of joint movement, such as holding a dumbbell

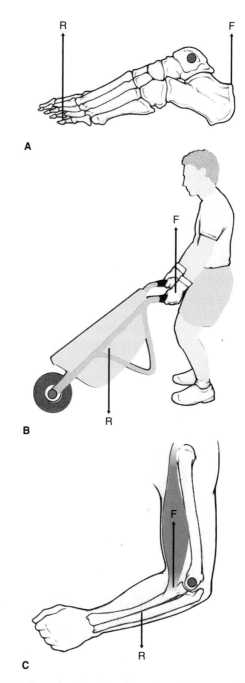

FIGURE 1-31. Examples of level systems, where *F* is he exerted force, *R* is the reaction force, and the *red dot* (●) is the center of rotation. Most musculoskeletal joints behave as third class lever. **A.** First-class lever. **B.** Second-class lever. **C.** Third-class lever.

in a biceps curl without movement. An action in which the muscle length changes is often called *dynamic*. Concentric and eccentric actions are dynamic muscle actions. A *concentric action* occurs when the muscle force being generated exceeds the resistance and the muscle shortens in length, such as the upward phase of a biceps curl. *Eccentric actions* occur when the force generated by the muscle is less than the resistance being encountered.

This results in the active muscle's being lengthened rather than shortened. Eccentric actions are often used when muscles have to slow down body parts or oppose external resistances. Using the biceps curl example, the downward phase of this exercise requires eccentric action of the biceps muscle.

Muscle Roles.   Movements of the human body generally require several muscles working together rather than a single muscle doing all the work. Also keep in mind that muscles cannot push, they can only pull; therefore, most skeletal muscles are arranged in opposing pairs such as flexor–extensor, internal–external rotators, and so on. Muscles can be classified according to their roles during movement. When a muscle or group of muscles is responsible for the action or movement, it is called a *prime mover* or **agonist**. For example, during a biceps curl, the prime movers are the elbow flexors, which include the biceps, brachialis, and brachioradialis muscles. The opposing group of muscles is called the **antagonist** (triceps and anconeus). In addition, most movements also involve other muscles called **synergists**. The role of these muscles is to prevent unwanted movement, which helps the prime movers perform more efficiently. Synergist muscles can also act as fixators or stabilizers. In this role, the muscles stabilize a portion of the body against a force. For example, the scapular muscles (e.g., rhomboids, serratus anterior, trapezius) must provide a stable base of support for the upper extremity muscles during the throwing motion.

Muscles and Exercise.   Muscle actions produce force that causes joint movement during exercise. Exercise science and other health care professionals should have a good knowledge and understanding of which large muscles are involved in the movements of the joints. This knowledge is the basis for the development of exercise programs to use in training and rehabilitation[43]. Tables 1-5 and 1-6 give a list of common resistance training exercises and the muscles involved[43].

Summary

Besides contributing to body shape and form, bones perform several important functions, including support, protection, movement, and storage of essential nutrients and blood cell formation. Skeletal muscle is responsible for bodily movement, body stabilization, and heat production. It is composed of varying amounts of types I, IIA, and IIB muscle fibers whose quantity and distribution are largely genetic. Physical activity patterns and sports performance characteristics develop from the varying properties of muscle fibers; the organization and integration of fiber recruitment patterns; and the levers, bones, and joints through which the fibers act. Although the conversion of muscle fiber types through either disuse or training and the splitting and generation of muscle fibers are somewhat controversial, what is certain about exercise training and fiber type is that specific training significantly enhances metabolic adaptations.

Acknowledgments
Portions of this chapter are adapted from the excellent work of the authors of previous editions of the Resource Manual.

REFERENCES

1. McArdle WD, Katch FI, Katch VL: Essentials of Exercise Physiology, 2nd ed. Philadelphia: Lippincott Williams & Wilkins; 2000.
2. Martini F: Fundamentals of Anatomy and Physiology, 6th ed. San Francisco: Benjamin & Cummins; 2003.
3. Human Anatomy & Physiology. Menlo Park, CA: Benjamin/Cummings; 1998.
4. Spence AP, Mason EB: Human Anatomy and Physiology, 4th ed. St. Paul: West Pub Co.; 1992.
5. Anthony CP, Thibodeau GA: Textbook of Anatomy & Physiology, 11th ed. St. Louis: Mosby; 1983.
6. Gray H, Williams PL, Bannister LH: Gray's Anatomy: The Anatomical Basis of Medicine and Surgery, 38th ed. New York: Churchill Livingstone; 1995.
7. Hole JW: Essentials of Human Anatomy and Physiology, 2nd ed. Dubuque, IA: WC Brown; 1986.
8. McArdle WD, Katch FI, Katch VL: Exercise Physiology: Energy, Nutrition, and Human Performance, 5th ed. Philadelphia: Lippincott Williams & Wilkins; 2001.
9. Brooks GA, Fahey TD, White TP, Baldwin KM: Exercise Physiology: Human Bioenergetics and Its Applications, 3rd ed. Mountain View, CA: Mayfield Pub.; 2000.
10. DeVries HA, Housh TJ: Physiology of Exercise for Physical Education, Athletics, and Exercise Science, 5th ed. Madison, WI: WCB Brown & Benchmark; 1994.
11. Fox EL, Bowers RW, Foss ML: The Physiological Basis for Exercise and Sport, 5th ed. Madison, WI: Brown Pub.; 1993.
12. Powers SK, Howley ET: Exercise Physiology: Theory and Application to Fitness and Performance, 5th ed. New York: McGraw-Hill; 2003.
13. Hall-Craggs ECB: Anatomy as a Basis for Clinical Medicine, 3rd ed. Baltimore: Williams & Wilkins; 1995.
14. Williams M: cardiovascular and respiratory Anatomy and Physiology: Responses to exercise. In Baechle TR, Earle RW, eds. Essentials of Strength Training and Conditioning, 2nd ed. Champaign, IL: Human Kinetics; 2000:115–136.
15. Montgomery RL: Basic Anatomy for the Allied Health Professions. Baltimore: Urban & Schwarzenberg; 1981.
16. Thibodeau GA, Patton KT: Anatomy & Physiology, 5th ed. St. Louis: Mosby; 2003.
17. Sokolow M, McIlroy MB, Cheitlin MD: Clinical Cardiology, 6th ed. Norwalk, CT: Appleton & Lange; 1993.
18. Wilmore JH, Costill DL: Physiology of Sport and Exercise, 3rd ed. Champaign, IL: Human Kinetics; 2004.
19. Nilsestuen J: Pulmonary physiology. In Berghuis P, Cohen N, Decker M, eds. Respiration. Redmond, WA: SpaceLabs; 1992:1–11.
20. Carrin B: Development and structure of the normal human lung. In Turner-Warwick M, Hodson M, Corrinm B, Kerr I, eds. Clinical Atlas: Respiratory Diseases. Philadelphia: J.B. Lippincott;Gower Medical Pub.; 1989:1–14.
21. Staub N, Albertine K: Anatomy of the lungs. In Murray JF, Nadel JA, eds. Textbook of Respiratory Medicine, vol 1, 2nd ed. Philadelphia: WB Saunders; 1994:3–25.
22. Light RW: Pleural Diseases, 2nd ed. Philadelphia: Lea & Febiger; 1990.
23. Moore KL: Clinically Oriented Anatomy, 4th ed. Baltimore: Williams & Wilkins; 2004.
24. Olson TR, Pawlina W: A.D.A.M. Student Atlas of Anatomy. Baltimore.: Williams & Wilkins; 1996.

25. Agur AMR, Lee MJ, Anderson JE: Grant's Atlas of Anatomy, 9th ed. Baltimore: Williams & Wilkins; 1991.

26. Moore KL, Agur AMR: Essential of Clinical Anatomy. Baltimore: Williams & Wilkins; 2002.

27. Huxley HE: The structural basis of muscular contraction. Proc R Soc Lond B Biol Sci 178:131–149, 1971.

28. Coggan AR, Spina RJ, King DS, et al: Skeletal muscle adaptations to endurance training in 60- to 70-yr-old men and women. J Appl Physiol. May72:1780–1786, 1992.

29. Jansson E, Kaijser :. Muscle adaptation to extreme endurance training in man. Acta Physiol Scand.100:315–324, 1977.

30. Armstrong RB: Muscle fiber recruitment patterns and their metabolic correlates. In Horton ES, Terjung RL, eds. Exercise, Nutrition, and Energy Metabolism. New York: Macmillan; 1988:265.

31. Chi MM, Hintz CS, Coyle EF, et al: Effects of detraining on enzymes of energy metabolism in individual human muscle fibers. Am J Physiol 244:C276–287, 1983.

32. Gollnick PD, Armstrong RB, Sembrowich WL, Shepherd RE, Saltin B: Glycogen depletion pattern in human skeletal muscle fibers after heavy exercise. J Appl Physiol.34:615–618, 1973.

33. Jacobs I, Esbjornsson M, Sylven C, Holm I, Jansson E: Sprint training effects on muscle myoglobin, enzymes, fiber types, and blood lactate. Med Sci Sports Exerc 19:368–374, 1987.

34. Jansson E, Sjodin B, Tesch P: Changes in muscle fibre type distribution in man after physical training. A sign of fibre type transformation? Acta Physiol Scand104:235–237, 1978.

35. Brooke MH, Kaiser KK. Muscle fiber types: how many and what kind? Arch Neurol 23:369–379, 1970.

36. Edstrom L, Nystrom B: Histochemical types and sizes of fibres in normal human muscles. A biopsy study. Acta Neurol Scand 45:257–269, 1969.

37. Fox EL, Bowers RW, Foss ML: The Physiological Basis of Physical Education and Athletics, 4th ed. Dubuque, IA: WC Brown; 1989.

38. Burke ER, Cerny F, Costill D, Fink W: Characteristics of skeletal muscle in competitive cyclists. Med Sci Sports 9:109–112, 1977.

39. Costill DL, Daniels J, Evans W, Fink W, Krahenbuhl G, Saltin B: Skeletal muscle enzymes and fiber composition in male and female track athletes. J Appl Physiol 40:149–154, 1976.

40. Vrbova G: Influence of activity on some characteristic properties of slow and fast mammalian muscles. Exerc Sport Sci Rev 7:181–213, 1979.

41. Komi PV, Karlsson J: Skeletal muscle fibre types, enzyme activities and physical performance in young males and females. Acta Physiol Scand 103:210–218, 1978.

42. Knudson DV, Morrison CS: Qualitative Analysis of Human Movement, 2nd ed. Champaign, IL: Human Kinetics; 2002.

43. DeLavier F: Strength Training Anatomy. Champaign, IL: Human Kinetics; 2001.

SELECTED REFERENCES FOR FURTHER READING

Aaberg E: Muscle Mechanics. Champaign, IL: Human Kinetics; 1998.

Calais-Germain B: Anatomy of Movement. Seattle: Eastland Press; 2003.

Delavier F: Strength Training Anatomy. Champaign, IL: Human Kinetics; 2001.

Floyd RT, Tompson CW: Manual of Structural Kinesiology, 15th ed. New York: McGraw-Hill Co.; 2003.

Hamill J, Knutzen KM: Biomechanical Basis of Human Movement 2nd ed. Philadelphia: Lippincott, Williams & Wilkins; 2003.

Jenkins DB, Hollinshead WH: Hollinshead's Functional Anatomy of the Limbs and Back. Philadelphia: WB Saunders; 1998.

Knudson DV, Morrison CS: Qualitative Analysis of Human Movement, 2nd ed. Champaign, IL: Human Kinetics; 2002.

Neuman, DA: Kinesiology of the Musculoskeletal System. St. Louis: Mosby; 2002.

INTERNET RESOURCES

American Association of Anatomists: http://www.anatomy.org

Anatomy on the Internet: http://www.meddean.luc.edu/lumen/ MedEd/GrossAnatomy/anatomy.htm

The Digital Anatomist Information System: http://sig.biostr.washington.edu/projects/da/

Human Anatomy Online: http://www.innerbody.com/htm/body.html

Integrated Medical Curriculum: http://www.imc.gsm.com

NISMAT Exercise Physiology Corner: A Primer on Muscle Physiology: http://www.nismat.org/physcor/muscle.html

Scottish Radiological Society: http://www.radiology.co.uk/srs-x/index.htm

University of California San Diego: Muscle Physiology Home Page: http://muscle.ucsd.edu/musintro/jump.shtml

University of Washington Diagnostic Radiology Residency Programs Anatomy Modules: http://www.rad.washington.edu/anatomy/index.html

Vesalius: The Internet Resource for Surgical Education: http://www.vesalius.com/

Virtual Hospital: http://www.vh.org

2 Biomechanics

DUANE KNUDSON

This chapter addresses KSAs from the following content areas:

1 **Exercise Physiology and Related Exercise Science**
2 Pathophysiology and Risk Factors
3 Health Appraisal, Fitness, and Clinical Exercise Testing
4 Electrocardiography and Diagnostic Techniques
5 Patient Management and Medications
6 Medical and Surgical Management
7 Exercise Prescription and Programming
8 Nutrition and Weight Management
9 Human Behavior and Counseling
10 Safety, Injury Prevention, and Emergency Procedures
11 Program Administration, Quality Assurance, and Outcome Assessment

Exercise and sports medicine professionals often advise clients regarding modifying movement technique and in using exercise or rehabilitation equipment. The discipline primarily involved in describing and understanding the mechanical causes of human movement is biomechanics. **Biomechanics** is the study of the motion of living things using the branch of physics known as mechanics. The study of forces and torques that cause movement is called **kinetics**, and describing the resulting motion is called **kinematics**. This chapter summarizes how understanding the causes of human motion (kinetics), the effects of forces on human tissues, and how kinematic measurements of human motion can be used by professionals to modify exercise prescriptions.

Kinetics

Understanding the causes of human movement requires an understanding of several kinetic variables. This section discusses the forces and torques that create motion; introduce Newton's Laws of Motion, which describe the creation of motion; and summarize major forces that affect human movement.

FORCES AND TORQUES

For a body segment to change its state of motion, a force must be applied. A **force** is a linear effect that can be defined as a push, pull, or tendency to distort. Forces can be represented by **vectors**. Forces have four important characteristics, two of which are its vector quantities of magnitude (size) and direction. The other two characteristics are a line of action and point of application.

Forces and the vectors used to represent them can be drawn as arrows with the length representing magnitude and direction indicated by the arrowhead (Fig. 2-1). The SI units of force magnitude are Newtons (N). The point of application of a force is the location at which the force acts on an object. The line of action is an imaginary line extending in both directions from the force vector (see Fig. 2-1). In most situations, multiple forces act on body segments, so vector addition techniques are needed to take into account the interacting magnitudes and directions. Adding vectors together determines a resultant vector. A vector can be also broken up into equivalent parts called *components*. For example, the forces between a runner's foot and the ground are usually resolved into right-angle components (Fig. 2-2).

Depending on how forces are applied to an object, they may cause three kinds of motion called a) translation or linear motion; b) rotation or angular motion; or c) general motion, which is a combination of translation and rotation. A force acting through the center of mass of an object creates translation. Forces with a line of action not acting though the object's center of mass tend to create rotation or general motion (see Fig. 2-2).

The measure of the rotary effect of a force is called a **moment of force** (M), which is commonly referred to as **torque**. A moment can be calculated as the product of the force and its **moment arm**, which is the perpendicular distance from the line of action of the force to the axis of rotation. The most common unit of a moment of force is Newton meters (Nm). Moments are also vector quantities that can be added to determine the net rotary effect of forces acting on an object. For instance, typical changes in the moment arm or leverage of the long head of the biceps brachii at the elbow during flexion are illustrated in Figure 2-3.

KEY TERMS

Base of support: The area of the supporting surface of an object such as between the feet in standing or between the hands in a handstand

Biomechanics: The study of the motion and causes of motion of living things

Buoyancy: The floating force on an object immersed in a fluid

Center of gravity: The location of a theoretical point that can be used to represent the total weight of an object

Drag: The fluid force that acts parallel to the relative flow of fluid past an object

Force: A push or pull that tends to modify motion or the shape of an object

Friction: The force that acts parallel to and opposes sliding between surfaces in contact

Kinematics: The branch of mechanics that describes motion

Kinetics: The branch of mechanics that explains the causes of motion

Lift: The fluid force that acts at right angles to the relative flow of fluid past an object

Moment arm: The leverage of a force creating a torque or moment of force; the perpendicular distance between the line of action of the force and the axis of rotation

Moment of force: The rotating effect of a force

Normal reaction: The force acting at right angles between two surfaces in contact

Stiffness: The measure of the elasticity of a material, defined as the slope of the stress/strain graph in the elastic region

Strain: A measure of the deformation of a material when acted upon by a force

Stress: The force per unit area in a material

Torque: Another term used to refer to a rotating effect of a force. Mechanics of materials uses *torque* to refer to torsional (twisting about a longidutinal) moments.

Vector: A variable that requires knowledge of both magnitude (size) and direction

NEWTON'S LAWS OF MOTION

Sir Isaac Newton developed three laws of motion that explain how forces create movement. The first law is the *law of inertia*, which states "a body continues in its state of rest, or uniform motion in a straight line, unless a force acts upon it." All objects have this innate property (inertia) that resists changes in state of motion. To move a motionless object, force must be applied to overcome its inertia and thus set it into motion. Likewise, the iner-

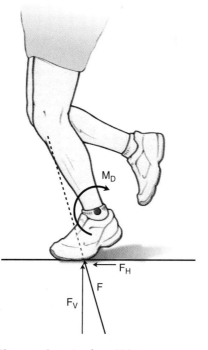

FIGURE 2-2. The ground reaction force (F) between a runner's foot in stance can be broken up into horizontal (F_H) and vertical (F_V) components. This ground reaction force acts off center to the ankle joint axis and creates a dorsiflexing (M_D) moment of force or torque.

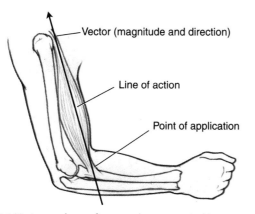

FIGURE 2-1. Vectors such as a force can be represented by an *arrow*. The four characteristics of a force are illustrated.

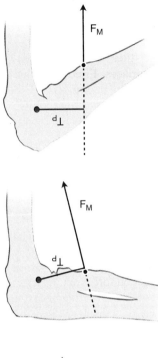

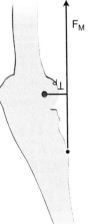

FIGURE 2-3. Schematic of the changes in the moment arm ($d_\perp$) at the elbow for the biceps brachii. The torque or moment of force the muscle can create is affected by both changes in force and moment arm ($T = F_M \cdot d_\perp$). The moment arm at the elbow for the long head of biceps would be affected by both shoulder and elbow joint rotation (note variation in the muscle angle of pull and the resulting moment arm).

tia of the moving object tends to keep it moving, so a force must be applied to either stop it or modify its motion.

The second law is usually called the *law of acceleration* and is represented by the mathematical formula $\Sigma F = ma$, where "ΣF" equals the sum of forces in a direction, m equals mass, and a equals acceleration in the same direction. This formula illustrates the relationship between kinetics and the resulting kinematics. The law says that "the acceleration an object experiences is proportional to the resultant force acting on the object in that

direction and is inversely proportional to the object's mass." This formula specifies the cause-and-effect relationship between forces and linear motion.

In angular motion, the law of acceleration is written as $\Sigma M = I\alpha$, where ΣM equals the sum of the moments acting on the object, I equals the moment of inertia of the object, and α equals the angular acceleration of the object. Newton's second law may be the most important because it defines the relationship between kinetics and kinematics, includes the inertia of objects (m and I), and provides for units of force. For example, a Newton of force is the linear effect that will accelerate 1 kg of mass (m) 1 m/s/s (a). These two formulas are applied in biomechanical models to estimate the net forces and torques acting in linked segment models. This is called *inverse dynamics* because measures of kinematics (α) and body segment inertial properties (I) are used to calculate the net moments (ΣM) or forces creating the movement.

Newton's third law is called the *law of action–reaction*. This says that "for every force there is an equal and opposite force." In other words, forces do not act only on one body but are an interaction between two bodies. The law can be expressed mathematically as: $F_{AB} = -F_{BA}$. When objects A and B interact, object A produces an equal and opposite effect on B. In turn, the second object, B, produces an equal and opposite effect on A. Positive and negative signs in mechanics refer to the direction of vector quantities. For example, during locomotion, the foot exerts a force every time it contacts the ground. The ground, however, exerts an equal and opposite force on the foot (see Fig. 2-2). This is an important law of kinetics that shows that forces and torques are mutual interactions between objects.

IMPORTANT FORCES IN HUMAN MOVEMENT

Forces that create human motion can be external forces between parts of the body and the environment (i.e., the ground reaction forces in Fig. 2-2) or internal forces created by the musculoskeletal system. These forces can be classified many ways, but the forces that are most often considered in biomechanical analyses are described in this section.

Gravity is the vertical, attraction force between the earth and an object. The magnitude of this force is the body weight (BW) of the object. BW is proportional to mass from Newton's second law. Because gravitational acceleration is fairly constant on the earth (9.81 m/s/s), a 50-kg barbell weighs 490.5 Newtons ($F_w = 50(9.81)$). Skeletal muscles must skillfully balance the weight of body segments and external objects such as dumbbells to move in even the simplest exercise. Standing in the anatomical position, the weight force of the body interacts with the supporting force from the floor.

Contact between the human body and another object (e.g., catching a ball, jumping, wearing ankle weights)

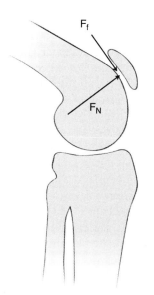

FIGURE 2-4. The contact force between two objects, such as at the patellofemoral joint, are often broken into friction (F_F) and normal reaction (F_N) components.

results in external forces that are often resolved into two important components: the **normal reaction** and **friction**. Friction (F_f) is the force acting parallel to the two surfaces in contact and it acts in the opposite direction of the motion or impending motion (Fig. 2-4). The force acting perpendicular to the surfaces of contact is called the normal reaction (F_N) or normal force. In dry conditions, the size of these two forces are related by the simple formula: $F_f = \mu F_N$, where μ is the coefficient of static friction. The coefficient of static friction is a dimensionless ratio that is experimentally determined and describes the frictional properties between the two interacting surfaces. When the two surfaces start to slide past each other, the friction force decreases, and a kinetic coefficient of friction must be used. For example, tennis shoes on sports surfaces typically have coefficients of static friction ranging from 0.4 to nearly 2.0[1]. Rotational friction can also be determined by how much moment of force must be applied to cause the surfaces to rotate against the other.

Some of the most important external forces in human movement are *ground reaction forces*. Ground reaction forces act between a person and the support surface on which they move, such as the foot of a runner shown in Figure 2-2. A force platform can be used to measure the changes in magnitude, direction, and point of application of the ground reaction forces during the period the foot is in contact with the platform. These ground reaction forces are resolved into three components relative to the person's direction of motion: the vertical (normal reaction) and two frictional components (anteroposterior and mediolateral). In running, the peak vertical ground reaction forces occur in midstance and are about 3 BW, and the peak anteroposterior forces are about 0.4 BW[2]. If the

coefficient of friction between this shoe and the platform surface was 0.8, then the maximum horizontal force that could be made before sliding would be 2.4 BW ($F_f = 0.8(3.0)$). As such, there is little danger of slipping while running on dry surfaces. Frictional forces in wet conditions are much smaller than in similar dry conditions. A child running on a wet pool deck might only have 0.15 BW of friction ($F_f = 0.05(3.0)$) because of the very low coefficient of friction.

Examples of internal forces are *joint reaction forces*. In linked segment biomechanical models, these forces between adjacent segments are modeled using Newton's laws of motion. In a squat exercise, for example, the downward force on an intervertebral disk from the weight of the upper body has an equal and opposite (acting upward) force from the lower body. The most common methods of inverse dynamics use Newton's laws to determine net joint reaction forces and moments of force from measurements of segment acceleration and inertial parameters. Unfortunately, the joint reaction forces are a combination of joint, muscle, and ligament forces and do not represent the true bone-on-bone forces at joints[3]. Actual bone-on-bone forces and contact pressures at joint surfaces are very difficult to calculate.

Other important internal forces are elastic forces. Elastic forces often contribute to many movements and are created by the tendency of a deformed material to return to its original shape. The size of the elastic force in a deformed material is called **stiffness** and is defined as the ratio of mechanical **stress** (σ) to **strain** (ϵ) in the linear (elastic) region of the curve. Figure 2-5 shows an idealized stress/strain curve. The slope of the linear portion of the graph (σ/ϵ) up to the yield point gives an indication of the stiffness of the material. Stress is defined as the

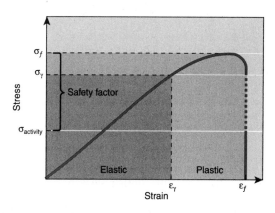

FIGURE 2-5. An idealized stress/strain curve. The elastic region is bounded by the yield point (designated by ϵ_y, σ_y). The plastic region is bounded by the yield point and the failure point (designated by ϵ_f, σ_f). The stress in musculoskeletal tissues in normal activity is much less than the yield point. The difference between the stress/strain of normal activities and the failure point is the safety factor. (Adapted with permission from Biewener AA, ed: Biomechanics: Structures and Systems. Oxford, UK: Oxford University Press; 1992.)

force per unit area of the material, and strain is usually defined as the percentage change in length. For example, the maximal muscular strength of muscle is usually reported as a stress of 25 to 40 N/cm^2, and the typical elongation of the Achilles tendon in a maximal voluntary contraction is a strain of about 5%[5]. Because the area of a deformed material changes, it is easier to ignore these small deformations and approximate stress/strain graphs with force/deformation graphs.

A stiff material is hard to deform (high force for small deformation) and, therefore, has high elasticity, tending to quickly return to its normal shape when an external force is removed. A material with low stiffness is called *compliant* because small forces can create larger deformations. Materials loaded in the elastic region of the curve return to their normal shape with minimal permanent change in shape. Stressing a material beyond the yield point into the plastic region of the curve results in permanent change in the material's structure. Materials have an ultimate mechanical strength or failure point that represents the maximum force or stress a material can withstand before breaking. Stresses in the musculoskeletal system in normal activities are much lower than the yield point for these tissues, so there is a large safety factor[6] in most physical activities. Sometimes the mechanical strength of a material is documented as the total energy absorbed. Note that the mechanical strength of materials is different from muscular strength. This chapter refers to muscular strength as "strength" and uses "mechanical strength" to avoid confusion in terminology.

Most tissues have more complex stress/strain curves than the one shown in Figure 2-5. The curves are nonlinear, and the stiffness depends on the timing of force loading. This rate dependence of mechanical behavior is called *viscoelasticity.* Tissues of the musculoskeletal system have greater stiffness when they are loaded rapidly. This is a major reason why static stretching is preferred over ballistic stretching because a greater level of musculotendinous elongation can be reached using a smaller and safer amount of force. In normal and vigorous movements, however, muscles and tendons can be stretched like a spring, and a large percentage of this elastic energy can be recovered in subsequent shortening[7]. This storage and recovery of elastic forces is just one mechanism of the important neuromuscular strategy called the *stretch–shortening cycle.* Many powerful movements are naturally initiated with a countermovement that is stopped with an eccentric muscle action and immediately reversed to a concentric action in the intended direction of motion[8]. For example, in the stance phase of sprinting, the plantar flexors are essentially eccentrically active in early stance that serves to increase the force of the following concentric action in push-off.

Maybe the most important and complex internal forces affecting human movement are muscle forces. Muscles exert forces on the skeleton to create motion, stabilize posture, dampen vibration, or decrease the stress in bones created by other forces. Muscles create only tensile forces that pull on all attachments. Muscle forces also create torques about joints. The torques are always changing as the joint moves through the range of motion (ROM) because the moment arms change as joints rotate and because muscle force production is related to muscle length and velocity. Therefore, the torque a muscle group can make is a complex phenomenon that is a combination of tension variations attributable to contractile conditions and geometric/moment arm changes for muscles.

The amount of tension a muscle can create depends on excitation and mechanical factors related to muscle length and velocity. The *force–velocity relationship* dictates that the magnitude of muscle force depends on the rate of length change or muscle velocity[9]. The faster a muscle shortens (concentric action), the less muscle force that can be created for the same level of excitation. On the other hand, the faster the active lengthening of muscle (eccentric action), the greater the muscle force. This relationship is illustrated in Figure 2-6. Note that the force potentials for all three muscle actions (eccentric, isometric, concentric) are defined by the graph. Training shifts the force/velocity graph upward but cannot change the pattern of decreased or increased force potential as muscle velocity changes.

The *force–length relationship* indicates how the isometric force a muscle can create varies with its length[10]. At intermediate lengths, muscles can produce the greatest force. Less force can be created in shortened conditions. Less active tension can also be created in lengthened conditions, but this is offset by increases in passive tension. In other words, the elastic force of stretched connective tissue and structural proteins within muscle generates tension that can be used to create subsequent motion. This passive tension is the discomfort that is felt in a vigorous stretch.

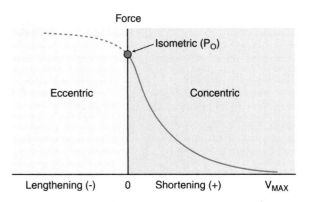

FIGURE 2-6. The force/velocity relationship of skeletal muscle illustrates skeletal muscle force potential for the rate of change of muscle length (velocity), so all three muscle actions can be visualized on the graph. (Adapted with permission from Knudson D: Fundamentals of Biomechanics. New York: Kluwer; 2003).

Muscles rarely work in isolation because there are multiple muscles crossing most joints with similar and opposing anatomical actions. Clinicians and researchers most often assess muscle group strength using measurements from handheld or isokinetic dynamometers. A dynamometer is a machine that measures force or torque. Isokinetic dynamometers measure torque in conditions of nearly constant joint angular velocity. Isokinetic dynamometers allow muscle group strength to be defined for all points in the ROM isometrically or at various constant speeds of shortening or lengthening. The torque-angle or moment-angle curves created by these machines illustrate the strength curves of muscle groups integrating the many mechanical factors affecting muscle force (Fig. 2-7). Extensive normative data are available for most joints of the body[11], and these data are usually normalized to body mass and categorized for a variety of populations (e.g., age, gender, sport).

Determining the contribution of individual muscles to movements is very difficult. The reason is that muscles have actions at all joints, not just the joints they cross, because of the linked segments of the human body[12]. The joint reaction forces acting at joints allow energy from a muscle to be transferred to segments quite distant from the segments the muscle attaches to. Computer simulations of complex biomechanical models have begun to determine these complex actions of muscles in movements[13]. Biomechanics uses a variety of research to validate these observations, including electromyography (EMG), movement kinematics, and direct measurements of forces in tendons. The use of EMG was one of the first technologies to show that muscular contributions to movement are more complex than hypothesized by anatomy[14]. The use of implanted force transducers in the tendons of animals and humans[15–18] and bright mode ultrasound images of muscle and tendon length changes[19] are recent developments in helping confirm the complex actions of muscles in movement. Often the hypothesized actions of muscles made in functional anatomy are incorrect, so the integration of several kinds of biomechanical research is needed to develop a good understanding of how muscles create movement.

Other important forces affecting human movement are fluid forces. Fluid forces arise when people are submerged and move in water or air. There are three fluid forces: **buoyancy**, **lift**, and **drag**. Buoyancy is the supporting or flotation force of a fluid. Water exercise programs use the upward force of buoyancy to decrease the vertical loading in the joints of the lower extremities. This is an effective exercise modality for persons with arthritis and persons in rehabilitation programs.

When there is relative flow of a fluid past an object, the flow forces are resolved into two components: lift and drag. Lift acts at right angles to the relative flow, and drag acts parallel to and opposing the flow. Both of these forces increase with the square of the velocity of flow, so the resistance to body movements in water exercises increases dramatically with faster speeds of movement. There are a variety of assistive devices that increase buoyancy, lift, and drag to adjust resistance during water exercise. For example, a life vest increases a person's buoyancy so he or she can float in an upright position. Attaching fins to the feet would increase the lift provided by kicking movements, and specialized suits can decrease drag forces, thereby increasing swimming speed. Cyclists ride directly behind other cyclists (draft) to decrease the drag forces of the air rushing past them.

Kinematics

Biomechanics has a long history of studies documenting the kinematics of human movements. Although most of these studies have been two-dimensional analyses, more and more research has focused on documenting the three-dimensional movements of the body. Precise three-dimensional measurement of the motion of human segments and joints has been labor intensive and involves considerable technical complexity[20]. However, kinematic studies have provided useful descriptive data in many areas of human movement. Kinematic data can be used to

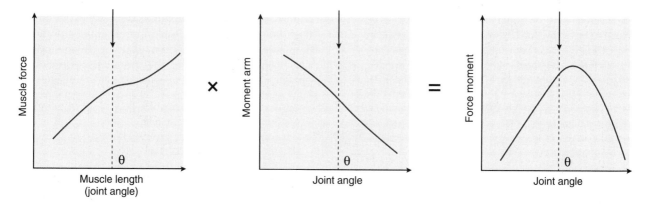

FIGURE 2-7. The joint moment–angle curve represents the strength curves of muscle groups. The shape of these curves is a combination of muscular properties (similar to the force–length relationship) and muscle moment arms. (Adapted with permission from Zatsiorsky V: Science and Practice of Strength Training. Champaign, IL: Human Kinetics; 1995).

profile the technique of athletes[21,22], help workers avoid potentially injurious work movements[23], and document normal patterns of movement such as locomotion[24,25].

There are several limitations in modifying client movement to match normal, skilled, or elite kinematics. First, there is within- and between-person variability in movement technique. Despite the precision of kinematic measurements, there is subjectivity in determining what is considered normal or desirable given the variability of human movement. One example is the variation in running economy (mass normalized steady state oxygen consumption for a given speed) that is fairly resistant to modifications in running technique[26–28]. Runners naturally tend to select kinematics that maximize economy, so it is difficult to effectively modify running technique based on kinematics alone unless there is extreme deviation from normative technique. Second, kinematics measurements do not, in and of themselves, explain the causes of motion. In other words, nearly identical movements can have different muscular causes[29]. For example, a physical therapist may help a patient with some muscular paralysis achieve a cosmetically normal walking pattern using other lower extremity muscles or orthotics. Therapists have been warned not to infer too much of the kinetic causes of walking from the kinematics of the patient's gait[30], and other exercise science professionals should also bear this in mind when qualitatively analyzing the kinematics of movements.

Despite the lack of explanatory power of kinematic measurements, useful information in kinematic studies can improve human movement. For example, the position and horizontal velocity of the whole-body center of mass relative to the base of support are important variables in theoretical models of stability and balance[31]. The clinical value of static and dynamic measures of stance, however, is more controversial because these tests may not correlate with regaining postural control when body position is unexpectedly disturbed[32]. More research on the kinematics of postural, locomotion, sport, and exercise movements may help improve the specificity of conditioning programs. The decreasing cost and greater automation of these calculations from video or position sensors may allow for the documentation of typical kinematics for more movements and with a wider variety of people (ages, skill levels, and disabilities). More examples of how kinematic data can be useful in improving human

movement are summarized in the next section on the application of biomechanics in sports and exercise.

Application to Human Movement Exercise Prescription

KINETICS

In prescribing exercise, professionals select the resistance and intensity of movements to match the fitness level and goals of clients. It has been hypothesized that there is an optimal window of loading that healthy people should maintain, with loading above this window presenting a greater risk of injury[33]. The idea can be viewed as a continuum (Fig. 2-8) between too little loading (resulting in musculoskeletal atrophy) and too much loading (resulting in injury). Unfortunately, this window has not been defined, and it is difficult to estimate the desirable loads in body tissues in various activities. Recently, some prospective studies have begun to address his issue. Fuchs et al.[34], for example, have shown that drop jump training can significantly increase bone mass in young children. More research on the forces involved in typical physical education activities could then help in the development of programs that not only build aerobic and muscular fitness but also promote long-term skeletal health. Research has also begun to link the exercise resistances used by older adults in weight training to increases in bone mass[35] and the kinds of training that create the largest increases in bone mechanical strength[36].

The mechanical variables related to external forces that have been measured to examine potential injury are the magnitude of the peak force, the rate of force development, and the repetition of loading. Figure 2-9 illustrates the difference in the vertical ground reaction force between heel–toe (rearfoot) and midfoot footstrike[2] patterns in running. The heel–toe running pattern has a passive peak or impact peak within the first 50 ms of contact from the heel striking the ground. The second peak force is the active peak force that corresponds to the reversal point of the down–up motion of the body. Note how the magnitude of the active peak force is about the same in both footstrike conditions, but there is usually a higher rate of force development in the heel–toe pattern compared with the midfoot pattern.

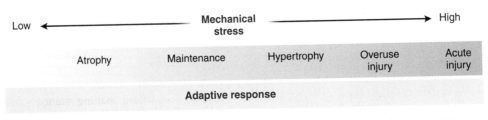

FIGURE 2-8. The continuum of mechanical stress imposed on tissue and the likely adaptive response.

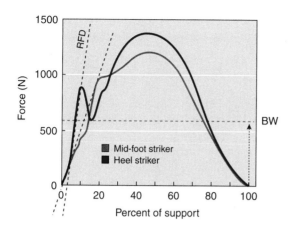

FIGURE 2-9. The vertical ground reaction force for heel and midfoot footstrike patterns. The heel–toe (rearfoot) footstrike pattern typically had a larger rate of force development (RFD) than the midfoot pattern. BW = body weight. (Adapted with permission from Hamill J, Knutzen KM: Biomechanical Basis of Human Movement. Philadelphia: Lippincott Williams & Wilkins; 2003).

During normal physical activities, the magnitude of the peak ground reaction forces usually creates stresses in lower extremity tissues within the elastic range and, therefore, do not cause trauma or injury. The rate of force development is an important variable because of the viscoelastic nature of tissues. The greater the rate of loading, the more stiff the tissue and the greater the load reached before failure. The rate of force development is also clinically relevant because it determines the kind of failure or fracture if loading goes beyond the elastic limit of the tissue. Studies of the kinetics of landing in Olympics gymnastics have been instrumental in changing rules and equipment that may help decrease the risk of injury to athletes[37].

Load repetition generally does not result in injury in normal physical activity. It is possible, however, for long-term repeated impacts to result in accumulation of microtrauma and the development of an overuse injury. *Overuse injuries* are usually the result of high-intensity activity over an extended period without adequate rest between training sessions. Because the long-term result of the mechanical stress of exercise can be either positive or negative, it is important for exercise professionals to be knowledgeable about symptoms of overtraining (see Section 3, Chapter 28) to reduce the risk of overuse injuries.

A promising area of biomechanics research involves the computer simulation of movements. In movements with simple performance criteria, computer simulations of biomechanical models can provide important information to optimize performance[38] and determine the effect of modifications in technique[39,40]. One study found that increasing the strength of a muscle group did not automatically improve vertical jump performance unless the coordination of the model was adjusted to take advantage of the added strength[41]. In the future, the integration of biomechanics and sports medicine research may enable professionals to define general guidelines for resistances and external force loading that results in desirable hypertrophy in tissues without elevated risk of injury.

KINEMATICS

Kinematics measurements of human movement may also have some use in defining desirable exercise and sports technique. Remember that earlier in the chapter, it was noted that documenting what movement occurs (kinematics) cannot explain how the movement was created (kinetics). There are, however, several ways that kinematic measurements can be used to help improve human movement.

There is some inherent value in documenting the kinematics of normal and skilled movement technique. This basic improvement in our understanding of what movements actually occur is important because many human movements are fast and difficult for professionals to see[42]. Kinematic information on how movement changes with motor development[43] or learning[44] also helps the professional know what movements to look for with growth or practice. For example, kinematics measurements of walking gait have yielded data that is used (clinical gait analysis) to assist medical professionals in treating and monitoring progress for many conditions[24]. Knowing how much trunk lateral bending there is in normal walking helps therapists judge how much a patient has recovered. In sports, kinematic studies have improved the coaching of cricket bowling techniques and has significantly reduced intervertebral disk degeneration in athletes[45]. Qualitative and quantitative kinematic analysis has also been used to remediate injuries and swing mechanics in golf[46,47]. The kinematic prescription of maintaining approximately normal lordosis (lumbar curvature) without transverse plane twisting is likely the safest spinal alignment in golf and most activities. Coaching this spinal position in lifting and sports movements evenly loads intervertebral disks and likely reduces the risk of injury (Fig. 2-11a).

Two more areas in which kinematic measurements have been applied in human movement are locomotion and lifting. Walking and running speed is a kinematic variable that is often used in modifying the intensity of exercise. Speed of locomotion is also strongly related to the biomechanical variables of gait, so coaches and therapists comparing walking or running technique over time need to evaluate clients at similar speeds. Locomotion is a highly skilled activity that requires considerable kinematic control to maintain balance. Weightlifting activities are often much slower and use more stable postures. A wide **base of support** and lower **center of gravity** increases stability. Whereas a squatting position favors stability over mobility, the upright, forwarding leaning stance phase of running favors mobility. Both lifting and running require balance (the control over positioning the body), but the kinematics and geometry of the postures favor different objectives (stability vs. mobility).

An object's center of gravity is a theoretical point where the weight force of the object can be considered to act. The kinematics (variation in height and horizontal distance) of the center of gravity relative to the base of support are often studied to examine the balance exhibited by performer. In a sit-to-stand movement, the body weight is shifted over the base of support where there is a transition from primarily horizontal motion to a vertical or lifting motion (Fig. 2-10).

Kinematics provides useful information for defining safe lifting technique. When lifting boxes from the ground, the lifter should squat with a wide base of support. Spreading the feet apart helps maintain stability and allows the load to be carried close to the body, minimizing the moment arm and resistance torques for the lower back. The lifter should also keep the trunk straight (normal lordosis) and avoid exaggerated trunk lean. Performing the lift slowly with the legs and without axial trunk twisting are also important mechanical factors that minimize the risk of injury. Unfortunately, people unconsciously tend to stoop lift (lean over) probably because small weights can be lifted with passive back muscle and ligament forces and, therefore, less metabolic cost (Fig. 2-11b). Repetitive use of this lifting technique is dangerous because of the large moment

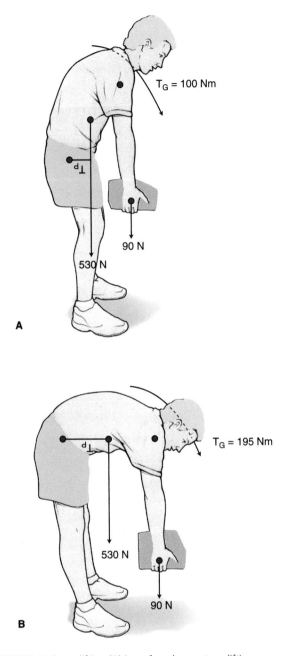

A

B

FIGURE 2-11. Squat lifting (**A**) is preferred over stoop lifting (**B**) because it decreases the gravitational torque (T_G) the lower back and hip extensors must balance. The kinematic variable of trunk lean is an important focus of observation because the angle of the trunk relative to gravity directly affects the moment arm ($d_\perp$) for the weight forces of the trunk and the box. A typical man decreases the gravitational torque about the hip from 195 Nm in the stoop lift to 100 Nm in the squat lift positions illustrated.

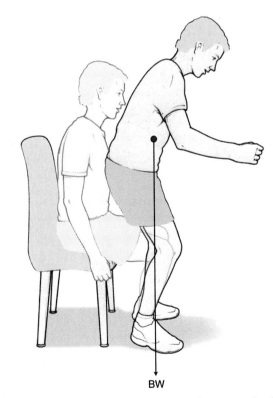

FIGURE 2-10. The initial phase of the sit-to-stand movement involves trunk lean and horizontal weight shift to position the center of gravity over the new base of support (feet). The movement of the center of gravity in several directions is often used to study balance. BW = body weight.

arm for the resistances and uneven spinal loading. The 30° of trunk lean in the squat lift illustrated in Figure 2-11 decreases the moment arms for weight forces of the box and upper body by one half (cos60 deg = 0.5) from the stoop position decreasing the gravitational torque loading on the lower back.

Statistical analysis of biomechanical data (including kinematics) has also been used to identify links between technique variables and performance[22]. Therefore, kinematic measurements do hold promise in confirming the clinical observations of therapists and coaches, and these data may play a role in identifying key technique factors that can be used to improve human movement or reduce the risk of injury. Kinematic data should, however, be integrated with other studies (kinetics, EMG, training) to confirm that certain technique points are important and causative factors in performance or injury prevention.

Summary

The study of biomechanics is essential to sports medicine and exercise science professionals because it forms the basis for documenting human motion (kinematics) and understanding the causes of that motion (kinetics). The key mechanical variables that explain the creation of motion are force and moment of force (torque). Newton's three laws of motion are critical to understanding how human movement is created and how it can be improved. Key forces that affect human motion are gravity; friction; normal reaction; joint reactions; ground reactions; and elastic, muscular, and fluid forces. Biomechanics also provides information to help modify exercise through studies of the kinematics of human movement. These studies precisely document the motion of the body for a variety of movements and mover characteristics that professionals serve. The application of biomechanics in the prescription of exercise through the use of kinetic and kinematic data is being increasingly used to define desirable exercise intensities and movement amplitudes that create musculoskeletal adaptions with less risk of injury.

Acknowledgments
Portions of this chapter are adapted from the excellent work of the authors of previous editions of the Resource Manual.

REFERENCES

1. Nigg BM, Luthi SM, Bahlsen HA: The tennis shoe—Biomechanical design criteria. In Segesser B, Pforringer W, eds. The Shoe in Sport. Chicago: Year Book Medical Publishers; 1989:39–52.
2. Munro CF, Miller, DI. Fuglevand AJ: Ground reaction forces in running: A reexamination. J Biomech 20:147–155, 1987.
3. Zatsiorsky VM: Kinetics of Human Motion. Champaign, IL: Human Kinetics; 2002.
4. Herzog W: Force-sharing among synergistic muscles: theoretical considerations and experimental approaches. Ex Sport Sci Rev 24:173–200, 1996.
5. Muramatsu T, Muraoka T, Takeshita D, Kawakami Y, Hirano Y, Fukunaga T: Mechanical properties of tendon and aponeurosis of human gastrocnemius muscle in vivo. J Appl Physiol 90:1671–1678, 2001.
6. Biewener AA, Ed: Biomechanics: Structures and Systems. Oxford, UK: Oxford University Press; 1992.
7. Alexander RM: Tendon elasticity and muscle function. Comp Biochem Physiol Part A 133:1001–1011, 2002.
8. Komi PV, Nicol C: Stretch-shortening cycle of muscle function. In Zatsiorsky V, ed. Biomechanics in Sport. Oxford, UK: Blackwell; 2000:87–102.
9. Hill AV: The heat of shortening and the dynamic constants of muscle. Proc R Soc 126:136–195, 1938.
10. Gordon AM, Huxley AF, Julian JF: The variation in isometric tension with sarcomere length in vertebrate muscle fibers. J Physiol 184:170–192, 1966.
11. Brown LE, Ed: Isokinetics in Human Performance. Champaign, IL: Human Kinetics; 2000.
12. Zajac FE, Gordon ME: Determining muscle's force and action in multi-articular movement. Exerc Sport Sci Rev 17:187–230, 1989.
13. Zajac FE: Understanding muscle coordination of the human leg with dynamical simulations. J Biomech 35:1011–1018, 2002.
14. Hellebrandt FA: Living anatomy. Quest 1:43–58, 1963.
15. Komi PV, Salonen M, Jarvinen M, Kokko O: In vivo registration of Achilles tendon forces in man. I. Methodological development. Int J Sports Med 8:3–8, 1987.
16. Komi PV, Belli A, Huttunen V, Bonnefoy R, Geyssant A, Lacour JR: Optic fibre as a transducer of tendomuscular forces. Eur J Appl Physiol 72:278–280, 1996.
17. Roberts TJ, Marsh RL, Weyand PG, Taylor DR: Muscular force in running turkeys: the economy of minimizing work. Science 275:1113–1115, 1997.
18. Finni T, Komi PV, Lukkariniemi J: Achilles tendon loading during walking: Application of a novel optic fiber technique. Eur J Appl Physiol 77:289–291, 1998.
19. Kawakami Y, Abe T, Fukunaga T: Muscle-fiber pennation angles are greater in hypertrophied than in normal muscles. J Appl Physiol 74:2740–2744, 1993.
20. Zatsiorsky VM: Kinematics of Human Motion. Champaign, IL: Human Kinetics; 1998.
21. Fleisig GS, Barrentine SW, Zheng N, Escamilla RF, Andrews JR: Kinematic and kinetic comparison of baseball pitching among various levels of development. J Biomech 32:1371–1375, 1999.
22. Lees A: Biomechanical assessment of individual sports for improved performance. Sports Med 28:299–305, 1999.
23. Hsiang SM, Brogmus GE, Courtney TK: Low back pain (LBP) and lifting technique—A review. Int J Industr Ergonomics 19:59–74, 1997.
24. Whittle M: Gait Analysis: An Introduction, 2nd ed. Oxford, UK: Butterworth-Heinemann; 1996.
25. Novacheck, TF: The biomechanics of running. Gait Posture 7:77–95, 1998.
26. Morgan DW, Martin PE, Craig M, et al: Effect of stride length variation on oxygen uptake during distance running. Med Sci Sports Exerc 14:30–35, 1982.
27. Messier SP, Cirillo, KJ: Effects of a verbal and visual feedback system on running technique, perceived exertion and running economy. J Sports Sci 7:113–126, 1989.
28. Lake MJ, Cavanagh PR: Six weeks of training does not change running mechanics or improve running economy. Med Sci Sports Exerc 28:737–743, 1996.
29. Winter DA: Kinematic and kinetic patterns of human gait: Variability and compensating effects. Hum Mov Sci 3:51–76, 1984.
30. Herbert R, Moore S, Moseley A, Schurr K, Wales A: Making inferences about muscles forces from clinical observations. Aust J Physiother 39:195–202, 1993.
31. Pai YC: Movement termination and stability in standing. Exerc Sports Sci Rev 31:19–25, 2003.
32. Owings TM, Pavol MJ, Foley KT, Grabiner MD: Measures of postural stability are not predictors of recovery from large postural disturbances in healthy older adults. J Am Geriatr Soc 48:42–50, 2000.
33. Nigg BM, Cole GK, Bruggeman GP: Impact forces during heel-toe running. J Appl Biomech 11:407–432, 1995.
34. Fuchs RK, Bauer JJ, Snow CM: Jumping improves hip and lumbar spine bone mass in prepubescent children: A randomized control trial. J. Bone Min Res 16:148–156, 2001.
35. Cussler EC, Lohman TG, Going SB, et al: Weight lifted in strength training predicts bone change in postmenopausal women. Med Sci Sports Exerc 35:10–17, 2003.

36. Turner CH, Robling AG: Designing exercise regimens to increase bone strength. Exerc Sport Sci Rev 31:45–50, 2003.

37. Bruggemann G-P: Improving performance and reducing injuries through biomechanics. Olympic Rev 22:9–10, 1998.

38. Hatze H: Biomechanical aspects of a successful motion optimization. In Komi PV, ed. Biomechanics VB. Baltimore: University Park Press; 1976:5–12.

39. Yeadon MR. The biomechanics of human flight. Am J Sports Med 25:575–580, 1997.

40. Holvoet P, Lacouture P, Duboy J: Practical use of airborne simulation in a release-regrasp skill on the high bar. J Appl Biomech 18:332–344, 2002.

41. Bobbert MF, van Soest AJ: Effects of muscle strengthening on vertical jump height: A simulation study. Med Sci Sports Exerc 26:1012–1020, 1994.

42. Knudson D, Morrison C: Qualitative Analysis of Human Movement, 2nd ed. Champaign, IL: Human Kinetics; 2002.

43. Roberton MA, Konczak J: Predicting children's overarm throw ball velocities from their developmental levels in throw. Res Quart Exerc Sport 72:91–103, 2001.

44. Southard D: Change in throwing pattern: Critical values for control parameter of velocity. Res Quart Exerc Sport 73:396–407, 2002.

45. Elliott BC, Kahangure M: Disk degeneration and fast bowling in cricket: An intervention study. Med Sci Sports Exerc 34:1714–1718, 2002.

46. Grimshaw PN, Burden AM: Case report: Reduction of low back pain in a professional golfer. Med Sci Sports Exerc 32:1667–1673, 2000.

47. Parziale JR: Healthy swing: A golf rehabilitation model. Am J Phys Med Rehabil 81:498–501, 2002.

SELECTED REFERENCES FOR FURTHER READING

Chaffin, BD, Andersson, GBJ, Martin, BJ: Occupational Biomechanics, 3rd ed. New York: Wiley; 1999.

Dvir Z, ed: Clinical Biomechanics. New York: Churchill Livingstone; 2000.

Hamill J, Knutzen K: Biomechanical Basis of Human Movement, 2nd ed. Baltimore: Lippincott Williams & Wilkins; 2003.

Hay JG: The Biomechanics of Sports Techniques, 4th ed. Englewood Cliffs, NJ: Prentice-Hall; 1993.

Knudson D: Fundamentals of Biomechanics New York: Kluwer/Plenum Publishers; 2003.

Whiting WC, Zernicke RF: Biomechanics of Musculoskeletal Injury. Champaign, IL: Human Kinetics; 1998.

INTERNET RESOURCES

American College of Sports Medicine Approved Interest Groups: http://www.asu.edu/clas/kines/biomechlab/ACSM

American Society of Biomechanics: http://www.asb-biomech.org

Clinical Gait Analysis: http://guardian.curtin.edu.au/cga

Coaches' Infoservice: http://www.coachesinfo.com

Exploratorium: Sport Science: http://www.exploratorium.edu/sport

ExploreLearning: Motion and Force: http://www.explorelearning. com/index.cfm?method=cResource.dspResourcesForCourse&CourseI D=330&CFID=461259&CFTOKEN=47919187

The Hosford Muscle Tables: Skeletal Muscles of the Human Body: http://ptcentral.com/muscles

International Society of Biomechanics: http://www.isbweb.org

The International Society of Biomechanics in Sports: http://www. uni-stuttgart.de/External/isbs

Exercise Physiology

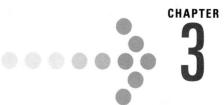

CHAD HARRIS, KENT J. ADAMS, AND NICOLE KEITH

This chapter presents a review of the acute responses of the body to the exercise stressor. Among the topics covered are the metabolic aspects of acute exercise, the acute cardiorespiratory responses to exercise, neuromuscular responses during exercise, the mechanisms of muscular fatigue, and the acute responses to exercise in varied environmental conditions.

Fundamentals of Exercise Metabolism

At rest, a 70-kg human has an energy expenditure of about 1.2 kcal·min^{-1}; less than 20% of resting energy expenditure is attributed to skeletal muscle. However, almost all changes that occur in the body during exercise are related to the increase in energy metabolism, largely within the contracting skeletal muscle. For example, cardiac output increases as a direct linear function of whole-body metabolism. To meet the demands on the heart, a fourfold increase in myocardial blood flow and oxygen consumption takes place.

During intense exercise, total energy expenditure may increase 15 to 25 times above resting values, resulting in a caloric expenditure of approximately 18 to 30 kcal·min^{-1}. Most of this increase is used to provide energy for exercising muscles, which may increase energy requirement by a factor of 200[1]. Therefore, daily caloric expenditure can be changed dramatically by simply altering the amount of physical activity performed during a day. Muscle fibers contain the metabolic machinery to produce adenosine triphosphate (ATP) by three systems: creatine phosphate (CP), rapid glycolysis, and aerobic oxidation of nutrients to carbon dioxide and water (oxidative phosphorylation).

The importance of the interaction of the aforementioned metabolic systems in the production of ATP during exercise should be emphasized. In reality, the energy to perform most types of exercise does not come from a single source but from a combination of anaerobic and aerobic sources (Fig. 3-1 and Table 3-1). The contribution of anaerobic sources (CP system and glycolysis) to exercise **energy metabolism** is inversely related to the duration and positively related to the intensity of the activity. The shorter and more intense the activity, the greater the contribution of anaerobic energy production; the longer the activity and the lower the intensity, the greater the contribution of aerobic energy production. Although proteins can be used as a fuel for aerobic exercise, carbohydrates and fats are the primary energy substrates during exercise in healthy, well-fed individuals. In general, carbohydrates are used as the primary fuel at the onset of exercise and during high-intensity work[2–4]. However, during prolonged exercise of low to moderate intensity (longer than 30 minutes), a gradual shift from carbohydrate toward an increasing reliance on fat as a substrate occurs (Fig. 3-2)[4,5]. The greatest amount of fat use occurs at about 60% of maximal aerobic capacity ($\dot{V}O_{2max}$). This chapter focuses on muscle bioenergetics and exercise metabolism. A detailed review of bioenergetics and exercise metabolism is provided in the suggested reading section of this chapter. A detailed discussion outlining the interplay of substrates during exercise is available from several sources[2–9]. A brief discussion of the energy pathways and the metabolic response to various types of exercise follows.

KEY TERMS

Acute mountain sickness (AMS): A sickness characterized by headaches, nausea, and lethargy that is related to acute exposure to altitude

Cardiorespiratory: The collective systems of the heart, blood vessels, and lungs that function to circulate blood in the body and exchange gasses

Central fatigue: The progressive reduction in voluntary drive to motor neurons during exercise

Cold stress: The loss in heat either from the core or locally that is brought on by environment, metabolism, and clothing

Concentric: When muscle length decreases during contraction

Eccentric: When muscle length increases during contraction

Electron transport chain: A series of chemical reactions in the mitochondria during which electrons from the hydrogen atoms of nicotinamide adenine dinucleotide (NADH) and flavin adenine dinucleotide (FADH) are transferred to oxygen. The electrochemical energy in this process is used production of adenosine triphosphate (ATP) from adenosine diphosphate (ADP) and inorganic phos-phate (Pi).

Energy metabolism: The net effect of chemical reaction in the body resulting in ATP production

Glycolysis: A series of chemical reactions for the conversion of glucose to pyruvate and the anaerobic production of ATP

Heat stress: An increase in core temperature collectively brought about by the environment, metabolism, and clothing

Hemodynamics: The acute response of the blood flow and blood composition to changes in the activity state of the body

Hypoxic ventilatory response: The increase in ventilation seen with acute altitude exposure as a result of reduced barometric pressure and lowered arterial oxygen pressure

Krebs cycle: A series of chemical reactions in the mitochondria in which acetyl-coenzyme A (CoA) is oxidized resulting in the production of 3 NADH, 1 FADH, 1 GTP, and 2 CO_2.

Maximal oxygen consumption ($\dot{V}O_{2max}$): The maximum rate of oxygen that can be used for production of ATP during exercise

Motor unit: The motor neuron and the muscle fibers it innervates

Muscle fatigue: The loss of force or power output in response to voluntary effort leading to reduced performance

Peripheral fatigue: The loss of force and power that is independent of neural drive

Primary pollutant: A direct source of pollution

Secondary pollutant: A pollutant formed from the interaction of a primary pollutant with an environmental factor

Size principle: The recruitment of motor units in order from smallest to largest according to recruitment thresholds and firing rates, resulting in a continuum of voluntary force

ENERGY FOR SHORT-TERM EXERCISE

Adenosine Triphosphate

The energy released through hydrolysis of the high-energy compound ATP to form adenosine diphosphate (ADP) and inorganic phosphate (Pi) powers skeletal muscle contractions. This reaction is catalyzed by the enzyme myosin ATPase:

$$(Myosin\ ATPase)$$
$$ATP \rightarrow ADP + Pi + energy$$

The amount of ATP directly available in muscle at any time is small, so it must be resynthesized continuously if exercise lasts for more than a few seconds.

Creatine Phosphate

The CP system transfers high-energy phosphate from CP to rephosphorylate ATP from ADP as follows:

$$(Creatine\ kinase)$$
$$ADP + CP \rightarrow ATP + C$$

This system is rapid because it involves only one enzymatic step (i.e., one chemical reaction); however, CP exists in finite quantities in cells, so the total amount of ATP that can be produced is limited. Oxygen is not involved in the rephosphorylation of ADP to ATP in this reaction, so the CP system is considered anaerobic (without oxygen).

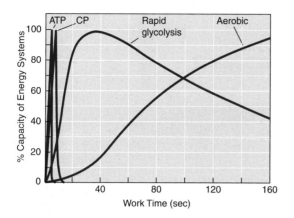

FIGURE 3-1. Interaction between anaerobic and aerobic energy sources during exercise, including adenosine triphosphate (ATP), creatine phosphate (CP), rapid glycolysis, and aerobic (oxidative phosphorylation). Note that whereas the energy to perform short-term high-intensity exercise comes primarily from anaerobic sources, the energy for muscular contraction during prolonged exercise comes from aerobic metabolism.

Rapid Glycolysis

When **glycolysis** is rapid, it is capable of producing ATP without involvement of oxygen. Glycolysis, the degradation of carbohydrate (glycogen or glucose) to pyruvate or lactate, involves a series of enzymatically catalyzed steps (Fig. 3-3). The net energy yield of glycolysis, without further oxidation through aerobic metabolism, is two or three ATPs through substrate level phosphorylation. The net production is two ATPs when glucose is the substrate and three ATPs when glycogen is the substrate. Although glycolysis does not use oxygen and is considered anaerobic, pyruvate can readily participate in aerobic production of ATP when oxygen is available in the cell. Therefore, in addition to being an anaerobic pathway capable of pro-ducing ATP without oxygen, glycolysis can also be considered the first step in the aerobic degradation of carbohydrate.

ENERGY FOR LONGER DURATION EXERCISE

Oxidative Phosphorylation

The final metabolic pathway for ATP production combines two complex metabolic processes, the **Krebs cycle** and **electron transport chain**; it resides inside

TABLE 3-1. Characteristics of the Two Mechanisms by Which ATP is Formed[130]

Mechanism	Food or Chemical Fuel	Oxygen Required?	Relative ATP Yield
Anaerobic phosphocreatine	Phosphocreatine	No	Extremely limited
Glycolysis	Glycogen (Glycogen)	No	Extremely limited
Aerobic Krebs cycle and electron transport system	Glycogen, fats, proteins	Yes	Large

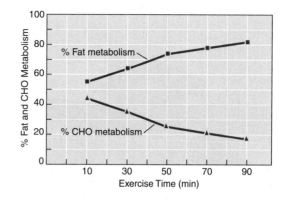

FIGURE 3-2. Alterations in substrate utilization during prolonged submaximal ($<60\%$ $\dot{V}O_{2max}$) exercise. CHO = carbohydrate. (Adapted with permission from Powers S, Byrd R, Tulley R, et al: Effects of caffeine ingestion on metabolism and performance during graded exercise. Eur J Appl Physiol 50:301, 1983.)

the mitochondria. Oxidative phosphorylation uses oxygen as the final hydrogen acceptor to form water and ATP. Unlike glycolysis, aerobic metabolism can use fat, protein, and carbohydrate as substrates to produce ATP. The interaction of these nutrients is illustrated in Figure 3-4.

Glucose
> Hexokinase

Glucose 6 – Phosphate
> Glucose 6 – Phosphate Isomerase

Fructose 6 – Phosphate
> Phosphofructokinase

Fructose 1,6 – Diphosphate
> Aldolase

Glyceraldehyde 3 – Phosphate + Dihydroxyacetone Phosphate
> Triophosphate Isomerase

Glyceraldehyde 3 – Phosphate
> Glyceraldehyde 3 – Phosphate Dehydrogenase

1,3 – Diphosphoglycerate
> Phosphoglycerate Kinase

3 – Phosphoglycerate
> Phosphoglucomutase

2 – Phosphoglycerate
> Enolase

Phosphoenolpyruvate
> Pyruvate Kinase

Pyruvate
> Lactate Dehydrogenase

Lactate

FIGURE 3-3. Enzymatic steps of glycolysis.

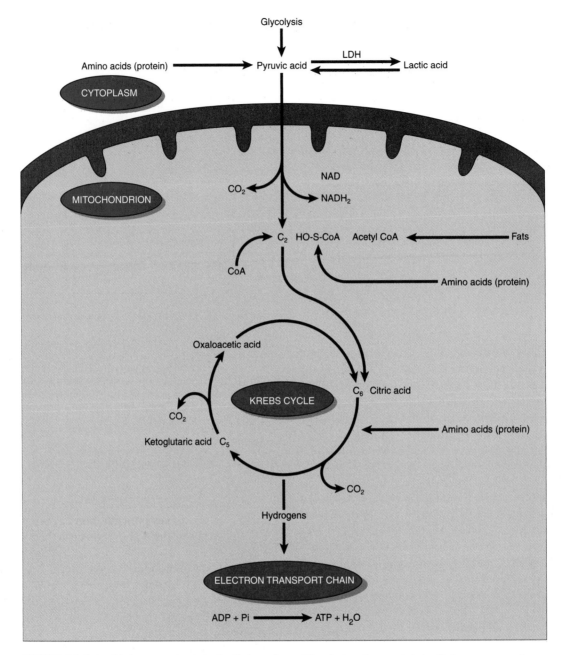

FIGURE 3-4. Relationship between glycolysis, the Krebs cycle, and the electron transport chain. CoA = coenzyme A; LDH = lactate dehydrogenase; NAD = nicotinamide adenine dinucleotide.

Conceptually, the Krebs cycle can be considered a primer for oxidative phosphorylation. Entry into the Krebs cycle begins with the combination of acetyl-coenzyme A (CoA) and oxaloacetic acid to form citric acid. The primary function of the Krebs cycle is to remove hydrogens from four of the reactants involved in the cycle. The electrons from these hydrogens follow a chain of cytochromes (electron transport chain) in the mitochondria, and the energy released from this process is used to rephosphorylate ADP to form ATP. Oxygen is the final acceptor of hydrogen to form water, and this reaction is catalyzed by cytochrome oxidase (see Fig. 3-4)

Oxidation of carbohydrates via the Krebs cycle and the electron transport chain results in a total of 36 ATPs per unit of glucose substrate or 38 ATPs per unit of glycogen substrate. A more detailed review of oxidative phosphorylation can be found in other sources[10].

Fat Metabolism

Oxidation of fat, which provides acetyl-CoA as substrate for the Krebs cycle, is possible through aerobic metabolism. Glycolysis can also interact with the Krebs cycle in the presence of oxygen by the conversion of pyruvate to form acetyl-CoA. Fats or triglycerides are lipids broken down to glycerol and fatty acids by hormone-sensitive lipase, which is inhibited by insulin and activated by catecholamines (epinephrine and norepinephrine) and growth hormone. Glycerol can be metabolized through glycolysis or used to make glucose. Free fatty acids enter the blood to be used as fuel in a process known as beta-oxidation, or they may be used as a precursor in the production of many substances such as cholesterol. Fatty acids must be activated using ATP and CoA and transported via the carnitine shuttle system to enter the mitochondria for oxidation. In the mitochondrial matrix, beta-oxidation proceeds sequentially by cleaving off two carbon atoms at a time, forming acetyl-CoA, the substrate for the Krebs cycle. A 16-carbon fatty acid such as palmitate yields 129 ATPs.

METABOLIC RESPONSE TO EXERCISE

Transition from Rest to Light Exercise

In the transition from rest to light exercise, oxygen uptake kinetics follow a monoexponential pattern, reaching a steady state generally within 1 to 4 minutes (Fig. 3-5)[11]. The time required to reach a steady state increases at higher work rates and is longer in untrained individuals than in aerobically trained individuals. Because oxygen uptake does not increase instantaneously to steady state at the onset of exercise, it is implied that anaerobic energy sources contribute to the required $\dot{V}O_2$ at the beginning of exercise. Indeed, evidence suggests that both the CP system and rapid glycolysis contribute to the overall production of ATP at the onset of muscular work[12]. As soon as a steady state is obtained, however, the ATP requirements are met by aerobic metabolism. The term *oxygen deficit* has been used to describe inadequate oxygen consumption at the onset of exercise (see Fig. 3-5). Similar to short-term heavy exercise, the principal fuel used during the transition from rest to light exercise is muscle glycogen[8].

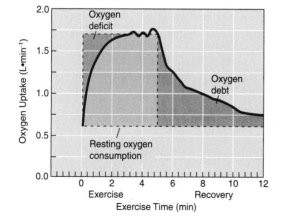

FIGURE 3-5. Oxygen uptake dynamics at onset and offset of exercise. See text for details.

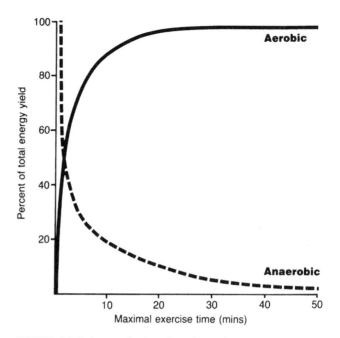

FIGURE 3-6. Relative contribution of aerobic and anaerobic metabolism during physical activity of increasing duration. In intense activities lasting 1.5 to 2.0 minutes, the ATP-CP and lactic acid energy systems generate approximately 50% of the energy, and aerobic metabolism supplies the remainder. A distance runner, on the other hand, derives essentially 98% of his or her energy from aerobic metabolism during a 50-minute training run.

Short-term, High-intensity Exercise

The energy to perform short-term, high-intensity exercise (5 to 60 seconds' duration), such as weightlifting or sprinting 400 meters, comes primarily from anaerobic systems (Fig. 3-6). Whether the ATP–CP system or glycolysis dominates the ATP production depends on the duration of the muscular effort. In general, energy for all activities lasting less than 5 seconds comes from the ATP–CP system. In contrast, energy to perform a 20-meter sprint (30 seconds) would come from a combination of the ATP–CP system and anaerobic glycolysis, with glycolysis predominating. The transition from the CP system to glycolysis is not abrupt but rather a gradual shift from one pathway to another as the duration of the exercise increases.

As illustrated in Figure 3-1, exercise bouts lasting longer than 45 seconds use a combination of the CP system, rapid glycolysis, and aerobic systems. For example, the energy required to sprint 400 meters (60 seconds) comes primarily (about 70%) from anaerobic sources (i.e., ATP, CP, rapid glycolysis), and the remaining ATP production is provided by aerobic metabolism. The principal fuel used during this type of exercise is carbohydrate (glycogen) stored in muscle[13].

Prolonged Submaximal Exercise

Steady-state $\dot{V}O_2$ can usually be maintained during 10 to 60 minutes of submaximal continuous exercise. This rule has two exceptions. First, prolonged exercise in a hot and humid environment results in a steady drift upward of $\dot{V}O_2$ during the course of exercise[14]. Second, continuous exercise at a high relative workload results in a slow rise in $\dot{V}O_2$ across time similar to that observed during exercise in a hot environment. In both cases, this drift probably occurs because of a variety of factors, such as rising body temperature and increasing blood catecholamines[15,16].

As depicted in Figure 3-2, both carbohydrate and fat are used as substrates during prolonged exercise. During prolonged low- and moderate-intensity exercise, there is a gradual shift from carbohydrate metabolism to the use of fat as a substrate. Explanations for this metabolic shift include the following: fatty acids inhibit the Krebs cycle, leading to accumulation of citrate, which lowers phosphofructokinase (PFK) activity. This causes reduced uptake and oxidation of glucose. Carbohydrate metabolism regulates fat metabolism during exercise[17]. The onset of exercise of low to moderate intensity produces a high glycolytic flux that slowly diminishes. The resulting glycolytic intermediates inhibit the carnitine transport system, thus preventing long-chain fatty acids from entering mitochondria for oxidation. Other factors that can affect the relative contribution of fat versus carbohydrate as energy substrate during prolonged exercise are nutritional status of the individual and the state of training.

Progressive Incremental Exercise

Figure 3-7 illustrates the oxygen uptake during a progressive incremental exercise test. Note that oxygen uptake increases linearly with work rate until $\dot{V}O_{2max}$ is reached. After reaching a steady state, ATP used for muscular contraction during the early stages of an incremental exercise test comes primarily from aerobic metabolism. However, as the exercise intensity increases, blood levels of lactate increase (Fig. 3-8). Although much controversy surrounds this issue, many investigators believe that this lactate inflection point is a point of increasing reliance upon anaerobic metabolism brought about by the increased recruitment of nonoxidative fast-twitch muscle fibers.

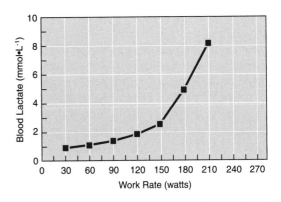

FIGURE 3-8. Changes in blood lactate concentrations as a function of work rate during incremental exercise.

Although the precise terminology is controversial, this sudden increase in blood lactate levels—termed the *anaerobic threshold* or *lactate threshold*—has important implications for the prediction of performance and perhaps exercise prescription. For example, it has been shown that the anaerobic threshold, used in combination with other physiological variables (i.e., $\dot{V}O_{2max}$), is a useful predictor of success in distance running[18,19]. The lactate threshold may also prove to be a marker of the transition from moderate to heavy exercise for subjects and, thus, useful in exercise prescriptions.

Recovery from Exercise

Oxygen uptake remains elevated above resting levels for several minutes during recovery from exercise (see Fig. 3-5). This elevated post-exercise oxygen consumption has traditionally been termed the *oxygen debt*, but more recently the term *elevated post-exercise oxygen consumption* (EPOC) has been applied[15]. In general, post-exercise metabolism is higher after high-intensity exercise than after light or moderate work. Furthermore, post-exercise $\dot{V}O_2$ remains elevated longer after prolonged exercise than after shorter-term exertion. The mechanisms to explain these observations are probably linked to the fact that both high-intensity and prolonged exercise result in higher body temperatures, greater ionic disturbance, and higher plasma catecholamines than in light or moderate short-term exercise[15].

METABOLIC OCCURRENCES DURING EXERCISE

Lactic Acid Threshold

Historically, increasing blood lactate levels during exercise have been considered an indication of increased anaerobic metabolism within the contracting muscle because of a lack of oxygen. If oxygen is not available in the mitochondria to accept hydrogen released during glycolysis, pyruvate must accept hydrogen to form lactate as an end product so that glycolysis can proceed. However,

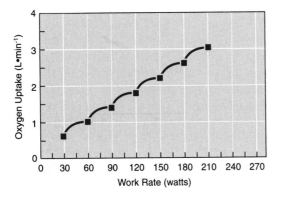

FIGURE 3-7. Changes in oxygen uptake as a function of work rate during incremental exercise.

the hypoxia theory is controversial. Whether the end product of glycolysis is pyruvate or lactate also depends on other factors, including muscle fiber type and how rapid glycolysis is proceeding. If glycolytic flux is extremely rapid, hydrogen production may exceed the transport capability of the shuttle mechanisms that move hydrogen from the cytoplasm (called *sarcoplasm* in muscle) into the mitochondria, where oxidative phosphorylation occurs without true hypoxia. When glycolytic hydrogen production exceeds the mitochondrial transport capability, pyruvate must again accept the hydrogens to form lactate so glycolysis can continue. During exercise, epinephrine (adrenaline) levels in the blood are elevated, which stimulates muscle *glycogenolysis* (breakdown of glycogen for fuel), increasing the rate of glycolysis. At rest and during low exercise intensities (<40% of maximal aerobic capacity), slow-twitch muscle fibers are recruited predominantly. As the exercise intensity increases, more fast-twitch fibers are recruited. This recruitment pattern has an important influence on lactic acid production. Conversion of pyruvate to lactate and vice versa is catalyzed by the enzyme lactate dehydrogenase (LDH), which exists in several forms (isozymes). Whereas fast-twitch muscle fibers contain an LDH isozyme that favors the formation of lactate, slow-twitch fibers contain an LDH form that promotes less conversion of pyruvate to lactate or even conversion of lactate to pyruvate. Therefore, more lactate formation occurs in fast-twitch fibers during exercise simply because of the type of LDH isozyme present, independent of oxygen availability in the muscle. Finally, fast-twitch fibers have higher activities of glycolytic enzymes than do slow-twitch fibers, indicating a greater potential of substrate flux through glycolysis.

In summary, debate over the mechanism or mechanisms responsible for muscle lactate production during exercise continues. It seems possible that any one or a combination of these possibilities (or lack of oxygen) may provide an explanation for muscle lactate production during exercise. The most important consequence of elevated lactic acid levels is the contribution to muscle fatigue. However, blood lactate can also be used as a fuel by muscles and other tissues during and after exercise. Lactate concentrations can increase in the blood only when the rate of lactate production begins to exceed its removal. A detailed discussion of this topic is available from other sources[20–23].

Anaerobic (Ventilatory) Threshold

The onset of metabolic acidosis during exercise, traditionally determined by serial measurements of blood lactate, can be non-invasively determined by assessment of expired gases during exercise testing, specifically pulmonary ventilation ($\dot{V}_E$) and carbon dioxide production ($\dot{V}CO_2$)[24]. Theoretically, gas exchange anaerobic threshold (AT) signifies the peak work rate or oxygen

consumption at which the energy demands exceed circulatory ability to sustain aerobic metabolism. The physiology underlying the AT may be attributed, at least in part, to buffering of lactic acid by sodium bicarbonate in the blood, so that carbon dioxide is released in excess of that produced by muscle metabolism, providing an additional stimulus for ventilation. These biochemical alterations are summarized by the following reaction:

$$HLa + Na\ HCO_3 \rightarrow Na\ La + H_2CO_3 \rightarrow H_2O + CO_2$$
(Lactic acid) (sodium bicarbonate) (sodium lactate) (carbonic acid)

Accordingly, values for $\dot{V}_E$ and carbon dioxide production increase out of proportion to the intensity of exercise performed (Fig. 3-9), suggesting an abrupt increase in serum lactate[25]. This method correlates well with the lactate method and obviates measurement of lactate in repeated blood samples. An increase in the ventilatory equivalent for oxygen ($\dot{V}_E/\dot{V}O_2$) during exercise without a corresponding change in the ventilatory equivalent for carbon dioxide ($\dot{V}_E/\dot{V}CO_2$) has also been reported to be sensitive and reliable for determining the AT[26]. There is, however, controversy surrounding the mechanisms responsible for the AT[27]. Increased lactate production may result from mechanisms not related to inadequate oxygen delivery. Another theory is that inflections in $\dot{V}_E$ and $\dot{V}CO_2$ are attributable to inadequate buffering at a fixed metabolic intensity, even when lactate production and oxygen uptake continue to increase linearly.

The AT from respiratory gas measurements is often expressed as a percentage of the $\dot{V}O_{2max}$. For example, a highly trained athlete with a $\dot{V}O_{2max}$ of 4.25 L·min^{-1} whose break point in $\dot{V}_E$ occurs at 3.20 L·min^{-1} has an AT corresponding to 75% of aerobic capacity (Fig. 3-10). This athlete should be able to maintain exercise intensities below 75% of $\dot{V}O_{2max}$ using a predominance of aerobic processes. Moreover, such exertion should be

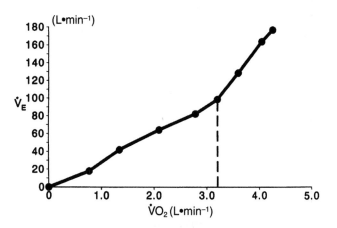

FIGURE 3-9. Relationship between intensity of exercise ($\dot{V}O_2$) and simultaneous, abrupt nonlinear increase in minute ventilation, signifying the anaerobic threshold. In this subject, the break point occurred at 3.20 L·min^{-1}, corresponding to 75% of measured $\dot{V}O_{2max}$ (4.25 L·min^{-1}).

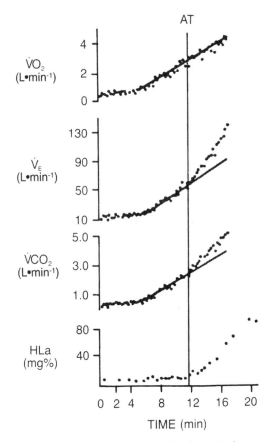

FIGURE 3-10. Relationship between intensity of exercise (oxygen consumption, $\dot{V}O_2$) and simultaneous, abrupt nonlinear increases in serum lactate (HLa), carbon dioxide production ($\dot{V}CO_2$), and pulmonary ventilation ($\dot{V}_E$) occurring at the anaerobic threshold (AT). Exercise was initiated at minute 4. (Adapted with permission from Davis JA, Vodak P, Wilmore JH, et al: Anaerobic threshold and maximal aerobic power for three modes of exercise. J Appl Physiol 41:544–550, 1976.)

accomplished without inducing a significant increase in blood lactic acid and muscle fatigue. Although the AT typically corresponds to $55\% \pm 8\%$ of the $\dot{V}O_{2max}$ in healthy untrained individuals, it normally occurs at a higher percentage of the $\dot{V}O_{2max}$ (i.e., 70–90%) in physically trained subjects[25,28].

The $\dot{V}O_{2max}$ is recognized as an important predictor of performance in endurance events. However, several studies now suggest that the highest percentage of the $\dot{V}O_{2max}$ that can be used over an extended duration without incurring significant increase in arterial lactate may be an even more important determinant of cardiorespiratory performance[28,29]. This suggests that the AT may be critical in determining optimal pace during endurance events.

REGULATION OF BIOENERGETIC PATHWAYS

Allosterism

The bioenergetic pathways that result in production of cellular ATP are under precise control. This control is achieved by regulation of one or more regulatory (allosteric) enzymes, which catalyze one-way reactions. Allosterism changes the conformation of an enzyme, which thereby changes the enzyme's activity. In positive allosterism, the enzyme is made more active; in negative allosterism, the enzyme is made less active. Rate-limiting enzymes in each of the aforementioned bioenergetic pathways can be upregulated or downregulated, depending on demand for ATP. In other words, cellular modulators regulate the catalytic activity of allosteric enzymes. Two of the most important modulators of bioenergetic regulatory enzymes are cellular concentrations of ATP and ADP. This type of negative feedback control is common among bioenergetic pathways in the muscle fiber.

Controlling Enzymes in the ATP–CP System

As it relates to the metabolic pathways, allosteric control is a process by which either an intermediate or the product of the pathway regulates the activity of the allosteric enzyme. One of the simplest examples of this type of control is the feedback inhibition exhibited by ATP on creatine kinase. Creatine phosphate breakdown is regulated by creatine kinase activity. Creatine kinase activity is elevated when cytoplasmic concentrations of ADP increase and ATP levels decrease. Conversely, high cellular ATP levels inhibit creatine kinase activity.

Controlling Enzymes in Glycolysis

The rate-limiting enzyme in glycolysis is PFK. PFK decreases early in the glycolytic pathway and catalyzes a committed step (fructose 6 phosphate to fructose 1–6 bisphosphate). In a committed step, the product of the reaction catalyzed by the allosteric enzyme is committed to the metabolic pathway from which it was produced. For example, fructose 1–6 bisphosphate must be used in glycolysis for the ultimate production of either pyruvate or lactate and ATP. Similar to the regulation of creatine kinase, PFK activity is increased by an increase in cellular ADP concentration and a decrease in ATP levels (i.e., low cellular energy levels). PFK activity is inhibited by a variety of factors, including high cellular concentrations of hydrogen ions, citrate, and ATP. These factors result in a downregulation of PFK and reduce the amount of committed intermediate (fructose 1–6 bisphosphate) that is formed.

Controlling Enzymes in Oxidative Phosphorylation

Nicotinamide adenine dinucleotide (NADH) and citrate control citrate synthase (CS) activity through negative allosteric inhibition early in the Krebs cycle. NADH also inhibits both isocitrate dehydrogenase (ICDH) and alpha-ketoglutarate dehydrogenase (α-KGDH) through allosteric inhibition. Calcium (Ca^{2+}) upregulates ICDH and α-KGDH. (Although oxidative phosphorylation is under complex control, it is clear that cellular energy levels of Ca^{2+} regulate key enzymes in the Krebs cycle (i.e., ICDH and α-KGDH) and electron transport chain (i.e., cytochrome oxidase). A decrease in cellular energy levels promotes oxidative phosphorylation, and high concentrations of ATP inhibit this process, which is similar to the control schemes presented for the CP system and glycolysis. A more detailed discussion of oxidative phosphorylation is available[30].

MEASUREMENT OF METABOLISM AND OXYGEN CONSUMPTION

Traditionally, whole-body metabolism is measured using one of two strategies: direct or indirect calorimetry[24]. The principles behind these two strategies can be explained by the following relationship:

$$Foodstuffs + O_2 \rightarrow Heat + CO_2 + H_2O$$
(Indirect calorimetry) (Direct calorimetry)

Heat is liberated as a consequence of cellular respiration and cell (e.g., muscular) work. Thus, heat production by the body allows a direct assessment of metabolism.

Direct calorimetry requires that a subject be placed in an airtight chamber. As heat is released, the temperature inside the chamber increases. Typically, a circulating jacket of water used to transfer heat to the environment allows a means of determining the metabolic rate in joules or kilocalories.

Although direct calorimetry is a precise technique, construction of large chambers for measurement of metabolic rate in humans is prohibitively expensive. Also, heat produced by exercise equipment can complicate measurements using direct calorimetry. The principle of indirect calorimetry uses the measurement of oxygen consumption ($\dot{V}O_2$) to determine metabolic rate. Using this method, metabolic rate in kilocalories can be estimated using the following formula:

$$Metabolic\ rate\ (kcal{\cdot}min^{-1}) = \dot{V}O_2\ (L{\cdot}min^{-1}) \times [4.0 + RQ]$$

The most common method of measuring oxygen consumption uses open-circuit spirometry (Fig. 3-11). The volume of inspired oxygen is measured using a dry gas meter, turbine, or pneumotach. A one-way valve directs air through the mouth. Gas fractions are sampled and measured by oxygen and carbon dioxide analyzers on the expired side. Typically, analog voltages from the gas meter and analyzers are converted to digital information and fed

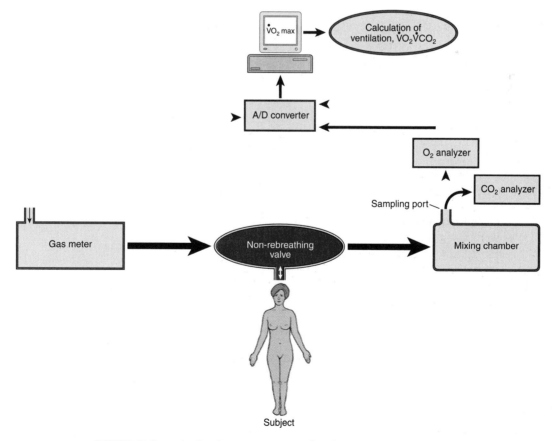

FIGURE 3-11. Open-circuit spirometry system interfaced with computer technology.

into a microcomputer with $\dot{V}O_2$ calculated using the Haldane transformation of the Fick equation:

$$\dot{V}O_2 = \dot{V}_I \times F_IO_2 \; \dot{V}_I \times ([1 - F_EO_2 - F_ECO_2] / [1 - F_IO_2 - F_ICO_2]) \times F_EO_2$$

Where $\dot{V}_I$ = inspired ventilation

F_IO_2 = Inspired oxygen fraction = 0.2093

F_ICO_2 = Inspired carbon dioxide fraction = 0.0003

F_EO_2 = Expired oxygen fraction

F_ECO_2 = Expired carbon dioxide fraction

ENERGY COST OF ACTIVITIES

The energy cost of many types of physical activity has been established. Appendix A lists some physical activities and their associated energy expenditures expressed in kilocalories per minute. Activities that are vigorous and involve large muscle groups usually result in more energy expended than activities that use small muscle mass or require limited exertion. The estimates of energy expenditure listed in Appendix A were obtained by measuring oxygen cost of these activities in an adult population.

Clinicians often use the term *metabolic equivalent* (MET) to describe exercise intensity. A single MET is equivalent to the amount of energy expended during 1 minute of rest. Therefore, exercise at a metabolic rate that is five times the resting $\dot{V}O_2$ rate is equivalent to 5 METs. In a strict sense, the absolute energy expenditure during exercise at a 5-MET intensity depends on the body size of the individual (i.e., a large person is likely to have a larger resting $\dot{V}O_2$ than a small person). For simplicity, individual differences in resting energy expenditures are often overlooked, and 1 MET is considered equivalent to a $\dot{V}O_2$ of 3.5 mL $O_2 \cdot kg^{-1} \cdot min^{-1}$; hence, 1 MET represents an energy expenditure of approximately 1.2 kcal·min^{-1} for a 70-kg person.

SUMMARY

Exercise metabolism is a reflection of each metabolic pathway as it contributes to the increased energy demands of activity and work. Substrates for energy production include carbohydrate, fat, and protein. The mix of these substrates during exercise metabolism depends on the intensity and duration of exercise and the conditioning of the individual.

Normal Cardiorespiratory Responses to Acute Aerobic Exercise

The energy requirements of exercising human muscle may increase substantially in the transition from rest to maximal physical exertion. Because the available stores of ATP are limited and capable of providing energy to maintain vigorous activity for only several seconds, ATP must be constantly resynthesized to provide continuous energy production. Therefore, exercising muscle must possess a large capacity for increasing metabolic rate to produce sufficient ATP so that increased activity can continue. Energy production relies heavily on the respiratory and cardiovascular systems for the delivery of oxygen and nutrients and for the removal of waste products to maintain the internal equilibrium of cells.

The purpose of this section is to review the normal **cardiorespiratory** responses to acute aerobic exercise with specific reference to energy systems, **hemodynamics**, posture, **maximal oxygen consumption ($\dot{V}O_{2max}$)**, the anaerobic threshold, dynamic versus isometric exertion, arm versus leg exercise, myocardial oxygen consumption, and the effects of physical conditioning. This information is vital to the understanding of the role of exercise physiology in the interpretation of diagnostic and functional exercise testing and the prescription of exercise in health and disease.

ACUTE CARDIORESPIRATORY RESPONSES TO EXERCISE

Many cardiorespiratory and hemodynamic mechanisms function collectively to support increased aerobic requirements of physical activity. The overall effect of changes in heart rate (HR), stroke volume (SV), cardiac output, blood flow, blood pressure (BP), arteriovenous oxygen difference, and pulmonary ventilation is to oxygenate the blood ensure that it is delivered to the active tissues.

Heart Rate

Heart rate increases in a linear fashion with the work rate and oxygen uptake during dynamic exercise. The increase in HR during exercise occurs primarily at the expense of diastole (filling time), rather than systole (Fig. 3-12)[31]. Thus, at high exercise intensities, diastolic time may be so short as to preclude adequate ventricular filling. The magnitude of the HR response is related to age, body position, fitness, type of activity, the presence of heart disease, medications, blood volume, and environmental factors such as temperature and humidity. In contrast to systolic BP (SBP), which usually increases with age, maximum attainable HR decreases with age. The equation, 220 − age provides an approximation of the maximum HR in healthy men and women, but the variance for any fixed age is considerable (standard deviation about ± 10 bpm).

Stroke Volume

The SV (volume of blood ejected per heart beat) is equal to the difference between end diastolic volume (EDV) and end systolic volume (ESV). Whereas the former is determined by HR, filling pressure, and ventricular compliance, the latter depends on two variables: contractility and afterload. Thus, a greater diastolic filling (preload) increases SV. In contrast, factors that resist ventricular outflow (afterload) result in a reduced SV.

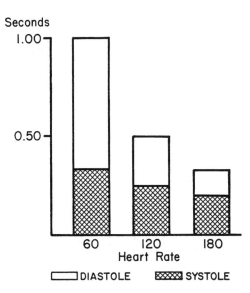

FIGURE 3-12. Relationship of systolic and diastolic time to heart rate (HR). Because coronary blood flow predominates during diastole, with increased HR, as during exercise, diastolic (perfusion) time is disproportionately shortened. (Adapted with permission from Dehn MM, Mullins CB: Physiologic effects and importance of exercise in patients with coronary artery disease. J Cardiovasc Med 2:365–387, 1977.)

Stroke volume at rest in the upright position generally varies between 60 and 100 mL·beat^{-1} among healthy adults, and maximum SV approximates 100 to 120 mL·beat^{-1}. During exercise, SV increases curvilinearly with the work rate until it reaches near maximum at a level equivalent to approximately 50% of aerobic capacity, increasing only slightly thereafter[32]. Within physiological limits, enhanced venous return increases EDV, stretching cardiac muscle fibers and increasing force of contraction (*Frank-Starling mechanism*); thus, ejection fraction (EF) may increase. EF is defined by the following:

$$EF = [SV/EDV] \times 100$$

Ejection fraction is normally 65% ± 8%, resulting from both the Frank-Starling mechanism and decreased ESV (Fig. 3-13)[33]. The latter is attributable to increased ventricular contractility, secondary to catecholamine mediated sympathetic stimulation. The magnitude of these changes depends on several variables, including ventricular function, body position, and the intensity of exercise. Moreover, at a higher HR, SV may actually decrease because of the disproportionate shortening in diastolic filling time (Fig. 3-12)[31,34].

Cardiac Output

The product of SV and HR determines cardiac output. Cardiac output in healthy adults increases linearly with increased work rate, from a resting value of approximately 5 L·min^{-1} to a maximum of about 20 L·min^{-1} during upright exercise. However, maximum values of cardiac output depend on many factors, including age, posture, body size, presence of cardiovascular disease, and the level of physical conditioning. At exercise intensities up to 50% $\dot{V}O_{2max}$, the increase in cardiac output is facilitated by increases in HR and SV[32]. Thereafter, the increase results almost solely from the continued increase in HR.

Blood Flow

At rest, 15% to 20% of the cardiac output is distributed to the skeletal muscles; the remainder goes to the visceral organs, the heart, and the brain[35]. With exercise, myocardial blood flow may increase four to five times; blood supply to the brain is maintained at resting levels[36]. As much as 85% to 90% of the cardiac output is selectively delivered to working muscle and shunted away from the skin and the splanchnic, hepatic, and renal vascular beds. This redistribution of blood away from the visceral organs during exercise is caused by the sympathetic and hormonal (i.e., norepinephrine) influences on arterial smooth muscle and the resulting vasoconstriction. In active skeletal muscle, the exercise hyperemia is partly caused by local factors influenced by the increase in metabolism. Decreases in PO_2 and increases in norepinephrine and endothelial cell shear stress in the arterial intima cause the release of *nitric oxide*, which was formerly termed *endothelial-derived relaxing factor* (EDRF). Nitric oxide exerts a vasodilatory effect on arteries and arterioles that supply the working muscles. In addition, it appears that venules paired to arterioles may release EDRFs in response to ATP release from red blood cells (RBCs). These venular EDRFs diffuse to arterioles and influence vasodilation and, therefore, blood flow[37].

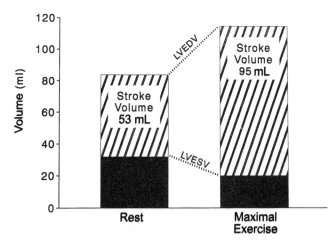

FIGURE 3-13. Changes in stroke volume from rest to maximal upright exercise is shown in young, healthy men. LVEDV = left ventricular end-diastolic volume; LVESV = left ventricular end-systolic volume. (Adapted with permission from Poliner LR, Dehmer GJ, Lewis SE, et al: Left ventricular performance in normal subjects: A comparison of the responses to exercise in the upright and supine position. Circulation 62:528–534, 1980.)

Blood Pressure

There is a linear increase in SBP with increasing levels of exercise, approximating 8 to 12 mm Hg per MET, where 1 MET = 3.5 mL $O_2 \cdot kg^{-1} \cdot min^{-1}$. Maximal values typically reach 190 to 220 mm Hg[38]. Nevertheless, maximal SBP should not be greater than 260 mm Hg[39]. Diastolic BP (DBP) may decrease slightly or remain unchanged; thus, pulse pressure (SBP minus DBP) generally increases in direct proportion to the intensity of exercise.

Because BP is directly related to cardiac output and peripheral vascular resistance, it provides a non-invasive way to monitor the inotropic performance, or pumping capacity, of the heart. Until automated devices are adequately validated, the BP response to exercise should be taken manually with a cuff and a stethoscope[39]. A SBP that fails to increase or decreases with increasing work loads may signal a plateau or decrease in cardiac output, respectively[40]. Exercise testing should be terminated in persons demonstrating exertional hypotension (SBP toward the end of a test decreasing below baseline standing level or SBP decreasing 20 mm Hg or more during exercise after an initial increase). This response has been shown to correlate with myocardial ischemia, left ventricular dysfunction, and an increased risk of cardiac events during follow-up[41]. In one study, men with a maximal SBP below 140 mm Hg had a 15-fold increase in the annual rate of sudden death compared with those whose pressures exceeded 200 mm Hg[42].

Arteriovenous Oxygen Difference (a-VO$_2$ diff)

Oxygen extraction by tissues reflects the difference between oxygen content of arterial blood (about 20 mL $O_2 \cdot 100^{-1}$ mL$\cdot dL^{-1}$ at rest) and the oxygen content of venous blood (about 15 mL $O_2 \cdot dL^{-1}$), yielding a typical arteriovenous oxygen difference ($CaO_2 - CvO_2$) at rest of 5 mL $O_2 \cdot dL^{-1}$. This approximates a use coefficient of 25%. During exercise to exhaustion, the mixed venous oxygen content typically decreases to 5 mL$\cdot dL^{-1}$ blood or lower, thus widening the arteriovenous oxygen difference from 5 to 15 mL$\cdot dL^{-1}$ blood, corresponding to a use coefficient of 75%[32].

Pulmonary Ventilation

Pulmonary ventilation ($\dot{V}_E$), the volume of air exchanged per minute, generally approximates 6 L$\cdot min^{-1}$ at rest in the average sedentary adult man. At maximal exercise, however, $\dot{V}_E$ often increases 15- to 25-fold over resting values. During mild to moderate exercise intensities, whereas $\dot{V}_E$ is increased primarily by increasing tidal volume, increases in the respiratory rate are more important to augment $\dot{V}_E$ during vigorous exercise. For the most part, the increase in pulmonary ventilation is directly proportional to the increase in somatic oxygen consumed ($\dot{V}O_2$) and carbon dioxide produced ($\dot{V}CO_2$). However, at

a critical exercise intensity (usually 47% to 64% of the $\dot{V}O_{2max}$ in healthy untrained individuals and 70–90% of the $\dot{V}O_{2max}$ in highly trained subjects), $\dot{V}_E$ increases disproportionately relative to $\dot{V}O_2$, paralleling the abrupt nonlinear increases in serum lactate and $\dot{V}CO_2$[43,44]. This suggests that pulmonary ventilation is perhaps regulated more by the requirement for carbon dioxide removal than by oxygen consumption and that ventilation is not normally a limiting factor to aerobic capacity. However, in highly trained male athletes exercising at high intensities (>80% $\dot{V}O_{2max}$), reductions in PaO_2 have been documented. Furthermore, female athletes have exhibited reduction in PaO_2, and the reductions began to occur at lower exercise intensities than with the male athletes. The exact mechanisms leading to the hypoxemic conditions are still being investigated. However, diffusion limitations, ventilation–perfusion inequalities, and limits to maximal flow rates may contribute to the occurrence of hypoxemia[45,46].

Cardiovascular Drift

Steady-state upright exercise is characterized by changes in cardiovascular response despite the constant work rate. SV and mean arterial pressure progressively decrease, and HR progressively increases. Traditionally, it was thought that the increase in HR may be attributed, at least in part, to alterations in sympathetic blood flow control mechanisms, increased shunting of blood to the periphery (skin) for cooling, and decreased central blood volume (particularly in warm environments). However, it now appears that there is not a strong association between cutaneous blood flow and SV. Rather, the decrease in SV results from increased HR whereby diastolic filling time and end-diastolic volume is reduced. Exercise during which dehydration occurs also contributes to cardiovascular drift, particularly if the dehydration leads to hypovolemia and hyperthermia. These conditions contribute to decreased SV and increased HR, respectively, thereby influencing the cardiovascular drift[47].

FACTORS INFLUENCING ACUTE CARDIORESPIRATORY RESPONSES TO EXERCISE

Posture

Posture has an effect on venous return and preload, particularly during brief bouts of physical exertion. At rest, EDV is highest when the body is recumbent. It decreases progressively as one shifts into sitting and standing postures, respectively. During exercise in the supine position, EDV remains largely unchanged. Thus, alterations in preload have little influence in increasing SV in this type of exercise. During exercise in the upright posture, EDV increases at intensities less than 50% $\dot{V}O_{2max}$.

However, at higher exercise intensities, end-diastolic and SVs may decrease in some subjects[48,49].

Dynamic Versus Static Exertion

Dynamic, or isotonic, activity (physical exertion characterized by rhythmic, repetitive movements of large muscle groups) results in increased oxygen consumption and HR that parallels the intensity of activity, as well as an increase in SV. There is a concomitant progressive increase in SBP with maintenance of or a slight decrease in DBP; thus, pulse pressure increases.

Blood is shunted from the viscera to working skeletal muscle, where increased oxygen extraction increases systemic a-vDO$_2$. Thus, dynamic exercise imposes a volume load on the myocardium, which is the basis for a cardiac training effect. In contrast, isometric exertion involves sustained muscle contraction against a fixed load or resistance with no change in length of the involved muscle group or joint motion. The cardiovascular response to isometric exertion is apparently mediated by a neurogenic mechanism[50]. Activities that involve less than 20% of the maximum voluntary contraction (MVC) of the involved muscle group evoke a modest increase in SBP, DBP, and HR. During contractions greater than 20% of the MVC, HR increases in relation to the tension exerted, and there is an abrupt and precipitous increase in SBP. The SV remains essentially unchanged except at high levels of tension (>50% MVC), where it may decrease. The result is a moderate increase in cardiac output, which is nevertheless high for the accompanying magnitude of increased metabolism. Despite the increased cardiac output, blood flow to the non-contracting muscle does not significantly increase, probably because of reflex vasoconstriction. The combination of vasoconstriction and increased cardiac output causes a disproportionate increase in SBP, DBP, and mean BP. Thus, a significant pressure load is imposed on the heart, presumably to increase perfusion to the active (contracting) skeletal muscle. A comparison of the relative hemodynamic responses to dynamic and isometric exercise is shown in Table 3-2.

The magnitude of the pressor response to isometric exertion depends on tension exerted relative to the greatest possible tension in the muscle group (% MVC), as well as muscle mass involved[51,52]. Thus, a relatively mild isometric contraction by weakened upper extremities may evoke an excessive pressor response. The increased myocardial demands are camouflaged by the relatively low aerobic requirements, so the usual warning signs of overexertion (tachycardia, sweating, dyspnea) may be absent. In persons who have an ischemic left ventricle, a marked pressure increase may lead to threatening ventricular arrhythmias; significant ST-segment depression; angina pectoris; ventricular decompensation; and in rare instances, sudden cardiac death[53].

TABLE 3-2. Comparison of the Relative Hemodynamic Responses to Dynamic and Static Exertion

	Dynamic (Isotonic)	Static (Isometric)
Cardiac output	++++	+
Heart rate	++	+
Stroke volume	++	0
Peripheral resistance	−	+++
Systolic blood pressure	+++	++++
Diastolic blood pressure	0−	++++
Mean arterial pressure	0+	++++
Left ventricular work	Volume load	Pressure load

+ = increase; − = decrease; 0 = unchanged.

Arm Versus Leg Exercise

At a fixed power output (kgm·min^{-1} or watts [W]), HR, SBP, and DBP, the product of the HR times SBP (rate times pressure), $\dot{V}_E$, $\dot{V}O_2$, respiratory exchange ratio, and blood lactate concentration are higher, and SV and AT (the latter expressed as a percentage of aerobic capacity) are lower during arm exercise than leg exercise[54]. Because cardiac output is nearly the same in arm and leg exercise at a fixed oxygen uptake, elevated BP during arm exercise is believed to reflect increased peripheral vascular resistance. During maximal effort, physiological responses are usually greater during leg exercise than arm exercise, except when subjects are limited in their ability to perform leg work by neurological, vascular, or orthopedic impairment of the lower extremities[55].

The disparity in cardiorespiratory and hemodynamic response to arm exercise versus leg exercise at identical work rates appears to be attributable to several factors. Mechanical efficiency (i.e., the ratio between the output of external work and caloric expenditure, or $\dot{V}O_2$) is lower during arm exercise than leg exercise[55]. This may reflect the involvement of smaller muscle groups and the static effort required with arm work, which increases $\dot{V}O_2$ but does not affect the external work output. The higher rate–pressure product and estimated myocardial oxygen consumption at a fixed external work rate for arm work compared with leg work (Fig. 3-14) is believed to reflect increased sympathetic tone during arm exercise, perhaps mediated by reduced SV with compensatory tachycardia, concomitant isometric contraction, vasoconstriction in the non-exercising leg muscles, or all of these factors[56].

$\dot{V}O_{2max}$ during arm exercise in men and women generally varies between 64% and 80% of leg $\dot{V}O_{2max}$[54]. Similarly, although maximal cardiac output is lower during arm exercise than leg exercise, the maximal HR, SBP, and rate–pressure product are comparable or slightly lower during arm exercise. The latter, however, has relevance to arm exercise training recommendations, particularly training intensity. Accordingly, an arm exercise prescription that assumes a maximal HR equivalent to leg

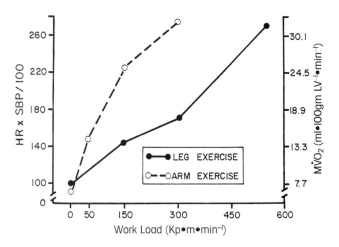

FIGURE 3-14. Mean rate–pressure product and estimated myocardial oxygen consumption (MVO_2) during arm (*broken line*) and leg (*solid line*) exercise. MVO_2 is estimated from its hemodynamic correlates, heart rate (HR) multiplied by systolic blood pressure (SBP). (Adapted with permission from Schwade J, Blomqvist CG, Shapiro W: A comparison of the response to arm and leg work in patients with ischemic heart disease. Am Heart J 94:203–208, 1977.)

exercise testing may result in an overestimation of the training HR. As a general guideline, the prescribed HR for leg training should be reduced by approximately 10 bpm for arm training[57].

MAXIMAL OXYGEN CONSUMPTION

The most widely recognized measure of cardiopulmonary fitness is maximal oxygen consumption or $\dot{V}O_{2max}$. This variable is defined physiologically as the highest rate of oxygen transport and use that can be achieved at maximal physical exertion. Somatic oxygen consumption ($\dot{V}O_2$) may be expressed mathematically by a rearrangement of the Fick equation:

$$\dot{V}O_2 = HR \times SV \times (a\text{-}vO_2 \text{ diff})$$

Where $\dot{V}O_2$ = oxygen consumption ($mL\ O_2 \cdot kg^{-1} \cdot min^{-1}$)

HR = Heart rate (bpm)

SV = Stroke volume ($mL \cdot beat^{-1}$)

($a\text{-}vO_2$ diff) = Arteriovenous oxygen difference

Thus, it is apparent that both central (i.e., cardiac output) and peripheral (i.e., arteriovenous oxygen difference) regulatory mechanisms affect the magnitude of body oxygen consumption.

Typical circulatory data at rest and during maximal exercise in a healthy, sedentary 30-year-old man and a similarly aged world-class endurance athlete are shown in Table 3-3. The absolute resting oxygen consumption (250 $mL \cdot min^{-1}$) divided by body weight (70 kg) gives the resting energy requirement, 1 MET (about 3.5 $mL \cdot kg^{-1} \cdot min^{-1}$). This expression of resting $\dot{V}O_2$, believed to originate from the work of Balke[58], is extremely important in exercise physiology, independent of body weight and aerobic fitness. Furthermore, multiples of this value are often used to quantify respective levels of energy expenditure. For example, running at a 6-mph pace requires 10 times the resting energy expenditure; thus, the aerobic cost is 10 METs, or 35 $mL\ O_2 \cdot kg^{-1} \cdot min^{-1}$.

The 10-fold increase in oxygen transport and use in the sedentary individual is contrasted by a 23-fold increase in the endurance athlete, corresponding to a $\dot{V}O_{2max}$ of 35 $mL \cdot kg^{-1} \cdot min^{-1}$ and 80 $mL \cdot kg^{-1} \cdot min^{-1}$, respectively. Increased aerobic capacity in trained athletes appears primarily as the result of increased maximal cardiac output because of a greater increment in HR and SV rather than an increased peripheral extraction of oxygen. Because there is little variation in maximal HR and maximal systemic arteriovenous oxygen difference with training, $\dot{V}O_{2max}$ virtually defines the pumping capacity of the heart. Therefore, it is of major importance in the cardiovascular evaluation of the individual.

$\dot{V}O_{2max}$ may be expressed on an absolute or relative basis, that is, in liters per minute, reflecting total body energy output and caloric expenditure (i.e., 1 L ≈ 5 kcal) or by dividing this value by body weight in kilograms. Because large persons usually have a large absolute oxygen consumption by virtue of larger muscle mass, the latter allows a more equitable comparison between individuals of different body mass. This variable, when expressed as milliliters of oxygen per kilogram of body weight per minute or as METs, is widely considered the single best index of physical work capacity or cardiorespiratory fitness[59].

TABLE 3-3. Hypothetical Circulatory Data at Rest and During Maximal Exercise for a Sedentary Man and a World-class Endurance Athlete: 30-Year-Old Subjects

Condition	Oxygen Consumption (L·min⁻¹)	Oxygen Consumption (mL·kg⁻¹·min⁻¹)	Cardiac Output (L·min⁻¹)	Heart Rate (bpm)	Stroke Volume (mL·beat⁻¹)	Arteriovenous oxygen difference (mL·dL⁻¹ blood)
Sedentary man (70 kg)						
Rest	0.25	3.5	6.1	70	87	4.0
Maximal exercise	2.50	35.0	17.7	190	93	14.0
World-class endurance athlete (70 kg)						
Rest	0.25	3.5	6.1	45	136	4.0
Maximal exercise	5.60	80.0	35.0	190	184	16.0

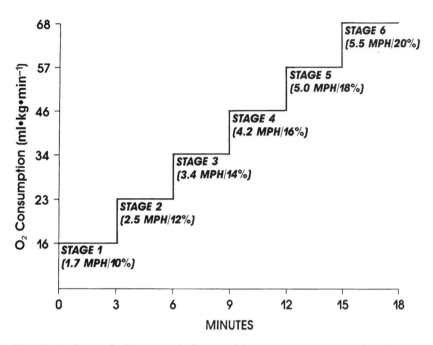

FIGURE 3-15. The standard Bruce treadmill protocol showing progressive stages (speed, percentage grade) and the corresponding aerobic requirement, expressed as mL·kg·min^{-1}.

Determination of the Maximal Oxygen Consumption

Maximal oxygen consumption is usually determined by measuring the volume and oxygen content of expired air, corrected to standard temperature and pressure dry (STPD), using the following equation:

$$\dot{V}O_2 = \dot{V}_E (F_IO_2 - F_EO_2)$$

Where $\dot{V}_E$ = Expired air (L·min^{-1})

F_EO_2 = Directly measured fraction oxygen in expired air

F_IO_2 = Directly measured fraction oxygen in inspired air (normally 0.2093)

Traditionally, $\dot{V}O_2$ has been measured using an open circuit or Douglas bag technique. However, several automated systems are available to measure $\dot{V}O_2$ and related respiratory variables during exercise testing.

Because it is often inconvenient to measure the $\dot{V}O_{2max}$ directly, physiologists have sought to estimate aerobic capacity from the peak treadmill speed and grade, or cycle ergometer work rate, expressed as kilogram·meters per minute (also see Chapter 14 and GETP7 Chapter 5). The conventional Bruce test is perhaps the most familiar and widely used treadmill protocol with normative data on oxygen consumption so that aerobic capacity may be estimated from the workload attained (Fig. 3-15)[60]. However, when a multistage protocol, such as the Bruce test, is used to predict the $\dot{V}O_{2max}$, aerobic capacity may be markedly overestimated[61]. One recent advance in test methodology that can overcome many of the limitations of incremental exercise is ramping[62,63]. Ramp protocols involve a nearly continuous and uniform increase in aerobic requirements that replaces the staging used in conventional exercise tests. With ramping, the gradual increase in demand allows a steady increase in cardiopulmonary responses.

MYOCARDIAL OXYGEN CONSUMPTION

Determinants of myocardial oxygen consumption (MVO$_2$) include HR, myocardial contractility, and the tension or stress developed in the ventricular wall. Wall tension reflects a combination of SBP and ventricular volume and is inversely related to myocardial wall thickness (Fig. 3-16). During exercise, increased HR is the major contributor to increased myocardial oxygen demand. In contrast, oxygen supply is primarily facilitated by increased coronary blood flow (see Chapter 29) enabled by decreased coronary vascular resistance with only a modest increase in an already substantial myocardial oxygen difference.

Several investigators have reported excellent correlations between measured MVO$_2$, (expressed as milliliters of oxygen per 100 g of left ventricle per minute), HR and rate–pressure product, where MVO$_2$ = 0.28 HR − 14 (r = 0.88) or MVO$_2$ = ([0.14 × HR × SBP]/100) − 6.3) (r = 0.92)[64,65]. HR alone is limited in ability to assess MVO$_2$, especially when SBP is markedly elevated; this may occur during upper extremity work involving isometric or isodynamic efforts.

Exercise-induced angina and significant ST-segment depression ($\geq$1 mm) usually occur at the same rate–pressure product in an individual with ischemic heart disease. This suggests the existence of an ischemic

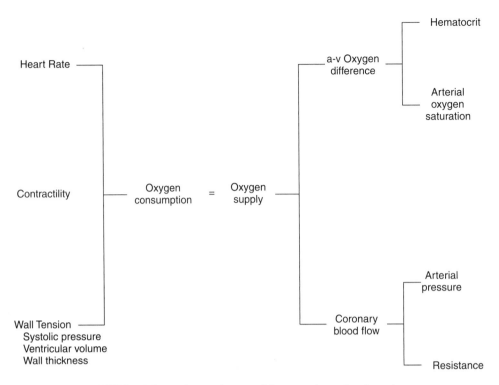

FIGURE 3-16. Determinants of myocardial oxygen demand and supply.

heart disease. This suggests the existence of an ischemic threshold at which myocardial oxygen demand exceeds myocardial oxygen supply. The rate–pressure product also provides an estimate of maximal workload that the left ventricle can perform. It has been suggested that an adequate rate–pressure product during maximal exercise is greater than 25,000; however, this may be influenced by age; clinical status; and medications, especially beta-blockers[39].

Factors Affecting the Acute Neuromuscular Responses to Resistance Exercise

Resistance training is repeated exposure to an acute exercise stimulus that is specific and characterized by various factors that define the physiological and biomechanical demands. Understanding the factors that affect acute resistance exercise stimuli is important in gaining insight into different resistance training protocols. Acute physiological changes are directly related to the configuration of external demands of resistance exercise, so resistance exercise protocols must be specific to the physiological systems targeted.

PHYSIOLOGY OF RESISTANCE EXERCISE

Neuromuscular Activation

The stimulus for muscle activation comes from a high-level central control command signal originating from the premotor cortex and the motor cortex. The signal is relayed through a lower-level controller (brainstem and spinal cord) and transformed into a specific motor unit activation pattern. To perform a specific task, the required motor units meet specific demands for force production by activating associated muscle fibers[66,67]. Various feedback loops modify force production and provide communication to other physiological systems, such as the endocrine system. The high- and low-level commands can be modified by feedback from peripheral sensory or higher central command.

Motor Unit Activation

The functional unit of the neuromuscular system is the **motor unit**[68]. It consists of the motor neuron and the muscle fibers it innervates. Motor units range in size from a few to several hundred muscle fibers. Muscle fibers from different motor units can be anatomically adjacent to each other; therefore, a muscle fiber may be actively generating force while the adjacent fiber moves passively with no direct neural stimulation. When maximal force is required, all available motor units are activated. Another adaptive mechanism affected by heavy resistance training is the muscle force affected by different motor unit firing rates and frequencies.

Motor unit activation is also influenced by the **size principle**. This principle is based on the observed relationship between motor unit twitch force and recruitment threshold. Specifically, motor units are recruited in order according to recruitment thresholds and firing rates, resulting in a continuum of voluntary force.

Whereas type I motor units are the smallest and possess the lowest recruitment thresholds, type IIa and IIb motor units are larger in size and have higher activation thresholds. Therefore, as force requirements of an activity increase, the recruitment order progresses from type I to IIa to IIb motor units. Thus, most muscles contain a range of motor units (type I and II fibers), and force production can span wide levels. Maximal force production requires not only the recruitment of all motor units, including high-threshold motor units, but also recruitment at a sufficiently high firing rate. It has been hypothesized that untrained individuals cannot voluntarily recruit the highest-threshold motor units or maximally activate muscles. Furthermore, electrical stimulation has been shown to be more effective in eliciting gains in untrained muscle or injury rehabilitation scenarios, suggesting further inability to activate all available motor units. Thus, training adaptation develops the ability to recruit a greater percentage of motor units when required.

Few exceptions to the size principle have been identified; however, some advanced weight lifters and other athletes may not require the order of recruitment stipulated by the size principle. It may be possible to inhibit low-threshold motor units yet activate high-threshold ones to enhance rate of force development and power production. This hypothesis emerged from observations during rapid, stereotyped movements and voluntary eccentric muscle action in humans. The central nervous system (CNS) can also limit force by engaging protective inhibitory mechanisms. Thus, training may result in changes in fiber recruitment order or reduced inhibition, which assists in the performance of certain types of muscle actions.

Muscle Fiber Types

Several nomenclatures have been used to classify skeletal muscle fibers, including color (red or white), contraction speed (fast or slow twitch), oxidative or glycolytic enzyme content (fast glycolytic, fast oxidative glycolytic, or oxidative), combination schemes (fast glycolytic), and myosin adenosine triphosphatase (ATPase) content (type I, IIa, IIb).

It is evident that exercise-induced changes in muscle have great plasticity[69–71]. This is caused partly by a complex yet readily adaptable group of contractile and regulatory proteins. Studies have focused on the myosin molecule and examination of fiber types. Fiber typing by myosin ATPase has been the most popular classification system[69–71]. Figure 3-17 illustrates the continuum of human muscle fiber types from the most oxidative (type I) to the least oxidative (type IIB) fibers.

Three major types of polypeptide chains, including a heavy chain and two types of light chains, constitute the myosin molecule. The complexity of the system allows for different expression of isomyosin forms with different heavy and light chain compositions. The differential myosin expression is of interest because it is related to muscle function and adaptation. A link between the myosin ATPase fiber type distribution and myosin heavy chain content in skeletal muscle has been investigated by examining relationships for entire biopsy samples or single fibers. The relative percentage of myosin heavy chain (MHC I, MHC IIa, MHC IIb) is highly correlated with the corresponding percentage of muscle fiber types (I, IIA, IIB) in both men and women[72].

Muscle Soreness

Muscle soreness may occur after an acute resistance training session. The exact mechanisms of muscle soreness remain speculative. Soreness is typically observed after excessively intense resistance training. It is most dramatic in relatively inexperienced or novice weight lifters. However, experienced weight lifters have soreness with novel exercise or excessive progression of intensity.

Several investigations demonstrate that eccentric exercise precipitates delayed-onset muscle soreness (DOMS). Eccentric contractions may damage the basic ultrastructure of the muscle cell. The focal point of the damage is the Z-disk, a structural component that anchors the contractile protein actin.

The loss of structural integrity of the Z-disks may be the stimulus leading to the associated symptoms. The appearance of DOMS ranges from 24 to 48 hours after exercise and may last up to 10 days. Symptoms of DOMS include local muscular stiffness; tenderness; local edema; limited range of motion caused by edema; and pain, which varies from low-grade ache to severe pain. Severity and location of discomfort specifically relate to the muscles used. The reason for increased soreness associated with eccentric training is unclear. However, one bout of eccentric exercise appears to result in protection from excessive soreness from another bout for up to 5 to 6 weeks in untrained or novice individuals. Thus, a slow progression in intensity is critical to limit soreness. It appears that excessive soreness develops from using resistance greater than the concentric 1 repetition maximum (RM).

HEMODYNAMIC RESPONSES TO ACUTE RESISTANCE EXERCISE

Heart Rate and Blood Pressure

Heart rate and BP increase during dynamic resistance exercise using machines, free weights, or isokinetics. Peak BP response is higher during weight training in which a concentric and an eccentric phase occur than during isokinetic exercise[73]. BP and heart rate may increase quite dramatically, with peak BPs of 320/250 mm Hg and heart rates of 170 bpm for a two-legged leg press at 95%

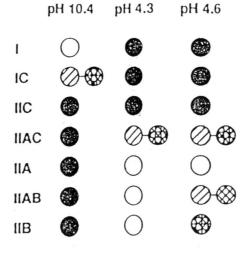

Human Muscle

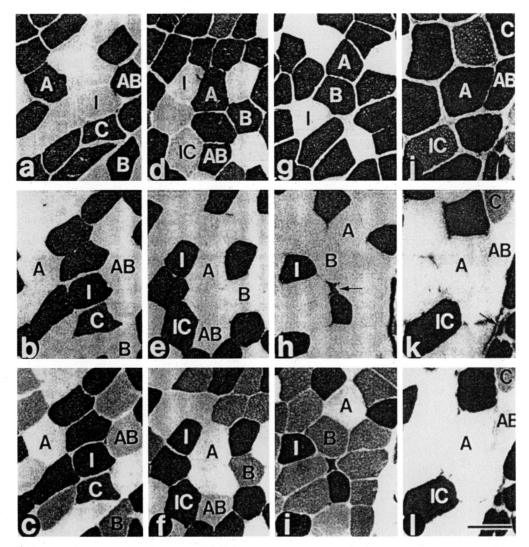

FIGURE 3-17. Myosin ATPase classification system. Staining profile and example fiber micrograph at 4.6 pH$^+$. (Courtesy of Dr. Robert Staron, Ohio University, Athens, OH.)

of 1 RM to voluntary concentric failure with a Valsalva maneuver. HR and BP responses are also significant when the Valsalva maneuver is limited.

Peak BP and HR normally occur during the last several repetitions of a set to voluntary concentric failure. BPs are higher during sets at submaximal resistance to voluntary failure than at 1 RM. In dynamic resistance exercise, BP but not HR increases during the concentric rather than the eccentric portion of a repetition. In addition, BP increases with active muscle mass, but the increase is not linear[73].

Stroke Volume and Cardiac Output

Stroke volume (determined by electrical impedance) is not significantly elevated above resting during the **concentric** phase of resistance training exercise with or without a Valsalva maneuver. However, during the **eccentric** phase, SV is significantly increased above rest (with or without a Valsalva maneuver) and is significantly greater than during the concentric phase of a repetition[73].

During both the concentric and eccentric phases of a repetition, cardiac output may be increased. For example, cardiac output during squatting exercise may increase to approximately 20 L during the eccentric phase but be only 15 L during the concentric phase. However, during exercise involving smaller muscle mass (e.g., knee extension), cardiac output may be elevated above rest only during the eccentric phase. The differing response between eccentric and concentric phases may result in no overall change from rest in mean cardiac output and SV during exercise involving a small muscle mass. Heart rate is not significantly different between the concentric and eccentric phases. Because SV is significantly greater during the eccentric than the concentric phase of a repetition, the higher cardiac output during the eccentric phase is caused by increased SV.

CALORIC COST OF RESISTANCE EXERCISE

The caloric cost of resistance exercise can be increased both during and after exercise. The caloric costs of an acute exercise session have been studied in a variety of protocols from single exercises to multiple exercise circuits. The caloric cost ranges from 14 to 75 $kcal \cdot kg^{-1} \cdot day^{-1}$. It appears that the caloric cost of resistance exercise is related to the amount of muscle mass activated (choice of exercises), the length of the rest period, the intensity of the exercise, and the ability to tolerate higher volumes of total work[74].

SUMMARY

The acute physiological stress of the neuromuscular system during resistance exercise is related to external demands. These demands are created by acute program variables that dictate the acute resistance exercise

protocol. Careful consideration of these variables affecting the demands allows optimization of the exercise prescription for resistance exercise (see Chapter 24).

Mechanisms of Muscular Fatigue

The causes of muscle fatigue has interested exercise scientists for more than a century, yet definitive fatigue agents have yet to be identified. **Muscle fatigue** is the loss of force or power output in response to voluntary effort leading to reduced performance. It is accepted that both central and peripheral fatigue factors contribute to fatigue. Whereas **central fatigue** is the progressive reduction in voluntary drive to motor neurons during exercise, **peripheral fatigue** is the loss of force and power that is independent of neural drive. The nature and extent of muscle fatigue clearly depend on the type, duration, and intensity of exercise; the fiber type composition of the muscle; individual fitness level; and environmental factors. For example, fatigue experienced in high-intensity, short-duration exercise depends on factors that differ from those precipitating fatigue in endurance activity. Similarly, fatigue during tasks involving heavily loaded contractions (e.g., weight lifting) probably differs from that produced during relatively unloaded movement (running and swimming). This section focuses primarily on muscle fatigue resulting from two general types of activity: short-duration, high-intensity exercise and longer duration, endurance exercise.

SHORT-DURATION, HIGH-INTENSITY EXERCISE

Fatigue during short-duration, high-intensity exercise may result from impairment anywhere along the chain of command from upper brain areas to contractile proteins (Fig. 3-18). Although the preponderance of evidence suggests that a dysfunction within the muscle itself (peripheral mechanisms) is the most likely cause of fatigue under these circumstances, central deficits in motor drive (central mechanisms) may also occur.

Peripheral Mechanisms

During heavy exercise, the high level of anaerobic metabolism occurring results in decreases of ATP, and CP, and increases in the levels of hydrogen ion (H^+), (Pi), ADP, and lactate. Theoretically, decreases in ATP level could contribute to fatigue because ATP supplies immediate energy for force generation in the muscles as well as provides for normal sodium–potassium pump and sarcoplasmic reticulum (SR) functioning. However, cell ATP concentration rarely decreases below 60% to 70% of the pre-exercise level, even in cases of extensive fatigue,[75] and it is likely that fatigue produced by other factors reduces the ATP use rate before ATP becomes limiting[76,77]. Furthermore, the

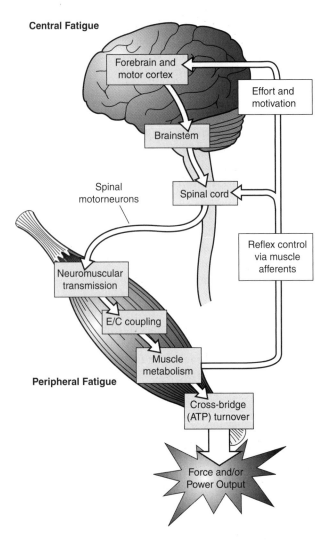

FIGURE 3-18. The chain of command for muscular contraction. Impairment along this pathway may be associated with fatigue. ATP = adenosine triphosphate. E/C = excitation-contraction.

declines in CP concentration and tension during contractile activity follow different time courses, making a causal relationship between CP and fatigue unlikely[76].

Although the increase in ADP, Pi, and H^+ ions during intense contractile activity may cause fatigue by direct inhibition of ATP hydrolysis[78–80], the majority of evidence points to the effects of elevated H^+[81]. More specifically, H^+ appears to produce fatigue via the following mechanisms:

1. Inhibition of crossbridge actomyosin ATPase and ATP hydrolysis
2. Inhibition of phosphofructokinase and thus the glycolytic rate
3. Competitive inhibition of Ca^{2+} binding to troponin C, reducing crossbridge activation
4. Inhibiting the SR ATPase, reducing Ca^{2+} reuptake and subsequently Ca^{2+} release[82]
5. Increasing the threshold of free Ca^{2+} required for contraction, particularly in fast-twitch fibers[83,84]

As evidenced by the preceding discussion, the primary sites of fatigue are within the muscle and do not generally involve peripheral nerves or the neuromuscular junction (NMJ). The observation that fatigued muscles generate the same tension whether stimulated directly or by the motor nerve argues against NMJ fatigue. However, there are several possible sites within the excitation–contraction (E-C) coupling sequence of a muscle cell where disruptions during heavy exercise may induce fatigue. Specifically, the resting membrane potential is frequently altered resulting in a reduced action potential (AP) amplitude and an increased AP duration that may ultimately effect Ca^{2+} release and contractile strength[75,85–87].

Central Mechanisms

The possibility that specific brain mechanisms can reduce the magnitude of descending motor drive has received the least attention as a possible mediator of muscular fatigue even though willingness to maintain central motor drive (e.g., willingness to maintain a maximal effort) probably contributes to fatigue in most people during activities of daily life. It has been postulated that because failure to produce the necessary force during fatigue is usually preceded by increased perceived effort, the central nervous system (CNS) processes are at least as likely to contribute to fatigue as are those that lie within the muscle[88].

During fatiguing contractions, there is inhibition of central motor drive[89–92]. Using a technique called transcranial magnetic stimulation (TMS)[93], it has been shown that the electrical stimulus reaching the muscle after magnetic stimulation of the motor cortex (motor-evoked potential) is suppressed after fatiguing exercise. Furthermore, a prolonged silent period after TMS has been demonstrated[91]. These changes are not influenced by muscle afferent feedback and can result from altered voluntary drive to the motor cortex as well as intrinsic cortical processes[90,91]. The genesis of central fatigue may involve inadequate neural drive by the motor cortex at the highest levels of the brain.

ENDURANCE EXERCISE

Numerous factors have been linked to fatigue resulting from prolonged endurance activity, including depletion of muscle and liver glycogen, decreases in blood glucose, dehydration, and increases in body temperature. Undoubtedly, each of these factors contributes to fatigue to a varying degree, the relative importance depending on environmental conditions and the nature of the activity. Mechanisms that involve various neurotransmitters and neuromodulators have also recently been proposed to explain possible CNS involvement in fatigue during prolonged exercise. This section reviews some of these factors. In particular, carbohydrate depletion, alterations in SR function, and increased brain serotonin are discussed.

Glycogen Depletion

It has long been suggested that the rate of carbohydrate use depends on the intensity of work. This belief was based on the observation that the respiratory exchange ratio (RER) increases from rest to exercise. The early theories have been confirmed by direct measurements of glycogen use at different work intensities[94,95]. The rate of body carbohydrate usage depends not only on intensity but also on the state of fitness. At a fixed workload, trained individuals have lower RERs, deplete glycogen more slowly, and can work longer than untrained individuals[95]. High-carbohydrate diets and ingestion of carbohydrate drinks during exercise can delay fatigue by increasing the availability and oxidation of carbohydrates[96]. These observations support the hypothesis that depletion of carbohydrate stores causes muscular fatigue during endurance activity. However, the exact mechanism is not known. Low muscle glycogen concentration may reduce NADH production and electron transport, drain intermediates of the Krebs cycle, or reduce fat oxidation, the effects of which would be to inhibit ATP production and cause fatigue[85,97].

It is also possible that central fatigue occurs in conjunction with carbohydrate depletion during prolonged exercise. Carbohydrate ingestion throughout exercise may attenuate the onset of negative CNS changes involving serotonin (discussed in more detail later in this section)[98]. However, the effects of carbohydrate feedings on central fatigue mechanisms and the well-established beneficial effects on the contracting muscle are difficult to distinguish[96]. It seems apparent that future efforts should focus on the mechanisms by which glycogen depletion causes fatigue.

Other Factors

Glycogen depletion is probably not an exclusive fatigue factor during endurance exercise. Other potential candidates include disruption of important intracellular organelles, such as the mitochondria, the SR, or the myofilaments[85]. The role of mitochondrial damage in fatigue is controversial[85,99].

The contractile proteins and, particularly, myofibril ATPase activity appear relatively resistant to change with endurance exercise[85,100]. Ca^{2+} uptake by the SR vesicles, however, is depressed in the slow- and fast-twitch red region of the vastus lateralis, which suggests uncoupling of the transport or a leaky membrane allowing Ca^{2+} flux back into the intracellular fluid. In addition to these functional changes, it has been demonstrated that exhaustive endurance exercise structurally damages the SR[85,101]. The exact nature of this change and its effect on muscle function has not been elucidated.

In one study, a prolonged swim produced a significant decrease in glycogen concentration in slow type I, fast type IIA, and fast type IIB fibers of muscles, but the type IIB fibers exhibited no fatigue and no change in any of the contractile or biochemical properties measured[100]. The apparent explanation is that the type IIB (fast white glycolytic) fiber is recruited less frequently during endurance activity, but glycogen use is similar to other fiber types despite fewer total contractions. It is apparent that muscle fatigue during endurance activity is somehow related to the degree of muscle use and is not entirely dependent on glycogen depletion.

In some cases, fatigue is characterized by a period of prolonged recovery during which force may be depressed for days. This low-frequency fatigue (LFF)[102] is caused by disruption of the E-C coupling process, perhaps because of excessive production of reactive oxygen species or prolonged exposure to high levels of intracellular Ca^{2+}[103,104].

The long recovery period after LFF may be related to the time required for refolding of damaged proteins or the replacement of degraded proteins[103]. Protein degradation could produce swelling and thus lead to muscle soreness. The time course of recovery from muscle soreness (i.e., days) exceeds that observed for most forms of fatigue but correlates well with recovery from LFF and reflects the time required to synthesize new muscle proteins.

Of the many proposed causes of central fatigue during prolonged exercise, the role of brain serotonin has generated the most interest. A review of the mechanisms involved in the control of brain serotonin synthesis and turnover at rest and during exercise (Fig. 3-19), along with its well-known influence on depression, sleepiness, mood, and pain make it a particularly attractive candidate[105].

Concentrations of serotonin and 5-hydroxyindole acetic acid (5-HIAA) (a major metabolite) increase in several brain regions during prolonged exercise and peak at fatigue[106,107]. The administration of serotonin agonist and antagonist drugs decreases and increases, respectively, run times to fatigue in the absence of any apparent peripheral markers of muscle fatigue[106,108,109].

SUMMARY

Both CNS and muscle mechanisms are likely to contribute to fatigue. After short-duration, high-intensity exercise, recovery in force production usually occurs in two components that are probably caused by separate mechanisms: (a) a rapidly reversible non–H^+-mediated perturbation, perhaps related to changes in E-C coupling and (b) A slower change that is probably mediated by H^+ and Pi. Reduction in central motor drive that occur at the highest levels of the brain can also accompany fatigue, but this aspect is much less well studied, and the mechanisms have not been elucidated.

In prolonged endurance exercise, the depletion of skeletal muscle carbohydrate stores frequently occurs, and it appears that muscle glycogen depletion is an important factor in fatigue. Additionally, minimal levels of muscle

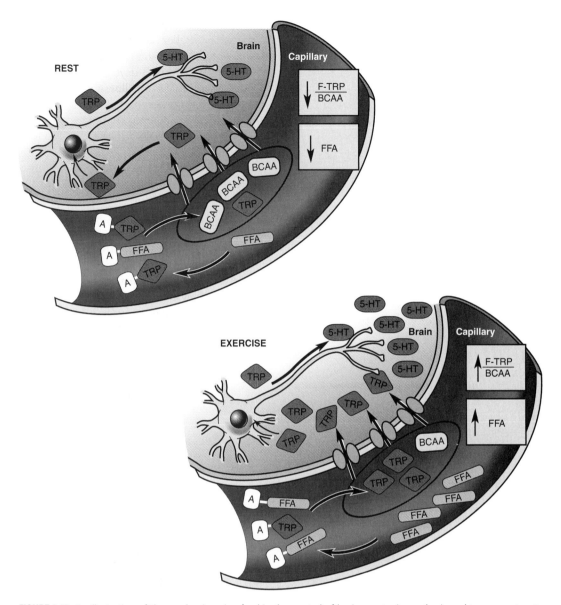

FIGURE 3-19. An illustration of the mechanisms involved in the control of brain serotonin synthesis and turnover at rest and during exercise. The well-known influence of these mechanisms on depression, sleepiness, mood, and pain make this a likely candidate for a center of fatigue. BCAA = branched chain amino acid, TRP = tryptophan, 5-HT = 5-hydroxytryptamine, FFA = free fatty acids.

glycogen metabolism may be important in maintaining essential Krebs cycle intermediates. Undoubtedly, other factors are involved because muscle glycogen depletion can exist without fatigue and vice versa. Disruption of muscle protein, particularly the E-C coupling complex, has been shown to be associated with LFF. This process may be mediated by elevated levels of reactive oxygen species (free radicals) or intracellular Ca^{2+}. Increased brain serotonin metabolism has also been implicated in central fatigue under these circumstances.

Environmental Considerations: Heat and Cold

The prevailing thermal environment can profoundly change the physiological response to exercise and increase

the risk of an environment-related disorder. In healthy individuals, a limited core temperature range (36.1 to 37.8°C) is maintained. With this narrow temperature range, an understanding of the interrelationships between thermal environment and exercise allows better management of risk for heat or cold disorders during exercise (see Chapter 28 and GETP7 Appendix E). The physiological response to heat and cold are different, and the disorders associated with these two stressors differ fundamentally. This chapter presents the interaction between the environment and exercise and disorders that may occur.

HEAT STRESS

Heat stress is the combination of environmental conditions, metabolic rate, and clothing that increases core temperature. The traditional approach to the study and assessment of heat stress is to describe the balance that must be achieved between all sources of heat gain and heat loss[110–112]. If a balance cannot be achieved, risk of excessive core temperature increases. A basic understanding of heat exchange is necessary to appreciate the interactions of environment, exercise, and clothing. The risk of a serious heat-related disorder is associated with the level of heat stress, and control of risk is based on maintaining health and managing exposure to heat stress (see Box 28-4).

Heat Balance

The major source of heat gain is internal heat generated by energy metabolism. Approximately 25% of metabolic energy expenditure is actually translated to mechanical work during locomotion (i.e., walking, biking); the remaining 75% is released as heat in contracting muscles[110]. As the metabolic rate increases to meet increasing demands of exercise, the rate of internal heat generation also increases. The rate of energy expenditure can be estimated using tables or equations[110,113]. An average man (73 kg) walking on a level surface at 1.6 m·sec^{-1} (3.5 mph) has a metabolic rate of about 350 watts[110].

Sweat Evaporative Cooling

The major avenue of heat loss is evaporation of sweat from the skin surface. Evaporative cooling by secreting water onto the skin surface through the eccrine sweat glands is one response to heat stress. As water absorbs heat from the skin, it changes from liquid to vapor. Surrounding air carries the vapor away. Because the heat of vaporization is quite high, small amounts of sweat remove relatively large amounts of heat. Specifically, the evaporation of 0.5 L of sweat per hour is sufficient to remove the 350 watts of excess heat in the preceding walking example[111].

If sufficient volumes of sweat are produced quickly enough and evaporation is not impeded, thermal balance is maintained and core temperature does not increase. However, this scenario does not occur for several reasons. First, there are physiological limits to sweat evaporation. In the short term, it is not reasonable to expect a sustained sweat rate above 1 L·hour^{-1}. In the long term (several hours), the rate of evaporation may be reduced by dehydration[114].

The physiological limit to volume of sweat produced varies by state of acclimation, by aerobic fitness, and genetically among individuals[111]. Acclimation (also known as acclimatization) is a physiological adjustment that occurs naturally with repeated exposures to heat stress during exercise. Acclimation increases rate of sweating, shortens onset time, and conserves sodium. Resulting benefits include reduced cardiovascular strain and lower core temperature for the same level of heat

stress. Most improvement occurs over the initial 3 to 5 days, with smaller additional improvements over the subsequent 2 to 7 days[110,111]. As a rule, 1 day of acclimation is lost for every 3 days away from exercise in heat stress, or in the case of illness, 1 day is lost per day of illness. Aerobic fitness is the single best indicator of a person's ability to tolerate heat stress. On the other hand, about one in 20 people are heat intolerant for unknown reasons[115].

Second, the physical limits to rate of evaporative cooling are caused by environmental conditions and clothing[110,112,116]. The primary drive for evaporative cooling is the difference in water vapor pressures on the skin and in the air. If the difference is small, the rate of evaporative cooling decreases; if the difference is large, the evaporation rate can be sufficient to balance even high rates of metabolic heat. Water vapor pressure on the skin is relatively constant. The vapor pressure of water in air is the primary source of differences in environmental contribution to heat stress. It is for this reason that humidity is an important factor in heat stress. Air movement also modifies the rate of evaporative cooling. If air movement is 2 to 3 m·sec^{-1} (4–6 mph), the maximum rate of evaporative cooling is achieved; higher speeds do not appreciably increase evaporative cooling[117].

Clothing

Clothing further restricts the maximum rate of evaporative cooling. Clothing between skin and the environment decreases the possibility of evaporation caused by the absorption of sweat or the prevention of vapor passage[111,116]. Under some circumstances, the effect of clothing is negligible. For example, if the air is very dry (low humidity) or if the metabolic rate is low, the rate of sweat evaporation through clothing is sufficient to allow adequate cooling. The resistance of clothing to sweat evaporation depends on surface area covered, nature of the fabric, number of layers, and construction of the ensemble. The following are important to minimize the effect of clothing:

- The covered surface area should be as small as is reasonable.
- The fabric should be lightweight open weave or other material that freely allows water vapor to pass through.
- Trapped air spaces from multiple layers should be minimized.
- The construction should be loose, with openings to allow easy movement of air around and through the clothing.

At the other extreme is clothing that covers most of the body; is impermeable to water vapor (e.g., plastic or rubber rain clothing); and is tightly fitting around openings for arms, legs, and head. Little evaporative cooling can occur in a person wearing this type of clothing.

Convection and Radiation

Other factors that modify overall heat stress are convection and radiation. When the air temperature is greater than skin temperature (nominally 35°C or 95°F), heat is added by convection. Conversely, when air temperature is lower than 35°C, some heat is lost by convection. The rate of convection is enhanced by air movement and reduced by clothing insulation. Whereas infrared radiation from the sun and warm or hot surfaces increase heat stress, cool surfaces reduce heat stress. Clothing insulation reduces rate of heat flow (in either direction) by radiation. Convection and radiation combined usually account for less than 20% of either heat gain or heat loss during exercise.

Physiological Response

The physiological response to heat stress is reflected in body temperature, HR, and sweating. Metabolic heat increases the temperature of working muscles, and circulating blood transports heat to the central organs, causing an increase in core temperature. Additional blood flow carries excess heat to the skin. To move heat from working muscles to the skin, cardiac output increases and blood flow is shunted from the splanchnic and renal circulation[118].

HEAT-RELATED DISORDERS

The normal and acceptable response to heat stress includes elevated core temperature, increased HR, and water loss caused by sweating. Left unchecked, however, these responses may lead to heat-related disorders and psychomotor and cognitive performance decrements. The disorders of particular importance during exercise are the following:

- Heat cramps
- Heat syncope
- Dehydration
- Heat exhaustion
- Heat stroke[110–112]

Box 3-1 lists these disorders and describes signs, symptoms, and first aid (also see Tables 28-14 and 28-16). It is important for exercise professionals to understand these features of heat disorders. Preventive measures are described next.

Heat Cramps and Syncope

Heat cramps are most likely to occur during or after sustained exercise with profuse sweating. Cramps usually appear in fatigued calf or abdominal muscles. Heat syncope may result from dehydration or excessive pooling of

---

BOX 3-1   Heat-related Disorders, Including Symptoms, Signs, and First Aid

Disorder	Symptoms	Signs	First Aid
Heat cramps	Painful muscle cramps, especially in abdominal or fatigued muscles	Incapacitating pain in voluntary muscles	Rest in cool environment Drink salted water (0.5% salt solution) Massage muscles
Heat syncope	Blurred vision (gray out)	Brief fainting or near fainting	Lie on back in cool environment
	Fainting (brief; (blackout)	Normal temperature	Drink water
Dehydration	No early symptoms Fatigue, weakness Dry mouth	Loss of work capacity Increased response time	Fluid and salt replacement
Heat exhaustion	Fatigue Weakness Blurred vision Dizziness, headache	High pulse rate Profuse sweating Low blood pressure Insecure gait Pale face Collapse Body temperature normal to slightly increased	Lie flat on back in cool environment Drink water Loosen clothing
Heat stroke	Chills Restlessness Irritability	Red face Euphoria Shivering Disorientation Erratic behavior Collapse Unconsciousness Convulsions Body temperature >40°C (104°F)	Immediate, aggressive, effective cooling Transport to the hospital

blood in peripheral vascular beds. The consequent hypotension may cause familiar blackout symptoms. Recovery is relatively quick, and most people are generally aware of the occurrence. In addition to adequate hydration, risk of syncope can be reduced by avoiding prolonged standing or rapid transition to standing.

Dehydration and Heat Exhaustion

Dehydration and heat exhaustion are most likely to occur in unacclimated persons and in those who do not drink enough or ignore early warning signs. In competitive sports, a 5% loss of body weight is not unusual[110,111]. Losses greater than 1.5% should be followed by a period of recovery and rehydration.

Heat Stroke

Heat stroke is a medical emergency, and the least suspicion that it may be present justifies an immediate and aggressive response. The risk of heat stroke is greatest among those who abuse alcohol or drugs, who are highly motivated and ignore symptoms of heat exhaustion, or who are heat intolerant (i.e., do not acclimate).

COLD STRESS

Cold stress is the combination of environment, metabolic rate, and clothing that results in heat loss from the core as a whole or from local areas[111,112,119]. Cold-related disorders include hypothermia and varying degrees of local tissue damage[110–112,119]. Again, control of cold stress is accomplished through managing risk factors.

Heat Balance

Similar to heat stress, cold stress is described as an imbalance between heat gained from metabolism and heat lost to the environment by convection, radiation, evaporation, and conduction[112]. The problem, however, is net loss rather than net gain.

The sole source of heat gain during cold stress is metabolic heat released during muscular work along with basal biological processes. As exercise demands increase, the rate of heat gain from metabolism increases. If the rate of metabolic heat decreases because of fatigue or changes in demand, a disorder is more likely[119].

Heat Loss

Heat is lost primarily by convection owing to the difference between skin and ambient temperature[111,119,120]. The rate of convection increases with air movement from wind (see Table 28-17) or motion through the air (e.g., cycling or running). Sitting or lying on a cold, solid surface may cause heat loss by conduction. Cyclic exercise and rest in which heat accumulates and the person sweats under clothing may be associated with heat loss through evaporation. Additional loss by radiant heat flow to colder surfaces is also possible.

Clothing

Proper clothing is the primary mechanism for achieving thermal balance during cold stress[119,120]. The amount of insulation that clothing affords is described in units called *clo*. A wool business suit has an insulating value of approximately 1 clo. Generally, each quarter inch of clothing adds 1 clo of insulation. Figure 3-20 illustrates the relations among air temperature, metabolic rate, and clothing in maintaining thermal balance[120]. The insulating quality of clothing decreases precipitously when it becomes wet.

Sometimes clothing is sufficient to protect from hypothermia, but exposed skin is still at risk for excessive local cooling. The major method of heat loss is convection, but conduction via contact with cold objects can also occur. Adequate heating from circulating blood may not be available because of reductions in peripheral blood flow (vasoconstriction) that naturally occur as a mechanism for heat conservation.

COLD-RELATED DISORDERS

Normal physiological response to cold stress is directed toward heat conservation, decreasing peripheral circulation and increasing metabolic rate. These mechanisms, however, are not adequate for most cold stress, and behavioral thermal regulation is crucial for preventing cold-related disorders. Cold-related disorders can be systemic or local. Box 3-2 is a list of some common cold-related disorders along with symptoms, signs, and steps for first aid[110–112,119].

Systemic Cold

The systemic cold disorder is hypothermia. Mild cases are marked by shivering and cold sensation in the extremities. Progression is associated with unstable cardiac function followed by CNS depression. Mild cases can be

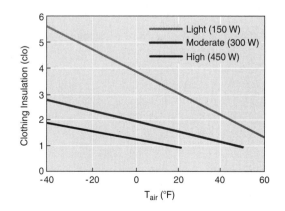

FIGURE 3-20. Relationship between air temperature and adequate clothing insulation for three levels of exercise. W = Watts

BOX 3-2	Cold-related Disorders, Including Symptoms, Signs, and First Aid		
Disorder	**Symptoms**	**Signs**	**First Aid**
Hypothermia	Chills	Euphoria	Move to warm area and remove wet clothing
	Fatigue or drowsiness	Slurred speech	Modest external warming
	Pain in the extremities	Slow, weak pulse	Drink warm carbohydrate-containing fluids
		Shivering	Transport to the hospital
		Collapse or unconsciousness	
		Body core temperature ≤35°C (95°F)	
Frostbite	Burning sensation at first	Skin color white or grayish yellow to reddish violet to black	Move to warm area and remove wet clothing
	Coldness, numbness, tingling		External warming (e.g., warm water)
		Blisters	Drink warm carbohydrate-containing fluids if conscious
		Response to touch depends on depth of freezing	Treat as a burn; do not rub affected area
			Transport to the hospital
Frost nip	Possible itching or pain	Skin turns white	Similar to that for frostbite
Trench foot	Severe pain	Edema	Similar to that for frostbite
	Tingling, itching	Blisters	
		Response to touch depends on depth of cooling	

addressed by simple first aid, but moderate to severe hypothermia requires medical attention.

Local Disorders

Acute local disorders are associated with local tissue freezing (frostbite) or cooling (frost nip and trench foot). Frostbite can occur only when ambient temperature is < −1°C (30°F): it is marked by actual crystallization of water in tissue and subsequent destruction of cells. Because of the risk of further complications, significant cases of frostbite should be referred to medical personnel. Frost nip and trench foot are skin disorders that result from extreme cooling of the skin and underlying tissue, but without actual freezing of water in the tissue. The distinguishing characteristic between frost nip and trench foot is the presence of damp clothing that has accelerated heat loss.

SUMMARY

Environmental stressors such as heat and cold can significantly affect exercise and can be dangerous if uncontrolled. Adequate preventive precautions for both heat and cold are possible and should be known by exercise professionals. Situations that require medical attention are fairly common, and immediate referral of such problems is important.

Exercise and the Environment: Altitude and Air Pollution

The condition of ambient air, which is inhaled into the lungs for respiratory gas exchange, has great importance for exercise capacity, physiological performance, and general health. This section discusses two main characteristics of ambient air: density, which changes with altitude, and contaminants, generally referred to as air pollution. It is necessary to be aware of hazards because exposure to altitude and polluted air can have profound effects on physical performance and can cause serious illnesses, even in well-trained individuals (see Chapter 28).

HIGH TERRESTRIAL ALTITUDE

Considerable evidence indicates that altitude training in preparation for competition at altitude is beneficial; therefore, many athletes spend considerable resources training at altitude. However, the value of this training for increasing performance at sea level is controversial. The lack of consensus may be attributed to differences in duration of exposure to altitude, elevations of training, initial fitness levels, and lack of a control group[121]. Recent studies indicate that under specific conditions, intermittent altitude exposure may have some beneficial effects for sea-level performance[122–124]. In this section, physiological responses that occur at altitudes up to 3000 m (11,800 feet) are discussed. Above 3000 m, the negative effects of prolonged exposure to hypoxia outweigh any positive training effects[125].

Physiological Responses

The amount of oxygen bound to hemoglobin in red blood cells depends on the partial pressure of oxygen in the inspired air (P_{IO_2}). P_{IO_2} decreases as a result of declines in barometric pressure with increasing altitude at constant oxygen percentage (Table 3-4). There is a decrease in the

TABLE 3-4. Barometric Pressure for a Standard Atmosphere and Inspired Partial Oxygen Pressure for Five Altitudes, Accounting for the Pressure of Water Vapor in the Lungs (47 mm Hg)

Altitude (m)	Barometric Pressure (mm Hg)	Inspired Oxygen Pressure (mm Hg)
0	760	149
1500	627	123
2000	596	115
2500	627	107
3000	522	100

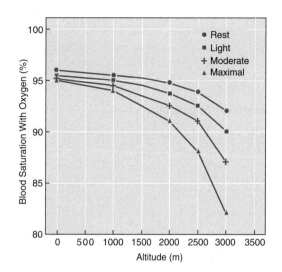

FIGURE 3-21. The effect of altitude and exercise levels on arterial oxygen saturation.

arterial oxygen saturation (Pa_{O_2}) with the decline in P_{Io2} and, thus, in the amount of oxygen available. Acute exposure to reduced oxygen saturation triggers several compensatory mechanisms to increase oxygen transfer to tissue. After these acute reactions, acclimation occurs with more fundamental adaptations.

Acute Physiological Responses

One of the most significant physiological compensatory reactions during acute exposure above 1200 m is increased pulmonary ventilation, or **hypoxic ventilatory response,** at rest and during exercise. Chemoreceptors in arterial blood vessels are stimulated, and signals are sent to the brain to increase ventilation. The increase in pulmonary ventilation is primarily associated with an increase in tidal volume, but with prolonged exposure or higher altitude, breathing frequency also increases. Hyperventilation substantially increases the arterial oxygen saturation. Increased ventilation also leads to washout of carbon dioxide in the blood. Therefore, uncompensated respiratory alkalosis (higher pH) may develop. This respiratory alkalosis can cause a left shift of the oxygen–hemoglobin dissociation curve, resulting in higher arterial oxygen saturation, a second compensatory mechanism[126]. Finally, early in exposure to altitude, reduced oxygen pressure is compensated for by small increases in cardiac output. This is primarily because of an increased HR because SV is constant or even slightly reduced at rest and during submaximal and maximal exercise.

Despite acute responses that compensate for lower oxygen tension at altitude, arterial oxygen saturation is decreased (Fig. 3-21). The magnitude of desaturation is directly related to altitude and exercise intensity. The primary pulmonary factor leading to increasing desaturation with increasing exercise intensity is limited alveolar end capillary diffusion. The result is an almost linear decrease of maximal oxygen uptake at a ratio of 10% per 1000 m altitude above 1500 m[127]. Because the oxygen uptake required by a fixed submaximal workload is not affected by altitude, the result is a higher relative exercise intensity for any given workload. Because of the nonlinear relationship between relative intensity (percent maximal

oxygen uptake) and endurance time, the magnitude of the performance decrement at altitude is not constant but varies in proportion to the duration of the activity. Therefore, the longer the running distance, the larger the relative decrement[128].

Muscular strength and muscular endurance seem unaffected during acute exposure to altitude. However, subtle neuropsychological effects associated with acute mountain sickness (AMS) can occur at altitudes of 3000 m within 6 hours of exposure. Above 4500 m, the deterioration in most mental functions may be considerable, although variations between individuals are large[129]. These neuropsychological effects may, in turn, affect muscular strength and endurance.

HIGH-ALTITUDE ILLNESS

Exposure to high altitude can lead to a number of illnesses that vary in seriousness. The speed of ascent and the absolute altitude are primary determinants of the incidence of altitude illness. Those exercising in or exposed to altitude (athletes and coaches) should anticipate the hazards and prepare through prevention and recognition of symptoms.

Acute Mountain Sickness

Acute mountain sickness is characterized by severe headache and often accompanied by nausea, vomiting, decreased appetite, weariness, and sleep disturbances[130]. AMS begins 6 to 12 hours after arrival, usually peaks on the second or third day, and disappears on the fourth or fifth day[131]. AMS normally appears above 2500 m, and the frequency of AMS increases with altitude and rate of ascent. Generally, above 3000 m, 24 hours of acclimation should be acquired for every 300-m altitude gain[131]. Although AMS is self-limiting, persistence of symptoms may require medical treatment. If AMS is not at least partially resolved within 2 to 3 days, descent is the only effective treatment. Supplemental oxygen and pharmacological treatment (acetazolamide, furosemide, analgesics) may be necessary for severe cases.

High-altitude Pulmonary Edema

High-altitude pulmonary edema (HAPE) is considered a progression in the severity of AMS, associated with pulmonary edema[131]. The onset may be subtle. Signs and symptoms include dyspnea, fatigue, chest pain, tachycardia, coughing, and cyanosis of the lips and extremities. As HAPE progresses, affected individuals may cough frothy or blood-tinged sputum[130]. This complication can be fatal if not treated promptly. Children and young adults are at higher risk of developing HAPE than adults, and immediate medical attention is necessary. Evacuation to a lower altitude is essential. Individuals with a history of HAPE appear to be particularly susceptible to subsequent bouts upon return to high altitudes.

High-altitude Cerebral Edema

High-altitude cerebral edema (HACE) may develop when the rate of ascent is too fast. The signs and symptoms of HACE include severe headache, fatigue, vomiting, nausea, ataxia, and changes of mental status[130]. The incidence of HACE is low (1%), but it can be fatal if untreated. In cases of symptoms of cerebral edema, direct medical care with immediate evacuation to a low altitude and supplemental oxygen is recommended[132].

Preventing Altitude Sickness

Acute mountain sickness can be prevented by adjusting the amount and rate of ascent. Options include an interrupted ascent with time (days) to acclimate at successive altitudes before reaching the final elevation or limiting daily gain in altitude to 300 m or less. Initially, unacclimated subjects should avoid vigorous exercise. Adequate hydration and a high-carbohydrate diet may aid prevention. Acetazolamide is the only drug for altitude sickness approved by the Food and Drug Administration (FDA). Because acetazolamide may affect exercise performance, it is contraindicated when training at high altitudes. Prophylactic administration of acetazolamide may be effective[130].

AIR POLLUTION

Air pollution can also affect exercise performance and health. Although nature contributes to pollution through ozone (O_3) from lightning, dust, sulfuric oxides from volcanic activity and other natural pollutants, modern industrialization has exacerbated the problem. Because of the severity of pollution in many areas, organizers of sporting events and exercisers are frequently confronted with problems related to exercising in polluted air. Both large sporting events and daily activity are performed in major cities, which are generally the sites with the highest pollution levels. Also, with indoor training and sports events, the infiltration of outdoor air pollution may be significant. Furthermore, the indoor environment may actually add to the problem with indoor air pollutants emitted by the occupants, activities, and building materials.

There are two major groups of pollutants: primary and secondary. **Primary pollutants** are directly attributable to a source of pollution, such as carbon monoxide (CO), sulfur oxides, nitrogen oxides, hydrocarbons, and particulates (dust, smoke, and soot). **Secondary pollutants** result from an interaction of the environment (sunlight, moisture, other pollutants) with primary pollutants. These include O_3, aldehydes, sulfuric acid (H_2SO_4), and peroxyacetyl nitrate (PAN). City air commonly contains both primary and secondary pollutants.

General Effector Mechanisms

The effect of pollutants is partly related to level of penetration. This "dosage" is determined by exposure time, concentration of pollutant in inspired air, ventilation rate, temperature and humidity of inspired air, and route of inspiration (the nose versus the mouth). Pollution primarily affects the respiratory tract. This tract provides a large surface area for contact by the pollutant. The mucous membranes of the nose effectively remove large particles and highly soluble gases (e.g., 99.9% of inhaled SO_2), preventing them from affecting deeper airways and lung tissue. However, smaller particles and agents with low solubility easily pass through this barrier. During exercise, when mouth breathing plays an important role, this air filtration is less efficient, and more pollutants reach the lungs, traverse the diffusion surface, and enter the blood and body tissues. Pollutants can have several effects during their course through the body, including the following:

- Irritation of the airways, which may lead to bronchoconstriction, hence increased airway resistance
- Reduction of alveolar diffusion capacity
- Reduction of oxygen transport capacity

Other effects of pollutants that can indirectly affect exercise performance are irritation of eyes (PAN and formaldehyde) and skin. Short-term effects of exposure to pollutants rather than long-term exposure is discussed in this section.

Outdoor Pollution

Geographical distribution of outdoor pollution is strongly related to industry and population density. Automobiles, trucks, buses, aircrafts, industrial sources, and combustion of fossil fuels are major sources of CO, sulfur and nitrogen oxides, hydrocarbons, and particles. Areas with equal production of pollutants do not necessarily have equally polluted air, or smog, because climate and topography play major roles. River and mountain valleys generally have greater smog levels than hilltops and plains. High temperature and humidity typically promote photochemical smog with associated high O_3 levels. For example, in the Los Angeles area, photochemical smog, trapped by summer winds blowing toward the surrounding mountains, is a common phenomenon[133]. Low temperature with a concomitant increase in fuel consumption for heating and high humidity (fog, rain) promote a different type of fog, in which high sulfur oxide concentrations combined with particulate matter are converted into sulfuric acid (acid rain) and sulfates. The most famous fog of this type is the London fog, which produced a large number of deaths in 1952 (4000 in a 4-day period)[134]. Such fog can be persistent when temperature inversion occurs, a condition brought about by little wind and a layer of cool polluted air trapped beneath a layer of warmer air.

Prevention

Avoidance of exposure is the primary method for preventing acute and long-term adverse effects of outdoor pollutants. Timing and selection of optimal location for exercise and moderating intensity and duration are key factors[135]. Knowledge of daily and seasonal patterns and fluctuations (Fig. 3-22) is important when planning an event involving high-intensity exercise. Avoiding periods and areas with heavy traffic can minimize CO exposure. Summer and early autumn afternoons can be unfavorable because of high O_3 exposure.

Information on air pollution can be acquired from local meteorological authorities, many of which provide a pollutant standards index (PSI) developed by the Environmental Protection Agency. The PSI converts

TABLE 3-5. National Ambient Air Quality Standards as Provided by the Environmental Protection Agency

Pollutant	Time Period	
	For Averaging	Standard Limit Level
Carbon monoxide	8 hr	9 ppm
	1 hr	35 ppm
Ozone	1 hr	0.12 ppm
	8 hr	0.08 ppm
Nitrogen dioxide (NO_2)	AAM	0.053 ppm
Sulfur dioxide (SO_2)	AAM	80 $\mu g \cdot m^{-3}$
	24 hr	365 $\mu g \cdot m^{-3}$
Particulates (PM-2.5)	AAM	15 $\mu g \cdot m^{-3}$
($\leq$2.5-μ diameter)	24 hr	65 $\mu g \cdot m^{-3}$
Particulates (PM-10)	AAM	50 $\mu g \cdot m^{-3}$
($\leq$10-micron diameter)	24 hr	150 $\mu g \cdot m^{-3}$

AAM = annual arithmetic mean.

For pollutants with high hourly or daily fluctuations, longer duration averages and short-term peak level limits are provided. The numbers correspond to a pollution standards index (PSI) of 100.

measured pollutant concentration to a number on a scale from 0 to 500. The critical number is 100, which corresponds to the threshold established under the Clean Air Act (Table 3-5)[136]. A PSI above 100 indicates pollution in an unhealthful range. PSI places maximum emphasis on acute health effects (24 hours or less), rather than chronic effects, making it useful for exercise planning. It does not incorporate interactions between pollutants. Table 3-6 has information on the PSI[136].

The important factors for controlling exposure to indoor pollution include selecting an optimal location for air intake, using low-emission building materials, regularly cleaning and use of low-dust floor coverings, clean ventilation and air conditioning systems, and sufficiently high fresh-air ventilation rate. More specifically, exercise centers and fitness facilities require higher ventilation rates than offices and living quarters. A CO_2 concentration limit of 1000 ppm at an outdoor concentration of 350 ppm is often used as an indicator of adequate ventilation. At that level, 80% of the users are satisfied with air quality. A level of 650 ppm CO_2 is needed to increase satisfaction to 90%[137]. Indoor exercise areas should maintain the lowest CO_2 concentration practically possible.

SUMMARY

The environmental effects of altitude and air pollution can affect exercise and athletic performance. Physiological adaptation or maladaptation (in the case of altitude sickness or exposure to air pollution) is often a factor in fitness, exercise, and training programs. Although some effects of altitude can be overcome with chronic adaptations to training at altitude, prevention of harmful effects of pollution is often a function of avoiding and minimizing exposure.

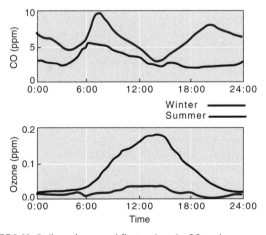

FIGURE 3-22. Daily and seasonal fluctuations in CO and ozone concentrations in the Los Angeles area. (Adapted with permission from McCafferty W: Air Pollution and Athletic Performance. Springfield, IL: Charles C Thomas; 1981.)

TABLE 3-6. The Pollutant Standards Index and Implications for Short-term Health Effects

Index Value	PSI Descriptor	General Health Effects	Cautionary Statements
Up to 50	Good	None for the general population	None required
51–100	Moderate	Few or none for the general population	None required
101–200	Unhealthful	Mild aggravation of symptoms among susceptible people, with irritation symptoms in the healthy population	Persons with existing heart or respiratory ailments should reduce physical exertion and outdoor activity; the general population should reduce vigorous outdoor activity
201–300	Very unhealthful	Significant aggravation of symptoms and decreased exercise tolerance in persons with heart or lung disease; widespread symptoms in the healthy population	Elderly and persons with heart or lung disease should stay indoors and reduce physical activity; general population should avoid vigorous outdoor activity
>300	Hazardous	Early onset of certain diseases in addition to significant aggravation of symptoms and decreased exercise tolerance in healthy persons. At PSI levels above 400, premature death of ill and elderly persons may result. Healthy people have adverse symptoms that affect normal activity	Elderly and persons with diseases should stay indoors and avoid physical exertion. At PSI levels above 400, the general population should avoid outdoor activity. All people should remain indoors, keeping windows and doors closed, and minimize physical exertion.

PSI = pollution standards index. Also see Table 28–18

Acknowledgments

The authors wish to confer sincere appreciation to the following individuals who contributed to the previous edition of this text. Their efforts greatly assisted our compilation of information for the current chapter: Thomas E. Bernard, Jill A. Bush, Mark Davis, Scott R. Demaree, Robert Fitts, Barry A. Franklin, George Havenith, Michael Holewijn, William J. Kraemer, John M. Lawler, and Scott K. Powers.

REFERENCES

1. Armstrong R: Biochemistry: Energy liberation and use. In Strauss RS, ed. Sports Medicine and Physiology. Philadelphia: WB Saunders; 1979.
2. Gollnick P, Riedy M, Quintinskie J, Bertocci L: Differences in metabolic potential of skeletal muscle fibres and their significance for metabolic control. J Exp Biol 115:191, 1985.
3. Gollnick P: Metabolism of substrates: Energy substrate metabolism during exercise and as modified by training. Fed Proc 44:353, 1985.
4. Newsholme E: The control of fuel utilization by muscle during exercise and starvation. Diabetes 28(suppl 1):1, 1979.
5. Powers S, Riley W, Howley E: Comparison of fat metabolism between trained men and women during prolonged aerobic work. Res Q Exerc Sport 51:427, 1980.
6. Holloszy J, Coyle E: Adaptations of skeletal muscle to endurance exercise and their metabolic consequences. J Appl Physiol 56:831, 1984.
7. Holloszy J: Utilization of fatty acids during exercise. In Taylor AW, Gollnick PD, Green HJ, et al, eds. Biochemistry of Exercise VII. Champaign, IL: Human Kinetics; 1990.
8. Stanley W, Connett R: Regulation of muscle carbohydrate metabolism during exercise. FASEB J 5:2155, 1991.
9. Bonen A, McDermott J, Tan M: Glucose transport in muscle. In Taylor AW, Gollnick PD, Green HJ, et al, eds. Biochemistry of Exercise VII. Champaign, IL: Human Kinetics, 1990.
10. Senior A: ATP synthesis by oxidative phosphorylation. Physiol Rev 68:177, 1988.
11. Powers S, Dodd S, Beadle R: Oxygen uptake kinetics in trained athletes differing in $\dot{V}O_{2max}$. Eur J Appl Physiol 54:306, 1985.
12. diPrampero P. Boutellier U, Pietsch P: Oxygen deficit and stores at onset of muscular exercise in humans. J Appl Physiol 55:146, 1983.
13. Powers S, Byrd R, Tulley R, et al: Effects of caffeine ingestion on metabolism and performance during graded exercise. Eur J Appl Physiol 50:301, 1983.
14. Powers S, Howley E, Cox R: Ventilatory and metabolic reactions to heat stress during prolonged exercise. J Sports Med 22:32, 1982.
15. Gaesser G, Brooks C: Metabolic bases of excess post-exercise oxygen consumption: A review. Med Sci Sports Exerc 16:29, 1984.
16. Powers S, Howley E, Cox R: A differential catecholamine response during prolonged exercise and passive heating. Med Sci Sports Exerc 14:435, 1982.
17. Coyle EF, Jeukendrup AE, Wagonmakers AJM, Saris WHM: Fatty acid oxidation is directly regulated by carbohydrate metabolism during exercise. Am J Physiol 273:E268, 1997.
18. Farrell PA, Wilmore JH, Coyle EF, et al: Plasma lactate accumulation and distance running performance. Med Sci Sports Exerc 11:338, 1979.
19. Powers S, Dodd S, Deason R, et al: Ventilatory threshold, running economy and distance running performance of trained athletes. Res Q Exerc Sport 51:179, 1983.
20. Graham T: Mechanisms of blood lactate increase during exercise. Physiologist 27:299, 1984.
21. Katz A, Sahlin K: Oxygen in regulation of glycolysis and lactate production in human skeletal muscle. Exerc Sport Sci Rev 18:1, 1990.
22. Richardsen RS, Noyszewsky EA, Leogh JS, Wagner PD: Lactate efflux from exercising human skeletal muscle: Role of intracellular P_{O_2}. J Appl Physiol 85:627, 1998.
23. Stainsby W, Brooks C: Control of lactic acid metabolism in contracting skeletal muscles during exercise. Exerc Sport Sci Rev 18:29, 1990.
24. Wasserman K, Whipp BJ, Koyal SN, et al: Anaerobic threshold and respiratory gas exchange during exercise. J Appl Physiol 35:236–243, 1973.

25. Davis JA, Vodak P, Wilmore JH, et al: Anaerobic threshold and maximal aerobic power for three modes of exercise. J Appl Physiol 41:544–550, 1976.

26. Davis JA, Frank MH, Whipp BJ, et al: Anaerobic threshold alterations caused by endurance training in middle-aged men. J Appl Physiol 46:1039–1046, 1979.

27. Brooks CA: Anaerobic threshold: Review of the concept and directions for future research. Med Sci Sports Exerc 17:22–31, 1985.

28. Costill DL: Physiology of marathon running. JAMA 221:1024–1029, 1972.

29. Costill DL, Thomason H, Roberts E: Fractional utilization of the aerobic capacity during distance running. Med Sci Sports Exerc 5:248–252, 1973.

30. Powers SK, Howley ET: Exercise Physiology. Madison, WI: Brown & Benchmark; 1994.

31. Dehn MM, Mullins CB: Physiologic effects and importance of exercise in patients with coronary artery disease. J Cardiovasc Med 2:365–387, 1977.

32. Mitchell JH, Blomqvist G: Maximal oxygen uptake. N Engl J Med 284:1018–1022, 1971.

33. Poliner LR, Dehmer CJ, Lewis SE, et al: Left ventricular performance in normal subjects: A comparison of the responses to exercise in the upright and supine position. Circulation 62:528–534, 1980.

34. Ferguson RJ, Faulkner JA, Julius S, et al: Comparison of cardiac output determined by CO₂ rebreathing and dye-dilution methods. J Appl Physiol 25:450–454, 1968.

35. Rowell IB: Circulation. Med Sci Sports 1:15–22, 1969.

36. Zobi EG, Talmers FN, Christensen RC, et al: Effect of exercise on the cerebral circulation and metabolism. J Appl Physiol 20:1289–1293, 1965.

37. Hester RL, Choi J: Blood flow control during exercise: role for the venular epithelium. Exerc Sport Sci Rev 30: 147–151, 2002

38. Naughton J, Haider R: Methods of exercise testing. In Naughton JP, Hellerstein HK, Mohler IC, eds. Exercise Testing and Exercise Training in Coronary Heart Disease. New York: Academic; 1973:79.

39. ACSM: Guidelines for Exercise Testing and Prescription, 5th ed. Baltimore: Williams & Wilkins; 1995:97.

40. Comess KA, Fenster PE: Clinical implications of the blood pressure response to exercise. Cardiology 68:233–244, 1981.

41. Franklin BA: Diagnostic and functional exercise testing: Test selection and interpretation. J Cardiovasc Nurs 10:8–29, 1995.

42. Irving JB, Bruce RA, DeRouen TA: Variations in and significance of systolic pressure during maximal exercise (treadmill) testing: Relation to severity of coronary artery disease and cardiac mortality. Am J Cardiol 39:841–848, 1977.

43. Davis JA, Vodak P, Wilmore JH, et al: Anaerobic threshold and maximal aerobic power for three modes of exercise. J Appl Physiol 41:544–550, 1976.

44. Costill DL: Physiology of marathon running. JAMA 221:1024–1029, 1972.

45. Powers SK, Martin D, Dodd, S: Exercise induced hypoxemia in elite endurance athletes: Incidence causes and impact on VO₂max. Sports Medicine 16:14–22, 1993.

46. Harms CA, McClaran SR, Nickele GA, Pegelow DF, Nelson WB, Dempsey JA: Exercise induced arterial hypoxemia in healthy young women. J Physiol 507:619–628, 1998.

47. Coyle EF, Gonzalez-Alonso J: Cardiovascular drift during prolonged exercise: New perspectives. Exerc Sport Sci Rev 29:88–92, 2001.

48. Ginzton LE, Conant R, Brizendine M, et al: Effect of long-term high intensity aerobic training on left ventricular volume during maximal upright exercise. J Am Coll Cardiol 14:364–371, 1989.

49. Concu A, Marcello C: Stroke volume response to progressive exercise in athletes engaged in different types of training. Eur J Appl Physiol 66:11–17, 1993.

50. Lind AR, Taylor SH, Humphreys PW, et al: The circulatory effects of sustained voluntary muscle contraction. Clin Sci 27:229–244, 1964.

51. Lind AR, McNichol GW: Muscular factors which determine the cardiovascular responses to sustained and rhythmic exercise. Can Med Assoc J 96:706–715, 1967.

52. Mitchell JH, Payne FC, Saltin B, et al: The role of muscle mass in the cardiovascular response to static contractions. J Physiol 309:45–54, 1980.

53. Atkins JM, Matthews OA, Blomqvist CG, et al: Incidence of arrhythmias induced by isometric and dynamic exercise. Br Heart J 38:465–471, 1976.

54. Franklin BA: Exercise testing, training and arm ergometry. Sports Med 2:100–119, 1985.

55. Fardy PS, Webb D, Hellerstein HK: Benefits of arm exercise in cardiac rehabilitation. Phys Sportmed 5:30–41, 1977.

56. Schwade J, Blomqvist CG, Shapiro W: A comparison of the response to arm and leg work in patients with ischemic heart disease. Am Heart J 94:203–208, 1977.

57. Franklin BA, Vander L, Wrisley D, et al: Aerobic requirements of arm ergometry: Implications for exercise testing and training. Phys Sportsmed 11:81–90, 1983.

58. Balke B: Experimental studies on the functional capacities of middle-aged and aging persons. J Okla Med Assoc 54:120–123, 1961.

59. Buskirk E, Taylor HL: Maximal oxygen intake and its relation to body composition, with special reference to chronic physical activity and obesity. J Appl Physiol 2:72–78, 1957.

60. Bruce RA, Kusumi F, Hosmer D: Maximal oxygen intake and nomographic assessment of functional aerobic impairment in cardiovascular disease. Am Heart J 85:546–562, 1973.

61. Franklin BA: Pitfalls in estimating aerobic capacity from exercise time or workload. Appl Cardiol 14:25–26, 1986.

62. Myers J, Buchanan N, Walsh D, et al: Comparison of the ramp versus standard exercise protocols. J Am Coll Cardiol 17:1334–1342, 1991.

63. Myers J, Buchanan N, Smith D, et al: Individual ramp treadmill: Observations on a new protocol. Chest 101:236S–241S, 1992.

64. Kitamura K, Jorgenson CR, Gobel FL, et al: Hemodynamic correlates of myocardial oxygen consumption during up-right exercise. J Appl Physiol 32:516–522, 1972.

65. Nelson RR, Gobel FL, Jorgensen CR, et al: Hemodynamic predictors of myocardial oxygen consumption during static and dynamic exercise. Circulation 50:1179–1189, 1974.

66. Edgerton VR, Roy RR, Gregor RJ, et al: Muscle fiber activation and recruitment. In Knuttgen HG, Vogel JA, Poortmans S, eds. Biochemistry of Exercise. Champaign, IL: Human Kinetics; 1983:31–49.

67. Faulkner J, Claflin D, McCully K: Power output of fast and slow fibers from human skeletal muscles. In Jones N, McCartney N, McComas A, eds. Human Muscle Power. Champaign, IL: Human Kinetics; 1986:81–90.

68. Noth J: Motor units. In Komi PV, ed. Strength and Power in Sport. Oxford, UK: Blackwell Scientific; 1992:21–28.

69. Staron RS, Hikida RS: Histochemical, biochemical, and ultrastructural analyses of single human muscle fibers with special reference to the C fiber population. J Histochem Cytochem 40:563–568, 1992.

70. Staron RS, Karapondo DL, Kraemer WJ, et al: Skeletal muscle adaptations during the early phase of heavy-resistance training in men and women. J Appl Physiol 76:1247–1255, 1994.

71. Staron RS, Leonardi MJ, Karapondo DL, et al: Strength and skeletal muscle adaptations in heavy-resistance trained women after detraining and retraining. J Appl Physiol 70:631–640, 1991.

72. Fry AC, Allemeier CA, Staron RS: Correlation between percentage fiber type area and myosin heavy chain content in human skeletal muscle. Eur J Appl Physiol 88:246–251, 1994.

73. Fleck SJ: Cardiovascular response to strength training. In Komi P, ed. Strength and Power in Sports: The Encyclopaedia of Sports Medicine. Oxford, UK: Blackwell Scientific, 1992:305–315.

74. Stone MH: Weight gain and weight loss. In Bacchle TR, ed. Essentials of Strength Training and Conditioning. Champaign, IL: Human Kinetics, 1994:231–237.

75. Bigland-Ritchie B, Rice CL, Garland SJ, et al: Task-dependent factors in fatigue of human voluntary contractions. In Gandevia SC, Enoka RM, McComas AJ, et al, eds. Fatigue: Neural and Muscular Mechanisms. New York: Plenum; 1995:361–380.

76. Davis JM, Bailey SP: Possible mechanisms of central nervous system fatigue during exercise. Med Sci Sports Exerc 29:45–57, 1997.

77. Enoka RM, Stuart DG: Neurobiology of muscle fatigue. J Appl Physiol 72:1631–1648, 1992.

78. Fitts RH: Cellular mechanisms of muscle fatigue. Physiol Rev 74:49, 1994.

79. Fitts RH: Cellular, molecular, and metabolic basis of muscle fatigue. In Rowell LB, Shephard JT, eds. Handbook of Physiology: Section 12: Regulation and Integration of Multiple Systems. New York: Oxford University; 1996.

80. Lannergren J, Westerblad H: Force and membrane potential during and after fatiguing, continuous high-frequency stimulation of single Xenopus muscle fibers. Acta Physiol Scand 128:359, 1986.

81. Metzger JM, Fitts RH: Fatigue from high and low frequency muscle stimulation: Role of sarcolemma action potentials. Exp Neurol 93:320, 1986.

82. Sjogaard G: Role of exercise-induced potassium fluxes underlying muscle fatigue: A brief review. Can J Physiol Pharmacol 69:238, 1990.

83. Fitts RH, Courtright JB, Kim DM, et al: Muscle fatigue with prolonged exercise: Contractile and biochemical alterations. Am J Physiol 242:C65, 1982.

84. Allen DG, Lee JA, Westerblad H: Intracellular calcium and tension in isolated single muscle fibers from Xenopus. J Physiol 415:433, 1989.

85. Westerblad H, Allen DG: Changes of myoplasmic calcium concentration during fatigue in single mouse muscle fibers. J Gen Physiol 98:615, 1991.

86. Bergstrom J: Muscle electrolytes in man. Scand J Clin Lab Invest 14(suppl 68), 1962.

87. Fitts RH, Holloszy JO: Lactate and contractile force in frog muscle during development of fatigue and recovery. Am J Physiol 231:430, 1976.

88. Fitts RH, Holloszy JO: Effects of fatigue and recovery on contractile properties of frog muscle. J Appl Physiol 45:899, 1978.

89. Sahlin K, Edstrom L, Sjoholm H: Force, relaxation and energy metabolism of rat soleus muscle during anaerobic contraction. Acta Physiol Scand 129:1, 1987.

90. Thompson LV, Fitts RH: Muscle fatigue in the frog semi-tendinosus: Role of high energy phosphates and P(I). Am J Physiol 263:C803, 1992.

91. Berstrom M, Hultman E: Energy cost and fatigue during intermittent electrical stimulation of human skeletal muscle. J Appl Physiol 65:1500, 1988.

92. Cooke R, Franko K, Luciana GB, et al: The inhibition of rabbit skeletal muscle contraction by hydrogen ions and phosphate. J Physiol 395:77, 1988.

93. Godt RE, Nosek TM: Changes of intracellular milieu with fatigue or hypoxia depress contraction of skinned rabbit skeletal and cardiac muscle. J Physiol 412:155, 1989.

94. Nosek TM, Fender KY, Godt RE: It is deprotonated inorganic phosphate that depresses force in skinned skeletal muscle fibers. Science 236:191, 1987.

95. Nakamura Y, Schwartz A: The influence of hydrogen ion concentration on calcium binding and release by skeletal muscle sarcoplasmic reticulum. J Gen Physiol 59:22, 1972.

96. Hill AV: The absolute value of the isometric heat coefficient T1/H in a muscle twitch, and the effect of stimulation and fatigue. Proc R Soc Lond B Biol Sci 103:163, 1928.

97. Sahlin K, Harris RC, Nylind B, et al: Lactate content and pH in muscle samples obtained after dynamic exercise. Plugers Arch 367:143, 1976.

98. Fabiato A, Fabiato F: Effects of pH on the myofilaments and the sarcoplasmic reticulum of skinned cells from cardiac and skeletal muscles. J Physiol 276:233, 1978.

99. Metzger JM, Moss RL: Greater hydrogen ion-induced depression of tension and velocity in skinned single fibres of rat fast rather than slow muscles. J Physiol 393:727, 1987.

100. Metzger JM, Fitts RH: Role of intracellular pH in muscle fatigue. J Appl Physiol 62:1392, 1987.

101. Thompson LV, Balog EM, Fitts RH: Muscle fatigue in frog semitendinosus: Role of intracellular pH. Am J Physiol 263:C1507, 1992.

102. Byrd SK, McCutcheon LJ, Hodgson DR, et al: Altered sarcoplasmic reticulum function after high-intensity exercise. J Appl Physiol 67:2072, 1989.

103. Wilkie DR: Muscular fatigue: Effects of hydrogen ions and inorganic phosphate. Fed Proc 45:2921, 1986.

104. Allen GM, Gandevia SC, McKenzie DK: Reliability of measurements of muscle strength and voluntary activation using twitch interpolation. Muscle Nerve 18:593–600, 1995.

105. Bigland-Ritchie B, Furbush B, Woods II: Fatigue of intermittent submaximal voluntary contractions: Central and peripheral factors. J Appl Physiol 61:421–429, 1986.

106. Garner SH, Sutton JR, Burse RL, et al: Operation Everest II: Neuromuscular performance under conditions of extreme simulated altitude. J Appl Physiol 68:1167–1172, 1990.

107. Westing SH, Cresswell AG, Thorstensson A: Muscle activation during maximal voluntary eccentric and concentric knee extension. Eur J Appl Physiol 62:104–108, 1991.

108. Bigland-Ritchie B: EMG/Force relations and fatigue of human voluntary contractions. Exer Sports Sci Rev 9:75–117, 1981.

109. Rube N, Secher NH: Paradoxical influence of encouragement on muscle fatigue. Eur J Appl Physiol 46:1–7, 1981.

110. McArdle D, Katch FI, Katch VL, eds: Exercise Physiology, 4th ed. Philadelphia: Lea & Febiger; 1996.

111. Pandolf B, Sawka MN, Gonzalez RG, eds: Human Performance Physiology and Environmental Medicine at Terrestrial Extremes. Carmel, IN: Cooper; 1986.

112. Bernard E. Thermal Stress. In Plog BA, ed. Fundamentals in Industrial Hygiene. Itasca, IL: National Safety Council, 1996.

113. Eastman Kodak Company: Ergonomic Design for People at Work, vol 2. New York: Van Nostrand Reinhold; 1986.

114. International Organization for Standardization: Hot environments: Analytical determination and interpretation of thermal stress using calculation of required sweat rate. Geneva: ISO 7933, 1989.

115. Wyndham CH, Strydom NB, Benade JS, et al: Heat stroke risk in unacclimatized and acclimatized men of different maximum oxygen intakes working under hot humid conditions. Chamber of Mines Research Report 12/72. Johannesburg: Chamber of Mines of South Africa: 1972.

116. Parsons KC: Human Thermal Environments. Bristol, PA: Taylor & Francis; 1993.

117. Kamon E, Avellini BD: Wind speed limits to work under hot environments for clothed men. J Appl Physiol 46:340–349, 1979.

118. Rowell LB: Human Cardiovascular Control. Cary, NC: Oxford University, 1994.

119. Holmer I: Cold Stress: 1.Guidelines for the practitioner. 2. The scientific basis (knowledge base) for the guide. Int J Indust Ergonom 14:139–159, 1994.

120. Holmer I: Assessment of cold stress in terms of required clothing insulation: IREQ. Int J Indust Ergonom 3:159–166, 1988.

121. Favier R, Spielvogel H, Desplanches D, et al: Training in hypoxia vs. training in normoxia in high-altitude natives. J Appl Physiol 78:2286–2293, 1995.

122. Levine BD, Roach RC, Houston CS: Work and training at altitude. In Sutton JR, Coates G, Houston CS, eds. Hypoxia and Mountain Medicine. Burlington, VT: Queen City Printers; 1992:192–201.

123. Levine BD, Stray-Gundersen J: A practical approach to altitude training. Int J Sports Med 13:S209–S212, 1992.

124. Rodriguez FA, Casa H, Casa M, et al: Intermittent hypobaric hypoxia stimulates erythropoiesis and improves aerobic capacity. Med Sci Sports Exerc 31:264–268, 1999.

125. Kayser B: Nutrition and energetics of exercise at altitude: Theory and possible practical implications. Sports Med 17:309–323, 1994.

126. Åstrand PO, Rodahl K: Textbook of Work Physiology: Physiological Bases of Exercise. Chicago: McGraw-Hill; 1986.

127. Buskirk ER: Decrease in physical working capacity at high altitude. In Hegnauer AH, Natick MA, eds. Biomedicine of High Altitude. US Army Res Inst Environ Med 1969:204–222.

128. Fulco CS: Maximal and submaximal exercise performance at altitude. Aviat Space Environ Med 69:793–801, 1998.

129. Cudaback DD: Four-KM altitude effects on performance and health. Pub Astronom Soc Pac 96:463–477, 1984.

130. Malconian MK, Rock PB: Medical problems related to altitude. In Pandolf KB, Swaka MN, Gonzalez RR, eds. Human Performance Physiology and Environmental Medicine at Terrestrial Extremes. Indianapolis: Benchmark; 1988.

131. Ward MP, Milledge JS, West JB: High Altitude Medicine and Physiology. New York: Chapman & Hall; 1989.

132. Hamilton AJ, Cymerman A, Black P: High altitude cerebral edema. Neurosurgery 19:841–849, 1986.

133. Haymes EM, Welss CL: Environment and Human Performance. Champaign, IL: Human Kinetics; 1986.

134. McCafferty W: Air pollution and athletic performance. Springfield, IL: Charles C Thomas; 1981.

135. Cedaro R: Environmental factors and exercise performance: A review. II. Air pollution. Excel 8:161–166, 1992.

136. Environmental Protection Agency: Public information provided on the World Wide Web server: http://www.epa.gov/1992.

137. Bienfait D, Fanger PO, Fitzner K, et al: European Concerted Action Report 11: Guidelines for ventilation requirements in buildings. Office for Publications of the European Communities, Brussels; 1992.

SELECTED REFERENCES FOR FURTHER READING

Astrand PO, Rodahl K, Dahl HA, Stromme SB: Textbook of Work Physiology: Physiological Basis of Exercise. Champagne, IL: Human Kinetics; 2003.

Baechle TR, Earle RW, eds Essentials of Strength and Conditioning. National Strength and Conditioning Association. Champagne, IL: Human Kinetics; 2000.

Brooks G, Fahey T, White T, Baldwin K: Exercise Physiology: Human Bioenergetics and its Applications. Mountain View, CA: Mayfield; 2000.

Fleck SJ, Kraemer WJ: Designing Resistance Training Programs. Champagne, IL: Human Kinetics; 2004.

Gleeson M, Maughan RJ: The Biochemical Basis of Sports Performance. Lavallette, NJ: Oxford University Press; 2004.

Hoffman J. Physiological Aspects of Sport Training and Performance. Champagne, IL: Human Kinetics; 2002.

Komi PV, ed: Strength and Power in Sport. Malden, MA: Blackwell Science; 2003.

Kraemer WJ, Hakkinen K, eds: Strength Training for Sport. Malden, MA: Blackwell Science; 2002.

Nieman DC: Exercise Testing and Prescription. Boston, MA: McGraw Hill; 2003.

Noakes T: Lore of Running. Champagne, IL: Human Kinetics; 2003.

Plowman SA, Smith DL: Exercise Physiology—for Health, Fitness, and Performance. San Francisco, CA: Benjamin Cummings; 2003.

Powers SK, Howley ET: Exercise Physiology—Theory and Application to Fitness and Performance. Boston, MA: McGraw Hill; 2004.

Saltin B, Boushel R, Secher N, Mitchell J, eds: Exercise and Circulation in Health and Disease. Champagne, IL: Human Kinetics; 2000.

Shephard RJ, Astrand PO, eds. Endurance in Sport. Malden, MA: Blackwell Science; 1992.

Whiting, WC, Zernicke, RF. Biomechanics of Musculoskeletal Injury Champaign, IL: Human Kinetics; 1998.

INTERNET RESOURCES

AACVPR: American Association of Cardiovascular and Pulmonary Rehabilitation:
http://www.aacvpr.org

American Academy of Pediatrics:
http://www.aap.org

American Cancer Society:
http://www.cancer.org

American College of Sports Medicine:
http://www.acsm.org

American Diabetes Association:
http://www.diabetes.org

American Heart Association:
http://www.americanheart.org

American Medical Association:
http://www.ama-assn.org

CHAA: Coalition for a Healthy & Active America:
http://www.chaausa.org

The Cooper Institute:
http://www.cooperinstitute.org

Gatorade Sports Science Institute:
http://www.gssiweb.com

Healthy People 2010:
http://www.healthypeople.gov

ISAPA: International Society for Aging and Physical Activity:
http://www.isapa.org

National Athletic Trainers' Association:
http://www.nata.org

NCPAD: The National Center on Physical Activity and Disability:
http://www.ncpad.org

National Heart, Lung, and Blood Institute:
http://www.nhlbi.nih.gov

National Heart, Lung, and Blood Institute: Clinical Guidelines on the Identification, Evaluation, and Treatment of Overweight and Obesity in Adults:
http://www.nhlbi.nih.gov/guidelines/obesity/ob_home.htm

National Institute on Aging:
http://www.nia.nih.gov

National Institutes of Health:
http://www.nih.gov

National Osteoporosis Foundation:
http://www.nof.org

NHLBI Healthy People 2010 Gateway:
http://hp2010.nhlbihin.net

NIOSH—The National Institute for Occupational Safety and Health:
http://www.cdc.gov/niosh
NSCA: National Strength & Conditioning Association:
http://www.nsca-lift.org

Nutrition Navigator:
http://www.navigator.tufts.edu

Sportscience:
http://www.sportsci.org

StrongWomen.com:
http://www.strongwomen.com

United States Department of Health & Human Services:
http://www.-os.dhhs.gov

The Weather Channel:
http://www.weather.com

Physiologic Effects of Aging and Deconditioning

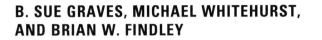

B. SUE GRAVES, MICHAEL WHITEHURST, AND BRIAN W. FINDLEY

This chapter addresses KSAs from the following content areas:

The Impact of Aging

As life span continues to increase, more and more consideration is being given to the changes in functional ability of the elderly and the contributions of the aging process versus inactivity to these changes[1]. Growth and development, maturation and degeneration are the inevitable processes involved in biological aging. Health care professionals often use intervention strategies that functionally categorize individuals based solely on chronological age. Table 4-1 lists these chronological stages of aging. However, caution is warranted because individual distinctions in activity level, aging, environment, and disease confound making generalizations with regard to health, fitness, and functional status. The purpose of this chapter is to identify the effects of aging and deconditioning on the systems most relevant to exercise testing and prescription (see GETP7 Chapter 10).

CARDIOVASCULAR SYSTEM

Heart

Although maximal cardiac output increases with growth in children, at any given level of submaximal work, cardiac output is somewhat lower in children than adults primarily because of lower stroke volume (SV)[2,3]. Lower sympathetic stimulation of the heart in children compared with adults has been suggested as a cause for the smaller SV[4]. However, during modest submaximal exercise, increases in SV do not seem to be related to aging. This phenomenon is a result of the Frank-Starling mechanism to compensate for a reduced number of pacemaker cells and impaired adrenergic chronotropic function[5,6]. In boys, SV is higher and heart rate (HR) lower than in girls at given absolute submaximal work rates[4].

Numerous physiological changes to the heart transpire with aging. It is imperative to differentiate between these normal biological changes and underlying pathologies that exist in cardiovascular disease. The aging heart shows decreases in intracellular transportation and pacemaker cells as well as sensitivity to beta-receptor, baroreceptor, and chemoreceptor stimulation. Furthermore, interstitial fibrosis within the myocardium and calcification of heart's connective tissue skeleton results in collagen crosslinking and elasticity loss. The heart is attenuated by an increase in arterial stiffness, systolic blood pressure (SBP), and left ventricular afterload and hypertrophy. Further changes in the left ventricle result in extended diastolic relaxation[7].

Maximal cardiac output in a 65-year-old person is 10% to 30% less than in a young adult. Decreases in both maximal HR and maximal SV contribute to decreased maximal cardiac output of older adults. By contrast, in the period immediately after high-intensity exercise, HR recovery, return of oxygen uptake to baseline, and muscular power recovery occur faster in children than in young adults and adults[8-10].

Several studies over the past 25 years have shown resting cardiac output and SV decrease with age[11-13]. Results

KEY TERMS

Anaerobic capacity: The ability to generate high peak blood lactate levels

Deconditioning: Partial or complete reversal of physiological adaptations to exercise caused by cessation of training

Detraining: Returning to a sedentary lifestyle after formalized exercise training

Muscle atrophy: Reduction in muscle size

Sarcopenia: The loss of muscle cross-sectional area and mass associated with the aging process

Specific tension: Force per unit muscle cross-sectional area

suggest cardiac output decreases about 1% per year, from a mean of 6.5 L per minute in the third decade to a mean of 3.9 L per minute in the ninth decade. From 25 to 85 years resting SV decreases 30%, from 85 mL to 60 mL[12]. However, in subjects who have been carefully screened for coronary artery disease, investigators have demonstrated overall left ventricular function, using resting ejection fraction as an index, does not decline between 25 and 80 years[13]. Estimates of volume made by echocardiography and radionuclide scintigraphy demonstrate resting SV also does not decline with age. Since resting HR is also not age related, these data suggest that resting cardiac output does not decline with age in healthy individuals.

Heart Rate

In children, HR is often high at rest (80 to 100 bpm), apparently as a result of reduced SV relative to body size[14]. This reduced SV generally vanishes with growth and increased levels of physical activity, thus it is not age specific. In combination with an increase in the oxygen carrying capacity of the blood secondary to hemoglobin increases that occur through the late teens, resting HR decreases to approximately 65–75 bpm by adulthood.

Resting HR is relatively unchanged throughout adulthood. However, maximal attainable HR declines

proportionally with age (predicted maximum HR = 220 − age)[15]. A decrease in myocardial sensitivity to catecholamines and the effect of prolonged diastolic filling appear to be responsible for this decline in maximal HR. In addition, as aging occurs through adulthood, a greater than normal increase in HR response occurs[15]. A decrease of 5 to 10 bpm per decade also appears during strenuous exercise independent of training level. However, increases in end-diastolic volume as a result of the training response can offset the decrease in exercise HR. As a result, recovery HR remains higher, and recovery takes longer after maximal exercise[11].

Maximal Oxygen Uptake

Aerobic capacity, assessed by maximal oxygen uptake ($\dot{V}O_{2max}$) appears to remain constant throughout childhood. However, some controversy exists concerning an apparent loss of $\dot{V}O_{2max}$ beginning at about age 12 years, perhaps related to decreased levels of physical activity[16]. During adulthood, a steady age-related decline in $\dot{V}O_{2max}$, averaging about 1% per year between 25 and 75 years (about 5 mL $O_2 \cdot kg^{-1} \cdot min^{-1}$ with each decade of aging) has been observed[17,18]. However, the degree to which this decline occurs is significantly affected by amount and intensity of physical activity. The decline in $\dot{V}O_{2max}$ parallels reduced maximum work capacity and is attributed to decreased maximal cardiac output and reduced arterial-venous oxygen difference (a-vDO_2) as well as a loss of skeletal muscle mass[19,20]. Microstructual changes, including myofilament disorganization and changes in mitochondrial structure and distribution resulting in reduced oxidative capacity, may explain the reduced maximal a-vDO_2[21]. Additionally, physical limitations resulting from sedentary lifestyles, loss of coordination, lack of familiarity of required skills, and disabling diseases such as arthritis and obesity may also play a role in limiting $\dot{V}O_{2max}$[22,23].

Blood Vessels

Vascular stiffness occurs with aging and is the result of worn elastin and changes in collagenous properties in the arterial walls. As a result, peripheral vascular resistance

TABLE 4-1. Stages of Aging

Neonatal	Birth to 3 weeks
Infancy	3 weeks to 1 year
Childhood	
Early	1–6 years
Middle	7–10 years
Later	**Prepubertal**
	Girls 9–15 years
	Boys 12–16 years
Adolescence	6 years after puberty
Adulthood	
Early	20–29 years
Middle	30–44 years
Later	45–64 years
Senescence	
Elderly	65–74 years
Older elderly	75–84 years
Very old	85 years and older

increases with age. Loss of plasticity of the aorta impedes pulsatile ejection, which delays the arteries in accepting SV. In turn, this results in an increase in SBP and mean arterial pressure[11, 24].

PULMONARY SYSTEM

Lung compliance increases with age, and the ability to expand the chest cavity becomes limited[25]. This is particularly evident by age 65 years. Starting in adulthood, a progressive decrease occurs in both maximal expiratory flow and lung volume reserve with aging. Residual volume increases by 30% to 35%, and vital capacity decreases by 40% to 50% by age 70 years[26], possibly because of a loss of elastic recoil of the lungs[15]. Furthermore, during exertion, increased ventilation is accomplished via greater frequency of breathing than depth of breathing in adulthood. The overall net effect is a 20% increase in the work of respiratory muscles[27]. Despite these changes, respiratory function does not limit exercise capacity or the ability to benefit from exercise training unless lung function is severely impaired. However, because of the increased work imposed on the respiratory muscles, elderly individuals may complain of breathing discomfort owing to the increased ventilatory demand caused by physical exertion, despite having normal cardiopulmonary function[28].

MUSCULOSKELETAL SYSTEM

Bone

Bone, or "osseous tissue," is continuously remodeling as a result of osteoblastic (formation) and osteoclastic (reabsorption) activity[11,15,29]. This dynamic, efficacious process of remodeling acts as a source of stored bone and calcium and is a result of the ever-changing mechanical stresses placed on the body as individuals pass through the various stages of life[11,15]. Genetics plays a major role in prepubescent bone maturation and is highly correlated to the loading factor imposed by the muscle mass in accordance with Wolff's law[30].

Bone growth during childhood presents two primary problems because the epiphysis is not united with the bone shaft. First, overuse can result in epiphysitis during this growth period. Second, fracture may pass through the epiphyseal plate, sometimes leading to abnormal growth[14]. Peak bone mass is posited to occur by the end of the second decade of life, although others claim that bone can continue to mature up to age 30 years[11,15]. Senescence generally occurs at the beginning of the sixth decade and is characterized by predominant osteoclastic activity, or "uncoupling"[11]. As a result, decreases in bone density manifested by decreases in calcium regulatory mechanisms, hormone levels, and metabolic activity occur[29]. Lifestyle factors such as physical activity level, calcium intake, and nutritional status play a major role as well, making it difficult to determine the intrinsic contribution of aging itself

on bone loss[29,31]. The rate of bone loss is site specific (e.g., the calcaneus shows significant bone loss earlier than other bones)[11]. Women tend to begin losing bone mass between 30 and 35 years of age at a rate of 0.75% to 1.0% per year[29]. Bone loss in men generally commences between 50 to 55 years of age at an initial rate of 0.4% per year[29]. In addition, women lose 36 g of bone mineral density (BMD) per decade compared with 30 g·decade in men[29]. These gender differences are attributable to the fact that women possess less initial bone calcium content and have reduced calcium intake during menopause[11,29]. By age 80 years, the trend has reversed somewhat. Men have shown a 55% decrease from their peak bone mineral content, and women only drop 40%[29]. This is at least partially responsible for the 1.5-cm height loss that occurs for every 30 years past the fifth decade of life[15]. This marked reduction of bone loss precipitates normal and pathological fractures causing increased morbidity and mortality[15]. Thus, clinical osteoporosis exposes a vulnerability to accommodate bone health and is a precursor to disability[31].

Muscle

The number and proportion of muscle fiber types are predetermined at birth and classified by pH sensitivity of myofibrillar ATPase[29,32]. Type I slow-twitch fibers are more resistant than type II fast-twitch fibers to atrophy until the seventh decade. Hence, the percentage of type I fibers increases because of the atrophy and degeneration of type II fibers. The selective loss of type II fibers, however, may be more a function of disuse given that activity patterns suggest less muscle contraction against resistance occurs from adulthood to senescence.

Muscle function is determined by muscle force per unit of cross-sectional area[33]. Twenty-five percent of muscle function as determined by force generating capacity is lost by the age of 65 years and up to 40% over a lifetime[34–36]. The loss of muscle mass and strength that accompanies the aging process has been termed **sarcopenia**. Declines in muscle fiber number and area, motor unit size and recruitment, innervation, capillarization, protein synthesis, and growth factor alterations are to some degree responsible for sarcopenia[37,38]. Whereas the decline in muscle strength in men and women is primarily the result of muscle mass losses, neural factors are responsible for additional functional decrements[33]. The etiology of sarcopenia is characterized by dual myopathic and neuropathic changes that result in functional limitations in gait and activities of daily living[39–41]. Additionally, sarcopenia impairs thermoregulation, metabolism, and glucose sensitivity[38]. There exists some agreement, however, that sarcopenia is primarily a result of diminishing stimulus secondary to sedentary lifestyles[15]. Furthermore, changes in the architecture of muscle (pennation angle, muscle thickness, fascicle length) may be additional factors worthy of consideration in muscle function[42].

Anaerobic capacity, which is described as the ability to generate high peak blood lactate levels, also develops through young adolescence. Ironically, anaerobic capacity in children has not been well documented, although their activity patterns are exemplified by short-term anaerobic activities[43]. Anaerobic power is lower in children than adults in both absolute power and when corrected for body mass as a consequence of differences in adenosine triphosphate (ATP), creatine phosphate (CP), glycolytic capacity, acidosis, and other factors[44]. Motivation and neuromuscular coordination factor into diminished anaerobic capacity in children. Both genders maintain a plateau in anaerobic capacity through about age 35 years, at which time it begins to decline. By age 65 years, anaerobic capacity declines to essentially the level of late childhood, even when subjects are highly motivated for testing. The aged anaerobic system does not work as quickly to produce energy, and when lactic acid is produced, it is not cleared as quickly. The probable reasons for the decline in the anaerobic system is the loss of large muscle mass and the decrease in the size and number of glycolytic fast-twitch fibers, which are known to rely more on glycolysis. Intramuscular blood flow is also lower in older people, which contributes to a slower recovery and lactate removal. Even in power-trained or endurance-trained master's athletes, anaerobic power declines 50% by age 75 years[11].

Body Composition

Approximately one third of the population of the United States is obese, escalating the risk of chronic disease[45,46]. Body fat percentages are independent of gender in prepubescent children but are highly influenced by genetics as well as environmental factors. Acceptable body fat percentages for prepubescent children are between 10% and 15%[47]. Gender differences begin to show during puberty and extend through adulthood with acceptable limits of 20% in men and 30% in women. Distribution of body fat is gender specific from the third to seventh decade. Whereas women tend to exhibit greater increases in internal body fat after age 45 years, men accumulate greater subcutaneous fat. Basal metabolic rate decreases approximately 5% per decade throughout adulthood and is a contributing factor along with genetics in fat gain. However, an accumulating body of knowledge points to lifestyle changes that includes increased physical inactivity as the underlying culprit. In elderly subjects, increased levels of fat mass contribute to slower gait speed and functional limitations[48].

Joints and Flexibility

A progressive loss of flexibility, resulting from a number of factors, including disease, deterioration of joint structures, and progressive degeneration of collagen fibers, begins during young adulthood. Increased incidence of knee and back problems from osteoarthritis has been observed beginning with middle age and progressing through old age[14]. Degeneration of joints, especially the spine, is often found in elderly persons. Excessive weight-bearing activity may accelerate this onset. Along with loss of strength, loss of flexibility plays a significant role in increase risk of falls and other injuries. The rate of deterioration accelerates beyond age 65 years, but few specific findings are available for this age group.

NERVOUS SYSTEM

Infants and very young children undergo intensive learning to develop motor skills for function and performance. The central nervous system (CNS) is recognized as the predominant center for determining the outcomes of this learning. The learning process includes the integration of movement patterns that minimize physiological cost, asymmetry, and variability of body segment coordination[49]. The improvement in economy of movement may actually decrease oxygen consumption at given velocities and improve reaction times, which can decrease 15% by age 70 years[50].

Detrimental changes in neurotransmitters, nerve conduction velocities, and fine motor control are all indicative of normal CNS aging[51]. The increased incidence of sensory deficits, particularly hearing and vision, and higher thresholds of perception for many stimuli may be related to the 35% to 40% increase in falls by persons older than age 60 years[52,53].

IMMUNE SYSTEM

Aging and environmental factors (e.g., pollutants, electromagnetism, environmental tobacco smoke) are responsible to varying degrees for decreased immune system function[14]. From peak immune system activity around puberty, an overall decline of 5% to 30% over a normal life span is expected, with some functional indices decreasing to 5% to 10% of early adulthood function. The major reason for the immune system loss is a fall off of suppressor T-cell function, which leads to an inability to fight pathogens[15]. The end result is reduced resistance to pathogens and increased incidence of both tumors and autoimmune disorders.

RENAL FUNCTION, FLUID REGULATION, AND THERMOREGULATION

Renal function declines approximately 30% to 50% between ages 30 and 70 years[14]. Along with this decline, acid-based control, glucose tolerance, and drug clearance decrease. A general reduction in total cellular water occurs with aging, with a decline of 10% to 50% in total body water compared with cellular water levels in early adults.

The primary maturational characteristics related to exercise in heat occur in late puberty or early adulthood.

Before that time, children have a consistently lower sweat rate characterized by lower absolute and relative sweat volumes along with a higher core temperature required to start sweating. Thus, children tend to rely more on radiation and convection for heat dissipation than adults. The composition of children's sweat also differs, particularly in regard to chloride[54,55]. Aging is also associated with attenuated skin blood flow, which may contribute to a reduced ability to thermoregulate. Furthermore, the effects of aging predispose older individuals to rapidly dehydrate. This may become particularly important during exercise through evaporative water loss and perspiration[56]. In addition, many older adults take a variety of medications that may further confound hydration levels, placing further limitations on thermoregulation.

Children have a greater ratio of surface area to mass than adults, which enhances convective and radiant heat transfer between skin and the environment, making tolerance to cold more difficult[57]. However, it has been suggested that other factors that occur with aging, such as thermogenic and vasoconstrictive responses, may also limit thermoregulation to cold in children. Beyond childhood, it has been demonstrated that the ability to regulate core temperature is affected by aging[55,58,59].

SUMMARY

Growth, development, maturation, and degeneration have profound effects on the body's capability to respond to the external stresses placed on it through exercise. Lifestyle factors associated with aging make it difficult to distinguish between degeneration attributable to normal physiological aging and alterations in habitual physical activity. Gerontological investigations reveal that reduction of activity is predictive of life span and attributable at least partly to altered neurotransmission in dopamine activity[60]. Table 4-2 highlights selected age-related changes and the possible effect of exercise compliance on those changes. The interrelationships between biological aging and physical activity warrant further investigation.

Impact of Deconditioning

A significant reduction or cessation of exercise results in **deconditioning**, a partial or complete reversal of physiological adaptations to exercise[61]. Almost everyone is affected by reductions in physical activity. One must understand musculoskeletal adaptations to reduced physical activity so that changes in functional ability can be predicted and appropriate exercise can be prescribed after disuse or in the rehabilitation process not only of elite or weekend athletes but also of diseased and disabled populations. Deconditioning can result from detraining, bed rest, casting, use of crutches, paralysis, aging, or even exposure to microgravity during space flight (Table 4-3). Following is a brief description of each of the modes of deconditioning that have yielded information regarding the effects of inactivity on the musculoskeletal system.

MODES OF DECONDITIONING

Decreased muscle activity is defined as a reduction in intensity or in amount of regularly performed daily activity by a muscle or muscle group. Detraining (returning to a sedentary lifestyle after formalized exercise training) does not suggest the same adaptive response as a sedentary individual would have with 1 month of bed rest. For example, bed rest for 1 month, which constitutes a dramatic change in the daily amount of muscle activity, even for a previously sedentary individual, causes greater skeletal muscle atrophy than for an individual who ceases resistance training for the same period but continues

TABLE 4-2. System Changes

	Neonatal	Infancy	Childhood	Adolescence	Adulthood	Senescence
Cardiovascular System						
Cardiac output			↑	↑	↔	↔
Stroke volume			↑	↑	↔	↓
HR_{max}			↑	↔	↓	↓
$\dot{V}O_{2max}$		↑		↑	↓	↓
Pulmonary System						
Vital capacity		↑	↑	↑	↓	↓
Musculoskeletal System						
Bone mineral density		↑	↑	↑	↔	↓
Muscle mass		↑	↑	↑	↑	↓
Anaerobic capacity			↑	↑	↑	↓
Flexibility			↑	↑	↓	↓
% Body fat			↑	↑	↑	↔
Nervous System						
Motor control		↑	↑	↑	↔	↓
Immune System						
Immune system function			↑	↑	↔	↓

↑ = increases; ↔ = no change; ↓ = decreases.

TABLE 4-3. Types of Deconditioning

Type	Noted Changes	References
Detraining	Muscle atrophy	78
	Decrease in muscle size	73
	Decrease in fiber numbers	139
	Capillaries undamaged	134
	Fiber type reverts to composition before training	66
Bedrest	Muscle atrophy (greater than in exercising individuals)	66
	Considerable atrophy of fast- and slow-twitch fibers	62
	No change in myonuclear number per mm of fiber length	138
Casting	Decrease in strength attributed to neural factors if short-term	141
	Severe atrophy if muscles in shortened position	136,142
	Neuromuscular transmission defects	143
Crutches	Reduction of strength by 20% in non–weight-bearing limb	137
	No changes in contralateral weight-bearing muscle	77,137
Paralysis	Reduced mitochondrial content	76,77
	Poor fatigue resistance	75,76
	Fast-twitch fibers greater atrophy after 6 months	77
	Proportion of type II B increases, and type II A decreases	77
	Actomysin ATPase activity not elevated	76
	Exercise activities generally limited to motor units above SCI	144
	Activities of daily living improved by strength and conditioning	145
	Atrophy of 50% or more after 6 months of injury	77,79
Space Flight	Muscle atrophy	146
	Muscle strength decreases	130,147
	Greater loss in fast-twitch than slow-twitch fibers	146
	Bone loss[7] to 12%	148
	Reduced $\dot{V}O_{2max}$	149
	Decreased work capacity and fatigued earlier	146
	Exercise counteracts harmful effects	146

daily physical activity[62,63]. Thus, the magnitude of the adaptive response to decreased activity depends on relative change in an individual's muscle use, which may be caused by injury, illness, or cessation of exercise program. **Muscle atrophy** (reduction in muscle size) from disuse in this case is a normal response, not a maladaptation. Table 4-3 indicates noted changes in the various modes used to study deconditioning.

Detraining

Detraining is defined as the process that occurs after the cessation of training in which adaptations to exercise are gradually reduced or lost[64–66]. Detraining in athletes often occurs during the off-season or because of an injury when normal training routines are interrupted. Detraining is most often observed in previously sedentary individuals who exercise for several weeks or months and then discontinue the practice.

Bed Rest

In the clinical setting, periods of bed rest are usually associated with some underlying disease, so differentiating musculoskeletal changes caused by inactivity versus disease process is often difficult. However, bed resting healthy individuals has been used as an experimental model of muscle unloading to rule out disease complica-

tions and has yielded results similar to casting or the use of crutches[62,67–71].

Casting

A cast typically places a joint in a fixed position with the objective of immobilizing injured tissue or bone. When a cast is used, it not only decreases muscle activity but also fixes the joint position such that the muscles are held at a relatively constant length. As a result, casting has been shown to cause skeletal muscle adaptations.

Crutches

The use of crutches may or may not be associated with casting. Although a lower limb in a cast often requires crutches, minor injuries (sprains and strains) may not require casting but may require non–weight bearing. Human lower limb suspension via the use of crutches has also been used as an experimental technique to study adaptations to unloading[72,73].

Paralysis

Many diseases and spinal cord injuries (SCIs) can lead to partial or total paralysis. Automobile accidents, sports (football, diving, and gymnastics), and gunshot wounds have been reported as the most common causes of

SCIs[74]. Although it is often difficult to distinguish how a disease process interacts with muscle disuse to produce functional changes, SCIs are unique in that affected muscles may still be innervated yet receive no input from higher nervous centers. Thus, muscles are innervated by intact motor neurons but are seldom activated except during spasm[75–81].

Space Flight

On a limited basis, researchers have been able to scientifically study the body's response to muscle unloading in the unique microgravity environment of outer space. However, with minimum flights and small numbers of crew members who repeat space missions, reproducibility of results has been difficult[82]. Therefore, simulations of microgravity have been used and involve water immersion and head-down tilt protocols[83].

EFFECTS ON BONE

Exercise that promotes skeletal loading induces a compensatory adaptation in the structure and functional integrity of bone (see Chapter 35). The processes underlying the adaptive mechanisms of bone to loading represent a complex interaction of endocrine and musculoskeletal systems. Exercise serves as a stimulus for skeletal adaptation that includes the maintenance or addition of bone mass. Conversely, inactivity as in bed rest because of injury or partly caused by inactivity associated with aging reduces bone mass by adversely affecting calcium metabolism and the bone formation process.

Bone formation may be described as a dynamic lifelong process. As such, bone health has been studied in young and old subjects under conditions of short-term immobilization, prolonged bed rest, exposure to microgravity associated with space flight, and clinical conditions such as paralysis. Although results from studies are similar, comparisons across subject populations regarding bone loss and genesis are made difficult by underlying pathologies.

Depending upon the length of enforced inactivity as well as underlying pathologies, recovery of lost bone or osteogenesis may be protracted. Health care practitioners need to know that extended periods of deconditioning and disuse not only result in bone loss but also compromise future bone health by increasing the patient's susceptibility to fracture and promoting early-onset osteoporosis.

The discussion that follows includes information from studies aimed at revealing the effects of inactivity, bed rest, and immobilization on bone mass and calcium metabolism in adult humans. Evidence of changes in bone mass and structural integrity has been inferred from radiologic measurements. Assays of endocrine regulators indicative of calcium absorption from the gut and deposition of calcium in bone are used in conjunction with urinary and fecal excretion of calcium to reveal the role of calcium metabolism in bone health. Several review articles offer additional detail[84–87].

Bone Mineral Density (BMD)

Whereas removal of the exercise stimulus has been shown to reverse gains in lumbar spine BMD in postmenopausal women[88,89], reducing the level of activity in habitually active middle-aged persons was associated with significant losses of bone mineral content in trabecular bone[90]. Similarly, elderly patients who must drastically reduce their level of activity because of hip fractures show significant decreases in BMD in the unaffected hip up to 13 months after the fracture[91]. Alfredson et al.[92] reported that male athletes who underwent Achilles tendon surgery showed significant calcaneal bone loss on the surgically repaired side compared with the non-injured side at 52 weeks after surgery with no signs of bone recovery 1 year after surgery.

Transcient bone mass changes, as a consequence of seasonal loads versus no load associated with the off season, have been reported in female collegiate gymnasts[93]. A recent investigation revealed greater BMD in premenarcheal gymnasts compared with inactive control subjects[94], owing to speculation that the active subjects' more robust skeletal architecture provides protection later in life. Contrary to the notion that above average BMD early in life protects individuals in the later years, Magnusson et al.[91] reported that young adult soccer players with above average BMD experienced a gradual decline in bone mass over the years with follow-up observations at age 70 years revealing no significant differences in bone mass between the former soccer players and control subjects.

In the absence of mechanical stress produced by weight-bearing activity, bed rest negatively affects the homeostatic mechanisms that underlie bone health. Without weight-bearing activity calcium balance is disturbed and, ultimately, bone mass is lost.

Calcium Balance

To preserve bone mass, there must be a balance between resorption of existing bone and the formation of new bone. Prolonged inactivity, such as bed rest, is known to upset this balance, resulting in excessive resorption of calcium from bone, as manifested in elevated levels of serum calcium or hypercalcemia and a concurrent increase in urinary and fecal calcium[95]. During periods of increased resorption, serum, urinary, and fecal levels of calcium fluctuate in response to hormonal regulation and decreased absorption of calcium from the intestines. Within weeks of inactivity, negative calcium balance has been observed in healthy persons subjected to bed rest[95], persons experiencing weightlessness[96], and individuals with SCIs[97].

Hormonal regulation of calcium metabolism, although

altered during periods of bed rest, plays a less prominent role in the maintenance of bone mass than the influences of mechanical load. That is, reduction in mechanical load or stress appears to trigger an ordered response of bone resorption and endocrine activity, including the regulation of calcium absorption from the gut by 1,25 dihydroxyvitamin D (1,25-D). Whereas the other prominent calcium regulator, parathyroid hormone (PTH), is unchanged or decreases slightly during periods of negative calcium balance in healthy subjects experiencing bed rest; 1,25-D decreased or does not change[95,98–100]. Conversely, during the acute phase, individuals with SCIs who are immobilized show low PTH and 1,25-D levels[97].

Bone Mass

Site-specific losses in BMD of 1% to 2% per month have been reported based on animal models, microgravity experienced by astronauts, and as a result of bed rest[101–104]. The rate and, ultimately, the amount of bone loss may be tied to health status. Based on ultrasound calcaneal measures, healthy men lost approximately 0.017% to 0.11% of bone mass per week during a 120-day bed rest study. Persons with SCIs, however, lose as much as 33% of calcaneus bone volume within 6 months of the injury[97].

Susceptibility to bone loss increases as a function of the proximity to mechanical load and type of bone. LeBlanc et al.[103] observed a 10% loss in BMD in the calcaneus compared with 4% at the femoral neck and spine; however, no significant reduction in bone mass occurred in the radius of the forearm after 17 weeks of bed rest. During periods of unloading, trabecular bone, lying inside cortical bone, with its high surface-to-volume area, is targeted by bone-absorbing osteoclasts. Under conditions of disuse, trabecular bone loss is greatest at load-bearing sites (e.g., proximal tibia) and occurs more rapidly than cortical bone loss[103,105].

Biochemical markers of bone turnover are used extensively in bed rest studies to assess the metabolic activity of bone. A recent study of healthy male subjects subjected to 120 days of bed rest showed increased bone resorption by day 7 and a decrease in bone formation by day 50[106]. Other investigators have also reported excessive bone resorption in healthy subjects during disuse[100,107], as well as in paraplegic subjects[108]. However, Palle et al.[109] reported only transient changes in bone resorption early in the course of bed rest, with values returning to baseline by the fourth and final month of the study. It appears that the bone loss may be explained as a disproportionate increase in osteoclast cell activity[110]. Moreover, osteoclast activity is noticeably localized in the lower body (e.g., calcaneus, tibia), ultimately compromising the structural components (e.g., matrix, collagen) of bone and increasing the risk of fracture.

An uncoupling of the bone resorption and formation process is evidenced by the fact that biochemical markers of bone formation do not increase during unloading. Investigators have reported that biochemical markers of bone resorption remain elevated for weeks upon resumption of activity[99,111,112]. Thus, individuals with a history of bone loss who subsequently undergo forced unloading are particularly vulnerable to injury caused by fracture as they regain their mobility.

Remobilization: Can Lost Bone Be Regained?

The timeline for regaining bone lost caused by disuse has been studied in animals and humans. Jaworski and Uhthoff[113] evaluated the osteogenic activity of old and young dogs after immobilization of the forelimbs for 32 weeks. At 28 weeks into remobilization, there was a 40% and 70% recovery of bone mass in old and young dogs, respectively. Significant deficits in bone mass were still apparent in horses who remobilized for 8 weeks after 7 weeks of disuse[114]. In contrast, the restoration of bone architecture in young rats after 3 weeks of hind limb immobilization was nearly complete after several weeks of exercise[115]. Similarly, Kaneps et al.[116] found the cancellous and cortical mechanical properties of immobilized forelimbs in dogs to be significantly less than controls at 16 weeks. However, at 32 weeks, including 16 weeks of treadmill running, no significant difference between immobilized and control limbs was observed.

Although limited, recovery of bone mass and the associated architectural integrity in humans is protracted with evidence that deficits can persist indefinitely. Bone mineral deficits induced by multiple space flights could still be observed in astronauts 5 years later[117]. Similarly, lumbar and femoral neck bone mass lost during 17 weeks of bed rest was not regained in healthy subjects after 6 months of normal remobilization[103]. Lower extremity bone density (calcaneus and proximal tibia), however, was regained in this study sample. Although tibial bone mass may take 1 to 1.5 years to recover after periods of non–weight bearing associated with hip surgery[103], permanent losses in BMD were reported in the lower limbs and spines of men who suffered tibial fractures 9 years earlier[118].

Implications and Considerations

After immobilization, the bone restoration process may be particularly difficult in certain populations (elderly, those with SCIs). Depending on baseline levels and the amount of bone loss, elderly individuals may be at greater risk of fracture after immobilization. Similarly, men older than age 60 years and postmenopausal women may be predisposed to accelerated bone loss, a condition that may exacerbate bone loss during immobilization. As such, an intervention strategy might be used that includes brief periods of assisted mobility during forced inactivity followed by remobilization at the earliest possible time.

Considering that bone mass restoration is outpaced by muscle strength, practitioners must be careful not to induce fracture by overly aggressive exercise programs. Clearly, the individual may possess normal strength while at the same time having bone that is close to the fracture threshold. A conservative approach, including range of motion exercises, a gradual overload of balance and stability challenges, site-specific muscle strengthening (Box 4-1), as supported by clinical evaluations and bone scans, is recommended.

Summary

Exercise that promotes skeletal loading stimulates compensatory adaptations, resulting in structural changes and healthier bones. Inactivity, regardless of the reason, is detrimental to maintaining bone health. It is difficult to distinguish between effects of normal physiological aging and alterations in exercise and physical activity patterns. Transient bone mass changes have been observed in athletes, persons with mobility issues, and individuals experiencing unloading for brief periods. Bone loss is greatest at distal points of loading and areas associated with postural integrity and mobility (e.g., vertebra, hip). Accelerated bone loss is associated with age, menopause, space flight, SCI, and extended periods of unloading. Although hormonal regulation of calcium balance is altered during periods of inactivity, the most salient feature of bone health is the influence of mechanical loading. Recovery of lost bone is at best protracted with evidence that deficits can persist indefinitely. Depending on baseline levels and amount of bone loss, practitioners must be careful not to rush rehabilitation because the risk of fracture is likely to increase after immobilization.

BOX 4-1	Guidelines for Exercise Professionals Working with Severely Detrained or Bed-Rested Individuals*

- Emphasize strength training of back and lower limb postural muscle groups:
  - Back extensors
  - Quadriceps
  - Hip extensors
  - Ankle plantar flexors (soleus and gastrocnemius)
- Start with low-intensity training
  - To accommodate potential neuromuscular deficits
  - To minimize potential for muscle damage
- Use gradual, progressive overload
- Be aware of increased risk of bone fracture
  - Particularly in estrogen-deficient women and the elderly
  - Even after muscle strength has returned to normal
- Incorporate training for postural stability and dynamic balance

*Refer to Chapter 23 for cardiovascular exercise guidelines.

EFFECTS ON SKELETAL MUSCLE

Morphological Consequences

Regardless of the method of unloading (see Table 4-3), the predominant adaptive response to decreased use is skeletal muscle atrophy[77,78]. Atrophy is the process whereby muscle size is reduced, almost exclusively because of reductions in the contractile proteins actin and myosin[119].

For the first several weeks of disuse, atrophy is almost linearly related to duration and extent of unloading and differs among muscles depending on function. Generally, atrophy is most severe in the muscles involved in weight bearing and postural control; extensor muscles are typically more severely affected than flexor muscles[69,73,77]. Likewise, it has recently been shown that the atrophic response of thigh adductor muscles to unloading is intermediate to that of extensor and flexor muscles[70,73]. Of particular concern are muscles of the thigh and calf. These are critical in normal walking and show marked atrophy in non–weight-bearing conditions[77].

In lower mammals, fiber type composition may influence the atrophic response to unloading; however, this has not been demonstrated in humans[79]. Human skeletal muscle generally does not present the clear segmentation of fiber type found in lower mammals[120].

Fast subtypes, unlike fast versus slow fibers, appear to show transformation with several months of unloading or after detraining[63,66,77]. Type IIB fibers in human muscle appear to serve as the default expression of the fast myosin gene. These transformations would not be expected to markedly alter energy demand of contraction, unlike slow to fast fiber movement, because actomyosin adenosine triphosphatase (ATPase) activity is more different between slow and fast fibers than between fast subtypes[121].

Metabolic Consequences

The influence of unloading on metabolic characteristics of human skeletal muscle has received less attention than atrophy and reduced strength. Whereas homogenates of muscle biopsies show decreased concentrations of enzyme markers of aerobic oxidative capacity after unloading, anaerobic enzymes of energy supply do not seem to change[62,122]. Reduced enzymes associated with aerobic capacity may reflect preferential loss of contractile protein with unloading; that is, aerobic oxidative enzyme content per fiber volume may not change, and the anaerobic enzyme content may actually increase[81,119]. Nonetheless, fiber atrophy results in lower total mitochondrial content, so unloading compromises absolute muscular endurance[122,123]. This also suggests that relative muscular endurance is not significantly affected by unloading[122]. However, preferential loss of contractile protein requires the remaining muscle to work against greater absolute load. This work is accomplished with reduced total capacity for aerobic–oxidative energy supply because mitochondrial content is lower.

Strength and Local Muscular Endurance

Unloading reduces muscular strength, regardless of the type of action or movement performed or the method of strength expression[63,67–70,122,124–126]. Strength reduction is nearly linearly related to the duration of unloading and extent of muscle atrophy for the first few weeks. Atrophy accounts for a large part but not all of decreased force production, suggesting the ability to activate muscle is also compromised by unloading (discussed later). This is interesting because marked force reduction during eccentric, isometric, and slow-speed concentric muscle contraction is believed to be controlled by some neural inhibitory mechanisms[127,128]. However, the relative decline in strength is comparable across speeds and types of muscle actions, so increased inhibition is not responsible for reduced voluntary activation, or if it is, the reduction is uniform across speeds and types of muscle actions[67,125,126,129].

The lack of shape change in the force–velocity relationship (see Chapter 3) with short-term unloading may suggest muscle fiber type composition is not altered. However, as transformation to a faster muscle occurs with long-term extreme unloading, an increased ability to maintain force as speed increases during concentric actions should be evident[127]. This finding has been reported after long-term space flight[130]. However, 120 days of unloading of otherwise healthy individuals did not alter relative rise time during surface electrical stimulation of the triceps surae muscle group, suggesting that myofibrillar actomyosin ATPase activity is not altered by 3 months of disuse[131]. Likewise, time to peak tension for a twitch of tibialis anterior muscle has been reported comparable between SCI patients and healthy control subjects, suggesting that long-term unloading does not markedly alter calcium kinetics[75]. Comparable twitch mechanics in SCI patients and healthy controls may be interpreted to imply that fiber type composition of muscle and, thereby, myofibrillar actomyosin ATPase activity is not altered by SCI[76,81,121]. Thus, a muscle appears faster in chronic SCI patients than control subjects yet is comparable to those of healthy individuals for myofibrillar actomyosin ATPase activity and mechanical function.

The magnitude of strength reduction is also specific to muscle group, with weight-bearing muscles most affected. For knee extensors, the decline in strength averages about 0.6% per day. In contrast, the first dorsal interosseus hand muscle is relatively resistant to adaptation after 3 to 5 weeks of immobilization[132].

Muscular endurance associated with disuse has not been widely studied. One recent report suggests that after 4 weeks of casting of the elbow flexors, endurance time was increased in female but not male subjects. Furthermore, the electromyography (EMG) activity during the endurance test was altered in the female subjects. The EMG was associated with intermittent motor unit activity instead of the continuous activity typically observed. This suggests that motor unit activation patterns are altered after disuse, at least in women[133]. The ability to maintain force over repeat contractions is not altered within 6 months of SCI but is markedly compromised in chronic SCI patients[75,77,78].

Neuromuscular Consequences

Decreased strength with reduced use has consistently been shown to be greater than that explained by muscle atrophy[134]. An exception to this concept has been reported after short-term space flight. Muscle strength decreases in proportionately similar amounts, or perhaps less than fiber size, after 5 or 11 days of unloading (about 15% versus 20%)[69,130]. This implies increased ability to recruit muscle or greater **specific tension** (force per unit muscle size. Neither has been reported in studies of unloading at normal gravity[70,71,135]. Thus, neuromuscular impairment may occur after unloading.

Electromyographic studies demonstrate that maximal firing rate and maximal integrated EMG activity are decreased and periods of silent EMG activity appear during maximal voluntary contractions after unloading[135]. The ability to recruit high-threshold motor units also seems to be compromised[136]. The greater relative decline in strength than in size suggests that more muscle may be used to perform a given submaximal task. This has recently been reported using magnetic resonance imaging (MRI), supporting EMG analyses in which greater numbers of motor units are required to develop submaximal force[70,129,134,137].

The exercise professional should account for these neuromuscular adaptations to unloading in exercise prescriptions for subjects recovering from reduced muscular activity. Submaximal loads that were once easily borne require more absolute muscle involvement. In addition, individuals may not have visible muscle atrophy but may be particularly weak because of irregularities in motor control.

Vulnerability of Muscle Damage

Unloading lower limb skeletal muscle for 5 weeks has demonstrated increased vulnerability to eccentric exercise-induced dysfunction and muscle injury[137]. MRI obtained 3 days after eccentric exercise demonstrated muscle damage over the unloaded cross-sectional area, but none was evident in the contralateral weight-bearing limb.

These results have practical importance to the exercise professional. Dysfunction and injury during reloading may be sufficient to prolong recovery. In the previous study, 10 days after the eccentric exercise, strength remained reduced by 20% (before unloading). Low-intensity exercise should be used with care initially during renewal of walking to minimize muscle dysfunction and injury.

Increased vulnerability to exercise-induced muscle injury has also been reported in elderly individuals[119]. Whether this is caused by aging, low physical activity, or both is not known, but when starting an exercise program for an elderly person, it is important to be cautious.

Possible Counter Measures

Few data exist regarding the efficacy of various countermeasures designed to prevent muscle atrophy and dysfunction or to enhance recovery during disuse. Endurance activity enhances fatigue resistance of skeletal muscle during unloading. Electrical stimulation of tibialis anterior muscle for 45 minutes to 2 hours/day in complete SCI patients evoked a marked increase in ability to maintain force during contraction. This response is partly attributed to increased muscle fiber aerobic–oxidative enzyme content[75,76]. Resistance-like exercise (high-force intermittent stimulation) in patients with SCIs or ladder climbing in hindlimb-suspended rats has been shown to increase muscle size[80], the former to near pre-injury levels. One recent report using only four subjects suggests that wearing a Penguin antigravity suit for 10 hours a day and performing resistance exercise for 15 minutes each hour can prevent muscle atrophy associated with bed rest[138]. However, this strategy is probably not practical for use in the bulk of the population.

Although it is not clear to what extent disuse is responsible for neuromuscular dysfunction in elderly patients, resistance exercise training can certainly be used by individuals to increase strength and muscle mass[139]. This may enhance performance of activities of daily living, decrease severity and occurrence of fall-related injuries, and delay onset of disease.

Retraining

Short-term retraining after detraining appears to return muscle strength and size to those of the previously trained state[66]. However, less deconditioning appears to exist than expected in previously trained individuals during detraining in the previously mentioned study and more rapid adaptation after resuming training than expected. In a 30-year follow-up of the Dallas bed rest study, a 6-month endurance training program reversed the age-related decline in aerobic power that was attributed to peripheral adaptation. However, no subject reached the same $\dot{V}O_{2max}$ as in the initial test[140].

Summary

Muscles atrophy regardless of the method of unloading (decreased training, bed rest, space flight), resulting in decreased strength and possible dysfunction and muscle injury. Therefore, individuals need to continue with activities that increase strength and are weight bearing.

REFERENCES

1. Freedman VA, Martin LG: Contribution of chronic conditions to aggregate changes in old-age functioning. Am J Pub Health 90: 1755–1760, 2000.
2. Falk B, Bar-Or O, McDougall JD: Aldosterone and prolactin response to exercise in the heat in circumpubertal boys. J Appl Physiol 71:1741–1745, 1991.
3. Rowland T, Popowski B, Ferrone L: Cardiac responses to maximal upright exercise in healthy boys and men. Med Sci Sports Exerc 29:1146–1151, 1997.
4. Turley KR, Wilmore JH: Cardiovascular responses to submaximal exercise in 7–9 year-old boys and girls. Med Sci Sports Exerc 29: 824–832, 1997.
5. Lakatta EG: Cardiovascular regulatory mechanisms in advanced age. Physiol Rev 73:413–467, 1993.
6. Tate CA, Hyek MF, Taffett GE: Mechanisms for the responses of cardiac muscle to physical activity. Med Sci Sports Exerc 26:561–567, 1994.
7. Cheitlin MD: Cardiovascular physiology—Changes with aging. Am J Geriatri Carsiol 12:9–13, 2003.
8. Heberstreet H, Mimura KI, Bar-Or O: Recovery of muscle power after high intensity short-term exercise: Comparing boys and men. J Appl Physiol 74:2875–2880, 1993.
9. Baraldi E, Cooper DM, Zanconato S, et al: Heart rate recovery from 1 minute of exercise in children and adults. Pediatr Res 29:575–578, 1991.
10. Zancanato S, Cooper DM, Armon Y: Oxygen cost and oxygen uptake dynamics and recovery with 1 minute of exercise in children and adults. J Appl Physiol 71:993–998, 1991.
11. Spirduso WW: Physical Dimensions of Aging. Champaign, IL: Human Kinetics; 1995.
12. Schulman SP, Lakatta EG, Fleg JL, et al: Age related decline in left ventricular filling at rest and exercise. Am J Physiol 263:H1932–H1938, 1992.
13. Rodeheffer RJ, Gerstenblith G, Becker LC et al: Exercise cardiac output is maintained with advancing age in healthy human subjects: Cardiac dilation and increased stroke volume compensate for a diminished heart rate. Circulation 69:203–213, 1984.
14. Shephard RJ: Physiologic changes over the years. In ACSM's Resource Manual for Guidelines for Exercise Testing and Prescription, 2nd ed. Philadelphia: Lea & Febiger; 1993.
15. Christiansen JL, Grzybowski JM: Biology of Aging. New York: McGraw-Hill; 1999.
16. Shephard RJ: Maximal oxygen intake. In Shephard RJ, Astrand PO, eds. Sports and Human Endurance. Oxford: Blackwell Scientific; 1992.
17. Jackson AS, Wier LT, Ayers GW, et al: Changes in aerobic power of women ages 20, 64 yr. Med Sci Sports Exerc 28:844–891, 1996.
18. Shvartz E, Reibold RC: Aerobic fitness norms for males and females aged 6, 75 years: A review. Aviat Space Environ Med 61:3–11, 1990.
19. Granath A, Johnson B, Strandell T: Circulation in healthy old men studied by right heart catheterization at rest and during exercise in a supine and sitting position. Acta Med Scand 176:425–446, 1964.
20. Julius S, Amery A, Whitlock LS, et al: Influence of age on a hemodynamic response to exercise. Circulation 36:222–230, 1967.
21. Shock NW: Physiological aspects of aging in man. Ann Rev Physiol 23:97–122, 1961.
22. Fitzgerald PL: Exercise for the elderly. Med Clin North Am 69: 189–196, 1995.
23. Ike RW, Lampman RM, Castor CW: Arthritis and aerobic exercise. Phys Sportsmed 17:128–139, 1989.
24. Schneider EL, Rowe JW: Biology of Aging. San Diego, CA: Academic Press; 1990.
25. Babb TG: Mechanical ventilatory constraints in aging, lung disease, and obesity: Perspectives and a brief review. Med Sci Sports Exerc 31:S12–S22, 1999.

26. Smith EL, Serfass RC: Exercise and Aging: The Scientific Basis. Hillside, NJ: Enslow; 1981.

27. DeVries HA, Adams GM: Comparison of exercise responses in old and young men. J Gerontol 27:344–348, 1972.

28. Babb TG: Ventilatory response to exercise in subjects breathing CO_2 or HcO_2. J Appl Physiol 82:746–754, 1997.

29. Shephard RJ: Aging, Physical Activity and Health. Champaign, IL: Human Kinetics; 1997.

30. Wang J, Horlick M, Thornton JC: Correlations between skeletal muscle mass and bone mass in children 6–18 years: Influences of sex, ethnicity, and pubertal status. Growth Dev Aging 63:99–109, 1999.

31. O'Flaherty EJ: Modeling normal aging bone loss, with consideration of bone loss in osteoporosis. Toxicological Science 55:171–188, 2000.

32. Staron RS: The classification of human skeletal muscle fiber types. J Strength Cond. Res 11:67, 1997.

33. Akima H, Kano Y, Enomoto Y: Muscle function in 164 men and women aged 20–84 yr. Med Sci Sports Exerc 33:220–226, 2001.

34. Shephard RJ: Body Composition in Biological Anthropology. London: Cambridge University; 1991.

35. Shephard RJ, Montelpare W, Plyley M et al: Handgrip dynamometry, Cybex measurements and lean mass as markers of the ageing of muscle. Br J Sports Med 25:204–208, 1991.

36. Aoyahi Y, Shephard RJ: Aging and muscle function. Sports Med 14:376–396, 1992.

37. Bemben, MG, Miccalip GA: Strength and power relationships as a function of age. J Strength Cond Res 13:330–338, 1999.

38. Mazzeo RS: Exercise and the older adult. ACSM Current Comment, 2000.

39. Bales CW, Ritchie CS: Sarcopenia, weight loss, and nutritional frailty in the elderly. Ann Rev Nutr 22:309–323, 2002.

40. Bemben MG: The physiology of aging. ACSM Current Comment, 2001.

41. Melton LJ, Khosia S, Crowson CS: Epidemiology of sarcopenia. J Am Geriatrics Soc 48:625–630, 2000.

42. Kubo K, Kanehisa H, Azuma K et al: Muscle architecture characteristics in women aged 20–79 years. Med Sci Sports Exerc 35: 39–44, 2003.

43. Armstrong N, Welsman JR, Williams C: Longitudinal changes in young people's short-term power output. Med Sci Sports Exerc 32:1140–1145, 2000.

44. Inbar O, Bar-Or O, Skinner JS: The Wingate Anaerobic Test. Human Kinetics: Champaign, IL; 1996.

45. Dal S, Labarthe DR, Grunbaum JA. Longitudinal analysis of changes in indices of obesity from age 8 years to age 18 years. Am J Epidemiology 156(8):720–729, 2002.

46. DiPietro L: Exercise and age-related weight gain. Current comment from the American College of Sports Medicine, 1999.

47. Müller MJ, Grund A, Kraus H: Determinants of fat mass in prepubertal children. Br J Nut 88:545–554, 2002.

48. Sternfeld B, Ngo L, Satariano WA: Associations of body composition with physical performance and self-reported functional limitation in elderly men and women. Am J Epidemiology 156:110–121, 2002.

49. Jeng SF, Liliao HF, Lai JS, Hou JW: Optimization of walking in children. Med Sci Sports Exerc 29:370–376, 1997.

50. Elia EA: Exercise and the elderly. Clin Sports Med 10:141–155, 1991.

51. Schut L: Motor system changes in the aging brain: what is normal and what is not. Geriatrics 53:S16–S19, 1998.

52. Ogawa T, Spina RJ, Martin WH, et al: Effects of aging, sex and physical training on cardiovascular response to exercise. Circulation 86:494–503, 1992.

53. Shock NW: Physiological aspects of aging in man. Ann Rev Physiol 23:97–122, 1961.

54. Meyer F, Bar-Or O, MacDougall D, et al: Drink composition and electrolyte balance of children exercising in the heat. Med Sci Sports Exerc 27:882–887, 1995.

55. Falk B, Bar-Or O, Smolander J. et al: Response to rest and exercise in the cold: effects of age and aerobic fitness. J Appl Phyisol 76: 72–78, 1994.

56. Kenney WL: Control of heat-induced vasodilatation in relation to age. Eur J Appl Physiol 57:120–125, 1988.

57. Kenny WL, Tankersley CG, Newswanger DL, et al: Age and hydrohydration independently influence the peripheral vascular response to heat stress. J Appl Physiol 68:1902–1908, 1990.

58. Tankersley CG, Smolander J, Kenney WL, et al: Sweating and skin blood flow during exercise: effects of age and maximal oxygen uptake. J Appl Physiol 71:236–242, 1991.

59. Young A: Effects of aging on human cold tolerance. Exp Aging Res 17:205–213, 1991.

60. Ingram DK: Age-related decline in physical activity: generalization to nonhumans. Med Sci Sports Exerc 32:1623–1629, 2000.

61. Mujika I, Sabino S: Muscular characteristics of detraining in humans. Med Sci Sports Exerc 33:1297, 2001.

62. Hikida RS, Gollnick PD, Dudley GA, et al: Structural and metabolic characteristics of human skeletal muscle following 30 days of simulated microgravity. Aviat Space Environ Med 60:664, 1989.

63. Hather BM, Bruce M, Tesh PA, et al: Influence of eccentric actions on skeletal muscle adaptations to resistance training. Acta Physiol Scand 143:177, 1991.

64. Narici MV, Roi GS, Landoni L, et al: Changes in force, cross-sectional area and neural activation during strength training and detraining of the human quadriceps. Eur J Appl Physiol 59:310, 1989.

65. Houston ME, Froese EA, Valeriote P, et al: Muscle performance, morphology and metabolic capacity during strength training and detraining: A one leg model. Eur J Appl Physiol 51:25, 1983.

66. Staron RS, Leonardi MJ, Karapondo DL, et al: Strength and skeletal muscle adaptations in heavy-resistance-trained women after detraining and retraining. J Appl Physiol 70:631, 1991.

67. Dudley GA, Duvoisin MR, Convertino VA, et al: Alterations of the in vivo torque-velocity relationship of human skeletal muscle following 30 days exposure to simulated microgravity. Aviat Space Environ Med 60:659, 1989.

68. Gogia PP, Schneider VS, LeBlanc AD, et al: Bed rest effect on extremity muscle torque in healthy men. Arch Phys Med Rehabil 69:1030, 1988.

69. LeBlanc A, Gogia P, Schneider V, et al: Calf muscle area and strength changes after five weeks of horizontal bed rest. Am J Sports Med 16:624, 1988.

70. Berg HE, Larsson L, Tesch PA. Lower limb skeletal muscle function after 6 weeks of bedrest. J Appl Physiol 82:182–188, 1996.

71. Duchateau J: Bed rest induces neural and contractile adaptations in triceps surae. Med Sci Sports Exerc 27:1581, 1995.

72. Ploutz-Snyder LL, Tesch PA, Crittenden DJ, et al: Effect of unweighting on skeletal muscle use during exercise. J Appl Physiol 79:168, 1995.

73. Hather BM, Adams GR, Tesch PA, et al: Skeletal muscle responses to lower limb suspension in humans. J Appl Physiol 72:1493, 1992.

74. Gordon T, Mao J: Muscle atrophy and procedures for training after spinal cord injury. Physical Therapy 74:1, 1994.

75. Stein RB, T Gordon T, Jefferson J, et al: Optimal stimulation of paralyzed muscle after human spinal cord injury. J Appl Physiol 72:1393, 1992.

76. Martin TP, Stein RB, Hoeppner PH, et al: Influence of electrical stimulation on the morphological and metabolic properties of paralyzed muscle. J Appl Physiol 72:1401, 1992.

77. Castro MJ, Apple DF Jr, Staron RS, et al: Influence of complete spinal cord injury on skeletal muscle within six months of injury. J Appl Physiol 86:350–358, 1999.

78. Hillegass EA, Dudley GA: Surface electrical stimulation of skeletal muscle after spinal cord injury. Spinal Cord 37:251–257, 1999.

79. Castro MJ, Apple DF Jr, Hillegass EA, Dudley GA: Influence of complete spinal cord injury on skeletal muscle morphology within six months of injury. Eur J Appl Physiol 80:373–378, 1999.

80. Dudley GA, Castro MJ, Rogers S, Apple DF Jr: A simple means of increasing muscle size after SCI: A pilot study. Eur J Appl Physiol 80:394–396, 1999.

81. Castro MJ, Apple DF Jr, Rogers S, Dudley GA: Influence of complete spinal cord injury on skeletal muscle mechanics within six months of injury. Eur J Appl Physiol 81:128–131, 2000.

82. Convertino VA: Insight into mechanisms of reduced orthostatic performance after exposure to microgravity: comparison of ground-based and space flight data. J Gravit Physiol 5:P85–88, 1998.

83. Prisk, GK: Physiology of a microgravity environment, Invited review: Microgravity and the lung. J Appl Physiol 89:385, 2000.

84. Bloomfield SA: Changes in musculoskeletal structure and function with prolonged bed rest. Med Sci Sports Exerc 29:197, 1997.

85. Uebelhart D, Demiaux-Domenech B, Roth M, et al: Bone metabolism in spinal cord injured individuals and in others who have prolonged immobilization: A review. Paraplegia 33:669, 1995.

86. Bikle DD, Halloran BP: The response of bone to unloading. J Bone Miner Metab 17:233, 1999.

87. Ehrlich PJ, Lanyon LE: Mechanical strain and bone cell function: A review. Osteoporosis Int 13:688, 2002.

88. Iwamoto J, Takeda T, Ichimura S: Effect of exercise training and detraining on bone mineral density in postmenopausal women with osteoporosis. J Orthop Sci 6:128, 2001.

89. Dalsky G, Stocke KS, Ehsani AA, et al: Weight-bearing exercise training and lumbar bone mineral content in postmenopausal women. Ann Intern Med 108:824, 1988.

90. Michel BA, Lane NE, Bloch DA, et al: Effect of changes in weight-bearing exercise on lumbar bone mass after age fifty. Ann Med 23:387, 1991.

91. Magnusson HI, Linden C, Obrant KJ, et al: Bone mass changes in weight loaded and unloaded skeletal regions following a fracture of the hip. Calcif Tissue Int DOI:10.1007/s002230020034,2001.

92. Alfredson H, Nordstrom P, Lorentzon R: Prolonged progressive calcaneal bone loss despite early weightbearing rehabilitation in patients surgically treated for Achilles tendinosis. Calcif Tissue Int 62:166, 1998.

93. Snow CM, Williams DP, LaRiviere J, et al: Bone gains and losses follow seasonal training and detraining in gymnasts. Calcif Tissue Int DOI: 10.1007/s00223-001-0014-5, 2001.

94. Nichols-Richardson SM, Modlesky CM, O'Connor PJ, Lewis RD: Premenarcheal gymnasts possess higher bone mineral density than controls. 32:63, 2000.

95. LeBlanc A, Schneider V, Spector E, et al: Calcium absorption, endogenous excretion, and endocrine changes during and after long-term bed rest. Bone 16:301S, 1995.

96. Smith SM, Wastney ME, Morukov BV, et al: Calcium metabolism before, during, and after a 3-mo spaceflight: kinetic and biochemical changes. Am J Physiol 277:R1, 1999.

97. Bloomfield SA, Mysiw WJ, Jackson RD: Bone mass and endocrine adaptations to training in spinal cord injured individuals. Bone 19:61, 1996.

98. RumL LA, Dubois SK, Roberts ML, et al: Revention of hypercalciuria and stone-forming propensity during prolonged bedrest by alendronate. J Bone Miner Res 10:655, 1995.

99. Van der Wiel HE, Lips P, Nauta J, et al: Biochemical parameters of bone turnover during ten days of bed rest and subsequent mobilization. Bone Miner 13:123, 1991.

100. Zerwekh JE, RumL LA, Gottchalk F, et al: The effects of twelve weeks of bed rest on bone histology, biochemical markers of bone turnover, and calcium homeostasis in eleven normal subjects. J bone Miner Res 13:1594, 1998.

101. Carmeliet G, Vico L, Bouillon R: Space flight: A challenge for normal bone homeostasis. Crit Rev Eukaryot Gene Expr 11:131, 2001.

102. Jee S, Wronski TJ, Morey ER, et al: Effects of spaceflight on trabecular bone in rats. Am J Physiol 244:310, 1983.

103. LeBlanc AD, Schneider VS, Evans HJ, et al: Bone mineral loss and recovery after 17 weeks of bed rest. J Bone Miner Res 5:843, 1990.

104. Barou O, Valentin D, Vico L, et al: High-resolution three-dimensional micro-computed tomography detects bone loss and changes in trabecular architecture early: Comparison with DEXA and bone histomorphometry in a rat model of disuse osteoporosis. Invest Radiol 37:40, 2002.

105. Young DR, Niklowitz WJ, Brown RJ, et al: Immobilization-associated osteoporosis in primates. Bone 7:109, 1986.

106. Inoue M, Tanaka H, Moriwake T, et al: Altered biochemical markers of bone turnover in humans during 120 days of bed rest. Bone 26:281–286, 2000.

107. Vico L, Chappard D, Alexandre C, et al: Effects of a 120 day period of bed rest on bone mass and bone cell activities in man: attempts at countermeasure. Bone Miner 2:383, 1987.

108. Minaire P, Meunier P, Edouard C, et al: Quantitative histological data on disuse osteoporosis: comparison with biological data. Calcif Tissue Res 17:57, 1974.

109. Palle S, Vico L, Bourrin S, et al: Bone tissue response to four-month antiorthostatic bed rest: a bone histomorphometric study. Calcif Tissue Int 51:189–194, 1992.

110. Laugier P, Novikov V, Elmann-Larsen B, et al: Quantitative ultrasound imaging of the calcaneus: Precisions and variations during 120-day bed rest. Calcif Tissue Int 66:16, 2000.

111. Lueken SA, Arnaud SB, Taylor AK, et al: Changes in markers of bone formation and resorption in a bed rest model of weightlessness. J Bone Miner Res 8:1433, 1993.

112. Uebelhart D, Bernard J, Hartmann DF, et al: Modifications of bone and connective tissue after orthostatic bedrest. Osteoporos Int 11:59, 2000.

113. Jaworski ZF, Uhthoff HK: Reversibility of nontraumatic disuse osteoporosis during its active phase. Bone 7:431, 1986.

114. van Harreveld PD, Lillich JD, Kawcak CE, et al: Effects of immobilization followed by remobilization on mineral density, histomorphometric features, and formation of the bones of the metacarpophalangeal joint in horses. Am J Vet Res 2:276, 2002.

115. Bourrin S, Palle S, Genty C, et al: Physical exercise during remobilization restores normal bone trabecular network after tail suspension-induced osteopenia in young rats. J Bone Miner Res 10:820,1995.

116. Kaneps AJ, Stover SM, Lane NE: Changes in canine cortical and cancellous bone mechanical properties following immobilization and remobilization with exercise. Bone 5:419, 1997.

117. Tilton FE; Degioanni JJ; Schneider VS: Long-term follow-up of Skylab bone demineralization. Aviat Space Environ Med 51 1209–1213, 1980.

118. Ito M, Matsumoto T, Enomoto H, et al: Effect of nonweight bearing on tibial bone density measured by QCT in patients with hip surgery. J Bone Miner Metab 17:45, 1999.

119. Manfredi TG, Fielding RA, O'Reilly KP, et al: Plasma creatine kinase activity and exercise-induced muscle damage in older men. Med Sci Sports Exerc 23:1028, 1991.

120. Roy RR, Baldwin KM, Edgerton VR: The plasticity of skeletal muscle effects of neuromuscular activity. Exerc Sports Sci Rev 19:269, 1991.

121. Castro MJ, Apple DF Jr, Rogers S, Dudley GA: Muscle fiber-type specific Ca2+ actomyosin ATPase activity after complete spinal cord injury. Muscle Nerve 23:119–121, 2000.

122. Berg HE, Dudley GA, Hather BM, et al: Work capacity and metabolic and morphologic characteristics of the human quadriceps muscle in response to unloading. Clin Physiol 13:337, 1993.

123. Duchateau J, Hainaut K: Effects of immobilization on contractile properties, recruitment and firing rates of human motor units. J Physiol 422:55, 1990.

124. Adams GR, Hather BM, Dudley GA: Effect of short-term unweighting on human skeletal muscle strength and size. Aviat Space Environ Med 65:1116, 1994.

125. Berg HE, Dudley GA, Haggmark T, et al: Effects of lower limb unloading on skeletal muscle mass and function in humans. J Appl Physiol 70:1882, 1991.

126. Dudley GA, Duvoisin MR, Adams GR, et al: Adaptations to unilateral lower limb suspension in humans. Aviat Space Environ Med 63:678, 1992.

127. Harris RT, Dudley GA: Factors limiting force during slow, shortening actions of the quadriceps femoris muscle group in vivo. Acta Physiol Scand 152:63, 1994.

128. Westing SH, Seger H, Thorstensson A: Effects of electrical stimulation on eccentric and concentric torque-velocity relationships during knee extension in man. Acta Physiol Scand 140:17, 1990.

129. Berg HE, Tesch PA: Changes in muscle function in response to 10 days of lower limb unloading in humans. Acta Physiol Scand 157:63–70, 1996.

130. Edgerton VR, Zhou MY, Ohira Y, et al: Human fiber size and enzymatic properties after 5 and 11 days of spaceflight. J Appl Physiol 78:1733, 1995.

131. Koryak Y: Contractile properties of the human triceps surae muscle during simulated weightlessness. Eur J Appl Physiol 70:344, 1995.

132. Fuglevand AJ, Bilodeau M, Enoka RM: Short-term immobilization has a minimal effect on the strength and fatigability of a human hand muscle. J Appl Physiol 78:847, 1995.

133. SemmLer JG, Kutzscher DV, Enoka RM: Gender differences in the fatigability of human skeletal muscle. J Neurophysiol 82:3590–3593, 1999.

134. Ploutz-Snyder LL, Tesch PA, Crittenden DJ et al: Effect of unweighting on skeletal muscle use during exercise. J Appl Physiol 79:168, 1995.

135. Kandarin SC, Boushel RC, Schulte LM: Elevated interstitial fluid volume in rat soleus muscles by hindlimb unweighting. J Appl Physiol 71:910, 1991.

136. Goldspink DF, Morton AJ, Loughna P, et al: The effect of hypokinesia and hypodynamia on protein turnover and the growth of four skeletal muscles of the rat. Pflugers Arch 407:333, 1986.

137. Ploutz-Snyder LL, Tesch PA, Hather BM, et al: Vulnerability to dysfunction and muscle injury after unloading. Arch Phys Med Rehabil 77:773–777, 1996.

138. Ohira Y, Yoshinaga T, Ohara M, et al: Myonuclear domain and myosin phenotype in human soleus after bed rest with or without loading. J Appl Physiol 87:1776–1785, 1999.

139. Tseng BS, Marsh DR, Hamilton MT, et al: Strength and aerobic training attenuate muscle wasting and improve resistance to the development of disability with aging [special issue]. J Gerontol Series A 50A:113, 1995.

140. McGuire DK, Levine BD, Williamson JW, et al: A 30 year follow-up of the Dallas bedrest and training study, Circulation 104:1358, 2001.

141. Deschenes, M, Giles, JA, McCoy, RW, et al: Neural factors account for strength decrements observed after short-term muscle unloading. Am J Physiol Regulatory Integrative Comp Physio 282:578, 2001.

142. Pattullo MC, Cotter MA, Cameron NE, et al: Effects of lengthened immobilization on functional and histochemical properties of rabbit tibialis anterior muscle. Exp Physiol 77:433, 1992.

143. Grana EA, Chiou-Tan F, Jaweed M: Endplate dysfunction in healthy muscle following a period of disuse. Muscle Nerve 19:989–993, 1996.

144. Jacobs PL, Mahoney, ET: Peak exercise capacity of electrically induced ambulation in persons with paraplegia. Med Sci Sports Exerc 34:1551, 2002.

145. Jacobs PL, Nash MS, Rusinowski JW: Circuit training provides cardiorespiratory and strength benefits in persons with paraplegia. Med Sci Sports Exerc 33:771, 2001.

146. Convertino, VA: Planning strategies for development of effective exercise and nutrition countermeasures for long-duration space flight. Nutrition 18:880, 2002.

147. LeBlanc A, Rowe R, Schneider V, et al: Regional muscle loss after short duration spaceflight. Aviat Space Environ Med 66:1151, 1995.

148. Vico L, Collet P, Guignandon A, et al: Effects of long-term microgravity exposure on cancellous and cortical weight-bearing bones of cosmonauts. Lancet 355:1607, 2000.

149. Levine BD, Lane LD, Watenpaugh DE, et al: Maximal exercise performance after adaptation to microgravity. J Appl Physiol 81:686, 1996.

SELECTED REFERENCES FOR FURTHER READING

Christiansen JL, Grzybowski JM: Biology of Aging. New York: McGraw-Hill; 1999.

Shephard RJ: Aging, Physical Activity and Health. Champaign, IL: Human Kinetics; 1997.

Spirduso WW: Physical Dimensions of Aging. Champaign, IL: Human Kinetics; 1995.

INTERNET RESOURCES

ISAPA: International Society for Aging and Physical Activity: http://www.isapa.org

National Institute on Aging: http://www.nia.nih.gov

Tufts University Health & Nutrition Newsletter: http://healthletter.tufts.edu

WebMD: http://www.webmd.com

Lifestyle Factors Associated with Health and Disease

SECTION EDITOR: HAROLD W. KOHL III, PhD, FACSM

Factors Associated with Increased Risk of Coronary Heart Disease

NEIL F. GORDON, RICHARD F. LEIGHTON, AND ARYAN MOOSS

This chapter addresses KSAs from the following content areas:

1   Exercise Physiology and Related Exercise Science
2   **Pathophysiology and Risk Factors**
3   Health Appraisal, Fitness, and Clinical Exercise Testing
4   Electrocardiography and Diagnostic Techniques
5   **Patient Management and Medications**
6   **Medical and Surgical Management**
7   Exercise Prescription and Programming
8   Nutrition and Weight Management
9   Human Behavior and Counseling
10   Safety, Injury Prevention, and Emergency Procedures
11   Program Administration, Quality Assurance, and Outcome Assessment

Cardiovascular disease (CVD) is the leading cause of death in developed countries and is a major component of the global burden of disease. In the United States in the year 2000, CVD was a primary or contributing cause in 60% of all deaths and 14.2 million patients had a history of myocardial infarction (MI) or angina. Many times that number are at risk for developing coronary heart disease[1]. Although, the age-adjusted rate of cardiovascular mortality has decreased by 40% in the past 30 years, apparently because of better treatment options and more effective primary and secondary prevention strategies[2], CVD remains the number 1 killer in the United States[1,2].

Coronary Risk Factors

Coronary heart disease results from atherosclerosis of the coronary arteries. Coronary atherosclerosis is multifactorial in origin. The process begins in childhood and results from an atherogenic milieu, which is the clustering of several genetic, biological, behavioral, and environmental factors collectively known as **coronary risk factors**. The term *risk factor*, proposed by the Framingham investigators, came with the realization that no known single factor is the sole cause of coronary atherosclerosis, but a combination of factors can be correlated with an increased risk for the development of coronary heart disease[3]. For a risk factor to be clinically useful, it must satisfy the following criteria: strength of association (high odds ratio), consistency (multiple studies confirming the association), temporal relationship (the risk factor must precede the disease over many years), gradient (the greater the level of the risk factor, the higher the risk), biological plausibility, and experimental and clinical evidence from human primary and secondary prevention studies[4]. From a practical standpoint, modifiability of a risk factor is also a clinically significant attribute.

Two important concepts in risk factor evaluation must be emphasized. First, risk factors, such as elevated **cholesterol** and **hypertension**, typically function in a continuum of increasing risk rather than through all-or-none cutoff values (e.g., a cholesterol level of ≥ 200 mg·dL^{-1} or blood pressure [BP] $\geq 140/90$ mm Hg). Individuals with cholesterol levels more than 300 mg·dL^{-1} are at three to five times higher risk for coronary heart disease than those with cholesterol levels of 200 mg·dL^{-1}, although only 3% to 5% of the Framingham population has cholesterol levels of 300 mg·dL^{-1} or more[5]. Similar data for hypertension prove that there is, indeed, a risk pyramid[6]. Those at the top of the pyramid are at the highest risk for disease, but those at the lower levels of the pyramid account for the largest number of cases in the community because they constitute a larger segment of the population. The second important consideration is the multiplicative effect of risk factors (i.e., the greater the number of risk factors, the greater the level of risk; Fig. 5-1). For example, a smoker with modest elevation of cholesterol or BP is at much higher risk for developing coronary heart disease than a nonsmoker with severe hypercholesterolemia or hypertension. Therefore, a comprehensive risk evaluation of an individual is an essential prerequisite to developing strategies for primary prevention of coronary heart disease.

Over the years, various coronary risk factor classification schemes have been proposed (also see GETP7 Chapters 2 and 3. In this Chapter, coronary risk factors will be discussed according to the classification used in the Adult Treatment Panel (ATP III) report of the National Cholesterol Education Program (NCEP)[7]. Thus, the chapter

KEY TERMS

Cholesterol: A fatlike substance (lipid) that is present in cell membranes and is a precursor of bile acids and steroid hormones

Coronary risk factors: Genetic, biological, behavioral, and environmental factors associated with an increased risk for the development of atherosclerosis in the coronary arteries and other vascular beds

Diabetes: As defined by the American Diabetes Association, as a fasting plasma glucose level of 126 mg·dL^{-1} or greater; individuals with a fasting plasma glucose level of 100 to 125 mg·dL^{-1} should be considered prediabetic

Emerging risk factors: Newly identified factors that currently do not qualify as a major coronary risk factor but are thought to be associated with an increased risk for atherosclerosis

Hypertension: As defined by the Seventh Report of the Joint National Committee on Prevention, Detection, Evaluation, and Treatment of High Blood Pressure, a blood pressure ≥ 140 mm Hg systolic or ≥ 90 mm Hg diastolic;

individuals with a systolic blood pressure of 120–139 mm Hg or a diastolic blood pressure of 80–89 mm Hg should be considered prehypertensive.

Lipoproteins: Cholesterol travels in the blood in distinct particles containing both lipid and proteins (lipoproteins). In order of decreasing density, the three major classes of lipoproteins are high-density lipoprotein, low-density lipoprotein, and very low-density lipoprotein

Metabolic syndrome: Syndrome characterized by a constellation of metabolic risk factors, including abdominal obesity, insulin resistance or glucose intolerance, atherogenic dyslipidemia, hypertension, and a prothrombotic and proinflammatory state

Obesity: As defined by the National Institutes of Health, a body mass index (weight in kg divided by height in meters squared) of ≥ 30 kg·m^{-2}

Overweight: As defined by the National Institutes of Health, a body mass index (weight in kg divided by height in meters squared) of 25 to 29.9 kg·m^{-2}

considers lipid, nonlipid, and **emerging** (which may be either lipid or nonlipid) **risk factors.** Finally, subclinical atherosclerosis and plaque burden and the **metabolic syndrome,** a common entity that incorporates lipid, nonlipid, and emerging risk factors, is considered separately (Box 5-1).

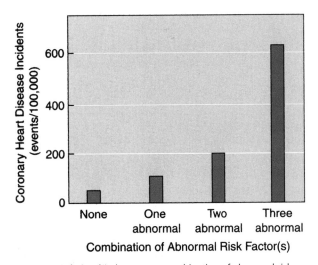

FIGURE 5-1. Relationship between a combination of abnormal risk factors (cholesterol = 250 mg·dL^{-1}, systolic blood pressure = 160 mm Hg, smoking = 1 pack of cigarettes/day) and incidence of coronary heart disease. (From Kannel WB, Gordon T: The Framingham Study: An epidemiological investigation of cardiovascular disease. Section 30. Washington, DC: Public Health Service, NIH, DHEW Publication [NIH] 74:599, 1974.)

LIPID RISK FACTORS

Low-density Lipoprotein Cholesterol

The relationship between serum cholesterol levels and coronary heart disease is continuous and graded (Fig. 5-2)[8]. Evidence from animal studies, experimental investigations, epidemiological studies, and clinical trials indicates conclusively that a high serum cholesterol is a major risk factor for coronary heart disease and that lowering cholesterol levels reduces the risk[9]. About 42 million Americans are estimated to have high total cholesterol levels (i.e., ≥ 240 mg·dL^{-1})[1]. Cholesterol circulates in the plasma in three major sizes of **lipoprotein** particles, namely, very low-density lipoprotein (VLDL) cholesterol, low-density lipoprotein (LDL) cholesterol, and high-density lipoprotein (HDL) cholesterol. Total cholesterol is equal to the sum of these three fractions. Coronary heart disease is directly and linearly related to the levels of total cholesterol and LDL cholesterol and inversely related to the level of HDL cholesterol. In MRFIT (Multiple Risk Factor Intervention Trial0, for each 50 mg·dL^{-1} increase in total cholesterol above 200 mg·dL^{-1}, coronary heart disease rates doubled[10]. Most of the risk attributed to total cholesterol is explained by the LDL cholesterol concentration[11]. Oxidized LDL cholesterol is considered to be a major factor in the pathogenesis of atherosclerosis (see Chapter 29).

The ATP III report set a high priority on LDL cholesterol management (Box 5-2) and established the most

| **BOX 5-1** | **Classification of Coronary Risk Factors** |

1. Modifiable lipid risk factors
   - LDL cholesterol
   - HDL cholesterol
   - Triglycerides[a]
   - Non-HDL cholesterol
   - Atherogenic dyslipidemia
2. Modifiable nonlipid risk factors
   - Hypertension
   - Cigarette smoking
   - Diabetes
   - Overweight or obesity
   - Physical inactivity
   - Atherogenic diet
3. Nonmodifiable nonlipid risk factors
   - Age
   - Male gender
   - Family history of premature coronary heart disease
4. Emerging risk factors
   a. Emerging lipid risk factors
      - Lipoprotein (a)
      - Lipoprotein remnants
      - Small LDL particles
      - HDL subspecies
      - Apolipoproteins B and A-1
      - Total cholesterol-to-HDL cholesterol ratio
   b. Emerging nonlipid risk factors
      - Homocysteine
      - Thrombogenic and hemostatic factors
      - Inflammatory markers
      - Impaired glucose tolerance
5. Subclinical atherosclerosis and plaque burden
6. The metabolic syndrome

HDL= high-density lipoprotein; LDL = low-density lipoprotein.

[a] Because of questions about their independence as a risk factor, triglycerides may also be considered an emerging risk factor.

Adapted from 7. Third Report of the National Cholesterol Education Program (NCEP) Expert Panel on Detection, Evaluation, and Treatment of High Blood Cholesterol in Adults. (Adult Treatment Panel III): Bethesda, MD: National Institutes of Health, National Heart, Lung, and Blood Institute, NIH Publication No. 02-5215; September 2002.

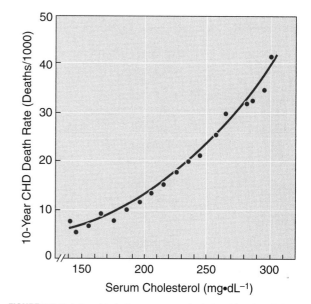

FIGURE 5-2. Relationship between serum cholesterol level and coronary heart disease death rate. (From Expert Panel on Detection, Evaluation, and Treatment of High Blood Cholesterol in Adults [Adult Treatment Panel II]: Second report of the National Cholesterol Education Program [NCEP] Men Screened for MRFIT Program. NIH Publication No. 93, 361:662, 1993.)

High-density Lipoprotein Cholesterol

A low level of serum HDL cholesterol is an important predictor of coronary heart disease. Several large epidemiological studies suggest that for each 1 mg·dL^{-1} increase in HDL cholesterol, there is an accompanying 2% decrease in coronary heart disease risk in men and a 3% decrease in women[21]. Furthermore, a low LDL cholesterol level does not eliminate the risk imparted by a low HDL cholesterol, but a high HDL cholesterol appears to offset some of the risk of a high LDL cholesterol (Fig. 5-3)[22]. HDL cholesterol plays a critical role in reverse cholesterol transport[23]. In addition, HDL cholesterol may retard atherogenesis through prevention of LDL cholesterol oxidation and monocyte adhesion to endothelial cells[24] and by maintaining endothelial function[25]. The Framingham risk prediction model incorporates HDL cholesterol and the ATP III report designates an HDL cholesterol of 60 mg·dL^{-1} or more as a "negative" risk factor (i.e., its presence removes one risk factor from the total count when determining a person's major risk factors that modify LDL cholesterol goals). In the ATP III report, low HDL cholesterol was defined as a level below 40 mg·dL^{-1} [7]. Low HDL cholesterol levels may be part of the metabolic syndrome and are also more prevalent in smokers and individuals taking certain drugs. Therapeutic options to increase HDL cholesterol levels include nonpharmacologic approaches, such as regular exercise, avoidance of very high carbohydrate intakes (i.e., > 60% of total daily energy intake), weight management, and cigarette smoking cessation as well pharmacologic agents (see GETP7 Appendix A), including

stringent goal levels for persons with coronary heart disease or coronary heart disease risk equivalents (i.e., other forms of atherosclerotic disease, **diabetes**, and multiple risk factors that confer a 10-year risk for coronary heart disease > 20%)[7]. The Framingham risk prediction model (Box 5-3) uses total cholesterol along with other major risk factors in estimating the 10-year risk of coronary events in persons without known atherosclerotic CVD[12]. The ATP III report (Box 5-2) used a modified Framingham risk score to set LDL cutpoints and goals for individuals with risk factors but without known CVD or diabetes. Several large randomized trials have proved the benefits of LDL cholesterol reduction with statin drug therapy in primary and secondary prevention[13–20].

BOX 5-2	ATP III Guidelines : Quick Desk Reference

STEP 1 DETERMINE LIPOPROTEIN LEVELS IN ALL ADULTS AGE 20 YEARS AND OVER; OBTAIN COMPLETE LIPOPROTEIN PROFILE (I.E., TOTAL CHOLESTEROL, LDL CHOLESTEROL, HDL CHOLESTEROL, AND TRIGLYCERIDES) AFTER 9- TO 12-HOUR FAST:

ATP III Classification of LDL, Total, and HDL Cholesterol (mg·dL^{-1})

LDL Cholesterol: Primary Target of Therapy

< 100 mg·dL^{-1}	Optimal
100–129 mg·dL^{-1}	Near optimal or above optimal
130–159 mg·dL^{-1}	Borderline high
160–189 mg·dL^{-1}	High
≥ 190 mg·dL^{-1}	Very high

Total Cholesterol

< 200 mg·dL^{-1}	Desirable
200–239 mg·dL^{-1}	Borderline high
≥ 240 mg·dL^{-1}	High

HDL Cholesterol

< 40 mg·dL^{-1}	Low
≥ 60 mg·dL^{-1}	High

STEP 2 IDENTIFY THE PRESENCE OF CLINICAL ATHEROSCLEROTIC DISEASE AND OTHER CONDITIONS THAT CONFER HIGH RISK FOR CHD EVENTS (I.E., CHD OR CHD RISK EQUIVALENTS):
- Clinical CHD
- Symptomatic carotid artery disease
- Peripheral arterial disease
- Abdominal aortic aneurysm
- Diabetes

STEP 3 DETERMINE THE PRESENCE OF MAJOR RISK FACTORS (OTHER THAN LDL):

Major Risk Factors (Exclusive of LDL Cholesterol) That Modify LDL Goals
- Cigarette smoking
- Hypertension (BP ≥ 140/90 mm Hg or on antihypertensive medication)
- Low HDL cholesterol (< 40 mg·dL^{-1})
- Family history of premature CHD (CHD in male first-degree relative < 55 years; CHD in female first-degree relative < 65 years)
- Age (men ≥ 45 years; women ≥ 55 years)
- HDL cholesterol ≥ 60 mg·dL^{-1} counts as a "negative" risk factor; its presence removes one risk factor from the total count

STEP 4 IF TWO OR MORE RISK FACTORS (OTHER THAN LDL) ARE PRESENT WITHOUT CHD OR CHD RISK EQUIVALENT, ASSESS 10-YEAR (SHORT-TERM) CHD RISK (SEE BOX 3-2).

Three levels of 10-year risk:
- >20% = CHD risk equivalent (= high risk)
- 10% to 20% = Moderately high risk
- < 10% = Moderate risk

STEP 5 DETERMINE RISK CATEGORY:
- Establish LDL goal of therapy
- Determine need for TLC
- Determine level for drug consideration

(continues)

BOX 5-2 | **ATP III Guidelines : Quick Desk Reference *(continued)***

LDL Cholesterol Goals and Cutpoints for TLC and Drug Therapy in Different Risk Categories and Proposed Modifications Based on Recent Clinical Trial Evidence.

Risk Category	LDL Goal	LDL Level at Which to Initiate TLC	LDL Level at Which to Consider Drug Therapy
High risk: CHD or CHD risk equivalents (10-year risk > 20%)	< 100 mg·dL^{-1} (optional goal: < 70 mg·dL^{-1})[b]	≥ 100 mg·dL^{-1} [c]	≥ 100 mg·dL^{-1} [e] (< 100 mg·dL^{-1}: consider drug options)[d]
Moderately high risk: 2+ (10-year risk 10% to 20%)	< 130 mg·dL^{-1} (optional goal: < 100 mg·dL^{-1})	≥ 130 mg·dL^{-1} [c]	≥ 130 risk factors mg·dL^{-1} (100 to 129 mg·dL^{-1}; consider drug options)[f]
Moderate risk: 2+ risk factors (10-year risk < 10%)	< 130 mg·dL^{-1}	≥ 130 mg·dL^{-1}	≥ 160 mg·dL^{-1}
Lower risk: 0 to 1 risk factor[a]	< 160 mg·dL^{-1}	≥ 160 mg·dL^{-1}	≥ 190 mg·dL^{-1} (160 to 189 mg·dL^{-1}: LDL-lowering drug optional)

STEP 6 INITIATE THERAPEUTIC LIFESTYLE CHANGES (TLC) IF LDL IS ABOVE GOAL[f]:

TLC Features
- TLC Diet:
  Saturated fat < 7% of calories, cholesterol < 200 mg·day^{-1}
  Consider increased viscous (soluble) fiber (10 to 25 g·day^{-1}) and plant stanols or sterols (2 g·day^{-1}) as therapeutic options to enhance LDL lowering
- Weight management
- Increased physical activity.
  Moderate risk: two or more risk factors (10-year risk < 10%).

STEP 7 CONSIDER ADDING DRUG THERAPY IF LDL EXCEEDS LEVELS SHOWN IN STEP 5:
- Consider drug simultaneously with TLC for CHD and CHD equivalents
- Consider adding drug to TLC after 3 months for other risk categories

STEP 8 IDENTIFY THE METABOLIC SYNDROME AND TREAT, IF PRESENT, AFTER 3 MONTHS OF TLC:

Clinical Identification of the Metabolic Syndrome: Any Three of the Following:

Risk Factor	Defining Level
Abdominal obesity	Waist circumference
Men	≥ 102 cm (> 40 in)
Women	≥ 88 cm (≥ 35 in)
Triglycerides	≥ 150 mg·dL^{-1}
HDL Cholesterol	
Men	< 40 mg·dL^{-1}
Women	< 50 mg·dL^{-1}
BP	≥ 130 ≥ 85 mm Hg
Fasting Glucose	≥ 100 mg·dL^{-1}

(continues)

BOX 5-2   **ATP III Guidelines : Quick Desk Reference** *(continued)*

Treatment of the Metabolic Syndrome
- Treat underlying causes (overweight, obesity, and physical inactivity):
  Intensify weight management
  Increase physical activity
- Treat lipid and nonlipid risk factors if they persist despite these lifestyle therapies:
  Treat hypertension
  Use aspirin for CHD patients to reduce prothrombotic state
  Treat elevated triglycerides or low HDL (as shown in Step 9)

STEP 9   TREAT ELEVATED TRIGLYCERIDES (AND LOW HDL CHOLESTEROL):

ATP III Classification of Serum Triglycerides (mg·dL^{-1})

<150	Normal
150–199	Borderline high
200–499	High
≥ 500	Very high

Treatment of elevated triglycerides (< 150 mg·dL^{-1})
- If triglycerides ≥ 500 mg·dL^{-1}, first lower triglycerides to prevent pancreatitis
- Primary aim of therapy is to reach LDL goal
- Intensify weight management
- Increase physical activity
- If triglycerides are ≥ 200 mg·dL^{-1} after LDL goal is reached, set secondary goal for non-HDL cholesterol (total HDL) 30 mg·dL^{-1} higher than LDL goal. If triglycerides are 200 to 499 mg·dL^{-1} after LDL goal is reached, consider adding drug if needed to reach non-HDL goal.

Treatment of low HDL cholesterol (> 40 mg·dL^{-1})
- First reach LDL goal, then:
- Intensify weight management and increase physical activity
- If triglycerides 200 to 499 mg·dL^{-1}, achieve non-HDL goal
- If triglycerides < 200 mg·dL^{-1} (isolated low HDL) in CHD or CHD equivalent, consider nicotinic acid or fibrate.

BP = blood pressure; CHD = coronary heart disease; HDL= high-density lipoprotein; LDL = low-density lipoprotein; TLC = therapeutic lifestyle changes.

[a] Almost all people with zero or one risk factor have a 10-year risk < 10%; thus, 10-year risk assessment in people with zero or one risk factor is not necessary.

[b] Very high risk favors the optional LDL cholesterol goal of < 70 mg·dL^{-1}, and in patients with high triglycerides, non-HDL cholesterol < 100 mg·dL^{-1}.

[c] Any person at high risk or moderately high risk who has lifestyle-related risk factors (e.g., obesity, physical inactivity, elevated triglycerides, low HDL cholesterol, or metabolic syndrome) is a candidate for therapeutic lifestyle changes to modify these risk factors regardless of LDL cholesterol level.

[d] When LDL-lowering drug therapy is used, it is advised that intensity of therapy be sufficient to achieve at least a 30% to 40% reduction in LDL cholesterol levels.

[e] If baseline LDL cholesterol is < 100 mg·dL^{-1}, institution of an LDL-lowering drug is a therapeutic option on the basis of available clinical trial results. If a high-risk person has high triglycerides or low HDL cholesterol, combining a fibrate or nicotinic acid with an LDL-lowering drug can be considered.

[f] For moderately high-risk persons, when LDL cholesterol level is 100 to 129 mg·dL^{-1}, at baseline or on lifestyle therapy, initiation of an LDL-lowering drug to achieve an LDL cholesterol level < 100 mg·dL^{-1} is a therapeutic option on the basis of available clinical trial results.

Adapted from Third Report of the National Cholesterol Education Program (NCEP) Expert Panel on Detection, Evaluation, and Treatment of High Blood Cholesterol in Adults. (Adult Treatment Panel III): Bethesda, MD: National Institutes of Health, National Heart, Lung, and Blood Institute, NIH Publication No. 02-5215; September 2002 and Grundy SM, Cleeman JI, Bairey Merz N, et al. Implication of recent clinical trials for the National Cholesterol Education Program Adult Treatment Panel III Guidelines. Circulation 110: 227-239, 2004.

---

niacin, fibrates, HMG-CoA reductase inhibitors (statins), and hormone replacement therapy (HRT). The results of trials using fibrates to increase low HDL cholesterol have been mixed. The Veterans Affairs High Density Lipoprotein Cholesterol Interventional Trial reported that in men with coronary heart disease and an HDL cholesterol level of 40 mg/dL or above, treatment with gemfibrozil resulted in a significant 24% reduction in death, nonfatal MI, and stroke[26]. In the Bezafibrate Infarction Prevention trial, however, treatment of patients with coronary heart disease and an HDL level below 45 mg/dL with bezafibrate resulted in a significant reduction in fatal or nonfatal MI and sudden death only in a small subgroup of study participants who had elevated baseline triglyceride levels[27].

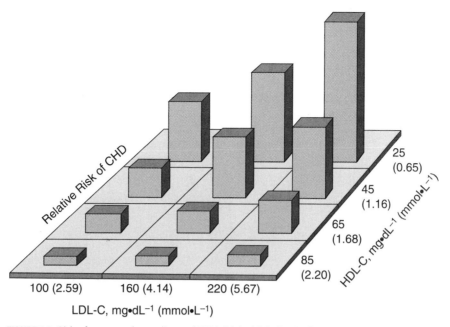

FIGURE 5-3. Risk of coronary heart disease (CHD) risk by high-density lipoprotein cholesterol (HDL-C) and low-density lipoprotein cholesterol (LDL-C) levels. (Adapted from Kannel WB, Gordon T: The Framingham Study: An epidemiological investigation of cardiovascular disease. Section 30. Washington, DC: Public Health Service, NIH, DHEW Publication [NIH] 74:599, 1974.)

Triglycerides and Non–High-density Lipoprotein Cholesterol

The relationship of elevated serum triglyceride levels to coronary heart disease is complex. Similar to low HDL cholesterol, elevated triglyceride levels are a part of the metabolic syndrome and, thus, are interrelated with other lipid fractions as well as with nonlipid risk factors. In addition, the atherogenic remnant lipoproteins that make up the VLDL fraction of serum cholesterol are rich in triglycerides. Finally, meta-analyses have revealed that elevated levels of triglycerides constitute an independent risk factor for coronary heart disease[28]. Although genetic influences, disease states, smoking, alcohol excess, and use of certain drugs may result in hypertriglyceridemia, the most common causative factors are **obesity** and physical inactivity. The ATP III report classified triglyceride levels as normal (< 150 mg·dL^{-1}), borderline high (150 to 199 mg·dL^{-1}), high (200 to 499 mg·dL^{-1}), and very high (≥ 500 mg·dL^{-1}) and recommended that patients with triglyceride levels of 150 mg·dL^{-1} or above be counseled to reduce body weight, increase exercise, decrease fat intake, quit smoking, and limit alcohol intake[7]. A review of studies has revealed that approximately 4 g·day^{-1} of omega-3 fatty acids from fish oil also can induce a 25% to 30% decrease in serum triglyceride levels[29]. Although LDL cholesterol remains the primary target for lipid-lowering therapy, the ATP III report also recommends that non-HDL cholesterol (the sum of VLDL and LDL cholesterol) be considered a secondary therapeutic target. Non-HDL cholesterol is calculated by subtracting the HDL cholesterol value from the total cholesterol value and is considered to be elevated when its level is 30 mg·dL^{-1} higher than the LDL cholesterol goal (see Box 5-2).

Atherogenic Dyslipidemia

Small, dense particles of LDL cholesterol, along with raised triglyceride and low HDL cholesterol levels, constitutes a triad that has been termed *atherogenic dyslipidemia* because it is commonly found in individuals with premature coronary heart disease[30]. This triad is the predominant dyslipidemia found in the metabolic syndrome[31] and is a common finding in patients with type 2 diabetes[32]. In epidemiologic studies, it has been difficult to separate the contribution of each component of the triad to coronary heart disease risk but some prospective population studies have suggested that the role of small dense LDL may be partly independent of other lipid risk factors[33,34]. Because their independence as a risk factor remains partly unresolved and standard, inexpensive methods for their measurement are not currently widely available, the NCEP Expert Panel has not recommended routine measurement of small LDL particles in all adults. Rather, the panel has suggested that their presence may be best used to reinforce therapy aimed at improving atherogenic dyslipidemia and the metabolic syndrome[7].

MODIFIABLE NONLIPID RISK FACTORS

Hypertension

Nearly 50 million adult Americans have high BP (i.e., systolic BP ≥ 140 mm Hg or diastolic BP ≥ 90 mm Hg)[35]. The relationship between BP and risk for cardiovascular events is continuous, consistent, and independent of other coronary risk factors. For individuals age 40 to 70 years, each increment of 20 mm Hg in systolic BP or 10 mm Hg in diastolic BP doubles the risk of CVD across the entire BP range from 115/75 to 185/115 mm Hg[36]. Elevation of BP causes vascular endothelial dysfunction and injury as well as adverse effects on the myocardium, which include increased wall stress, increased myocardial oxygen demand, and left ventricular hypertrophy (LVH). The major randomized trials of antihypertensive therapy have demonstrated a 35% to 40% reduction in the incidence of

stroke, a 20% to 25% reduction in MI, and a more than 50% reduction in heart failure[37]. Isolated systolic hypertension, defined as a systolic BP of ≥ 140 mm Hg and diastolic BP < 90 mm Hg, is common in men and women older than age 65 years and is an independent risk factor for coronary heart disease. A recent meta-analysis suggests that for patients with hypertension and additional risk factors, a sustained 12-mm reduction in systolic BP would prevent one death for every 11 patients treated[38]. The guidelines from the Joint National Committee on Prevention, Detection, Evaluation, and Treatment of High Blood Pressure (JNC 7) recommend an aggressive approach in the treatment of hypertension, especially in the presence of target organ damage, diabetes, or clinical CVD[35].

Blood pressure may be classified and managed as outlined in Figure 5-4 and GETP7 Table 3–1. Lifestyle

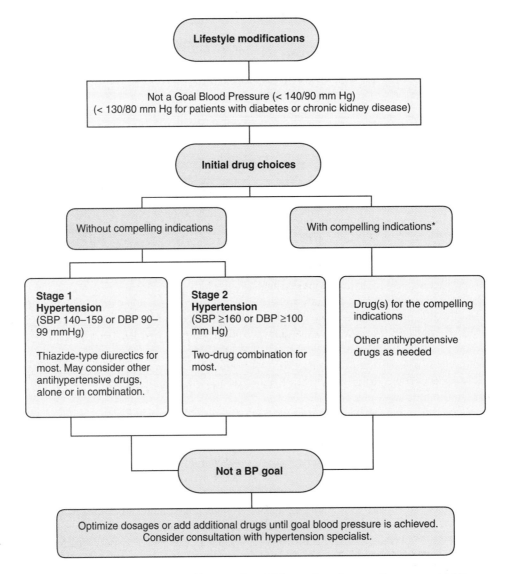

FIGURE 5-4. Algorithm for the treatment of hypertension. ACEI = angiotensin-converting enzyme inhibitor; ARB = angiotensin receptor blocker; BB = beta-blocker; CCB = calcium channel blocker; DBP = diastolic blood pressure; SBP = systolic blood pressure.

modification, including weight reduction, a DASH eating plan (i.e., a diet rich in fruits, vegetables and low-fat dairy products with a reduced content of saturated and total fat), dietary sodium reduction (no more than 2.4 g·day^{-1} of sodium), physical activity, and moderation of alcohol consumption, remains the cornerstone of antihypertensive therapy[35]. For patients who require drug therapy in addition to lifestyle modification, low-dose diuretics are the most effective initial treatment for preventing cardiovascular events and mortality[39]. The JNC 7 report emphasized that most patients will require two or more antihypertensive medications to achieve their BP goal (i.e., < 140/90 mm Hg or < 130/80 mm Hg for patients with diabetes or chronic kidney disease)[35].

Cigarette Smoking

Cigarette smoking is the most preventable cause of death in the United States[40]. Autopsy studies have shown that the extent of atherosclerosis is linearly related to the number of cigarettes smoked (Fig. 5-5)[41]. The risk also increases in accordance with the number of years of smoking and the depth of inhalation. Nearly 40% of cardiovascular deaths are attributable to cigarette smoking. Smokers have twice the risk of developing coronary heart disease and a twofold to fourfold increased risk of

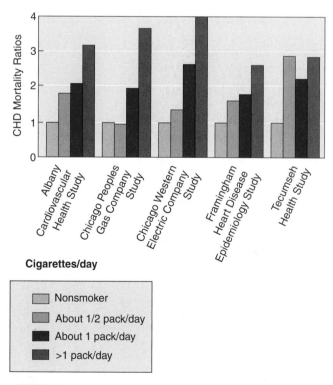

FIGURE 5-5. Coronary heart disease (CHD) mortality ratios according to the amount of cigarettes smoked in five populations. (Reprinted with permission from The Pooling Project Research Group: Relationship of blood pressure, serum cholesterol, smoking habit, relative weight, and ECG abnormalities to incidence of major coronary events: Final report of the Pooling Project. J Chron Dis 31:202, 1978.)

sudden death. The deleterious effects of smoking are particularly noteworthy in younger adults. In MI survivors who younger than age 40 years, the most common accompanying risk factor is cigarette smoking. As in men, women who smoke are at increased risk for coronary heart disease[42]. Risk doubles in women who smoke as few as one to four cigarettes per day. Acutely, cigarette smoking accentuates risk by elevating the myocardial oxygen demand (through increases in heart rate and BP), reducing oxygen transport, increasing susceptibility to malignant ventricular arrhythmias, predisposing the coronary artery to spasm, and increasing platelet adhesiveness. Smoking also leads to endothelial dysfunction[43]. The resultant vasoconstriction and loss of endothelial cell integrity facilitates transport of atherogenic lipoproteins and scavenger cells across the endothelial barrier. Cigarette smokers have increased levels of fibrinogen and reduced systemic fibrinolytic activity[44] as well as impaired coronary release of tissue plasminogen activator (tPA), resulting in a reduced fibrinolytic capacity[45]. Smoking also has a direct effect on serum lipids, decreasing HDL cholesterol levels and increasing LDL cholesterol and triglyceride levels[46].

Evidence shows that stopping smoking substantially reduces the cardiovascular risk, affecting both initial and recurrent coronary heart disease event rates. A recent meta-analysis of 20 clinical trials revealed that smoking cessation resulted in a 36% decrease in all-cause mortality in patients with CVD[47]. Finally, it has been estimated that 50,000 deaths per year in the United States are caused by passive smoke, and most of these deaths are attributable to CVD[48]. A meta-analysis of epidemiological studies related to passive smoking concluded that overall, nonsmokers exposed to environmental smoke had a relative risk of coronary heart disease of 1.25 compared with that of nonsmokers not exposed to environmental smoke[49].

Diabetes

Coronary heart disease is the most common cause of death in patients with diabetes, and the mortality rate in diabetics with coronary heart disease is higher than in nondiabetics[1]. The risk for coronary heart disease is significantly increased with both type 1 and type 2 diabetes[50,51]. The importance of diabetes as a major coronary risk factor is further recognized in the ATP III report, which considers the presence of diabetes equivalent in risk to the presence of clinical CVD[7]. Both microvascular and macrovascular disease are strongly associated with diabetes and appear to be major components of the pathogenesis of atherosclerosis in diabetics.

Diabetes is defined as a fasting blood glucose level of 126 mg or above[52], but the risk for cardiac death increases continuously from impaired fasting glucose (100 to 125 mg/dL, also known as prediabetes) through previously diagnosed diabetes[53]. The increased risk of diabetics can be partially attributed to hyperglycemia, independent of accompanying obesity and atherogenic dyslipidemia.

Thus, in The Diabetes Control and Complication Trial aggressive management of diabetes with tight glycemic control reduced the rate of microvascular complications in type 1 diabetics and reduced major cardiovascular events by 41%[54]. The United Kingdom Prospective Diabetes Study Group reported that intensive blood glucose control reduced diabetes-related microvascular disease in persons with type 2 diabetes, with a strong trend in favor of reduced risk of MI[55] and a significant reduction in diabetes-related death, MI, and all-cause mortality in obese patients[56]. Management of other risk factors has been shown to reduce the incidence of coronary events in diabetics. In particular, aggressive control of BP,[57,58] serum lipids, and lipoproteins has been shown to result in less morbidity and mortality in patients with type 2 diabetes[17,18,26,56,59–62]. With the increasing prevalence of obesity in the United States, the prevalence of diabetes has increased dramatically. The estimated prevalence of 7.3% among U.S. adults in 2000, from the Centers for Disease Control and Prevention Behavioral Risk Factor Surveillance System, represents a 49% increase in prevalence of diabetes in the decade from 1990 to 2000[63]. Nevertheless, recent studies have shown that in patients with impaired fasting glucose, an intensive program of lifestyle change can reduce the incidence of diabetes, even more effectively than use of the antihyperglycemic drug metformin[64,65].

Overweight and Obesity

Obesity is defined as a body mass index (BMI) (weight in kg/height in meters squared) of 30 kg·m^{-2} or above and **overweight** as a BMI of 25 to 29.9 kg·m^{-2} (see Chapter 12). The prevalence of overweight and obesity in the United States has increased substantially in the past decade. The age-adjusted prevalence of overweight and obesity increased from 55.9 in the 1988 to 1994 National Health and Nutrition Examination Survey (NHANES) III to 64.5% in 1999 to 2000. During the same period, the prevalence of obesity increased from 22.9% to 30.5%[66]. Thus, two in three adult Americans are now considered overweight or obese.

Obesity contributes to many adverse health outcomes, and obesity-related conditions are estimated to contribute to 300,000 deaths annually in the United States[67]. Obesity is associated with an accentuated risk of CVD (Fig. 5-6). Analysis of the relationship between obesity and coronary heart disease is difficult because of its association with other risk factors, particularly physical inactivity, hypertension, hyperlipidemia, and diabetes. However, reports from the Framingham study support the independence of obesity as a risk factor for coronary heart disease[68].

No studies have specifically evaluated the effect of weight loss on coronary heart disease events. Comprehensive programs that incorporate behavioral modalities to increase physical activity and improve diet have been shown to induce weight loss sufficient to produce significant cardiovascular health benefits in many obese individuals. In this respect, even modest weight losses of 5% to 10% of initial body weight has positive benefits on coronary heart disease risk factors, and weight loss of this magnitude may be realistic for many individuals[69].

Unfortunately, improvements in coronary heart disease risk factors are not maintained if weight is regained, and most of those who lose a significant amount of weight regain the lost weight within a relatively short period of time. Recognition of the need for long-term and perhaps lifelong treatment has led certain experts to embrace the concept of long-term drug therapy, as is used in other chronic diseases. A national task force on the prevention and treatment of obesity, however, has concluded that until more long-term data are available, pharmacotherapy cannot be recommended for routine use in obese individuals, although it may be helpful in carefully selected patients[70].

Physical Inactivity

Physical inactivity is associated with an increased risk for CVD, and physical activity has been shown to reduce the risk[71–75]. The precise mechanism by which physical inactivity predisposes persons to coronary heart disease has yet to be fully elucidated. Beneficial results of increased physical activity include the following:

1. Improvement of the balance between myocardial oxygen supply and demand at a given submaximal exercise intensity
2. Decreased platelet aggregation and enhanced fibrinolysis
3. Reduced susceptibility to malignant ventricular arrhythmias
4. Improved endothelial function
5. Reduction in obesity

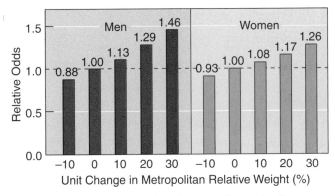

FIGURE 5-6. The relative odds of developing cardiovascular disease corresponding to degree of change in relative weight between age 25 years and entry into the Framingham Study. The odds ratios reflect adjustments for the effects of relative weight at age 25 years and risk factor levels at examination 1. (With permission from Hubert HB, et al: Obesity as an independent risk factor for cardiovascular disease: A 26-year follow-up of participants in the Framingham Heart Study. Circulation 67:968, 1983.)

6. Direct effects (i.e., independent of improvement in body weight and composition) on other coronary risk factors, including lowering of BP, reduction in serum triglyceride levels, increase in serum HDL cholesterol levels, and enhanced glucose tolerance and insulin sensitivity[74–76].

Despite this evidence, millions of adult Americans remain essentially sedentary. Indeed, the number of individuals who are inactive is substantially greater than the number who smoke cigarettes, have hypercholesterolemia, or have hypertension. Thus, the overall effect of stimulating Americans to lead more physically active lifestyles could lower coronary heart disease rates more than by reducing any other single risk factor[77].

Atherogenic Diet

Prospective epidemiologic studies have demonstrated that dietary patterns modify the baseline risk for coronary heart disease of populations[78,79]. Although some of the adverse effects of diet composition undoubtedly relate to established risk factors (e.g., increases in LDL cholesterol and BP with high intakes of dietary saturated fat and sodium, respectively), dietary patterns appear to influence risk beyond the known risk factors. For example, populations that eat diets high in fruits, vegetables, whole grains, and unsaturated fatty acids appear to be at a lower risk for coronary heart disease than can be explained by standard risk factors. Further research is needed to fully clarify the precise nutrients that impact this lower risk for coronary heart disease. Strong candidates are thought to include antioxidant nutrients, folic acid and other B vitamins, omega-3 fatty acids, and other micronutrients[7,79–82].

NONMODIFIABLE NONLIPID RISK FACTORS

Age, male gender, and family history of premature coronary heart disease are nonmodifiable risk factors. At any level of cholesterol, the risk of developing coronary heart disease is greater in older individuals, and at any age, the risk is higher in men than in women[12]. As indicated in Box 5-2, the ATP III considers increased risk to begin at age 45 years in men and age 55 years in women. Age and gender are prominent components in calculating risk using the Framingham risk prediction model. Over age 65 years, women accumulate more points for age than do men[12]. Several prospective studies have established a family history of premature coronary heart disease as an independent risk factor[83,84]. The ATP III report defines a family history as clinical coronary heart disease or sudden death in a first-degree male relative younger than age 55 years or in a first-degree female relative younger than age 65 years[7].

EMERGING RISK FACTORS

Because the major risk factors that appear in Box 5-1 do not predict all cases of coronary heart disease, there has been considerable interest in newer factors that have been termed *emerging risk factors*. Recently, however, analyses of 14 randomized clinical trials[85] and three observational studies[86] have indicated that 80% to 90% of cases of coronary heart disease can be related to one or more of the major risk factors. In addition, a Medline database search for citations on four emerging risk factors has failed to support their use in routine screening for CVD[87]. Nevertheless, because the emerging risk factors appear to identify some otherwise unexplainable cases of CVD and may enhance the predictive capacity of the major coronary risk factors, they continue to be of interest. Similar to the major coronary risk factors, emerging risk factors may be classified as lipid and nonlipid risk factors.

EMERGING LIPID RISK FACTORS

Lipoprotein(a)

Lipoprotein(a), or Lp(a), is formed by linkage of a unique protein, apo(a) to the apolipoprotein B-100 site of LDL cholesterol. Data regarding the risk of CVD associated with elevated lipoprotein(a) levels conflict. Although a meta-analysis of prospective investigations has suggested an independent role for Lp(a) in predicting major coronary events[88], in some prospective studies, Lp(a) levels have failed to identify individuals at risk[89,90]. Lp(a) levels are higher in African Americans than in whites but do not appear to be associated with increased risk in this population[91]. There is some evidence that Lp(a) may act synergistically with LDL cholesterol[92] or with apolipoprotein B[93] to provide a higher degree of cardiovascular risk for these lipid factors. There are a large number of apo(a) isoforms. Their heterogeneity complicates measurement of Lp(a) levels, and they appear to differ in the strength of their association with coronary atherosclerosis[94]. Lifestyle interventions are not effective in reducing Lp(a) levels, and niacin is the only conventional lipid agent known to lower Lp(a)[95]; however, when LDL cholesterol is lowered to target levels, Lp(a) no longer appears to exert an atherogenic effect[92].

Other Emerging Lipid Risk Factors

We have previously discussed triglycerides, lipoprotein remnants, and small LDL particles, which may be considered emerging risk factors because of questions concerning their independence. Apolipoprotein B, the principal protein component of LDL cholesterol, has been proposed as a potentially superior predictor of coronary events, but no convincing body of evidence has been developed to recommend replacement of LDL cholesterol as a therapeutic target. When both LDL cholesterol and triglyceride levels are elevated, apolipoprotein B is disproportionally elevated, but this possibility may be pursued by using non-HDL cholesterol as a secondary target in patients with hypertriglyceridemia[7]. Likewise, apolipoprotein A-1 is the principal protein component of HDL cholesterol, but its measurement, as well as determination of HDL subspecies, does not appear to have added significantly to the value of measuring HDL cholesterol as a coronary risk factor.

Many studies show that the total cholesterol-to-HDL cholesterol ratio is a powerful predictor of risk for coronary heart disease[7]. The Framingham risk score used by ATP III uses both the total cholesterol and HDL cholesterol and, in this way, incorporates the concept of total cholesterol-to-HDL cholesterol ratios into risk assessment. ATP III does not define the total cholesterol-to-HDL cholesterol ratio as a specified lipid target of therapy. According to ATP III, the treatment of ratios will divert priority from specific lipoprotein fractions as targets of therapy[7].

EMERGING NONLIPID RISK FACTORS

Homocysteine

Homocysteine is an amino acid formed during methionine metabolism. In the normal individual, the fasting plasma homocysteine level is 5 to 15 μmol·L^{-1}. Homocysteine levels increase with aging; menopause; smoking; chronic renal insufficiency; vitamin B6, B12, and folate deficiency; hypothyroidism; pernicious anemia; certain carcinomas; and in response to several drugs[96]. In the rare homozygous form of cystathionine B-synthase deficiency seen in children, marked elevations of plasma homocysteine are associated with premature coronary heart disease and thromboemboli. In adults, high levels of homocysteine are associated with endothelial dysfunction, enhanced platelet aggregation, and vascular smooth muscle proliferation. A meta-analysis of 27 studies indicated that increased homocysteine levels are associated with an increased risk of coronary heart disease, peripheral arterial disease, stroke, and venous thromboembolism[97]. Increased homocysteine levels seem to predict mortality in patients with known coronary heart disease[98]. Folate supplementation has been shown to be effective in reducing homocysteine levels[99], but it has not been shown that folate administration will reduce coronary events by reducing homocysteine levels. In fact, a low folate intake has been shown to be associated with coronary events[100], and folate administration has been shown to improve endothelial function independent of any change in plasma homocysteine levels[101]. The clinical usefulness of measuring homocysteine levels as part of cardiovascular risk evaluation remains uncertain.

Thrombogenic and Hemostatic Factors

Because thrombosis is an inherent part of acute coronary events and stroke, evidence of impaired fibrinolysis has been pursued as a potential risk factor. Fibrinolytic activity is regulated by a balance between plasminogen activators (e.g., tPA) and inhibitors (e.g., plasminogen activator inhibitor-1 [PAI-1]). In a meta-analysis of prospective studies, fibrinogen has been shown to have a consistent, statistically significant association with coronary heart disease[102]. Fibrinogen has also been found to be associated with the traditional coronary risk factors[103]. PAI-1 levels have been correlated with risk of coronary events, principally related to insulin resistance as part of the metabolic syndrome[104,105]. Routine measurement of fibrinogen and PAI-1 in risk assessment has not been recommended[7].

Inflammatory Markers

Although other inflammatory markers have been studied, high sensitivity C-reactive protein (hs-CRP) has emerged as the most reliable. CRP is released from the liver in response to inflammation. Because inflammatory cells are present in coronary plaques, it has been postulated that the coronary endothelium may be the source of interleukin-6 and other mediators that stimulate CRP release in patients with coronary heart disease[106]. The stability of hs-CRP in frozen serum has allowed its measurement in stored blood samples of participants in the major epidemiologic studies. The blood level of CRP has been shown to be comparable or superior to other risk factors in its ability to predict coronary events[107] and to add to the predictive capacity of lipid factors such as the cholesterol-to-HDL ratio in both men (Fig. 5-7)[108] and women[109]. CRP levels are increased in smokers, obese and physically inactive individuals, diabetics, and users of HRT[110–112]. The initiation of lifestyle changes has been shown to reduce CRP levels[113]. Finally, CRP levels may be lowered by aspirin[114] or statin[115,116] therapy. As a result, it is not clear that measurement of CRP is useful in patients with CVD who have already initiated lifestyle changes and are taking aspirin and a statin. Rather, measuring CRP may be of benefit when added to other risk factor assessment in the primary prevention of vascular disease. Comprehensive guidelines on the application of hs-CRP to clinical and public health practice were recently published by a joint panel of the American Heart Association and the Centers for Disease Control and Prevention[117].

IMPAIRED FASTING GLUCOSE

As earlier mentioned, the risk for cardiac death increases continuously from impaired fasting glucose (i.e., fasting glucose = 100 to 125 mg·dL^{-1}) through previously diagnosed diabetes[53]. Although some researchers view impaired fasting glucose to be an independent risk factor for coronary heart disease, the strong association between impaired fasting glucose and other risk factors of the metabolic syndrome casts doubt on the independent predictive power of impaired fasting glucose[7]. Thus, the ATP III identifies impaired fasting glucose as one component of the metabolic syndrome that signifies the need for more intensive lifestyle intervention, namely, weight reduction and increased physical activity[7].

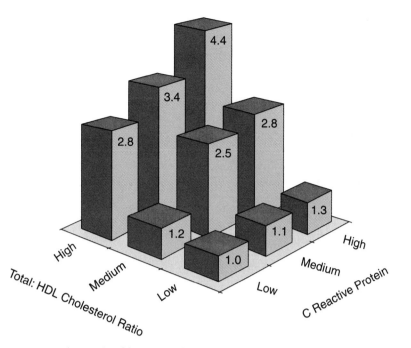

FIGURE 5-7. Relative risks of first myocardial infarction among apparently healthy men associated with high, middle, and low tertiles of the total cholesterol-to-high-density lipoprotein (HDL) ratio and high, middle, and low tertiles of C-reactive protein. (Adapted with permission from Ridker PM, Glynn RJ, Henneckens CH: C-reactive protein adds to the predictive value of total and HDL cholesterol in determining risk of first mycoardial infarction. Circulation 97:2007–2011, 1998.)

Subclinical Atherosclerotic Disease and Plaque Burden

Individuals with advanced subclinical atherosclerosis are at greater risk for coronary events than are those with less severe atherosclerosis. Thus, subclinical evidence of plaque formation may be considered a risk factor for development of coronary events. In the conventional sense, plaque burden is not a risk factor for the disease; rather, it is the disease. However, disease demonstrated in extra-coronary vascular beds (e.g., in the carotid arteries) and coronary calcium score measured by electron beam computed tomography (EBCT) may be used as surrogate markers of plaque burden. There is a high correlation between the severity of atherosclerosis in the coronary and carotid arteries[118]. Thus, measurement of the thickness of the carotid intima by ultrasonography predicts major coronary events independent of other risk factors[119]. EBCT may be used to measure the amount of calcium in the coronary arteries, and the calcium score reflects the extent of disease[120]. A recent prospective study suggests that EBCT may be highly effective in predicting cardiovascular events[121]. Although neither carotid ultrasound nor EBCT is recommended for routine screening, their use may complement risk assessment using the conventional risk factors. According to ATP III, other diagnostic tests that can be used to identify persons at high risk for coronary heart disease include the ankle–brachial BP index and various tests for myocardial ischemia[7]. Regarding the latter, in the ATP III guidelines, the presence of myocardial ischemia appropriately identified by stress testing qualifies as a diagnosis of coronary heart disease[7].

The Metabolic Syndrome

The metabolic syndrome, first identified in the 1980s[122] consists of a constellation of metabolic risk factors, namely, abdominal obesity, insulin resistance or glucose intolerance, atherogenic dyslipidemia, hypertension, and a prothrombotic and proinflammatory state. The ATP III report defined the syndrome as having at least three of the five characteristics that are listed in Box 5-2[7]. The age-adjusted prevalence of the metabolic syndrome was estimated from the NHANES III survey for the years 1988 to 1994 was 23.7%, or one in four of adult Americans[123]. The risk of having the metabolic syndrome increases steeply among individuals classified as being overweight or obese[124]. As a result, given the marked increase in the prevalence of overweight and obesity in the United States that has occurred in recent years[63,66], the prevalence of the metabolic syndrome is likely to be even greater than previously estimated. The metabolic syndrome brings together multiple known coronary risk factors and, thus, is a potent predictor of cardiovascular risk. In the West of Scotland Coronary Prevention Study, risk increased as the number of metabolic syndrome factors increased so that men with four of five factors had a 3.7-fold increased risk of coronary events and a 24-fold increased risk of developing diabetes[125]. The coronary event risk for men with the metabolic syndrome in this trial was intermediate between that for men with diabetes and those without the metabolic syndrome. Follow-up studies show both increased cardiovascular and all-cause mortality rates for men with the metabolic syndrome[126].

Elevated CRP levels have been found in men and women with the metabolic syndrome and have been shown to add independently to the risk of coronary events and of developing diabetes[125,127,128]. A recent study of various ethnic groups has emphasized the contribution to increased cardiovascular risk in individuals with the metabolic syndrome of fibrinolytic dysfunction, as manifested by elevated PAI-1 levels[129]. Elevation of both PAI-1 and CRP levels in patients with the metabolic syndrome may be attributed to their excess of adipose tissue, which can secrete PAI-1 as well as inflammatory cytokines[130], and to recent evidence that CRP may stimulate the expression and activity of PAI-1[131].

The basic therapeutic approach to patients with the metabolic syndrome should be an organized program of lifestyle change, focusing on increased physical activity and weight reduction. Lifestyle management has been shown to improve insulin resistance and prevent the onset of diabetes[64,65]. A secondary approach is pharmacologic treatment of hypertension and the metabolic components, including atherogenic dyslipidemia. For patients who also have elevated LDL cholesterol levels in addition to the atherogenic dyslipidemia of the metabolic syndrome, statin therapy has been shown to reduce cardiovascular risk to a greater extent than for patients with isolated LDL cholesterol elevations[132].

Other Possible Risk Factors

Although not included in the ATP III risk factor classification scheme, psychosocial factors and postmenopausal status or use of HRT have been linked to the risk for coronary heart disease. The psychosocial factors associated with risk of coronary heart disease include the type A personality, hostility, depression, chronic stress produced by situations with high demand and low control, and social isolation (Fig. 5-8)[4]. Psychosocial factors are postulated to accentuate the risk via two major mechanisms. First, they may exert a detrimental influence by direct mechanisms that primarily include neuroendocrine effects, such as changes in catecholamine and serotonin levels. Second, they may indirectly accentuate risk by influencing adherence to lifestyle recommendations and compliance with drug therapy. Interventions of potential benefit include behavior modification, meditation, exercise, and (when indicated) pharmacotherapy.

Coronary heart disease manifests itself approximately a decade later in women than in men. Nevertheless, it remains the leading cause of death among women in the United States. The role of HRT in postmenopausal

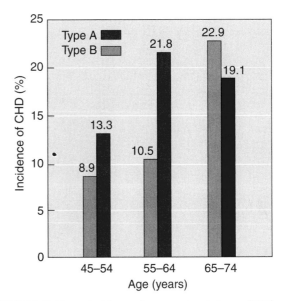

FIGURE 5-8. Eight-year incidence of coronary heart disease (CHD) among men by the Framingham types A and B behavior patterns. (With permission from Haynes SG, Feinleib M, Kannel WB: The relationship of psychosocial factors to coronary heart disease in the Framingham Study. III. Eight-year incidence of coronary heart disease. Am J Epidemiol 111:37, 1980.)

women is uncertain. The postmenopausal estrogen–progesterone intervention trials have established the efficacy of HRT in increasing HDL cholesterol levels and decreasing levels of LDL cholesterol, total cholesterol, and fibrinogen[133]. However, trials of HRT have shown no benefit for coronary heart disease endpoints and have even suggested detrimental effects[134,135]. As a result, the use of HRT is not recommended as a treatment strategy for the primary or secondary prevention of coronary heart disease or coronary events[136].

Global Risk Assessment in Asymptomatic Individuals

Patients with known coronary heart disease are at heightened risk for future coronary events, and this risk can be substantially reduced by well-accepted secondary prevention strategies[137]. In contrast to secondary prevention, primary prevention aims to prevent new-onset coronary heart disease. If efforts at prevention are delayed until advanced coronary atherosclerosis has developed, the U.S. public will continue to suffer from a heavy burden of coronary heart disease[7]. In particular, waiting until a diagnosis of coronary heart disease is made before initiating risk factor modification will miss the immense opportunity to prevent coronary heart disease in individuals whose first presentation is sudden death or disability. Approximately one third of people who suffer an acute MI die within 24 hours, and many survivors have serious residual morbidity, including congestive heart failure, angina, and an increased risk of sudden death. According to ATP III, this

BOX 5-3 | **Framingham Tables**

Estimate of 10-Year Risk for Men
(Framingham Point Scores)

A.

Age, y	Points
20–34	−9
35–39	−4
40–44	0
45–49	3
50–54	6
55–59	8
60–64	10
65–69	11
70–74	12
75–79	13

B.

Total Cholesterol, mg·dL^{-1}	Age 20–39	Age 40–49	Age 50–59	Age 60–69	Age (y) 70–79
< 160	0	0	0	0	0
160–199	4	3	2	1	0
200–239	7	5	3	1	0
240–279	9	6	4	2	1
≥ 280	11	8	5	3	1

C.

	Age 20–39	Age 40–49	Age 50–59	Age 60–69	Age (y) 70–79
Nonsmoker	0	0	0	0	0
Smoker	8	5	3	1	1

D.

HDL, mg·dL^{-1}	Points
≥ 60	−1
50–59	0
40–49	1
< 40	2

E.

Systolic BP, mmHg	If Untreated	If Treated
< 120	0	0
120–129	0	1
130–139	1	2
140–159	1	2
≥ 160	2	3

Point Total	10-Year Risk, %
< 0	< 1
0	1
1	1
2	1
3	1
4	1
5	2
6	2
7	3
8	4
9	5
10	6
11	8
12	10
13	12
14	16
15	20
16	25
≥ 17	≥ 30

Estimate of 10-Year Risk for Women
(Framingham Point Scores)

A.

Age, y	Points
20–34	−7
35–39	−3
40–44	0
45–49	3
50–54	6
55–59	8
60–64	10
65–69	12
70–74	14
75–79	16

B.

Total Cholesterol, mg·dL^{-1}	Age 20–39	Age 40–49	Age 50–59	Age 60–69	Age (y) 70–79
< 160	0	0	0	0	0
160–199	4	3	2	1	1
200–239	8	6	4	2	1
240–279	11	8	5	3	2
≥ 280	13	10	7	4	2

C.

	Age 20–39	Age 40–49	Age 50–59	Age 60–69	Age (y) 70–79
Nonsmoker	0	0	0	0	0
Smoker	9	7	4	2	1

D.

HDL, mg·dL^{-1}	Points
≥ 60	−1
50–59	0
40–49	1
< 40	2

E.

Systolic BP, mmHg	If Untreated	If Treated
< 120	0	0
120–129	1	3
130–139	2	4
140–159	3	5
≥ 160	4	6

Point Total	10-Year Risk, %
< 9	< 1
9	1
10	1
11	1
12	1
13	2
14	2
15	3
16	4
17	5
18	6
19	8
20	11
21	14
22	17
23	22
25	27
≥ 25	≥ 30

Source: Third Report of the National Cholesterol Education Program (NCEP) Expert Panel on Detection, Evaluation, and Treatment of High Blood Cholesterol in Adults. (Adult Treatment Panel III): Bethesda, MD: National Institutes of Health, National Heart, Lung, and Blood Institute, NIH Publication No. 02-5215; September 2002.

observation argues strongly for primary prevention of coronary heart disease[7].

It should be noted, however, that in the setting of primary prevention, some experts consider the precise role of aggressive strategies to reduce risk to be less clear in some instances. The controversy regarding intensive primary prevention strategies can be attributed to two major observations: First, the absolute cardiovascular risk in many asymptomatic individuals with coronary heart disease risk factors is relatively low, making aggressive prevention strategies less cost effective than in higher risk individuals. Second, most coronary events in a community occur in individuals with only mild to moderate elevation of risk factors. The individuals with marked elevation of risk factors, such as cholesterol or BP, constitute only a minority of the total population. Therefore, strategies aimed at identifying and aggressively managing high-risk individuals have a beneficial effect for the individual but only minimal usefulness in preventing cardiovascular events for the community. It is for this reason that the ATP III guidelines support two complementary approaches to primary prevention, namely, population strategies and clinical strategies[7].

By using the concept of assessment of global risk (i.e., risk for coronary heart disease based on multiple risk factors), risk prediction models can provide a quantitative estimate of the risk of coronary events. For example, patients with stable angina have an average risk of nonfatal MI or death of approximately 20% over the next 10 years[138]. Such individuals, whose event rate is expected to be 20% or greater in 10 years, are considered high risk, and aggressive secondary prevention strategies are clearly appropriate. Thus, in an individual with no known coronary heart disease but in whom the risk prediction model suggests a 10-year event rate of 20% or greater, it is logical to consider the same aggressive strategies in an attempt at primary prevention. Clinical guidelines for the primary and secondary prevention of coronary heart disease using a combination of lifestyle modification and, if clinically indicated, appropriate drug therapy have been published by the American Heart Association[137,139,140].

A global risk prediction model takes into account multiple major risk factors for coronary heart disease and gives a quantitative estimate of coronary event rate. The most widely used global risk prediction instrument is the Framingham model, which incorporates age, gender, BP, diabetes, total cholesterol, HDL cholesterol, and cigarette smoking[12]. In the original Framingham risk prediction model, LVH was also included[141]. However, in the more recent Framingham prediction model, LVH was excluded because it was thought that hypertension is a confounding variable for LVH and that adding LVH and BP might overpredict risk[12]. Although the Framingham model was derived from the white population of Framingham, Massachusetts, its accuracy has been verified in other populations in the United States, including Hispanics, African

Americans, and Hawaiians. The Framingham prediction model has most recently been revised for use as part of the ATP III cholesterol management guidelines (Box 5-3)[7].

Summary

Coronary heart disease has been and continues to be a major public health problem in the United States and other Western countries. Even though there are many risk factors for coronary heart disease, the major risk factors continue to be highly prevalent, and aggressive primary and secondary prevention (see Table 30–1) strategies aimed at controlling these risk factors are likely to lead to further decreases in the mortality and morbidity from this lethal disease. Aggressive primary prevention strategies may be most appropriate for individuals at high risk for coronary heart disease, as indicated by the presence of vascular disease in noncoronary vascular beds, asymptomatic coronary atherosclerosis detected by EBCT, type 2 diabetes, and a 20% or higher risk of having coronary events based on Framingham prediction models. The universal strategy of lifetime primary prevention can be applied at a community level irrespective of the individual coronary risk profile; this strategy includes smoking cessation, correct nutrition, weight management, and moderate-intensity aerobic exercise for at least 30 minutes on most days of the week.

REFERENCES

1. American Heart Association: Heart Disease and Stroke Statistics Update. Dallas: American Heart Association; 2003.
2. Miller M, Vogel RA: The practice of coronary artery disease prevention, 1st ed. Baltimore: Williams & Wilkins; 1996:2.
3. Kannel WB, Dawber TR, Kagan A, et al: Factors of risk in the development of coronary heart disease: Six-year follow-up experience. Ann Intern Med 55:33–50, 1961.
4. Pasternak RC, Grundy SM, Levy D, Thompson PD: Spectrum of risk factors for coronary heart disease. J Am Coll Cardiol 27:978–990, 1996.
5. Castelli WB, Anderson K, Wilson PW, Levy D: Lipids and risk of coronary heart disease: The Framingham Study. Ann Epidemiol 2:23–28, 1992.
6. Stamler J, Stamler R, Neaton JD: Blood pressure, systolic and diastolic, and cardiovascular risk: Years population data. Arch Intern Med 153:598–615, 1993.
7. Third Report of the National Cholesterol Education Program (NCEP) Expert Panel on Detection, Evaluation, and Treatment of High Blood Cholesterol in Adults. (Adult Treatment Panel III): Bethesda, MD: National Institutes of Health, National Heart, Lung, and Blood Institute, NIH Publication No. 02-5215; September 2002.
8. MRFIT Research Group: Multiple risk factor changes and mortality results. JAMA 248:1465–1477, 1982.
9. American Heart Association, National Heart, Lung and Blood Institute: The cholesterol facts: A summary of the evidence relating to dietary fat, serum cholesterol and coronary heart disease. Circulation 81:1721–1733, 1990.
10. Stamler J, Wentworth D, Neaton JD: Is relationship between serum cholesterol and risk of premature death from coronary heart disease continuous and graded? JAMA 256:2823–2828, 1986.
11. Lloyd-Jones DM, Larson MG, Beiser A, Levy D: Lifetime risk of developing coronary heart disease. Lancet 353:89–92, 1999.

12. Wilson PWF, D'Agostino RB, Levy D, et al: Prediction of coronary heart disease using risk factor categories. Circulation 97:1837–1847, 1998.

13. Sacks F, Pfeffer M, Moye L, et al: Effect of pravastatin on coronary events after myocardial infarction in patients with average cholesterol levels. N Engl J Med 335:1001–1009, 1996.

14. Tonkin AM: Management of the long term intervention with pravastatin in ischemic heart disease study. Am J Cardiol 76:107C–112C, 1995.

15. Scandinavian Simvastatin Survival Study Group: Baseline serum cholesterol and treatment effect in the Scandinavian Simvastatin Survival Study. Lancet 345:1274–1275, 1995.

16. Shepherd J: The West of Scotland Coronary Prevention Study: A trial of cholesterol reduction in Scottish men. Am J Cardiol 76:113C–117C, 1995.

17. Bowns JR, Clearfield M, Weiss S, et al: Primary prevention of acute coronary events with lovastatin in men and women with average cholesterol levels. Results of AFCAPS/TEXCAPS. JAMA 279: 1615–1622, 1998.

18. Long-Term Intervention with Pravastatin in Ischaemic Disease (LIPID) Study Group: Prevention of cardiovascular events and death with pravastatin in patients with coronary heart disease and a broad range of initial cholesterol levels. N Engl J Med 339:1349–1357, 1998.

19. Heart Protection Study Collaborative Group: MRC/BHF Heart Protection Study of cholesterol lowering with simvastatin in 20, 536 high-risk individuals: a randomized placebo-controlled trial. Lancet 360:7–22, 2002.

20. Sever PS, Dahlof B, Poulter NR, et al: Prevention of coronary and stroke events with atorvastatin in hypertensive patients who have average or lower-than-average cholesterol concentrations, in the Anglo-Scandinavian Cardiac Outcomes Trial-Lipid Lowering Arm (ASCOT-LLA): A multicentre randomized controlled trial. Lancet 361: 1149–1158, 2003.

21. Harper CR, Jacobson TA: New prospective on the management of low levels of high density lipoprotein cholesterol. Arch Intern Med 159:1049–1057, 1999.

22. Gordon T, Castelli WP, Hjortland MC, et al: High density lipoprotein as a protective factor against coronary heart disease. Am J Med 62:707–714, 1997.

23. Tall AR: Plasma high density lipoproteins. J Clin Invest 86:379–384, 1990.

24. Maier JA, Barcengi HL, Pagan IF, et al: The protective role of high density lipoprotein on oxidized low density lipoprotein induced U937/endothelial cell interactions. Eur J Biochem 221:35–41, 1994.

25. Bisoendial RJ, Hoving GK, Levels JHM, et al: Restoration of endothelial function by increasing high-density lipoprotein in subjects with isolated low high-density lipoprotein. Circulation 107:2944–2948, 2003.

26. Rubins HB, Robins SJ, Collins D, et al: Gemfibrozil for the secondary prevention of coronary heart disease in men with low levels of HDL cholesterol. N Engl J Med 341:410, 1999.

27. The BIP Study Group: Secondary prevention by raising HDL cholesterol and reducing triglycerides in patients with coronary artery disease: the Bezafibrate Infarction Prevention (BIP) study. Circulation 102:21–27, 2000.

28. Austin MA, Hokanson JE, Edwards KL: Hypertriglyceridemia as a cardiovascular risk factor. Am J Cardiol 81:7B–12B, 1998.

29. Kris-Etherton PM, Harris WS, Appel LG for the Nutrition Committee: AHA scientific statement: Fish consumption, fish oil, omega-3 fatty acids, and cardiovascular disease. Circulation 106:2747–2757, 2002.

30. Austin MA, King M-C, Vranizan KM, Krauss RM: Atherogenic lipoprotein phenotype: a proposed genetic marker for coronary heart disease risk. Circulation 82:495–506, 1990.

31. Grundy SM: Hypertriglyceridemia, atherogenic dyslipidemia, and the metabolic syndrome. Am J Cardiol 81(suppl 4A):18B–25B, 1998.

32. Kreisberg RA: Diabetic dyslipidemia. Am J Cardiol 82:67U–73U, 1998.

33. Gardner CD, Fortmann SP, Krauss RM: Association of small low-density lipoprotein particles with the incidence of coronary artery disease in men and women. JAMA 276:875–881, 1996.

34. Lamarche B, Tchernof A, Moorjani S, et al: Small, dense low-density lipoprotein particles as a predictor of the risk of ischemic heart disease in men. Prospective results from the Quebec Cardiovascular Study. Circulation 95:69–75, 1997.

35. Chobanian AV, Bakris GL, Black HR, et al: The Seventh Report of the Joint National Committee on Prevention, Detection, Evaluation, and Treatment of High Blood Pressure. The JNC 7 Report. JAMA 289:2560–2572, 2003.

36. Lewington S, Clarke R, Qizilbash N, et al: Age-specific relevance of usual blood pressure to vascular mortality. Lancet 360:1903–1913, 2002.

37. Neal B, MacMahon S, Chapman N: Effects of ACE inhibitors, calcium antagonists, and other blood pressure-lowering drugs. Lancet 356:1955–1964, 2000.

38. Ogden LG, He J, Lydick E, Whelton PK: Long-term absolute benefit of lowering blood pressure in hypertensive patients according to the JNC VI risk stratification. Hypertension 35:539–543, 2000.

39. Psaty BM, Lumley T, Furberg CD, et al: Health outcomes associated with various antihypertensive therapies used as first-line agents. A network meta-analysis. JAMA 289:2534–2544, 2003.

40. McGinnis JM, Foege WH: Actual causes of death in the United States. JAMA 270:2207–2212, 1993.

41. McGill HC Jr: The cardiovascular pathology of smoking. Am Heart J 115:250–257, 1988.

42. Willett WC, Green A, Stampfe MJ, et al: Relative and absolute excess risk of coronary heart disease among women who smoke cigarettes. N Engl J Med 317:1303–1309, 1987.

43. Reinders JH, Brinkman HA, VanMourik JA, DeGroot PG: Cigarette smoke impairs endothelial cell prostacyclin production. Atherosclerosis 6:15–23, 1986.

44. Allen RA, Klauf TC, Brommer EJ: Effect of chronic smoking on fibrinolysis. Atherosclerosis 5:443–450, 1985.

45. Newby DE, McLeod AL, Uren NG, et al: Impaired coronary tissue plasminogen activator release is associated with coronary atherosclerosis and cigarette smoking. Direct link between endothelial dysfunction and atherothrombosis. Circulation 103:1936–1941, 2001.

46. Craig WY, Palomaik GE, Haddow JE: Cigarette smoking and serum lipid and lipoprotein concentrations: An analysis of published data. BMJ 298:784–788, 1989.

47. Critchley JA, Capewell S: Mortality risk reduction associated with smoking cessation in patients with coronary heart disease. JAMA 290:86–97, 2003.

48. Glantz SA, Parmley WW: Passive smoking and heart disease: Epidemiology, physiology and biochemistry. Circulation 83:1–12, 1991.

49. He J, Vupputuri S, Allen K, et al: Passive smoking and the risk of coronary heart disease—a meta-analysis of epidemiologic studies. N Engl J Med 340:920–926, 1999.

50. Kannel WB, McGee DL: Diabetes and cardiovascular disease: The Framingham Study. JAMA 241:2035–2038, 1979.

51. Haffner SM, Lehto S, Ronnemaa T, et al: Mortality from coronary heart disease in subjects with type II diabetes and nondiabetic subjects with and without prior myocardial infarction. N Engl J Med 339:229–234, 1998.

52. Gavin JR III, Alberti KGMM, Davidson MB, et al: Report of the Expert Committee on the Diagnosis and Classification of Diabetes Mellitus. Diabetes Care 21(suppl):S5–S19, 1998.

53. Muhlestein JB, Anderson JL, Horne BD, et al: Effect of fasting glucose levels on mortality rate in patients with and without diabetes mellitus and coronary artery disease undergoing percutaneous coronary intervention. Am Heart J 146:351–358, 2003.

54. DCCT Research Group: The effect of intensive treatment of diabetes on the development and progression of long term complications of insulin dependent diabetes mellitus. N Engl J Med 329: 977–986, 1993.

55. UKPDS Group: Intensive blood glucose control with sulfonylureas or insulin compared with conventional treatment and risk of complications in patients with type II diabetes. Lancet 352:837–853, 1998.

56. UKPDS Group: Effect of intensive glucose control with metformin on complications in overweight patients with type II diabetes. Lancet 352:854–865, 1998.

57. UKPDS Group: Tight blood pressure control and risk of macro and microvascular complications in type II diabetes. BMJ 317:703–713, 1998.

58. Hanson I, Jarchett A, Carruths SG, et al: Effects of intensive blood pressure lowering and low dose aspirin in patients with hypertension, the HOT Study Group. Lancet 351:1755–1762, 1998.

59. Haffner SM, Alexander CM, Cook TJ, et al. for the Scandinavian Simvastatin Survival Study Group: Reduced coronary events in simvastatin-treated patients with coronary heart disease and diabetes or impaired fasting glucose levels: Subgroup analyses from the Scandinavian Simvastatin Survival Study. Arch Intern Med 159:2661–2667, 1999.

60. Goldberg RB, Mellies MJ, Sacks FM, et al. for the CARE Investigators: Cardiovascular events and their reduction with pravastatin in diabetic and glucose-intolerant myocardial infarction survivors with average cholesterol levels: subgroup analyses in the Cholesterol and Recurrent Events (CARE) trial. Circulation 98:2513, 1998.

61. Hoogwerf BJ, Waness A, Cressman M, et al: Effects of aggressive cholesterol lowering and low-dose anticoagulation on clinical and angiographic outcomes in patients with diabetes: The Post Coronary Artery Bypass Graft trial. Diabetes 48:1289–1294, 1999.

62. Koskinen P, Manttari M, Manninen V, et al: Coronary heart disease incidence in NIDDM patients in the Helsinki Heart Study. Diabetes Care 15:820–825, 1992.

63. Makdad AH, Bowman BA, Ford ES, et al: The continuing epidemic of obesity and diabetes in the United States. JAMA 286:1195–1200, 2001.

64. Tuomilehto J, Lindstrom J, Eriksson JG, et al. for the Finnish Diabetes Prevention Study Group: Prevention of type 2 diabetes mellitus by changes in lifestyle among subjects with impaired glucose tolerance. N Engl J Med 344:1343–1350, 2001.

65. The Diabetes Prevention Program Research Group: Reduction in the incidence of type 2 diabetes with lifestyle intervention or metformin. N Engl J Med 346:393–403, 2002.

66. Flegal KM, Carroll MD, Ogden CL, Johnson CL: Prevalence and trends in obesity among U.S. adults, 1999–2000. JAMA 288:1723–1727, 2002.

67. Allison DB, Fontaine KR, Stevens J, VanItallie TB: Annual deaths attributable to obesity in the United States. JAMA 282:1530–1538, 1999.

68. Hubert HB, Feineib M, McNamara PM, et al: Obesity as an independent risk factor for cardiovascular disease: A 26-year follow-up of participants in the Framingham Heart Study. Circulation 67:968–977, 1983.

69. Blackburn GL, Rosofsky W: Making the connection between weight loss, dieting, and health: The 10% solution. Weight Control Dig 2: 121–127, 1992.

70. National Task Force on the Prevention and Treatment of Obesity. Long-term pharmacotherapy in the management of obesity. JAMA 276:1907–1915, 1996.

71. Leon AS, Connett J, Jacobs DR Jr, Rauramaa R: Leisure-time physical activity levels and risk of coronary heart disease and death: the Multiple Risk Factor Intervention Trial. JAMA 258:2388–2395, 1987.

72. Paffenbarger RS Jr, Hyde RT, Wing AL, et al: The association of changes in physical activity level and other lifestyle characteristics with mortality among men. N Engl J Med 328:538–545, 1993.

73. Hu FB, Stampfer MJ, Colditz GA, et al: Physical activity and risk of stroke in women. JAMA 283:2961–2967, 2000.

74. Pate RR, Pratt M, Blair SN, et al: Physical activity and public health: A recommendation from the Centers for Disease Control and Prevention and the American College of Sports Medicine. JAMA 273: 402–407, 1995.

75. Thompson PD, Buchner D, Pina IL, et al: AHA scientific statement: Exercise and physical activity in the prevention and treatment of atherosclerotic cardiovascular disease. Circulation 107:3109–3116, 2003.

76. LaMonte MJ, Eisenman PA, Adams TD, et al: Cardiorespiratory fitness and coronary heart disease risk factors. The LDS Hospital Fitness Institute Cohort. Circulation 102:1623–1628, 2000.

77. Caspersen CJ, Heath GW: The risk factor concept of coronary heart disease (pp. 151–167). In ACSM's Resource Manual for Guidelines for Exercise Testing and Prescription, 2nd ed. Philadelphia: Lea & Febiger; 1993

78. U.S. Department of Agriculture and U.S. Department of Health and Human Services: Nutrition and Your Health: Dietary Guidelines for Americans, 5th ed. Home and Garden Bulletin no. 232. Washington, D.C.: U.S. Department of Agriculture; 2000.

79. Krauss RM, Eckel RH, Howard B, et al: AHA Dietary Guidelines: Revision 2000: A statement for healthcare professionals from the Nutrition Committee of the American Heart Association. Circulation 102:2284–2299, 2000.

80. DeLogeril M, Salen P, Martin JL, et al: Mediterranean diet, traditional risk factors and the rate of cardiovascular complications after myocardial infarction: final report of the Lyon Diet Heart Study. Circulation 99:779–785, 1999.

81. Kris-Etherton P, Daniels SR, Eckel RH, et al: Summary of the scientific conference on dietary fatty acids and cardiovascular health. Conference summary from the Nutrition Committee of the American Heart Association. Circulation 103:1034–1039, 2001.

82. Kromhout D, Menotti A, Kesteloot H, Sans S. Prevention of coronary heart disease by diet and lifestyle. Evidence from prospective cross-cultural, cohort, and intervention studies. Circulation 105:893–898, 2002.

83. Pankow JS, Folsom AR, Province MA, et al. on behalf of the Atherosclerosis Risk in Communities Investigators and Family Heart Study Research Group: Family history of coronary heart disease and hemostatic variables in middle-aged adults. Thromb Haemost 77: 87–93, 1997.

84. Williams RR, Hunt SC, Heiss G, et al: Usefulness of cardiovascular family history data for population-based preventive medicine and medical research (the Health Family Tree Study and the NHLBI Family Heart Study). Am J Cardiol 87:129–135, 2001.

85. Khot UN, Khot MB, Bajzer CT, et al: Prevalence of conventional risk factors in patients with coronary heart disease. JAMA 290: 898–904, 2003.

86. Greenland P, Knoll MD, Stamler J, et al: Major risk factors as antecedents of fatal and nonfatal coronary heart disease events. JAMA 290:891–897, 2003.

87. Hackam DG, Anand SS: Emerging risk factors for atherosclerotic vascular disease. A critical review of the evidence. JAMA 290: 932–940, 2003.

88. Danesh J, Collins R, Peto R: Lipoprotein(a) and coronary heart disease. Circulation 102:1082–1085, 2000.

89. Ridker PM, Henneken CM, Stampfer MJ: Prospective study of lipoprotein-a and the risk of myocardial infarction. JAMA 270: 2195–2199, 1993.

90. Marcovina SM, Koschinsky ML: Lipoprotein(a) as a risk factor for coronary artery disease. Am J Cardiol 82:57U–66U, 1998.

91. Moliterno DJ, Jokinen EV, Miserez AR, et al: No association between plasma lipoprotein(a) concentrations and the presence or absence of coronary atherosclerosis in African Americans. Arterioscler Thromb Vasc Biol 15:850–855, 1995.

92. Maher VMG, Brown BG, Marcovina SM, et al: Effects of lowering elevated LDL cholesterol on the cardiovascular risk of lipoprotein(a). JAMA 274:1771–1774, 1995.

93. Cantin B, Gagnon F, Moorjami S, et al: Is lipoprotein(a) an independent risk factor for ischemic heart disease in men? The Quebec Cardiovascular Study. J Am Coll Cardiol 31:519–525, 1998.
94. Kronenberg F, Kronenberg MF, Kiechl S, et al: Role of lipoprotein(a) and apolipoprotein(a) phenotype in atherogenesis: prospective results from the Bruneck study. Circulation 100:1154–1160, 1999.
95. Carlson LA, Hamsten A, Asplund A: Pronounced lowering of serum levels of lipoprotein Lp(a) in hyperlipidaemic subjects treated with nicotinic acid. J Intern Med 226:271–276, 1989.
96. Welch GN, Loscalzo J: Homocysteine and atherothrombosis. N Engl J Med 338:1042–1050, 1998.
97. Boushey CJ, Beresford AS, Omenn GS, Motulsky AG: A quantitative assessment of plasma homocysteine as a risk factor for vascular disease. JAMA 274:1049–1057, 1995/
98. Nygar DO, Nordrehaug JE, Refsum H, et al: Plasma homocysteine levels and mortality in patients with coronary artery disease. N Engl J Med 337:230–236, 1997.
99. Jacques PF, Selhub J, Bostom AG, et al: The effect of folic acid fortification on plasma folate and total homocysteine concentrations. N Engl J Med 340:1449–1454, 1999.
100. Voutilainen S, Rissanen TH, Virtanen J, et al: Low dietary folate intake is associated with an excess incidence of acute coronary events. The Kuopio Ischemic Heart Disease Risk Factor Study. Circulation 103:2674–2680, 2001.
101. Doshi SN, McDowell IFW, Moat SJ, et al: Folic acid improves endothelial function in coronary artery disease via mechanisms largely independent of homocysteine lowering. Circulation 105:22–36, 2002.
102. Danesh J, Collins R, Appleby P, Peto R: Association of fibrinogen, C-reactive protein, albumin, or leucocyte count with coronary heart disease. Meta-analyses of prospective studies. JAMA 279:1477–1482, 1998.
103. Stec JJ, Silbershatz H, Tofler GH, et al: Association of fibrinogen with cardiovascular disease in the Framingham offspring population. Circulation 102:1634–1638, 2000.
104. Juhan-Vague I, Pyke SDM, Alessi MC, et al. on behalf of the ECAT Study Group: Fibrinolytic factors and the risk of myocardial infarction or sudden death in patients with angina pectoris. Circulation 94:2057–2063, 1996.
105. Kohler HP, Grant PJ: Plasminogen-activator inhibitor type 1 and coronary artery disease. N Engl J Med 342:1792–1801, 2001.
106. Rader DJ: Inflammatory markers of coronary risk. N Engl J Med 343:1179–1182, 2000.
107. Ridker PM, Rifai N, Rose L, et al: Comparison of C-reactive protein and low-density lipoprotein cholesterol levels in the prediction of first cardiovascular events. N Engl J Med 347:1557–1565, 2002.
108. Ridker PM, Glynn RJ, Hennekens CH: C-reactive protein adds to the predictive value of total and HDL cholesterol in determining risk of first myocardial infarction. Circulation 97:2007–2011, 1998.
109. Ridker PM, Hennekens CH, Buring JE, Rifai N: C-reactive protein and other markers of inflammation in the prediction of cardiovascular disease in women. N Engl J Med 342:836–843, 2000.
110. Tracy RP, Psaty BM, Macy E, et al: Lifetime smoking exposure affects the association of C-reactive protein with cardiovascular disease risk factors and subclinical disease in healthy elderly subjects. Arterioscler Thromb Vasc Biol 17:2167–2176, 1997.
111. Ford ES: Body mass index, diabetes, and C-reactive protein among U.S. adults. Diabetes Care 22:1971–1977, 1999.
112. Ridker PM, Hennekens CH, Rifai N, et al: Hormone replacement therapy and increased plasma concentration of C-reactive protein. Circulation 100:713–716, 1999.
113. Ford ES: Does exercise reduce inflammation? Physical activity and C-reactive protein among U.S. adults. Epidemiology 13:561–568, 2002.
114. Ridker PM, Cushman M, Stampfer MJ, et al: Inflammation, aspirin, and the risk of cardiovascular disease in apparently healthy men. N Engl J Med 336:973–979, 1997.
115. Ridker PM, Rifai N, Pfeffer MA, et al: Inflammation, pravastatin, and the risk of coronary events after myocardial infarction in patients with average cholesterol levels. Circulation 98:839–844, 1998.
116. Albert MA, Danielson E, Rifai N, Ridker PM for the PRINCE Investigators: Effect of statin therapy on C-reactive protein levels. The Pravastatin Inflammation/CRP Evaluation (PRINCE): A randomized trial and cohort study. JAMA 286:64–70, 2001.
117. Pearson TA, Mensah GA, Alexander RW, et al: AHA/CDC scientific statement: Markers of inflammation and cardiovascular disease. Circulation 107:499–511, 2003.
118. Crouse JR: Carotid and coronary atherosclerosis: What are the connections? Postgrad Med 90:175–179, 1991.
119. Hodis HN, Mack WJ, LaBree I, et al: The role of carotid arterial intima-media thickness in predicting clinical coronary events. Ann Intern Med 128:262–269, 1998.
120. Rumberger JA, Schwartz RS, Simons DB: Relation of coronary calcium determined by EBCT and lumina narrowing determined by autopsy. Am J Cardiol 74:1169–1173, 1994.
121. Arad Y, Spadaro LA, Goodman K, et al: Predictive value of EBCT of the coronary arteries. Circulation 93:1951–1953, 1996.
122. Reaven GM: Banting lecture 1988: Role of insulin resistance in human disease. Diabetes 37:1595–1607, 1988.
123. Ford ES, Giles WH, Dietz WH: Prevalence of the metabolic syndrome among US adults. Findings from the Third National Health and Nutrition Examination Survey. JAMA 287:356–359, 2002.
124. Park Y-W, Zhu S, Palaniappan L, et al: The metabolic syndrome. Prevalence and associated risk factor findings in the U.S. population from the Third National Health and Nutrition Examination Survey, 1988–1994. Arch Intern Med 163:427–436, 2003.
125. Sattr N, Gaw A, Scherbakova O, et al: Metabolic syndrome with and without C-reactive protein as a predictor of coronary heart disease and diabetes in the West of Scotland Coronary Prevention Study. Circulation 108:414–419, 2003.
126. Lakka H-M, Laaksonen DE, Lakka TA, et al: The metabolic syndrome and total and cardiovascular disease mortality in middle-aged men. JAMA 288:2709–2716, 2002.
127. Festa A, D'Agostino R Jr, Howard G, et al: Chronic subclinical inflammation as part of the insulin resistance syndrome. The Insulin Resistance Atherosclerosis Study (IRAS). Circulation 102:42–47, 2000.
128. Ridker PM, Buring JE, Cook NR, Rifai N: C-reactive protein, the metabolic syndrome, and the risk of incident cardiovascular events. Circulation 107:391–397, 2003.
129. Anand SS, Yi Q, Gersteom H, et al: Relationship of metabolic syndrome and fibrinolytic dysfunction to cardiovascular disease. Circulation 108:420–425, 2003.
130. Grundy SM: Obesity, metabolic syndrome, and coronary atherosclerosis. Circulation 105:2696–2698, 2002.
131. Devaraj S, Xu DY, Jialal I: C-reactive protein increases plasminogen activator inhibitor-1 expression and activity in human aortic endothelial cells. Implications for the metabolic syndrome and atherothrombosis. Circulation 107:398–404, 2003.
132. Ballantyne CM, Olssson AG, Cook TJ, et al. for the Scandinavian Simvastatin Survival Study (4S) Group: Influence of low high-density lipoprotein cholesterol and elevated triglyceride on coronary heart disease events and response to simvastatin therapy in 4S. Circulation 104:3046–3051, 2001.
133. Writing Group for the PEPI Trial: Effects of estrogen and estrogen-progesterone regimen on heart disease risk factors in postmenopausal women. JAMA 273:199–208, 1995.
134. Grady D, Herrington D, Bittner V, et al: Cardiovascular disease outcomes during 6.8 years of hormone therapy: Heart and Estrogen/Progestin Replacement Study Follow-up (HERS II). JAMA 288:49–57, 2002.

135. Manson JE, Hsia J, Johnson KC, et al. for the Womens' Health Initiative Investigators: Estrogen plus progestin and the risk of coronary heart disease. N Engl J Med 349:533–534, 2003.

136. Mosca L, Collins P, Herrington DM, et al: Hormone replacement therapy and cardiovascular disease: A statement for Healthcare Professionals from the American Heart Association. Circulation 104:499, 2001.

137. Smith SC, Blair SN, Bonow RO, et al: AHA/ACC guidelines for preventing heart attack and death in patients with atherosclerotic cardiovascular disease: 2001 update. Circulation 104:1577–1579, 2001.

138. Grundy SM: Primary prevention of coronary heart disease. Circulation 100:988–998, 1990.

139. Pearson TA, Blair SN, Daniels SR, et al: AHA guidelines for primary prevention of cardiovascular diseases and stroke: 2002 update. Circulation 106:388–391, 2002.

140. Mosca L, Appel LJ, Benjamin E, et al: AHA guidelines. Evidence-based guidelines for cardiovascular disease prevention in women. Circulation 109:672–693, 2004.

141. Wilson PW: Established risk factors in coronary artery disease, the Framingham Study. Am J Hypertension 7:7S–12S, 1994.

SELECTED REFERENCE FOR FURTHER READING

Smith SC, Blair SN, Bonow RO, et al. AHA/ACC guidelines for preventing heart attack and death in patients with atherosclerotic cardiovascular disease: 2001 update. Circulation 104:1577–1579, 2001.

Pearson TA, Blair SN, Daniels SR, et al. AHA guidelines for primary prevention of cardiovascular diseases and stroke: 2002 update. Circulation 106:388–391, 2002.

Mosca L, Appel LJ, Benjamin E, et al. AHA guidelines. Evidence-based guidelines for cardiovascular disease prevention in women. Circulation 109:672–693, 2004.

Third Report of the National Cholesterol Education Program (NCEP) Expert Panel on Detection, Evaluation, and Treatment of High Blood Cholesterol in Adults. (Adult Treatment Panel III). National Institutes of Health, National Heart, Lung, and Blood Institute, NIH Publication No. 02-5215, September, 2002.

Chobanian AV, Bakris GL, Black HR, et al. The Seventh Report of the Joint National Committee on Prevention, Detection, Evaluation, and Treatment of High Blood Pressure. The JNC 7 Report. JAMA 289:2560–2572, 2003.

INTERNET RESOURCES

American College of Cardiology:
http://www.acc.org

American Diabetes Services:
http://www.americandiabetes.org

American Heart Association:
http://www.americanheart.org

Centers for Disease Control and Prevention:
http://www.cdc.gov

National Heart, Lung, and Blood Institute:
http://www.nhlbi.nih.gov

General Overview of Preparticipation Health Screening and Risk Assessment

TIMOTHY CHURCH

This chapter addresses KSAs from the following content areas:

1 Exercise Physiology and Related Exercise Science
2 **Pathophysiology and Risk Factors**
3 **Health Appraisal, Fitness, and Clinical Exercise Testing**
4 Electrocardiography and Diagnostic Techniques
5 Patient Management and Medications
6 Medical and Surgical Management
7 Exercise Prescription and Programming
8 Nutrition and Weight Management
9 Human Behavior and Counseling
10 Safety, Injury Prevention, and Emergency Procedures
11 Program Administration, Quality Assurance, and Outcome Assessment

It is clear that a physically active lifestyle provides protection against several major chronic diseases. Regular physical activity has been shown to be beneficial in the primary prevention of coronary artery disease (CAD), stroke, diabetes, and some cancers[1]. Given the high prevalence of a sedentary lifestyle[2], there is little doubt that considerable public health benefit would accrue if inactive individuals became more active.

The many health-related benefits, as well as the responsible physiological mechanisms, of a physically active lifestyle are well documented. However, it is essential to realize that to be most effective, regular exercise must be combined with other positive lifestyle interventions and, when applicable, with appropriate medical therapy. Furthermore, although exercise is extremely safe for most individuals, it is prudent to take certain precautions to optimize the benefit-to-risk ratio. The two most common risks associated with starting a new physical activity program or performing an exercise test are sudden cardiac events and orthopedic injury. The risks associated with physical activity and exercise testing are detailed in Chapter 1 of GETP7.

To ensure an optimal benefit-to-risk ratio, exercise professionals should incorporate some form of health appraisal before performing fitness testing or initiating an exercise program. Although Chapter 2 of the GETP7 provides a thorough description of proper **preparticipation health screening and risk stratification,** this chapter provides a general overview of this process as well as addressing medical conditions that demand special considerations. The purpose of preparticipation health screening is to provide information relevant to the safety of fitness testing or beginning exercise training and to identify known diseases and risk factors for CAD so that appropriate lifestyle interventions can be initiated. Furthermore, it is important to identify additional factors that require special consideration when developing an appropriate exercise prescription and programming that optimize adherence, minimize risks, and maximize benefits. The purposes of the preparticipation health screen include the following:

- Identification and exclusion of individuals with medical contraindications to exercise (see GETP7 Box 3-5)
- Identification of individuals who should undergo a medical evaluation and exercise testing before stating an exercise program because of increased risk for disease because of age, symptoms, or risk factors (see GETP7 Table 2-1)
- Identification of persons with clinically significant disease who should participate in medically supervised exercise programs
- Identification of individuals with other special needs

The precise nature and extent of the appraisal should be determined by the age, gender, and perceived health

KEY TERMS

AHA/ACSM Health/Fitness Facility Preparticipation Screening Questionnaire: Slightly most complex then the Physical Activity Readiness Questionnaire, this questionnaire was designed for fitness professionals to help assess readiness of starting a physical activity program; developed jointly by the American Heart Association and the American College of Sports Medicine

Medical screening examination: A thorough medical examination performed by a health care professional, often a physician, to assess readiness of starting a physical activity program; often the need of obtaining a medical screening examination is identified during the pre-participation health screening and risk assessment

Physical Activity Readiness Questionnaire (PAR-Q): A widely used and simple prescreening health assessment questionnaire developed by the British Columbia Ministry of Health for assessing readiness of starting a physical activity program

Preparticipation health screening and risk assessments: Standardized tools for identifying existing medical conditions with the goal of assessing the risks associated with starting a new exercise program or performing an exercise test

status characteristics of the participants, as well as the available economic, personnel, and equipment resources. Most prospective participants in exercise programs conducted in non-medical settings are sedentary individuals who consider themselves "generally healthy" and whose goals are to improve their fitness and well being, reduce weight, and reduce risk of chronic disease. For such individuals, the primary safety goal of a pre-participation health appraisal is to identify individuals who should receive further medical evaluation to determine whether there are contraindications to exercise testing or training or whether referral to a medically supervised exercise program is necessary.

Health appraisals can range from a short questionnaire to interviews and sophisticated computerized evaluations. Also, many appraisals include common screening measurements including height and weight, waist circumference, blood pressure (BP), and blood testing (cholesterol and glucose) [see GETP7 Chapter 3]. The most common form of method of prescreening health assessment is the use of standardized forms, and a number of standardized forms are available that can be used to risk stratify individuals. Standardized forms should be viewed as a minimal standard for entry into a new exercise program. In general, these forms are aimed at identifying individuals at moderate to high risk who should receive medical advice before beginning or increasing their level of physical activity. Two of the more reputable standardized forms are the **Physical Activity Readiness Questionnaire (PAR-Q)** and AHA/ACSM (American Heart Association/American College of Sports Medicine) Health/Fitness Facility Preparticipation Screening Questionnaire. The PAR-Q is well developed, has been used and tested extensively[3] . The PAR-Q is designed to be used when a person wants to begin a program of light to moderate physical activity. One of the benefits of the PAR-Q is simplicity, so much so that in

some circumstances in which there is no alternative, the PAR-Q can be self administered by the participant. The **AHA/ACSM Health/Fitness Facility Preparticipation Screening Questionnaire** is designed to be completed when the participant registers at a health or fitness facility or program[4] (see Box 28-5). This form is slightly more complex than the PAR-Q and uses history, symptoms, and risk factors (including age) to assess the need for physician evaluation before beginning a new exercise program. This form was specifically designed for prescreening in health and fitness facilities. It can be completed in a few minutes, identifies moderate- and high-risk individuals, documents the results of the screening, educates the consumer and staff, and encourages appropriate use of the health care system. The use of the of the PAR-Q and AHA/ACSM Health/Fitness Facility Preparticipation Screening Questionnaire are explained in detail, and sample forms are provided in Chapter 2 of GETP7. Both of these forms have limitations and should only be interpreted by qualified staff, who should always document the results. Again, it needs to be emphasized that many sedentary individuals can safely begin a *light- to moderate-intensity* physical activity program without the need for extensive medical screening.

No form or set of guidelines for preparticipation screening can cover all situations. Furthermore, the use of forms such as the PAR-Q can only identify those who are at high risk; they do not differentiate between those at low, moderate, and high risk. Additionally, most forms do not make recommendations based on intensity of the proposed exercise program. The ACSM's recommendations for medical examinations and exercise testing before participation in a new exercise program both stratify individuals into categories of low, moderate, and high risk and combine this with proposed exercise intensity to assess need of medical evaluation before the start of a new exercise program.

Although a variety of risks are associated with exercise participation, the most important is precipitation of sudden cardiac death. Several studies clearly demonstrate that the transiently increased risk of cardiac arrest occurring during vigorous exercise results largely from the presence of preexisting cardiac abnormalities, particularly CAD. The importance of identifying individuals at high risk of CAD or demonstrating symptoms associated with CAD cannot be overstated for ensuring the safe participation in a physical activity program. Thus, it is critically important for exercise professionals to have a good understanding of the medical history, signs, and symptoms that require evaluation by a physician before a client starts a new physical activity program. Important medical history includes any heart conditions such as heart attack, cardiac catheterization, abnormal rhythms, valve disease, or congenital conditions. As described in GETP7 Table 2-2, the common CAD risk factors are all deserving of attention and include age, impaired fasting glucose, sedentary lifestyle, obesity, high cholesterol, smoking, hypertension, and family history of CAD. Important signs and symptoms (see GETP7 Table 2-3) include any form of chest discomfort or unreasonable shortness of breath with exertion, dizziness, fainting, blackouts, or cramping or burning in the legs. Limitations attributable to bone or joint issues or previous injuries should also be addressed. This is brief overview of the medical history, signs, and symptoms that should raise concern in the exercise professional and are usually associated with referral for physician clearance. Both the ACSM (GETP7) and the AHA[5] provide guidance on when a medical referral is recommended. It should also be noted that detection of elevated BP, cholesterol, or glucose should also trigger a medical referral[6–8]. Prescreening forms have been recommended as a minimum pre-exercise screening standard for entry into a light to moderate-intensity physical activity program. After an individual has been provided with medical clearance to participate in an exercise program (as a recommended follow-up to either the AHA/ACSM Health/Fitness Facility Preparticipation Screening Questionnaire or a more comprehensive health appraisal), it is important for the exercise professional to determine whether there are any additional health-related factors that require special consideration.

Overview of the Medical Screening Examination

A **medical screening examination** to evaluate the risk of starting a new physical activity program can range in complexity from a simple clinical examination to extensive diagnostic testing depending on the age, medical history, risk factors, and symptoms of the individual. At a minimum, the medical prescreening examination should include a detailed medical history and thorough physical examination. In obtaining the medical history, every effort should be made to acquire specific information about pre-

vious medical diagnoses, particularly those pertaining to cardiac and vascular disease, as well as the associated risk factors such as hypertension, diabetes, high cholesterol, tobacco use, and family history. Particular attention should also be given to reviewing past skeletal and muscular injuries and current physical limitations caused by either acute injury or chronic conditions such as arthritis or osteoporosis. A review of the individual's medications is an important part of the medical history, to identify medical problems that may have been missed during the interview and also to identify any medications that may alter the exercise prescription. Although a review of symptoms should be standard part of the examination, any symptoms of chest discomfort or shortness of breath associated with exertion should be probed in detail (see GETP7 Box 3-1).

A standard physical examination should be performed with particular importance placed on the assessment of the cardiovascular and respiratory systems as well as the skeletal muscular system. BP and heart rate (HR) should be measured, and an ausculatory examination of the heart and lungs should be performed. Weight and height should be measured to classify the individual as normal weight, overweight, or obese but also to assess the potential impact of excess weight on joint health. Joint mobility should be checked as well as range of motion (ROM) and strength. A neurological examination that includes a balance tested should be administered. Examining the feet, looking for open wounds, is particularly important in elderly individuals and those with diabetes (see GETP7 Box 3-2).

Based on the information obtained during the history and examination combined with the participant's exercise goals and in accordance with published recommendations, the examining physician may elect to order or perform more advanced diagnostic or screening tests. These include exercise stress test with or with nuclear imaging (technetium or thalium), radiographs, magnetic resonance imaging, or even cardiac catheterization if symptoms warrant (see GETP7 Box 3-3).

Common Risk Stratification Schema and Their Use

The use of national guidelines to stratify risk of adverse health events, usually cardiac, can be very useful. Common sources of risk stratification schema include the National Cholesterol Education Program Expert Panel on Detection, Evaluation, and Treatment of High Blood Cholesterol in Adults (NCEP ATP III); the Seventh Report of the Joint National Committee on Prevention, Detection, Evaluation, and Treatment of High Blood Pressure (JNC 7); and the American Heart Association Scientific Statement on Exercise Standards for Testing and Training[5–7]. Although these references serve as excellent resources for risk stratification, they can also serve as a point of confusion, both in terms of using different schema to define low, moderate, and high risk and by occasionally having different thresholds of risk for the same risk factor. These differences are may be caused by a number reasons, but the two most obvious are the dates when guidelines were produced and the specific focus of the individual guidelines. Even a 1- or 2-year gap between when different sets of guidelines were released allows for new information to evolve that may affect acceptable risk factor thresholds. For example, the NCEP ATP III guidelines define hypertension as systolic BP of 140 mm Hg or above, and although JNC 7 generally agrees with this threshold, it also suggests that systolic BP above 130 mm Hg should be treated like hypertension in individuals with diabetes. This example is also a good illustration of how each set of guidelines has a specific focus such as cholesterol or BP that is addressed in great detail but other important risk factors are only briefly mentioned or oversimplified. Although the treatment guidelines from respected national organizations may have small inconsistencies in content, they all put a premium on the value of screening for the most common risk factors and leave the decision to treat with medication or not up to the physician. Furthermore, they all recognize that value of exercise as part of the lifestyle changes for individuals with borderline abnormalities and as an adjunct treatment for those needing drug therapy.

Medical Conditions That Complicate the Exercise Prescription

There are number of issues that warrant special consideration when assessing the need of further screening before a client begins a physical activity program. There are varieties of conditions that may affect the exercise prescription; a few of the more common ones are discussed here. However, a safe strategy when a complicating medical condition is present is to assure that the individuals' health care provider is aware of the individuals desire to become physically active and that the provider has approved this change in behavior.

ELDERLY INDIVIDUALS

Special consideration must be made in elderly individuals (> 65 years of age) when assessing the need for medical clearance before they start exercise programs as well as in developing the exercise prescription[5,9]. A number of physiological changes occur with aging, and they affect how elderly individuals respond to acute exercise and training. Maximal HR, left ventricular (LV) function, and cardiac output decrease with age, and there is general loss of muscle mass (see Chapter 4). This is further complicated by compromised balance and mobility in elderly individuals. Given these concerns, the referral of elderly individuals to their primary care doctors for clearance is most often the prudent course of action. Furthermore, many elderly individuals will benefit from medically supervised exercise sessions, and although some may graduate to unsupervised sessions, many may not. For most elderly individuals who

have been sedentary for an extended period, there needs to be an extended building-up period, in terms of both the intensity and duration as they begin a new exercise program (see GETP7 Chapter 10). This building-up period could take weeks to months. Furthermore, given the high prevalence of functional limitations in this population, low-impact simple activities such as walking or stationary bike riding are recommended. Additional information about exercise prescription is provided in Chapter 10 of the GETP7 and in American College of Sports Medicine position stand[9]. The American Association of Retired People's website is another good resource for recommendations on exercise in elderly individuals.

DIABETES

Diabetes is a strong and independent contributor to the risk of developing cardiovascular disease (CVD). This excessive risk includes CAD, peripheral vascular disease, and congestive heart failure. Diabetes is a metabolic disease that requires specific diet and exercise therapy alone or in combination with prescribed medications. Regular physical activity greatly reduces both the risk of developing diabetes and the medical complications associated with diabetes. However, given the large CVD risk associated with having diabetes, the prescription of exercise for individuals with the disorder must be done with great thought and care[8,10]. Virtually every individual with diabetes who wants to start an exercise programs needs to be referred to his or her primary care doctor for clearance. This is important not only to assess risk based on history and symptoms but also because glucose-related medication requirements are likely to change with participation in an exercise program.

Many individuals with diabetes are at risk for foot ulceration attributable to peripheral neuropathy, peripheral vascular disease, or other reasons. For these individuals, it may be advisable to limit their physical activity to non–weight-bearing exercises such as swimming or bicycling. Also, some acute issues related to blood sugar must be addressed when an individual with diabetes starts a new exercise program. For example, blood sugar should be checked before and after each exercise session, and blood glucose levels lower than 100 and above 300 $mg \cdot dL^{-1}$ should preclude exercise. Furthermore, hypoglycemia may occur hours after the exercise session. For more details related to exercise and diabetes, see American College of Sports Medicine[10], Chapter 9 of GETP7, Chapter 33, or the American Diabetes Association's recommendations[8].

ARTHRITIS AND OTHER RHEUMATIC DISEASES

Regular exercise can reduce joint pain and stiffness and increase flexibility, muscle strength, cardiac fitness, and endurance in individuals with arthritis. It also helps with weight reduction and contributes to an improved sense of well being. Exercise is considered by many to be one part of a comprehensive arthritis treatment plan. Individuals with arthritis should discuss exercise options with their doctors and other health care providers. A doctor may refer the patient to a physical therapist who can help design an appropriate exercise program and teach clients about pain relief methods, proper body mechanics, and joint protection. There are many types of arthritis. Experienced doctors, physical therapists, and occupational therapists can recommend exercises that are particularly helpful for specific types of arthritis. Doctors and therapists also know specific exercises for particularly painful joints. There may be exercises that are off limits for people with a particular type of arthritis or when the joints are swollen and inflamed. Many people with arthritis begin with easy, ROM exercises and low-impact aerobics. People with arthritis can participate in a variety of, but not all, exercise programs. The three types of exercise often cited as best for people with arthritis are ROM exercises (e.g., dance), resistance training, and aerobic exercises. Weight control can be important to people who have arthritis because extra weight puts extra pressure on many joints. Some studies show that aerobic exercise can reduce inflammation in some joints. For more details related to exercise and arthritis, refer to Chapter 9 of GETP7, Chapter 35, or the Arthritis Foundation's website.

OSTEOPOROSIS

Weight-bearing exercise and resistance training have an important role in both the prevention and treatment of osteoporosis. However, the diagnosis of osteoporosis has it own set of safety concerns, and the start of any new exercise in an individual with osteoporosis should not be undertaken without physician approval[11]. Particular attention must be given to frail individuals, those who have had a fracture, and those who fall frequently. Certain movements (e.g., twisting of the spine, high-impact aerobics, and bending from the waist) should be avoided in individuals with osteoporosis. A primary concern in individuals with osteoporosis is avoiding fractures, and preventing falls is essential to this goal. Thus, when working with individuals with osteoporosis, helping prevent opportunities to fall should always be a top priority. For more detailed information, refer to American College of Sports Medicine position stand[11], Chapter 9 of GETP7, or Chapter 35.

CARDIOVASCULAR DISEASE

It is well documented that regular exercise has powerful benefits for both preventing and treating CVD. However, it is also well known that an acute bout of exercise, particularly in sedentary individuals, can precipitate and cardiac event in those with preexisting CVD. Thus, exercise prescription in individuals with CVD must be done with both physician approval and input[5]. Often, individuals with CVD need to start their program under medically supervised conditions, and some individuals may never progress to unsupervised exercise. Although a good strategy in all sedentary individuals starting a new exercise program, it is especially important for individuals with CVD to start slowly and progress gradually in exercise intensity and duration. All individuals with CVD who wish to start an exercise program must be taught the warning signs of acute cardiac events such as chest pain, unreasonable shortness of breath, and tingling in jaw or left hand. For more detailed discussion related to exercise for individuals with CVD, see Chapter 8 of GETP7, Chapter 31, or Fletcher et al[5].

CHRONIC LUNG DISEASE

Chronic lung disease is a general term used to describe long-term illnesses of the respiratory system, including such diseases as asthma, chronic bronchitis, and emphysema. Regular exercise is an important part of rehabilitation for chronic lung disease and can help improve endurance and feelings of shortness of breath[12]. As with most chronic diseases, it is important to have permission from the individual's health care provider before starting a program. Furthermore, it is likely that a respiratory therapist or other health care professional will have to be involved during the initial stages for individuals who have been sedentary for an extended period of time. This is another group that stands to benefit from starting slowly and progressing gradually in exercise intensity and duration. One important safety considerable when working with anyone with a breathing disorder is making sure the individual always has enough "rescue" medication available when exercising. This is particularly true for individuals with asthma. For more detailed discussion related to exercise for individuals with CVD, see Chapter 9 of GETP7, Chapter 32, or the American Lung Association's website.

CANCER

Evidence suggests that physical exercise can improve various quality of life parameters, including fatigue and depression, both during and after cancer treatment. Given the complexities of cancer treatment and both the long- and short-term side effects of the treatment, this is an area in which the individual's physician must approve of and regularly be updated about the individual's exercise prescription[13,14]. Furthermore, research suggests that physicians who prescribe exercise improve motivation and adherence in their patients who have cancer. Cancer treatment, particularly chemotherapy and radiation, can make exercise prescription a challenge and must be given great consideration. Although exercise may be an effective quality of life intervention for many cancer patients and survivors, mitigating factors may make exercise unwise or dangerous for some. Cancer patients who have such conditions may benefit from appropriately designed and supervised exercise programs, but the risk-to-benefit ratio may be higher and close medical supervision may be required. In brief, conditions that warrant prescription modification include fatigue during treatment, acute or chronic physical impairments that may have resulted from surgery or adjuvant therapy, and the presence of bone cancer. Contraindications to exercise include severe anemia, immune-compromised conditions, low platelet count, severe nausea, severe balance issues, fever, and bone pain. For more detailed discussion related to exercise for individuals with cancer, see Chapter 38.

PREGNANCY

Regular exercise can play an important role in the health and well being of pregnant women. Women who exercise during pregnancy have reduced weight gain, more rapid weight loss after pregnancy, improved mood, and improved sleep patterns. However, it must be emphasized that regular exercise in pregnant women should only be done with the physician's knowledge and approval[15]. A woman's overall health, including obstetric and medical risks, should be evaluated before prescribing an exercise program. In the absence of either medical or obstetric complications, 30 minutes or more of moderate exercise a day on most, if not all, days of the week is recommended for pregnant women. If the individual has been following a regular exercise program before the pregnancy, she should be able to maintain that program to some degree throughout the pregnancy. If she is just starting an exercise program as a way of improving her health during her pregnancy, she should start very slowly and be careful not to overexert. Activities with a high risk of falling or those with a high risk of abdominal trauma (e.g., ice hockey, kickboxing, soccer, and horseback riding) should be avoided during pregnancy. Scuba diving should also be avoided throughout pregnancy because the fetus is at an increased risk for decompression sickness during this activity. For more details related to exercise and pregnancy, please refer to Chapter 9 of the GETP7 and to American College of Obstetricians and Gynecologists[15].

Special Safety Considerations for Resistance Training

Numerous investigations in healthy adults and low-risk cardiac patients have reported few orthopedic complications or cardiovascular events associated with resistance training[16]. The safety of resistance testing and training in moderate- to high-risk cardiac patients requires additional study. Contraindications to resistance training are similar to those used assess readiness to start an aerobic exercise program. Contraindications to resistance training include unstable angina, uncontrolled hypertension, uncontrolled dysrhythmias, a recent history of congestive heart failure that has not been evaluated and effectively treated, severe stenotic or regurgitant valvular disease, and hypertrophic cardiomyopathy. Because patients with myocardial ischemia or poor LV function may develop wall motion abnormalities or serious ventricular arrhythmias during resistance training exertion, moderate to good LV function and cardiorespiratory fitness (> 5 or 6 metabolic equivalents) without anginal symptoms or ischemic ST-segment depression have been suggested as additional prerequisites for participation in traditional resistance training programs, with cardiac medications maintained as clinically indicated.

Low- to moderate-risk cardiac patients who wish to initiate mild to moderate resistance training should first participate in a traditional aerobic exercise program for a minimum of 2 to 4 weeks. Although scientific data to support this recommendation are lacking, this time period permits sufficient surveillance of the patient in a supervised setting and allows the cardiorespiratory and musculoskeletal adaptations that may reduce the potential for complications to occur.

A preliminary orientation should establish appropriate weight loads and instruct the participant on proper lifting techniques, ROM for each exercise, and correct breathing patterns to avoid straining and the Valsalva maneuver. Because systolic BP measurements taken by the standard cuff method immediately after resistance exercise may significantly underestimate true physiological responses, such measurement is usually not recommended. For more details related to resistance training and health see GETP7 Chapter 7, Pollock et al.,[16] and American College of Sports Medicine[17].

Summary

The purpose of preparticipation health screening is to provide information relevant to the safety of fitness testing or beginning exercise training to identify known diseases and risk factors for CAD so that appropriate lifestyle interventions can be initiated. Furthermore, it is important to identify additional factors that require special consideration when developing an appropriate exercise prescription and programming that optimize adherence, minimize risks, and maximize benefits. The precise nature and extent of the appraisal should be determined by the age, gender, and perceived health status characteristics of the participants, as well as the available economic, personnel, and equipment resources. The primary safety goal of a preparticipation health appraisal is to identify individuals who should receive further medical evaluation to determine whether there are contraindications to exercise testing or training or whether referral to a medically supervised exercise program is necessary.

REFERENCES

1. U.S. Department of Health and Human Services: Physical Activity and Health: A Report of the Surgeon General, Atlanta, GA. U.S. Department of Health and Human Services, Centers for Disease

Control and Prevention, National Center for Chronic Disease Prevention and Health Promotion, 1996.

2. Ham SA, Yore MM, Sapkota S, Kohl HW: Trends in physical activity during leisure-time. 35 States and District of Columbia, United States 1988–2002. Morbid Mortal Weekly Rep 53:76–81, 2004.

3. Shephard RJ, Thomas S, Weller I: The Canadian home fitness test: 1991 update. Sports Med 11:358, 1991.

4. Balady GJ, Chaitman B, Driscoll D, et al: Recommendations for cardiovascular screening, staffing, and emergency policies at health/ fitness facilities. Circulation 97:2283–2293, 1998.

5. Fletcher GF, Balady GJ, Amsterdam EA, et al: Exercise Standards for Testing and Training: A Statement for Healthcare Professionals from the American Heart Association. Circulation 104:1694–1740, 2001.

6. National High Blood Pressure Education Program: The Seventh report of the Joint National Committee on Detection, Evaluation, and Treatment of High Blood Pressure (JNC VII). JAMA 289:2560–2572, 2003.

7. Expert Panel on Detection, Evaluation, and Treatment of High Blood Cholesterol in Adults: Executive Summary of The Third Report of The National Cholesterol Education Program (NCEP) Expert Panel on Detection, Evaluation, And Treatment of High Blood Cholesterol In Adults (Adult Treatment Panel III). JAMA 285:2486–2497, 2001.

8. American Diabetes Association: Physical activity/exercise and diabetes mellitus. Diabetes Care 27(suppl 1):S58–S62, 2004.

9. American College of Sports Medicine: Position stand: Exercise and physical activity for older adults [review]. Med Sci Sports Exerc 30:992–1008, 1998.

10. Albright A, Franz M, Hornsby G, et al: American College of Sports Medicine position stand. Exercise and type 2 diabetes. Med Sci Sports Exerc 32:345–1360, 2000.

11. American College of Sports Medicine position stand. Osteoporosis and exercise. Med Sci Sports Exerc 4:i–vii, 1995.

12. ACCP/AACVPR Pulmonary Rehabilitation Guidelines Panel: Pulmonary rehabilitation: Joint ACCP/AACVPR evidence-based guidelines [review]. American College of Chest Physicians. American Association of Cardiovascular and Pulmonary Rehabilitation. Chest 112:1363–1396, 1997.

13. Lucia A, Earnest C, Perez M: Cancer-related fatigue: Can exercise physiology assist oncologists? Lancet Oncol 4:616–625, 2003.

14. Courneya KS: Exercise in cancer survivors: An overview of research. Med Sci Sports Exerc 35:1846–1852, 2003.

15. American College of Obstetricians and Gynecologists: Exercise during pregnancy and the postpartum period. Clin Obstet Gynecol 46:496–499, 2003.

16. Pollock ML, Franklin BF, Balady GF, et al: Resistance exercise in individuals with and without cardiovascular disease: Benefits, rationale, safety and prescription. Circulation 101:828–833, 2000.

17. American College of Sports Medicine: Position stand. Progression models in resistance training for healthy adults. Med Sci Sports Exerc 34:364–380, 2002.

SELECTED REFERENCES FOR FURTHER READING

American Association of Cardiovascular and Pulmonary Rehabilitation. Guidelines for Pulmonary Rehabilitation Programs (3rd ed). Champaign, IL: Human Kinetics, 2004.

American Association of Cardiovascular and Pulmonary Rehabilitation, Guidelines for Cardial Rehabilitation and secondly prevention programs (4th ed.). Champaign, IL: Human Kinetics, 2004.

INTERNET RESOURCES

AARP: American Association of Retired People:
http://www. aarp. org/ health-active

American Diabetes Association:
http://www.diabetes.org

American Heart Association:
http://www.americanheart.org

American Lung Association:
http://www.lungusa.org

Arthritis Foundation:
http://www.arthritis.org

Physical Activity Status and Chronic Diseases

PETER T. KATZMARZYK

An increasing volume of scientific evidence implicates physical inactivity as a major modifiable risk factor for several chronic diseases and premature mortality[1-3]. Given the high prevalence of physical inactivity observed in many developed and developing nations, the burden of physical inactivity on public health is substantial[4-6]. The purpose of this chapter is to review the current state of the evidence linking physical activity status to the risk of selected chronic diseases.

Physical Activity or Physical Fitness?

A question currently of interest to physical activity epidemiologists is whether physical activity or physical fitness best predicts the risk of chronic disease. Whereas **physical activity** is a behavior that is any bodily movement produced by the contraction of skeletal muscles that substantially increases energy expenditure, **physical fitness** is an attained set of attributes (i.e., cardiorespiratory endurance; flexibility; agility; reaction time; body composition; and skeletal muscle endurance, strength, and power) that relates to the ability to perform physical activity[7]. Although physical fitness has several components, as de-

scribed, the majority of the studies discussed in this chapter have relied on an index of cardiorespiratory fitness in assessing relationships with chronic disease. An important area of future research is the degree to which other components of physical fitness, such as musculoskeletal fitness, are associated with the risk of chronic diseases.

A recent review[8] and a meta-analysis[9] concluded that both physical activity and cardiorespiratory fitness are related to the risk of coronary heart disease (CHD) and other health outcomes in a **dose–response relationship** (see GETP7 Table 1-2). In other words, for any increase in physical activity or fitness, there was a corresponding reduction in the risk of chronic diseases and all-cause mortality. However, the relationships across categories of cardiorespiratory fitness were different than for physical activity. In general, the dose response relationship across categories of cardiorespiratory fitness is steeper than the relationship across categories of physical activity. It has been suggested that the more robust findings with some indicators of physical fitness by comparison with physical activity is that physical fitness is measured more objectively than physical activity, which is generally assessed using questionnaires or other methods of self-report[8]. Thus, the finding that physical fitness may be a better predictor of health outcomes is to be expected because of the more objective and reliable nature of the measurements. Whatever the outcome of the continuing scientific discourse around the issue of physical activity versus physical fitness as predictors of chronic disease, it is clear that public health initiatives should target increasing physical activity levels of the population rather than increasing physical fitness[10]. Through an increase in physical activity levels, there should be a consequent increase in physical fitness levels. Although up to 50% of the variation in cardiorespiratory fitness levels can be explained by familial factors (genetic and shared lifestyle factors)[11], the most logical way to increase physical fitness levels is through an increase in physical activity.

The Scientific Evidence

This chapter describes scientific evidence from the field of physical activity epidemiology. **Epidemiology** is the study of the distribution and determinants of disease or injury, and physical activity epidemiologists place a partic-

KEY TERMS

Confidence interval (CI): A range around a relative risk estimate that refers to the probability that the range includes the true value of the relative risk estimate

Dose–response relationship: A relationship between two variables in which any increase or change in one variable is associated with a corresponding change in the other variable. A dose–response relationship does not have to be linear, but it can follow a number of patterns (e.g., curvilinear, quadratic).

Epidemiology: The study of the distribution and determinants of disease or injury

Physical activity: A behavior that is any bodily movement produced by the contraction of skeletal muscles that substantially increases energy expenditure

Physical fitness: An attained set of attributes (i.e., cardiorespiratory endurance; flexibility; agility; reaction time; body composition; and skeletal muscle endurance, strength, and power) that relates to the ability to perform physical activity

Relative risk (RR): The risk of disease or injury in one group compared with another group. The two groups usually differ in terms of one or more key factors (e.g., physical activity levels). RR is usually expressed as a risk ratio comparing incidence or prevalence rates among two groups.

ular emphasis on physical inactivity and poor physical fitness as risk factors for disease and injury. The studies described in this chapter use mainly observational prospective designs in which a group of people are evaluated for a given set of characteristics (age, gender, physical activity, physical fitness, obesity) and followed over time to describe the incidence of disease, injury, or mortality. In most studies, the incidence of chronic disease in two or more groups that differs from one another in their level of physical activity or fitness are compared with one another using a ratio called the **relative risk (RR)**. The confidence we have in the point estimate of the RR (i.e., the precision) is generally expressed as a 90% or 95% **confidence interval (CI)** around the RR. If the 95% CI crosses the value of "1", one would generally say that the RR is not statistically significant. For an in-depth description of the study designs used in epidemiology with reference to research in exercise science, readers are referred to the reviews of Heath[12] and Paffenbarger[13].

The idea that physically active individuals are generally healthier than their sedentary peers has been around for centuries; however, modern physical activity epidemiology arguably began with the classic studies of occupational physical activity and the incidence of CHD conducted by Jeremy Morris et al. in the 1950s. Briefly, these early studies demonstrated that men in physically demanding occupations (bus conductors and postmen) had lower incident CHD rates than men in less demanding occupations (bus drivers and office workers)[14]. Over the subsequent 50 years, the field of physical activity epidemiology has progressed greatly by extending and expanding upon the work of Morris et al.[15].

Physical Activity and All-cause Mortality

Although the purpose of this chapter is to outline the relationships between physical activity levels and chronic diseases, it is useful to start with a discussion of all-cause mortality. Among the major causes of mortality in the United States are heart disease (30.3%), cancer (23.0%), stroke (7.0%), and diabetes mellitus (2.9%)[16]. Thus, discussions of physical activity and all-cause mortality largely reflect the relationship between physical activity and these major chronic diseases. However, deaths caused by other causes such as suicide, homicide, infectious diseases, and accidents are included under the rubric of "all-cause mortality," so the results are diluted by these causes of death that are not linked with physical activity by a pathway of biological plausibility.

For detailed reviews of the role of physical activity in averting premature mortality, readers are referred to two excellent reviews of the topic[17,18]. Two classic studies are used here to illustrate the relationships between physical activity and cardiorespiratory fitness and all-cause mortality. First, the Aerobics Center Longitudinal Study (ACLS) is a prospective observational study of physical activity, physical fitness, and health outcomes among men and women receiving a preventative medical examination, including a graded exercise treadmill test, at the Cooper Clinic in Dallas, TX. The results depicted in Figure 7-1 are from an analysis of approximately 10,000 men and 3000 women followed for 8 years for all-cause mortality in relation to initial level (quintiles) of cardiorespiratory fitness (see Fig. 7-1, top panel)[19]. A salient inverse relationship between cardiorespiratory fitness and all-cause mortality was observed in both men and women. Men and women in the lowest fitness quintile were 3.44 (95% confidence interval [CI]: 2.05–5.77) and 4.65 (95% CI: 2.22–9.75) times more likely to die of any cause compared with men and women in the upper quintile, respectively. The greatest decrease in the risk of mortality occurred when moving between the first and second quintiles.

Second, the Harvard Alumni Study is a prospective observational study of approximately 17,000 men who

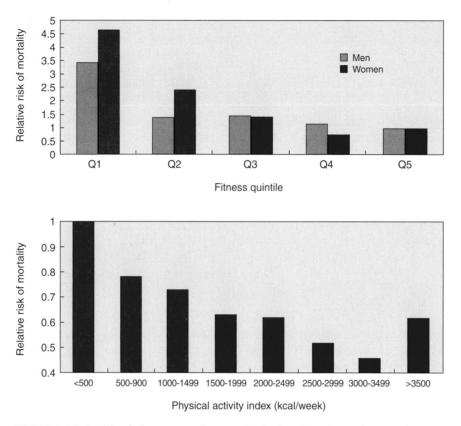

FIGURE 7-1. Relative risks of all-cause mortality across levels of cardiorespiratory fitness in the Aerobics Center Longitudinal Study[19] (*top panel*) and physical activity in the Harvard Alumni Study[20] (*bottom panel*).

attended Harvard University between 1916 and 1950. The results of a 16-year follow-up of physical activity levels and all-cause mortality revealed an inverse dose–response relationship between physical activity levels and all-cause mortality (see Fig. 7-1, bottom panel)[20]. Greater levels of physical activity were associated with a lower risk of death from all causes, and men who expended more than 2000 kcal·week^{-1} (8372 kJ·week^{-1}) of energy in physical activity had a 27% lower risk of mortality compared with men expending less than 2000 kcal·week^{-1} [20]. For an average person walking at 4 mph, approximately 400 kcal are expended each hour. Thus, an energy expenditure of 2000 kcal can be accumulated in about 5 hours of brisk walking per week. A clear dose–response relationship between physical activity or physical fitness and all-cause mortality has been observed in these and many other studies.

Changes in Physical Activity or Fitness and All-cause Mortality

Some of the strongest evidence for an effect of physical activity or physical fitness on mortality rates comes from studies of changes over time and their relationship with mortality. Although there is consistent evidence from intervention studies that increases in physical activity result in improvements in risk factors for chronic disease[21–24], it

is much more difficult to demonstrate changes in *actual risk of disease* caused by *changes* in physical activity levels. A minimum requirement for these types of studies is an assessment of physical activity or fitness at two times separated by a significant period of time along with a subsequent follow-up period for ascertainment of mortality.

Only eight published studies have related natural changes in physical activity or changes in physical fitness over time to changes in the risk of all-cause mortality[25–32]. Figure 7-2 presents the results of studies that used comparable fitness or physical activity change groups. Participants who maintain persistently high physical activity or fitness levels over a period of times are less likely to die than those who maintain consistently low physical activity or fitness levels. Additionally, those who increase their level of physical activity or fitness over time have a decreased risk of mortality compared with those who were consistently physically inactive or unfit. In general, a reduced risk of mortality is also observed in participants who decreased their physical activity over time compared with those who were persistently unfit. These results suggest that there are some short-term benefits of physical activity that may persist for a period of time after a change in physical activity levels. Given that physical activity and fitness were assessed at only two time points in these studies, it is impossible to determine when the changes actually occurred during the interval between the two measurements.

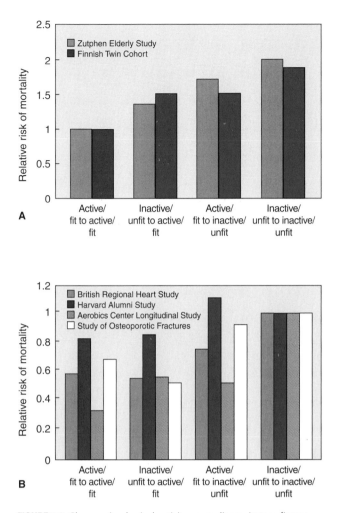

FIGURE 7-2. Changes in physical activity or cardiorespiratory fitness and relative risks of all-cause mortality. **A** presents the results of two studies that used the active/fit to active/fit group as the reference group; results in *left bars* are from the Zutphen Elderly Study,[30] and results in *right bars* are from a Finnish twin cohort[31]. **B** presents the results of four studies that used the inactive/unfit to inactive/unfit group as the reference group; results *from left to right bars* are from the British Regional Heart Study,[29] results in *red* are from the Harvard Alumni Study,[25] results in *yellow* are from the Aerobics Center Longitudinal Study,[26] and results in *white* are from the Study of Osteoporotic Fractures[32]. The average time between successive measurements of physical activity or cardiorespiratory fitness ranged from approximately 6 years to 11 to 15 years.

In addition to the studies presented in Figure 7-2, two other studies have examined the effects of changes in physical activity or fitness and all-cause mortality. Swedish women who decreased their physical activity levels over 6 years had approximately double (RR = 2.07) the risk of dying over a subsequent 20-year follow-up period compared with women who maintained consistent physical activity levels over the same time period[27]. Finally, a study of changes in physical fitness over 7 to 10 years among men 20 to 60 years of age demonstrated an inverse relationship between changes in physical fitness and all-cause mortality, regardless of initial level of fitness[28]. Taken to-

gether, all of the available studies show a consistently lower risk of all-cause mortality in people who maintain high levels of physical activity or physical fitness over a period of years compared with those who decreased or maintained low levels of physical activity or physical fitness over the same time period.

Physical Activity and Coronary Heart Disease

The most studied chronic disease in relation to physical activity and physical fitness is CHD, largely because of the fact that CHD is a leading cause of death in many developed countries and there is biological plausibility linking physical activity with CHD risk. Several excellent reviews and meta-analyses have been written on the topic of physical activity and CHD, and readers are referred to the most recent ones for more specific details about individual studies because it is not possible to summarize them all here[33–35]. Beginning with the classic studies of Morris et al. in the 1950s[14], a large body of evidence linking physical inactivity to the risk of CHD has accumulated, and the cardioprotective effects of physical activity are now being acknowledged by the medical community. For example, the most recent guidelines for the primary prevention of cardiovascular disease and stroke from the American Heart Association emphasize regular, appropriate physical activity as an integral part of maintaining a healthy lifestyle, a cornerstone of primary prevention[36].

The results of a meta-analysis of the results from published studies of physical activity and CHD estimated a summary (four studies) RR of 1.4 (95% CI: 1.0–1.8) comparing sedentary versus active occupations and a summary (five studies) RR of 1.6 (95% CI: 1.3–1.8) for low versus high non-occupational physical activity[34]. The corresponding analysis for CHD death produced a summary (five studies) relative risk of 1.9 (95% CI: 1.6–2.2) comparing sedentary and active occupations and a summary (two studies) RR of 1.9 (95% CI: 1.0–3.4) for low versus high non-occupational physical activity[34]. A review of the rigorous principles of epidemiology as they relate to the relationship between physical activity and CHD suggests that physical activity is linked with CHD in a causal manner[13]. Likewise, a more recent review supports the notion that the relationship between physical activity and CHD is causal and that it follows a dose–response pattern[35]. In other words, higher levels of physical activity result in an incrementally reduced risk of CHD.

Physical Activity and Stroke

Studies of physical activity and risk of stroke have produced interesting results. Table 7-1 presents the available prospective studies of physical activity or physical fitness and risk of stroke that reported estimates of RR[37–51]. The trends reported in Table 7-1 are also supported by two case-control studies[52,53] that demonstrated significant

TABLE 7-1. Results of Prospective Longitudinal Studies of Physical Inactivity or Physical Fitness and Risk of Stroke that Provided Relative Risk Estimates

Population	Sample Size	Stroke Classification	Activity/Fitness Classification	RR (95% CI)
Finnish women[37]	3688	Incident stroke (ICD 430–437)	None vs some LTPA	1.30 (0.73–2.16)*
Finnish men[37]	3978	Incident stroke (ICD 430–437)	None vs some LTPA	1.00 (0.65–1.62)*
Swedish Men[38]	7495	Total stroke mortality	PA score 1 vs scores 2–4	1.2 (0.8–1.8)
		Subarachnoid hemorrhage mortality	PA score 1 vs scores 2–4	1.8 (0.6–5.5)
		Intracerebral hemorrhage mortality	PA score 1 vs scores 2–4	1.1 (0.4–3.7)
		Cerebral infarction mortality	PA score 1 vs scores 2–4	1.2 (0.7–2.0)
		Unspecified stroke mortality	PA score 1 vs scores 2–4	1.2 (0.6–2.2)
Seventh-day Adventist men[39]	9484	Stroke mortality	Low vs moderate PA	1.28 (1.00–1.64)
			Low vs high PA	1.06 (0.74–1.54)
British Men[40]	7630	Incident stroke (ICD 430–438)	None vs occasional PA	1.25 (0.59–2.50)
			None vs light PA	1.67 (0.77–5.00)
			None vs moderate PA	1.67 (0.67–5.00)
			None vs moderately vigorous PA	1.67 (0.63–5.00)
			None vs vigorous PA	5.00 (0.67–> 10)
Asian American men[41]	7530	Incident hemorrhagic stroke	Middle vs high tertile PA	2.2 (0.8–6.4)
			Low vs high tertile PA	3.7 (1.3–10.4)
		Incident thromboembolic stroke	Nonsmokers	
			Middle vs high tertile PA	1.7 (1.0–2.8)
			Low vs high tertile PA	1.8 (1.1–3.1)
			Smokers	
			Middle vs high tertile PA	0.6 (0.4–1.0)
			Low vs high tertile PA	1.2 (0.8–1.8)
Framingham Study men[42]	1228	Incident stroke	Tertile 1 vs tertile 2 PA	2.44 (1.45–4.17)
			Tertile 1 vs tertile 3 PA	1.89 (1.19–2.94)
Framingham Study women[42]	1676	Incident stroke	Tertile 1 vs tertile 2 PA	1.03 (0.68–1.56)
			Tertile 1 vs tertile 3 PA	0.83 (0.51–1.33)
U.S. white women[43]	1473	Incident stroke	Moderate vs high LTPA	1.80 (0.52–6.22)
			Low vs high LTPA	3.13 (0.95–10.32)
		Incident nonhemorrhagic stroke	Moderate vs high LTPA	1.54 (0.44–5.42)
			Low vs high LTPA	2.89 (0.87–9.55)
U.S. white men[43]	1285	Incident stroke	Moderate vs high LTPA	1.17 (0.61–2.27)
			Low vs high PA	1.24 (0.63–2.41)
		Incident nonhemorrhagic stroke	Moderate vs high LTPA	1.16 (0.58–2.32)
			Low vs high LTPA	1.10 (0.54–2.23)
U.S. black men and women[43]	771	Incident stroke	Moderate vs high LTPA	1.33 (0.63–2.79)
			Low vs high PA	1.33 (0.67–2.63)
		Incident nonhemorrhagic stroke	Moderate vs high LTPA	1.34 (0.61–2.94)
			Low vs high LTPA	1.43 (0.70–2.94)
Swedish men[44]	7142	Stroke mortality	Sedentary vs moderate/high PA	1.12 (0.61–2.04)
Dutch men[45]	802	Stroke mortality (ICD 430–438)	Low vs middle tertile PA	1.54 (0.80–3.03)
			Low vs upper tertile PA	1.82 (0.79–4.17)

Population	Sample Size	Stroke Classification	Activity/Fitness Classification	RR (95% CI)
Harvard University alumni[46]	11,130	Incident stroke	< 4184 vs 4,184–8,367 kJ/wk PA	1.32 (1.02–1.69)
			< 4184 vs 8,368–12,548 kJ/wk PA	1.85 (1.32–2.63)
			< 4184 vs 12,549–16,736 kJ/wk PA	1.28 (0.87–1.89)
			< 4184 vs ≥16,736 kJ/wk PA	1.22 (0.88–1.72)
Reykjavik men[47]	4484	Incident stroke (ICD 430–434,436)	None vs some PA after age 40	1.45 (0.99–2.13)
		Incident ischemic stroke	None vs some PA after age 40	1.61 (1.03–2.50)
ARIC study men and women[48]	14,575	Incident ischemic stroke	Low vs high quartile LTPA	1.12 (0.73–1.75)
U.S. male physicians[49]	21,823	Incident stroke	None vs vigorous PA 1 time/wk	1.27 (0.97–1.64)
			None vs vigorous PA 2–4 times/wk	1.25 (1.01–1.54)
			None vs vigorous PA ≥ 5 times/wk	1.27 (0.97–1.64)
		Incident ischemic stroke	None vs vigorous PA 1 time/wk	1.18 (0.88–1.56)
			None vs vigorous PA 2–4 times/wk	1.19 (0.93–1.49)
			None vs vigorous PA ≥ 5 times/wk	1.15 (0.86–1.52)
		Incident hemorrhagic stroke	None vs vigorous PA 1 time/wk	1.69 (0.85–3.33)
			None vs vigorous PA 2–4 times/wk	1.45 (0.86–2.44)
			None vs vigorous PA ≥ 5 times/wk	1.82 (0.89–3.70)
U.S. female nurses[50]	72,488	Incident stroke	Quintile 1 vs 2 PA	1.02 (0.78–1.33)
			Quintile 1 vs 3 PA	1.22 (0.91–1.64)
			Quintile 1 vs 4 PA	1.35 (0.99–1.85)
			Quintile 1 vs 5 PA	1.52 (1.10–2.13)
		Incident ischemic stroke	Quintile 1 vs 2 PA	1.15 (0.81–1.61)
			Quintile 1 vs 3 PA	1.20 (0.84–1.72)
			Quintile 1 vs 4 PA	1.32 (0.90–1.92)
			Quintile 1 vs 5 PA	1.92 (1.25–3.03)
		Incident hemorrhagic stroke	Quintile 1 vs 2 PA	1.09 (0.62–1.89)
			Quintile 1 vs 3 PA	1.12 (0.63–2.00)
			Quintile 1 vs 4 PA	1.45 (0.76–2.78)
			Quintile 1 vs 5 PA	0.98 (0.55–1.72)
U.S. men[51]	16,877	Stroke mortality (ICD 430–438)	Low vs moderate aerobic fitness	2.70 (1.20–5.88)
			Low vs high aerobic fitness	3.13 (1.22–8.33)

ARIC = Atherosclerosis Risk In Communities, ICD = International Classification of Diseases, PA = Physical Activity, LTPA = Leisure-Time Physical Activity

*95% confidence interval calculated from 90% confidence interval reported in study.

associations between physical activity and stroke risk. In most studies, there is a trend towards an increased risk of stroke among those who are physically inactive, but a dose–response relationship between physical activity levels and stroke risk is generally not found[35]. It has been pointed out that whereas studies with more cases and a more detailed assessment of physical activity have found an inverse dose–response relation between physical activity and stroke, studies with less stringent designs have produced weaker results[54]. Only one study has examined an objective measure of cardiorespiratory fitness in relation to the risk of mortality from stroke. A sample of 16,878 men from the ACLS was followed prospectively for 10 years to evaluate the relationship between baseline cardiorespiratory fitness level and stroke mortality. Men in the low fitness category had 2.70 (95% CI: 1.20–5.88) and 3.13 (95% CI: 1.22–8.33) times the risk of developing a stroke during the follow-up period compared with men in the moderate and high fit categories, respectively[51]. These results support the notion that studies that use more objective measures of physical activity or physical fitness may produce stronger results than those that use less objective measures.

Because of methodological constraints, most studies have reported relationships with total stroke incidence or mortality rather than examining ischemic or hemorrhagic stroke separately. Given the strong inverse relationship between physical activity and CHD, it seems logical that physical inactivity should be related to ischemic stroke because it shares the same underlying pathophysiologic mechanisms[35]. However, studies that examined the effects of physical activity on both ischemic and hemorrhagic stroke have found mixed results. For example, whereas data from the U.S. Nurses' Health Study demonstrated a significant inverse dose–response relationship between physical activity and both total stroke ($P = 0.005$) and ischemic stroke ($P = 0.003$) incidence, the trend for hemorrhagic stroke was less clear and not significant ($P =$

0.88)[50]. On the other hand, results from the Physicians' Health Study demonstrated a significant inverse trend between physical activity and total stroke incidence ($P = 0.04$), and the relationships appeared stronger for hemorrhagic stroke than for ischemic stroke in subgroup analyses[49]. Thus, there is a need for more research addressing the protective effects of physical activity, specifically on hemorrhagic versus ischemic stroke.

In summary, physical activity provides protection against stroke. It is unclear whether a dose–response or a threshold relationship exists, but better designed studies tend to show stronger results. There is a need for more studies of physical activity, fitness and stroke, particularly in women and minority groups, and for those that test hypotheses regarding dose–response issues.

Physical Activity and Hypertension

Hypertension is a prevalent chronic disease in developed nations. For example, it is estimated that in the year 2000, approximately 50 million Americans had hypertension[55]. Given the high prevalence of hypertension, it is interesting that there have been relatively few prospective studies of physical activity and incident hypertension[56–59]. Figure 7-3 presents the RRs from available studies. The first epidemiological investigation of physical activity levels and hypertension was published using data from 14,998 men from the Harvard Alumni Study who were followed prospectively for 6 to 10 years. The risk of developing hypertension was 1.30 (95% CI: 1.09–1.55) times higher in men expending less than 2000 kcal·week^{-1} in physical activity versus those expending more than 2000 kcal·week^{-1} [56]. Similarly, Iowa women with "low" physical activity levels were 1.43 (95% CI: 1.11–1.67) times more likely to develop hypertension compared with women with "high" physical activity levels over a 2-year follow-up period[57]. Two more recent population-based studies that included

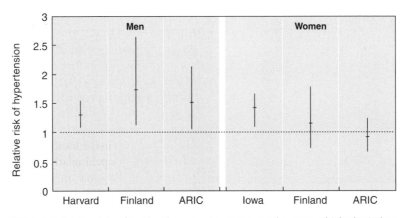

FIGURE 7-3. Relative risks of incident hypertension comparing low versus high physical activity levels in published studies. Data for Harvard alumni are from Paffenbarger et al.[56], Finnish men and women are from Haapanen et al.[58], and Atherosclerosis Risk in Communities (ARIC) study men and women are from Pereira et al.[59]. Error bars denote 95% confidence intervals.

both men and women as participants have also shown a protective effect of physical activity on the risk of hypertension[58,59] (see Fig. 7-3). Thus, although there have been few prospective studies of hypertension risk, the results are consistent in showing a protective effect of physical activity in both men and women.

Physical Activity and Type 2 Diabetes

Like many of the chronic diseases associated with modern living, type 2 or adult-onset diabetes mellitus is a multifactorial disease with no established single cause. Rather, a host of risk factors *predisposes* individuals to develop the disease. The traditional risk factors for type 2 diabetes include older age, obesity, a family history of diabetes, history of gestational diabetes, physical inactivity, and race or ethnicity[60]. Whereas older age, a family history of diabetes, race or ethnicity, and a history of gestational diabetes are *nonmodifiable risk factors*, physical inactivity and obesity are *modifiable risk factors*, ones over which individuals have some control. There is consistent evidence that a physically active lifestyle provides protection against the development of type 2 diabetes, and the relationship follows a clear dose–response pattern. The results of available prospective studies of physical activity and incident type 2 diabetes are presented in Figure 7-4. Three of the major epidemiological investigations of physical activity and type 2 diabetes are described below.

The Nurses' Health Study is a prospective cohort study of 121,700 U.S. female nurses aged 30 to 55 years, established in 1976. Manson et al.[61] presented the results relating physical activity levels to incident type 2 diabetes using 8 years of follow-up data on 87,253 participants.

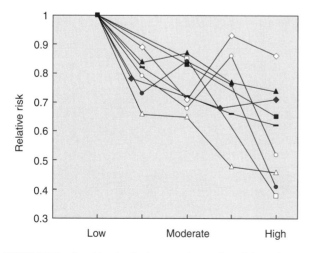

FIGURE 7-4. Results of longitudinal prospective studies of physical activity and incident type 2 diabetes. Physical activity levels are defined in the individual studies. Data are from Manson et al. (61) ◇ (women), Manson et al. (63) ◆ (men), Haapanen et al. (58) □ (women) ■ (men), Hu et al.[62] ▲ (men), Wannamethee et al.[102] △ (men), Helmrich et al.[103] ○ (men), Burchfiel et al.[104] ● (men), and Hu et al.[64] − (men).

Women who engaged in no physical activity had 1.45 (95% CI: 1.00–2.08) times the risk of developing diabetes compared with women who engaged in vigorous exercise at least once a week. More recently, Hu et al.[62] reported that over 8 years of follow-up, women in the low quintile of physical activity were 1.35 (95% CI: 1.12–1.61) times more likely to develop diabetes compared with women in the upper quintile of physical activity.

The Physicians' Health Study is a prospective, randomized, double-blind, placebo-controlled trial of the effects of low-dose aspirin and beta-carotene on cardiovascular diseases and cancer. A total of 22,271 male physicians aged 40 to 84 years at entry in 1982 participated. Manson et al.[63] reported the results relating physical activity and incident type 2 diabetes after 5 years of follow-up. Similar to the results from the Nurses' Health Study, men who reported no physical activity had 1.41 (95% CI: 1.10–1.79) times the risk of developing diabetes compared with men who engaged in vigorous activity at least once a week.

The Health Professionals' Follow-up Study started in 1986 when 51,529 male health professionals, including dentists, optometrists, pharmacists, podiatrists, osteopaths, and veterinarians, enrolled in the study. Hu et al.[64] recently reported the results for physical activity and incident diabetes in the 10-year follow-up of 37,918 of the men aged 40 to 75 years at baseline. Men in the low versus the high quintile were 1.61 (95% CI: 1.32–2.00) times more likely to develop diabetes.

Taken together, the available prospective studies indicate a protective effect for physical activity and type 2 diabetes. There is a dose–response relationship (see Fig. 7-4) in which greater levels of physical activity result in a lower risk for the development of type 2 diabetes. However, further research is required to better delineate the relationship between physical activity and type 2 diabetes among different ethnic groups.

In addition to the epidemiological evidence, two recent large-scale intervention studies have highlighted the importance of physical activity in the prevention of type 2 diabetes in high-risk people[65,66]. The Finnish Diabetes Prevention Study (DPS) was a trial that randomized 522 middle-aged, overweight adults with impaired glucose tolerance to either a control group or a lifestyle intervention that was aimed at reducing body weight, improving diet, and increasing physical activity[65]. After an average of 3.2 years of follow-up, the risk of developing type 2 diabetes was 58% lower in the lifestyle intervention compared with the control group. Similarly, the U.S. Diabetes Prevention Program (DPP) was an intervention that randomized 3234 participants into one of three groups: a) placebo control, b) metformin drug therapy (850 mg twice daily), or c) lifestyle-modification program. The lifestyle program in this study also reduced the risk of developing type 2 diabetes by 58% compared with the control group over an average of 2.8 years of follow-up and was significantly more effective than the metformin drug therapy (31% reduction in incidence)[66]. Thus, the weighted evidence indicates that leading a healthy lifestyle, including being physically active, is an effective prevention strategy for type 2 diabetes.

Physical Activity and Cancer

Cancer is a group of diseases characterized by the uncontrolled growth of abnormal cells. Given the wide range of possible cancer causes and potential anatomic sites, risk factors for specific cancers vary widely. Physical activity has the potential to influence cancer risk through a number of mechanisms, including improved circulation, ventilation, energy balance, immune function, and possibly DNA repair processes[67]. Physical activity has been studied in relation to incident cancers at many sites; however, the available evidence for a protective effect is strongest for overall cancer risk and for cancers of the colon and breast, specifically. Other cancer sites that have been investigated in relation to physical activity include endometrial, ovarian, prostate, testicular, and lung; however, the evidence for a protective effect is less clear[67]. Thus, reviewed here is the available evidence for a relationship between physical activity and cancers of the colon and breast.

A large body of evidence links a sedentary lifestyle to an increased risk of colon cancer. Men and women in sedentary occupations have an elevated risk of colon cancer, as do men and women who are physically inactive in their leisure time[67–69]. However, a relationship between physical activity and rectal cancer has not been consistently observed. Whether physical activity differentially affects cancers of the ascending, transverse, or descending colon is an area for future investigation. It has been hypothesized that a lower risk of colon cancer may be conferred by a decreased transit time for fecal matter through the colon of physically active individuals, leading to decreased exposure of the intestinal wall to carcinogens.

Table 7-2 summarizes the available prospective studies of physical activity and incident breast cancer[70–86]. There is now sufficient epidemiological evidence that physical activity reduces the risk of breast cancer[87], and the association follows a dose–response pattern[67]. Two studies that illustrate the dose–response relation are outlined below.

A 10-year follow-up of 77,024 women from the Nurses' Health Study yielded valuable information on the dose–response relationship between physical activity and breast cancer risk[78]. Compared with women accumulating less than 1 hour per week in moderate or vigorous physical activity, women who accumulated 1.0 to 1.9 hours, 2.0 to 3.9 hours, 4.0 to 6.9 hours, and 7 hours or more had 0.88 (95%CI: 0.79–0.98), 0.89 (95% CI: 0.81–0.99), 0.85 (95% CI: 0.77–0.94), and 0.82 (95% CI: 0.70–0.97) times the risk of incident breast cancer (P for trend = 0.04), respectively[78]. Similarly, a 13.7-year follow-up of 25,625 Norwegian women also demonstrated a significant dose–response relationship between physical activity and incident breast cancer[74]. Compared with women who were sedentary in their leisure time, women who were moderately active or regular exercisers had 0.93 (95% CI: 0.71–1.22) and 0.63 (95% CI: 0.42–0.95) times the risk of breast cancer, respectively (P for trend = 0.04). A similar trend was observed for occupational physical activity.

TABLE 7-2. Results of Prospective Longitudinal Studies of Physical Inactivity or Physical Fitness and Risk of Breast Cancer that Provided Relative Risk Estimates

Population	Sample Size	Activity/Fitness Classification	RR (95% CI)
U.S. college alumni[70]	5398	College non-athletes vs athletes	1.86 (1.00–3.47)
U.S. women[71]	7407	Little to no exercise vs much exercise	1.00 (0.60–1.60)
Framingham Heart Study women[72]	2307	Low vs high quartile PA	1.60 (0.90–2.90)
Seventh-day Adventist women[73]	20,341	Low vs moderate exercise	1.46 (1.11–1.92)
Norwegian women[74]	25,624	Sedentary vs regular exercise	1.59 (1.05–2.38)
University of Pennsylvania alumni[75]	1566	< 2092 vs ≥4186 kJ/wk PA	1.37 (0.88–2.17)
Iowa women[76]	1,806	Inactive vs moderate PA	2.00 (0.91–3.33)
U.S. female nurses[77]	104,468	<1 vs ≥7 h/wk moderate to vigorous PA	0.91 (0.67–1.25)
U.S. female nurses[78]	85,364	<1 vs ≥7 h/wk moderate to vigorous PA	1.22 (1.03–1.43)
Swedish women[79]	253,336	Sedentary vs high/very high occupational PA	1.30 (1.20–1.40)
Iowa women[80]	37,105	No moderate PA vs > 4 times/wk	1.18 (0.98–1.41)
U.S. college alumni[81]	3940	College non-athletes vs athletes	1.65 (1.20–2.28)
Finnish women[82]	30,548	< Once/wk vs daily LTPA	0.99 (0.70–1.39)
U.S. women[83]	39,322	< 840 vs ≥6300 kJ/wk PA	1.49 (1.00–2.27)
U.S. women[84]	6160	Consistently high vs low PA	1.72 (0.93–3.23)
Danish women[85]	2924	< 30 vs > 90 min/day LTPA	1.32 (1.01–1.72)
Swedish twins[86]	9539	Sedentary vs regular LTPA	1.67 (1.00–2.50)

LTPA = Leisure-Time Physical Activity; PA = Physical Activity.

The biologically plausible mechanisms whereby physical activity may affect breast cancer risk include the alteration of menstrual cycle patterns and exposure to sex hormones, enhancement of immune function, better energy balance, and changes in insulin and insulinlike growth factors[88].

Physical Activity and Mortality in Unhealthy Participants

The majority of the prospective studies on physical activity or physical fitness and chronic diseases or mortality has relied on asymptomatic or healthy participants at baseline in order to better quantify the relationships with incident disease. However, another area of interest is the effects of physical activity or fitness on mortality among those with existing chronic conditions. There are fewer prospective studies of this type; however, several examples are presented here. The prospective relationship between cardiorespiratory fitness and mortality was examined in healthy men and men with cardiovascular disease using 8.5-year follow-up data from the Lipid Research Clinics Study[89]. The RRs of all-cause mortality for physical fitness (per 2 standard deviation lower treadmill time) in healthy men and men with cardiovascular disease were 1.8 (95% CI: 1.2–2.6] and 2.9 (95% CI: 1.7–4.9), respectively. These results support the notion that maintaining physical fitness is important for preventing premature mortality in healthy men and particularly in those with diagnosed cardiovascular disease.

The relationship between cardiorespiratory fitness and all-cause mortality was examined in men without hypertension ($n = 15,726$), with hypertension ($n = 3,184$), and without a history of hypertension but an elevated laboratory blood pressure measurement at baseline (white-coat hypertension; $n = 3,257$) in the ACLS[90]. The RR of all-cause mortality in high fit versus low fit men was similar in the normotensives (RR = 0.50 [95% CI: 0.37–0.68]), hypertensives (RR = 0.42 [95% CI: 0.27–0.66]), and those with an elevated clinic blood pressure measurement (RR = 0.44 [95% CI: 0.29–0.68]). Similar results were also seen for cardiovascular disease mortality in all three groups[90]. Similarly, Wei et al.[91] examined the relationship between cardiorespiratory fitness and mortality in men with type 2 diabetes (n = 1,263) in the ACLS. Compared with men in the low fit group, men in the high fit group had a RR of all-cause mortality of 0.48 (95% CI: 0.34–0.67) after adjustment for age, examination year, and traditional lifestyle and conventional risk factors. Thus, there is consistent evidence that physically fit men with existing chronic conditions such as cardiovascular disease, hypertension, or type 2 diabetes have a lower risk of mortality compared with men who are unfit. More research is required to confirm these findings in women and different ethnic groups.

Musculoskeletal Fitness and All-cause Mortality

All of the studies of the relationship between physical fitness and mortality or incidence of chronic diseases described in this chapter to this point have been concerned with the effects of cardiorespiratory fitness. An important area for future research is the relation between musculoskeletal fitness and various health outcomes. Musculoskeletal fitness includes aspects of bone health; joint flexibility; and muscular strength, power, and endurance. Musculoskeletal fitness is related to health-related quality of life and mobility[92], and lower body function has been shown to be predictive of disability and death in elderly individuals[93, 94]. On the other hand, there is relatively little research on the effects of musculoskeletal fitness on the incidence of chronic diseases or premature mortality. There are apparently only eight studies that have examined the relationship between musculoskeletal fitness and mortality[95–101], and all but two[96,100] relied on an index of muscular strength (usually grip strength) only when examining the relationship with mortality. In general, higher levels of musculoskeletal fitness are associated with a lower risk of mortality; however, the nature of the relationship varies from indicator to indicator and from study to study (Table 7-3). More research on the relationships between different aspects of musculoskeletal fitness and the incidence of chronic diseases and premature mortality is required. Studies that examine the effects of gender, ethnicity, and age on the relationships would be particularly timely.

Summary

There is abundant evidence that physical activity and physical fitness levels are inversely associated with the risk of premature mortality and many chronic diseases, including CHD, stroke, hypertension, type 2 diabetes, and some cancers (particularly of the colon and breast). Furthermore, dose–response relationships have been observed in many studies that have used multiple physical activity or physical fitness categories, and better-designed studies tend to produce stronger results. It is also important to note that individuals can *change* their risk of chronic disease or premature mortality by *changing* their level of physical activity. These results have several important public health implications. First, given the high prevalence of physical inactivity in many developed nations, the burden of sedentary living on health care associated with the treatment of chronic diseases is substantial. Second, measures of physical activity or physical fitness should be incorporated into assessing an individual's global risk of developing chronic diseases. Third, the knowledge that increasing an individual's physical activity level results in a reduction in disease

TABLE 7-3. Prospective Longitudinal Studies of Musculoskeletal Fitness and Mortality

Population	Sample Size	Age Range (y)	Follow-up Length (y)	Indicators of Musculoskeletal Fitness	Results
American men and women[95]	9105	20–82	14	Sit-ups, bench press, and leg press	Mortality rates were lower in men and women with moderate and high muscular fitness compared with those with high
Canadian men and women[96]	8116	20–69	13	Grip strength, sit-ups, push-ups, trunk flexibility	Sit-ups (men and women) and grip strength (men) inversely related to mortality
American men[97]	1071	NR	17.5	Grip strength	Grip strength related to mortality in total sample and in men $\geq$ 60 y old in particular
Australian men and women[98]	1464	70–84	6	Grip strength	Grip strength inversely relate to mortality in combined sample of men and women
Japanese-American men[105]	6040	45–68	30	Grip strength	Grip strength inversely related to mortality within several body mass index categories
Danish men and women[106]	406	75	5	Knee extension and body extension strength	Knee extension strength inversely related to mortality in women only
Japanese men and women[100]	7286	40–85	6.1	Grip strength, sit-ups, side step, vertical jump, trunk flexion	Grip strength, side step, and vertical jump inversely related to mortality in men only
Finnish men and women[101]	463	75 and 80	4.0–4.8	Grip strength and knee extension strength	Grip strength and knee extension strength inversely related to mortality in combined sample of men and women

NR = not reported.

risk should be highlighted in public health campaigns designed to increase the physical activity levels of the population.

REFERENCES

1. Bouchard C, Shephard RJ, Stephens T: Physical Activity, Fitness, and Health. Champaign, IL: Human Kinetics; 1994.
2. U.S. Department of Health and Human Services: Physical Activity and Health: A Report of the Surgeon General. Atlanta: Department of Health and Human Services, Centers for Disease Control and Prevention, National Center for Chronic Disease Prevention and Health Promotion; 1996.
3. Kesaniemi YK, Danforth E Jr, Jensen MD, Kopelman PG, Lefebvre P, Reeder BA: Dose-response issues concerning physical activity and health: an evidence-based symposium. Med Sci Sports Exerc 33:S351–S358, 2001.
4. Powell KE, Blair SN: The public health burdens of sedentary living habits: Theoretical but realistic estimates. Med Sci Sports Exerc 26:851–856, 1994.
5. Colditz GA: Economic costs of obesity and inactivity. Med Sci Sports Exerc 31:S663–S667, 1999.
6. Katzmarzyk PT, Gledhill N, Shephard RJ: The economic burden of physical inactivity in Canada. Can Med Assoc J163:1435–1440, 2000.
7. Howley ET: Type of activity: resistance, aerobic and leisure versus occupational physical activity. Med Sci Sports Exerc 33:S364–S369, 2001.
8. Blair SN, Cheng Y, Holder JS: Is physical activity or physical fitness more important in defining health benefits? Med Sci Sports Exerc 33:S379–S399, 2001.
9. Williams PT: Physical fitness and activity as separate heart disease risk factors: A meta-analysis. Med Sci Sports Exerc 33:754–761, 2001.
10. Blair SN, Jackson AS: Physical fitness and activity as separate heart disease risk factors: A meta-analysis. Med Sci Sports Exerc 33: 762–764, 2001.
11. Bouchard C, Daw EW, Rice T, et al: Familial resemblance for $\dot{V}O_{2max}$ in the sedentary state: The HERITAGE family study. Med Sci Sports Exerc 30:252–258, 1998.
12. Heath GW: Epidemiologic research: A primer for the clinical exercise physiologist. Clin Exerc Physiol 2:60–67, 2000.
13. Paffenbarger RS Jr: Contributions of epidemiology to exercise science and cardiovascular health. Med Sci Sports Exerc 20:426–438, 1988.
14. Morris JN, Heady JA, Raffle PAB, Roberts CG, Parks JW: Coronary heart-disease and physical activity of work. Lancet ii:1053–1057, 1111–1120, 1953.
15. Paffenbarger RS Jr, Blair SN, Lee IM: A history of physical activity, cardiovascular health and longevity: The scientific contributions of Jeremy N Morris, DSc, DPH, FRCP. Int J Epidemiol 30:1184–1192, 2001.
16. Hoyert DL, Arias E, Smith BL, Murphy SL, Kochanek KD: Deaths: Final data for 1999. National Vital Statistics Reports 49; 2001.
17. Lee IM, Skerrett PJ: Physical activity and all-cause mortality: what is the dose-response relation? Med Sci Sports Exerc 33:S459–S471, 2001.
18. Lee IM, Paffenbarger RS Jr: Do physical activity and physical fitness avert premature mortality? Exerc Sport Sci Rev 24:135–171, 1996.
19. Blair SN, Kohl HW, et al. Physical fitness and all-cause mortality: A prospective study of healthy men and women. JAMA 1989;262: 2395–2401.
20. Paffenbarger RS Jr, Hyde RT, Wing AL, Hsieh CC: Physical activity, all-cause mortality, and longevity of college alumni. N Engl J Med 314:605–613, 1986.

21. Durstine JL, Grandjean PW, Davis PG, Ferguson MA, Alderson NL, DuBose KD: Blood lipid and lipoprotein adaptations to exercise: A quantitative analysis. Sports Med 31:1033–1062, 2001.

22. Fagard RH: Exercise characteristics and the blood pressure response to dynamic physical training. Med Sci Sports Exerc 33:S484–S492, 2001.

23. Kelley DE, Goodpaster BH: Effects of exercise on glucose homeostasis in Type 2 diabetes mellitus. Med Sci Sports Exerc 33:S495–S501, 2001.

24. Leon AS, Sanchez OA: Response of blood lipids to exercise training alone or combined with dietary intervention. Med Sci Sports Exerc 33:S502–S515, 2001.

25. Paffenbarger RS Jr, Hyde RT, Wing AL, Lee I-M, Jung DL, Kampert JB: The association of changes in physical-activity level and other lifestyle characteristics with mortality among men. N Engl J Med 328:538–545, 1993.

26. Blair SN, Kohl HW, Barlow CE, Paffenbarger RS Jr, Gibbons LW, Macera CA: Changes in physical fitness and all-cause mortality. A prospective study of healthy and unhealthy men. JAMA 273: 1093–1098, 1995.

27. Lissner L, Bengtsson C, Bjorkelund C, Wedel H: Physical activity levels and changes in relation to longevity. A prospective study of Swedish women. Am J Epidemiol 143:54–62, 1996.

28. Erikssen G, Liestol K, Bjornholt J, Thaulow E, Sandvik L, Erikssen J: Changes in physical fitness and changes in mortality. Lancet 352:759–762, 1998.

29. Wannamethee SG, Shaper AG, Walker M: Changes in physical activity, mortality, and incidence of coronary heart disease in older men. Lancet 351:1603–1608, 1998.

30. Bijnen FC, Feskens EJ, Caspersen CJ, Nagelkerke N, Mosterd WL, Kromhout D: Baseline and previous physical activity in relation to mortality in elderly men: The Zutphen Elderly Study. Am J Epidemiol 150:1289–1296, 1999.

31. Kujala UM, Kaprio J, Koskenvuo M: Modifiable risk factors as predictors of all-cause mortality: The roles of genetics and childhood environment. Am J Epidemiol 156:985–993, 2002.

32. Gregg EW, Cauley JA, Stone K, et al: Relationship of changes in physical activity and mortality among older women. JAMA 289: 2379–2386, 2003.

33. Powell KE, Thompson PD, Caspersen CJ, Kendrick JS: Physical activity and incidence of coronary heart disease. Ann Rev Public Health 8:253–287, 1987.

34. Berlin JA, Colditz GA: A meta-analysis of physical activity in the prevention of coronary heart disease. Am J Epidemiol 132:612–628, 1990.

35. Kohl HW 3rd: Physical activity and cardiovascular disease: Evidence for a dose response. Med Sci Sports Exerc 33:S472–S483, 2001.

36. Pearson TA, Blair SN, Daniels SR, et al: AHA Guidelines for Primary Prevention of Cardiovascular Disease and Stroke: 2002 Update: Consensus Panel Guide to Comprehensive Risk Reduction for Adult Patients Without Coronary or Other Atherosclerotic Vascular Diseases. American Heart Association Science Advisory and Coordinating Committee. Circulation 106:388–391, 2002.

37. Salonen JT, Puska P, Tuomilehto J: Physical activity and risk of myocardial infarction, cerebral stroke and death: A longitudinal study in Eastern Finland. Am J Epidemiol115:526–537, 1982.

38. Harmsen P, Rosengren A, Tsipogianni A, Wilhelmsen L: Risk factors for stroke in middle-aged men in Goteborg, Sweden. Stroke 21:223–229, 1990.

39. Lindsted KD, Tonstad S, Kuzma JW: Self-report of physical activity and patterns of mortality in seventh-day adventist men. J Clin Epidemiol 44:355–364, 1991.

40. Wannamethee G, Shaper AG: Physical activity and stroke in British middle aged men. BMJ 304:597–601, 1992.

41. Abbott RD, Rodriguez BL, Burchfiel CM, Curb JD: Physical activity in older middle-aged men and reduced risk of stroke: The Honolulu Heart Program. Am J Epidemiol 139:881–893, 1994.

42. Kiely DK, Wolf PA, Cupples LA, Beiser AS, Kannel WB: Physical activity and stroke risk: The Framingham Study. Am J Epidemiol 140:608–620, 1994.

43. Gillum RF, Mussolino ME, Ingram DD: Physical activity and stroke incidence in women and men. The NHANES I Epidemiologic Follow-up Study. Am J Epidemiol 143:860–869, 1996.

44. Rosengren A, Wilhelmsen L: Physical activity protects against coronary death and deaths from all causes in middle-aged men. Evidence from a 20-year follow-up of the primary prevention study in Goteborg. Ann Epidemiol 7:69–75, 1997.

45. Bijnen FCH, Caspersen CJ, Feskens EJM, Saris WHM, Mosterd WL, Kromhout D: Physical activity and 10-year mortality from cardiovascular diseases and all causes: The Zutphen Elderly Study. Arch Intern Med 158:1499–1505, 1998.

46. Lee IM, Paffenbarger RS Jr: Physical activity and stroke incidence: The Harvard Alumni Health Study. Stroke 29:2049–2054, 1998.

47. Agnarsson U, Thorgeirsson G, Sigvaldason H, Sigfusson N: Effects of leisure-time physical activity and ventilatory function on risk of stroke for men: The Reykjavik Study. Ann Intern Med 130:987–990, 1999.

48. Evenson KR, Rosamond WD, Cai J, et al: Physical activity and ischemic stroke risk. The atherosclerosis risk in communities study. Stroke 30:1333–1339, 1999.

49. Lee IM, Hennekens CH, Berger K, Buring JE, Manson JE: Exercise and risk of stroke in male physicians. Stroke 30:1–6, 1999.

50. Hu FB, Stampfer MJ, Colditz GA, et al: Physical activity and risk of stroke in women. JAMA 283:2961–2967, 2000.

51. Lee CD, Blair SN: Cardiorespiratory fitness and stroke mortality in men. Med Sci Sports Exerc 34:592–595, 2002.

52. Herman B, Schmitz PIM, Leyten ACM, et al: Multivariate logistic analysis of risk factors for stroke in Tilburg, the Netherlands. Am J Epidemiol 118:514–525, 1983.

53. Sacco RL, Gan R, Boden-Albala B, et al: Leisure-time physical activity and ischemic stroke risk: The Northern Manhattan Stroke Study. Stroke 29:380–387, 1998.

54. Batty GD, Lee I-M: Physical activity for preventing strokes. BMJ 325:350–351, 2002.

55. NHLBI: Fact Book, Fiscal Year 2002. Bethesda, MD: National Heart Lung and Blood Institute, National Institutes of Health; 2003.

56. Paffenbarger RS Jr, Wing AL, Hyde RT, Jung DL: Physical activity and incidence of hypertension in college alumni. Am J Epidemiol 117:245–257, 1983.

57. Folsom AR, Prineas RJ, Kaye SA, Munger RG: Incidence of hypertension and stroke in relation to body fat distribution and other risk factors in older women. Stroke 21:701–716, 1990.

58. Haapanen N, Miilunpalo S, Vuori I, Oja P, Pasanen M: Association of leisure time physical activity with the risk of coronary heart disease, hypertension and diabetes in middle-aged men and women. Int J Epidemiol 26:739–747, 1997.

59. Pereira MA, Folsom AR, McGovern PG, et al: Physical activity and incident hypertension in black and white adults: The Atherosclerosis Risk in Communities Study. Prev Med 28:304–312, 1999.

60. Centers for Disease Control and Prevention: National diabetes fact sheet: General information and national estimates on diabetes in the United States, 2000. Atlanta: U.S. Department of Health and Human Services, Centers for Disease Control and Prevention; 2002.

61. Manson JE, Rimm EB, Stampfer MJ, et al: Physical activity and incidence of non-insulin-dependent diabetes mellitus in women. Lancet 338:774–778, 1991.

62. Hu FB, Sigal RJ, Rich-Edwards JW, et al: Walking compared with vigorous physical activity and risk of type 2 diabetes in women: A prospective study. JAMA 282:1433–1439, 1999.

63. Manson JE, Nathan DM, Krolewski AS, Stampfer MJ, Willett WC, Hennekens CH: A prospective study of exercise and incidence of diabetes among US male physicians. JAMA 268:63–67, 1992.

64. Hu FB, Leitzmann MF, Stampfer MJ, Colditz GA, Willett WC, Rimm EB: Physical activity and television watching in relation to risk

for type 2 diabetes mellitus in men. Arch Intern Med 161:1 542–1548, 2001.

65. Tuomilehto J, Lindstrom J, Eriksson JG, et al: Prevention of type 2 diabetes mellitus by changes in lifestyle among subjects with impaired glucose tolerance. N Engl J Med 344:1343–1350, 2001.

66. Knowler WC, Barrett-Connor E, Fowler SE, et al: Reduction in the incidence of type 2 diabetes with lifestyle intervention or metformin. N Engl J Med 346:393–403, 2002.

67. Thune I, Furberg AS: Physical activity and cancer risk: Dose-response and cancer, all sites and site-specific. Med Sci Sports Exerc 33:S530–S550, 2001.

68. Sternfeld B: Cancer and the protective effect of physical activity: The epidemiological evidence. Med Sci Sports Exerc 24:1195– 1209, 1992.

69. Shephard RJ, Futcher R: Physical activity and cancer: How may protection be maximized? Crit Rev Oncogenesis 8:219–272, 1997.

70. Frisch RE, Wyshak G, Albright NL, et al: Lower lifetime occurrence of breast cancer and cancers of the reproductive system among former college athletes. Am J Clin Nutr 45:328–335, 1987.

71. Albanes D, Blair A, Taylor PR: Physical activity and risk of cancer in the NHANES I population. Am J Public Health 79:744–750, 1989.

72. Dorgan JF, Brown C, Barrett M, et al: Physical activity and risk of breast cancer in the Framingham Heart Study. Am J Epidemiol 139:662–669, 1994.

73. Fraser GE, Shavlik D: Risk factors, lifetime risk, and age at onset of breast cancer. Ann Epidemiol 7:375–382, 1997.

74. Thune I, Brenn T, Lund E, Gaard M: Physical activity and the risk of breast cancer. N Engl J Med 336:1269–1275, 1997.

75. Sesso HD, Paffenbarger RS Jr, Lee IM: Physical activity and breast cancer risk in the College Alumni Health Study (United States). Cancer Causes Control 9:433–439, 1998.

76. Cerhan JR, Chiu BC-H, Wallace RB, et al: Physical activity, physical function, and the risk of breast cancer in a prospective study among elderly women. J Gerontol 53A:M251–M256, 1998.

77. Rockhill B, Willett WC, Hunter DJ, et al: Physical activity and breast cancer risk in a cohort of young women. J Natl Cancer Inst 90:1155–1160, 1998.

78. Rockhill B, Willett WC, Hunter DJ, Manson JE, Hankinson SE, Colditz GA: A prospective study of recreational physical activity and breast cancer risk. Arch Intern Med 159:2290–2296, 1999.

79. Moradi T, Adami HO, Bergstrom R, et al: Occupational physical activity and risk for breast cancer in a nationwide cohort study in Sweden. Cancer Causes Control10:423–430. 1999.

80. Moore DB, Folsom AR, Mink PJ, Hong CP, Anderson KE, Kushi LH: Physical activity and incidence of postmenopausal breast cancer. Epidemiology 11:292–296, 2000.

81. Wyshak G, Frisch RE: Breast cancer among former college athletes compared to non-athletes: A 15-year follow-up. Br J Cancer 82:726–730, 2000.

82. Luoto R, Latikka P, Pukkala E, Hakulinen T, Vihko V: The effect of physical activity on breast cancer risk: A cohort study of 30,548 women. Eur J Epidemiol 16:973–980, 2000.

83. Lee IM, Rexrode KM, Cook NR, Hennekens CH, Burin JE: Physical activity and breast cancer risk: The Women's Health Study (United States). Cancer Causes Control 12:137–145, 2001.

84. Breslow RA, Ballard-Barbash R, Munoz K, Graubard BI: Long-term recreational physical activity and breast cancer in the National Health and Nutrition Examination Survey I epidemiologic follow-up study. Cancer Epidemiol Biomarkers Prev 10:805–808, 2001.

85. Dirx MJ, Voorrips LE, Goldbohm RA, van den Brandt PA: Baseline recreational physical activity, history of sports participation, and postmenopausal breast carcinoma risk in the Netherlands Cohort Study. Cancer 92:1638–1649, 2001.

86. Moradi T, Adami HO, Ekbom A, et al: Physical activity and risk for breast cancer: A prospective cohort study among Swedish twins. Int J Cancer 100:76–81, 2002.

87. Friedenreich CM, Thune I, Brinton LA, Albanes D: Epidemiologic issues related to the association between physical activity and breast cancer. Cancer 83:600–610, 1998.

88. Hoffman-Goetz L, Apter D, Demark-Wahnefried W, Goran MI, McTiernan A, Reichman ME: Possible mechanisms mediating an association between physical activity and breast cancer. Cancer 83:621–628, 1998.

89. Ekelund L-G, Haskell WL, Johnson JL, Whaley FS, Criqui MH, Sheps DS: Physical fitness as a predictor of cardiovascular mortality in asymptomatic North American men: The Lipid Research Clinics Mortality Follow-up Study. N Engl J Med 319:1379–1384, 1988.

90. Church TS, Kampert JB, Gibbons LW, Barlow CE, Blair SN: Usefulness of cardiorespiratory fitness as a predictor of all-cause and cardiovascular disease mortality in men with systemic hypertension. Am J Cardiol 88:651–656, 2001.

91. Wei M, Gibbons LW, Kampert JB, Nichaman MZ, Blair SN: Low cardiorespiratory fitness and physical inactivity as predictors of mortality in men with type 2 diabetes. Ann Intern Med 132: 605–611, 2000.

92. Warburton DE, Gledhill N, Quinney A: Musculoskeletal fitness and health. Can J Appl Physiol 26:217–237, 2001.

93. Guralnik JM, Simonsick EM, Ferrucci L, et al: A short physical performance battery assessing lower extremity function: association with self-reported disability and prediction of mortality and nursing home admission. J Gerontol 49:M85–M94, 1994.

94. Guralnik JM, Ferrucci L, Simonsick EM, Salive ME, Wallace RB: Lower-extremity function in persons over the age of 70 years as a predictor of subsequent disability. N Engl J Med 332:556–561, 1995.

95. Fitzgerald SL, Barlow CE, Kampert JB, Morrow JR, Jackson AW, Blair SN: Muscular fitness and all-cause mortality: Prospective observations. J Phys Act Health1:7–18, 2004.

96. Katzmarzyk PT, Craig CL: Musculoskeletal fitness and risk of mortality. Med Sci Sports Exerc 34:740–744, 2002.

97. Metter EJ, Talbot LA, Schrager M, Conwit R: Skeletal muscle strength as a predictor of all-cause mortality in healthy men. J Gerontol A Biol Sci Med Sci 57:B359–B365, 2002.

98. Anstey KJ, Luszcz MA, Giles LC, Andrews GR: Demographic, health, cognitive, and sensory variables as predictors of mortality in very old adults. Psychol Aging 16:3–11, 2001.

99. Rantanen T, Harris T, Leveille SG, et al: Muscle strength and body mass index as long-term predictors of mortality in initially healthy men. J Gerontol A Biol Sci Med Sci 55:M168–M173, 2000.

100. Fujita Y, Nakamura Y, Hiraoka J, et al: Physical-strength tests and mortality among visitors to health-promotion centers in Japan. J Clin Epidemiol 48:1349–1359 1995.

101. Laukkanen P, Heikkinen E, Kauppinen M: Muscle strength and mobility as predictors of survival in 75–84-year–old people. Age Ageing 24:468–473, 1995.

102. Wannamethee SG, Shaper AG, Alberti KG: Physical activity, metabolic factors, and the incidence of coronary heart disease and type 2 diabetes. Arch Intern Med 160:2108–2116, 2000.

103. Helmrich SP, Ragland DR, Leung RW, Paffenbarger RS Jr: Physical activity and reduced occurrence of non-insulin-dependent diabetes mellitus. N Engl J Med 325:147–152, 1991.

104. Burchfiel CM, Sharp DS, Curb JD, et al: Physical activity and incidence of diabetes: the Honolulu Heart Program. Am J Epidemiol 141:360–368, 1995.

105. Rantanen T, Masaki K, Foley D, Izmirlian G, White L, Guralnik JM: Grip strength changes over 27 yr in Japanese-American men. J Appl Physiol 85:2047–2053, 1998.

106. Schroll M, Avlund K, Davidsen M: Predictors of five-year functional ability in a longitudinal survey of men and women aged 75 to 80. The 1914-population in Glostrup, Denmark. Aging (Milano) 9:143–152, 1997.

SELECTED REFERENCES FOR FURTHER READING

Blair SN, Kohl HW, Barlow CE, Paffenbarger RS Jr, Gibbons LW, Macera CA: Changes in physical fitness and all-cause mortality. A prospective study of healthy and unhealthy men. JAMA 273: 1093–1098, 1995.

Blair SN, Kohl HW, Paffenbarger RS Jr, Clark DG, Cooper KH, Gibbons LW: Physical fitness and all-cause mortality: A prospective study of healthy men and women. JAMA262:2395–2401, 1989.

Kohl HW 3rd: Physical activity and cardiovascular disease: Evidence for a dose response. Med Sci Sports Exerc 33:S472–S483, 2001.

Paffenbarger RS Jr, Blair SN, Lee IM: A history of physical activity, cardiovascular health and longevity: the scientific contributions of Jeremy N Morris, DSc, DPH, FRCP. Int J Epidemiol 30:1184–1192, 2001.

Paffenbarger RS Jr, Hyde RT, Wing AL, Hsieh CC: Physical activity, all-cause mortality, and longevity of college alumni. N Engl J Med 314:605–613, 1986.

Thune I, Furberg AS: Physical activity and cancer risk: Dose-response and cancer, all sites and site-specific. Med Sci Sports Exerc 33: S530–S550, 2001.

Whaley MH, Blair SN: Physical activity, physical fitness and coronary heart disease. J Cardiovascular Risk 2:289–295, 1995.

INTERNET RESOURCES

Health Canada Physical Activity Unit:
http://www.hc-sc.gc.ca/hppb/fitness/about.html

National Center for Disease Prevention and Health Promotion, Nutrition and Physical Activity:
www.cdc.gov/nccdphp/dnpa/physical/index.htm

National Coalition for Promoting Physical Activity
http://www.ncppa.org/physactfactsheets.asp

United States Department of Health & Human Services
http://aspe.hhs.gov/health/reports/physicalactivity/

World Health Organization
http://www.who.int/hpr/physactiv/index.shtml

Physical Activity Assessment

SHANNON J. FITZGERALD AND JAMES R. MORROW, JR.

This chapter addresses KSAs from the following content areas:

1 **Exercise Physiology and Related Exercise Science**
2 Pathophysiology and Risk Factors
3 **Health Appraisal, Fitness, and Clinical Exercise Testing**
4 Electrocardiography and Diagnostic Techniques
5 Patient Management and Medications
6 Medical and Surgical Management
7 Exercise Prescription and Programming
8 Nutrition and Weight Management
9 Human Behavior and Counseling
10 Safety, Injury Prevention, and Emergency Procedures
11 Program Administration, Quality Assurance, and Outcome Assessment

Physical activity has been defined as bodily movement generated by skeletal muscles resulting in energy expenditure. The physical activity portion of energy expenditure can be further divided into spontaneous activities such as fidgeting and voluntary physical activity. Voluntary physical activity includes those of daily living and those that require amounts of energy above that necessary to perform activities of daily living. It is this component of physical activity that varies most among individuals.

The benefits of a physically active lifestyle are widely known[4,5]. Physical activity recommendations given by organizations have evolved over time[4-7]. Early recommendations focused on higher intensity physical activities to achieve high levels of physical fitness (the "product"). Now the impetus is getting individuals to participate in moderate-intensity lifestyle physical activities (the "process") to improve health. The understanding is that those engaging in the process of physical activity will achieve the product of physical fitness. Given the health implications of physical activity, it is important to assess the type, frequency, and intensity of physical activities. Specific reasons to measure physical activity include the ability to investigate the direct relationship between physical activity and disease endpoints as well as the indirect relationship with disease through the effects of activity on diet or body weight[8]. Additional reasons include being able to study physical activity patterns, determinants, and barriers and to evaluate physical activity interventions[9,10].

Various **subjective methods** and **objective methods** can be used to measure physical activity. When using subjective methods such as questionnaires or diaries, the physical activity assessment is based on the individual's perception of his or her level of activity. With objective methods, physical activity assessment is determined by an instrument, and the individual's interpretation and perception of physical activity are not taken into account.

Several of the advantages and disadvantages of using subjective and objective methods of assessment are listed in Table 8-1. The main advantages of using subjective measures such as questionnaires or diaries include the ability to administer the assessment relatively inexpensively to a large number of individuals in a short amount of time. Disadvantages of subjective assessment include inaccurate recall that results in the over- or under-reporting of physical activity and the inability to accurately capture all types of physical activity (e.g., moderate, lifestyle, occupational). Unlike subjective assessment methods, recall error is not an issue for objective methods such as **pedometers**, **accelerometers**, and **heart rate monitors**. These objective monitors, for the most part, are small, lightweight, and unobtrusive. The disadvantages of this type of assessment include the expense, the inability to assess specific types of activities, and the potential effect of extraneous factors on the physical activity assessment results.

Regardless of the technique, because of day-to-day and seasonal variation, the method should reflect physical activity participation on the weekends and weekdays as well as each season of the year[11]. It is also important to use a reliable and valid evaluation method. A reliable method is reproducible, giving the same results for a given amount of physical activity. A valid method is one that accurately measures what it is intended to measure. Establishing validity of a physical activity measure is difficult because no true gold standard of physical activity exists[12]. Methods of energy expenditure (i.e., doubly labeled water, indirect and direct calorimetry) are often used to validate physical activity assessments. These measures are not gold standards for physical activity validation because physical activity encompasses movement, and energy expenditure takes into account movement and body mass[11]. Given these limitations, validity is indirectly established by comparing results with other physical activity measures as well as physiological variables. To determine if a physical activity assessment tool is reliable, the reproducibility should be examined with a test–retest period of 2 to 4 weeks. This is a short enough time period that behaviors should not change, but it is long enough that the initial administration is not influencing the second test[13]. The following sections describe various valid and reliable subjective and objective methods of physical activity assessment as well as the various criteria to consider when deciding on the appropriate method to use.

Subjective Assessment: Self-report Measures of Physical Activity

Subjective physical activity measurements include questionnaires and diaries. The complexity of the questionnaire can vary from a single, physical activity–related question to a more thorough, detailed account regarding physical activity patterns[3,14–17]. Even though a single-item question cannot provide a complete account of one's physical activity, it may be an adequate measure for classifying individuals into crude activity categories. A more comprehensive questionnaire takes into account the type of activity, how frequently it is performed over a certain time period, and the duration and intensity of the activity session[3]. A physical activity diary can also range in complexity from one that has participants record every activity every minute of the day to those that have participants record activities in 4-hour time periods and can be as general as including only the intensity of the activity. One example is the ACTIVITYGRAM, a component of the FITNESSGRAM assessment[18]. Children are asked to record their activities in 30-minute time blocks for this component. However, this may be further divided into 15-minute intervals depending on whether the activity was performed "all of the time" (given credit for entire 30 minutes) during the 30-minute segment or "some of the time" (given credit for 15 minutes). Other examples of popular questionnaires and diaries are found in resources by Montoye[11] and Periera et al[3]. The following sections describe questionnaires and diaries as well as several advantages and disadvantages to using each (Table 8-2).

TABLE 8-1. Advantages and Disadvantages of Subjective and Objective Physical Activity Measures

Subjective		Objective	
Advantages	**Disadvantages**	**Advantages**	**Disadvantages**
Relatively inexpensive	Inaccurate recall	Not subject to recall error	Specific types of activity not assessed
Easy to administer	Fails to accurately capture all types of activity (e.g., moderate, lifestyle, and occupational activity)	Small and lightweight	Extraneous variables may affect results
Data collected for a large number of individuals	Not recommended for children younger than age 10 years	Unobtrusive	Usually more expensive than questionnaires
Can be ascertained with a few questions			

TABLE 8-2. Subjective Measurement of Physical Activity

	Advantages	Disadvantages
Diary	• Suitable for large populations • Little expense • No observer or interviewer • Collected in many subjects at the same time • Specific activities and patterns can be recorded	• Large amount of data to process, increasing the time and expense • Participants' cooperation and motivation required • Longer collection period can result in less accurate data • Need to record throughout the year to get typical physical activity
Questionnaire	• Suitable for large populations • Specific activities can be recorded • Patterns of behavior not affected • Total energy expenditure may be estimated • Applicable to wide age range	• Inaccurate recall • May be burdensome • Must be age appropriate • Interviewer may be necessary for accuracy • Limited use with younger children (younger than age 10 years)

QUESTIONNAIRES

A physical activity questionnaire usually can be administered quickly and inexpensively, is reliable, and does not cause a person's normal daily activity habits to change[19]. This type of instrument does not provide an absolute measurement of energy expenditure, but it allows estimates of energy expenditure and for individuals to be ranked from least to most active[17]. As soon as a person's relative activity level is known, it is possible to examine the associations between physical activity and various disease endpoints such as heart disease, diabetes, various types of cancer, and obesity[17].

Self-report measures, such as questionnaires, can be used by various age groups and may be modified based on the study purpose or population[17,20]. When using a questionnaire to assess physical activity in young children, a proxy report (e.g., time spent playing outside[21]) can be used. Assessing physical activity level in women is an example of the importance of questionnaire modification based on the population. According to national data from the year 2000, women were almost 7% less active than men[22]. This discrepancy may be partly attributable to the nature of the physical activity questions asked by national surveys rather than women's actual activity levels. Some women may spend a large part of their day involved in household, family, and transportation activities, which are not captured by national survey questions[23].

Limitations of questionnaires include recall bias, individuals' problems with accurately recalling information, and differing recollection based on factors such as the person's age and disease status. Sedentary and high-intensity activities are the most reliably recalled using self-reported methods[16,20,24]. Difficulties remembering and accurately recording moderate physical activities, especially lifestyle activities, offer another challenge to using questionnaires to assess physical activity. Finally, individuals may feel compelled to give socially desirable answers to physical activity questions when responding directly to an interviewer. Overall, the evidence suggests that adults tend to overestimate their physical activity levels[20].

DIARIES

Collecting physical activity information with a diary allows for data collection from many participants at the same time and eliminates the expense associated with an interviewer or observer. With this method of assessment, specific activities are usually recorded on the diary; therefore, physical activity patterns can be determined. Given that participants are asked to record their activities throughout the day, it is important that they are cooperative and willing to perform the task accurately. Recording all activities can be quite tedious. Therefore, keeping a diary over long periods of time can result in inaccurate data collection. Three days of diary collection—2 weekdays and 1 weekend day—are adequate to accurately assess physical activity patterns[25]. The short, 3-day assessment timeframe limits participant burden.

A limitation to using a diary is the time and expense it takes to process large amounts of data. In addition, the diary process should be completed at various times (seasons) throughout the year to help ensure that regular activity patterns are being ascertained. For example, in some areas of the country, physical activity levels may be higher in the summer than in the winter.

SUMMARIZING DATA

After the data have been collected with a diary or questionnaire, they can be summarized in several different ways. Ways to express physical activity summary scores include time, metabolic equivalents (METs), and kilocalories (kcals)[3]. Figure 8-1 illustrates three potential ways to derive a physical activity summary score[3]. The most basic way is to calculate total time spent in physical activity. This is done by multiplying the number of sessions per week of the activity by the time spent performing the activity each session. A second calculation weighs the time spent in the activity by an estimated metabolic cost of each activity (MET). A MET is an estimate of intensity based on the ratio of working metabolic rate to resting metabolic rate. One MET is equivalent to oxygen uptake of 3.5 $mL \cdot kg^{-1} \cdot min^{-1}$ and represents energy expended at rest;

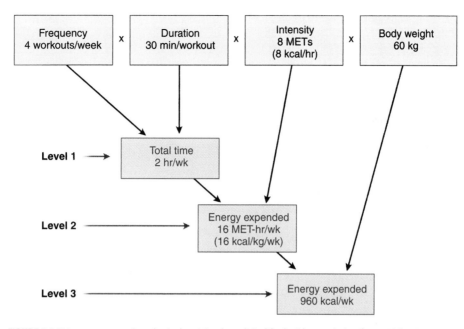

FIGURE 8-1. Ways to summarize physical activity data. (Modified with permission from Kriska AM, Caspersen CJ: A collection of physical activity questionnaires for health related research. Med Sci Sports Exerc 6:S7, 1997.)

an activity that expends eight times the resting energy expenditure such as running is 8 METs. The Compendium of Physical Activities compiled by Ainsworth et al. is a popular resource for obtaining MET values for a wide range of physical activities[9,26,27]. A copy of the compendium can be found in the Appendix. An example of a calculation using METs (see Fig. 8-1) follows. An individual reported running four times a week for 30 minutes a session. As shown at level 1 in the figure, this equates to 2 hours a week spent running. Multiplying the total time spent in running by its MET value, or 8 METs, results in an estimated energy expended from running of 16 MET-hr·wk^{-1} (level 2; see Fig. 8-1). Finally, if the individual's body weight is known, one can calculate the kilocalories per week expended in physical activity. The results from this calculation are provided at level 3 (see Fig 8-1). An individual weighing 60 kg equates to 960 kcal·wk^{-1}. Assumptions made when using these calculations include a) MET values are representative of the way an activity is performed, regardless of the skill level of the individual or pace of the activity, and b) the metabolic cost of performing activities is constant among individuals, regardless of body weight[3].

Objective Assessment: Direct Measurement of Physical Activity

Physical activity monitors such as pedometers, accelerometers, and heart rate (HR) monitors provide objective estimates of one's physical activity. Other objective measures of physical activity and energy expenditure such as direct observation, doubly labeled water, and indirect calorimetry are often used to estimate physical activity level; however, these costly methods may not always be practical with large groups of individuals. Direct observation is primarily used for physical activity assessment in children over short periods of time. Examples of direct observation systems include the System for Observing Play and Leisure Activity in Youth (SOPLAY) and the Children's Activity Rating Scale (CARS)[28,29]. Total energy expenditure measures such as doubly labeled water are limited because they do not allow for the determination of physical activity patterns[30]. Different activity combinations or patterns (e.g., a small amount of strenuous activity versus a larger amount of moderate intensity activity) can result in the same amount of energy expenditure[11]. Many energy expenditure methods do not provide accurate estimates of absolute amount of physical activity[20].

Accelerometers and pedometers can accurately determine baseline and small changes in activity level[12]. The cost of the instruments make these measures potentially more expensive to administer than questionnaires. Unlike questionnaires, they are not subject to recall bias or inaccurate recall by participants. Physical activity monitors are also relatively easy to use, and participant language and reading ability are not issues. However, the monitors are designed to record ambulatory activity and cannot be worn while performing water activities. Therefore, they may not accurately detect movement from activities such as bicycling, weight lifting, or swimming[30]. Monitors appear to be reasonable measures of ambulatory activity[11]. Several methods of objective assessment of physical activity as well as the advantages and disadvantages of each are described below and listed in Table 8-3.

TABLE 8-3. Objective Measurement of Physical Activity

	Advantages	Disadvantages
Pedometer	• Instrument low to moderate expense • Small and lightweight • Unobtrusive • With proper instruction, is easy to use	• Detects only ambulatory activity • Cannot determine type, intensity, or pattern of activity • Cannot detect changes in terrain • Cannot be worn in the water or when cycling
Accelerometer	• Total energy expenditure may be estimated • Applicable to wide age range • Enjoyable	• Detects only ambulatory activity • Cannot detect changes in terrain • Cannot be worn in the water or when cycling • Expense of instrument and hardware or software to process data • Cannot determine type of activity
Heart rate monitor	• Physiological marker • Can record and store heart rate data over an extended period of time • Can detect different intensities of activity	• Influenced by factors not related to physical activity participation • Cannot determine type of activity • Hard to detect low-intensity activities • Time and cost of processing data

PEDOMETERS

Pedometers detect vertical accelerations of the body and record a "step" when vertical acceleration exceeds a threshold value[31]. These monitors are small and relatively inexpensive but do not provide information as extensive as accelerometers. Some pedometers have proven to be quite accurate for recording the number of steps taken and distance walked at various walking paces[32–34]. Pedometers are more reliable for faster walking and running paces compared with slower ones[31,32]. It has been shown that a pedometer records a higher number of steps for walking compared with running for the same distance[31]. This is not surprising given that the stride length is shorter when walking compared with running. The accuracy of the pedometer does not appear to differ based on the type of walking or running surface[31,32]. Welk et al. extended the pedometer research to compare step counts with energy expenditure estimated from self-reported physical activities[31]. They found that the relationship between pedometer step counts and energy expended in moderate intensity activities was stronger than the relationship with energy expended in vigorous activities[31]. Finally, some pedometers express energy expenditure in kilocalories; however, these functions have not been as well validated as actual step counting.

Limitations to using a pedometer for physical activity assessment include the insensitivity to changes in walking speed and the inability to determine intensity or duration of the activity being performed[31]. Even though the pedometer does not give a complete picture of physical activity patterns, step count results are related to physical activity assessments from various accelerometers, which provide a more thorough pattern of activity[30,35]. Therefore, a pedometer is a practical and accurate means of assessing physical activity[36].

ACCELEROMETERS

Accelerometers can be worn on the trunk or limbs and measure movement based on acceleration and deceleration of the body. These measurements are proportional to muscular forces[11]. Given this principle, most results from accelerometers are in proportion to energy expenditure and are used to ascertain the time, frequency, and duration of physical activity performed at various intensities[11,23]. These types of activity patterns cannot be determined from other methods of energy expenditure, such as doubly labeled water[30].

Single plane accelerometers, such as the Caltrac (Muscle Dynamics, Torrence, CA) accelerometer and Acti-Graphs (formerly known as CSA; MTI Health Services, Ft Walton Beach, FL), measure movement in the vertical plane. Triaxial monitors, such as the Tritrac-R3D (Hemokinetics Inc., Madison, WI), measure movement in the vertical, horizontal, and mediolateral planes[37].

Advantages of the accelerometer include its small size and ability to record data over long periods of time (e.g., several days or weeks) as well as the ability to download data and to segment physical activity time periods[38]. To reduce the expense of using this type of device, the same accelerometer can be worn repeatedly by different participants. When using one monitor worn at different times for multiple participants, only small amounts of data can be collected at one time[12].

This type of objective assessment requires more time and resources than a pedometer because technical expertise, hardware, and software are needed to calibrate, input, download, and analyze data[12,39]. Single-plane accelerometers may not accurately detect movement from activities such as bicycling, weight lifting, or swimming[30]. In addition, when worn on the hip, certain accelerometers may not accurately identify activity level on other areas of the body[10]. None are able to detect increased activity level resulting from upper body movement, carrying a load, or variations in the surface (e.g., climbing uphill)[38]. Given the limitation of type of movement detected, Swartz et al. had participants wear monitors on the hip and wrist simultaneously and determined the extra monitor slightly increased the accuracy of estimating the energy expenditure necessary to perform various physical activities[40]. The small increases in accuracy reported with the additional monitor need to be weighed against the time, cost, and effectiveness of an additional monitor[40].

An additional limitation of this mode of measuring physical activity is the potential to misclassify one's activity levels. The accelerometer equations that estimate energy expenditure are derived from specific laboratory activities; therefore, they may not be applicable to free-living situations, resulting in over- or underestimating physical activity level[38]. When assessing lifestyle activities such as gardening and housework, there is a moderate relationship between the results measured with an accelerometer and those measured with indirect calorimetry (considered the gold standard)[10,30]. The relationship between treadmill walking or running measured in a laboratory with an accelerometer and indirect calorimetry is stronger than that reported for moderate lifestyle activities[10]. Explanations for the weaker relationship between accelerometers and indirect calorimetry for lifestyle activities include the limited range of data from those activities and the nature of the lifestyle activities compared with those measured in a laboratory[10].

According to Welk et al., accelerometers give the most objective and detailed physical activity data for research purposes[10]. Overall, accelerometers provide a useful measure of physical activity and by themselves are less accurate for determining total energy expenditure[10,38]. This is partly attributable to limitations of physical activity monitors mentioned earlier (e.g., primarily detecting ambulatory movement). Ways to improve estimations of physical activity include supplementing accelerometer data with questionnaire data to address these limitations and improving the energy estimation equations these devices use[10,38].

HEART RATE MONITORING

Heart rate is linearly related to $\dot{V}O_2$ consumption; therefore, HR monitoring is another reasonable method of physical activity assessment[37]. It is one of the most practical physiologically based ways to estimate energy expenditure in the field[11]. HR monitoring is "low cost, noninvasive and able to give information of the pattern of physical activity[41]." As with accelerometers, HR recorders can store data, which allows for the estimation of frequency, duration, and intensity of physical activity for days and weeks. Strath et al. reported a correlation of 0.87 when comparing the relationship between energy expenditure for lifestyle activities measured with indirect calorimetry

and estimates from HR monitoring[40]. This correlation is stronger than those reported between energy expenditure measured with indirect calorimetry and accelerometers for lifestyle activities[42].

Strath et al. suggested that when subjects wear an accelerometer and a HR monitor simultaneously, energy expenditure estimation and classification of time spent in light, moderate, and hard activity were more accurate[42]. Further research needs to be conducted, but it appears that HR monitors with additional types of activity assessment may be effective means of assessing physical activity[11,42].

The primary limitation to using HR monitors to assess physical activity includes its sensitivity to factors such as ambient temperature, emotional state, hydration status, type of contraction, and size of muscle mass, which affect HR regardless of physical activity level[11]. In addition, the specific type of activity can not be determined, and low-intensity activities are hard to detect.

Other Potential Methods

There are several other types of technologically advanced objective measures, such as task-specific monitoring sensors and the global positioning system (GPS), which may be helpful for improving physical activity assessment in the future. Eventually, it may be possible to have sensors located on clothing and accessories that can monitor physiological responses such as HR and respiration and transmit the information to a computer[43]. This information, along with that provided by a wearable digital camera that can provide pictures of the day's activities, could give an accurate, objective account of an individual's physical activities throughout the day[43]. GPS is a satellite-based navigational system that uses signal information between satellites and receivers, worn by individuals, to ascertain the velocity and duration of displacement[44]. Research studies to date support the ability of GPS to provide accurate assessments of speed, ranging from slow walking to fast running as well as other biomechanical parameters[44,45]. Currently, there are relatively inexpensive ($100) units available that are lightweight; can be worn on the wrist; and provide speed, distance, and pace information while walking or running. As these methods continue to become more feasible and their cost is reduced, they have the potential to expand our ability to accurately assess physical activity.

Choosing a Method

Various types of subjective and objective physical activity assessments have been described. There are several criteria to consider when choosing an assessment method. These criteria include the purpose of the assessment, cost, characteristics of the population being assessed, and the endpoints being evaluated. The method chosen should be valid and reproducible in a representative population and reflect the study aim[8]. There are also additional considerations such as the assessment time frame and method of administration that should be taken into account when administering questionnaires.

PURPOSE

Regardless of your health or fitness profession, at least one of the tools described in this chapter can help you achieve the purpose of assessing physical activity. For example, if you are a health and fitness specialist in a fitness center, are working with a new participant, and would like to assess his or her past physical activity habits, you may want to use a past year assessment tool such as the Modifiable Activity Questionnaire[3]. This type of questionnaire allows you to determine the frequency and duration of an individual's specific activities performed over the past year to ascertain his or her usual physical activity habits. Knowing an individual's physical activity patterns is also helpful in developing an appropriate exercise program. If your purpose is monitoring a participant's physical activity level or change in physical activity level, you could use an objective measure or an activity log. If ambulatory activity is primarily being performed, then a participant could wear a pedometer and record the number of steps taken. For this method to be effective, the baseline number of steps the participant takes should be established. Then the monitor should be worn continuously or at various intervals over time to evaluate the maintenance or change in physical activity. If the activities primarily involve weight training, it is important to use a log that includes the exercise performed, the amount of weight lifted, and the number of sets and repetitions performed. For monitoring general activity, logs can be completed by participants through the Internet at no cost. An example of this type of log can be found at the following site: http://www.presidentschallenge.org/activity_log/track_progress.aspx. Versions of this log can either be printed out and completed or completed online. This type of log allows participants to record the type of physical activity as well as intensity and duration. Alternatively, there is an option for recording the number of pedometer steps taken each day.

COST

With all these measures, it is necessary to weigh the cost of assessment against the quality of data obtained. More expensive techniques usually provide more precise data. Self-report methods to assess physical activity typically involve low to moderate costs, mostly for printing and data processing. Higher costs with diary administration relate to the large amounts of data to process. Interviewer administered questionnaire expenses are predominantly attributable to personnel costs. The cost of using physical activity monitors depends on the expense associated with the instrument. Pedometers are less expensive than accelerometers and HR monitors. Data storage capabilities with accelerometers and HR monitors also result in the additional cost of downloading, preparing, and analyzing the data.

STUDY POPULATION

As discussed previously, there are issues with accurately measuring moderate and lifestyle physical activities and physical activity in women. Therefore, it is crucial that methods used to assess physical activity levels accurately capture these types of activities. Similar issues exist when assessing physical activity in various minority ethnic or racial groups. It important to determine the types of activities that contribute the most to energy expenditure in the study population[46]. For some minority groups, the activities include occupational activities, transportation, household chores, and caretaking, rather than sports and high-intensity leisure activities[46]. Therefore, physical activity assessment tools should validly and reliably measure physical activity common to the population under study.

Age should also be a consideration, especially in questionnaire administration. This method may not be appropriate for children younger than age 10 years old. For older individuals, it has been suggested that effective questionnaire administration should involve an interviewer. This mode of administration is important to clarify questions individuals may have. The type of domains assessed should be age appropriate (i.e., in older adults activities such as walking, light to moderate housework, and yard work should be the focus of the assessment), and recall timeframes should be short[11]. Older adults also tend to handle short, specific questions involving specific activities and time periods (e.g., minutes spent in an activity, times per week an activity is done) better than general, open-ended questions[11]. If using an objective measure, pedometers may be as effective as accelerometers in older individuals if the activities predominantly involve walking rather than jogging, running, and upper body motion. These instruments also appear to be appropriate in children[47].

ENDPOINTS

The endpoint being evaluated is also an important consideration when choosing a method to assess physical activity. For example, measuring lifetime patterns of physical activity may be important when examining the relationships between cancer and bone health[48–50]. If the focus of the study is to establish a dose–response relationship with a health-related endpoint, a questionnaire, accelerometer, or HR monitor that allows for physical activity pattern determination is necessary. Finally, if the study goal is to determine the effectiveness of a physical activity intervention, comparing pre- and postdata from questionnaires with shorter timeframes (e.g., past week or 3-day diary) or physical activity monitors should be appropriate. Exceptions to using a monitor include the evaluation of interventions that involve strength training or another type of non-ambulatory activity not accurately assessed with a monitor.

CONSIDERATIONS FOR QUESTIONNAIRE AND DIARY USE

Time Frames

Time frames used when assessing physical activity vary from a diary that segments the day and has participants record their activities in 15-minute intervals to questionnaires that ask about lifetime physical activity. The time-frame assessed depends on the population and endpoint of interest to the researcher.

Shorter timeframes are the easiest to recall; however, they may not give an accurate picture of typical physical activity patterns. There are certain endpoints that rely on recent physical activity to accurately predict risk because it may affect the outcome more than the history of physical activity. This is reflected in studies by Paffenbarger et al. and Blair al. that demonstrated that changes in physical activity or fitness levels predict mortality risk[51,52]. For example, a person may be unfit at one point in time, but if her fitness level improves, her mortality risk is lower than someone who remained unfit. One's relatively recent physical activity level, rather than one's physical activity history, was related to mortality. Questionnaires that cover shorter periods of time, however, may not provide an adequate representation of a person's normal activity level (e.g., during bad weather, assessment of activities from the past week or past month may substantially underestimate one's activity level for the remainder of the year)[19]. Physical activities performed over the past year may not be remembered as accurately, but they do provide a more complete physical activity profile. Lifetime physical activity may be important to assess for its relationship to certain types of cancer as well as bone health[48–50]. Although this timeframe might be the most difficult to recall accurately, several studies have reported reasonable reliability results for long-term physical activity recall[53–55]. In addition, research has examined the validity of long-term recall (i.e., 10–15 years) and have found results comparable to that of questionnaires with shorter recall time frames[56–58].

Administration Techniques

Questionnaires are administered in a variety of ways. Questionnaires that are interviewer administered, either in person or over the telephone, take more time and are more costly than those that are self-administered. This method allows participants to clarify any issues and uncertainties about the questions, thereby reducing response errors.

Self-administered questionnaires are inexpensive and provide information comparable to that from interviewer-administered questionnaires[59]. Using this method of administration, the questionnaire can either be given to participants or sent to them through the mail. These questionnaires can be easily administered to large groups of individuals in a short amount of time.

More recent advances in technology have made the Internet a viable means of questionnaire administration. With the popularity and widespread availability of computers and Internet access, this may be a cost-effective way to monitor activity levels. Potential uses include online questionnaire administration and continuous monitoring of physical activity (e.g., online physical activity diaries). Further validation is needed for this potentially valuable method of recording and tracking physical activity behaviors.

Summary

It is important to use a valid and reliable method that is appropriate for the population as well as the study endpoint. The advantages and disadvantages of each type of subjective and objective physical assessment have been introduced. Given these strengths and weaknesses, a combination of physical activity assessment methods may provide the most accurate estimate of physical activity. This combination approach to assessment has not been widely examined[58]. However, based on the conclusion of various reports regarding the assessment of physical activity, using more than one method of ascertainment should increase the accuracy of the measurement[12,36,39,44,58]. Treuth recently recommended that additional research should focus on applying different combinations of assessment techniques to larger samples as well as various age groups and special populations[60].

REFERENCES

1. Caspersen CJ, Powell KE, Christenson GM: Physical activity, exercise, and physical fitness: Definitions and distinctions for health-related research. Pub Health Rep 100:126–131, 1985.
2. Ravussin E, Swinburn BA: Pathophysiology of obesity. Lancet 340:404–408, 1992.
3. Pereira MA, FitzGerald SJ, Gregg EW, et al: A collection of physical activity questionnaires for health-related research. Med Sci Sports Exerc 29:S1–S205. 1997
4. Pate RR, Pratt M, Blair SN, et al: Physical activity and public health: A recommendation from the Centers for Disease Control and Prevention and the American College of Sports Medicine. JAMA 273:402–407, 1995.
5. U.S. Department of Health and Human Services: Physical activity and health: A report of the Surgeon General, Atlanta: U.S. Department of Health and Human Services, Centers for Disease Control and Prevention, National Center for Chronic Disease Prevention and Health Promotion; 1996.
6. American College of Sports Medicine: The recommended quantity and quality of exercise for developing and maintaining fitness in healthy adults. Medicine and Science in Sports 10:vii–x, 1978.
7. American College of Sports Medicine: The recommended quantity and quality of exercise for developing and maintaining cardiorespiratory and muscular fitness in healthy adults. Med Sci Sports Exerc 22:265–274, 1990.
8. Pols MA, Peeters PH, Kemper HC, Grobbee DE: Methodological aspects of physical activity assessment in epidemiological studies. Eur J Epidemiol 14:63–70, 1998.
9. Ainsworth BE, Haskell WL, Leon AS et al: Compendium of physical activities: classification of energy costs of human physical activities. In ACSM's Resource Manual for Guidelines for Exercise Testing

and Prescription. Philadelphia: Lippincott Williams & Wilkins; 2001:673–686.

10. Welk GJ, Blair SN, Wood K, Jones S, Thompson RW: A comparative evaluation of three accelerometry-based physical activity monitors. Med Sci Sports Exerc 32:S489–S497, 2000.

11. Montoye HJ: Measuring physical activity and energy expenditure. Champaign, IL: Human Kinetics; 1996.

12. Tudor-Locke CE, Myers AM: Challenges and opportunities for measuring physical activity in sedentary adults. Sports Med 31:91–100, 2001.

13. Washburn RA, Heath GW, Jackson AW: Reliability and validity issues concerning large-scale surveillance of physical activity. Res Q Exerc Sport 71:S104–S113, 2000.

14. Haskell WL, Taylor HL, Wood PD, Schrott H, Heiss G: Strenuous physical activity, treadmill exercise test performance and plasma high-density lipoprotein cholesterol. The Lipid Research Clinics Program Prevalence Study. Circulation 62:IV53–IV61, 1980.

15. Weiss TW, Slater CH, Green LW, et al: The validity of single-item, self-assessment questions as measures of adult physical activity. J Clin Epidemiol 43:1123–1129, 1990.

16. Sallis JF, Haskell WL, Wood PD, et al: Physical activity assessment methodology in the Five-City Project. Am J Epidemiol 121:91–106, 1985.

17. Kriska AM, Bennett PH: An epidemiological perspective of the relationship between physical activity and NIDDM: From activity assessment to intervention. Diabetes Metab Rev 8:355–372, 1992.

18. Welk GJ, Morrow JR: Physical activity assessments. In Meredith MD, Welk GJ, eds. The Fitnessgram Test Administration Manual. Champaign, IL: Human Kinetics; 1999:55–65.

19. LaPorte RE, Montoye HJ, Caspersen CJ: Assessment of physical activity in epidemiologic research: Problems and prospects. Public Health Rep 100:131–146, 1985.

20. Sallis JF, Saelens BE: Assessment of physical activity by self-report: Status, limitations, and future directions. Res Q Exerc Sport 71:S1–S14, 2000.

21. Sallis JF, Nader PR, Broyles SL, et al: Correlates of physical activity at home in Mexican-American and Anglo-American preschool children. Health Psychol 12:390–398, 1993.

22. Barnes PM, Schoenborn CA: Physical activity among adults: United States, 2000. Advance Data (from Vital and Health Statistics of the CDC)333:1–23, 2003.

23. Ainsworth BE: Issues in the assessment of physical activity in women. Res Q Exerc Sport 71:S37–S42, 2000.

24. Kimsey CD, Ham SA, Macera CA, Ainsworth BE, Jones DA: Reliability of moderate and vigorous physical activity questions in the Behavioral Risk Factor Surveillance System (BRFSS) [abstract]. Medicine and Science in Sports 35:S114, 2003.

25. Bouchard C, Tremblay A, Leblanc C, et al: A method to assess energy expenditure in children and adults. Am J Clin Nutr 37:461–467, 1983.

26. Ainsworth BE, Haskell WL, Whitt MC, et al: Compendium of physical activities: An update of activity codes and MET intensities. Med Sci Sports Exerc 32:S498–S516, 2000.

27. Ainsworth BE: The compendium of physical activities. The President's Council on Physical Fitness and Sports Research Digest Series 4:1–8, 2003.

28. McKenzie TL, Marshall SJ, Sallis JF, Conway TL: Leisure-time physical activity in school environments: An observational study using SOPLAY. Prev Med 30:70–77, 2000.

29. Puhl J, Greaves K, Hoyt M, Baranowski T: Children's Activity Rating Scale (CARS): Description and calibration. Res Q Exerc Sport 61:26–36, 1990.

30. Bassett DR Jr, Ainsworth BE, Swartz AM, et al: Validity of four motion sensors in measuring moderate intensity physical activity. Med Sci Sports Exerc 32:S471–S480, 2000.

31. Welk GJ, Differding JA, Thompson RW, et al: The utility of the Digi-walker step counter to assess daily physical activity patterns. Med Sci Sports Exerc 32:S481–S488, 2000.

32. Bassett DR Jr, Ainsworth BE, Leggett SR, et al: Accuracy of five electronic pedometers for measuring distance walked. Med Sci Sports Exerc 28:1071–1077, 1996.

33. Crouter SE, Schneider PL, Karabulut M, Bassett DR: Validity of 10 electronic pedometers for measuring steps, distance, and energy cost. Med Sci Sports Exerc 35:1455–1460, 2003.

34. Schneider PL, Crouter SE, Lukajic O, Bassett DR: Accuracy and reliability of 10 pedometers for measuring steps over a 400-m walk. Med Sci Sports Exerc 35:1779–1784, 2003.

35 Leenders NYJM, Sherman WM, Nagaraja HN: Comparisons of four methods of estimating physical activity in adult women. Med Sci Sports Exerc 32:1320–1326, 2000.

36. Tudor-Locke CE: Taking steps toward increased physical activity: using pedometers to measure and motivate. The President's Council on Physical Fitness and Sports Research DigestSeries 3:1–8; 2002.

37. Freedson PS, Miller K: Objective monitoring of physical activity using motion sensors and heart rate. Res Q Exerc Sport 71:S21–S29, 2000.

38. Hendelman D, Miller K, Baggett C, Debold E, Freedson P: Validity of accelerometry for the assessment of moderate intensity physical activity in the field. Med Sci Sports Exerc 32:S442–S449, 2000.

39. Tudor-Locke C, Ainsworth BE, Thompson RW, Matthews CE: Comparison of pedometer and accelerometer measures of free-living physical activity. Med Sci Sports Exerc 34:2045–2051, 2002.

40. Swartz AM, Strath SJ, Bassett DR Jr, et al: Estimation of energy expenditure using CSA accelerometers at hip and wrist sites. Med Sci Sports Exerc 32:S450–S456, 2000.

41. Strath SJ, Swartz AM, Bassett DR Jr., et al: Evaluation of heart rate as a method for assessing moderate intensity physical activity. Med Sci Sports Exerc32:S465–S470, 2000.

42. Strath SJ, Bassett DR Jr, Thompson DL, Swartz AM: Validity of the simultaneous heart rate-motion sensor technique for measuring energy expenditure. Med Sci Sports Exerc 34:888–894, 2002.

43. Healey J: Future possibilities in electronic monitoring of physical activity. Res Q Exerc Sport 71:S137–S145, 2000.

44. Schutz Y, Herren R: Assessment of speed of human locomotion using a differential satellite global positioning system. Med Sci Sports Exerc 32:642–646, 2000.

45. Terrier P, Ladetto Q, Merminod B, Schutz Y: High-precision satellite positioning system as a new tool to study the biomechanics of human locomotion. J Biomech 33:1717–1722, 2000.

46. Kriska A: Ethnic and cultural issues in assessing physical activity. Res Q Exerc Sport 71:S47–S53, 2000.

47. Welk GJ, Corbin CB, Dale D: Measurement issues in the assessment of physical activity in children. Res Q Exerc Sport 71:S59–S73, 2000.

48. Matthews CE, Shu XO, Jin F, et al: Lifetime physical activity and breast cancer risk in the Shanghai Breast Cancer Study. Br J Cancer 84:994–1001, 2001.

49. Nieves JW, Grisso JA, Kelsey JL: A case-control study of hip fracture: evaluation of selected dietary variables and teenage physical activity. Osteoporos Int 2:122–127, 1992.

50. Vuillemin A, Guillemin F, Jouanny P, Denis G, Jeandel C: Differential influence of physical activity on lumbar spine and femoral neck bone mineral density in the elderly population. J Gerontol A Biol Sci Med Sci 56:B248–B253, 2001.

51. Paffenbarger RS Jr, Hyde RT, Wing AL, et al: The association of changes in physical-activity level and other lifestyle characteristics with mortality among men. N Engl J Med 328:538–545, 1993.

52. Blair SN, Kohl HW III, Barlow CE, et al: Changes in physical fitness and all-cause mortality: A prospective study of healthy and unhealthy men. JAMA 273:1093–1098, 1995.

53. Kriska AM, Sandler RB, Cauley JA, et al: The assessment of historical physical activity and its relation to adult bone parameters. Am J Epidemiol 127:1053–1063, 1988.

54. Kriska AM, Knowler WC, LaPorte RE, et al: Development of questionnaire to examine relationship of physical activity and diabetes in Pima Indians. Diabetes Care 13:401–411, 1990.

55. Chasan-Taber L, Erickson JB, McBride JW, et al: Reproducibility of a self-administered lifetime physical activity questionnaire among female college alumnae. Am J Epidemiol 155:282–289, 2002.

56. Bowles HR, FitzGerald SJ, Morrow JR, Jackson AW: Construct validity of self-reported historical physical activity [abstract]. Med Sci Sports Exerc 34:S206, 2003.

57. Winters-Hart CS, Brach JS, Storti KL, Kriska AM: Validity of a questionnaire to assess historical leisure physical activity in postmenopausal women [abstract]. Med Sci Sports Exerc 35:S339, 2003.

58. Kohl HW III, Kampert JB, Mâasse LC, Fulton JE, Tortolero SR, Blair SN: The accuracy of historical physical activity recall among middle- aged women and men [abstract]. Med Sci Sports Exerc 29:S242, 1997.

59. Jacobs DRJ, Ainsworth BE, Hartman TJ, Leon AS: A simultaneous evaluation of 10 commonly used physical activity questionnaires. Med Sci Sports Exerc 25:81–91, 1993.

60. Treuth MS: Applying multiple methods to improve the accuracy of activity assessments. InWelk GJ, ed. Physical Activity Assessments for Health-Related Research. Champaign, IL: Human Kinetics; 2002:213–225.

SELECTED REFERENCES FOR FURTHER READING

Measurement of Physical Activity: The Cooper Institute Conference Series. Proceedings from the 9th Measurement and Evaluation Symposium. Research Quarterly for Exercise and Sport, 71(suppl 2) 2000.

Montoye HJ, Kemper HCG, Saris WHM, Washburn RA: Measuring Physical Activity and Energy Expenditure. Champaign, IL: Human Kinetics; 1996.

National Center for Health Statistics: Assessing Physical Fitness and Physical Activity in Population-Based Surveys. Drury TF, ed. DHHS Pub. No. (PHS) 89-1253. Public Health Service. Washington, D.C: U.S. Government Printing Office; 1989.

Pereira MA, FitzGerald SJ, Gregg EW, Joswiak ML, Ryan WJ, Suminski RR, et al: A collection of physical activity questionnaires for health related research. Kriska AM, Caspersen CJ,(eds.). Med Sci Sports Exerc 6:S3–S205, 1997.

Welk, GJ, ed: Physical Activity Assessments for Health-Related Research. Champaign, IL: Human Kinetics; 2002.

INTERNET RESOURCES

CDC: Nutrition & Physical Activity: http://www.cdc.gov/nccdphp/dnpa/index.htm

The Cooper Institute: http://www.cooperinst.org

PACE Projects: http://www.paceproject.org

The President's Challenge: http://www.presidentschallenge.org/activity_log/track_progress.aspx

USC PRC Reports and Tools: http://prevention.sph.sc.edu/tools/index.htm

Relationship of Nutrition to Chronic Diseases

JESSICA KRENKEL, SACHIKO ST. JEOR, AND DOINA KULICK

This chapter addresses KSAs from the following content areas:

1 Exercise Physiology and Related Exercise Science
2 **Pathophysiology and Risk Factors**
3 Health Appraisal, Fitness, and Clinical Exercise Testing
4 Electrocardiography and Diagnostic Techniques
5 Patient Management and Medications
6 **Medical and Surgical Management**
7 Exercise Prescription and Programming
8 **Nutrition and Weight Management**
9 Human Behavior and Counseling
10 Safety, Injury Prevention, and Emergency Procedures
11 Program Administration, Quality Assurance, and Outcome Assessment

Compelling evidence proves that lifestyle changes (including diet, physical activity, and behavior) prevent or delay major chronic diseases, including cardiovascular disease (CVD), cancer, obesity, diabetes, and osteoporosis. Importantly, recent research[5] confirms that the effects of diet and other lifestyle changes may be additive. At the same time that clinical and population studies support the importance of diet, the understanding of the effects of nutrients and foods on genome stability, imprinting, expression, and viability correlated diet factors at the molecular level to prevention[6]. Because of this evidence, a paradigm shift in health care approaches has occurred toward early and aggressive prevention strategies. Thus, a greater proportion of the population will need behavioral strategies for lifestyle changes that positively impact chronic disease risk. The purpose of this chapter is to examine the relationship of diet and nutrition to chronic disease and to encourage health care professionals to promote healthier lifestyles.

Chronic diseases and their dietary recommendations are often intertwined. For example, obesity is associated with the comorbidities of CVD, diabetes, and the metabolic syndrome. Risk factors for obesity, CVD, and diabetes converge in the metabolic syndrome, which is characterized by increased morbidity and mortality risk from insulin resistance and its consequences[7]. Increased levels of circulating free fatty acids from excess stored fat contribute to insulin resistance, although the mechanisms are still debated[8]. The prevalence of metabolic syndrome in the United States is 22.8% and 22.6% in men and women, respectively[9].

The criteria for the metabolic syndrome (or the dysmetabolic syndrome) include any three of the following: large waist circumference above 102 cm or 40 inches in men and >88 cm or 35 inches in women, high triglycerides ($\geq$150 mg·dL^{-1}), low serum high-density lipoprotein (HDL) level (<40 mg·dL^{-1} for men and <50 mg·dL^{-1} for women), high blood pressure (BP; systolic $\geq$130 mm Hg or diastolic $\geq$85 mm Hg), and fasting plasma glucose concentration above 110 mg·dL^{-1}.

The prospective Insulin Resistance Atherosclerosis Study found that the best predictor for developing the metabolic syndrome in adults with no diabetes was waist circumference[10]. The authors conclude that obesity may precede the development of other metabolic syndrome components. In other research supporting this relationship, the development of insulin resistance in young adulthood was strongly predicted from childhood adiposity and serum insulin levels and from being the offspring of a parent with type 2 diabetes[11–13]. These studies underscore the need to address obesity in children.

There is no agreement about the optimal diet for preventing and treating chronic diseases, but recommendations from professional organizations and government institutes or agencies provide evidence-based guidelines, such as the guidelines for diabetes, cancer, obesity, and CVD in Table 9-1. The American Dietetic Association advocates the terminology, medical nutrition therapy

KEY TERMS

Antioxidants: Dietary components such as vitamins C and E, selenium, carotenoids, and other phytochemicals (chemicals from plants with antioxidant or hormone-like actions) that can protect DNA and cell membranes against oxidative damage from carcinogens

Body mass index (BMI): Body weight in kg·[Height in meters]^2 is an expression used to evaluate weight in the context of the distribution of mass over an individual's height[1]

Glycemic index: The increase in blood sugar after ingestion of a food or food component compared with the increase after ingestion of white bread. White bread is assigned an index of 100, with foods being assigned higher and lower relative values. The glycemic response varies with type of sugar, other food components, the amount of carbohydrate, the nature of the starch, and cooking or food processing.

High-density lipoproteins (HDLs): Compounds that transport body cholesterol to other lipoproteins for disposal, contain a high proportion of phospholipids (30%) and protein (45–50%), and decrease the risk of coronary artery disease

Impaired fasting glucose (IFG): A prediabetic condition in which the fasting blood sugar is elevated (100 to 125 mg·dL^{-1}) after an overnight fast[2]

Impaired glucose tolerance (IGT): A prediabetic condition in which the blood sugar level is elevated (140 to 199 mg·dL^{-1}) after a 2-hour glucose tolerance test[2].

Low density lipoproteins (LDLs): Substances that are taken up by receptor and scavenger pathways in blood vessels, contain a high proportion of cholesterol (45%), and increase the risk of coronary artery disease

Metabolic syndrome: A condition characterized by insulin resistance and a high risk of developing cardiovascular disease or diabetes.

Monounsaturated fats: Fatty acids with one double bond between the carbon atoms that are prevalent in olive oil, canola oil, and high oleic acid oils. These fats are neutral or only slightly increase serum low-density lipoprotein cholesterol levels.

Obesity: As defined by the National Institutes of Health, a body mass index of greater than 30 kg·m^2

Omega-3 fatty acids: Fatty acids with the first double bond between carbon atoms located between the third and fourth carbon, including alpha linolenic acid (ALA) and the three series such as eicosapentaenoic acid (EPA) and docosahexenoic acid (DHA). These fats decrease the risk of cardiovascular disease and are prevalent in fish and flaxseed, walnut, canola, and soybean oils[3].

Omega-6 fatty acids: Fatty acids with the first double bond between carbon atoms located between the sixth and seventh carbons, which are converted to hormone-like substances called eicosanoids. Sources of omega-6 fatty acids are corn, safflower, peanut, cottonseed, soybean, sesame, rapeseed, borage, and primrose oils[3].

Osteoporosis: A condition characterized by microarchitectural deterioration of bone tissue leading to decreased bone mass and increased bone fragility

Overweight: As defined by the National Institutes of Health, a body mass index of 25 to 29.9 kg·m^{-2}

Polyunsaturated fats: Fatty acids with two or more double bonds between carbon atoms. These fats decrease serum low-density lipoprotein cholesterol levels. Foods with a high percentage of polyunsaturated fats include corn, safflower, peanut, cottonseed, soybean, fish, walnut, and flaxseed oils[3].

Prehypertensive: Systolic blood pressure of 120 to 139 mm Hg or a diastolic blood pressure of 80 to 89 mm Hg[4]

Saturated fats: Fatty acids with single bonds between the carbons atoms. These fats increase serum low-density lipoprotein cholesterol levels and are prevalent in animal fats; butter; meats; milk fat; cheeses; and tropical oils such as palm, coconut, and palm kernel oil[3].

Trans fats: Fatty acids with a rearrangement of the bond between some of the carbon atoms to a form rarely found in natural foods. The change occurs because of processing such as the hydrogenation (the addition of hydrogen to change texture and improve shelf life). Foods containing these fats include margarine, shortening, processed foods, and commercially baked or fried foods[3].

(MNT), for the nutritional diagnostic, therapeutic, and counseling services to accomplish the following:

- Effectively treat and manage disease conditions
- Reduce or eliminate the need for prescription drug use
- Help reduce complications in patients with disease
- Improve patients' overall health and quality of life[14]

The MNT recommendations for obesity, diabetes, cancer, and CVD specify dietary proportions of macro-

TABLE 9-1. Medical Nutrition Therapy for Obesity/Metabolic Syndrome, Hypertension, Cardiovascular Disease, and Diabetes

Diagnostic Criteria & Risk Factors	Nutrition & Lifestyle Recommendations	Therapeutic Objectives	Practice Guidelines (References)
Obesity/Metabolic Syndrome Criteria for dysmetabolic syndrome include any 3 of the following: Waist Circumference: Men >102 cm (>40 in) Women >88 cm (>35 in) BP: ≥130 / ≥85 mm Hg Trig: ≥150 mg·dL^{-1} HDL: Men <40 mg·dL^{-1}, Women <50 mg·dL^{-1} FPG: ≥100 mg·dL^{-1} Other Risk Factors: BMI ≥30, sleep apnea, elevated CRP levels Hyperinsulinemia & insulin resistance may also be present	**Low Calorie Step I Diet & Referral to Dietitian** (for individuals at lower risk) 500–1,000 Kcal·d^{-1} reduction, ≤30% Fat, 8–10% SFA, <300 mg Chol, ~2.4 g Na, 1,000–1,500 mg Ca, 20–30 g fiber **TLC Diet & Referral to Dietitian** (for individuals at higher risk) Establish appropriate Kcal Rx 50–60% CHO ~15% Protein 25–35% Total Fat <7% SFA, <200 mg Chol **[same in Step II Diet]** PUFA (up to 10% of total kcals) MUFA (up to 20% of total kcals) 10–25 g viscous (soluble) fiber 2 g Plant stanols/sterols **Weight reduction & longterm control** 1–2 pounds wt loss/wk and gradually reach healthy BMI (<30 initially, then <25) **Increase physical activity (~200 Kcal/d)** **Smoking cessation**	1) Reasonable weight loss of 5–10%, maintain healthy BMI, prevent weight gain 2) Primary: ↓LDL to ↓CHD risk Secondary: recognize & treat metabolic syndrome for further risk reduction Optimal BMI range: 18.5–24.9 Target Total Chol: <200 mg·dL^{-1} Target TG: <150 mg·dL^{-1} Target LDL: <100 mg·dL^{-1} Target HDL: ≥40 (Men), ≥50 (Women) mg·dL^{-1} Target BP: <130 / <85 mm Hg Target FPG: <100 mg·dL^{-1}	NHLBI, NIH - Classification of Overweight & Obesity, Weight Loss Goals, and Low-Calorie Step I & Step II Diets (1) NCEP ATP III - Metabolic Syndrome Criteria and Therapeutic Lifestyle Changes (3) www.nhlbi.nih.gov/guidelines/obesity/ www.nhlbi.nih.gov/guidelines/cholesterol/ www.surgeongeneral.gov/topics/obesity
Hypertension BP Classification: normal: <120 / 80 mm Hg pre HTN: 120–139 / 80–89 mm Hg stage 1 HTN: 140–159 / 90–99 mm Hg stage 2 HTN: ≥160 / ≥100 mm Hg *Risk of CVD, beginning at 115 / 75 mm Hg, doubles with each increment of 20 / 10 mm Hg	**Dash Diet & Referral to Dietitian** Establish appropriate Kcal Rx ≤2400 mg Na, <30% Total Fat Limit Alcohol: Men ≤2 drinks/d, Women ≤1drink/d Reduce dietary sodium & red meat intake. Increase dietary calcium, magnesium, potassium & fiber via fruits, vegetables, whole grains, reduced fat dairy & lean protein. Include fish, nuts, seeds & dry beans weekly. Choose plant fats & oils. **Achieve & maintain healthy body weight** **Increase physical activity** **Smoking cessation**	1) Prevent progression to HTN in pre-hypertensive population 2) Decrease CVD complications & reduce cardiovascular & renal morbidity and mortality in hypertensive population Optimal BP: <120 / <80 mm Hg Goal of tx: BP <130 / <80 (for patients with diabetes or chronic kidney disease) Goal of tx: BP <140 / <90 (for patients with HTN)	NHLBI, NIH - Prevention, Detection, Evaluation, and Treatment of High Blood Pressure and Dash Eating Plan (4). www.nhlbi.gov/guidelines/hypertension/ www.nhlbi.nih.gov/health/public/heart/hbp/dash/index/htm

Cardiovascular Disease

Abnormal Blood Lipid Profile:
Total Cholesterol: ≥200 mg·dL⁻¹
Triglyceride: ≥150 mg·dL⁻¹
LDL: ≥100 mg·dL⁻¹
HDL: Men <40 mg·dL⁻¹, Women <50 mg·dL⁻¹

Other major CVD risk factors include:
Obesity, inactive lifestyle, atherogenic diet
Elevated BP, blood glucose & homocysteine levels
Hyperinsulinemia & insulin resistance may also be present

AHA Dietary Guidelines & Referral to Dietitian
Establish appropriate Kcal Rx
<6 g NaCl (<2400 mg Na)
<30% Total Fat, Limit TFA's
[AHA population-wide recommendations for individuals at lower risk]
<10% SFA, <300 mg Chol
[AHA MNT for individuals at higher risk]
<7% SFA, <200 mg Chol
Limit Alcohol: Men ≤2 drinks/d, Women ≤1drink/d
Limit high caloric / low nutrient dense foods & beverages.
Increase intake of antioxidants, omega fatty acids & fiber via variety of fruits, vegetables, whole grains, reduced fat dairy, fish, legumes, nuts, plant fats & oils.

Achieve & maintain healthy body weight
Increase physical activity- 30 minutes daily of moderate intensity exercise using large muscle groups (i.e. walking or swimming)
Smoking cessation

1) Reduce CVD risk, morbidity & mortality by preventing or reducing the development of atherosclerotic disease & stroke
2) For overweight / obese patients, ↓ weight by 10% in 1st year of therapy
Target Total Chol: <160 mg·dL⁻¹ (optimal)
Total Chol: 160–199 mg·dL⁻¹ (low risk profile)
Target LDL: <100 mg·dL⁻¹ if ≥2 CHD risk factors
Target HDL: >40 (Men), >50 (Women) mg·dL⁻¹
Goal BP: <140 / <90 or <130 / <85 mm Hg for patients with renal insufficiency, heart failure or <130 / <80 mm Hg for patients with diabetes

AHA Dietary Guidelines, Revision 2002 (23)
AHA Dietary Guidelines, 2000 (22)
www.americanheart.org

Diabetes

Normoglycemia:
FPG <100 mg·dL⁻¹
2-h PG <140 mg·dL⁻¹

IFG (Impaired Fasting Glucose):
FPG ≥100 and <126 mg·dL⁻¹

IGT (Impaired Glucose Tolerance):
2-h PG ≥140 and <200 mg·dL⁻¹

Diabetes:
FPG ≥126 mg·dL⁻¹
2-h PG ≥200 mg·dL⁻¹
Casual PG ≥200 mg·dL⁻¹ (symptoms present)

ADA Dietary Guidelines & Referral to Dietitian
Establish appropriate Kcal Rx
CHO & MUFA together should provide 60–70% total kcal
15–20% protein
<30% total fat, Minimize TFA's
<10% SFA, <300 mg chol if LDL <100 mg·dL⁻¹
<7% SFA, <200 mg chol if LDL ≥100 mg·dL⁻¹
Limit Alcohol: Men ≤2 drinks/d, Women ≤1drink/d
*Appropriate Rx's may integrate any of the following established regimens:
Low Calorie Step I or Step II, TLC, DASH, AHA, or Mediterranean Diets

Goals of MNT & Self Management Education:
*Attain and maintain recommended metabolic outcomes, including glucose, A1c, LDL, HDL, TG levels; BP; and body weight.
*Modify nutrient intake and lifestyle as appropriate for the prevention and treatment of obesity, dyslipidemia, HTN, CVD, depression, and nephropathy.
*Structured, intensive lifestyle programs involving participant education, individualized counseling, regular physical activity, and SMBG.
*Smoking cessation

1) Diabetes prevention: ↓risk by encouraging physical activity and food choices that facilitate moderate weight loss (5–7%) or at least prevent weight gain
2) Prevent and treat chronic complications and comorbidities of diabetes
Target HbA1c: <7.0%
Target FPG: 80–120 mg·dL⁻¹
Target Bedtime BG: 100–140 mg·dL⁻¹
Target BP: <130 / 80 mm Hg
Target Blood Lipids (mg·dL⁻¹):
TG <150
LDL <100
HDL ≥40 (Men), ≥50 (Women)
Target Microalbumin: <30 µg·mg⁻¹ creatinine

American Diabetes Association: Clinical Practice Guidelines (2, 17, 152)
American Dietetic Association: Nutrition Practice Guidelines at www.eatright.org
www.diabetes.org

* Table used by permission of Loredo G and Herzog H, Division of Medical Nutrition and Center for Nutrition and Metabolic Disorders. Department of Internal Medicine. University of Nevada School of Medicine, Reno, NV. 2004.

nutrients: carbohydrate, fat, and protein. The average diet in the United States for individuals older than 20 years currently consists of 34% kcal from total fat, 49% kcal from carbohydrates, 15% to 16% kcal from protein, and 2% to 3% of kcal from alcohol[15]. When a diet low in one macronutrient is promoted, other macronutrients are concomitantly increased at a given energy level; for example, a low-carbohydrate diet usually results in a higher fat and protein dietary intake[16]. Therefore, frequent monitoring of fasting lipid panels may be indicated for persons at risk of chronic disease who choose a low-carbohydrate diet[17]. Usually slight to moderate changes in macronutrient proportions have little effect on the short-term health parameters, such as serum lipids, but deleterious, long-term health effects are often unknown.

The greatest similarities across national diet recommendations (see Table 9-1) for obesity, hypertension, CVD, diabetes, and cancer are the recommendations to maintain a healthy weight and to consume total dietary fat of approximately 30% kcal. the National Cholesterol Education Program (NCEP) Therapeutic Lifestyle Changes (TLC) recommends a dietary fat intake of 25% to 35% of daily kcalocalories[3]. The specified purpose of the TLC diet is for prevention and treatment of obesity, metabolic syndrome, and CVD. Although recommendations for specific diet components vary with disease risk, a healthy weight is a primary step toward decreasing chronic disease risk. All calorie-restricted diets can be balanced to result in weight loss, regardless of their composition, but some diets meet nutrition needs with less health risk and should be the preferred choice for health professionals. A reasonable guide is the Institutes of Medicine, National Academy of Sciences' 2002 recommendation of Acceptable macronutrient ranges of 20% to 35% fat, 45% to 60% carbohydrate, and 10% to 35% protein[18].

Cardiovascular Disease and Diet

Cardiovascular diseases leading to heart attacks and strokes are the leading causes of death and disability in the United States and worldwide[19,20]. The World Health Organization currently attributes one third of all global deaths to CVD. This ongoing and increasing health problem underlines the need to improve our communication of improved diet and lifestyle interventions. Disease progression occurs over a lifetime and, thus, dietary changes need to be maintained to be effective. Public health and clinical approaches alone have limitations. Therefore, a recent American Heart Association (AHA) community health guide[21] for community health advocates for complementary public health and clinical approaches. The guide identifies public health problems, including limited access to screening; limited long-term and effective strategies for diet and physical activity changes; poor identification of healthy food choices at grocery stores and restaurants; and a lack of safe, attractive sites for physical activity in many communities. Clinical set-

tings provide a complementary focus on individuals with high disease risk, but diet counseling and nutrition education are often inadequate and highly variable[21]. Diverse and interdisciplinary diet and lifestyle changes are required to address the CVD risk.

CORONARY HEART DISEASE

Coronary heart disease (CHD) includes the development of atherosclerosis with the potential negative outcome of clot formation, resulting in a myocardial infarction (MI) or heart attack (see Chapter 29). Risk factors for CHD include an abnormal lipid profile, obesity, inactive lifestyle, atherogenic diet, elevated blood glucose and homocysteine levels, and hyperinsulinemia and insulin resistance. The preferred lipid profile includes a total cholesterol of 200 mg·dL^{-1} or less with a target of 160 mg·dL^{-1} with high CHD risk, triglycerides 150 mg·dL^{-1} of less, low-density lipoprotein (LDL) 100 mg·dL^{-1} or less, and an HDL equal to or greater than 40 for women and 50 for men[3,22,23].

The primary dietary factors that prevent atherosclerotic lesions and abnormally elevated serum lipid levels include diets moderate or low in saturated fat and cholesterol, decreased transfatty acids, increased omega-3 fatty acids, and shifted sources of fat to more monounsaturated fats[22–24] (see Table 9-1). Vitamins decrease cardiovascular risk if patients consume an adequate food intake of antioxidants and dietary vitamins (B12, B6, folate) to maintain normal serum homocysteine levels. In addition, the recommended intake of fruits, vegetables, breads, cereals, nuts, seeds, and other plant foods provides fiber, plant sterols, and phytochemicals, such as flavonoids, that decrease cardiovascular risk. A variety of other foods and food components, such as alcohol and soy protein, have been investigated to decrease cardiovascular risk[3]. Similar dietary factors that are important for CVD risk decrease clot formation (e.g., regular consumption of fish sources containing high concentrations of omega-3 fatty acids and alcohol intake). Also, a habitual high-fat diet may increase the activity of the blood clotting factor, factor VII, and increase cardiovascular risk[25].

Fats and Cholesterol

Saturated and Unsaturated

Saturated fatty acids, cholesterol, and high-fat diets are strongly associated with increased risk of CHD in susceptible persons. Changes in dietary cholesterol can dramatically alter serum LDL in a select segment of the population. Genetic explanations, such as apoprotein E and E4 variants, have been explored, but the results have been variable and remain unclear[3,26]. Egg yolks are a rich source of cholesterol but are low in saturated fatty acids. The role of eggs has been controversial, but current approaches emphasize limiting dietary intake to achieve 200 to 300 mg per day of dietary cholesterol[3,24]. Dietary saturated fat can be decreased by changing total fat intake to moderate- (<30% kcal) or low-fat (20% kcal) levels while altering the sources and types of fat to increase monounsaturated and polyunsaturated fats. Saturated fatty acids that need reduction include those with the greatest effect on increasing serum cholesterol and LDL: myristic and palmitic acids found in dairy products and meat[27] and transfatty acids found in margarine, processed foods, and commercially baked or fried foods containing hydrogenated oils[28]. The primary dietary monounsaturated fatty acid is oleic (abundant in olive and canola oils and nuts), and the primary dietary polyunsaturated fatty acid is linoleic (abundant in soybean and sunflower oils)[22].

Omega-3 Fatty Acids

Omega-3 fatty acids exert a cardioprotective effect and reduce CHD risk by reducing elevated triglyceride levels, inhibiting platelet aggregation and formation of blood clots, lowering BP, preventing plaque formation, and promoting the health of the vascular epithelium in the coronary arteries[29]. Omega-3 fatty acids are found in plant foods (flaxseed, canola oil, soybean oil, walnuts, mustard seed oil, and some leafy vegetables) as alpha linolenic acid (ALA) and in cold water fish as the eicosanoids (eicosapentaenoic acid [EPA] and docosahexanoic acid [DHA]). About 10% of the ALA that is consumed is converted in the body to EPA and DHA depending on the presence of omega-6 fatty acids that compete for the same enzymes.

The evidence for benefits of omega-3 fatty acids from the diet and supplements has been mixed[30], but a recent meta-analysis supports a strong association of CHD and fish intake[31]. The meta-analysis consisted of 228,864 adult participants from 14 cohort and five case-control studies in which fish was consumed on a regular basis in the experimental group while the comparison group consumed little or no fish. Overall, fish consumption was associated with a 20% reduction in the risk of fatal CHD and a 10% reduction in total CHD. The reduction in fatal CHD was hypothesized to be related to omega-3 fatty acid intake. In addition to the meta-analysis, a systematic review of prospective cohort studies found that high-risk populations had the most benefit from fish consumption, with an average of 1.5 to 2.0 oz of fish per day being associated with a 50% reduction in CHD death[32]. In 1989, the randomized, controlled, secondary prevention trial, Diet and Reinfarction Trial (DART), found a 2-year, 29% decrease in mortality for survivors of a first MI in the group advised to consume fatty fish two times per week[33]. Supplemental omega-3 fatty acids have similar benefits as fish consumption to reduce CVD mortality, stroke, and all-cause mortality[34–36]. The largest supplement trial included 11,324 patients who were survivors of MIs[34,35]. The fish oil supplement group had a 20% reduction in total mortality, a 30% reduction in cardiovascular death, and a 45% decrease in sudden death 3.5 years after supplementation began.

The AHA guidelines recommend at least two servings of fish (preferably oily: tuna, salmon, and mackerel) per week

for adult, nonpregnant or nursing patients without documented CHD[30]. For patients with documented CHD, the recommendation is to consume a diet rich in ALA and 1 g of EPA and DHA per day, preferably from fish, but an omega-3 fatty acid supplement may be needed to meet this level. The use of supplements requires review by the patient's physician. Patients who need omega-3 fatty acids for triglyceride lowering are recommended to take 2 to 4 g of EPA and DHA under their physician's care[30]. The American Diabetes Association guidelines indicated the usefulness of supplemental omega-3 fatty acids for the population of patients with diabetes and severe hypertriglyceridemia but recommended monitoring for increases in LDL[17].

Transfatty Acids

Transfatty acids behave similarly to saturated fat in many ways, including increasing LDL cholesterol level. But they are even more destructive than saturated fat because they also lower HDL cholesterol level[31]. The Food and Drug Administration (FDA) will require that food labels have the content of transfatty acids by January 2006, but there is insufficient information regarding the effects of various intake levels to establish a Daily Reference Value of transfatty acids[37].

Recommended Diets

Patients who are at high risk of CHD or who have been diagnosed with CHD benefit from a nutrition plan that is consistent with the AHA Dietary Guidelines, including Step I and Step II diets[22,23] or the NCEP ATP III guidelines that use the TLC diet[3] (also see Chapter 30). The TLC diet is comparable to the Step II AHA diet with the exception that the range of calories from fat is greater to accommodate evidence that CHD risk can be reduced with a variety of dietary patterns (see Table 9-1). The Step II AHA and the TLC diets have the lower saturated fat recommendation of 7% versus 10% on Step I and the lower cholesterol recommendation of 200 mg·day^{-1} versus 300 mg·day^{-1} on Step I. A meta-analysis of 37 studies[38] found that the stricter Step II or TLC diets versus the Step I reduced total serum cholesterol by 15% (32 mg·dL^{-1} average reduction) versus 10% (24 mg·dL^{-1} average reduction) and reduced LDL cholesterol by 16% (25 mg·dL^{-1} average reduction) versus 12% (19 mg·dL^{-1} average reduction), but both diets reduced triglycerides 8% (15 to 17 mg·dL^{-1} average reductions). One caveat was that whereas the Step I diet maintained HDL levels, the Step II and TLC diets decreased HDL by 7%. The AHA recommends the Step II diet for individuals who have CHD or who have not met the LDL cholesterol goals with Step I.

Low-fat diets have an additional positive benefit when they contribute to weight loss, but the diet should be coupled with activity recommendations to maintain or improve the serum HDL level. Obesity decreases HDL levels, so the net effect of weight loss, when coupled with increased activity, is to improve cardiovascular health by decreasing LDL and increasing or maintaining HDL[3].

The Mediterranean diet may be useful for individuals who prefer a moderate fat intake with more added monounsaturated fats than the AHA or TLC diets[39, 40]. The Mediterranean diet also has positive cardiovascular benefits and approximates the Step I AHA diet with higher levels of monounsaturated fatty acids, such as oleic acid and a polyunsaturated fatty acid, ALA. The traditional Mediterranean diet is composed of higher amounts of fruits, vegetables, bread and other cereals, potatoes, poultry, beans, nuts, fish, grains, dairy products, and moderate amounts of alcohol as well as olive oil. It is low in red meat. This yields a diet low in saturated fat and high in monounsaturated fat (mainly because of olive oil), complex carbohydrates, fiber, beta carotene, vitamin C, and tocopherols.

In the CARDIO2000 study, hypercholesterolemic participants who were taking statins were placed in control and diet groups[40]. The Mediterranean diet group ate fruits, vegetables, dairy products, potatoes, and bread and used olive oil in cooking on a daily basis. Fish, poultry, and eggs, olives, and legumes were consumed two to three times per week. Red meat was only consumed one to two times per month, and wine was drunk in moderation (one to two glasses per day). The subjects adhering to the Mediterranean diet had a 17% greater reduction in coronary event risk compared with participants who did not adopt the Mediterranean diet. These results demonstrate the potential benefit of dietary interventions combined with statin therapy.

A population-based study examined the effects of the Mediterranean diet on total mortality, cardiac mortality, and cancer mortality in 22,043 adults in Greece[39]. The median follow-up was 44 months, and adherence to the Mediterranean diet positively correlated with a reduction in total mortality, death caused by coronary artery disease, and death caused by cancer. Interestingly, the individual food groups contributing to the Mediterranean diet did not have a significant effect on total mortality unless they were integrated together into a diet. A secondary prevention trial, the Lyon Diet Heart Study, with subjects who had a history of an initial MI incorporated the Mediterranean diet with increased levels of ALA[41]. ALA was increased by adding it to margarine, monounsaturates were increased with olive oil, and polyunsaturated omega-6 fatty acids were increased with rapeseed oil. The participants following the Mediterranean-style diet had 50% to 70% lower risk of recurrent heart disease with risk reductions of the same size as those typically associated with statin drug therapy. This multifactorial dietary intervention study demonstrated a positive effect of decreasing the ratio of omega-6 to omega-3 fatty acids to four to one versus the typical Western diet ratio of 14 to 20 to one.

Vitamins

Antioxidants

Food sources of antioxidant vitamins, instead of supplements, are advised because of the positive potential health effects of other associated food components such as flavones. Epidemiological studies of vitamin supplementation with antioxidant vitamins, particularly vitamins C, E, and A as well as beta-carotene, had supported their possible role in reducing risk, but recent randomized, placebo-controlled trial results have challenged the benefits for vitamins A and E and beta-carotene supplementation. Over a 5-year period, the Heart Protection Collaborative Group[42] studied the effects of supplementation with vitamins E and C and beta-carotene versus placebo on mortality and coronary events. There were no significant differences in any parameters for the 20,536 adults other than increased blood vitamin concentrations. The investigators reviewed the results for their 6000 patients with diabetes and the results for 7000 patients with no evidence of CHD before randomization and found no evidence of benefit for vitamin supplementation. These results are in agreement with the Age-Related Eye Diseases (ARED) placebo-controlled trial of the same vitamins in a sample with 4500 older adults without any recent cardiovascular events[43]) Similarly, the Primary Prevention Project[44] studied the effects of vitamin E and the alpha-tocopherol beta-carotene[45] by investigating low-dose vitamin E and beta-carotene supplementation, with results indicating no significant differences in CHD outcomes. Likewise, natural vitamin E as opposed to synthetic products produced no significant difference for CHD[46]. These studies indicated that, despite previously encouraging results from nonrandomized, observational studies and small clinical trials, the preponderance of evidence from well-designed, large studies found that there was no clear evidence of CHD benefits for antioxidant supplementation.

Homocysteine

Elevated serum homocysteine levels are a CHD risk factor that may be related to other risk factors rather than being an independent risk[47]. Homocysteine, a highly reactive sulfur containing amino acid, may be damaging to health because of toxic effects that damage endothelial cells, increase cholesterol oxidation, modify apolipoproteins, promote platelet adhesion and aggregation, scavenge nitric oxide, and inhibit vascular motility. Homocysteine decreases nitric oxide, the smooth muscle relaxant in the arterial wall that decreases the tendency of platelets to aggregate and adhere to the vascular endothelium. Increased serum homocysteine is most often caused by a combination of a genetic variant of an enzyme in homocysteine metabolism or suboptimal nutritional status for folate and vitamins B12 and B6. The conversion of the amino acid methionine to homocysteine is limited when adequate folic acid is available, and the conversion of homocysteine to less toxic compounds is promoted when vitamin B6 is available. B12 is another cofactor in the metabolism of homocysteine, and it interacts with folic acid or substitutes for folic acid in some cases[48]. A meta-analysis by Wald et al.[49] concluded that a folic acid intake of 800 $\mu g \cdot day^{-1}$ would reduce the risk of ischemic heart disease by 16% and stroke by 24%. Data from the Nurses' Health Study showed that folate and vitamin B6 from the diet and supplements protected against CHD[50]. Increased serum homocysteine level has been associated with obesity in children in relation to folate intake and to hyperinsulinism with insulin resistance[51].

Plant Sources

Plant sources combined in a dietary plan, the "Portfolio," have produced significant reductions in LDL cholesterol compared with the traditional TLC diet and statin cholesterol lowering drugs[52]. The diet consists of 1 oz of almonds; 2 g of plant sterols from enriched margarine; 35 g of soy protein; and 15 g of viscous fiber from sources such as oats, barley, eggplant, and okra. A study of 25 hyperlipidemic patients had a 35% reduction of LDL in 2 weeks of consuming the prepared diet compared with a 12% LDL reduction for those consuming the TLC diet[52]. The benefit of these plant sources individually has been identified, and their inclusion is advocated in the TLC diet.

Fiber and Plant Sterols

Recommendations for dietary changes to decrease serum cholesterol include increased intake of dietary fiber and plant sterols. The TLC diet recommends a total of 20 to 30 g of fiber each day[3]. Soluble fiber increases the excretion of cholesterol in the bile, and an intake of 10 to 25 $g \cdot day^{-1}$ is suggested. To increase intake of soluble fiber, include or increase servings of fruits (especially those with high pectin content, such as apples, strawberries, and citrus), vegetables, oats, oat bran, and beans. The remainder of daily fiber intake is insoluble fiber that is not digested, adds bulk to the stool, and contributes to correcting diarrhea and constipation. Wheat bran is a good source of insoluble fiber[3].

The plant kingdom contains a number of sterols that differ from cholesterol because of their ethyl or methyl groups or unsaturation in the side chain. The major plant sterols—itosterol, stigmasterol, and campesterol—can be present in Western diets in amounts almost equal to dietary cholesterol. Sitosterol, the most prominent dietary sterol, with the saturated stanol derivative, sitostanol, reduces the absorption of cholesterol and decreases blood cholesterol level. In 1999, several companies began marketing margarine, salad dressings, and other products containing either stanols or sterols made from soy and corn.

An intake of 2 to 3 g per day or about 2–3 servings a day of products containing plant stanols and sterols decreased both dietary and biliary cholesterol absorption. Serum cholesterol levels decreased by 10%, and LDL serum cholesterol decreased by 13%[53].

Sitosterols and a sterol precursor, squalene, are present in both monounsaturated and polyunsaturated vegetable oils and, thus, may be responsible for some of the variable cholesterol-lowering effects found in studies using these products. The levels of these sterols may explain differences in study results seen between various sources and degrees of refinement of olive oil[54,55].

Flavonoids

Flavonoids are chemically varied compounds present in fruits, vegetables, nuts, and seeds that have been inversely linked with CHD. In the Zutphen Elderly Study[56], the Seven Countries Study[57] and a cohort study in Finland[58], people with low intakes of flavonoids had a higher death rate from CHD than did those who consumed more flavonoids. The amounts of foods rich in flavonoids, such as intake of about five to six cups of tea per day, that have been effective in these studies are at levels greater than usual dietary intake.

The major flavonoid categories are flavones (apple skins, berries, broccoli, celery, cranberries, grapes, lettuce, olives, onions, parsley), catechins (red wine, tea), flavanones (citrus fruits, citrus peel), isoflavones (soy), and anthocyanins (berries, cherries, red wine, grapes, tea). Subdivisions of flavonoids include quercetin glucoside in onions and quercetin rutinoside in tea. Some flavonoids have toxic effects (gastrointestinal or allergic), especially if taken in large amounts[59].

Additionally, flavonoids have antioxidant properties. For example, the phenolic substances in red wine inhibit oxidation of human LDL. Flavonoids have also been shown to inhibit the aggregation and adhesion of platelets in the blood, which may be another way they lower the risk of CHD. Isoflavones in soy foods have been reported to lower plasma cholesterol level and to have effects similar to estrogen[59].

Soy Protein

The FDA approved the CVD health claim for soy protein, noting that when it is included in a low-fat and low-cholesterol diet, soy protein can lower total blood cholesterol and LDL cholesterol levels (about 5% with 25 $g \cdot day^{-1}$ of soy protein) without adversely affecting HDL cholesterol levels[6]. The mechanism is not known, but soy isoflavones, fiber, phytic acid, and saponins in combination with soy protein are probably involved[23,60]. Protein was identified as the active component rather than isoflavones, fiber, phytic acid, or saponins. The FDA stated, "In order to claim the health effects of soy, a product must contain 6.25 g of soy protein or more, be low fat (less than 3 g), be low in saturated fat (less than 1 g) and low in cholesterol (less than 20 mg)"[61]. Food sources of soy protein (serving size and grams of protein) include soybeans (1/2 cup = 30 g), soy flour (1/2 cup = 15 g), textured soy protein (1 cup dry = 12 g), soy milk (1/2 cup = 3 g), tofu (1/2 cup = 20 g), and tempeh (1/2 cup = 16 g), but soy sauce and soy oil do not contain protein[62,63].

Alcohol

The AHA's Dietary Guidelines: Revision 2000[22] concluded that moderate alcohol consumption (one drink per day for women and two drinks a day for men) reduces the overall risk of CHD, but the basis for the protective effect of alcohol remains unclear. Alcohol consumption beginning in middle age (ages 35 to 69 years) might suffice for cardioprotective effects while averting much of the risk of accidents and cancer associated with drinking alcohol[64,65]. The phenolic compounds in red wine contribute to a greater coronary risk reduction than other alcohol sources, but other wines, beer, and spirits also reduce CHD risk. Alcohol has potentially negative consequences for patients with diabetes, hypertension, cancer risk, and liver disease. Additional recommendations for alcohol consumption suggest that those who do not consume alcohol should not be encouraged to begin the practice and that medications need to be reviewed by their physicians for potential interactions[66,67].

HYPERTENSION

Hypertension is the third leading cause of death in the world, with 1 billion individuals worldwide affected and approximately 50 million individuals affected in the United States[19,20]. High BP increases the risk of MI, heart failure, stroke, and kidney disease. Kottke et al.[68] identified high BP as a symptom of the "lifestyle syndrome," a cluster of conditions and diseases that result from consuming too many calories and too much saturated fat, sodium, and alcohol; not balancing intake with physical activity; and using tobacco. Obesity is a major risk factor for hypertension that is addressed later in this chapter and book. Current knowledge about the prevention and treatment of hypertension with lifestyle changes and other effective early interventions has not been adequately translated to the public and to high-risk individuals. For example, Greenlund et al.[69] found that more than one third of persons with established stroke did not receive advice from a health care professional on dietary or exercise changes.

The Seventh Report of the Joint National Committee on Prevention, Detection, Evaluation, and Treatment of High Blood Pressure established the optimal BP as a systolic BP of 115 mm Hg and a diastolic of 75 mm Hg with the need to begin treatment when the patient has a systolic BP of 120 to 139 mm Hg or a diastolic BP of 80 to 89 mm Hg[4]. The prehypertensive state initially requires

health-promoting lifestyle modifications, not medications, to prevent CVD (see Chapters 5 and 30).

For children, especially those with a higher risk of hypertension because of obesity, prevention is an ideal intervention approach. In the Bogalusa Heart Study, hypertension and obesity in parents and relatives increased the risk of the child's developing hypertension[11,70]. The prevalence of increased BP in elementary school children found that high systolic BP was 4.5 times more likely and high diastolic pressure 2.4 times more likely among obese children. Figeroa-Colon et al.[71] found 20% to 30% of obese children ages 5 to 11 years from a high-risk population had hypertension. The response to dietary sodium may vary with the degree of adiposity in children and adolescents. Obese adolescents who changed from a high- to a low-salt diet had a significantly larger decrease in BP compared with an insignificant change among non-obese adolescents[72].

Recommendations for dietary minerals that positively influence hypertension include limiting the daily sodium intake to less than 2400 mg (6 g salt) and increasing the food sources of calcium, magnesium, and potassium[3,4]. The preponderance of the evidence for a benefit from increasing minerals is for potassium[73]. Healthy food choices to provide the preferred mineral balance include an intake of five or more servings fruits and vegetables, consumption of six or more servings of grains, and daily low fat dairy product intake of two to four servings[4]. The effect of dietary modifications varies among individuals because of genetic factors, age, medications, and other host factors. Two recent systematic reviews of the effects of reductions in dietary sodium or salt found minimal effects for normal and hypertensive patients, particularly whites, but greater effects were seen for Asians and blacks[74] and for maintenance of a lower BP after antihypertensives were discontinued[75].

Benefits of Comprehensive Diet Changes

Changes encompassing several dietary factors have lowered BP in hypertensive and normotensive individuals with systolic BPs of less than 160 mm Hg and diastolic BPs of 80 to 95 mm Hg. The lifestyle modifications to manage hypertension[4] provided decreases in systolic BP of 5 to 20 mm Hg per 10 kg of weight loss, 8 to 14 mm Hg for adopting the Dietary Approaches to Stop Hypertension (DASH) diet high in fruits and vegetables, 2 to 8 mm Hg for dietary sodium restriction, 4 to 9 mm Hg for 30 min·day^{-1} of physical activity, and 2 to 4 mm Hg for moderate alcohol consumption. In particular, the DASH diet significantly reduced systolic and diastolic BP by 5.5 and 3.0 mm Hg more than the control diet for participants whose BPs were normotensive[76]. In participants with hypertension, the DASH diet without a specific salt restriction reduced systolic and diastolic BP by 11.4 and 5.5 mm Hg more, respectively, than the control diet. The DASH diet was lower in fat and higher in vegetables, fruits, and low-fat dairy foods and includes whole grains, poultry, fish, and nuts. The diet was also rich in calcium, magnesium, and potassium. The control group had a diet composition typical of the average individual in the United States (low in fruits, vegetables, and dairy products, with an average fat content). The addition of a lower salt intake (1500 mg·day^{-1}), lowered the mean systolic BP by 7.1 mm Hg for participants without hypertension and by 11.5 mm Hg in participants with hypertension[76–78].

The PREMIER Collaborative Research Group[5] compared the implementation of three interventions in a population of 810 adults at four clinical centers: (a) "established" (a behavioral intervention that implemented established recommendations), (b) "established" + DASH, and (c) advice only. Both the established and the established + DASH interventions resulted in significant weight reduction, improved fitness, and lowered sodium intake. Decreases in the prevalence of hypertension, and increases in optimal BP were highly significant ($P <$ 0.001) for the "established" + DASH intervention. Combining lifestyle interventions had an additive effect with significant results and significant implications for counseling patients.

Obesity and Diet

The prevalence of obesity and overweight in the United States has increased dramatically with obesity (body mass index [BMI] ≥ 30) increasing from 13.4% in 1960 to 30.9% in 2000 among adults[79]. Additionally, the incidence of severe obesity (BMI ≥ 35 with comorbidities or BMI ≥ 40) based on U.S. 1999 to 2000 population data is 3.1% for men and 6.7% for women. Poor diet coupled with physical inactivity is the second leading cause of preventable death, underscoring the depth of this major public health challenge[80,81]. In 1999, Allison et al.[80] reported ~300,000 deaths from overweight and obesity. Mokdad et al.[81] used the hazard ratios of Allison et al.[80] and the Centers for Disease Control and Prevention's 1999 and 2000 National Health and Nutrition Examination Surveys[82] to estimate the 400,000 U.S. deaths in 2000 attributable to being overweight, having a poor diet, and being inactive[81].

Obesity-related diseases that increase morbidity include CHD, hypertension, stroke, sleep apnea, type 2 diabetes, and certain types of cancer (i.e., endometrial, breast, prostate, and colon)[1,83]. The risks of obesity on health begin during pregnancy and extend throughout childhood into adulthood. Some of the obstetric and gynecological risks include menstrual abnormalities, polycystic ovary syndrome, and shoulder dystopia in childbirth. Orthopedic problems are a common health consequence of obesity, with Dietz[84] reporting that 30–50% of children with slipped capital epiphyses and bilateral slipped capital epiphyses were obese. Likewise, Blount's disease (i.e., severe bowing of the legs) is greatly increased with childhood obesity. Adult musculoskeletal problems may include increased joint pain and back pain[85]. Obesity stimulates biliary excretion of cholesterol that increases the likelihood of gallstone formation. Childhood and adult obesity are associated with up to 33% of the cases of gallstones[86–89].

The impact of childhood obesity on the progression of the metabolic syndrome as adults is alarming. Pinhas-Hamiel et al.[90] reported that about one third of diabetes diagnosed in 10- to 19-year-old children and young adults was related to obesity. A 1999 review of dyslipemia in adults aged 27 to 31 years who were previously Bogalusa Heart Study participants reported that adult hyperinsulinemia was 12.6 times more likely for children who had been obese[91]. In another study, participants identified as overweight adolescents had a 2.4 times increase in the prevalence of total cholesterol values above 240 mg·dL^{-1}, a three times increase in LDL values above 160 mg·dL^{-1}, and an eight times increase in HDL levels below 35 mg·day^{-1}[55]. The importance of modest weight losses of 5% to 15% have beneficial effects on serum triglycerides, total cholesterol, BP, degenerative joint disease, gynecological problems, insulin sensitivity, and glucose control and may lead to improvement or resolution of other comorbidities for both children and adults[92].

Obesity is a chronic, multifactorial problem caused by factors over which the individual has no control (e.g., genetics, gender, age, developmental stages) and those that can be modified for weight loss (e.g., diet, physical activity, medications, environmental contributions, social considerations). The increased prevalence of obesity in the United States reflects a change in lifestyle patterns influenced by an overabundance of food choices, large portion sizes, and fast foods; industrialization, technology, and conveniences, which decrease opportunities and motivation for physical activity; and a decline in cigarette smoking[83,93,94]. Approximately 24% of American adults are completely sedentary, and 54% spend inadequate time in physical activity[95].

The 1998 Behavioral Risk Factor Surveillance Survey found that about one third of U.S. adults were trying to lose weight and another third were trying to maintain weight at any one time[96]. Many types of weight loss and weight management programs are available, including balanced deficit diets, very low-calorie diets, gastric bypass surgery, and pharmacotherapy. It has been estimated that $30 billion to $50 billion dollars is spent annually on weight loss gimmicks and remedies[97]. Even with programs that result in weight loss, the results are often short term, and regaining weight is a significant problem for most individuals who initially lose weight. The key to sustaining weight loss is to adopt permanent diet and physical activity changes. A more conservative means for achieving healthy body weight recommended by the American Dietetic Association's guidelines includes adoption of a healthful eating style with an energy intake that does not exceed expenditure[98].

Cancer

Dietary exposures that cause cancer include food mutagens with the formation of carcinogen-DNA adducts as the most common process; epigenetic factors including changes in DNA methylation patterns; oxidative DNA damage; and genetic susceptibility related to polymorphisms of enzymes involved in detoxification, DNA repair, cell cycle control, and apoptosis (cell death). Dietary intervention is more effective in the early stages of cancer—initiation and promotion—because diet and lifestyle over a lifetime may determine if there are multiple DNA mutations leading to the development of a precancerous lesion. Dietary interventions may also be effective for preventing reoccurrence of cancer and risk for other cancers after an initial cancer site has been identified[20,99,100].

Food mutagens and carcinogens affect specific organs, but determining the effect of a specific compound is difficult. Well-studied compounds, such as polycyclic aromatic hydrocarbons, are complex chemical mixtures that have both environmental and food sources. Many other potential metabolic and carcinogenic consequences are often unpredictable. Food sources of known carcinogens, polycyclic aromatic hydrocarbons, n-nitrosamines, heterocyclic amines (HCAs), and aflatoxin B1 are given in Table 9-2 [101].

Foods also contain anticarcinogens or chemoprotective agents, such as antioxidants or phytosterols, that provide a balance to decrease the risk of cancer from foods. Phytochemical compounds in foods, such as organosulfur compounds in onions, garlic, and leeks and isothiocyanates in broccoli, cauliflower, cabbages, watercress, and radishes, affect phase 2 enzymes in the liver that conjugate activated carcinogens and promote excretion, which decreases cancer risk. Food substances can influence cancer growth through hormone-like activity (e.g., vitamins A and D, estrogens, and the phytoestrogen in soybeans, genistein). Examples of phytochemical rich foods are provided in Box 9-1 [102].

NATIONAL DIET RECOMMENDATIONS

The American Institute of Cancer Research (AICR) and the American Cancer Society (ACS) recommend dietary increases in plant-based foods (especially fruits and vegetables), weight maintenance, regular physically activity, low-fat food choices, and alcohol consumption in moderate amounts[103,104]. The guidelines differ in the definitions for alcohol intake and physical activity, and the AICR adds low-salt foods and safe food preparation to their recommendations (see Box 9-1) [also see Chapter 38].

The dietary factor with the highest overall risk for cancer is excessive energy intake from all sources. The cancer guideline for a healthy weight reflects this fact[103–105]. Controversies continue about recommendations for macronutrients, especially fat intake. The references to decreasing total fat and increasing total fiber have been eliminated from most national guidelines. A study of increasing fruit and vegetable intake without decreasing fat intake led to an increase of 6 lbs, and women with increased fruit and vegetable intake and decreased fat led to a decrease of 5 lbs in a year[106]. Also, specific fatty acids may have protective or carcinogenic effects. For example, in colorectal cancer, short chain fatty acids (SCFAs) and eicosanopentaenoic acid (EPA) are protective but increased medium chain fatty acids (MCFAs) and arachidonic acid (AA) are associated with increased risk[107].

OBESITY AND CANCER

A consequence of prolonged excessive energy intake is obesity, and obesity has a high association with many cancers. The National Cancer Institute identifies the cancers associated with obesity as those of the breast, endometrium, colon, kidney, esophagus, stomach, and gallbladder, but there are only links between obesity and cancers of the prostate, ovaries, and pancreas[99]. In the Nurses Health Study of 95,256 nurses aged 30 to 55 years, the researchers reported weight gain after the age of 18 years was

TABLE 9-2. Carcinogens in Foods and Related Cancers

Carcinogens	Food or Nutrient	Evidence Supporting Human Association	Possible Association
Polycyclic aromatic hydrocarbons (charbroiled foods)	Decreased charbroiling	Colon cancer	Lung Breast Oropharynx GI
N-Nitrosamines (cured meats and fish products)	Vitamin C minimizes gastric nitrosamines	Esophageal cancers GI cancers	Lung cancer
Heterocyclic amines (high temperature pyrolysis of proteins, amino acids or creatine)			Colon cancer Breast cancer
Aflatoxin B1 (mold-contaminated corn, peanuts, and animal feed)		Liver cancer	

GI = gastrointestinal.

.BOX 9-1 | **Dietary Recommendations for Cancer Prevention**

1. Body mass index should be maintained between 18.5 and 25. Weight gain during adulthood should remain less than 11 lbs.
2. Consume year-round a variety of vegetables and fruits other than roots, tubers, legumes, and grains (see next item), providing 7% or more of calories or totaling 15 to 30 oz or five portions per day.
3. Consume 20 to 30 oz or seven servings per day of other plant foods, minimally processed (including roots, tubers, legumes, and grains), providing 45% to 60% of total calories. Refined sugars should be limited to less than 10% of total calories.
4. Alcohol consumption is not recommended. If consumed, alcohol should be limited to one serving for women and two servings for men per day. A serving is 3 oz wine, 1 oz distilled spirits, or 8 oz beer.
5. Limit red meat to less than 3 oz·day^{-1}. Fish, poultry, and nondomesticated meats are preferable.
6. Limit total fat to 15% to 30% of calories.
7. Limit intake of fatty foods.
8. Salt from all sources should amount to less than 6 g·day^{-1}.
9. Perishable foods should be safely stored or refrigerated to minimize fungal contaminants and mycotoxins.
10. When levels of food additives, contaminants, or other residues are properly regulated in food and drinks, their presence is not known to be harmful. In economically developing countries where there may be insufficient regulation, these may be health hazards.
11. Cook meat and fish at low temperatures. Do not eat charred food or burned meat juices. Only occasionally consume meat or fish that has been grilled over direct flame.

associated with increased breast cancer incidence after menopause[108]. The researchers found that weight gain independently accounted for 16% of postmenopausal breast cancers, but the association increased to 30% when hormone replacement therapy use was combined with weight gain. After menopause, obese women who were not taking supplemental estrogen had a 1.5 times greater risk of developing breast cancer than postmenopausal women with a healthy BMI[109–111]. The mechanism is suspected to be estrogen production from fat tissue as the ovaries stop producing estrogen[112, 113]. The complexity of the relationship of weight to breast cancer was emphasized by a recent Swedish study of breast cancer risk for 7303 women who were hospitalized for anorexia nervosa before age 40 years[114]. The overall incidence of breast cancer was 53% of the predicted incidence, with parous women having a 76% lower incidence. Also, obesity increases the risk of breast cancer reoccurrence. In addition, overweight is estimated to contribute 34% to 56% of the risk for endometrial can-

cer[115] with a two to four times greater risk compared with women with healthy BMIs[116-118]. The contribution of excess weight to endometrial cancer is attributed to higher insulin and estrogen levels[116].

LUNG CANCER

Lung cancer is now the leading cause of cancer in both genders. Beta-carotene (see Table 9-3 for foods rich in beta-carotene) supplementation trials have shown that pharmacologic doses increase lung cancer incidence and mortality in relatively high-intensity smokers[119,120] or have no effect on the risk of lung cancer in current and former smokers[121]. Contradictory results from observational studies have shown an association of increased serum beta-carotene level with decreased cancer risk. Investigations to clarify these differences include focusing on the other carotenoids in fruits and vegetables versus supplements. Holick et al.[122] analyzed the relationship between lung cancer risk and dietary beta-carotene, lutein/zaexanthin, lycopene, beta-cryptoxanthin, vitamin A, serum beta-carotene, and serum retinal in the 27,084 male smokers of the Alpha-Tocopherol, Beta Carotene Cancer Prevention Study. In 1985, these subjects completed a 276-item dietary questionnaire, and lung cancer development was determined in 1993. A high-fruit and high-vegetable intake, particularly carotenoids, tomatoes, and tomato-based products, reduced the relative risk of lung cancer to 0.73.

COLORECTAL CANCER

Colorectal cancer is the second most common malignant neoplasm in the United States[123]. About 6% of Americans are expected to develop the disease, with a doubling of risk for each decade after ages 50 to 55 years. Epidemiologic and clinical investigations support an association of diets high in fat, protein, calories, alcohol, and meat (both

TABLE 9-3. Examples of Phytochemical Rich Foods

Phytochemical	Food Sources
Ascorbic acid	Citrus, leafy green vegetables, broccoli, tomatoes, strawberries, melons
Beta-carotene	Carrots, sweet potatoes, pumpkin, winter squash, cantaloupe, mango, papaya
Courmarin	Citrus
d-Limonene	Oil from peel of citrus fruit
Ellagic acid	Blueberries, strawberries
Isothiocyanates, indole-3-carbinol	Cruciferous vegetables
Lutein	Green vegetables
Lycopene	Tomatoes
Organosulfur compounds	Onions, garlic, leeks, chives
Quercetin	Red wine, tea
Selenium	Plant foods from high-selenium soil
Vitamin E	Vegetable oils, whole grains

red and white) and diets low in calcium and folate with increased rates of colorectal cancer. The interaction of these components may be significant because the study of individual factors have produced inconsistent results[99]. Willett et al.'s[124] prospective study of nurses reported an increased risk of colon cancer for high intakes of red meat and saturated and monounsaturated fat intake. These results contrast with two other large prospective studies, the American Cancer Society's Cancer Prevention Study II[125] and the Iowa Women's Health Study[126], in which there were no increases in risk with meat or fat consumption. A prospective cohort study of Seventh Day Adventists who ate no meat versus those who had one or more servings per week found a relative risk of 1.85 for meat consumption ($P = 0.01$[127]. The theory that HCAs from cooking at high temperatures explained the increased colorectal cancer risk attributable to meat consumption was not confirmed in a Swedish study that measured total HCA intake[128,129]. Conversely, diets high in fiber, fruits, and vegetables and low in fat (20% of total calories) did not reduce the rate of colorectal adenoma (premalignant lesions) recurrence over a 3- to 4-year period in a multicenter, randomized, controlled trial[130].

OTHER CANCERS

Diets high in vegetables and fruits, vitamin C, and a carotenoids are associated with a decreased risk of esophageal cancer, and a high alcohol intake is associated with an increased risk of esophageal cancer[99].

Breast cancer has a lifetime risk for women of one in eight and is the second cause of cancer mortality in women. Genetic changes accumulate over time and the genes identified with breast cancer risk, such as *BRCA1* and *BRCA2*, only explain a small percentage of all breast cancer cases. The wide variation in worldwide incidence of breast cancer also indicates that there are modifiable environmental and lifestyle determinants of breast cancer[99].

The pooled analysis of cohort studies for low-fat diets[131] and for fruit and vegetable consumption[132] have not supported an association with decreased breast cancer risk, although there have been mixed results from case, epidemiologic, and cohort studies. The dietary association included in cancer guidelines is for limited alcohol intake because of a moderate increase breast cancer risk, and there is considerable interest in the interaction of folate, beta-carotene, vitamin A, and vitamin C to decrease the risk associated with alcohol use[99].

Osteoporosis

Osteoporosis contributes to 1.3 million fractures annually in the United States. American women aged 50 years and older have an incidence of osteoporosis affecting 13% to 18% of women with early decreases in porosity, osteopenia, being present in another 37% to 50% of

BOX 9-2	Risk Factors for Osteoporosis[134,144]
Female gender	High caffeine intake
Petite body frame	High carbonated soda intake
White or Asian ancestry	Excessive alcohol use
Sedentary lifestyle or immobilization	Low body weight
Family history of osteoporosis	Anorexia nervosa
Nulliparity	Premenopausal amenorrhea (>1 yr)
Increasing age	Smoking
Lifelong low calcium intake	Postmenopausal status
Impaired calcium absorption	Long-term use of certain drugs
High protein intake	Renal disease
Vitamin A supplementation >3 mg·day^{-1}	Bariatric surgery

women[133]. Although the incidence is less in men, men older than 65 years have approximately 30% of the hip fractures. Peak bone mass is usually achieved by age 30 years for both men and women. The risk factors for osteoporosis include genetics, diet, activity, lifestyle, hormone status, medication use, and some diseases (Box 9-2)[134] [see also Chapter 35]. Genetic and environmental factors contribute to poor bone mass acquisition during adolescence and accelerated bone loss in perimenopausal women and men in the sixth decade and older. Contributing factors for reduced bone mass include hormone deficiencies such as estrogen; inadequate calcium and vitamin D intake; tobacco and alcohol abuse; decreased physical activity; comorbidities such as renal failure, hyperparathyroidism, and athletic amenorrhea; and medication effects such as chronic steroid use. The recent follow-up of the Nurses' Health Study found that whereas women with diets high in calcium and vitamin D tended to use more multivitamin, calcium, and estrogen supplements, women with the lowest intakes were more likely to smoke and consume alcohol[135].

CALCIUM BALANCE AND VITAMIN D

The FDA allowed a bone health claim for calcium-rich foods, and the National Institutes of Health Consensus Development Panel stated that a prolonged high calcium intake decreases osteoporosis[60,134]. A high calcium intake does not protect a person against bone loss caused by hormone changes, physical activity, or other causes but does prevent osteoporosis caused by low calcium intake. Calcium supplementation in bone remodeling studies has shown an assimilation of additional calcium to increase bone density by about 2%, but density does not continue to increase, and losses occur after supplementation ends[136–138].

A systematic review of 15 randomized, controlled trials with 1806 participants evaluated the use of calcium supplements versus usual dietary intake with placebo for at least 1 year[138]. The review confirmed that the percent change from baseline was 2.05% for total body bone density. There were smaller increases for bone density for the lumbar spine (1.66%), hip (1.60%), and distal radius (1.91%). The data for a reduction in vertebral fractures showed a trend, but the nonvertebral fracture effects were inconclusive. Peacock et al.[139] investigated the effects of supplementation with 750 mg·day^{-1} of calcium and 15 μg oral 25-hydroxyvitamin D on hip bone density in men and women age 60 years or older over a 4-year trial. The calcium group lost 1% in bone density, the placebo group lost 3%, and the vitamin D group lost 2.7%. Feskanich et al.[135] reported a lower risk of hip fracture with a higher calcium intake when there was a concurrent high intake of vitamin D. They confirmed the lack of a relationship between risk of fractures and calcium intake but concluded that adequate vitamin D intake was associated with a lower occurrence of osteoporotic hip fractures. Decreased risk of fractures has been consistently shown for women who have higher milk or dairy food intake at age 30 years or younger but not necessarily for women older than age 50 years[140].

Even after full skeletal growth is completed, the body loses calcium every day that must be replaced. The National Academy of Sciences recommends 1000 to 1200 mg/day of calcium for adult men and women[141]. Calcium supplements from unrefined oyster shell, bone meal, coral calcium or dolomite without the United States Pharmacopeia (USP) symbol may contain higher levels of lead or other toxic metals and should be avoided, especially during pregnancy. Calcium from food and supplements is absorbed best when taken several times a day in amounts of 500 mg or less. Calcium carbonate is absorbed best when taken with food; calcium citrate can be taken at any time[142].

Vitamin D, phosphorus, magnesium, zinc, boron, and fluoride are nutrients that are important for bone growth and maintenance, but they do not have to be consumed with calcium for absorption nor do they require supplementation unless the diet is inadequate in these nutrients. Vitamin D increases calcium absorption in the gastrointestinal tract, and an adequate vitamin D intake reduces nonvertebral fracture rates[143]. Vitamin D intake (1 μg cholecalciferol = 40 IU Vitamin D) as recommendations increase with age (5 μg·day^{-1} for those ages 19 to 50 years; 10 μg·day^{-1} for those ages 51–70 years, and 15 μg·day^{-1} for those older than age 70 years) because of changes in absorption and utilization; a four times decrease in skin synthesis of vitamin D; and decreased exposure to sunlight, particularly in the winter[141,142]. Nutrient needs and osteoporosis may be affected by medications such as glucocorticoids, anticonvulsants, long-term heparin therapy, and excessive thyroxine therapy[144].

Dietary factors may alter calcium balance by decreasing calcium bioavailability or increasing urinary calcium excretion. Foods high in oxalates (e.g., spinach, rhubarb, almonds) or in phytates (e.g., legumes and wheat bran) contain calcium that is unavailable for absorption and may bind with calcium in the gut to reduce absorption. Dietary advice includes eating calcium-rich foods before or several hours after foods with phytates and oxalates or compensate for their reduced absorption with a higher calcium intake for the day. Protein, alcohol, and sodium may increase calcium excretion through the kidneys. Protein intakes of 2 g·kg^{-1} of body weight used by some athletes have the potential to decrease calcium balance. Alcohol also has a negative impact on osteoblast function[112].

OTHER FACTORS AND OSTEOPOROSIS

Several studies have found a relationship between increased hip fracture and excessive supplemental use of vitamin A[135,145,146]. In the Nurses' Health Study, vitamin A intake of 1.5 mg·day^{-1} or more retinal (most common form of vitamin A) was associated with a relative risk of 1.64 for hip fracture and 21% of subjects exceeded 3 mg·day^{-1}[135]. Screening for multiple sources of supplementation or large single doses of vitamin A is recommended for individuals at a high risk of developing osteoporosis.

Eating disorders and the inability to maintain body mass promote osteoporosis. In addition to the impact of body mass, low-calorie diets and, particularly, low-carbohydrate diets that promote ketosis have the potential to leach cationic minerals such as calcium from the bones[147]. Patients who have recovered from anorexia nervosa require many years to improve their bone density but may never have complete recovery[134].

Diabetes

Diabetes is a major cause of mortality and morbidity, with 213,062 annual deaths in 2000 attributable to diabetes in the United States and 2002 estimates of 13 million Americans diagnosed with diabetes. Approximately 5.2 million Americans have diabetes and have not been diagnosed, and 10 million Americans are at risk of developing diabetes ([148, 149]). The prevalence of diabetes in the United States has increased by 50% from 1990 to 2000. An increased risk of developing diabetes or prediabetes is estimated to be a concern for 41 million U.S. adults with **impaired glucose tolerance (IGT)** and **impaired fasting glucose (IFG)**. Prediabetes has also become a concern in the pediatric population. Conditions of hyperinsulinemia and impaired glucose have been directly related to weight in children and adolescents[150].

Diabetes results from inaction or impairment of insulin secretion and defects in insulin action that may occur simultaneously in the same patient[2,151]. Autoimmune processes with an absolute deficiency of insulin secretion characterize the less common type 1 diabetes, but insulin resistance and an inadequate insulin secretion response characterize the more prevalent type 2 diabetes. Acute symptoms include hyperglycemia with polyuria, polydipsia, weight loss, sometimes polyphagia, and often blurred vision. Chronic hyperglycemia may lead to retarded growth and to increased incidence of infections. An asymptomatic period and impaired glucose tolerance with slightly abnormal blood glucose level (i.e., IFG) and potential organ changes without clinical symptoms may precede overt symptoms. The incidence of retinopathy, peripheral neuropathy, foot ulcers, lower limb amputation, gastroparesis, sexual dysfunction, peripheral vascular disease, MI, hyperlipidemia, periodontal disease, cerebrovascular disease, hypertension, and psychological dysfunction increase with a history of diabetes.

Symptoms associated with insulin resistance include acanthosis nigricans (dark, thickened skin at the back of the neck or under the breasts), hypertension, dyslipidemia, and polycystic ovarian syndrome. The visible presence of acanthosis nigricans correlated with higher insulin needs in a study of newly diagnosed type 2 diabetes[152]. The study found 36.1% of the 216 patients with newly diagnosed type 2 diabetes and 54% of patients with a BMI of 30 or above manifested the skin changes.

Type 2 diabetes has many different forms, but obesity, especially abdominal distribution, may increase insulin resistance and contribute to diabetes development when coupled with genetic predisposition (family history, high-risk ethnic group), increasing age (steep increase after age 45 years), and a lack of physical activity[153]. Other risk factors for diabetes include previously identified IFG or IGT, history of gestational diabetes mellitus or delivery of a baby weighing more than 9 lbs, hypertension ($\geq$140/90 mm Hg in adults), HDL cholesterol of 35 mg·dL^{-1} or less or a triglyceride level of 250 mg·dL^{-1} or more, polycystic ovary syndrome, and a history of vascular disease[2,151]. Nutrient intake, both specific macronutrients and micronutrients, does not contribute to the development of diabetes. Type 2 diabetes has been increasing in children and adolescents with combinations of risk factors, especially increasing rates of excessive weight and obesity. Screening for diabetes in high-risk groups has been recommended as a cost-effective practice.

LIFESTYLE MODIFICATION

Recent large, well-designed, randomized controlled studies have supported the value of lifestyle changes that include diet and physical activity to prevent diabetes in high-risk persons[154–156] (also see Chapter 33). Tuomilehto et al.[154] found that intensive individualized diet and exer-

cise instruction had a 58% relative reduction in the incidence of diabetes compared with brief diet and exercise counseling in 522 middle-aged men with IGT and obesity (mean BMI, 31 kg·m^{-2}). The average follow-up time was 3.2 years. Halting the progression toward diabetes was strongly correlated with the subject's ability to accomplish one of the following goals: 5% weight reduction, fat intake less than 30% of calories, saturated fat less than 10% of calories, fiber intake 15 g·1000 kcal or more, and exercise more than 150 minutes·week^{-1}.

The Da Qing, China, study of 520 normal weight participants over 6 years found significant reductions in diabetes for a diet group (31%), exercise group (46%), and diet plus exercise (42%)[155]. Overall, the lifestyle intervention groups lost 3.4 kg more than the control subjects in the first year. The study underlines the value of lifestyle changes, especially exercise, for leaner subjects.

The Diabetes Prevention Program results supported the value of intensive diet and exercise interventions (58% relative reduction in progression to diabetes) compared with metformin (31% relative reduction in progression to diabetes) or placebo medication interventions with standard diet and exercise[156]. The 3,234 ethnically and racially diverse subjects with a mean age of 51 years were followed for weight and glucose intolerance for an average of 2.8 years. The weight reduction goal of a loss of more than 7% of initial weight at 6 months was met by 38% of the lifestyle change group. The exercise goal of achieved 7% more than 150 min·week^{-1} was maintained by 74% of the lifestyle change group.

Lifestyle interventions to prevent type 2 diabetes are recommended for all patients with prediabetes and possibly all patients who meet the criteria for the metabolic syndrome[153,154]. Diabetes management includes balancing diet, exercise, and medications to achieve treatment goals associated with diabetes[16]. Total carbohydrate intake is the dietary component that is the most important determinant of blood sugars. However, contrary to popular belief, studies have shown that simple or complex carbohydrates yield similar glycemic responses, and there is considerable variability in the results. There is presently no evidence-based research conclusion supporting improved blood sugar control with the use of the glycemic index[16]. The American Diabetes Association's Nutrition Principles Position Statement suggests that people with type 2 diabetes can substitute carbohydrates with monounsaturated fats to reduce postprandial glycemia and triglyceridemia[16]. A liberal intake of monounsaturated fat can promote weight gain, so this substitution should only be advised when carbohydrate calories are replaced by fat calories. Saturated fats should be limited to 7% to 10% of total daily energy intake, and total fat intake should be less than 30% of total calories. Cholesterol should be less than 200 mg·day^{-1} if the LDL level is above 100 mg·dL^{-1}. Protein intake is also a concern in the setting of diabetes because of the potential of promoting nephropathy. If renal function is normal, a protein intake of 15% to

20% of total daily energy intake is acceptable, but high-protein diets are not recommended.

Microalbuminuria, small amounts of albumin in the urine, is the first evidence of damage to the kidneys[16,151]. About 30% of people with type 1 diabetes develop kidney disease. In contrast, ethnicity is the primary determinant of the incidence of kidney disease for people with type 2 diabetes. Kidney disease develops in 40% to 50% Native Americans, 20% to 30% African Americans and Latinos, and 10% whites with type 2 diabetes. High-protein diets cause hyperfiltration in the kidneys and may potentially contribute to kidney failure for high-risk individuals. The American Diabetes Association's Standards of Medical Care currently recommend protein intakes of 0.8 to 1.0 $g \cdot kg^{-1}$ of body weight$\cdot$day^{-1} for prevention of kidney disease and 0.8 $g \cdot kg^{-1}$ or about 10% of kilocalories for treatment of overt kidney disease.

A primary principle of diabetes management is the relationship of medication dosage, selection, and timing to dietary intake, especially carbohydrates, and physical activity[16]. Patient preferences and lifestyle can be incorporated into a plan that typically focuses on consistency of dietary intake and exercise patterns balanced with medications. Patients who are willing to become educated and monitor themselves can increase their diet and physical activity options.

Summary

Prevention of chronic disease with dietary interventions is one tool in the arsenal of lifestyle changes that combine to effectively improve disease risk. Dietary treatment of the diet-related chronic diseases—CVD, cancer, obesity, diabetes, and osteoporosis—improves morbidity, mortality, and quality of life. Prevention efforts for children need to be increased if the potential benefits of healthy lifestyles are to be realized.

REFERENCES

1. Expert Panel on the Identification, Evaluation, and Treatment of Overweight and Obesity in Adults: Clinical Guidelines on the Identification, Evaluation, and Treatment of Overweight and Obesity in Adults. Washington, DC: National Heart, Lung, and Blood Institute Obesity Education Initiative; 1998.
2. The Expert Committee on the Diagnosis and Classification of Diabetes Mellitus. Report of the expert committee on the diagnosis and classification of diabetes mellitus. Diabetes Care 27:S5–S10, 2004.
3. NCEP Expert Panel: Executive summary of the third report of the National Cholesterol Education Program (NCEP) Expert Panel on Detection, Evaluation, and Treatment of High Blood Cholesterol in Adults (Adult Treatment Panel III). JAMA 285:2486–2497, 2001.
4. Chobanian AV, Bakris GL, Black HR, et al: The seventh report of the joint national committee on prevention, detection, evaluation, and treatment of high blood pressure: JNC 7 report. JAMA 289:2560–2572, 2003.
5. PREMIER Collaborative Research Group: Effects of comprehensive lifestyle modification on blood pressure control: main results of the PREMIER clinical trial. JAMA 289:2083–2093, 2003.
6. Stover PJ: Nutritional genomics. Physiol Genom 16:161–165, 2004.
7. American College of Endocrinology: Position statement of insulin resistance syndrome. Endocrinol Pract 9:240–252, 2003.
8. Shulman G: Cellular mechanisms of insulin resistance. J Clin Invest 106:171–176, 2000.
9. Park YW, Zhu S, Palaniappan L, et al: The metabolic syndrome: Prevalence and associated risk factor findings in the US population from the Third National Health and Nutrition Examination Survey, 1998–1994. Arch Intern Med 163:427–436, 2003.
10. Palaniappan L, Carnethod MR, Wang Y, et al: Predictors of the incident metabolic syndrome in adults. Diabetes Care 27:788–793, 2004.
11. Srinivasan SR, Frontini MG, Berenson GS: Longitudinal changes in risk variables of insulin resistance syndrome from childhood to young adulthood in offspring of parents with type 2 diabetes: The Bogalusa Heart Study. Metabolism 52:443–450, 2003.
12. Srinivasan SR, Meyers L, Berenson GS: Predictability of childhood adiposity and insulin for developing insulin resistance syndrome (syndrome x) in young adulthood. The Bogalusa Heart Study. Diabetes 51:204–209, 2002.
13. Pankow JS, Jacobs DR, Steinberger J, et al: Insulin resistance and cardiovascular disease risk factors in children of parents with the insulin resistance (metabolic) syndrome. Diabetes Care 27:775–780, 2004.
14. American Dietetic Association: http://www.eatright.org/Public/GovernmentAffairs/98_8723.cfm
15. McDowell MA, et al: Energy and Macronutrient Intakes of Persons Ages 2 Months and Over in the United States: Third National Health and Nutrition Examination Survey, Phase I, 1998–1991. Washington, DC: US Government Printing Office; 1994.
16. Scott BJ, Permumean-Chaney S, St Jeor ST: Relationship of body mass index to energy density and diet composition in a free-living population. Top Clin Nutr 17:38–46, 2002.
17. American Diabetes Association: Nutrition principles and recommendations in diabetes. Diabetes Care 27:S36–S46, 2004.
18. Institute of Medicine, National Academy of Sciences: Dietary Reference Intakes Energy, Carbohydrate, Fiber, Fat, Fatty Acids, Cholesterol, protein and Amino Acids. Washington, DC: National Academy of Sciences; September 2002.
19. American Heart Association: Heart Facts 2003. All Americans. Available at: http://www.americanheart.org
20. Report of a Joint WHO/FAO Expert Consultation: Diet, Nutrition and the Prevention of Chronic Diseases. WHO Technical Report Series #916. Geneva: World Health Organization; 2003.
21. Pearson TA, Bazzarre, TL, Daniels SR, et al: American Heart Association guide for improving cardiovascular health at the community level: A statement for public health practitioners, healthcare providers, and health policy makers from the American Heart Association expert panel on population and prevention science. Circulation 107:645–651, 2003.
22. Kraus RM, Eckel RH, Howard B, et al: AHA Dietary Guidelines: revision 2000: A statement for healthcare professionals from the Nutrition Committee of the American Heart Association. Circulation 102:2284–2299, 2000.
23. American Heart Association: Guidelines for primary prevention of cardiovascular disease and stroke: 2002 update. Circulation 106:388–391.
24. Kris-Etherton PM, Daniels SR, Eckel RH, et al: Summary of the scientific conference on dietary fatty acids and cardiovascular health: Conference summary from the nutrition committee of the American Heart Association. Circulation 103:1034–1039, 2001.
25. Lovejoy JC, Windhauser MM, Rood JC, et al: Effect of controlled high fat versus low-fat diet on insulin sensitivity and leptin levels in African-American and Caucasian women. Metabolism 47:1520–1524, 1998.
26. Ginsberg HN: Lipoprotein physiology. In Jeffrey Hoeg, ed. Endocrinology and Metabolism Clinics of North America. Philadelphia: W.B. Saunders; 1998.

27. Katan MJ, Zock PL, Mensink RP, et al: Dietary oils, serum lipoproteins, and coronary heart disease. Am J Clin Nutr 61(suppl 6): 1368–1373, 1995.

28. Katan MD: Trans fatty acids and plasma lipoproteins. Nutr Rev 58:188–191, 2000.

29. Harper CR, Jacobson TA: The fats of life: the role of omega-3 fatty acids in the prevention of coronary heart disease. Arch Intern Med 161:2185–2192, 2001.

30. Kris-Etherton PM, Harris WS, Appel LJ: Fish consumption, fish oil, omega-3 fatty acids, and cardiovascular disease. Circulation 106:2747–2465, 2002.

31. Whelton SP, He J, Whelton PK, et al: Meta-analysis of observational studies on fish intake and coronary heart disease. Am J Cardiol 93:1119–1123, 2004.

32. Marckmann P, Gronback M: Fish consumption and coronary heart disease mortality. A systematic review of prospective cohort studies. Eur J Clin Nutr 53:585–590, 1999.

33. Burr ML, Fehily AM, Gilbert JF, et al: Effects of changes in fat, fish, and fiber intakes on death and myocardial reinfarction trial (DART). Lancet 2:757–761, 1989.

34. GISSI-Prevenzione investigators: Dietary supplementation with n-3 polyunsaturated fatty acids and vitamin E after myocardial infarction: Results of the GISS-Prevenzione trial. Lancet 354:447–455, 1999.

35. Marchioli R, Barzi F, Bomba E, et al: Early protection against sudden death by n-3 polyunsaturated fatty acids after myocardial infarction: time course analysis of the results of the Gruppo Italiano per lo Studio della Sopravvivenza nell'Infarto Micocardico (GISSI)-Prevenzione. Circulation 105:1897–1903, 2002

36. Singh RB, Niaz MA, Sharma JP, et al: Randomized, double blind, placebo-controlled trial of fish oil and mustard oil in patients with suspected acute myocardial infarction: The Indian experiment of infarct survival—4. Cardiovasc Drugs Ther 11:485–491, 1997.

37. U.S. Food and Drug Administration: FDA Acts to provide better information to consumers on trans fats. Available at http://www.fda.gov/oc/initiatives/transfat

38. Yu-Poth S, Zhao G, Etherton T, et al: Effect of the National Cholesterol Education Program's Step I and Step II dietary intervention programs on cardiovascular disease risk factors: A meta-analysis. Am J Clin Nutr 68:632–646, 1999.

39. Trichopoulou A, Costacou T, Bamia C, Trichopoulous D: Adherence to a Mediterranean diet and survival in a Greek population. N Engl J Med 348:2599–608, 2003.

40. Pitsavos C, Panagiotakos DB, Chrysohoou C, et al: The effect of Mediterranean diet on the risk of the development of acute coronary syndromes in hypercholesterolemic people: A case control study (CARDIO2000). Coron Artery Dis 13:295–300, 2003.

41. de Lorgeril M, Salen P, Martin JL, et al: Mediterranean diet, traditional risk factors, and the rate of cardiovascular complications after myocardial infarction: final report of the Lyon Diet Heart Study. Circulation 99:779–785, 1999.

42. Heart Protection Study Collaborative Group: MRC/BHF Heart Protection Study of antioxidant vitamin supplementation in 20,536 high risk individuals: A randomized placebo controlled trial. Lancet 360:23–33, 2002.

43. Age-Related Eye Disease Study Research Group: A randomized, placebo controlled clinical trial of high-dose supplementation with vitamins C and E and beta-carotene for age-related cataract and vision loss: AREDS Report No. 9. Arch Ophthalmol 119:1439–1452, 2001.

44. Collaborative Group of the Primary Prevention Project (PPP): Low dose aspirin and vitamin E in people at cardiovascular risk: A randomized trial in general practice. Lancet 357:89–95, 2001.

45. The Alpha-Tocopherol, Beta Carotene Cancer Prevention Study Group: The effect of vitamin E and B-carotene on the incidence of lung cancer and other cancers in male smokers. N Engl J Med 330:1029–1035, 2000.

46. The Heart Outcomes Prevention Evaluation Study Investigators: Vitamin E supplementation and cardiovascular events in high-risk patients. N Engl J Med 342:154–160, 2000.

47. Ueland PM: The controversy over homocysteine and cardiovascular risk. Am J Clin Nutr 72:324–332, 2000.

48. Homocysteine Lowering Trialists' Collaboration: Lowering blood homocysteine with folic acid based supplements meta-analysis of randomized trials. BMJ 316:894–898, 1998.

49. Wald DS, Law M, Morris JK: Homocysteine and cardiovascular disease: Evidence on causality from a meta-analysis. BMJ 325:1202–1208, 2002.

50. Rimm EB, Willett WC, Hu FB: Folate and vitamin B6 from diet and supplements in relation to risk of coronary heart disease among women. JAMA 279:359–364, 1998.

51. Gallistl S, Sudi K, Mangge H, et al: Insulin is an independent correlate of plasma homocysteine levels in obese children and adolescents. Diabetes Care 23:1348–1352, 2000.

52. Jenkins JA, Kendall CWC, Marchie A, et al: The effect of combining plant sterols, soy protein, viscous fibers, and almonds in treating hypercholesterolemia. Metabolism 52:1478–1483, 2003.

53. Carter NB: Plant stanol ester: Review of cholesterol-lowering efficacy and implications for coronary heart disease risk reduction. Prev Cardiol 3:121–130, 2000.

54. Lichtenstein AH, Deckelbaum RJ: Stanol/sterol ester-containing foods and blood cholesterol levels. Circulation 103:1177–1179, 2001.

55. Patel S: Sitosterolemia: Dietary cholesterol absorption. Lancet 358(suppl):S63, 2001.

56. Hertog G: Dietary antioxidant flavanoids and risk of coronary heart disease: The Zutphen Elderly Study. Lancet 342:1007–1011, 1993.

57 Joshipura KJ, Hu FB, Manson JE, et al: The effect of fruit and vegetable intake on risk for coronary heart disease. Ann Intern Med 134:1106–1114, 2001.

58. Knekt P, Jarvinen R, ReunanenA, et al: Flavonoid intake and coronary mortality in Finland: a cohort study. BMJ 312:478–481, 1996.

59. Nijveldt RJ, van Nood E, van Hoorn DEC, et Al: Flavanoids: A review of probable mechanisms of action and potential applications. Am J Clin Nutr 74:418–425, 2001.

60. Erdman JW: Soy protein and cardiovascular disease. Circulation 102:2555–2559, 2000.

61. U.S. Food and Drug Administration: Label claims. Available at http://www.cfsan.fda.gov/~dms/lab-hlth.html

62. Stevens & Associates, Inc: Soy foods directory. Available at http://www.soyfoods.com

63. U.S. National Agricultural Library: Nutrient data laboratory Available at http://www.nal.usda.gov/fnic/foodcomp/search

64. Klatsky A, Armstrong M, Friedman G: Red wine, white wine, liquor and beer and the risk of coronary hospitalizations. J Am Coll Cardiol 29(suppl 76A)416–420, 1997.

65. Thun MJ, Peto R, Lopez AD, et al: Alcohol consumption and mortality among middle-aged and elderly US adults. N Engl J Med 337:1705–1713, 1997.

66. Goldberg IJ, Mosca L, Piano MR, et al: Wine and your heart: a science advisory for healthcare professionals from the Nutrition Committee, Council on Epidemiology and Prevention, and Council on Cardiovascular Nursing of the American Heart Association. Circulation 103:472–475, 2001.

67. Pearson TA: Alcohol and heart disease. Circulation 94:3023–3025, 2000.

68. Kottke TE, Stroebel RJ, Hoffman RS: JNC 7—It's more than high blood pressure. JAMA 289:2573–2574, 2003.

69. Greenlund KJ, Giles WH, Keenan NL, et al: Physician advice, patient actions, and health-related quality of life in secondary prevention of stroke through diet and exercise. Stroke 33:565–571, 2002.

70. Srinivasan SR, Bao W, Wattigney WA, Berenson, GS: Adolescent overweight is associated with adult overweight and related multiple cardiovascular risk factors: The Bogalusa Heart Study. Metabolism 45:235–240, 1996.

71. Figeroa-Colon R, Franklin FA, et al: Prevalence of obesity with increased blood pressure in elementary school-aged children. South Med J 90:806–813, 1997.

72. Rocchini AP, Key J, Bondie D, et al: The effect of weight loss on the sensitivity of blood pressure to sodium in obese adolescents. N Engl J Med 321:580–585, 1989.

73. Whelton PK, He J, Cutler JA, et al: Effects of oral potassium on blood pressure: meta-analysis of randomized clinical trials. Ann Intern Med 124:825–831, 1996.

74. Graudal JG: Effects of low sodium diet versus high sodium diet on blood pressure, renin, aldosterone, catecholamines, cholesterols, and triglyceride. Cochrane Database Syst Rev (1):CD004022, 2004.

75. Hooper L, Bartlett C, Davey SG, Ebrahim S: Advice to reduce dietary salt for prevention of cardiovascular disease. Cochrane Database Syst Rev (1):CD003656, 2004.

76. Appel LJ, Moore TJ, Obarzanek E, et al: A clinical trial of the effects of dietary patterns on blood pressure. DASH Collaborative Research Group. N Engl J Med 336:1117–1124, 1997.

77. Sacks FM, Svetkey LP, Vollmer WM, et al: Effects on blood pressure of reduced dietary sodium and the Dietary Approaches to Stop Hypertension (DASH) diet. DASH-Sodium Collaborative Research Group. N Engl J Med 344:3–10, 2001.

78. US Department of Health and Human Services: Facts about the DASH diet eating plan. National Heart, Lung, and Blood Institute Information Center. NIH Publication number 03-4082. Revised May 2003.

79. Flegal KM, Carroll MD, Ogden CL, Johnson CL: Prevalence and trends in obesity among US adults, 1999–2000. JAMA 288: 1723–1727, 2002.

80. Allison DB, Fontaine KR, Manson JE, et al: Annual deaths attributable to obesity in the United States. JAMA 282:1530–1538, 1999.

81. Mokdad, AH, Marks, JS, Stroup D, Gerberding JL: Actual causes of death in the United States, 2000. JAMA 291:1238–1245, 2004.

82. Centers for Disease Control and Prevention, National Center for Health Statistics: National Health Interview Survey. Available at http://www.cdc.gov/nchs/about/major/dvs/mortdata.htm

83. Plodkowski RA. St. Jeor ST: Diet in the treatment of obesity. Endocrinol Metab Clin N Am 32:935–965, 2003.

84. Dietz W: Health consequences of obesity in youth: Childhood predictors of adult disease. Am J Dis Child Pediatr 101:518–525, 1998.

85. Brown, WJ, Dobson AJ, Mishra G: What is a healthy weight for middle aged women. Int J Obes Relat Metab Disord 22:520–528, 1998.

86. Everhart JE: Contributions of obesity and weight loss to gallstone disease. Ann Intern Med 119:1029–1035, 1993.

87. Acalivschi MV, Blendes D, Pascu M. et al: Risk of asymptomatic and symptomatic gallstones in moderately obese women: A longitudinal follow-up study. Am J Gastroenterol 92:127–131, 1997.

88. Weinsier RL, Wilson LJ, Lee J: Medically safe rate of weight loss for the treatment of obesity: A guide based on risk of gallstone formation. Am J Med 98:115–117, 1995.

89. Barlow SE, Dietz WH: Obesity evaluation and treatment: Expert committee recommendations. Pediatrics 102:102–113, 1998.

90. Pinhas-Hamiel O, Dolan LM, Daniels SR, et al: Increased incidence of non-insulin-dependent diabetes mellitus among adolescents. J Pediatr 128:608–615, 1996.

91. Freedman DS, Dietz WH, Srinivasan SR, et al: The relation of overweight to cardiovascular risk factors among children and adolescents: The Bogalusa Heart Study. Pediatrics 103:1175–1182, 1999–

92. Deitel M: How much weight loss is sufficient to overcome major comorbidities? Obes Surg 11:659, 2001.

93. Pi-Sunyer FX: The fattening of America. JAMA 272:238–239, 1994.

94. Smiciklas-Wright H, Mithchell DC, Mickle SJ, et al: Foods commonly eaten in the United States, 1989–1991 and 1994–1996: Are portion sizes changing? J Am Diet Assoc 103:41–47, 2003.

95. Pate RR, Pratt M, Blair SN, et Al : Physical activity and public health: A recommendation from the Centers for Disease Control and Prevention and the American College of Sports Medicine. JAMA 273:402–407, 1995.

96. Serdula MK, Mokdad AH, Williamson DH, et al: Prevalence of attempting weight loss and strategies for controlling weight. JAMA 282:1353–1358, 1999.

97. The painful business of losing weight. Economist 344(8032):45–47: Aug 30, 1997.

98. American Dietetic Association: Position of the American Dietetic Association: Weight management. J Am Diet Assoc 102:1145–1155, 2000.

99. National Cancer Institute: PDQ Cancer Information Summaries: Prevention. Available at http://www.cancer.gov/cancerinfo/pdq/prevention

100. Watson WH, Cai J, Jones DP: Diet and apoptosis. Ann Rev Nutr 20:485–505, 2000.

101. Goldman R, Shields PG: Food mutagens. J Nutr 133:965S–973S, 2003.

102. Wildman REC: Handbook of nutraceuticals and functional foods. Boca Raton, FL: CRC Press,;2001.

103. American Institute for Cancer Research. Available at http://www.aicr.org

104. American Cancer Society. Available at http://www.cancer.org

105. National Cancer Institute. Available at http://cis.nih.gov

106. Djuirc Z, Poore KM, Depper JB, et. Al: Methods to increase fruit and vegetable intake with and without a decreased in fat intake: Compliance and effects on body weight in the nutrition and breast health study. Nutr Cancer 43:141–151, 2002.

107. Nkondjock A, Shatenstein B, Maisonneuve P, Ghadirian P: Specific fatty acids and human colorectal cancer: An overview. Cancer Detect Prev 27:55–66, 2003.

108. Huang Z, Hankinson SE, Cloditz GA, et al: Dual effects of weight and weight gain on breast cancer risk. JAMA 278: 1407–1411, 1997.

109. Van den Brandt PA, Spiegelman D, Yuan SS, et al: Pooled analysis of prospective cohort studies on height, weight, and breast cancer risk. Am J Epidemiol 152:514–527, 2001.

110. Friedenreich CM: Review of anthropometric factors and breast cancer risk. Eur J Cancer Prev 10:15–32, 2001.

111. Trentham-Dietz A, Newcomb PAA, Storer BE, et Al: Body size and risk of breast cancer. Am J Epidemiol 145:1011–1019, 1997.

112. Toniolo PG, Levitz M, Zeleniuch-Jacquotte A, et al: A prospective study of endogenous estrogens and breast cancer in postmenopausal women. J Natl Cancer Inst 87:190–197, 1995.

113. Yoo KY, Tajima K, Park SK, et al: Postmenopausal obesity as a breast cancer risk factor according to estrogen and progesterone receptor status. Cancer Letters 167:57–63, 2001.

114. Michels KB, Ekborn A: Caloric restriction and incidence of breast cancer. JAMA 291:1226–1230, 2004.

115. Ballard-Barbash R, Swanson CA: Body weight: estimation of risk for breast and endometrial cancers. Am J Clin Nutr 63(suppl): 4375–4341, 1996.

116. Weiderpass E, Persson I, Adami HO, et al: Body size in different periods of life, diabetes mellitus, hypertension, and risk of postmenopausal endometrial cancer. Cancer Causes Control 11:185–192, 2000.

117. Salazar-Martinez E, Lazcano-Ponce EC, Gonzalez Lira-Lira G, et al: Case-control study of diabetes, obesity, physical activity and risk of endometrial cancer among Mexican women. Cancer Causes Control 11:707–711, 2000.

118. Shoff SM, Newcomb PA: Diabetes, body size, and risk of endometrial cancer. Am J Epidemiol 148:234–240, 1998.

119. Omenn GS, Goodman GE, Thornquist MD, et al: Effects of a combination of beta carotene and vitamin A on lung cancer and cardiovascular disease. N Engl J Med 334:1150–1155, 1996.

120. The Alpha-Tocopherol, Beta Carotene Cancer Prevention Study Group: The effect of vitamin E and beta carotene on the incidence of lung cancer and other cancers in male smokers. N Engl J Med 330:1029–1035, 1994.

121. Hennekens CH, Buring JE, Manson JE, et Al : Lack of effect of long-term supplementation with beta carotene on the incidence of malignant neoplasms and cardiovascular disease. N Engl J Med 334:1145–1149, 1996.

122. Holick CN, Michaud DS, Stolzenberg-Solomon R, et al: Dietary carotenoids, serum beta-carotene, and retinal and risk of lung cancer in the alpha-tocopherol, beta-carotene cohort study. Am J Epidemiol 156:536–547, 2002.

123. American Cancer Society: Cancer facts and figures 2003. Atlanta: American Cancer Society; 2003.

124. Willett WC, Stampfer MJ, Colditz GA, et al: Relation of meat, fat, and fiber intake to the risk of colon cancer in a prospective study among women. N Engl J Med 323:1664–1672, 1990.

125. Thun MJ, Calle EE, Namboodiri MM, et al: Risk factors for fatal colon cancer in a large prospective study. J Natl Cancer Inst 84:1491–1500, 1992.

126. Bostick RM, Potter JD, Sellasts TA, et al: Relation of calcium, vitamin D, and dairy food intake to incidence of colon cancer among older women. The Iowa Women's Health Study. Am J Epidemiol 137:1302–1317, 1993.

127. Singh PN, Fraser GE: Dietary risk factors for colon cancer in a low-risk population. Am J Epidemiol 148:761–774, 1998.

128. Augustsson K, Skog K, JAugerstad M, et al: Dietary heterocyclic amines and cancer of the colon, rectum, bladder, and kidney: a population-based study. Lancet 353:703–707, 1999.

129. Forman D: Meat and cancer: a relation in search of a mechanism. Lancet 353:686–687, 1999.

130. Schatzkin A, Lanza E, Corle D, et al: Lack of effect of a low-fat, high-fiber diet on the recurrence of colorectal adenomas. Polyp Prevention Trial Study Group. N Engl J Med 342: 1149–1155, 2000.

131. Hunter DJ, Spielgelman D, Adami HO, et al: Cohort studies of fat intake and the risk of breast cancer—a pooled analysis. N Engl J Med 334:356–361, 1996.

132. Smith-Warner SA, Speigelman D, Yaun SS, et al: Intake of fruits and vegetables and risk of breast cancer: A pooled analysis of cohort studies. JAMA 285:769–776, 2001.

133. Looker AC, Wahner HW, Dunn WL, et al: Updated data on proximal femur bone mineral levels of US adults. Osteoporos Int 8:468–489, 1998.

134. NIH Consensus Development Panel on Osteoporosis Prevention, Diagnosis, and Therapy: Osteoporosis prevention, diagnosis, and therapy. JAMA 285:785–795, 2001.

135. Feskanich D, Willett WC, Colditz GA: Calcium, vitamin D, milk consumption, and hip fractures: A prospective study among postmenopausal women. Am J Clin Nutr 77:504–511, 2003.

136. Dawson-Hughes B: Calcium supplementation and bone loss: A review of controlled clinical trials. Am J Clin Nutr 54:274S–280S, 1991.

137. Elders PA, Netelenbos JC, Lips P, et al: Calcium supplementation reduces vertebral bone loss in perimenopausal women: A controlled trial in 248 women between 46 and 55 years of age. J Clin Endocrinol Metab 73:533–540, 1991.

138. Shea B, Wells, G, Cranney A., et al: Calcium supplementation on bone loss in postmenopausal women, Cochrane Database Syst Rev (1):CD004526, 2004.

139. Peacock M, Liu G, Carey M, et al: Effect of calcium or 25)H vitamin D3 dietary supplementation on bone loss at the hip in men and women over the age of 60. J Clin Endocrinol Metab 85:3011–3019, 2000.

140. Weinsier RL, Krumdieck CL: Dairy foods and bone health: examination of the evidence. Am J Clin Nutr 72:681–689, 2000.

141. Standing Committee on the Scientific Evaluation of Dietary Reference Intakes, Food and Nutrition Board, Institute of Medicine, National Academy of Sciences: Dietary reference intakes for calcium, phosphorus, magnesium, vitamin D, and fluoride. Washington, DC: National Academy Press; 2000.

142. National Osteoporosis Foundation: Prevention. Available at http://www.nof.org/prevention

143. Reid IR: The role of calcium and vitamin D in the prevention of osteoporosis. Endocrinol Metab Clin North Am 27:389–398, 1998.

144. ACOG Practice Bulletin: Clinical management guidelines for obstetrician-gynecologists. Osteoporosis. Obstet Gynecol 103:203–216, 2004.

145. Melhus H, Michaelsson K, Kindmark A, et al: Excessive dietary intake of vitamin A is associated with reduced bone mineral density and increased risk for hip fractures. Ann Intern Med 129:770–778, 1998.

146. Michaelsson K, Lithell H, Vessby B: Serum retinal levels and the risk of fracture. N Engl J Med 348:287–294, 2003.

147. Bray G: Low carbohydrate diets and realities of weight loss. JAMA 289:1853–1855, 2002.

148. American Diabetes Association: Diabetes by the numbers. Diabetes Forecast 6:78; 2003.

149. Centers for Disease Control and Prevention: National diabetes fact sheet. Available at http://www.cdc.gov/diabetes/pubs/estimates.htm

150. Mc Cance DR, Pettitt DJ, Hanson RL, et al: Glucose, insulin concentrations and obesity in childhood and adolescence as predictors of NIDDM. Diabetologia 37:617–623, 1994.

151. Franz MJ, Bantle JD, Beebe CA, et al: Standards of medical care for patients with diabetes mellitus. Diabetes Care 27:S15–S35, 2004.

152. Litonjua P, Pinero-Pilona A, Aviles-Santa L, Raskin P: Prevalence of acanthosis nigricans in newly-diagnosed type 2 diabetes. Endocrinol Pract 10:101–106, 2004.

153. Centers for Disease Control and Prevention Primary Prevention Working Group: Primary Prevention of type 2 diabetes mellitus by lifestyle intervention: implications for health policy. Ann Intern Med 140:951–957, 2004.

154. Tuomilehto J, Lindstron J, Eriksson JG, et al: Prevention of type 2 diabetes mellitus by changes in lifestyle among subjects with impaired glucose tolerance. N Engl J Med 344:1343–1350, 2001.

155. Pan XR, Li GW, Hu YH, et al: Effects of diet and exercise in preventing NIDDM in people with impaired glucose tolerance. The Da Qing IGT and Diabetes Study. Diabetes Care 20:537–544, 1997.

156. Diabetes Prevention Research Group: Reduction in the evidence of type 2 diabetes with life-style intervention or metformin. N Engl J Med 346:393–403, 2002.

SELECTED REFERENCE FOR FURTHER READING

Felson DT, Kiel DP, Anderson JJ, Kannel WB: Alcohol consumption and hip fractures: The Framingham Study. Am J Epidemiol 128:1102–1110, 1988.

Lichtenstein AH, Deckelbaum RJ: Stanol/sterol ester-containing foods and blood cholesterol levels. Circulation 103:1177–1179, 2001.

INTERNET RESOURCES

American Cancer Society
http://www.cancer.org/docroot/PED/content/PED_3_2X_Diet_and_Activity_Factors_That_Affect_Risks.asp?sitearea=PED

American Diabetes Association
http://diabetes.org/nutrition-and-recipes/nutrition/overview.jsp

American Heart Association
http://americanheart.org/presenter.jhtml?identifier=1200010

National Center for Chronic Disease Prevention
http://cdc.gov/nccdphp/pe_factsheets/pe_pa.htm

Assessment of Dietary Intake

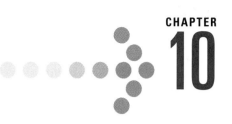

SUZANNE BRODNEY-FOLSE AND RUTH ANN CARPENTER

This chapter addresses KSAs from the following content areas:

1   Exercise Physiology and Related Exercise Science
2   Pathophysiology and Risk Factors
3   Health Appraisal, Fitness, and Clinical Exercise Testing
4   Electrocardiography and Diagnostic Techniques
5   Patient Management and Medications
6   Medical and Surgical Management
7   Exercise Prescription and Programming
8   **Nutrition and Weight Management**
9   **Human Behavior and Counseling**
10 Safety, Injury Prevention, and Emergency Procedures
11 Program Administration, Quality Assurance, and Outcome Assessment

Accurate **dietary assessment** is a challenge because of the day-to-day variation in the type and amount of foods and beverages consumed; the difficulty in describing and recalling these items; the lack of a single "best" method or gold standard to measure diet; the difficulty in estimating portion size; the cost and amount of time to collect and process the data; and the need to translate the foods, beverages, and amounts consumed using nutrient or food group databases to meaningful feedback[1]. Despite these challenges, dietary assessment can provide worthwhile information if the assessment is conducted with the appropriate tool for the question asked and the interviewer and client understand the level of detail required to assess intake.

The objectives of the chapter are to understand a) the purpose of dietary assessment; b) the steps of dietary assessment; c) the pros and cons of the various dietary assessment tools, when each should be used, and how to provide useful feedback to clients; and d) intra-individual variation of dietary intake and how it impacts dietary assessment. This chapter focuses on how fitness professionals can follow the steps of dietary assessment to obtain, assess, and evaluate their clients' dietary intake. Practical tips and case examples are used to illustrate main concepts.

The Steps of Dietary Assessment

Conducting a dietary assessment to estimate intake involves a) identifying the purpose of the dietary assessment, b) selecting the appropriate diet assessment tool, c) obtaining the dietary intake data from the individual, d) analyzing the dietary intake data, e) evaluating the diet, and f) providing useful feedback. Each of these steps is described in detail in this chapter.

Identifying the Purpose of Dietary Assessment

A dietary assessment is performed to evaluate the quality and quantity of foods and beverages consumed by individuals. It is one of several indicators of nutritional status; the others include anthropometrics, biochemical data, and clinical data[2]. Dietary assessment may be conducted for research purposes or to evaluate an individual's intake in a counseling setting. Many of the diet assessment tools may be used for both purposes; however, this chapter focuses on an individual's dietary assessment.

The benefits to assessing an individual's diet include the ability to identify food consumption patterns, inadequate or excessive intakes of certain foods or food groups, and issues related to portion size. An individual may seek a diet assessment for several reasons, such as to lose weight, lower fat intake, decrease calories, increase fruit and vegetable consumption, improve overall diet, or optimize dietary intake for athletic performance. In addition, when the diet assessment is used as a part of counseling, the individual may become more aware of his or her intake habits, and this information can be a useful teaching method.

Selecting the Appropriate Dietary Assessment Tool

Dietary assessment methods include observation, diet histories, **food frequency questionnaires (FFQs)**, **24-hour recalls**, and **diet records**. Each of these methods has advantages and disadvantages, and selection of the appropriate dietary assessment tool depends on whether the information collected will be for an individual or group and the reason for the assessment. Understanding the strengths and weaknesses of the tools used in each step of the dietary assessment process helps ensure that the appropriate method is used. Certain types of dietary assessment tools may not be appropriate to use in some populations such as children, those with memory problems, those with low literacy levels, or visually or hearing impaired individuals.

This section begins with the methods least likely to be used for assessing individual dietary intake in a fitness setting and concludes with the tools anticipated to be used more commonly, which are the 24-hour recall and diet record. A brief description of each tool, how it should be administered, and its benefits and limitations are discussed. The sections that follow provide specific information on analyzing the dietary intake data, evaluating the diet, and providing useful feedback to the client.

OBSERVATION

Description

Likely the best method to determine an individual's actual intake is to directly observe a client during a number of days and record all foods and beverages consumed; however, this is not a realistic option in a free-living population. Using this method, a trained observer records all foods, beverages, and amounts consumed by an individual or group during mealtime. In order to accurately determine the amount consumed, the observer must know the exact amount the individual or group is served, which is why this method works well in controlled situations, such as metabolic units, institutionalized populations, and schools. The interviewer does not interact with the individuals consuming the food. This method is more often used to assess intake of a group because it is typically conducted during one time period.

Benefits and Limitations

The benefit of the observation method is the accuracy of the dietary intake data collected for the time period assessed. The main limitations of this method are that it is very labor intensive and costly and is not appropriate for assessing usual intake.

DIET HISTORY

Description

The diet history is a combination of several diet assessment methods to provide a detailed assessment of health habits and usual eating patterns[3]. The diet history was originally used in human growth and development studies to assess an individual's usual meal patterns, food preparation practices, and intake over a certain time, such as a month or year. This method, which is an interviewer-administered tool, includes a 24-hour recall and a food checklist for the past month; a 3-day food record may be used as a cross-check of the data collected. Nutrition knowledge and training are generally necessary to probe for personal dietary habits and patterns, and a high level of respondent participation and cooperation is required.

Benefits and Limitations

A diet history can provide an accurate assessment of usual diet[4] and does not alter usual diet. A limitation of this method includes interviews that are time consuming and may last 1 to 2 hours. Also, after data are collected, they must be coded and analyzed, processes that are labor intensive, difficult, and expensive.

FOOD FREQUENCY QUESTIONNAIRE

Description

The food frequency questionnaire (FFQ) is a dietary assessment tool used to assess usual intake by inquiring about frequency of past consumption of selected foods or food groups over a specific time[5]. In research, this method is useful for assessing the relationship between diet and disease because it can be used to rank individuals by high and low intake. The FFQ may either be interviewer or self-administered; will not alter usual diet; and depending on the size of the questionnaire, takes between 20 and 30 minutes to complete.

The FFQ is composed of a food list, options for reporting the frequency of intake, and options for portion size. The food list used must be representative of the population being studied to ensure that the foods or food groups that are popular sources of nutrient intake are represented. This food list may be subdivided by food groups and typically contain 100 to 125 foods. The options used for collecting data about frequency of consumption include, daily, weekly, monthly, and yearly, and the options depend on the purpose for assessing the diet.

An FFQ may or may not contain portion size options. A nonquantitative FFQ only requires the individual to provide information about the frequency of consumption. For example, the individual would specify only if he or she ate or drank that item over a specified time period (day, week, or month). A semiquantitative FFQ inquires about the frequency of consumption of a prespecified amount of food or beverage. Prespecified amounts such as a slice of bread or glass of milk are easier to report than items not typically consumed as easily quantifiable, such as chicken. A quantitative FFQ asks the individual to complete information on a portion size, but the portion size options can range from small, medium, or large to open-ended questions[5].

Benefits and Limitations

The FFQ relies on memory and may be challenging for participants to estimate the foods and beverages consumed over a prespecified length of time. The FFQ may be less expensive and require less administrative time than other methods because answers to the FFQ can be entered on scan sheets and the data entered directly into a database.

24-HOUR RECALL

Description

The 24-hour recall is the most popular method to assess current dietary intake. In a structured interview, the respondent is asked to recall all foods and beverages consumed in the past 24 hours, including the amount consumed and details on the method of preparation. A single 24-hour recall provides an estimate of actual intake for a specific day but is not appropriate for estimating usual intake because of the daily variation in diet. In order to estimate usual intake, several 24-hour recalls would need to be collected, with the actual number depending on the

nutrient of interest. However, in a research setting, a single 24-hour recall collected from groups of individuals can be used to adequately assess average intake of the groups.

The 24-hour recall is the dietary assessment method used by the U.S. Department of Agriculture (USDA) to assess the nutrient intakes of Americans in the current national nutrition survey. In order to obtain the necessary level of detail on each recall, the USDA has developed a five-step multiple pass method to administer the tool[6]. The five steps include a quick list, a forgotten foods list, time and occasion, detail cycle, and the final review probe. The accuracy of the five-step method has been tested in normal, overweight, and obese women and was found to assess mean intake within 10% of actual intake that was measured by direct observation[6].

Benefits and Limitations

When used for counseling, the 24-hour recall is useful as a method to discuss general eating patterns, keeping in mind that a single day is not representative of overall diet. The 24-hour recall can be completed relatively quickly in about 20 minutes; however, coding the data can be costly. For some populations, this method may not be ideal because of poor memory or difficulty with estimating amounts. This method does not alter usual diet, although individuals may under- or overreport foods that are more "socially desirable" to appear healthier.

DIET RECORDS

Description

Diet records are based on the report of actual intake over a specific number of days, typically 3 to 4 days and not more than 7 days. When selecting days, it is ideal to include at least one weekend day. The individual records all foods and beverages consumed for a predetermined number of days in detail with the portion size[1]. The data are then coded and averaged over the number of days collected. The respondent may also be encouraged to write down information about where, when, and with whom the foods were eaten. This method may be used with nonliterate populations by using tape recorders to record intake.

It is critical to remember that 1 day of intake does not provide an accurate assessment of usual dietary intake. The number of days of intake necessary to assess an individual's intake varies by the nutrient. Collecting more than 1 day of intake allows estimations of the within-person error, which can assist in determining the number of days to estimate true intake[5]. The number of days necessary to estimate usual intake of energy and the macronutrients ranges from 3 to 10 days[7]; the number of days to estimate many of the micronutrients require even more days.

Benefits and Limitations

The strengths of the diet record are that it provides quantitatively accurate information for the time that the diet record is kept and that by recording foods when they are consumed, the participant does not rely on memory to recall the information[1]. Eating behaviors and patterns can also be addressed with this assessment tool. The limitations of this tool include a high respondent burden. Additionally, the process of recording the items consumed can alter eating behaviors, respondents must be motivated and literate, and coding of the data is costly and time consuming[7]. Collecting too few days of intake will not provide an accurate assessment of an individual's usual intake, and caution should be used when providing feedback to acknowledge the shortcomings of this assessment method.

Summary

As illustrated by the descriptions and benefits and limitations of each diet assessment tool, the choices for assessing diet are varied, and the best method depends on the reason for the assessment. Each dietary assessment tool has strengths and weaknesses, but we anticipate that fitness professionals will be more likely to use the 24-hour recall or diet record in counseling situations. Thus, the remaining sections in this chapter focus specifically on these two methods. It is important for fitness professionals to realize that the processes associated with assessing dietary intake are quite complicated and require a good bit of training and practice. We simply provide an overview in this chapter and encourage readers to work with dietitians or other nutrition specialists to hone skills in this area or assist by completing one or more of the following tasks.

Obtaining the Dietary Intake

This section focuses on the steps that can be incorporated into dietary assessment to optimize the data quality obtained from 24-hour recalls and diet records. These steps include providing detailed, verbal and written, easy-to-understand instructions to the client about recording intake and estimating portion size; probing either during the interview or after the completed recall has been received to elicit the necessary detail about intake and portion size; and scanning the completed assessment for missing values and outliers.

COMPLETING THE 24-HOUR RECALL AND DIET RECORD

Usually, the 24-hour recall is completed by the interviewer and does not require instructions for the client. The client is asked to recall all foods and beverages consumed in the past 24 hours and to estimate the portion size of each item. The interviewer is responsible for recording the intake and probing for as much detail as possible. It is important to ask

open-ended questions, as well as portray a nonjudgmental expression when inquiring about an individual's intake. If the interviewer expects the client to record all the items consumed in the previous 24 hours, then the interviewer should provide detailed instructions such as those used for diet records (see discussion below).

When a client is asked to keep a diet record for a predetermined number of days, detailed instructions are very useful because clients are typically sent home with the diet records. Box 10-1 provides a list of instructions for a client to record intake. Table 10-1 lists several probes to help elicit the necessary detail about the foods consumed. The instructions should include general information about how to complete the record as well as the contact information of an individual able to assist with the process, if necessary.

BOX 10-1 | **Instructions for Recording Intake**

GENERAL INSTRUCTIONS FOR KEEPING A DIET RECORD

Write legibly.

Record for the specific number of days.

Record each meal, snack, and beverage *immediately* after you eat it. See additional instructions below.

Record each food on a separate line.

Leave one or two blank lines after each meal or snack.

If additional space is required for the same day, continue on an extra page.

INSTRUCTIONS FOR RECORDING OF FOODS

Write down every bit of food and beverage that goes into your mouth—even snacks—for the entire day!

Fully describe everything you eat and drink *in detail* (e.g., chicken thigh, skin not eaten; decaffeinated coffee; low-calorie French dressing; low-fat mayonnaise; whole milk).

Specify preparation methods (e.g., whether meat is breaded and fried, broiled, baked; vegetables cooked with fat).

List each separate ingredient for mixed dishes (sandwiches, casseroles, salads) on a separate line.

Record exact amounts of food and beverages. If possible, weigh and measure your foods.

Attach food labels or recipes, if possible.

Include anything that you add to your food at the table (e.g., baked potato with 1 tb butter; coffee with 1 tsp sugar).

Try not to modify your eating habits.

Adapted with permission from the Cooper Institute, Dallas, Texas.

TABLE 10-1. Probes for Identifying Details of Foods

Type of Information	Did You Specify?
Grains and Cereals	
Bread or tortilla	Brand, type (e.g., diet, regular, wheat, whole wheat, rye, flour vs corn)
Bakery items	Brand, type (bran, blueberry), how prepared (cake, raised), toppings
Cereal	Brand, type, anything added during preparation or consumption (sugar, fat)
Pasta, rice, and other grains	Brand; fat or salt added
Vegetables and Fruits	
Vegetables and fruit	Fresh, frozen, canned, dried; brand name; cooked or raw; juice: added sugar; salads: what was in salad; added fats, oils, or other toppings (e.g., croutons, sauces, bacon)
Dairy	
Milk	Brand, percent fat, anything added
Cheese	Brand, type (cheddar, American, cottage), version (lite, low fat, low sodium)
Yogurt	Brand, version, frozen or regular
Non-dairy	Brand, powder or liquid
Other (ice cream, cream)	Brand, version, type, flavor
Meat, Poultry, and Fish	
Fresh cuts	Type of cut (e.g., T-bone, sirloin, thigh, breast, salmon, haddock)
	Fat trimmed or skin removed, before or after cooking
	Is reported weight for cooked or raw, with or without bone
	Percent lean (hamburger)
	How prepared (baked, grilled, fried, barbecue)
	Fat, sauces and seasonings used during cooking?
Cold cuts	Brand, version (e.g., lite hot dog, bun length, footlong.), type (e.g., beef, turkey)
Canned tuna and salmon	Type (solid white, chunk light), packed in oil or water, reduced salt
Oils, Spreads, and Dressings	
Margarine	Brand, type (stick, tub, liquid), version (whipped, diet, lite)
Oils	Brand, type (corn, canola, olive)
Mayonnaise/salad dressings	Brand, type or flavor; version (low fat, nonfat, cholesterol free)
Other	
Mixed dishes	Is recipe included, brand, principal components
Pizza	Brand, thin or thick crust, toppings, diameter (e.g., 16", 20"), how many pieces eaten
Soup	Brand or homemade, type or flavor, creamed, water or milk added
Other	Brand; include recipe, if possible; principal components; gravies and sauces
Beverages	Brand, sweetened or unsweetened, alcohol, diet or low cal, decaffeinated
Eggs	Whole, egg substitute, brand, how prepared
Crackers, snacks, chips	Brand, type, how prepared (e.g., microwave popcorn), size, handfuls, bowls (vitamins B1 and B2 food models, cups or ounces if they read it of the bag)
Pies, cakes,	Brand, type, one or two crusts or layers, type of frosting

In addition, instructions for keeping the diet record should be reviewed with the client to reinforce the importance of the exercise, answer questions, explain the level of detail needed for accurate assessment, and remind the client not to omit foods or beverages or change intake.

RECORDING PORTION SIZE

The estimation of portion size is one of the most challenging components of dietary assessment. Portion size can be determined by weighing food portions; visually estimating weights of foods; and visual estimates of size through the use of household measures, food models, or photographs[8]. The interviewer may suggest that the client use common household items, such as scales, measuring cups, or a ruler to assist with estimating portion size. Additionally, the client may be asked to bring in recipes and food labels. Given that portion size is difficult to estimate and mistakes are often encountered during this step, a list of probes to assist with estimating portion size has been provided (Table 10-2). Specific attention should be given to the common mistake of confusing fluid and weight ounces when describing portion size.

The importance of estimating portion size should be highlighted. The expanding portion sizes of foods and beverages coupled with the decrease in physical activity energy expenditure are likely contributors to the current epidemic of overweight and obesity in the United States[9]. Recent analyses from past national nutrition surveys indicate an increase in the portion size of several foods eaten inside and outside the home[10,11]. Because weight reduction is a common reason for seeking dietary advice, inaccurate assessment of portion size may not reveal opportunities for improvement or modification of diet.

TABLE 10-2. Portion Size Probes

Portion Sizes	
How many?	Discrete numbers
Food model	Usual kitchen measures (e.g., cup, tablespoon, teaspoon, ounces)
	Ounces—fluid or weighed
	Reasonable
	Portion of model
Thickness or ice in drink	Meat
	Cakes, brownies
	Unsliced bread
	Cubes or crushed
	A lot of ice, a little ice
	If the subject knows *exactly* how much he ior she drank (e.g., one 12-oz can), you do not need to know if ice was used

Inaccurate estimation of portion size has been documented in several populations. Underreporting of diet is a common problem and may be more prevalent in overweight and obese individuals[12]. Underreporting has been observed in men[13] and women,[14] and the amount of underreporting has ranged from 20% to 50%, depending on the nutrient.

Analyzing the Dietary Intake

After dietary intake has been recorded and reviewed, the contents of the diet need to be analyzed. The goal of this step is to translate the food and beverage consumption data to nutrient intake or food group information using nutrient composition or food group databases. Several resources are available to analyze dietary data, such as computerized databases, software, nutrient composition tables, and food manufacturer data.

Before the use of computerized databases, nutrition professionals looked up foods in published tables of nutrient composition, such as those found in *Bowes and Church's Food Values of Portions Commonly Used*[15]. Each item was looked up individually, the nutrient content of the food was calculated and adjusted based on the reported portion size, and the nutrient values for each item were added to get an estimate of intake. This is a very time-consuming and tedious process. The introduction of computerized nutrient databases has saved considerable time and effort. Several diet analysis software packages are available for purchase, and many may be downloaded free of charge from the Internet.

The authors of a recent article compared the functionality of several online diet analysis tools[16]. They conducted Internet searches using popular search engines to identify fee-based and non fee-based diet assessment websites and then compared the features. The authors compared the computer programs and Internet sites on several useful features, such as number of foods, database source, fee, and type of feedback. This useful review provides an

introduction to the types of computer programs available without having to invest in expensive software. In addition, in April 2003, the USDA made publicly available a user-friendly interface for downloading and using the Survey Nutrient Database, which is the most authoritative nutrient database available. The database includes more than 6000 foods and 117 nutrients as well as several options for coding portion size[17]. In addition, the USDA offers an online dietary and physical activity assessment site called the "Interactive Healthy Eating Index and Physical Activity Assessment Tool." We discuss this resource later in this chapter.

Evaluating Dietary Intake

After the results of a qualitative or quantitative analysis have been determined, the next step is to compare the results with dietary recommendations. Food and nutrient needs differ based on gender, age, physical activity level, life stage, and health status. Since the 1940s, the federal government has established guidelines for food and nutrient intake. Initially, the guidelines were designed to reduce the prevalence of nutrient deficiencies. As such, the dietary recommendations were used to establish policies for many federal aid programs such as the National School Lunch and the Women, Infants, and Children programs. Dietary recommendations are still used for this purpose, but as the prevalence of chronic diseases such as coronary heart disease, stroke, cancer (Box 10-2), diabetes, and obesity has grown in the past 50 years, the guidelines shifted to a dual focus of preventing deficiencies and promoting health.

In addition to providing the basis for many federal nutrition programs, current public health dietary recommendations are used as a basis for nutrition label information, military rations, the development of some food and nutritional products, and evaluation of the adequacy of intake for individuals and groups. The remainder of this section focuses on food and nutrient guidelines that fitness professionals would most likely use for evaluating dietary intake of individuals. Practical recommendations for using these guidelines are also provided.

CURRENT PUBLIC HEALTH RECOMMENDATIONS

The Dietary Guidelines for Americans[18] have been the cornerstone of federal nutrition policy and nutrition education since 1980. The guidelines reflect a consensus of the most current science and medical knowledge available. To account for ongoing research efforts in nutrition and health, the guidelines are updated every 5 years. The next revision is due in 2005. The government convenes a panel of nutrition, medical, and epidemiological experts to review the existing guidelines in light of new scientific data. The panel's recommendations are reviewed by

BOX 10-2 | **Dietary Recommendations for Cancer Prevention**

1. Body mass index should be maintained between 18.5 and 25. Weight gain during adulthood should remain less than 11 pounds.
2. Year-round, consume a variety of vegetables and fruits other than roots, tubers, legumes, and grains (see next item), providing 7% or more of calories or totaling 15 to 30 oz or five portions per day.
3. Consume 20 to 30 oz or seven servings per day of other plant foods, minimally processed (including roots, tubers, legumes and grains), providing 45% to 60% of total calories. Refined sugars should be limited to less than 10% of total calories.
4. Alcohol consumption is not recommended. If consumed, alcohol should be limited to one serving per day for women and two servings per day for men. A serving is 3 oz wine, 1 oz distilled spirits, or 8 oz beer.
5. Limit red meat to less than 3 oz/day. Fish, poultry and undomesticated meats are preferable.
6. Limit total fat to 15% to 30% of calories.
7. Limit intake of fatty foods.
8. Salt from all sources should amount to less than 6 g/day.
9. Perishable foods should be safely stored or refrigerated to minimize fungal contaminants and mycotoxins.
10. When levels of food additives, contaminants, or other residues are properly regulated in food and drinks, their presence is not known to be harmful. In economically developing countries where there may be insufficient regulation, these may be a health hazard.
11. Cook meat and fish at low temperatures. Do not eat charred food or burned meat juices. Only occasionally consume meat or fish that has been grilled over direct flame.

government agencies and then provided to the public for comment. In addition, testing is done to determine consumer understanding of the guidelines before they are finalized.

The current Dietary Guidelines are 10 basic principles for healthy eating for healthy Americans 2 years of age and older (see Box 10-3). The "Aim for Fitness" guidelines highlight the importance of attaining and maintaining a healthy weight and makes a specific physical activity recommendation. The "Build a Healthy Base" portion of the guidelines focuses on foods that should comprise the foundation of a healthy diet. It recommends that consumers use the Food Guide Pyramid[19] to ensure adequate intake of nutrients. The "Choose Sensibly" guidelines attempt to help consumers moderate their use of nutrients, foods, and beverages that are associated with common chronic diseases. The current and future versions of *Nutrition and Your Health: Dietary Guidelines for Americans* can be viewed and downloaded from http://www.usda.gov/cnpp.

Food Guide Pyramid

The Food Guide Pyramid was developed in 1992 as a graphical way to translate the Dietary Guidelines into practical recommendations for foods consumers need to eat daily to get the nutrients they need for good health (Fig. 10-1). Given the significant advances in nutrition research over the past 12 years, the USDA is currently updating the pyramid and will publish a revised practical guide to daily food intake in 2005. Whether the result is a remodeled pyramid or another graphical format, we believe the new approach will continue to provide a useful means by which to evaluate dietary intake.

Dietary Reference Intakes

Evaluating a client's diet using a food focus is a perfectly adequate and efficient way to determine the dietary needs of your clients and is especially useful if you do not have more sophisticated tools such as dietary analysis software available to you. However, some clients may want information regarding specific nutrients. For example, a man with a family history of early heart attacks who is trying to lower his blood cholesterol level may want to evaluate his total fat and saturated fat intake. A postmenopausal woman may want to know how much

BOX 10-3 | **Dietary Guidelines for Americans**

AIM FOR FITNESS
- Aim for a healthy weight.
- Be physically active every day.

BUILD A HEALTHY BASE
- Let the Food Guide Pyramid guide your food choices.
- Choose a variety of grains daily, especially whole grains.
- Choose a variety of fruits and vegetables daily.
- Keep food safe to eat.

CHOOSE SENSIBLY
- Choose a diet that is low in saturated fat and cholesterol and moderate in total fat.
- Choose beverages and foods to moderate your intake of sugars.
- Choose and prepare foods with less salt.
- If you drink alcoholic beverages, do so in moderation.

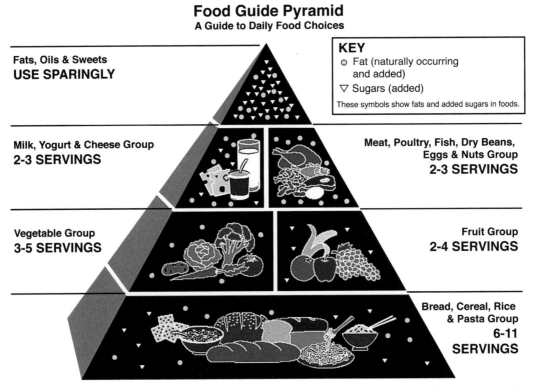

FIGURE 10-1. The Food Guide Pyramid. (From U.S. Department of Agriculture. The Food Guide Pyramid. Home and Garden Bulletin No. 252. Hyattsville (MD): Washington, DC: Government Printing Office; 1992.)

calcium she is getting to determine if she should take a calcium supplement.

In an effort to make public health recommendations based on the latest research on nutrient needs, the Federal government periodically commissions leading scientists in various areas of nutrient research to review the literature and establish estimates of nutrient intakes that can be used to assess and plan diets for generally healthy people. These are called the **Dietary Reference Intakes** (DRIs)[20-25]. For macronutrients such as carbohydrate, fat, protein, Acceptable Macronutrient Distribution Ranges (AMDRs) have recently been established[24].

The DRIs include three classifications that are of interest to fitness professionals. First, the Recommended Dietary Allowances (RDAs) and Adequate Intakes (AIs) can both be used as goals for clients. The RDAs are set to meet the nutrient needs of almost all individuals in a group. Second, when scientists establish an AI instead of an RDA for a nutrient, it is because they believe that the AI is adequate to meet the needs of all individuals in a group but there is not sufficient data to establish an RDA for that particular nutrient. For some nutrients, there is enough data that supports the setting of a Tolerable Upper Intake Level (UL). This is the maximum daily intake level that is likely to pose no risk or adverse effects. In most cases, the UL includes total daily intake from food, water, and supplements. Not all nutrients (e.g., thiamin, B_{12}, vitamin K) have a UL established for them, but that

does not mean that it is safe to take them in amounts above the RDA or AI for these nutrients.

Evaluating Dietary Intake

Diet can be evaluated at the food or nutrient level. For the former, you would use the Food Guide Pyramid or any dietary guidance system that replaces it when the dietary guidelines are updated in 2005. For the latter, you would use the DRIs. Regardless of the method you use, the steps are the same.

1. Convert foods and amounts eaten into food group servings or nutrients.
2. Determine the recommended intake of food groups or nutrients.
3. Compare the amount eaten with recommendations to determine dietary inadequacies.

Because it is unknown at the time of this writing what, if any, changes will be made to the Food Guide Pyramid, we will describe each of the steps, focusing on nutrients. Here again, we offer the caution that although these appear to be simple steps, the diet assessment process is not simplistic. It can be fraught with missing information, errors, and miscalculations, as described in earlier sections of this chapter. These can be compounded when dietary assessment is done by people with little or no training or experience. If fitness professionals feel uncomfortable with any part of this process, they should consult with or refer their clients to a registered dietitian.

CONVERTING FOODS AND AMOUNTS EATEN

You can calculate nutrient intake by hand or by using computer software. The former requires you to list out each food and the amount eaten. Then you need to use a reference guide such as Bowes and Church[15] to look up the amount of different nutrients in each food. Using computer software can be much faster and more accurate than the hand tabulation method. All you have to do is enter the foods and amount eaten into a dietary analysis software program, and it calculates the quantity consumed for dozens of nutrients for each food. It then sums the quantity of each nutrient for all foods to generate a total daily intake for each nutrient. Many programs calculate an average nutrient intake amount for multiple days of food data as well.

DETERMINE THE RECOMMENDED INTAKE

In step one, you determine nutrient intake either by hand calculation or by computer. Likewise, in step two, you can look up a client's intake need for most nutrients in reference. Please refer to the following website for the RDA's; AIs; and, where established, UIs, for adults: (http://www.nal.usda.gov/fnic/etext/000105). As you review this table, take note that nutrient needs sometimes differ from one age category to another or between genders. Computerized dietary analysis software contain DRI information for each nutrient.

COMPARE THE AMOUNT EATEN WITH RECOMMENDATIONS

Determining nutrient adequacy simply means comparing actual intake with nutrient recommendations for a person based on his or her age and gender. Most nutrient analysis software programs have a database of the DRIs against which nutrient intake is compared. These applications often provide a tabular and graphical presentation of the adequacy of a client's intake compared with the nutrient needs of someone of their gender and age. These are often given as percentages of recommended intake. For example, Figure 10-2 shows a graph that many applications may use.

You can see from this example that the client did not meet her nutrient needs 100% exactly for a single

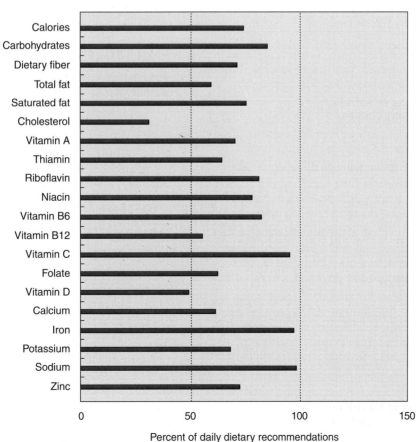

FIGURE 10-2. Sample nutrient analysis report.

nutrient. Does this mean she is nutritionally at risk? How should this be interpreted? There are several things to consider:

1. **Dietary assessment information is an estimate:** The report you generate from either a 24-hour recall or diet record is an estimate of nutrient intake. It is only as good as the completeness of the data provided to you, the quality of the analysis software you use to analyze the intake, and your data entry accuracy.
2. **Number of days recorded:** One day's food record can have a high degree of variability compared with another day's. What you eat today may be very different from what you eat tomorrow or the next day, and what you eat in a single day is not likely to impact your health positively or negatively. It is most useful to smooth out the highs and lows in the daily variability of nutrient intake by averaging the nutrient values across several days.
3. **Typical of usual intake:** If the day (or days) the client recorded were not very typical of his or her usual eating pattern, then the analysis may be skewed. For example, a client usually has a bowl of cereal and skim milk every morning, but on two of the days he recorded, he only ate a granola bar as he commuted to the courthouse for jury duty.
4. **Accurate portion descriptions:** Often people guess at the size of their portions or misinterpret information provided on their measuring tools.
5. **Data entry errors:** It is common to make a mistake in entering the many foods in a client's dietary intake record. For example, misplacement of a decimal point can make 0.75 cup of Brussels sprouts 75 cups of sprouts! When the results seem very skewed, review the data you entered to make sure you have selected the correct food option and entered the right portion amount.

If reviewing these issues does not at least somewhat account for any nutrient values below or above the recommended levels, it is rarely cause for alarm. Deficiency is not a concern until a client is chronically below 66% of recommended intake. In general, if a client is taking a multivitamin supplement, this is not usually included in the computer analysis, so it is likely the client is getting an adequate intake. Excessive intake can occur when a client chronically consumes levels above the UL from both diet *and* supplements.

In summary, this section has provided a step-by-step process for evaluating dietary intake. You can use a food-focused evaluation process using the Food Guide Pyramid or a nutrient-focused evaluation using the DRIs. The former is fairly simple and can be done without special software or references. The latter gives very specific information that may be important in some situations. A third, recommended method that combines a food and nutrient focus is the "Interactive Healthy Eating Index." This Web-based resource is available to you and your clients free of

---

BOX 10-4 | The Interactive Healthy Eating Index

The U.S. Department of Agriculture provides a website at which you or your clients can enter their daily food intake to receive a "score" on the overall quality of their diet for that day. The score compares food intake information against a person's recommendations for 10 important dietary factors: grains, vegetables, fruits, dairy, meat, total fat, saturated fat, cholesterol, sodium, and variety. The total score ranges from 0 to 100, with 100 being optimal. A helpful feature is that users can compare their scores with national the average. This educational website also analyzes the food intake for 25 different nutrients. In addition, it creatively provides feedback by building a Food Pyramid based on the person's intake. As such, it graphically shows how lopsided or aligned a person's diet is with the Pyramid. You can access the website at http://209.48.219.53.

---

charge (see Box 10-4). It has recently been updated to include a physical activity assessment tool. Regardless of the method you use, you must translate the dietary evaluation into practical recommendations for changing food intake, and you must work with clients to help them set attainable, personal goals for dietary improvement.

Giving Dietary Feedback

After you have analyzed and evaluated a client's diet, you are ready to educate the client about the aspects of his or her diet that need to be changed to improve dietary intake. There are two components of giving feedback. The first is the content, or, the information you want to give the client. The second component is the process or the way in which you give the information.

FEEDBACK CONTENT

Your task is to inform clients of the gaps that occur in their diets based on what they reported eating and what is recommended for them. These gaps can be characterized as under consumption or overconsumption of foods or nutrients. It is fairly easy to give feedback to close such gaps using foods and Food Guide Pyramid's food groups. Box 10-5 provides a list of practical recommendations for improving intake of foods in different food groups.

If you have evaluated a client's diet using a nutrient analysis, you need to convert nutrient needs to food-based recommendations. For example, if you determine that a client is eating too much saturated fat, you could recommend that the client reduce the intake of whole milk dairy products, including cheese; choose small portions of meat; choose lean meats only; choose red meats less often;

BOX 10-5 | **Dietary Feedback Tips**

BREAD, CEREAL, PASTA, AND RICE
Most people get adequate servings of the bread group. Because people often misjudge serving size (e.g., one bagel is equal to two to three servings), overconsumption is common.

Increase Servings
- Double up on servings of cereal, pasta, and rice.
- Enjoy low-fat breads as a snack. Choose whole-grain options whenever possible.

Decrease Servings
- Watch portion sizes. Measure cereal, rice, and pasta and weigh bread, muffins, and other bread foods to become familiar with the actual size of one serving.

Increase Whole Grains
- Start the day with a whole-grain breakfast cereal. Look for one that has at least 5 g of fiber per serving.
- Use 100% whole wheat bread.
- Make oatmeal a regular part of your diet.
- Double up on servings
- Try new whole grains such as bulgur (wheat berries), barley, amaranth, spelt, and quinoa in place of rice or pasta or as side dishes and salads.

VEGETABLES
Few people eat enough vegetables, and the vegetables they do eat are often limited to a few kinds such as potatoes, corn, and iceberg lettuce.

Increase Servings
- Double and triple up on servings at meals.
- Order a side of vegetables when eating out.
- Enjoy large salads as a meal instead of a sandwich or burger. They can often count as two to four servings, depending on the size.
- Try vegetable juices as a refreshing alternative to soda.
- Eat vegetables and low-fat dips as healthy snack.
- Add extra veggies to soups, stews, and casseroles.

Other Suggestions
- Choose a variety of vegetables. Challenge your taste buds with sweet potatoes, rutabagas, hubbard squash, kale, and other nutrient-packed veggies.
- Choose colorful vegetables such as carrots, melons, spinach, and tomatoes. Often, the more color, the more nutrients.
- Use canned or frozen vegetables to speed up the preparation process. Look for choices with no added sodium.

FRUITS
As with vegetables, fruits are underconsumed by most adults. They are packed with many nutrients.

Increase Servings
- Start your day with a glass of orange or grapefruit juice.

- Snack on fresh or dried fruits instead of chips or candy bars.
- Serve fruit as dessert and help yourself to seconds.

Other
- Like vegetables, choose a rainbow of colors.
- Pack frozen fruit in your lunch bag, and it will be thawed by the time the noon hour rolls around.

MEAT, POULTRY, FISH, EGGS, DRIED BEANS, AND MEAT ALTERNATES
Most people eat adequate amounts of meat and poultry, and some people eat these foods in excess.

Limit Meat Group Foods that are High in Total and Saturated Fat
- Choose lean cuts of meat. Cuts with the words "loin" or "round" in the name are usually good choices.
- Choose ground beef that is at least 90% lean.
- Trim visible fat from meat and poultry before cooking.
- Substitute two egg whites for one whole egg.
- Choose reduced-fat processed meats, cold cuts, and sausages. Check the Nutrition Facts label.

Choose Lean Meats and Meat Alternatives
- Go fishing for good nutrition by eating fish at least two servings of fish a week. If you do not like to cook fish, make it your choice when eating out.
- Give soy and other plant-based meat alternates a try. Sausages, burgers, and chicken tenders are all available in veggie versions, and many grocery stores carry them. Look in the freezer section. Remember, do not expect them to taste just like meat, but enjoy them for their own delicious flavor.
- Eat several meatless meals each week. Look in cookbooks or online for vegetarian recipes.
- Get a leg up with legumes. Try different types of dried beans, peas, and lentils as meat substitutes in soups, salads, or casseroles.

MILK, YOGURT, AND CHEESE
Dairy foods are often overlooked by many adults who think only children need milk. Even people who are lactose intolerant can (and should) enjoy dairy foods by using specially prepared dairy products.

Choose Low-fat and Nonfat Dairy Foods
- Use skim or 2% or 1% milk or yogurt.
- Use reduced fat cheese or use less of regular cheese.
- Go easy on regular ice cream. Try low-fat or fat-free versions. Sorbet and sherbet are other low-fat choices.

(continues)

BOX 10-5 | **Dietary Feedback Tips** *(continued)*

Increase Dairy Foods
- Make hot cereals and condensed soups with skim milk instead of water.
- Enjoy fruit and low-fat yogurt smoothies for a quick, delicious meal or snack.
- Drink low-fat milk with meals instead of soda.

FATS, OILS, AND SWEETS
Foods in this category are high in calories, and many do not provide much in the way of nutrients; that, is they provide essentially empty calories. So, these foods should be used sparingly.

Limit Empty Calories
- Choose fruits and vegetables as snacks instead of candy.
- Cut amount of fat or oil called for in a recipe by one quarter or one third.
- Replace regular soda or sweetened soft drinks with diet versions or fruit juices or low-fat milk.

Other Ideas
- When choosing a fat for cooking, select vegetable oils such as canola or olive oil instead of using lard, butter, or shortening.
- Retrain your sweet tooth by gradually removing high-sugar foods from your diet.

---

and limit butter and foods with hydrogenated fats. If a client needs to increase her fiber intake, you could advise that she eat more whole-grain products, fruits, vegetables, legumes, and nuts. The following website provides tables of the best food sources for each of the different nutrients to aid you in providing food-based feedback: http://www.nal.usda.gov/fnic/etext/000105.html.

THE PROCESS OF GIVING FEEDBACK

Identifying the gaps in what a client eats and what is recommended for him is the first step in providing dietary guidance. Working with the client to determine a plan for closing the gaps is the next step. This step requires an understanding about the behavior change process, and although this is covered elsewhere in this book, we have listed below several change strategies that fitness professionals can use to help clients succeed at improving their diets. It is important to note that the process is done collaboratively with clients. Simply telling clients what they need to change and then letting them figure out how to do it on their own is not an effective way of giving feedback.

Educate on Dietary Gaps

This is simply an instructive step in which you inform the client of her dietary needs. It is important to share all needs while being mindful not to overwhelm the client. Many clients are tempted to want to totally overhaul their eating habits based on the information you provide. Point out early on in the feedback process that it is best that they choose one or two areas that they want to work on at first. After they have had success making those changes, they can refocus their efforts to address other areas.

Assess Readiness to Change

Clients may be more ready to change some aspects of their diet than others. For example, a client may be more willing

to incorporate more whole grains than increase dairy foods. It is important that you determine which of the dietary improvement areas you have identified that the client is most ready to change. This strategy has been discussed as it relates to physical activity readiness in Chapter 38. It can easily be adapted to assessing readiness to change diet.

Set Goal(s)

People who are successful at changing habits challenge themselves by setting goals. However, it is not enough to simply state: "I want to eat better." Effective goals are those that are realistic (are within a client's reach), specific (defined in behavioral terms), and measurable (will be able to know whether or not it was attained). Ask clients to state some short-term (1-day to 1-month) and long-term (more than one-month) goals for the dietary improvement area (or areas) they are ready to change. Here is an example of a good goal: "On 5 of the next 7 days, I will eat at least five servings of fruits and vegetables." It is *realistic* because the client was already eating three servings on most, but not all days. In addition, the client recognizes that it is not likely that he is going to be able to get five servings every day, so he set the goal at 5 days. The goal is *specific* because it states what aspect of the diet (fruits and vegetables) he is going to change and to what extent. Finally, it is *measurable* because he defined a time frame (i.e., the next 7 days) and quantified the specific parameters of the goal.

Define an Action Plan

A goal is hollow unless it has an action plan to back it up. An action plan identifies the specific strategies the client is going to use to attain his goal. Using the example goal given previously, the client identified the following action plan: "Go to the store on my way home to buy orange juice, fresh strawberries, carrots, premixed salad, and frozen vegetables. Have orange juice for breakfast every morning. Take strawberries and carrots to work for snacks. Eat a big salad at lunch or dinner every weekday. Double up on servings of vegetables at dinner."

Identify a Self-monitoring Strategy

Daily logging helps clients identify whether they are on track toward their goals. Not only does self-monitoring help clients keep a record of what they are doing to attain their goals, it can also prompt clients to make better choices. Unlike keeping diet records for a dietary analysis, when clients are focusing on a specific goal, such as eating five or more servings of fruits and vegetables, they only need to focus on recording that specific behavior. This simplifies the recording process a great deal.

Arrange Follow-up

Before you end your feedback session with your client, set a follow-up appointment. The follow-up can be done face-to-face, by telephone, or by electronic means such as fax or email. The important thing is that clients know you will be available to discuss the success or difficulties they had with attaining is goals. This is a good time to praise clients for their attainment of goals, problem solve difficulties, and set new goals. Many clients find the accountability of a follow-up contact to be very motivating.

As stated earlier, this is a rather simplistic overview of the process for helping clients take the information you provide about their dietary needs and applying it to their particular lifestyle. The behavior change principles described in Chapter 38 give a much more thorough review of the change process.

When to Refer Clients

It is appropriate for fitness professionals to provide dietary guidance to clients who are generally healthy. Many of these clients are interested in improving their diets to lose weight, improve sports performance, or simply slow the development of age-related chronic diseases. There are however, circumstances under which you should refer clients to a registered or licensed dietitian. These include clients who have special dietary needs such as people with diabetes, renal problems, eating disorders, or other similar serious medical conditions. To locate dietitians in your area to whom you can refer clients, check with your local hospital to find out if they provide outpatient services. Also, you can go to the American Dietetic Association's website at http://www.eatright.org. Look for the "Find a Nutrition Professional" section and enter your client's zip code.

Summary

This chapter is intended to serve as a resource for fitness professionals interested in assessing diet by providing the descriptions of the diet assessment tools and their benefits and limitations. The steps to dietary assessment include identifying the purpose of diet assessment, selecting the appropriate diet assessment tool, obtaining the dietary intake from the individual, analyzing the data, evaluating the diet, and providing useful feedback. Assessing diet is a complex task and requires follow-through with each step in order to assist clients with reaching their goals.

REFERENCES

1. Thompson FE, Byers T: Dietary assessment resource manual. J Nutr 124:2245s–2317s, 1994.
2. Lee RD, Nieman DC: Measuring diet. In Nutritional Assessment, 3rd edition. New York: McGraw Hill; 2003.
3. Burke B: Dietary history as a tool in research. J Am Diet Assoc 23:1041–1047, 1947.
4. Byers TE, Marshall JR, Anthony E, Fiedler R, Zielezny M: The reliability of dietary history from the distant past. Am J Epidemiol 125:999–1011, 1987.
5. Willet WC: Nature of variation in the diet. Nutritional Epidemiology. New York: Oxford University Press; 1990:34–51.
6. Conway JM, Ingwersen LA, Vinyard BT, Moshfegh AJ: Effectiveness of the US Department of Agriculture 5-step multiple-pass method in assessing food intake in obese and non-obese women. Am J Clin Nutr 77:1171–1178, 2003.
7. Buzzard M: 24-hour dietary recall and food record methods. In Willett W, ed. Nutritional Epidemiology. New York: Oxford University Press; 1997:50–73.
8. Young LR, Nestle M: Portion sizes in dietary assessment: Issues and policy implications. Nutr Reviews 53:149–159, 1995.
9. Young LR, Nestle M: The contribution of expanding portion sizes to the US obesity epidemic. Am J Public Health 92:246–249, 2002.
10. Nielson SJ, Popkin BM: Patterns and trends in food portion sizes, 1997–1998. JAMA 289:450–453, 2003.
11. Smiciklas-Wright H, Mitchell D, Mickle SJ, Goldman JD, Cook A: Foods commonly eaten in the United States, 1989–1991 and 1994–1996: Are portion sizes changing? J Am Diet Assoc 103:41–47, 2003.
12. Heitmann BL: The influence of fatness, weight change, slimming history and other lifestyle variables on diet reporting in Danish men and women aged 35–65 years. Int J Obes 17:329–336, 1993.
13. Braam LA, Ocke MC, Bueno-de-Mesquita HB, Seidell JC: Determinants of obesity-related underreporting of energy intake. Am J Epidemiol 147:1081–1086, 1998.
14. Heitmann BL, Lissner L: Dietary underreporting by obese individuals—is it specific or non-specific. BMJ 311:986–989, 1995.
15. Pennington JAT: Bowes and Church's Food Values of Portions Commonly Used, 17th ed. Philadelphia: Lippincott-Raven Publishers; 1998.
16. Neighbors-Demberecky L, Painter J: Online diet analysis tools: A functional comparison. J Am Diet Assoc 102:1738–1740, 2002.
17. U.S. Department of Agriculture, Agricultural Research Service.: USDA National Nutrient Database for Standard Reference, Release 15. Nutrient Data Laboratory Home Page; 2002. http://www.nal.usda.gov/fnic/foodcomp.
18. U.S. Departments of Agriculture and Health and Human Services. Nutrition and your health: Dietary guidelines for Americans, 5th ed. Home and Garden Bulletin No. 232. Washington, DC: Government Printing Office; 2000.
19. U.S. Department of Agriculture: The food guide pyramid. Home and Garden Bulletin No. 252. Hyattsville (MD): Washington, DC: Government Printing Office; 1992.
20. Institute of Medicine: Dietary Reference Intakes for Calcium, Phosphorous, Magnesium, Vitamin D and Fluoride. Washington, DC: National Academy Press; 1997.

21. Institute of Medicine: Dietary Reference Intakes for Thiamin, Riboflavin, Niacin, Vitamin B6, Folate, Vitamin B12, Pantothenic Acid, Biotin and Choline. Washington, DC: National Academy Press; 1997.
22. Institute of Medicine: Dietary Reference Intakes for Vitamin C, Vitamin E, Selenium and Beta-Carotene, and other Carotenoids. Washington, DC: National Academy Press; 2000.
23. Institute of Medicine: Dietary Reference Intakes for Vitamin A, Vitamin K, Arsenic, Boron, Chromium, Copper, Iodine, Iron, Manganese, Molybdenum, Nickel, Silicon, Varadium and Zinc. Washington, DC: National Academy Press; 2001.
24. Institute of Medicine: Dietary Reference Intakes for Energy, Carbohydrate, Fiber, Fat, Fatty Acids, Cholesterol, Protein and Amino Acids. Food and Nutrition Board. Washington, DC: National Academy Press; 2002.
25. Institute of Medicine: Dietary Reference Intakes for Water, Potassium, Sodium, Chloride, and Sulfate. Food and Nutrition Board. Washington, DC: National Academy Press; 2004.

SELECTED REFERENCES FOR FURTHER READING

Charney P, Malone A: ADA Pocket Guide to Nutrition Assessment. Chicago: American Dietetic Association, 2004.
Pennington JA, Douglass JS: Bowe and Church's Food Values of Portions Commonly Used. Philadelphia: Lippincott Williams & Wilkins, 2004.

INTERNET RESOURCES

American Dietetic Association: http://www.eatright.org

Dietary Reference Intakes (DRI) and Recommended Dietary Allowances (RDA): http://www.nal.usda.gov/fnic/etext/000108.html and http://www.nal.usda.gov/fnic/etext/000108.html

Interactive Healthy Eating Index: http://www.forcevbc.com/good/food.htm

Nutrition and Your Health: Dietary Guidelines for Americans: : http://www.health.gov/dietaryguidelines

National Cancer Institute
htt://riskfactor.cancer.gov/DHQ/

The Influence of Emotional Distress on Chronic Illness

ROBERT SCALES, SIMON L. BACON, AND JAMES A. BLUMENTHAL

This chapter addresses KSAs from the following content areas:

1 Exercise Physiology and Related Exercise Science
2 Pathophysiology and Risk Factors
3 Health Appraisal, Fitness, and Clinical Exercise Testing
4 Electrocardiography and Diagnostic Techniques
5 Patient Management and Medications
6 Medical and Surgical Management
7 Exercise Prescription and Programming
8 Nutrition and Weight Management
9 Human Behavior and Counseling
10 Safety, Injury Prevention, and Emergency Procedures
11 Program Administration, Quality Assurance, and Outcome Assessment

Chronic diseases such as cardiovascular disease (CVD), cancer, chronic obstructive pulmonary disease (COPD), and diabetes account for more than 66% of deaths in the United States[1]. Consequently, the alleviation of chronic disease is a priority of the Year 2010 Health Objectives for the nation[2]. Chronic diseases typically progress through a series of stages characterized by increased morbidity and disability. Whereas the term *disease* is commonly used to describe pathological or physiological changes in the body, *illness* refers to the individual's ensuing adaptation to the disease. Physical limitations and emotional issues surrounding chronic illness can have a devastating effect on the patient's quality of life. The influence of emotional distress on chronic illness is often under recognized compared with other risk factors[3] despite a rapidly growing body of evidence showing a reciprocal relationship between psychosocial factors and chronic disease progression, in which emotional distress can be both a cause and consequence of chronic illness.

This chapter is directed to exercise specialists who may have a limited background in psychology and the mental health aspects of disease prevention. It is intended to serve as a quick reference guide for those who need relevant information for professional and public education. The chapter does not provide a comprehensive review of the psychosocial literature associated with chronic illness. Instead, it focuses on the major chronic illnesses that account for most of the morbidity and mortality in the United States adult population, including CVD, diabetes, COPD, asthma, cancer, HIV/AIDS, arthritis, and chronic pain.

The chapter reviews epidemiological and clinical research investigating the relationship between emotional distress and chronic illness. The evidence linking psychosocial factors to the onset and progression of chronic disease is examined. In addition to the three psychosocial domains identified in the Surgeon General's Report on Mental Health[4], **life stress**, **depression**, and **anxiety**, consideration is given to the role of low **social support** and **psychological states and traits** (e.g., **hostility**). The chapter also describes the impact of psychosocial and behavioral interventions on emotional distress. Particular attention is given to the role of cognitive behavioral therapy (CBT) because of its general application to numerous chronic conditions. This is a counseling method that is used by trained mental health specialists to change ineffective or unrealistic thought patterns and subsequently modify behavior. Consideration is also given to a style of communication called motivational interviewing, which has demonstrated success in the treatment of substance abuse and has more recently been adapted to improve a wide range of problem behaviors in medical settings[5,6]. Motivational interviewing is a patient-centered, directive method of communication that can be used by a wide variety of trained health care providers to enhance an individual's intrinsic motivation to change unhealthful behavior by exploring and resolving ambivalence[7]. Finally, the chapter briefly reviews the direct role exercise may have in the reduction of emotional distress.

KEY TERMS

Anxiety: A perception of fear or apprehension that is accompanied by a state of heightened physiological arousal that may include a surge in heart rate, sweating, and tensing of muscles

Depression: The presence of a depressed mood or a markedly decreased interest in all activities, persisting for at least 2 weeks and accompanied by at least four of the following additional symptoms: changes in appetite, sleep disturbance, fatigue, psychomotor retardation or agitation, feelings of guilt or worthlessness, difficulty concentrating, and suicidal thoughts

Hostility: An attitude of cynicism and mistrust that may provoke feelings of anger, irritation, and impatience

Life stress: A combination of negative physiological, cognitive, emotional, and behavioral responses that occur

in response to an individual's unique perception of life events

Psychological traits: Persistent and stable enduring attributes or predispositions of an individual (e.g. type A pattern, which may be characterized by an overcommitment to work or completing tasks, competitiveness, an exaggerated need to achieve, free-floating hostility and a propensity to become easily angered or annoyed)

Psychological states: Transient changes in mood that may reflect a person's circumstance at a particular point in time

Social support: An affiliation with social networks that provide emotional support and assistance with aspects of daily living

Chronic Disease and Illness

CARDIOVASCULAR DISEASE

Approximately 13 million Americans have coronary artery disease (CAD); 5 million have cerebrovascular disease, and 5 million have congestive heart failure[8]. Consequently, CVD is the most prevalent chronic illness in the United States[2]. In reviewing the literature, it is clear that there is more research investigating the relationship between psychosocial factors and CVD than any other chronic illness. Therefore, a large portion of this chapter focuses on the CVD literature.

Evidence indicates there is a relationship between chronic life stress at work and the development of CVD. Stressful life events include the breakup of intimate personal relationships, death of a family member or friend, economic hardship, role conflict, work overload, racism and discrimination, poor physical health, accidental injuries, and intentional assaults of physical safety[9–11]. Stressful life events may also reflect past events. Severe trauma in childhood, including sexual and physical abuse, may persist as stressors into adulthood or may make individuals more vulnerable to ongoing stress[12]. Each individual exhibits a unique response to stressful life events that includes some combination of physiological, cognitive, emotional, and behavioral characteristics that may be harmful to susceptible individuals.

In a meta-analysis of five different populations numbering over 12,000 individuals and covering an 18- to 30-year time period, work stress was associated with higher levels of cholesterol, systolic blood pressure (BP), and smoking behavior[13]. Monotonous work, high-paced

work, and job burnout have been correlated with an increased incidence of CAD[14]. High-demand jobs with low decision latitude have been associated with a fourfold increased risk of cardiovascular-related death[15]. Work stress associated with high demand and low reward has also resulted an increase in cardiac events[16–17] and the progression of carotid atherosclerosis[18]. Researchers have identified that in a working population compared with a nonworking population, there is 33% increase in relative risk of disease onset on Mondays[19]. In a more recent study involving a sample of 170,000 men and women, death from CVD was 20% above the daily average on Mondays for those younger than age 50 years[20]. In the 20-year follow-up of the Framingham Study, the incidence of angina was two times greater among those who exhibited higher levels of worry, dissatisfaction with work, feeling undue time pressure, and competitive drive[21]. Together, these studies indicate that there is strong association between this form of chronic stress and the development of CVD. Almost 4 decades ago, Holmes and Rahe[9] developed the Recent Life Change Questionnaire to assess the severity of typical stressful life events. Whereas the death of a spouse, divorce and loss of a job were considered high stress, vacations and holidays were given a lower weighting. A retrospective recall identified that elevated scores on the survey were associated with higher rates of myocardial infarction (MI) or sudden cardiac death at 6-month follow-up[19].

Acute stress has been implicated in the triggering of cardiovascular events. Epidemiological evidence has revealed that life-threatening situations such as earthquakes[23–26] and war[27–28] are associated with increased rates of MI and cardiac mortality. This observation does not appear to be limited to life-threatening situations. An increase in the rate of hospital admissions for MI and sudden cardiac death has been reported after important national soccer games[29,30]. In an examination of the acute effect of anger as a trigger of MI, retrospective interviews of 1623 post-MI patients identified a greater than twofold relative risk of MI after an episode of anger[32]. Cross-sectional studies have yielded evidence that acute negative emotional states, such as anger, anxiety, and frustration[33], are associated with myocardial ischemia. In a retrospective analysis, the MILIS study[31] found that 49% of patients identified a possible exogenous trigger for their MI, including emotional upsets. It has been hypothesized that acute psychological triggers increase sympathetic nervous system activation, which then leads to increases in heart rate and BP, greater endothelial injury, and heightened hemostatic and platelet activation[79].

Depression takes a monumental toll on human suffering, lost productivity, and death. Moreover, when unrecognized, depression can result in excessive health care utilization. Depression ranks among the top 10 causes of worldwide disability[34]. Major depression is the most well-known mood disorder, but there are others, including bipolar disorder (one or more episodes of mania) and dysthymia (a chronic but less severe form of major depression)[4]. Episodes of major depression are characterized by the presence of a depressed mood or a markedly decreased interest in all activities, persisting for at least 2 weeks and accompanied by at least four of the following additional symptoms: changes in appetite, sleep disturbance, fatigue, psychomotor retardation or agitation, feelings of guilt or worthlessness, problems concentrating, and suicidal thoughts. It is estimated that depression will rank as the second major cause of disability worldwide in the year 2020[35]. The causes of depression are not fully known. It may be triggered by stressful life events, enduring stressful social conditions (e.g., poverty and discrimination), neurochemical imbalance in the brain, maladaptive cognitions, or a combination of these factors. The 1-month community-based prevalence of major depression episodes is approximately 5%[36]. However, the prevalence is three times higher among CVD patients and the point prevalence of major depression in the general population is 6.6%[37]. Depression is twice as common in women as men. Depression tends to be underdiagnosed and treated in cardiac patients. Fewer than 25% of patients with major depression are recognized as being depressed by their cardiologists or general internists, and only about 50% of patients diagnosed as depressed receive treatment[38]. The reasons for this are not clear; it has been suggested that physicians may have difficulty differentiating between the symptoms of depression and those related to the disease[39]. Depression can reduce the sensitivity of standard tests for CVD. In a study of nearly 1400 patients undergoing standard SPECT exercise testing, depressed patients had a higher rate of false negative ECG ischemia compared to non-depressed patients[40]. Epidemiological evidence demonstrates a significant prospective relationship between the occurrence of depression, or depressive symptoms, and the incidence of future cardiac events among healthy[41,42] and CAD populations[43,45] in many, but not all, studies[46,47]. In a Finnish study of more than 95,000 individuals followed over 4–5 years, the highest risk of mortality occurred one month after bereavement, with more than a twofold risk for men and a threefold risk for women[48]. Hopelessness, which is a component of depression, has shown a particularly strong link with sudden death and the development of CAD[41] and carotid atherosclerosis[49].

Anxiety disorders are the most prevalent mental disorders in adults[50]. The anxiety disorders also affect twice as many women as men. These disorders include panic disorder, phobias, obsessive-compulsive disorder, posttraumatic stress disorder, and generalized anxiety disorder. Prevalence rates for all anxiety disorders in the general population are estimated to be 1% to 13%[51]. Underlying this heterogeneous group of disorders is a state of heightened arousal or fear in relation to stressful events or feelings. The biological manifestations of anxiety, which are grounded in the "fight-or-flight" response, are unmistakable: they include surge in heart rate, sweating, and tensing of muscles. The Harvard Mastery of Stress Study, one of the longest prospective studies ever conducted in this field, revealed that severe anxiety and conflict with hostility were significant predictors of CVD and risk of overall future illness[52].

Social support has been widely recognized as an independent predictor of health and well being in both general and clinical populations[53], especially among patients with cardiac disease. For example, low social support has been prospectively associated with poor clinical prognosis among patients with congestive heart failure[54] and stable CAD[55–58]. In addition, at least three relatively large-scale studies have found that low levels of support predicted an increased risk of mortality after an acute MI[59–61]. In two large studies involving CAD patients, those at higher risk had significantly more socioeconomic difficulties while simultaneously lacking social support or social connections to deal with stress[62,63].

There are two broad categories of social support *Structural support* refers to social networks and includes such indices as marital status, number of friends, and participation in church or civic organizations. *Functional support* refers to the perception of support and includes such elements as instrumental support (e.g., having someone that can assist in activities of daily living) and emotional support (e.g., having someone to talk to and whom you believe loves or cares for you)[53].

Studies on animals[64] and humans[65–71] have identified that psychological stress has an adverse impact on the cardiovascular system. The mechanism by which stress may influence atherogenesis involves a complex interaction of sympathetic arousal, hypothalamic stimulation, and adrenergic and neurohormonal responses that lead to increased BP, increased circulating catecholamine levels, and increased platelet activity[72–74]. The resulting increased shearing forces of blood on the arterial wall lead to endothelial injury and arterial wall damage. Thus, chronic exposure to psychological stress promotes the development of atherosclerosis that may result in vasospasm[75], myocardial ischemia[76], coronary artery occlusion, MI, and increased incidence of ventricular arrhythmia, a known risk factor for sudden coronary death[77]. These pathophysiological mechanisms have been schematized by Rozanski et al.[78] in Figure 11-1.

Although conclusions regarding the mechanisms by which more chronic psychosocial factors contribute to cardiac events are not definitive, considerable evidence points to several mechanisms likely to be involved in the impact of depression on the prognosis of patients with established CVD. For example, it has been shown that depressed patients exhibit increased sympathetic nervous system outflow and decreased parasympathetic function[79]. This can lead to ventricular arrhythmias, platelet activation and aggregation, and increased myocardial oxygen consumption. It is plausible that these kinds of reactions could contribute to the pathophysiologic processes involved in the development of both CAD and MI.

Increased activation of the pituitary adrenal axis in depressed patients has also been shown to produce high levels of cortisol[80], which can potentiate and prolong the effects of catecholamines[78].

Depression has been shown to be a predictor of poor adherence to a wide variety of medical treatments[81]. An electronic medication-monitoring device has demonstrated that elderly patients with major depression are less adherent to taking their medications than are nondepressed patients[82]. In patients recovering from MI, there is evidence that depression is associated with poor adherence to cardiac rehabilitation and risk factor modification[83]. Consequently, depression may indirectly promote the progression of chronic illness by preventing adherence to other treatment regimens such as healthy eating, physical activity and exercise, taking medications appropriately, abstaining from smoking, managing stress, and moderating alcohol consumption.

Psychosocial and Behavioral Interventions

Psychosocial and behavioral intervention trials in patients with CVD have reported mixed success. In a study of 107 cardiac patients with exercise-induced ischemia, a CBT-based approach to stress management was associated with improved psychosocial measures, a reduction in mental stress induced ischemia[84] and fewer clinical events after a 5-year follow-up when compared with exercise therapy

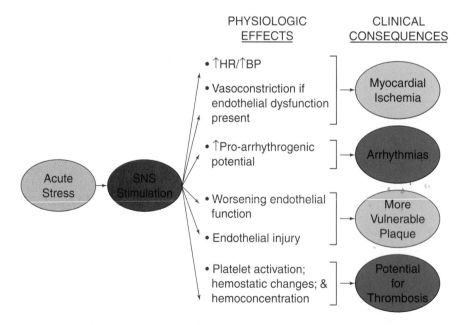

FIGURE 11-1. Pathophysiological effects of acute psychosocial stress. Sympathetic nervous system (SNS) stimulation emanating from acute stress leads to a variety of effects, ranging from heart rate (HR) and blood pressure (BP) stimulation to direct effects on coronary vascular endothelium. Clinical consequences of these effects include myocardial ischemia, cardiac arrhythmias, and fostering of more vulnerable coronary plaques and hemostatic changes. These changes form a substrate for development of acute myocardial infarction and sudden cardiac death. (Adapted with permission from Rozanski A, Blumenthal JA, Kaplan J: Impact of psychological factors on the pathogenesis of cardiovascular disease and implications for therapy. Circulation 99:2192–2217, 1999.)

alone or usual care[85]. In a review of other studies involving similar populations, CBT interventions have been reported to improve quality of life and reduce mortality in cardiac patients[86]. However, the ENRICHD Trial, a multicenter trial involving 2481 post-MI patients with depression or low social support, CBT reduced depression levels but failed to yield a significant reduction in all-cause mortality and cardiac morbidity[87]. Other trials[88,89] have also reported negative findings, and the failure of these brief interventions to alter psychosocial risk factors such as anxiety and depression may have been responsible for the lack of effect on "hard" clinical endpoints such as mortality and morbidity.

The role of exercise as a standalone intervention in the prevention and management of CVD is well documented[90,91]. However, it should be recognized that there is uncertainty about the extent to which clinical outcomes may have been directly or indirectly impacted by improved psychosocial status as a result of exercise. Regardless, it is safe to conclude that exercise therapy added to a multi-intervention approach that includes behavioral cardiac risk modification, education, and counseling may enhance the improvements in CVD outcomes reported in exercise only interventions[91]. This is exemplified by the Lifestyle Heart Trial, which demonstrated that an intervention comprised of exercise therapy, group support meetings, education and skills training in a low-fat diet, and daily stress management (i.e., yoga-derived stretching, breathing, meditation, imagery, and relaxation techniques) could assist a highly motivated group of cardiac patients to make comprehensive changes in lifestyle. Arteriographic data identified an average arterial stenosis regression from 40% to 37.8% in the intervention group compared with a progression from 42.7% to 46.1% in a usual care group at a 1-year follow-up[92]. A 5-year follow-up showed continued progression in the control group and regression in the intensive lifestyle intervention group[93]. Motivating CAD patients to adopt and maintain comprehensive changes in lifestyle is a challenge that faces health care professionals, and motivational interviewing is an innovative approach that has demonstrated efficacy in brief consultations. Scales et al.[94] found that compared with traditional cardiac rehabilitation, adding motivational interviewing coupled with brief skills-building sessions significantly lowers stress and enhances multiple health-related behaviors in CAD patients.

DIABETES

Diabetes is a chronic disease caused by insulin deficiency, or resistance to insulin action, or both. In the United States, approximately 800,000 people are newly diagnosed each year[95]. Diabetes is the leading cause of nontraumatic amputations (~157,000/year), blindness among working-age adults (~20,000/year), and end-stage kidney disease (~30,000/year)[96]. Stress, depression, and anxiety are more prevalent among diabetics than the general population[97–99].

Evidence suggests that stress may precipitate the onset of diabetes or compromise glucose control after the disease is established[99]. Glucose toxicity that results from chronic, intermittent, stress-induced elevations in blood glucose further compromise pancreatic secretary ability[100], leading to the progression of the disease. However, evidence characterizing the effects of stress in type I diabetes is inconsistent. Human studies have shown that stress can stimulate hyperglycemia or hypoglycemia, or have no effect at all on glycemic status in established diabetes. More consistent evidence supports the role of stress in type II diabetes. Animal and human studies suggest that individuals with type II diabetes have altered adrenergic sensitivity in the pancreas, which could make them particularly sensitive to stressful life events. However, although substantial data links stress to the expression or control of type II diabetes[101], further evidence is needed. Moreover, few studies have followed patients long enough to determine the long-term consequences of stress in diabetic patients.

Psychosocial and Behavioral Interventions

The few studies involving psychosocial and behavioral interventions in diabetic patients have involved CBT, coping skills, empowerment, and diabetes management training. These approaches have been found to decrease diabetes-related anxiety and avoidance behaviors; enhance quality of life, coping ability, and emotional well being; and, most importantly, improve self-care and glycemic control[101].

The Diabetes Prevention Program (DPP) Research Group[102] demonstrated the strong effect that physical activity and weight loss can exert in preventing the onset of diabetes in high-risk adults. Compared with usual care, there was a 58% reduction in the onset of diabetes over a period of approximately 3 years among individuals who were supported in their efforts to follow a healthful lifestyle. Although the intervention did not directly target stress management, these individuals received regular weekly support from a case manager and additional meetings with an exercise specialist, dietitian, and behavioral counselor. An intervention involving medication alone reduced the incidence of new cases by 31%. Therefore, individual or group support from a healthcare provider may help control the development of diabetes.

CHRONIC OBSTRUCTIVE PULMONARY DISEASE

Chronic obstructive pulmonary disease is characterized by the presence of airflow obstruction due to chronic bronchitis and emphysema; two diseases that can often coexist[2]. It is estimated that more than 16 million Americans have symptomatic COPD[1]. Chronic lower respiratory diseases rank as the fourth leading cause of death in the United States[103] and is the only major disease condition in the top 10 that is continuing to increase in prevalence[104].

Common psychological reactions among patients with COPD include anger, frustration, guilt, dependency, and embarrassment[105,106]. However, the most frequently observed psychological symptoms among patients with COPD are depression and anxiety. Studies have reported the prevalence of depression to be anywhere from 26% to 74%[106–108]. Anxiety is another common psychological consequence of COPD. Up to 37% of COPD patients may experience one or more panic attacks, which include bouts of intense anxiety, physiological arousal, temporary cognitive impairment, and a desire to flee the situation[109]. Dyspnea in conjunction with fear of suffocation and death is a source of significant anxiety in this population[106]. The emotional arousal of anxiety then increases ventilatory demands on the body, which may lead to hypoxia or hypercapnia. Increased physiological arousal, in turn, exacerbates anxiety symptoms, which then produce greater insufficiency, resulting in a circular pattern that is difficult to break[4]. The medical regimen of COPD patients is often complex, with an average of six medications per patient[101]. Consequently, nonadherence is high, with about 50% of the patients either over- or underutilizing their medications[110–111].

Psychosocial and Behavioral Interventions

Treatment studies involving COPD patients have shown that psychosocial intervention combined with exercise therapy improves mood, anxiety, and neurocognitive functioning[112]. Psychological interventions on their own have been shown to reduce breathlessness and general disability and improve quality of life[113]. In comparison, exercise-based interventions have tended to show additional benefits[114], with relief of dyspnea and improved functioning and control of the disease[115]. However, these studies have been limited with small sample sizes, and as such, large scale clinical trials are required before definitive conclusions can be drawn.

ASTHMA

Asthma is a lung disease with recurrent exacerbations of airflow constriction, mucous secretion, and chronic inflammation of the airways, resulting in reduced airflow that causes symptoms of wheezing, coughing, chest tightness, and difficulty breathing. An estimated 15 million Americans have asthma, with an 82% increase in the rate over the past 15 years. More than 500,000 hospitalizations, 5000 deaths, and more than 133 million days of restricted activity are caused by asthma each year[2].

Research has demonstrated an association between emotional stress and various indices of impaired airway function, including increased breathlessness (dyspnea) and bronchoconstriction[116]. As with COPD patients, anxiety is common in asthma patients, with panic disorder being particularly prevalent[117]. Anxiety appears to be related to excessive use of bronchodilators, greater prescriptions for corticosteroid medication, more frequent hospital readmissions, and more lengthy hospitalizations, independent of pulmonary impairment[118]. Autonomic dysfunction, irregular immune response, deleterious breathing patterns, and inappropriate symptom identification have all been proposed as mechanisms linking negative emotion and asthma, suggesting that the relationship is multifactorial[119].

Psychosocial and Behavioral Interventions

A limited number of psychological intervention studies have been done with asthma patients. Therapies such as training in CBT, stress management, yoga, biofeedback, and symptom perception have been show to reduce measures of asthma morbidity and improve patient quality of life[120]. In addition, because of its complex medication regimen, adherence has been one of the main foci of behavioral interventions[117]. The primary intervention used is asthma education and management, which has been shown to improve measures such as frequency of asthma attacks and symptoms, medication adherence, and self-management skills[117]. Although it is still unclear if exercise interventions in asthmatics improve pulmonary function and bronchial responsiveness, there is very good evidence that exercise training improves quality of life[121].

CANCER

Cancer is the second leading cause of death in the United States. Approximately 1.25 million Americans are newly diagnosed each year. The four major cancer sites—lung, female breast, prostrate, and colon—account for about 54% of these new diagnoses[122]. Some researchers believe that stressful life events[123–125] and chronic depression[126] are associated with the onset of cancer.

Ample evidence from human and animal studies demonstrates the downward modulation of immune function concomitant with a variety of stressors[127]. Depression has also been demonstrated to cause immune suppression by increasing the synthesis and release of adrenal corticosteroids[128] and by decreasing lymphocyte proliferation and natural killer cell activity[129,130]. It is estimated that 20% to 25% of cancer patients suffer often unrecognized and untreated long-term depression[131]. However, the evidence of an association between depression and cancer occurrence from prospective cohort studies is inconclusive[132], with findings of both a lack of association[133–135] and a weak positive relationship[136,137]. Therefore, better systematically designed research is needed to further elucidate the impact of psychological factors on cancer.

Psychosocial and Behavioral Interventions

Various psychosocial intervention trials, including CBT, relaxation training, and coping skills training in cancer patients have found reductions in anxiety and depression, with improvements in mood and quality of life[138]. In a landmark study, Spiegel et al. found that a yearlong CBT-based intervention decreased the death rate in women with breast cancer[139]. However, a more recent study involving a larger sample size and a comparable psychosocial group therapy intervention did not show prolonged survival in this population[140]. Currently, we know of no studies that have assessed the benefits of a joint psychosocial and exercise intervention. However, exercise-only interventions have been found to have short-term benefits, with reductions in psychological distress (e.g., anxiety and anger), as well as improvements in clinical measures (e.g., immune markers, infection rates, and reductions in hospitalization)[138].

HIV/AIDS

Approximately 712,000 Americans have been diagnosed with AIDS since the first reported case 20 years ago, with at least 40,000 continuing to contract the HIV infection each year[141]. The annual death rate from AIDS has declined within the United States since the introduction of highly active antiretroviral therapies in 1996[141]. However, this type of therapy remains expensive, and varying degrees of success have been reported[142]. It is suspected that chronic stress coupled with dysfunctional coping may explain the variability in survival[143].

The lifetime prevalence of depression in HIV patients has been estimated to be 22% to 52%[144–145]. In addition, HIV-infected persons have higher rates of stressful life events, such as abuse and bereavement, independent of their disease[143]. The Coping in Health and Illness Project found that in symptom-free HIV-positive men, prior stressful life events predicted worsening HIV disease stage at follow-up[146] and faster progression to AIDS[147]. In addition, increased levels of depressive symptoms has been associated with a higher 7-year mortality in HIV-positive men[145]. Although the potential immune mechanisms through which negative mood and stressful life events accelerates HIV remain to be fully understood, cortisol has been suggested as the most likely intermediary link. Stimulation of HIV viral replication, modifications in programmed cell death, and altered patterns of cytokine secretion have all been proposed as cortisol-driven mechanisms for deterioration in HIV-positive individuals[143].

Psychosocial and Behavioral Interventions

Much of the original work in this area focused on prevention in at-risk populations. Psychological, social, and situational factors associated with patterns of high-risk sexual or drug-use behavior were the basis for these original interventions[148]. More recently, interventions have been developed to improve emotional and immunological aspects of the disease in diagnosed individuals. A reduction in dysphoric mood[149], perceived stress, and improved coping in HIV-positive patients has been demonstrated with CBT[148]. Although there are no data on the effects of behavioral interventions on mortality in HIV patients, a variety of CBT interventions has been shown to increase CD4 and NK cell counts and decrease cortisol levels[143].

Although these results are promising, there is still a dearth of psychological and behavioral clinical trials. Most of the few studies of exercise interventions in HIV/AIDS patients have suffered from small sample sizes and high dropout rates[150]. However, beneficial effects of exercise in these patients include improved psychological state[151]. These improvements are found without any adverse effects on the patients' disease status.

ARTHRITIS

Arthritis is a chronic, systemic, autoimmune disorder with no known cause that is characterized by painful swelling and stiffness of joints. It is estimated that 37 million Americans have arthritis[152]. Approximately half of this population are older than age 70 years and suffer from osteoarthritis (OA). The overall prevalence of rheumatoid arthritis (RA) is approximately 1% in the total United States population. The prevalence of RA increases with age, and in those older than age 65 years, it may be as high as 5% to 7%. The severity of joint problems tends to fluctuate over time, with periods of mild activity punctuated by more intense flare-ups. For two thirds of affected patients, the overall course of the disease is one of progressive deformity and destruction of joints, accompanied by increasing disability[153]. RA is more common in women than in men, with a ratio of about 2.5 to 1.0[154]. The debilitating nature of this disorder, with its associated pain, can interfere with the patient's life in a number of ways. As arthritis progresses, patients may no longer be able to participate in recreational activities and may find their social lives curtailed. Not surprisingly, it has been found that arthritis has a negative impact on quality of life and satisfaction with life[155].

Studies to date have shown that arthritis can have a negative impact on patients' mental health[156,157]. Frank et al.[156] estimated that the prevalence of major depression and dysthymia in RA patients was around 18% and 41%, respectively, which is higher than that found in a general population. Depression in OA patients is not as high as that in RA patients, but is still higher than expected and has been estimated to be 10%[159]. Reviews of the literature indicate that methodological flaws in the research have weakened any evidence linking the various psychological factors with the cause of the disease[156,160–161]. However, in one study, which attempted to better understand the pathogenic mechanisms associated with the disease, Hendrie et al.[162] investigated the relationship between psychological stress, depressed immune system activity, and the initial manifestation of arthritic symptoms. These investigators compared immunoglobulin levels and life change scores in polyarthritis patients with a history of joint disease of less than 6 months' duration. Polyarthritis patients whose immunoglobin levels were elevated produced a mean life change score for the year preceding initial symptom manifestation that was almost three times greater than that of their counterparts without elevated immunoglobulin levels.

Other researchers have suggested that psychosocial factors could have a negative impact on compliance with the treatment of arthritis and consequently have an indirect link with the progression of the disease. Estimates of nonadherence with medication in RA patients have ranged from 22%[163] to 67%[164]. Patients with more severe arthritic disease or longer duration of illness may be more likely to be nonadherent than those with relatively mild or recent disease[165].

Psychosocial and Behavioral Interventions

Arthritis has been treated with CBT since the 1980s. Originally, these treatments focused on RA and were designed to help patients manage pain. However, more recent approaches have also targeted psychological disturbance, interpersonal distress, and physical function[166]. Psychological interventions for OA were not conducted until the early 1990s and have been effective in reducing pain and decreased psychological morbidity[167]. This includes an improvement in the severity and frequency of swollen joints, both in the short and long term, as well as reduced pain and increased self-efficacy during follow-up[166]. Evidence suggests that psychological interventions may reduce neuroendocrine and immune system markers in RA patients[168]. It has also been suggested that psychological treatments may provide significant cost savings (i.e., reduced medical resource use[169]), although more work is needed to support this claim. Exercise interventions in both RA[165] and OA[170] patients improves quality of life, as well as aerobic capacity, muscular strength, and joint mobility, with seemingly no adverse effect on pain and disease progression.

CHRONIC PAIN

Chronic pain is a demoralizing situation that confronts individual sufferers, not only with stress created by pain but also with many other continuing stressors that compromise all aspects of the patient's life. Living with chronic pain requires considerable emotional resilience and tends to deplete the individual's emotional reserves[171]. Gatchel[172] describes chronic pain as a complex psychophysiological behavior pattern that cannot be broken down into distinct psychosocial and physical components. Instead, pain includes elements of both components. Furthermore, as pain becomes more chronic, the psychosocial factors play an increasingly dominant role in the maintenance of pain behavior and suffering.

Although a relationship is usually found between pain and certain psychological problems such as depression[173], the nature of the relationship between the two variables remains inconclusive. Some, but not all, patients develop depression secondary to chronic pain. Others show depression as the primary syndrome, of which pain is a symptom. Moreover, factors that mediate the relationship between depression and pain remain largely unknown[174].

In a study initially evaluating one aspect of this "chicken-or-egg" question, Polatino et al.[175] assessed 200 patients with chronic low back pain (pain disability present for an average of well over 1 year) for current lifetime psychiatric syndromes. Results revealed that 77% of patients met lifetime diagnostic criteria and 59% demonstrated current symptoms for at least one psychiatric diagnosis. The most common of these were major depressive disorder, anxiety disorders, and substance abuse. All of these prevalence rates were significantly higher than in the general population. In patients with a lifetime history of psychiatric syndromes, 54% of those with depression, 95% of those with anxiety disorders, and 94% of those with a substance abuse had experienced these syndromes before the onset of their back pain. These are the first results to suggest that certain psychiatric syndromes appear to precede chronic low back pain. It appears that a prospective study is needed to substantiate these retrospective-recall results more clearly because the findings cannot definitively answer the question of whether psychopathological disorders in chronic pain patients are consequences of experiencing the chronic pain or whether preexisting disorders act as predispositions for pain to become chronic.

Psychosocial and Behavioral Interventions

A variety of psychological interventions have been used to help treat the various site specific pain disorders. This includes reported improvement in the treatment of lower back pain, noncardiac chest pain, arthritis, headaches, temporomandibular disorder, and whiplash-associated disorder. Additionally, CBT appears to inhibit the development of chronic disability in pain patients[176]. Psychosocial interventions have been found to be most effective when combined with other treatments. For example, the additions of physical therapy and education to CBT was found to reduce health care utilization and medication usage compared with no or mono intervention[177]. It has also been estimated that these kind of multifaceted interventions are nearly 21 times more cost effective than alternatives such as surgery[176].

Exercise Therapy to Reduce Emotional Distress

The association between regular exercise and mood has been recognized since the late 1970s; however, the role of exercise as a clinical treatment for psychiatric disorders has only been explored recently[178]. One of the original long-term prospective studies, the Alameda County Study[179], found that compared with individuals who were active at baseline, inactive participants were at a greater risk of high depression scores 9 years later. In addition, participants who increased their exercise levels across the first 9 years of the study were at no greater risk for depression after 18 years than those who exercised throughout the study. However, those who became inactive after the first 9 years were more likely to become depressed after 18 years relative to active participants. A recent meta-analysis of clinical trials[180] found that compared with no treatment, exercise reduced depression and was equally as effective as cognitive therapy. Also, evidence from cross-sectional and prospective studies suggests a dose–response effect of physical activity on depressive and anxiety disorders, although this relationship has not yet been found in clinical trials[181]. Exercise has been shown to improve stress management ability, general feelings of well being, self-esteem[182], and muscular tension[183]. Clinically, exercise training potentially offers a vehicle for nonspecific psychological therapy. It also offers a specific psychological treatment that may be particularly effective for patients for whom more conventional psychological interventions are less acceptable[184].

A variety of mechanisms has been suggested for the therapeutic effects of exercise; including alterations in the central monoamine systems, improved regulation of the hypothalamic-pituitary-adrenal axis, and increased β-endorphin levels. However, to date, there are no known studies that have directly assessed the mechanisms behind the exercise–mood relationship[178]. Exercise training has also been shown to attenuate the cardiovascular response to emotional stressors[185–188]. This includes a decreased β-adrenergic myocardial response to physical or behavioral challenges and an acute prophylactic effect in reducing BP response to psychological stressors[188,189]. Additionally, there may be indirect effects of exercise on emotional distress. For example, the addition of diagnostic exercise testing can reassure anxious patients of safety and improve self-confidence[190]. In summary, although good evidence suggests that increased physical activity and exercise training improve psychological distress, more high-quality studies are needed to identify if there is a dose–response relationship and to identify the mechanisms by which exercise exerts its antidepressant and anxiolytic effects.

Summary

Psychosocial factors such as depression, anxiety, and low perceived social support are common among patients living with chronic illness and appear to be both a cause and a consequence of a number of chronic medical conditions. However, future prospective studies that include valid measures to assess psychosocial factors and clinical outcomes associated with chronic illness are needed to further our understanding in this field of research.

Most people with psychosocial risk factors do not present themselves to mental health services for treatment. Therefore, systems need to be established to help non–mental health professionals, such as exercise specialists, to find ways to screen for emotional distress and recognize potential symptoms. Consideration should also be given to developing improved liaison relationships with psychological or behavioral specialists to facilitate more specialized interventions when appropriate. Individual or group CBT-based interventions have shown to be particularly effective in this regard. In addition, non–mental health specialists need to be encouraged and supported to develop skills that will enable them to better promote healthful behavior and emotional functioning in the overall treatment of individuals with chronic illness. For example, motivational interviewing is one of several useful approaches that can be used by exercise professionals to meet this challenge.

REFERENCES

1. National Center for National Health Statistics: United States, 2002 National Vital Statistics Report 53(No. 17) p. 9, 2005.
2. U.S. Department of Health and Human Services Office of Public Health and Science: Healthy People 2010 Objectives: Draft for public comment. U.S. Department of Health and Human Services Office of Public Health and Science, Washington, DC; 1998.
3. McKenna MT, Taylor WR, Marks JS, Koplan JP: Current issues and challenges in chronic disease control (pp. 1–26). In Brownson RC, Remington PL, Davis JR, eds. Chronic Disease Epidemiology and Control. Washington, DC: American Public Health Association; 1998.
4. U.S. Department of Health and Human Services: Mental Health: A Report of the Surgeon General. Rockville, MD: U.S. Department of Health and Human Services, Substance Abuse and Mental Health Services Administration, Center for Mental Health Services, National Institute for Mental Health, National Institute of Mental Health; 1999.
5. Dunn C, DeRoo L, Rivara, FP: The use of brief interventions adapted from motivational interviewing across behavioral domains: A systematic review. Addiction 96:1725–1742, 2001.
6. Burke, BL, Arkowitz H, Dunn C: The effectiveness of motivational interviewing and its adaptations: What we know so far (pp. 217–250). In Miller WR, Rollnick S, eds. Motivational Interviewing: Preparing People to Change Addictive Behavior, 2nd ed. New York: Guilford Press; 2002.
7. Miller WR, Rollnick S: Motivational Interviewing: Preparing People for Change, 2nd ed, New York: Guilford Press; 2002.
8. American Heart Association: Heart disease and stroke statistics–2005 update. Dallas: American Heart Association, 2005.
9. Holmes T, Rahe R: The social readjustment rating scale. J Psychosomat Res 11:213–218, 1967.
10. Krieger N, Rowley DL, Herman AA, et al: Racism, sexism, and social class: Implications for studies of health, disease, and well-being. Am J Prevent Med 9(suppl):82–122, 1993.
11. Lazarus RS, Folkman S: Stress, Appraisal and Coping. New York: Springer; 1984.
12. Browne A, Finkelhor D: Impact of child sexual abuse: A review of the research. Psychol Bull 99:66–77, 1986.
13. Pieper C, LaCroix A, Karasek R: The relationship of psychosocial dimensions on work with coronary heart disease. Am J Epidemiol 129:483–494.

14. Appels A, Schouten E: Burnout as a risk factor for coronary heart disease. Behav Med 17:53–59, 1991.

15. Karasek RA, Baker D, Marxer F, et al: Job decision latitude, job demands, and cardiovascular disease: A prospective study of Swedish men. Am J Publ Health 71:694–705, 1981.

16. Bosma H, Peter R, Siegrist J, Marmot M: Two alternative job stress models and the risk of coronary heart disease. Am J Publ Health 88:68–74, 1998.

17. Siegrist J, Peter R, Junge A, et al: Low status control, high effort at work and ischemic heart disease: Prospective evidence from blue-collar men. Soc Sci Med 331:1127–1134, 1990.

18. Lynch JJ, Krause N, Kaplan GA, Salonen R, Salonen JT: Work place demands, economic reward, and progression of carotid athersosclerosis. Circulation 96:302–307, 1997.

19. Willich S, Hannelore L, Lewis M, et al: Weekly variation of acute myocardial infarction. Circulation 90:87–93, 1994.

20. Evans C, Chalmers J, Capewell S, et al: "I don't like Mondays"—day of the week of coronary heart disease death in Scotland: Study of routine collected data. BMJ 320:218–219, 2000.

21. Eaker ED, Abbott RD, de Knell WB: Frequency of uncomplicated angina pectoris in Type A compared with Type B persons (the Framingham Study). Am J Cardiol 63:1042–1045, 1989.

22. Rahe RH, Romo M, Bennett L, Siltanen P: Recent life changes, myocardial infarction, and abrupt coronary death. Arch Intern Med 133:221–228, 1974.

23. Trichopoulus D, Katsouyanni K, Zavitsanos X, et al: Psychological stress and fatal heart attack: The Athens 1981 earthquake natural experiment. Lancet I:441–444, 1983.

24. Lear J, Kloner RA: The Northridge earthquake as a trigger for acute myocardial infarction. Am J Cardiol 77:1230–1232, 1996.

25. Katsouyanni K, Kogevinas M, Trichopoulos D: Earthquake related stress and cardiac mortality. In J Epidemiol 15:326–330, 1986.

26. Suzuki S, Sakamoto S, Miki S, Matsuo T: Hanshin-Awaji earthquake and acute myocardial infarction. Lancet 345:981, 1995.

27. Meisel SR, Kutz I, Dayan KI, et al: Effect of Iraq missile war on incidence of acute myocardial infarction and sudden death in Israeli civilians. Lancet 338:660–661, 1991.

28. Bergovec M, Mihatov S, Prpic H, et al: Acute myocardial infarction among civilians in the Zagreb city area. Lancet 339:303, 1992.

29. Carroll D, Ebrahim S, Tiling K, et al: Admissions for myocardial infarction at World Cup football: Database survey. BMJ 325:21–28, 2002.

30. Witte DR, Bots MI, Hoes AW, Grobbee DE: Cardiovascular mortality in Dutch men during the 1996 European football championship: Longitudinal population study. BMJ 321:1332–1334, 2000.

31. Tofler GH, Stone PH, MacLure M, et al: Analysis of possible triggers of acute myocardial infarction (The MILIS Study). Am J Cardiol 66:22–27, 1990.

32. Mittleman MA, MacLure M, Sherwood JB, et al. for the Determinants of Myocardial Infarction Onset Study Investigators: Triggering of acute myocardial infarction onset by episodes of anger. Circulation 92:1720–1725, 1995.

33. Gullette EC, Blumenthal JA, Babyak M, et al: Effects of mental stress on myocardial ischemia during daily life. JAMA 277:1521–1526, 1997.

34. Murray CJL, Lopez AD: Evidence-based health policy: Lessons from the Global Burden of Disease Study. Science 274:740–743, 1996.

35. Murray CJL, Lopez AD: Alternative projections of mortality and disability by cause 1990–2020: Global Burden of Disease Study. Lancet 349:1498–1504, 1997.

36. Blazer DG, Kessler RC, McGonagle KA, Swartz MS: The prevalence and distribution of major depression in a national community sample: The national co-morbidity survey. Am J Psychiatr 151:979–986. 1994.

37. Kessler RC, Berglund P, Demler O, et al: The epidemiology of major depressive disorder. Results from the National Comorbidity Survey Replication (NCS-R). JAMA 289:3095–3105, 2003.

38. Mayou R, Foster A, Williamson B: Medical care after myocardial infarction. J Psychosomat Res 23:23–26, 1979.

39. Clarke DM: Psychological factors in illness and recovery. N Z Med J 111:410–412, 1998.

40. Lavoie KL, Fleet PP, Lesperance F, et al: Are exercise stress tests appropriate for assessing myocardial eschemia in patients with major depressive disorder? Am Heart J 148:621–627, 2004.

41. Anda R, Williamson D, Jones D, et al: Depressed affect, hopelessness, and risk of ischemic heart disease in a cohort of U.S. adults. Epidemiology 4:285–294, 1993.

42. Barefoot JC, Schroll M: Symptoms of depression, acute myocardial infarction, and total mortality in a community sample. Circulation 93:1976–1980, 1996.

43. Barefoot JC, Helms MJ, Mark DB: Depression and long-term mortality risk in patients with coronary artery disease. Am J Cardiol 78:613–717, 1996.

44. Frasure-Smith N, Lesperance F, Talajic M: Depression and 18-month prognosis after myocardial infarction. Circulation 91:999–1005, 1995.

45. Frasure-Smith N, Lesperance F, Junea M, et al: Gender, depression, and one-year prognosis after myocardial infarction. Psychosomat Med 61:26–37, 1999.

46. Lane D, Carroll D, Ring C, et al: In-hospital symptoms of depression do not predict mortality 3 years after myocardial infarction. Int J Epidemiol 31:1179–1182, 2002.

47. Mayou R, Gill D, Thompson DR, et al: Depression and anxiety as predictors of outcome after myocardial infarction. Psychosomat Med 62:212–219, 2000.

48. Kaprio J, Koskenvuo M, Rita H: Mortality after bereavement: A prospective study of 95,647 persons. Am J Publ Health 77:283–287, 1987.

49. Everson SA, Kaplan GA, Goldberg, DE: Hopelessness and 4-year progression of carotid atherosclerosis: The Kuopio ischemic heart disease risk factor study. Arteriosclerosis and Thrombolytic Vascular Biology 17:1490–1495, 1997.

50. Regier DA, Farmer ME, Rae DS, et al: Comorbidity of mental disorders with alcohol and other drug abuse. Results from the Epidemiologic Catchment Area (ECA) Study. JAMA 264:2511–2518, 1990.

51. American Psychiatric Association: Diagnostic and Statistical Manual of Mental Disorders, 4th ed. Washington, DC: American Psychiatric Association; 1994.

52. Russek LG, King SH, Russek SJ, Russek HI: The Harvard Mastery of Stress Study—35 year follow-up: Prognostic significance of patterns of psychophysiological arousal and adaptation. Psychiatr Med 52:271–285, 1990.

53. Uchino BN, Cacioppo JT, Kiecolt-Glaser JK: The relationship between social support and physiological processes: A review with emphasis on underlying mechanisms and implications for health. Psychol Bull 119:488–531, 1996.

54. Murberg TA, Bru E: Social relationships and mortality in patients with congestive heart failure. J Psychosomat Res 51:521–527, 2001.

55. Brummett BH, Barefoot JC, Siegler IC, et al: Characteristics of socially isolated patients with coronary artery disease who are at elevated risk for mortality. Psychosomat Med 63:267–272, 2001.

56. Horsten M, Mittleman MA, Wamala SP, et al: Depressive symptoms and lack of social integration in relation to prognosis of CHD in middle-aged women. The Stockholm Female Coronary Risk Study. Eur Heart J 21:1072–1080, 2000.

57. Williams RB, Barefoot JC, Califf RM, et al: Prognostic importance of social and economic resources among medically treated patients with angiographically documented coronary artery disease. JAMA 267:520–524, 1992.

58. Orth-Gomer K, Unden AL, Edwards ME: Social isolation and mortality in ischemic heart disease. A 10-year follow-up study of 150 middle-aged men. Acta Medica Scandinavica 224:205–215, 1988.

59. Berkman LF, Leo-Summers L, Horwitz RI: Emotional support and survival after myocardial infarction. A prospective, population-based study of the elderly. Ann Intern Med 117:1003–1009, 1992.

60. Welin C, Lappas G, Wilhelmsen L: Independent importance of psychosocial factors for prognosis after myocardial infarction. J Intern Med 247: 629–639, 2000.

61. Gorkin L, Schron EB, Brooks MM, et al: Psychosocial predictors of mortality in the Cardiac Arrhythmia Suppression Trial-1 (CAST-1). Am J Cardiol 71:263–267, 1993.

62. Kaplan, GA, Salonsen JT, Cohen RD, et al: Social connections and mortality from all causes and from cardiovascular disease: Prospective evidence from eastern Finland. Am J Epidemiol 128:370–380, 1988.

63. Williams RB, Barefoot JC, Califf RM, et al: Prognostic importance of social and economic resources among medically treated patients with angiographically documented coronary artery disease. JAMA 267: 520–524, 1992.

64. Kaplan JR, Manuck SB, Clarkson TB, et al: Social status, environment and atherosclerosis in cynomolgus monkeys. Arteriosclerosis 2:359–368, 1982.

65. Blazer DG: Social support and mortality in an elderly community program. Am J Epidemiol 115: 684–694, 1984.

66. Deanfield JE, Shea M, Kensett M, et al: Silent myocardial ischemia due to mental stress. Lancet 2:1001–1005, 1984.

67. Jiang W, Babyak M, Krantz, DS, et al: Mental stress-induced myocardial ischemia and cardiac events. JAMA 25:1651–1656, 1996.

68. Krantz, DS, Helmers KF, Bairey NC, et al: Cardiovascular reactivity and mental stress-induced myocardial ischemia in patients with coronary artery disease. Psychosomat Med 53:1–12, 1991.

69. Orth-Gomer K, Johnson JV: Social isolation and mortality: A six-year follow-up study of a random sample of the Swedish population. J Chron Dis 40:949–957, 1987.

70. Rozanski A, Bairey N, Krantz, DS, et al: Mental stress and the induction of silent myocardial ischemia in patients with coronary artery disease. N Engl J Med 318:1005–1012, 1988.

71. Bacon SL, Watkins LL, Babyak M, et al: The effects of daily stress on autonomic cardiac control in coronary artery disease patients. Am J Cardiol 93:1292–1294, 2004.

72. Coumel P, Leenhardt A: Mental activity, adrenergic modulation, and cardiac arrhythmias in patients with heart disease. Circulation 83(suppl 4):58–70, 1991.

73. Naesh O, Haedersdal C, Hindberg I, Trap-Jensen J: Platelet activation in mental stress. Clinical Physiology, 13:299–307, 1993.

74. Verrier RL, Dickerson LW: Autonomic nervous system and coronary blood flow changes related to emotional activation and sleep. Circulation, 83(suppl 2):81–89, 1991.

75. Yeung AC, Vekshtein VI. Krantz DS, et al: The effect of atherosclerosis on the vasomotor response of the coronary arteries to mental stress. N Engl J Med 325:1551–1556, 1991.

76. Blumenthal JA, Jiang W, Waugh RA, et al: Mental stress-induced ischemia in the laboratory and ambulatory ischemia during daily life: Association and hemodynamic features. Circulation 8:2102–2108, 1995.

77. Davis A, Natelson B: Brain-heart interactions: Neurocardiology of arrhythmia and sudden death. Texas Heart Institute Journal, 20: 158–169, 1993.

78. Vieth RC, Lewis N, Linares OA, et al: Sympathetic nervous system activity in major depression: Basal and desipramine-induced alterations in plasma norepinephrine kinetics. Arch Gen Psychiatr 51:411–422. 1994

79. Rozanski P, Blumenthal JA, Kaplan J: Impact of psychological factors on the pathogenesis of cardiovascular disease and implications for therapy. Circulation 99:2197–2217, 1999.

80. Koetnansky R: Catecholamines-corticosteroid interactions (pp. 7). In Usdin E, Koetnansky R, Kopin IJ, eds. Catecholamines and Stress. Amsterdam: Elsevier/North Holland; 1980.

81. Dunbar J: Predictors of patient adherence: Patient characteristics (pp. 348–360). In Shumaker SA, Schron EB, Ockene JK, eds. The Handbook of Health Behavior Change. New York: Springer Publishing; 1990.

82. Carney RM, Freedland KE, Eisen SE, et al: Depression is associated with poor adherence to medical treatment regimen in elderly cardiac patients. Health Psychol 14:88–90, 1995.

83. Guiry E, Conroy, RM, Hickey N, Mulcahy R: Psychological response to an acute coronary event and its effect on subsequent rehabilitation and lifestyle change. Clin Cardiol 10:256–260, 1987.

84. Blumenthal JA, Jiang W, Babyak MA, Krantz, et al: Stress management and exercise training in cardiac patients with myocardial ischemia. Effects on prognosis and evaluation of mechanisms. Arch Intern Med 157:2213–2223, 1997.

85. Blumenthal JA, Babyak M, Wei J, et al: Usefulness of psychosocial treatment of mental stress-induced myocardial ischemia in men. Am J Cardiol 89:164–168, 2002.

86. Linden W: Psychological treatments in cardiac rehabilitation: Review of rationales and outcomes. J Psychosomat Res 48: 443–454, 2000.

87. Writing committee for the ENRICHD investigators: Effects of treating depression and low perceived social support on clinical events after myocardial infarction. JAMA 289:3106–3116, 2003.

88. Frasure-Smith N, Lesperance F, Prince RH, et al: Randomised trial of home-based psychosocial nursing intervention for patients recovering from myocardial infarction. Lancet 350:473–479, 1997.

89. Jones DA, West RR: Psychological rehabilitation after myocardial infarction: Multicentre randomised controlled trial. BMJ 313: 1517–1521, 1996.

90. U.S. Department of Health and Human Services: Physical Activity and Health: A Report of the Surgeon General. Atlanta: Centers for Disease Control and Prevention, National Center for Chronic Disease Prevention and Health Promotion; 1996.

91. Wenger NK, Froehlicher ES, Smith LK, et al: Cardiac rehabilitation: clinical practice guidelines. Rockville, MD: Agency for Health Care Policy and Research and the National Heart, Lung and Blood Institute; 1995.

92. Ornish D, Brown SE, Scherwitz LW, et al: Can lifestyle changes reverse coronary heart disease? The Lifestyle Heart Trial. Lancet 336:129–133, 1990.

93. Ornish D, Scherwitz LW, Billings JH, et al: Intensive lifestyle changes for reversal of coronary heart disease. JAMA 280:2001–2007, 1998.

94. Scales R, Lueker RD, Atterbom HA, et al: Motivational interviewing and skills-based counseling to change multiple lifestyle behaviors [abstract]. Ann Behav Med 22D, 20:68, 1998.

95. Centers for Disease Control and Prevention: National diabetes fact sheet: National estimates and general information on diabetes in the United States. Atlanta: U.S. Department of Health and Human Services, Centers for Disease Control and Prevention; 1997.

96. Centers for Disease Control and Prevention: Diabetes Surveillance. Atlanta: U.S. Department of Health and Human Services, Centers for Disease Control and Prevention; 1997.

97. Robinson N, Fuller JH: Role of life events and difficulties in the onset of diabetes mellitus. J Psychosomat Res 29:583–591, 1985.

98. Peyrot M, Rubin RR: Levels and risks of depression and anxiety symptomatology among diabetic adults. Diabet Care, 20:585–590, 1997.

99. Surwit RS, Schneider MS, Feinglos MN: Stress and diabetes mellitus. Diabet Care 15, 10:1413–1422, 1992.

100. Leahy JL: Natural history of beta-cell dysfunction in NIDDM. Diabet Care 13:992–1010, 1990.

101. Gonder-Frederick LA, Cox DJ, Ritterband LM: Diabetes and behavioral medicine: The second decade. J Consult Clin Psychol 70:611–625, 2002.

102. Diabetes Prevention Program Research Group: Reduction in the incidence of type 2 diabetes with lifestyle intervention or metformin. N Engl J Med 346:393–403, 2003.

103. Kochanek KD, Smith BL: Deaths: Preliminary Data for 2002. National vital statistics reports 52:13. Hyattsville, MD: National Center for Health Statistics; 2004.

104. Centers for Disease Control and Prevention: Mortality patterns: Preliminary data; United States—1996. Morbid Mortal Wkly Rep 46:941–944, 1997.

105. Guyatt GH, Townsend M, Berman LB, Pugsley SO: Quality of life in patients with chronic airflow limitation. Br J Dis Chest 81:45, 1987.

106. Sandhu HS: Psychosocial issues in chronic obstructive pulmonary disease. Clin Chest Med 7:629, 1986.

107. Agle DP, Baum GL: Psychological aspects of chronic obstructive pulmonary disease. Med Clin N Am 61:749, 1977.

108. Isoaho R, Puolijoki H, Huhti E, et al: Chronic obstructive pulmonary disease and cognitive impairment in the elderly. Int Psychogeriatr 8:113, 1996.

109. Porzelius J, Vest M, Nochomovitz, M: Respiratory function, cognitions, and panic in chronic obstructive pulmonary patients. Behav Res Ther 30:75,1992.

110. Dolce JJ, Crisp C, Manzella B, et al: Medication adherence patterns in chronic obstructive pulmonary disease. Chest 99:837, 1991.

111. James PNE, Anderson JB, Prior JG, et al: Patterns of drug taking in patients with chronic airflow obstruction. Postgrad Med J 61:7–10, 1985.

112. Kozora E, Tran ZV, Make B: Neurobehavioral improvement after brief rehabilitation in patients with chronic obstructive pulmonary disease. J Cardiopul Rehabil 22:426–430, 2002.

113. Rose C, Wallace L, Dickson R, et al: The most effective psychologically-based treatments to reduce anxiety and panic in patients with chronic obstructive pulmonary disease (COPD): A systematic review. Patient Education & Counseling 47:311–318, 2002.

114. Emery CF, Schein RL, Hauck ER, et al: Psychological and cognitive outcomes of a randomized trial of exercise among patients with chronic obstructive pulmonary disease. Health Psychol 17:232–240, 1998.

115. Berry MJ, Walschlager SA: Exercise training and chronic obstructive pulmonary disease: Past and future research directions. J Cardiopul Rehabil 18:181–191, 1998.

116. Affleck G, Apter A, Tennen H, et al: Mood states associated with transitory changes in asthma symptoms and peak expiratory flow. Psychosomat Med 62:61–68, 2000.

117. Lehrer P, Feldman J, Giardino N, et al: Psychological aspects of asthma. J Consult Clin Psychol 70:691–711, 2002.

118. Kaptein AA: Psychological correlates of length of hospitalization and rehospitalization in patients with acute, severe asthma. Soc Sci Med 16:725–729, 1982.

119. Rietveld S, Everaerd W, Creer TL: Stress-induced asthma: a review of research and potential mechanisms. Clin Exp Allergy 30:1058–1066, 2000.

120. Lehrer P, Smetankin A, Potapova T: Respiratory sinus arrhythmia biofeedback therapy for asthma: A report of 20 unmedicated pediatric cases using the Smetankin method. Applied Psychophysiology & Biofeedback 25:193–200, 2000.

121. Satta A: Exercise training in asthma. J Sports Med Phys Fit 40:277–283, 2000.

122. Landis S, Murray T, Bolden S, Eingo PA: Cancer statistics. A Cancer Journal for Clinicians 48:6–29, 1998.

123. Fras I, Litin EM, Pearson JS: Comparison of psychiatric symptoms in carcinoma of the pancreas with those in some other intra-abdominal neoplasms. Am J Psychiatr 123:1553–1556, 1967.

124. Horne RL, Picard RS: Psychosocial risk factors for lung cancer. Psychosomat Med 43:431–438, 1979.

125. Leherer S: Life change and gastric cancer. Psychosomat Med 42:499–502, 1980.

126. Penninx BWJH, Guralnik JM, Pahor M, et al: Chronically depressed mood and cancer risk in older persons. J Nat Cancer Inst 90:1888–1893, 1998.

127. Kiecolt-Glaser JK, Glaser R: Psychoneuroimmunology: Can psychological interventions modulate immunity? J Consult Clin Psychol 60, 4:569–575, 1992.

128. Caroll B, Curtis G, Mendels J: Cerebrospinal fluid and plasma free cortisol concentrations in depression. Psychosomat Med 6:235–244, 1976.

129. Petitto JM, Folds JD, Ozer H, et al: Abnormal diuranal variation in circulating natural killer cell phenotypes and cytotoxic activity in major depression. Am J Psychiatr 149:694–696, 1992.

130. Stein M, Miller AH, Trestman RL: Depression, the immune system, and health and illness: Findings in search of meaning. Arch Gen Psychiatr 48:171–177, 1991.

131. Bottomley A: Depression in cancer patients: A literature review. Eur J Cancer Care 7:181–191, 1998.

132. Levenson JL, Bemis C: The role of psychological factors in cancer onset and progression. Psychosomatics 32, 2:124–134, 1990.

133. Kaplan GA, Reynolds P: Depression and cancer mortality and morbidity: Prospective evidence from the Alameda County Study. J Behav Med 11:1–13, 1988.

134. Zonderman AB, Costa PT Jr, McCrae RR: Depression as a risk for cancer morbidity and mortality in a nationally representative sample. JAMA 262:1191–1195, 1989.

135. Bleiker MA, van der Ploeg HM: Psychosocial factors in the etiology of breast cancer: Review of a popular link. Patient Education 37:201–124, 1999.

136. Knekt P, Raitasalo R, Heliovaara M, et al: Elevated lung cancer risk among persons with depression mood. Am J Epidemiol 144:1096–2103, 1996.

137. Anderson BL: Biobehavioral outcomes following psychological interventions for cancer patients. J Consult Clin Psychol 70:590–610, 2002.

138. Linkins RW, Comstock GW: Depressed mood and development of cancer. Am J Epidemiol 132:962–972, 1990.

139. Spiegel D, Bloom JR, Kraemer HC, Gottheil E: Effect of psychosocial treatment on survival of patients with metastatic breast cancer. Lancet 2:888–891, 1989.

140. Goodwin PJ, Leszcz M, Ennis M, et al: The effect of group psychosocial support on survival in metastatic breast cancer. N Engl J Med 345:1719–1726, 2001.

141. CDC AIDS Community Demonstration Projects Research Group: Community-level HIV intervention in 5 cities: Final outcome data from the CDC AIDS Community Demonstration Projects. Am J Publ Health 89:336–345, 1999.

142. Deeks SG, Smith M, Holodniy M, Kahn JO: HIV-1 protease inhibitors. A review for clinicians. JAMA 277:145–153, 1997.

143. Leserman J: The effects of stressful life events, coping, and cortisol on HIV infection. CNS Spectrums 8:25–30, 2003.

144. Penzak SR, Reddy YS, Grimsley SR: Depression in patients with HIV infection. Am J Health-System Pharm 57:376–386, 2000.

145. Cruess DG, Petitto JM, Leserman J, et al: Depression and HIV infection: impact on immune function and disease progression. CNS Spectrums 8:52–58, 2003.

146. Evans DL, Leserman J, Perkins DO, et al: Severe life stress as a predictor of early disease progression in HIV infection. Am J Psychiatr 154:630–634, 1997.

147. Leserman J, Petitto JM, Gu H, et al: Progression to AIDS, a clinical AIDS condition and mortality: Psychosocial and physiological predictors. Psychol Med 32:1059–1073, 2002.

148. Kelly JA, Kalichman SC: Behavioral research in HIV/AIDS primary and secondary prevention: Recent advances and future directions. J Consult Clin Psychol 70:626–639, 2002.

149. Lutgendorf SK, Antonio MH, Ironson G, et al: Cognitive-behavioral stress management decreases dysphoric mood and herpes simplex virus-type 2 antibody titers in symptomatic HIV-seropositve gay men. J Consult Clin Psychol 65:31–43, 1997.

150. Nixon S, O'Brien K, Glazier RH, Tynan AM: Aerobic exercise interventions for adults living with HIV/AIDS. Cochrane HIV/AIDS Group Cochrane Database of Systematic Reviews, 1, 2003.

151. LaPerriere A, Klimas N, Fletcher MA, et al: Change in CD4+ cell enumeration following aerobic exercise training in HIV-1 disease: Possible mechanisms and practical applications. Int J Sports Med 18 (suppl 1):S56–S61, 1997.

152. Centers for Disease Control and Prevention: Arthritis prevalence and activity limitations: United States. Morbid Mortal Wkly Rep 43:433–438, 1990.

153. Walsh JD, Blanchard EB, Kremer JM, Blanchard CG: The psychosocial effects of rheumatoid arthritis on the patient and well partner. Behav Res Ther 37:259–271, 1999.

154. Schumacher HR: Primer on the Rheumatic Diseases, 8th ed. Atlanta: Arthritis Foundation; 1988.

155. Bendtsen P, Hornquist JO: Change and status in quality of life in patients with rheumatoid arthritis. Quality of Life Research 1:296–305, 1992.

156. Anderson KO, Bradley LA, Young LD, et al: Rheumatoid arthritis: Review of psychological factors related to etiology, effects and treatment. Psychol Bull 98, 2:358–387, 1985.

157. Young LD: Psychological factors in rheumatoid arthritis. J Consul Clin Psychol 60, 4:619–627, 1992.

158. Frank RG, Beck NC, Parker JC, et al:. Depression in rheumatoid arthritis. J Rheumatol 15:920–925, 1988.

159. Abdel-Nasser AM, Abd El-Azim S, Taal E, et al: Depression and depressive symptoms in rheumatoid arthritis patients: An analysis of their occurrence and determinants. Br J Rheumatol 37:391–397, 1998.

160. Baum J: A review of psychological aspects of rheumatic diseases. Sem Arthritis Rheumat 11:353–361, 1982.

161. Persson L-O, Berglund K, Sahlberg D: Psychological factors in chronic rheumatic diseases—A review. Scand J Rheumatol 28:137–144, 1999.

162. Hendrie HC, Paraskevas F, Baragar FD, Adamson J D: Stress, immunoglobin levels and early polyarthritis. J Psychosomat Res 15:337–343, 1971.

163. Ferguson K, Bole GG: Family support, health beliefs, and therapeutic compliance in patients with rheumatoid arthritis. Patient Couns Health Educ 1:101–105, 1979.

165. Geersten HR, Gray RM, Ward JR: Patient non-compliance within the context of seeking medical care for arthritis. J Chron Dis 26:689–698, 1973.

165. Lee P, Tan LJ: Current trends in the treatment of rheumatoid arthritis in general practice. N Z Med J 89:165–167, 1979.

166. Keefe FJ, Smith SJ, Buffington ALH, et al: Recent advances and future directions in the biopsychosocial assessment and treatment of arthritis. J Consult Clin Psychol 70:640–655, 2002.

167. Keefe FJ, Caldwell DS, Williams DA, et al: Pain coping skills training in the management of osteoarthritic knee pain: A comparative study. Behav Ther 21:49–62, 1990.

168. Nakajima A, Hirai H, Yoshino S: Reassessment of mirthful laughter in rheumatoid arthritis. J Rheumatol 26:512–513, 1999.

169. Young LD, Bradley LA, Turner RA: Decreases in health care resource utilization in patients with rheumatoid arthritis following a cognitive behavioral intervention. Biofeedback and Self-Regulation 20:259–268, 1995.

170. Rejeski WJ, Focht BC, Messier SP, et al: Obese, older adults with knee osteoarthritis: Weight loss, exercise, and quality of life. Health Psychol 21:419–426, 2002.

171. Turk DC: Biopsychosocial perspective on chronic pain (pp. 3–32). In Gatchel RJ, Turk DC, eds. Psychological Approaches to Pain Management: A Practitioner's Handbook. New York: Guilford Press; 1996.

172. Gatchel R. Psychological disorders and chronic pain: Cause-effect relationships (pp. 33–52). In Gatchel RJ, Turk DC, eds. Psychological Approaches to Pain Management: A Practitioner's Handbook.

New York: Guilford Press; 1996.

173. Romano JM, Turner JA: Chronic pain and depression: Does the evidence support a relationship? Psychol Bull 97:18–34, 1985.

174. Turk DC, Rudy TE: Toward an empirically derived taxonomy of chronic pain patients: Integration of psychological assessment data. J Consult Clin Psychol 56:233–238, 1988.

175. Polatino PB, Kinney RK, Gatchel RJ, et al: Psychiatric illness and chronic low back pain. Spine 18:66–71, 1993.

176. Turk DC, Okifudi A: Psychological factors in chronic pain: Evolution and Revolution. J Consult Clin Psychol 70:678–690, 2002.

177. Flor H, Fydrich T, Turk DC: Efficacy of multidisciplinary pain treatment centers: A meta-analytic review. Pain 49:221–230, 1992.

178. Brosse AL Sheets ES, Lett HS, Blumenthal JA: Exercise and the treatment of clinical depression in adults: recent findings and future directions. Sports Med 32, 12:741–60, 2002.

179. Camacho TC, Roberts RE, Lazarus NB, et al: Physical activity and depression: Evidence from the Alameda County study. Am J Epidemiol 134:220–231, 1991.

180. Lawlor DA, Hopker SW: The effectiveness of exercise as an intervention in the management of depression: systematic review and meta-regression analysis of randomised controlled trials. BMJ 322:763–767, 2001.

181. Dunn AL, Trivedi MH, O'Neal HA: Physical activity dose-response effects on outcome of depression and anxiety. Med Sci Sports Ex 6(suppl.):S587–S597, 2001.

182. Fillingim RB, Blumenthal JA: The use of aerobic exercise as a method of stress management (pp. 443–4620). In Lehrer PM, Woolfolk RL, eds. Principles and Practice of Stress Management. New York: Guilford Press; 1993.

183. DeVries H, Hams G: Electromyographic comparison of single dose of exercise and meprobamate as to effects on muscular relaxation. Am J Phys Med 51:130–141, 1972.

184. Salmon P: Effects of physical exercise on anxiety, depression, and sensitivity to stress: a unifying theory. Clin Psychol Rev 21:33–61, 2001.

185. Sothman M, Hart B, Horn T: Plasma catecholamine response to acute psychological stress in humans: Relation to aerobic fitness and exercise testing. Medicine & Science in Sports & Exercise 23:873–881, 1991.

186. Georgiades A, Sherwood A, Gullette ECD, et al: Effects of exercise and weight loss on mental stress-induced cardiovascular responses in individuals with high blood pressure. Hypertension 36:171–176, 2000.

187. Blumenthal JA, Fredrikson M, Kuhn CM, et al: Aerobic exercise reduces levels of cardiovascular and sympathoadrenal responses to mental stress in subjects without prior evidence of myocardial ischemia. Am J Cardiol 65:93–98, 1990.

188. Boone JB, Probst MM, Rogers MW, Berger R: Post-exercise hypotension reduces cardiovascular responses to stress. J Hypertens 11:449–453, 1993.

189. Light KC, Obrist PA, James SA, Strogatz DS: Cardiovascular responses to stress: II relationships to aerobic exercise patterns. Psychophysiology 24:79–85, 1987.

190. Ewart CK, Taylor CB, Reese LB, DeBusk RF: Effects of early postmyocardial infarction exercise testing on self-perception and subsequent physical activity. Am J Cardiol 51:1076–1080, 1983.

SELECTED REFERENCES FOR FURTHER READING

Behavioral Medicine and Clinical Health Psychology. J Consult Clin Psychol [special issue] 70:459–856.

INTERNET RESOURCES

Cognitive Behavior Therapy: http://www.cognitive-behavior-therapy.org

Mental Health: A Report of the Surgeon General: http://www.surgeon-general.gov/library/mentalhealth/home.html

Motivational Interviewing: http://www.motivationalinterviewing.org

Physical Fitness and Clinical and Diagnostic Assessments

SECTION EDITOR: LARRY F. HAMM, PhD, FACSM

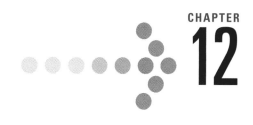

Body Composition

LEONARD KAMINSKY AND GREGORY DWYER

This chapter addresses KSAs from the following content areas:

1   Exercise Physiology and Related Exercise Science
2   Pathophysiology and Risk Factors
3   Health Appraisal, Fitness, and Clinical Exercise Testing
4   Electrocardiography and Diagnostic Techniques
5   Patient Management and Medications
6   Medical and Surgical Management
7   Exercise Prescription and Programming
8   Nutrition and Weight Management
9   Human Behavior and Counseling
10 Safety, Injury Prevention, and Emergency Procedures
11 Program Administration, Quality Assurance, and Outcome Assessment

Body composition is both a field of study and a component of physical fitness. Strictly speaking, body composition refers to the make up of the body. Body composition can be assessed on elemental (atomic), chemical, cellular, and tissue system levels[1]. It is possible to measure more than 30 components of human body composition[2]. In health and fitness environments, the principle interests are knowledge of the relative amount of body fat in proportion to lean tissue mass and the distribution of fat in the body, with additional interest in changes in these components. In clinical environments, many additional components of the body may be of interest and importance (e.g., bone density).

Rationale for Body Composition Assessment

The rationale for assessment of body composition is strong and continues to expand as improved assessment technology and research findings evolve. Knowledge of the relative amount of body fat is helpful in many regards. The associations between obesity (excess body fat), especially excessive intra-abdominal (visceral) fat and increased risk of many chronic diseases (type II diabetes,

hypertension, hyperlipidemia, the metabolic syndrome, coronary artery disease [CAD], and certain types of cancer), are strong with new scientific studies being published regularly[3]. Because of the epidemic of obesity in the United States (as discussed in Chapter 5), detection of obesity and its development (overweight) are of primary importance for many health and exercise science professionals. An excessively low level of body fat is also detrimental, as evidenced by the physiological dysfunction of chronically undernourished individuals and those with eating disorders. In addition, monitoring changes in body fat storage through growth, maturation, and aging is desirable for the detection of increased risk of disease development.

Assessment of muscle mass is also important in both health and fitness and clinical environments. The muscle wasting (sarcopenia) that occurs with certain diseases and with aging not only decreases muscle strength and the capacity for even routine activities but is also a strong correlate of mortality. Recently, there has been increased emphasis on the development of interventions to increase lean tissue mass in healthy aging and clinical populations as well as in athletes.

Other components of the body are also valuable to measure in clinical settings. Bone is one of primary importance. Low bone mass and density are primary predictors of the risk of osteoporotic fracture.

Health and exercise science professionals can obtain extremely valuable information from body composition assessments. These measurements are used for risk assessment, individualization of the exercise prescriptions, and evaluation of the efficacy of interventions.

Selection of Methodology

There are no direct in vivo methods available to measure the different components of the body. Clinical and fitness program professionals have many alternative indirect assessment methods available. Similar to other physical fitness and health risk measurements, the decision of which body composition assessment method to select depends on the purpose of the evaluation and the needs of the individual. Additionally, the cost of the measurements, their availability, the amount of technician

KEY TERMS

Body fat percentage: The amount, expressed as a percentage, of the body that is made up of fat tissue. This can only be estimated in the human body (i.e., no direct measurement methods are available for total body fat percentage)

Component-based methods: A system of detailed taxonomies that separates the body into different components (e.g., fat tissue, lean tissue, bone density, body water)

Property-based methods: Measurement of specific properties, such as body volume, decay properties of specific isotopes, or electrical resistance

Standard error of the estimate: A statistic used to express the amount of variability (error) from predictions. The prediction error of a test score can be expressed as the standard error of the estimate (SEE). Similar to the standard deviation, the SEE is generally expressed as a ± of the score. Using the bell-shaped curve for normal distribution, ± SEE unit refers to 68% of the population, or 68% of the population will be within the score ± the SEE.

training, and individual characteristics and performance requirements all affect the decision of which measurement is used.

HEALTH RISK ASSESSMENT

Anthropometry or body composition assessment is an important part of health risk screenings because obesity is now an accepted independent risk factor for CAD, as well as other conditions. Screening programs typically use measurements that can be done quickly (to allow testing of large numbers in a short period of time), economically (cost to individual or screening entity), and with limited technical training. Thus, the principle measurements recommended for assessing body composition in screening programs (see GETP7 Chapter 2) are body weight, body height, and waist circumference.

Measurements of body weight, height, and waist circumference are relatively simple to perform and rapid to complete. Each measure requires but a few simple standardizations to obtain reliable and accurate values[4]. Measurement procedures for circumferences are provided in GETP7 Box 4-1, which also describes the correct location for the waist site (two options). It is important to note that although the Dietary Advisory Committee has proposed a new description of the waist site for improved standardization of measurement (Fig. 12-1), most, if not all, of the research has used the narrowest part of the torso location when identifying health risks. Body weight is best measured on a calibrated scale with a beam and moveable weights. If other types of scales are used, it is recommended that they be calibrated using standardized weights or compared with measured weight from the beam-type scale. The major measurement issue for body weight assessment is clothing. The type and amount of clothing must be standard-

ized (Box 12-1). Ideally, measurement should be completed in the nude or with only a paper hospital gown. However, this requirement is not feasible in most circumstances. Thus, it is recommended that a facility adopt the most reasonable clothing standardization for their population. Minimally, this standard requires that individuals remove their shoes and any excess layers of clothing (e.g., coats), empty their pockets, and remove jewelry and cell phones. In many fitness environments, a

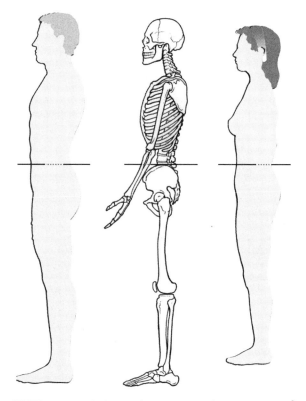

FIGURE 12-1. Standardization for waist circumference landmarks[3].

reasonable standard is shorts and a t-shirt. Height should be assessed with a stadiometer (vertical ruler [mounted on a wall] with a wide horizontal headboard). Although many commercial platform scales have a vertical ruler with a thin head bar, use of these devices to measure height is less reliable and, thus, is not recommended. Standards for height measurements are simple: individuals being measured need to remove their shoes, stand with their heels together, take and hold a deep inhalation, and stand with their head level. Failure to follow these standards results in reduced reliability and, thus, inaccuracy.

As presented in GETP7 Table 4.1, body mass index (BMI = weight [kg] · height [m^{-2}]) and waist circumference can be used to classify an individual's body weight and determine their risk of developing type II diabetes, hypertension, and CAD according to standards developed by the Expert Panel on the Identification, Evaluation, and Treatment of Overweight and Obesity in Adults[3]. Criticisms of the use of the BMI for body composition assessment are that it is a relatively poor predictor of **body fat percentage** and it results in inaccurate classifications (normal, overweight, obese) for some individuals. Table 4-2 in GETP7 provides a method of estimating body fat ranges for adult men and women in three different age categories from BMI classifications of underweight, normal, overweight, and obese. It is noted that the **standard error of the estimate (SEE)** for predicting percent body fat from BMI is ± 5%. Thus, from a prediction of body fat percentage perspective, the criticism of the BMI is valid. However, for non-athletic adult populations, misclassification of body weight is not that prevalent. Simply inquiring if the individual participates in resistance-type exercise (either occupationally or recreationally), particularly if he or she has had a stable body weight in adulthood, identifies those for whom the BMI is more likely to be inaccurate (most typically "overweight" or even "obese" classifications for an individual with an acceptable range of body fat percentage). For these individuals, BMI classifications should not be used; more advanced methods to estimate a body fat percentage should be used instead. In most other adults who are weight stable (nonresistance exercisers) or who have gained weight in their adult years (which is, unfortunately, the norm in the U.S. population), the BMI should provide a reasonably accurate classification of body weight status. Common sense suggests that except for the person who has begun a vigorous resistance-training program or has developed a condition that has resulted in excess fluid accumulation, essentially all of the weight gained in adult years is excess body fat. Thus, if the objective is to assess health risk, using the BMI and a waist circumference measurement would meet this objective in most adult populations (see GETP7 Tables 4-1 and 4-3). Clinical and fitness professionals can use additional body composition measurements for any individuals for whom they have concerns about the accuracy of the BMI classification.

	Standards for Basic Body Composition Measurements	
BOX 12-1		
MEASUREMENT	**INSTRUMENT**	**STANDARD-IZATION**
Waist Circumference	Tension-controlled tape	See GETP7 Box 4-1
Weight	Balance beam scale	Nude or hospital gown
		Or
		Facility-developed standard
Height	Stadiometer	No shoes, heels together, after a deep inhalation, head level

Advanced Body Composition Assessment

More advanced body composition assessment methodologies can be used in the assessment of this component of physical fitness (either as part of a clinical evaluation or in research settings). In these situations, more information about the amounts of certain components of the body, namely body fat and muscle mass, may be desired. Chapter 4 of GETP7 provides an overview of these advanced methods that can provide an estimate of body fat percentage and then, by mathematical manipulation, an estimate of fat-free mass (FFM). Additional information can be obtained from the sources listed in the "Selected References for Further Reading" section at the end of this chapter.

THEORETICAL ASPECTS: BODY COMPARTMENT MODELING

Body composition methods can be categorized as being direct, indirect, or doubly indirect[5,6]. A direct method, the chemical analysis of the whole body or cadaver, is obviously not suitable for "live" human body composition assessment. Therefore, body composition analysis in live (in vivo) humans is done using only indirect or doubly indirect methods. However, the direct method is central to all other assessment techniques because this method provides basic data (e.g., whole body and tissue density) that is the foundation from which indirect and doubly indirect methods were developed. Indirect methods (e.g., hydrodensitometry) were derived from the direct method of chemical analysis, and doubly indirect methods (e.g., skinfold analysis) were generally derived from an indirect method (e.g., hydrodensitometry). Therefore, doubly indirect methods are generally prone to greater error in measurement by adding their unique error to the error associated with indirect methods from which they are derived (e.g., Total error of skinfold technique = Skinfold measurement error + Hydrodensitometry error). Table 12-1 categorizes many of the popular body composition methods into indirect or doubly indirect.

Indirect methods can be based on either property or component[2]. **Property-based methods** involved the measurement of specific properties, such as body volume, decay properties of specific isotopes, or electrical resistance. The development of in vivo neutron activation analysis, for example, has made possible nondestructive chemical analysis by measuring the radiation given off during the decay of excited atoms[7]. An example of a more common property-based method is the estimation of total body water (TBW) from tritium dilution[8].

Component-based methods depend on well-established models, usually ratios of measurable quantities to components that are assumed constant both within and between individuals. With component-based methods, the measured quantity is first assessed using a property-based method, and the component is estimated by application of the model. Thus, FFM, one of the components of the two-component model described later, can be estimated from body water by use of tritium dilution to measure TBW, which is converted to FFM according to the relation between TBW and FFM.

Two types of mathematical functions or approaches are used to estimate composition with property- and component-based methods. The model approach, which depends on knowing the relation (ratio) between a particular constituent and the component of interest, was illustrated earlier. In the second approach, regression analysis

TABLE 12-1. Categorization of Common Body Composition Assessment Techniques

Assessment Technique	Method	Component Model
Skinfolds	Doubly indirect	Largely 2C (some multiple C equations)
Bioelectrical impedance	Doubly indirect	3C
Near-infrared interactance	Doubly indirect	2C
Hydrodensitometry	Indirect	2C
CT and MRI scans	Indirect	Multiple C
Plethysmography: air displacement	Indirect	2C
Dual-energy x-ray absorptiometry (DEXA)	Indirect	3C

Method = direct, indirect, or doubly indirect (see text for complete explanation).

Component model = 2C (two compartment), 3C (three compartment), multiple C (more than 2C) (see text for complete explanation).

is used with experimental data to derive an equation that relates a measured property or component to an unknown (estimated) component. Typically, measuring the unknown component and the known component in the same subjects develops the equation. Regression analysis is used to derive the equation relating the known component to the unknown component. Equations for estimating body fat from skinfold thickness or bioelectrical resistance are developed in this manner. Because they generally depend on a combination of methods used to estimate an unknown component, they are considered to be doubly indirect methods.

It is clear from the preceding discussion that a hierarchy of methods exists. Direct methods represent the most fundamental approach to assessment, property-based methods are one step removed, and component-based methods are two steps removed. Assessment methods are structured so that measurement errors or inaccurate assumptions are propagated from one level to the next. Thus, doubly indirect methods, furthest removed from direct methods, are most susceptible to inaccuracies unless precautions are taken to minimize measurement error.

Many models have been proposed for characterizing human body composition by dividing the sum into its parts (compartments). A feature of all these models is that the sum of the compartments closely approximates the whole, body weight. The two-compartment (2C) model of fat versus FFM was developed by many body composition pioneers, including Brozek et al.[9] and Siri[10] in the 1950s. Using previous human cadaver biochemical analysis (direct method), they determined the relationship between the density of the whole body to the percentage of body fat. The 2C model is limited by several assumptions. Two of these assumptions are that the water and mineral contents of the body remain constant throughout life and between all groups of individuals (e.g., age, gender, ethnicity) and that the density of the fat-free tissues (e.g., muscle, bone) is constant among all individuals. The assumption related to fat-free tissue composition is known to be violated by age, gender, and ethnicity differences. Many of the body composition techniques used today, including hydrodensitometry and plethsmyography, are based on the 2C model and, thus, contain some error in their estimates of percent body fat. Table 12-1 categorizes the models likely to be used with each body composition assessment technique listed.

Because of the violation of the inherent assumptions with the 2C model, multicompartment models have been developed. Multicompartment models for body composition divide the body into more than two compartments. These models require fewer assumptions about the composition of the FFM. For this reason, these models may give more accurate results. However, their application requires additional measurements (e.g., total body water, bone mineral content); thus, the theoretical reduction in total error by use of a multicompartment model may be offset by increased technical error in measuring multiple components. Multicompartment body composition models currently include the three-compartment (3C) and four-compartment (4C) models. It is important to consider the analytical accuracy of these multicompartment models when considering their use.

An example of the use of the 2C model is found in the Siri or the Brozek body density equations[9,10]. For instance, the Siri equation generally gives accurate estimates of fat and FFM in young to middle-aged white men. In contrast, systematic differences among children, various racial and ethnic groups, athletes, and the elderly lead to errors in estimation of body fat and invalidate the Siri equation in these groups. The choice of an appropriate model depends on the component of FFM (e.g., mineral content) that is expected to vary the most from the norms for that particular subpopulation. For example, young children may have proportionally less mineral content and more total body water than adults. Thus, a 4C model that adjusts for variability in both total body water and mineral content is ideal, although satisfactory results can be achieved with a 3C model that adjusts for only total body water. A 3C model that adjusts for differences in minerals is useful in African American men and women, the elderly, and many athletes, because race or ethnicity, age, and physical training differences are attributable primarily to systematic variation in bone mineral content (mass and density).

When instrumentation (for measuring these other components) is limited and 3C and 4C models are not feasible, population-specific equations (that use a 2C model) that are adjusted for systematic differences in the composition of the FFM (for various population groups) can be used to improve accuracy (see GETP7 Table 4-4). Population-specific equations appropriate for children and older adults, various racial or ethnic groups, athletic groups, and some clinical populations have been reviewed elsewhere[11-14]. Although estimation error is always a factor, when used appropriately, population-specific equations should result in more accurate estimates than generalized equations.

BODY FAT PREDICTION EQUATION SELECTION

Prediction equations are either population specific or generalizable. Population-specific equations are derived for use in a specific homogeneous population (e.g., prepubescent white boys or elderly African American women). Thus, the population-specific equations usually systematically underestimate or overestimate body composition if they are applied to individuals from other populations. In contrast, generalizable equations can be applied to individuals who differ greatly in physical characteristics. Generalizable equations are developed from diverse, heterogeneous samples, and they account for differences in age, gender, race or ethnicity, and other characteristics by including these variables as predictors in the equation.

To develop prediction equations, it is necessary to select a representative sample of the specific population to which the equations will be applied. The predictor variables (e.g., height and weight, gender, age, race or ethnicity, skinfolds, or bioelectrical impedance) and the criterion estimates of body composition (e.g., percent body fat) are measured in the same subjects, and the equation is developed using appropriate statistical methods. The usefulness of the equation depends on the strength of association between the variables and the accuracy with which the dependent variable is estimated. Useful equations give estimates of percent fat or FFM that are reasonably well correlated ($r > 0.80$) with the criterion estimate. Moreover, the means and standard deviations of the estimated and criterion scores should be nearly equal, and the SEE for predicting the criterion from the estimated values is between ± 2.5% to 3.5% for percent body fat[14].

To select the most appropriate equation, it is important to evaluate the relative merit of the various methods and equations. The following questions should be considered[14]:

1. **To whom is the specific percent body fat equation used applicable?** Factors such as age, race or ethnicity, gender, physical activity level, and estimated amount of body fat all may influence which specific equation should be used. Unless the equation has been shown to generalize to other groups, it should not be applied to groups with different characteristics.
2. **Was an appropriate compartment model used to develop the equation used?** Errors from the compartment model used contribute to the total error in the equation. For instance, multicompartment models require fewer assumptions and give more accurate reference measurements than methods based on the 2C model. Equations derived from reference measurements based on the 3C and 4C models should be used in populations for whom the assumptions underlying the 2C model are not valid.
3. **Was a representative sample of the population studied?** Large, randomly selected samples are needed to ensure that the data used to derive the equation are representative of the population. If random sampling is not possible and convenience samples are used, the prediction equation may be acceptable as long as a sufficient number of subjects are studied. With a large sample size, a more stable and valid equation will be derived.
4. **How were the predictor variables measured?** When any equation is applied, it is important that the predictor variables be measured in the same way as the original investigators, who developed the equation, measured. Although it is recommended that standard procedures and sites be used, this is not always done, and prediction errors may be too large if the original procedures are not followed[15].

5. **Was the equation cross-validated in another sample of the population?** Because of investigator- and laboratory-specific procedural differences, equations that sometimes give accurate validation results may not be accurate when used in a different laboratory or by a different investigator, and the equation should be tested in other samples of the same population.
6. **Does the equation give accurate estimates of percent body fat?** In validation studies, the multiple correlation between the variables should be $R^2 > 0.80$, and SEEs should range from 2.5% to 3.5% when estimating percent body fat[11].

GENERAL ERROR CONCEPTS IN BODY COMPOSITION ASSESSMENT

All indirect body composition techniques currently used predict a percent body fat rather that actually measuring fat. Although the specific procedure (i.e., skinfolds) measures a component of body composition (i.e., subcutaneous fat), a prediction is made from the component measured to the percent body fat. Because prediction is an important part of body composition assessment, it is worth a brief explanation.

You must accept that there is going to be some error in body fat prediction because no method is perfect. The measurement error in prediction of a test score can be expressed as the SEE. To understand how to apply the SEE, you should review the characteristics of the bell-shaped curve and the normal distribution of scores (standard deviation) in the population. The predicted value (in this case, for percent body fat) is the mean of the distribution of a population of individuals with the same measurement value (i.e., sum of skinfolds). The SEE is a measure of the variability of this population's actual percent body fat values (i.e., similar to the standard deviation of the scores in a bell-shaped distribution) and is expressed as $\pm$, reflecting scores both above and below the predicted value. Measurements obtained with a prediction method should be expressed as the predicted score $\pm$ the SEE (typically $\pm$ 1 SEE, which refers to 68% of the population). The SEE for one of the many commonly used Jackson and Pollock skinfold equations for percent body fat is SEE = $\pm$ 3.5%[15]. An application of using the SEE can be demonstrated by the following example using the above information. An individual's skinfold measurement resulted in a predicted percent body fat of 20 $\pm$ 3.5%. This means that 68% of similar individuals with the same sum of skinfolds (and same age and gender) actually have percent body fats between 16.5% to 23.5%. The remaining 32% of individuals with the same sum of skinfolds have percent body fats even greater than 3.5% different from the predicted value (i.e., <16.5 % or >23.5%). Thus, although you as a technician may calculate an individual's percent body fat as 20%, it is very possible (about one in every three cases) that this individual's actual percent body fat may be less that 16.5% or greater than 23.5%.

SKINFOLD ANALYSIS

The popular method of skinfold measurement to predict percent body fat can provide reasonable estimates if performed by a properly trained technician and with a quality skinfold caliper. However, it should be remembered that skinfold analysis is considered a doubly indirect method; is still an estimate or prediction of body density and, thus, percent body fat; and is largely based on the 2C model (there are a few multicompartment models that use skinfold analysis). Skinfold analysis is based on the principle that the amount of subcutaneous fat is directly proportional to the total amount of body fat. However, the proportion of subcutaneous to total fat varies with gender, age, race or ethnicity, and other factors. Numerous regression equations, using a combination of multiple skinfold sites, have been developed to predict body density or fat from skinfold measurements. These multiple regression equations are either generalizable or population-specific for gender, age, race or ethnicity, and activity or sport status.

Specific recommendations, including descriptions of standardized skinfold anatomical sites, are provided in GETP7 Box 4.2. It should be remembered that the specific skinfold regression equation used must match the author of the equation/technique's description of the skinfold sites and technique because there are differences in reported skinfold anatomical site descriptions and measurement techniques (GETP7 Box 4-3). Thus, major limitations to the skinfold analysis procedure for body composition are the amount of technician training in equation selection, skinfold site measurement accuracy, and measurement technique.

Information concerning the reliability and accuracy of skinfold determination of body composition is specific to the skinfold regression equation used. The variability in predictions of percent body fat from skinfold analysis is approximately $\pm$ 3.5% (SEE) assuming that appropriate techniques and equations have been used[11]. As reported previously, the age-generalized three-site skinfold equations for men from Jackson and Pollock have a SEE of 3.5%[15].

BIOELECTRICAL IMPEDANCE ANALYSIS

Bioelectrical impedance analysis (BIA) is a noninvasive and easy-to-administer method for assessing body composition. The basic premise behind this procedure is that the mass of fat-free tissue in the body is proportional to the electrical conductivity of the body[16]. Thus, in BIA, a small electrical current is passed into the body, and then the impedance (impedance is a combination of the electrical terms *resistance* and *reactance*) to that current is measured. The theory behind BIA is that whereas fat is a poor electrical conductor containing little water, lean tissue, containing mostly water and electrolytes, is a good electrical conductor. Thus, fat tissue acts as an impedance to electrical current. In actuality, BIA estimates total body water and uses equations for percent body fat (based on a

3C model) using assumptions about hydration levels of individuals and the exact water content of various tissues[14]. In the most common application of BIA, a single-frequency (50-kHz) low-level excitation current (500 mA) is used to measure whole-body impedance using a four-electrode system using the legs and arms. Unlike lower-frequency current (<50 kHz), which flows through the extracellular fluid, higher frequencies penetrate the cell membranes and flow through both the intracellular and extracellular fluid. Thus, total body impedance at the constant frequency of 50 kHz primarily reflects the volumes of water (intracellular and extracellular fluid) and muscle compartments constituting the FFM.

Most BIA machines use different equations that account for the differences in water content and body density between different genders, ages, and races or ethnicities as well as by physical activity status. These equations are specific to each manufacturer and are not generally available for analysis. The BIA technology has been validated against hydrodensitometry and skinfold analysis and has been shown to be affected by certain subject and environmental factors that affect hydration status (e.g., fluid intake or meal timing, bladder fullness, diuretic or caffeine use, and recent exercise). These conditions must be controlled for to ensure the subject is of normal hydration. The reported SEE for BIA is between ± 3.5% and 5 %, which is greater than that reported for skinfold analysis[16]. In addition, percent body fat from BIA appears to be consistently overestimated for lean individuals and underestimated for obese persons.

As with anthropometry, subject factors, technical skill, the prediction equation used to estimate FFM, and the instruments used affect the accuracy and precision of BIA. To reduce measurement error (and improve accuracy), analyzers should be calibrated before measurement (which is not commonly performed), and the same brand of analyzer (ideally the same instrument) should be used when following changes in body composition within an individual. Factors such as eating, drinking, and exercising must be controlled because hydration status, fluid distribution, and temperature are sources of error in resistance measurements. Technician error is minor if standard procedures for electrode positioning and subject positioning are followed. Finally, as with skinfold analyses, equation error can be reduced by selecting prediction equations according to age, gender, race or ethnicity, and level of physical activity.

Recent research suggests that with the newer multiple-frequency BIA, it may be possible to estimate extracellular and intracellular water compartments along with TBW[16]. As a result, this methodology may be less affected by hydration status and, therefore, may be a better estimate of FFM. Multiple-frequency BIA may also enhance the clinical application of BIA to assess changes and shifts between intracellular and extracellular fluid compartments associated with certain diseases as well as accurate hydration status. However, the multiple-frequency BIA is not currently commercially available.

NEAR-INFRARED INTERACTANCE

Near-infrared interactance (NIR) is based on the principles of light absorption and reflection using near-infrared spectroscopy to provide information about the chemical composition of the body. A light wand device is positioned on a body part, and the absorption of the infrared beam is measured. Research to date has reported unacceptable prediction errors for NIR[14]. Some commercial versions of NIR (e.g., Futrex-5000) are very portable and require minimal technician training, making them attractive to the health and fitness industry (and make measurement easy for subjects). However, a major limitation of the technology is the relatively small sampling area on the body for NIR absorption; some devices only sample over the biceps muscle of the dominant arm. The SEE reported for NIR varies more than ± 5.0 percent body fat[17].

UNDERWATER OR HYDROSTATIC WEIGHING: HYDRODENSITOMETRY

Underwater weighing or hydrostatic weighing is considered the criterion, or gold standard, method for body composition analysis and is also known as hydrodensitometry[12]. This method is based on Archimede's principle and can determine the body's density by the following equation: Density = Mass/Volume. Thus, the density of the body can be calculated from the mass of the body and the volume of the body. A volumetric analysis of the body is possible with underwater weighing (body volume can be measured by either hydrodensitometry or air displacement plethysmography). The density of the body is then converted to percent body fat using a 2C model equation, such as the Siri or Brozek body density equation[9,10]. In this technique, the body is divided into two components: fat and FFM. All other popular methods of body composition analyses (e.g., skinfolds, BIA) are validated against hydrodensitometry. Thus, all other body composition methods discussed thus far are less accurate than hydroden-sitometry.

Several variables must be known for the hydrodensitometry method, including (a) the residual volume (which can be measured or predicted using a combination of age, gender, and height), (b) density of the water (which varies with water temperature), (c) trapped gas in the gastrointestinal system (generally a predicted constant is used), (d) dry body weight, and (e) the body weight fully submerged in water. Next, the density of the body may be calculated and then converted to percent body fat using a 2C model prediction equation (see GETP7 Table 4-4).

The test–retest reliability of hydrodensitometry is reported to be excellent (r = 0.95)[11]. Certain groups of the population may realize more error in this measurement than others (e.g., African Americans, youths, elderly individuals). Although the density of lean tissue is assumed to be 1.10 g·cc^{-1} for all, African Americans (>1.11 g·cc^{-1}) and youths (< 1.09 g·cc^{-1}) may have significantly different densities for their lean tissue. The assumption of similar tissue density among different groups (e.g., African Americans and whites) is suspected to be the major problem with the hydrodensitometry method[18].

Major limitations to the practical use of the hydrodensitometry method include space and plumbing requirements, the cost and specialized use of the equipment needed, the time involved in each measurement, the need for an accurate residual volume measurement, and the inherent fear many adults have in staying fully submerged in water for a sufficient time to allow for the weight measurement. Because of these limitations, hydrodensitometry is not a standard part of the body composition assessment strategies used in the health and fitness field.

In addition, within any group of the same age, gender, and race or ethnicity, the density of the FFM varies from individual to individual, resulting in an SEE of about ± 2.7% body fat, even when the measurement technique is performed flawlessly[11].

CLINICAL ASSESSMENT PROCEDURES: COMPUTED TOMOGRAPHY SCANS AND MAGNETIC RESONANCE IMAGING SCANS

Cross-sectional imaging of the whole body is now an available technique for body composition analysis. All the major organs and tissues of the body can be viewed with computed tomography (CT) and magnetic resonance imaging (MRI). These imaging techniques can produce scans that can non-invasively quantify the volume of certain body tissues, such as fat. A total body composition analysis is possible with sequential "slicing" through the body and assumptions for tissue densities. Theses scans use a multicompartment model for body composition. There is a lack of statistical error data to compare these methods with other methods for body composition analysis. These scans may provide an additional benefit in that a relative analysis of muscle and bone density can be performed. Scanning is, thus, extremely useful in clinical settings and research. The use of radiation in CT scans may limit its usefulness for children and some adults. Scanning is typically associated with a high cost, making it impractical[14].

PLETHYSMOGRAPHY: AIR DISPLACEMENT

Body volume can be measured by air displacement rather than water displacement. Air displacement plethysmography is touted as an alternative technique to hydrodensitometry for the many individuals that may experience difficulty with the underwater weighing procedure. One commercial system (Bod Pod) uses a dual-chamber plethysmograph that measures body volume by changes in air pressure within a closed two-compartment chamber. This technology shows promise and generally reduces the anxiety associated with the technique of hydrodensitometry. After body density has been determined, percent

body fat can be calculated. However, most prediction equations used to convert body density to percent body fat using air displacement plethysmography are the same ones used in hydrodensitometry, with the same limitations as derived from the 2C model of body composition[14]. The range for the reported SEE varies from 2.2% to 3.7%[19].

Air displacement plethysmography equipment can be expensive. Body fat estimation requires the measurement or prediction of thoracic gas volume using single use antibacterial filters (additional expense per test), and the technique involves a unique breathing procedure. Also, clients should wear tight-fitting (i.e., Lycra) clothing for measurement.

DUAL-ENERGY X-RAY ABSORPTIOMETRY

Dual-energy x-ray absorptiometry (DXA) is based on a 3C model of total body mineral stores, mineral-free lean mass, and fat mass. DXA can be used to assess total bone mineral as well as regional estimates of bone, fat, and lean tissues. Individual variations in bone mineral are accounted for, and variations in total body water have only minimal effects on the outcome compared with other techniques. DXA uses low-level radiation and is safe, fast, and accurate[14]. The DXA machines are generally large and expensive, although the machines are becoming more accessible in number. Because of the expense of the DXA equipment, it is typically found in a clinical or research setting. Also, there is concern over the lack of standardization between DXA equipment manufacturers. DXA can also be used to measure total bone mineral content, an important variable associated with bone health and aging.

The DXA applies the use of a specialized x-ray device to take measurements (whole-body or segmental scanning) at certain places on the body. DXA is capable of quantification of bone mineral content, total fat mass, and fat-free body mass. Because of the difficulty of generating error statistics for DXA compared with other techniques (e.g., hydrodensitometry), there is a paucity of error data to use and compare. Lohman[17] reported a precision for the DXA technique of about 1% with a SEE of about 1.8% body fat.

A summary of all the discussed body composition techniques can be found in Box 12-2.

INTERPRETATION OF BODY FAT PERCENTAGE ESTIMATES

Interpretation of estimates of body fat percentage is complicated by two major factors. These factors are (a) there are no universal (national or international) standards (either criterion or normative) for percent body fat that have been established and accepted and (b) all methods of measurement are indirect, so the measurement error should be considered. Another important point is that there is no universally accepted criterion measurement method and, thus, for the many different standards that

| BOX 12-2 | Summary of Body Composition Techniques |

SKINFOLD ANALYSIS
- Highly regarded technique yet prone to many sources of error
- Technician training and anatomical site selection important
- Many skinfold formulas exist from single site up to 10 sites
- Not more accurate than hydrodensitometry
- SEE is approximately ± 3.5% (differs with each equation)

BIOELECTRICAL IMPEDANCE
- Less technician training required compared with skinfold measurement
- Numerous pretest control conditions need to be followed by the client (anything that affects body water status)
- SEE is approximately ± 3.5% to 5 % (differs with each equation)

HYDRODENSITOMETRY
- Procedure is time consuming
- Equipment is fairly expensive and requires adequate space and plumbing and high maintenance
- Criterion-reference (or gold) standard
- Some clients may not be able to perform the procedure (complete water submersion at full exhalation)
- Also requires measurement of residual lung volume (additional equipment needed)
- SEE is approximately ± 2.5 %

NEAR-INFRARED INTERACTANCE
- Limited research on this procedure compared with other techniques
- Very little technician training needed
- SEE is approximately ± 5 % (differs with each equation)

CLINICAL ASSESSMENT PROCEDURES: COMPUTED TOMOGRAPHY SCANS AND MAGNETIC RESONANCE IMAGING SCANS
- Procedures are time consuming
- Equipment is expensive and is generally accessible only in clinical facilities
- Has numerous clinical applications
- SEE is not yet fully developed (more research data are needed)

PLETHYSMOGRAPHY: AIR DISPLACEMENT
- Equipment is expensive and is generally accessible only in research facilities
- No physical performance requirements for client (advantage compared with hydrodensitometry)
- Does require special clothing (tight-fitting Lycra-type material)
- SEE is approximately ± 2.2% to 3.7 % (more research data are needed)

DUAL-ENERGY X-RAY ABSORPTIOMETRY
- Equipment is expensive and is generally accessible only in clinical or research facilities
- Has more clinical utility than just percent body fat (also bone density)
- Can provide regional measurements on the body
- SEE is approximately ± 1.8 % (more research data are needed)

have been proposed, many different body fat estimation methods have been used in their development.

Body Fat Percentage Standards

Although national standards have been developed and accepted for BMI and waist circumference (GETP7 Table 4-2), none exist for estimates of body fat percentage. Thus, interpreters of body fat estimates must choose from among the many classification schema that have been proposed by textbook authors, researchers, and programs. Standards may be based on a relationship with either health or with physical performance. From a criterion-based viewpoint, only gender is considered to be a differentiating factor in body fat levels. However, it is well known that body fat percentages also increase with age in the U.S. population. How much of the increase in body fat with age is associated with changes in lifestyle factors (affecting energy intake and energy expenditure) versus what would be considered normal physiological consequences of aging is not completely understood. Thus, all standards for body fat differ by gender and most also differentiate by age.

Since 1981, the *ACSM Guidelines for Exercise Testing and Prescription* has adopted the normative based standards developed by the Institute of Aerobics Research in Dallas, TX. The most current version of these norms was revised in 1994 and was developed using skinfold measurements to estimate body fat percentage in a population of predominately white and college-educated men and women (GETP7 Tables 4-5 and 4-6). These norms provide percentiles that differ by gender and age (ranging from 20 to 60+ years). The average (fiftieth percentile) for young (20 to 29 years) men and women is 15.9% and 22.1%, respectively. The average increases to 23.5% and 30.9% for old (60+ years) men and women, respectively. The difference from the tenth to the ninetieth percentile is approximately 16% points in men and 17% points in women within each of the age groupings.

The National Health and Nutrition Examination Survey (NHANES II)[21] measured triceps and subscapular skinfolds on a representative sample of approximately 20,000 men and women from the United States. These data provide a larger and more heterogeneous sample than what is available from the Institute of Aerobics Research data set. Lohman et al.[22] estimated body fat percentages from the NHANES data using established prediction equations[13,23] and observed that the average (fiftieth percentile) percent body fat for young (20 to 34 years) men and women was 12% and 28%, respectively. They also observed that body fat percentage increased with age. Based on their analyses, they proposed a set of standards for men and women, divided into three age groups, as shown in Figure 12-2. Some increase in body fat with age was allowed. This was done in consideration of recent studies showing that lower body fat or reduced body fat in middle-aged women was associated with a lower bone mineral content, putting women at increased risk for osteoporosis and bone fractures. Thus, the emphasis on lower body fat percentage to prevent heart diseases, especially in women, was balanced against the increased risk of bone fractures, especially if bone mineral content is already low.

Excess body fat has no benefit and is usually detrimental to health. Likewise, excess body fat impairs physical performance of most activities. Thus, from both health and performance perspectives, criterion-based standards are preferred. Unfortunately, here again, no national standards exist for what are considered normal and obese body fat percentages. The most typically used normal (average) values for young adults are 12% to 15% for young men and 22% to 25% for young women. Note that both the Institute of Aerobics Research and NHANES data averages for young adults fall into these ranges, with the exception of a slightly higher (28%) value for young women. Commonly, obesity is considered when body fat values exceed the normal range by at least 5%.

Because of the lack of national standards for body fat, a generalized approach to interpretation can be used. This approach uses the criterion values for young adults as representative of targets for good health. Normalization of the data based on age is obtained by adding 2% each decade, beginning in the thirties. Thus for example, an average value for a 55-year-old man would be 18% to 21% (12% to 15% [criterion value] +6% [2% increase ° 3 decades]).

Measurement Error Considerations

As reviewed earlier, all methods for human body fat percentage assessment are indirect, and the most common method, skinfold measurement, is considered doubly indirect. Because all methods only provide an estimate of body fat percentage, body fat percentage data should be presented and interpreted with the SEE term for the procedure used (ex. 22 ± 3.5%). Minimally, ± 1 SEE unit should be used; however, if the 95% confidence interval (CI) limits are desired, then ± 2 SEE units are required.

A major concern in interpreting body fat percentage values is the relatively large SEE of the measurements. This concern is easily demonstrated by an example using the SEE of ± 3.5% for the most commonly used skinfold equations. Consider a 45-year-old woman who had skinfold measurements taken and had a percent body fat estimated to be 28.5%. Use of the Institute of Aerobics Research standards (GETP7 Table 4-6) for this value would result in an interpretation that she is at the thirty-eighth percentile for women her age. However, when considering the 95% CI (± 2SEE), her body fat percentage may really be as low as 21.5% (eightieth percentile) or as high as 35.5% (<tenth percentile). Certainly, the recommendations by an allied health professional to this woman would be much different if she was 21.5% fat versus 35.5% fat.

Because of the lack of universally accepted national standards and the relatively large SEE, interpretation of percentage body fat estimates needs to be done with caution and with consideration of other known characteristics of the client. The best use of these estimates may be for serial measurement over time or to evaluate responses to lifestyle changes (e.g., diet or physical activity). In this case, the same measurement procedure (and ideally the same instrument and technician) should be used for all repeated measures. Additionally, consideration of the reasonableness of the estimate should be evaluated in light of the known characteristics of the client. For example, an estimated body fat percentage on client that suggests her body composition status is above average should be questioned if it is known that she has been sedentary in recent years and has gained 25 pounds in the past 20 years. Likewise, caution should be used in making recommendations for weight (fat) loss for a client whose estimated body fat suggests he is obese yet it is known that he has been weight stable in adult life and has normal blood pressure, blood lipids, and blood glucose. Obviously comparing the estimated body fat data with the BMI and waist circum-

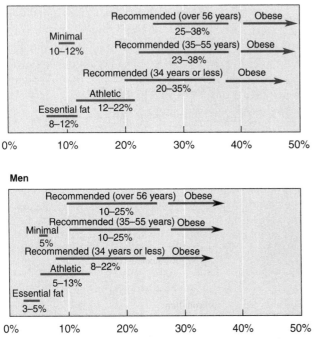

FIGURE 12-2. Percent body fat standards for men and women.

ference classifications would be advantageous for non-athletic adult population.

Acknowledgments
The authors wish to credit the writers of this topic in previous editions of the Resource Manual for their excellent work, specifically Scott Going and Rebecca Davis for their chapter from the 4th edition. Portions of this chapter were retained from the previous editions.

Summary

Excess body fat is detrimental to both health and physical performance. Measurement and quantification of excess fat is of importance to both allied health professionals and athletic personnel. In most non-athletic adults, a reasonable assessment of excess weight (fat) status can be determined from simple measurements of height, weight, and waist circumference. These measurements are easy to obtain, do not require extensive training to perform, and do not require expensive equipment. In clients and circumstances in which more specific information is desired, advanced body composition estimates can be made. It is important for users of these more advanced body fat estimation methods to understand the error associated with these measurements and use the SEE in reporting body composition results.

REFERENCES

1. Wang ZM, Pierson RN, Heymsfield SB: The five level model: A new approach to organizing body composition research. Am J Clin Nutr 56:19–28, 1992.
2. Heymsfield SB, Wang ZM, Withers RT: Multicomponent molecular level models of body composition. In Roche AF, Heymsfield SB, Lohman TG, eds. Human Body Composition. Champaign, IL: Human Kinetics; 1996:129–147.
3. National Heart, Lung, and Blood Institute: Clinical Guidelines on the Identification, Evaluation, and Treatment of Overweight and Obesity in Adults: The Evidence Report. Bethesda, MD: National Institutes of Health, National Heart, Lung, and Blood Institute. U.S. Department of Health and Human Services, Public Health Service; 1998.
4. Lohman TG, Roche AF, Martorell R, eds: Anthropometric Standardization Reference Manual. Champaign, IL: Human Kinetics; 1988.
5. Wang ZM, Heshka S, Pierson RN, et al: Systematic organization of body composition methodology: An overview with emphasis on component-based methods. Am J Clin Nutr 61:457–465, 1995.
6. Heymsfield SB, Wang J, Lichtman S, et al. Body composition in elderly subjects: A critical appraisal of clinical methodology. Am J Clin Nutr 50:1167–1175, 1989.
7. Ellis KJ: Whole-body counting and neutron activation analysis. In Roche AF, Heymsfield SB, Lohman TG, eds. Human Body Composition. Champaign, IL: Human Kinetics; 1996:45–61.
8. Schoeller DA: Hydrometry. In Roche AF, Heymsfield SB, Lohman TG, eds. Human Body Composition. Champaign, IL: Human Kinetics; 1996:25–43.
9. Brozek J, Grande F, Anderson J, et al: Densitometric analysis of body composition: revision of some quantitative assumptions. Am NY Acad Sci 110:113–140, 1963.
10. Siri WE: The gross composition of the body. Adv Biol Med Physiol 4:239–280, 1956.
11. Lohman TG: Advances in Body Composition Assessment. Champaign, IL: Human Kinetics; 1992.
12. Going SB, Williams DP, Lohman TG: Aging and body composition: Biological changes and methodological issues. Exerc Sport Sci Rev 23:411–458, 1995.
13. Going SB: Densitometry. In Roche AF, Heymsfield SB, Lohman TG, eds: Human Body Composition. Champaign, IL: Human Kinetics; 1996: 3–23.
14. Heyward VH, Wagner DR: Applied Body Composition Assessment. Champaign, IL: Human Kinetics; 2004.
15. Jackson AS, Pollock ML: Generalized equations for predicting body density of men. Br J Nutr 61:497–504, 1978.
16. Baumgartner RN: Electrical impedance and total body electrical conductivity. In Roche AF, Heymsfield SB, Lohman TG, eds. Human Body Composition. Champaign, IL: Human Kinetics; 1996:79–107.
17. Erickson JM, Stout JR, Eveertourch TK, et al: Validity of self-assessment techniques for estimating percent body fat in men and women. J Stren Cond Res 12:243–247, 1998.
18. Malina, RM: Regional body composition: Age, sex, and ethnic variation. In oche AF, Heymsfield SB, Lohman TG, eds. Human Body Composition. Champaign, IL: Human Kinetics, 1996:217–255.
19. Fields DA, Goran MI, McCory MA: Body composition assessments via air displacement plethysmography in adults and children: a review. Am J Clin Nutr 75:453–467. 2002.
20. Lohman TG: Dual energy x-ray absorptiometry. In Roche AF, Heymsfield SB, Lohman TG, eds. Human Body Composition. Champaign, IL: Human Kinetics; 1996:63–78.
21. U.S. Department of Health and Human Resources: Basic data on anthropometric measurements and angular measurements of the hip and knee joints for selected age groups 1–74 years of age (1971–1975). DHHS Publication No. (PHS) 81–1669, Series II, No. 219, 2003.
22. Lohman TG, Houtkooper LB, Going SB: Body composition assessment: Body fat standards and methods in the field of exercise and sports medicine. ACSM Health Fitness J 1:30–35, 1997.
23. Jackson AS, Pollock ML, Ward A: Generalized equations for predicting body density of women. Med Sci Sports Exerc 12: 175–182, 1980.

SELECTED REFERENCES FOR FURTHER READING

Heyward VH, Wagner DR: Applied Body Composition Assessment. Champaign, IL: Human Kinetics, 2nd ed.; 2004.
Lohman TG, Roche AF, Martorell R, eds: Anthropometric Standardization Reference Manual. Champaign, IL: Human Kinetics; 1988.
National Heart, Lung, and Blood Institute: Clinical Guidelines on the Identification, Evaluation, and Treatment of Overweight and Obesity in Adults: The Evidence Report. Bethesda, MD: National Institutes of Health, National Heart, Lung, and Blood Institute, U.S. Department of Health and Human Services, Public Health Service; 1998.
Roche AF, Heymsfield SB, Lohman TG. Human Body Composition, Champaign, IL: Human Kinetics; 1996.
Yasmura S, Wang J, Pierson RN, eds: In vivo body composition studies. Ann N Y Acad Sci 904, 1–631, 2000.

INTERNET RESOURCES

Body Fat Lab:
http://www.shapeup.org/bodylab/frmst.htm

National Heart Lung and Blood Institute: Clinical Guidelines on the Identification, Evaluation, and Treatment of Overweight and Obesity in Adults: http://www.nhlbi.nih.gov/guidelines/obesity/ob_home.htm

National Institutes Of Health : Calculate your body mass index:
http://www.nhlbisupport.com/bmi

National Center for Health Statistics. National Health and Nutrition Examination Survey. http://www.cdc.gov/nchs/nhanvs.htm

BRENDAN HUMPHRIES, ERIC L. DUGAN, AND TIM L.A. DOYLE

Muscular Fitness

The primary characteristics of muscular fitness are muscular strength and flexibility. Muscular strength further refines to the qualities of maximal strength, muscular endurance, muscle power, reactive strength, and functional strength. Both muscular strength and flexibility play an important role in the overall physical fitness and health of individuals. Other important fitness and health parameters include cardiorespiratory fitness, psychological health, and body composition. The assessment of muscular strength qualities can be achieved using both laboratory and field assessment measurements using a variety of muscular contractions. There are five basic types of muscle contraction: isotonic (constant load), isokinetic (velocity dependent), isometric (constant joint angle), concentric (shortening of a muscle), and eccentric (lengthening of a muscle)[1–4].

The most recognized quality of muscular strength is **maximal muscular strength**, and it represents the capacity of skeletal muscle to voluntarily develop forces in a single tetanic contraction at a specific velocity[1,3]. The "reference standard" for the laboratory assessment of maxi-

mal muscle strength may include (a) a maximal isotonic contraction[1,5], (b) a single maximal voluntary isometric contraction (MVC)[4], or (c) isokinetic peak torque[4,6]. There are no equivalent field tests for these laboratory techniques; however, because of the widespread use of strength training equipment, the isotonic **one repetition maximum (1RM)** assessment can be done in most weight training facilities.

Yet another quality of muscular strength is **muscular endurance**. This term refers to the ability of the muscle to delay the onset or minimize the effects of fatigue during repeated contractions using a relative (% of 1RM) or absolute (selected resistance) load at a given velocity[1,5]. The method of assessment for muscular endurance typically involves a series of repetitions using either isotonic or isokinetic contractions or a sustained isometric contraction (30 to 60 s). The assessment of muscle endurance can be conducted in both laboratory- and field-based settings. The field-based tests to assess muscular endurance typically involve repeated lifts using weight training equipment, an individual's own body weight (number of push-ups or sit-ups in a designated time), or the timed number of lifts or throws using a weighted object such as a medicine ball[5].

The muscular strength quality of power is determined by work and time. Power represents the ability of the muscle to contract and perform work either instantaneously or averaged for any portion of a single movement or a series of movements (ms to 3 s). The laboratory measures for power aim to measure the distance and time of an explosive isotonic, isokinetic, or isometric performance for either the upper or lower body. The field-based tests assess power as a single maximal movement for height (vertical jump) or distance (standing broad jump, five-hop test, medicine ball throw). The muscular strength quality of reactive strength is related to that of power but is based on the ability to react to a change in direction, load, and contraction. The functional measures of strength are designed to assess the strength of an individual under conditions that match everyday activities specific to movement velocity, action, and balance between the left and right sides of the body.

Another aspect of muscular fitness relates to the ability of the muscular system to maintain optimal movement

KEY TERMS

Dynamic flexibility: The ability to perform dynamic (or kinetic) movements of the muscles to bring a limb through its full range of motion in the joints

Free weight exercise (constant resistance): To use a constant load based on barbells or dumbbells throughout the range of motion

Machine weight exercise (variable resistance): To use a variable load based on cams, pulleys, and levers throughout the range of motion

Maximal muscular strength: The peak force developed during a maximal voluntary contraction

Muscular endurance: The body's ability to sustain submaximal muscular contractions with minimal local fatigue

One repetition maximum: The maximal amount of load that can be lifted in a single effort

Range of movement: The amount of motion available at a given joint (or joints)

Resistance training: Training the muscles of the body to increase strength, power, or muscular endurance through moving a load or weight; the most common form is weight training

Static flexibility: The ability to assume extended positions and then maintain them using only your weight, the support of your limbs, or some other apparatus

ranges and muscle suppleness at the intended site. The term used to address this aspect of muscular fitness is joint flexibility or, more precisely, range of motion (ROM) at the joint (or joints) of interest. An individual's flexibility is related to the structural limitations of the joint (or joints), the mechanical properties of the muscles and connective tissues of the joint (or joints), neuromuscular properties relating to length and rate of length change of the muscle (or muscles), agonist and antagonist interaction, and the ability of the subject to advance to the joint limits[3,7,8]. Improvements to joint flexibility help reduce muscle tension and may reduce the risk of muscle and tendon injuries. The assessment of joint flexibility requires the use of standard testing methods to ensure accuracy and reliability The evaluation of joint ROM can be made under conditions of passive (external control) or active (active muscular control) joint movements.

Physiological and Mechanical Factors of Muscles

The physiological and mechanical factors that contribute to the expression of strength include neurological, hormonal, muscle fiber type and size, and biomechanical characteristics. The neurological factors associated with strength have been well documented[7–10] and are responsible for making efficient use of the contractile elements of the musculature[10]. Neural adaptations contribute to the increase in strength, primarily during the early phases of a resistance training program as a result of learning and recognition of motor patterns[9,10]. The continued changes in strength after approximately 8 to 12 weeks of training are associated with hypertrophy resulting from changes in the muscle contractile elements such as increased muscle fiber size and cellular components (increased sarcomeres, enzymes, fuel stores)[1,2,9,10]. The continued changes in

muscular strength in response to resistance training are also influenced by hormonal factors.

The hormonal factors responsible for strength development are incredibly complex and predominately relate to anabolic hormones that increase protein synthesis[10,11]. The primary differences in hypertrophic changes with resistance training probably stem from gender-specific anabolic effects, testosterone (males), and estrogen (females). These hormonal responses can also be influenced by the frequency, intensity, and type of training a person performs[11]. Because of the complex nature of the endocrine system, much research is required to gain a thorough understanding of the interactions of hormones on the development of strength and the adaptations to muscle fiber type and size.

Muscle fiber type and size also contribute to the development of muscular strength (also see Chapter 3). Historically, skeletal muscle fibers were categorized as either type I slow oxidative (SO), type IIa fast oxidative glycolytic (FOG), or type IIb fast glycolytic (FG). Type I or SO fibers being innervated by small motor neurons belonging to the type S motor unit, which fire at low frequencies, have slow conduction velocities and are specialized for sustained contractions[11–14]. Type IIa and IIb fibers are innervated by slightly larger corresponding motor neurons, type FR and type FF motor units, that fire at high frequencies, have fast conduction velocities, and are specialized for short-duration contractions[12,13] The taxonomy of human skeletal muscle fibers may be better described as a continuum of fiber populations between typed I and II[14]. At present, the majority of subdivisions present in human skeletal muscle are found within the fast-twitch fiber group. These include intermediate type IIa, FG or type IIb, intermediate variable type IIab, and variable type IIc fibers[12,13] More recently, these subdivisions of fast-twitch fibers have been extended to include another category known as type IIx. Currently, the following seven different muscle fiber types have been identified: I, IC, IIA, IIB, IIAB, IIC, and IIX[14]. It is not unrealistic to assume that further subdivisions within the current classification of fiber types will be established as technology improves. Although muscle fiber type influences skeletal muscle strength, it is unclear whether this factor is genetically determined or is a direct result of strength training. Research studies have attempted to solve this issue; however, some studies report no changes in the proportion of muscle fiber type secondary to resistance training[2]. In contrast, other studies have shown proportional increases in the cross-sectional area (CSA) of type I and II muscle fibers and an increase in type IIa fibers after heavy resistance training programs[15–18].

Muscle size also plays a role in the expression of overall strength. It has been shown that increases in muscle CSA and overall muscle mass have been significantly correlated with improvements in strength[8,18]. Likewise, a decrease in CSA or muscle mass has been shown to accompany proportional strength decrements. A change in strength performance resulting from a decrease in muscle mass is evident in inactive and aging populations and as a result of joint immobilization. The biomechanical factors such as lever length, bone strength, and tendon insertions also contribute to the expression of muscle strength[19,20]. Although these factors are important for the expression of strength, they are not factors that can be quickly influenced as a result of training.

Resistance training encompasses various forms of conditioning modalities that require the muscle to contract against a load. The global term *resistance training* not only includes strength training, weight lifting, and circuit training but can also be associated with other forms of conditioning such as plyometrics, water workouts, body weight exercises, impact landings, resistive ball exercises, isokinetic or isometric modalities, and even activities of daily living. The essential purposes of resistance training programs are to improve maximal muscle strength, muscle endurance, power, and reactive and functional strength and as a prehabilitative means to prevent injury. Resistance training programs have been used across a wide range of populations and for a multitude of health-related purposes. Resistance training has been advocated to improve athletic performance; for injury rehabilitation; to improve health and fitness in industrial athletes, children, and aging populations; for conditions such as obesity, arthritis, diabetes, anorexia nervosa, osteoporosis, cardiovascular disease, and neuromuscular disorders; and for recipients of organ transplants, stroke victims, and others (see Chapter 25 and GETP7 Chapter 7). The common denominator for these programs is an accurate assessment of the appropriate muscular strength qualities before the initiation of the training program. This can be used as a benchmark to assess improvement and as the basis for establishing training intensities.

Measurement of Muscular Strength

Over the past 50 years, the scientific information available concerning the development of muscular fitness has increased dramatically. Muscular assessment has expanded into so many specific components that sometimes it becomes difficult to find specific application to training programs (Table 13-1). Under such circumstances, it becomes apparent that a set of standardized testing protocols and procedures is necessary so research findings easily transfer to training. However, considerable variation exists in research methodologies, experimental design, reporting of data, and the overall interpretation of test results.

In general, the assessment of strength is determined by the amount of weight or load that can be pushed or pulled in a standardized manner. Factors that should be a standard part of this assessment include a consistent ROM for each test, controlling excessive acceleration or deceleration of the load (unless instructed), and limiting any body movement (or movements) or muscle contributions not involved in the lift. These conditions must be strictly adhered to while maintaining the correct technique in order to provide useful results.

Muscular Strength Tests

ASSESSMENT OF MAXIMAL ISOTONIC STRENGTH

The most common term used to describe the eccentric and concentric muscular action used in resistance training is an *isotonic contraction*. However, this is a misnomer because an isotonic contraction is not commonly used in everyday activities or during standard resistance training. The application of the term *isotonic* may be criticized because the actual force applied to the external load rarely remains constant as it is lifted through a range of movement. Acceleration and deceleration phases, as well as changes in mechanical advantage, cause variations in the applied force. However, the term *isotonic* is widely used throughout the literature. The term *isoinertial* has also been used to describe the process of muscle contractions in standard resistance training. The term *isoinertial* represents an individuals ability to overcome the initial static resistance but thereafter as the load is moved throughout the range of the joint (or joints), the mechanical advantage is altered, so the relative force (mass and acceleration) required to move the resistance must vary[19–21]. Although both terms do not represent mechanically the contraction taking place when lifting a weight, both terms are frequently used to describe the contraction of muscle when lifting weights.

Maximal dynamic muscular strength is typically measured by the 1RM method for a particular movement (See GETP7 Tables 4-9 and 4-10). The 1RM is defined as the weight that can be successfully lifted no more than one time without failure through a specified ROM[4,21–23]. In

TABLE 13-1. Laboratory and Field Measures for the Various Strength Qualities

Strength Parameter	Test	Movement Pattern	Contraction Speed/Type	Test Equipment	Test Location
Maximal muscle strength	1RM	Isoinertial/isotonic	Slow, concentric	Free weights; machines	Laboratory, field
	MVC	Isometric	Slow, isometric	Load cells; dynamometers (hand, back)	Laboratory, field
	Maximal torque	Isokinetic	Slow, concentric	Isokinetic dynammometer	Laboratory
	Maximal eccentric	Isoinertial, isotonic	Slow, eccentric	Free weights (load cells; transducers)	Laboratory
Muscle endurance	Relative muscle endurance (% 1RM)	Isoinertial, isotonic	Slow, concentric	Free weights; machine	Laboratory, field
	Absolute muscle endurance (selected weight)	Isoinertial, isotonic	Slow, concentric	Free weights; machine	Laboratory, field
	Mean torque (# contractions; fatigue level)	Isokinetic	Slow, concentric	Isokinetic dynammometer	Laboratory
	Abdominal sit-up test	SSC	Controlled, concentric, eccentric	Timer; metronome	Field
	Push-up test	SSC	Controlled, concentric, eccentric	Timer; metronome	Field
	Chin-up test	SSC	Controlled, concentric, eccentric	Timer; metronome	Field
Muscle power	RFD	Isometric	Fast, concentric	Load cells; force plate	Laboratory
	Explosive power movements	SSC	Fast, eccentric/concentric	Smith machine and linear transducer	Laboratory
	Vertical jump	SSC	Fast, eccentric, concentric	Yardstick; linear transducer; force plate; video	Laboratory, field
	Standing broad jump	SSC	Fast, eccentric, concentric	Measuring tape; linear transducer; video	Laboratory, field
	Five-hop test	SSC	Fast, eccentric, concentric	Measuring tape; linear transducer; video	Laboratory, field
	Medicine ball throws	SSC	Fast, eccentric, concentric	Measuring tape; video; force plate	Laboratory, field
Reactive muscle Strength	Drop jump	SSC	Fast eccentric/concentric	Drop heights, timing mats	Laboratory, field
Functional muscle strength	Closed-chain functional tests (jumps; cutting; hops)	SSC	Fast, eccentric, concentric	Timing mats; timing gates	Laboratory, field
	Gait analysis	SSC	Controlled, eccentric, concentric	Timing mats; timing gates; load cells; foot pressure mats; force plates; NeuroCom Balance Master; video	Laboratory

MVC = maximal voluntary isometric contraction; RFD = rate of force development; SSC = stretch-short style.

this situation, the maximal force is high and the velocity of contraction is quite low. Typically, the performance of the 1RM is deemed unsuccessful under the following criteria: (a) any lift that does not incorporate the full ROM; (b) any lift not performed primarily by the specified muscle groups; and (c) any performance that compromises the in-tegrity of the lift, such as a shift in body position or the inclusion of body movement. The test and retest reliability for most 1RM lifts range between good to excellent. The small differences in reliability between various testing laboratories are caused partly by the populations being assessed, the variation in methodologies used in testing, the muscle groups being tested, and the fact that 1RM tests are multiarticular.

Standard testing parameters required when performing a 1RM assessment (see GETP7 p. 82) include a consistent contraction duration of 3 to 5 seconds to complete each lift; a minimum rest period of 3 to 5 minutes between repeat attempts to establish 1RM to minimize the effects of fatigue; reaching the maximal load with minimal trials (three to five trials); providing an adequate warm-up that incorporates gradual submaximal increments in load with reciprocal decreases in repetitions; maintaining the same motivation for all subjects; explaining all the conditions associated with a successful lift before testing; and implementing a set of homogeneous conditions for body, foot, and hand position.

The 1RM has been used as the gold standard of dynamic maximal isotonic muscle assessment since the early 1960s. Although the 1RM lift is recognized as the standard, it is common to see various hybrid strength measures developed from this measure. Over the past 10 years, there has been a trend to use various combinations of exercises to predict the 1RM. Common used predictors include the use of submaximal or repetition maximums (RM) such as 3RM, 6RM, and 10RM. These lifts are defined as the maximum number of repetitions performed before fatigue prohibits the completion of an additional repetition. The greater the number of repetitions used to estimate strength, the more the lift becomes reliant on muscular endurance and less on maximal strength, reducing its effectiveness to predict the 1RM. The predicted 1RM is based on the performance of submaximal loads, body mass, percentage loads, repetitions completed, or some combination of these factors.

Multiple repetitions of submaximal loads have been used to estimate the 1RM of various populations, including elite athletes, novices, specific sports groups, children, and elderly individuals[3,23,24]. The idea behind using submaximal lifts such as the 3RM to predict 1RM is to overcome motivational barriers of performing maximally, reduce the likelihood of injury, and overcome a lack of recent training. Although these are good reasons for performing submaximal lifts, the end result is that there is just as much motivation, if not more, required to perform for a longer period when completing three near-maximal lifts. Likewise, when performing a 3RM lift, the person is placed under a greater stress for a greater period of time, increasing the potential for injury. For example, whereas a 1RM lift at 100 kg (918 N) taking 4 seconds provides a 3924 N·s of load on the musculature, a 3RM at 85 kg (834 N) taking 4 seconds per repetition would equate to 10008 N·s of load on the musculature. Using estimates or predicted equations for the 1RM that incorporate multiple-RM lifts can underestimate or overestimate the actual 1RM lift. Another limitation of the multiple-RM lifts is that it can have a profound effect on an individual's results such that novice lifters are often underestimated and well-trained lifters are overestimated in their 1RM values.

Maximal muscular strength has also been assessed using maximal eccentric contractions where a maximum load selected as 130% to 150% of the maximum 1RM is lowered during a 4-second time frame. The most common lifts used for this type of testing are the bench press and squat. The test involves maintaining constant eccentric lowering force set between a force window of 10% to 20% above or below the actual lowering force, as monitored by a force plate. The bar movement is also tracked so a constant bar velocity is maintained during the descent of the lift, as measured by a linear transducer. It is important to closely monitor force and bar velocity to ensure that they fall within the test parameters.

In addition to performance assessment, the 1RM measure is also used to assist in developing training intensities using the 1RM or percentages of the 1RM. For example, a person who can lift 70 kg 10 times before exhaustion has completed a 10RM. The amount of weight that can be lifted based on a percentage of the 1RM value is referred to as percent RM. For example, if a 1RM lift is 100 kg and a person performs repetitions at 80% 1RM, he or she is lifting 80 kg. Training intensities are typically represented by either %RM or RM values[20–23,24,26], as presented in Table 13-2.

ASSESSMENT OF ISOTONIC MUSCULAR ENDURANCE

Almost all devices for measuring maximal muscular strength can be used to assess muscular endurance. Tests of muscular endurance are designed to evaluate the ability of muscle groups to produce submaximal force for an extended period. Measures of muscular endurance include time to fatigue, number of contractions, and percentage strength decline for a given time epoch. Similar to the maximal strength measure already discussed, the endurance measures can also be assessed under the same muscle contraction conditions[3,5,13].

The isotonic measurement of muscular endurance using free weights or machines can be achieved by measuring the relative or absolute strength of the person. The relative strength measure requires the person to lift a load that represents a percentage of his or her 1RM for as many con-

TABLE 13-2. Percentage of One Repetition Maximum and the Range of Repetitions That are Typically Used in Training

% One Repetition Maximum	Repetition Range
60	16–18
65	14–16
70	12–14
75	10–12
80	8–10
85	6–8
90	4–6
95	2–4
100	1

tractions as possible[25]. An example is to have a person attempt to perform as many repetitions as possible at 60% of his or her 1RM. A concern of selecting a relative load arises when using experienced or well-trained individuals because stronger individuals can perform more repetitions at a given RM percentage than weaker individuals. As a comparative test between groups of individuals, the relative endurance test becomes a reliable muscular endurance test when using standard guidelines for testing. These guidelines are based on those used for 1RM maximal lifting.

The absolute measure of muscular endurance requires the individual to perform as many repetitions as possible at an arbitrary load such as 45 or 60 kg[25]. As a comparative test, novice lifters may be disadvantaged because this load could exceed their capability or is much closer to their maximal lift (e.g., it is more of a strength test versus an endurance test). The relative endurance test, therefore, becomes a more reliable and equitable test than the absolute endurance test[25]. Another variation of the absolute strength test is to implement the YMCA model in which each individual is assessed using an individually assigned absolute load based on training background and occupational demands (see GETP7 Table 4-13).

Yet another variation of the muscle endurance test is to perform as many lifts as possible of the pretraining 1RM load at the completion of a training period. The primary limitation with this strategy is assuming that there will be an improvement in 1RM. Muscle endurance can also be assessed using an individual's own body mass in the form of push-ups (upper arm and shoulder musculature), chin-ups (back and arm musculature), or sit-ups (abdominal musculature). The objective of these tests is to determine the absolute number of lifts that can be performed or the number of lifts that can be performed in a set time frame such as 60 seconds. It is equally important to standardize the hand and arm position, body position, and depth of the body movement during these body weight lifts so an accurate assessment of endurance is obtained.

ASSESSMENT OF ISOMETRIC POWER, REACTIVE STRENGTH, AND FUNCTIONAL STRENGTH

The laboratory assessment for muscle power involves the use of transducer instrumented equipment such as a smith machine. The instrumented equipment is interfaced with a computer with which specialized software calculates the distance, time, velocity, and acceleration of the bar during a lift. The mass is also measured or entered into the software to determine force and power of the lift. The measurement of power can be calculated as the peak or average power of the lift. The field tests used to assess muscle power include the vertical jump, standing broad jump (long jump), and the five-hop test. Each of these field measures aims to determine the peak displacement of a single performance. The measurement of these variables

uses a tape measure and a set of stringent guidelines to perform each test. For a vertical jump, the maximal reach height of the dominant side is measured before the subject performs a single step followed by a jump or a countermovement jump. The standing broad jump involves the subject's standing with feet parallel and the toes at a starting line. The subject swings the arms backward and crouches and then immediately performs a forward arm swing and jump. The displacement is recorded at the back of the foot closest to the starting line. The five-hop test is performed similar to the standing broad jump in that the person propels the body as far forward using five consecutive hops on one side of the body and then the other. The test is measured in the same manner as the standing broad jump. Three trials for each test are performed, with the peak displacement recorded to represent the power of the lower limbs. A variation on the power measurements is the two-handed chest pass or a single arm put of a medicine ball for maximal distance. The displacement can be recorded on a tape measure or more accurately with a tape measure and video recorder to determine power.

The assessment of reactive strength has been assessed using a drop jump movement performed over a force-plate. The test involves the subject stepping off a box, between 20 and 120 cm; landing on a force plate; and immediately reacting by performing a vertical jump for maximal height. Values for reactive strength are based on peak force, peak height, and ratios between force and contact time.

The assessment of functional strength typically involves measuring the force, time, distance, or some combination of ratios between these values and the balance between the left and right sides of the body. The most common form of functional strength is the measurement of gait using force plates, video cameras, timing gates, and foot pressure mats. The data recorded are used to determine stride length and rate, step width, heel contact, toe off, foot pressure distribution, joint ROM and velocity, and gait velocity.

ASSESSMENT OF MAXIMAL ISOMETRIC STRENGTH

During an isometric contraction, the muscle is prevented from shortening by fixing both of its ends so that the muscle develops tension at its points of attachment. In everyday activities, isometric contractions contribute to the maintenance of posture, torso stabilization, and efforts against immovable objects. Muscular strength can be assessed using an MVC; this maximal contraction is performed at a specific joint angle against an immovable resistance[1,2,4,9,13]. It is important to remember that the peak strength and the rate at which that strength can be produced when performing an isometric contraction vary with joint position. These indices of muscle strength change as the elastic components of the muscle and tendinous tissue are placed under different levels of stretch and the angle of pull of the muscle on bone is altered.

Isometric testing is a useful, relatively inexpensive, and accurate mode of testing muscular strength that can be conducted using simple cable tensiometry or hand-grip and back-leg dynamometers. Alternatively, isometric strength can be assessed using a multitude of computerized dynamometers that are expensive and very accurate, provide an automatic correction for gravity, control for extraneous body movement, and allow for elaborate methods of data manipulation. The computerized methods of collecting data on isometric muscular contractions provide for a variety of data analysis options. The peak force recorded during the performance is used as the maximal isometric force. Peak isometric strength can also be measured using commercial isokinetic dynamometers such as Cybex, (Cybex International, Medway, MA) Kin-Com Chattanooga Group, Chattanooga, TN, and Biodex (Biodex Medical Systems, Shirley, NY) systems using a velocity setting at 0 degrees per second. These commercial isokinetic dynamometers also provide the ability to control the joint angle. The test and retest reliability of the isometric devices mentioned above has been shown to range from good to excellent.

Standard testing parameters required to perform a MVC lasting 3 to 5 seconds to assess strength and power include consistent instructions to all participants that reflect the intended assessment criteria; the contraction needs to be of maximal force and as rapid as possible; appropriate limb immobilization so only the joint of interest is assessed; and accurate joint positioning. Other considerations include a thorough warm-up, familiarization trials, consistent motivation, and 1 to 2 minutes of recovery between contractions lasting 10 seconds or less. Another important issue when collecting isometric force data using computerized methods is to select a reasonable sampling rate between 200 and 1000 Hz so as not to eliminate any data that may provide information about the contraction.

ASSESSMENT OF ISOMETRIC MUSCULAR ENDURANCE

The measurement of isometric muscular endurance requires the individual to maintain a single contraction over an extended period of time to so the rate at which strength declines can be examined. Similar to the maximal isometric strength measures, these tests can be performed using the computerized method or handheld dynamometer to track the decay in force production or simply the time to strength decline below a set level such as 50% of peak strength. Standard testing parameters required to perform a sustained MVC lasting between 10 to 30 s are similar to those of the MVC to assess strength and power. The exception for a fatigue decrement assessment is in the instructions provided to perform the contraction; the contraction needs to graduate to a peak force and be maintained. Likewise, recovery between repeat contractions requires between 3 and 5 minutes of rest. The computerized method of data collection provides a greater variation of calculated measures for the endurance test compared with the simple handheld dynamometers. The computerized method also allows for greater accuracy during this type of assessment compared with the handheld measures, which do not continuously record the information.

ASSESSMENT OF ISOMETRIC POWER

Following the guidelines for maximal isometric assessment as already discussed, isometric power is measured as the rate at which force or torque is developed or, more aptly, the rate of force development (RFD). The following variables are often assessed in association with the RFD: peak RFD; RFD at 30%, 60%, or 90% of peak force (PF); time (or times) to develop PF at 30%, 60%, or 90% of PF (or some other percentage); or the slope of the curve averaged over 5, 10, 20, or 30 ms bins. In the force time analysis, it is important to include measures early (30% PF) and later (90% PF) in the contraction because of requirements of sport, work, performance, and the effects of training that may be specific to a particular phase of the contraction. Some of the limitations of isometric testing include the following: (a) determining the baseline strength or contraction commencement, (b) determining initial PF on a smoothed curve, (c) determining PF on an uneven curve, and (d) using average rate of force rather than instantaneous rate of force such as over a 5-ms interval. An example of typical isometric force trace can be seen in Figure 13-1.

ASSESSMENT OF MAXIMAL ISOKINETIC STRENGTH

Another mode of muscular assessment that limits or maintains the velocity of the body segment at a preselected and constant level is referred to as *isokinetic muscular performance testing*. The term *isokinetic* is used to describe constant-velocity concentric and eccentric contractions. Isokinetic dynamometers measure the force or moment exerted by the muscle or muscle groups contracting against a controlled accommodating resistance. Isokinetic dynamometry can trace its origins back to the early 1970s but did not become a popular strength assessment device until 10 years later. Since the development of the isokinetic dynamometer, it has undergone many improvements, with the current devices using servo-controlled motors to move the lever arms at a constant preset speed as the subject exerts effort against the lever. The latest devices are also interfaced with high-quality computers and software to manipulate an array of measuring possibilities. In particular, the isokinetic devices typically can assess muscular contractions through a range of testing velocities spanning 0 to 500 degrees per second. It is important to be aware that the ability of a muscle to generate concentric force is greatest at slower velocities and decreases as the testing velocity is increased.

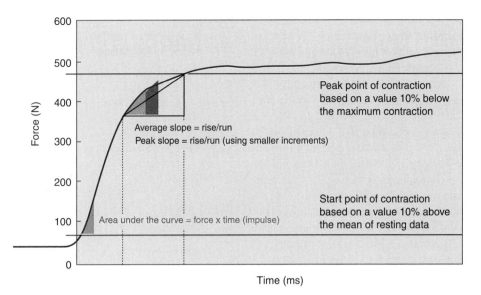

FIGURE 13-1. The isometric force trace indicates a standard technique for start and finish times, area under the curve, and slope of the curve values based on an arbitrary time frame.

The commercial isokinetic dynamometers provide valuable information about muscular assessments through numerous isokinetic, isotonic (concentric, eccentric), and isometric strength variables. In addition, these devices can be used to assess power and endurance. The data obtained from an isokinetic evaluation may be used to assess muscular strength in various populations, predict susceptibility to injury, monitor a rehabilitative program, or assist in developing a prehabilitative comparative tool for workers and athletes returning to normal activities after a therapeutic exercise program. The isokinetic muscular strength measurements possible from an isokinetic dynamometer include variables such as peak torque, average torque, angle specific torque, power and RFD (only from high testing speeds, i.e., 300 degrees per second and higher).

The range in test–retest reliability (Intra-Class Correlation [ICC]: r = 0.01 to 0.98), associated with isokinetic assessments have stemmed from problems such as a lack of proper instruction and familiarization of the patient with the testing procedure, type of contraction (concentric, eccentric, isometric, isokinetic, isotonic), contraction sequence (eccentric/concentric, eccentric/eccentric, concentric/concentric, concentric/eccentric), pretest procedures (warm-up, gravity correction, starting position, stabilization, axes alignment, lever-arm length, preload), limb dominance, test conditions (speed, test sequence, rest intervals, feedback), and type of data analysis[27–32].

The standard procedures for isokinetic muscular assessments should include sufficient familiarization of subjects, accurate placement and recording of lever arm placements, sufficient warm–up at submaximal speeds graduating to testing speed, and accurate aligning of the joint center to the machine pivotal axis.

ASSESSMENT OF ISOKINETIC MUSCULAR ENDURANCE

Isokinetic endurance measures are also possible and are based on the capacity of the muscle to produce force at a constant velocity over multiple contractions. Isokinetic endurance is assessed using multiple contraction fatiguing protocols and quantified as a contraction number, time, or a torque decline value that falls below 50% of the maximum value. Endurance has also been quantified as a percentage based on the average of three initial and final contractions in a series of 30 or 50 contractions. In terms of muscular assessment, isokinetic dynamometry has also been used to provide bilateral muscle group comparisons, usually between injured and uninjured limbs, and to determine muscular balance between flexor and extensor muscle groups. The test and retest reliability in isokinetic measures, as previously discussed, have been shown to provide good results based on normal populations[6]. Interestingly, there have been mixed results reported on the test–retest reliability when assessing individuals presenting with pathologies[27]. With all maximal and endurance muscular assessments, the results obtained are most valuable and reliable if the participants provide a full and maximum voluntary effort. Under these circumstances, the assessment produces reliable results. Assessments that are based on contractions that are less than a 100% effort produce less-than-desirable results.

Free Weights Versus Machines

A **free weight exercise** involves the application of constant resistance to a freely moving body using equipment such as barbells, dumbbells, medicine balls, and body mass. A **machine weight exercise** incorporates a guided application of variable resistance that follows the path of an elliptical, circular, or kidney bean–shaped track or a lever system. Machines include resistance based on loaded weight plates, pin-loaded stacks, pneumatic devices, electronically braked devices, springs, and rubber band devices. Both free weights and machines play a vital role in the development of muscular strength qualities.

Resistance training offers far greater potential rewards than it does possible safety concerns. Considering all the variations in resistance training and the populations using the benefits of resistance training, this form of training is relatively safe, with very few injuries reported from testing or training. Even considering the lack of injuries from resistance training programs, there is a long-standing argument that resistance training involving machine weights is safer than resistance training using free weights; however, there is no evidence to support this belief[33]. Each form of training has its own strengths and weaknesses, as reported in Box 13-1.

A concluding comment about the use of free weights and machines is that current information indicates that for most activities training with complex, multi-joint exercises using free weights can produce superior results compared with training with machine weights[34]. The underlying logic here is that free weights more closely mimic movement patterns and match muscular activation patterns associated with these movements. Based on the advantages listed above, the use of free weight exercises should dominate in resistance training programs. Machine weights should be implemented as an adjunct to free weight training.

Muscular Strength Assessment and Special Populations

AGING

Under normal conditions, muscle strength in women and men reaches its peak between the ages of 20 and 30 years, after which it remains virtually unchanged for another 20 years, if unaffected by injury[35]. After the age of 45 years, there is an accelerated loss in strength[13,35,36,37]. This deterioration of muscular performance occurs at a rate of about 5% per decade, amounting to a 30% to 40% loss of functional strength over the adult life span[13]. Some researchers have indicated a less severe loss of 18% to 20%[37], and still others have shown no change or significant deterioration in muscle strength before age of 60 years[38]. After age 60 years, the loss of muscle strength has been reported at a consistent rate of 1% to 2% per year for dynamic, isometric, and isokinetic contractions[37]. The variation in research concerning the decline in muscle strength of elderly populations may reflect the diversity of occupations, training backgrounds, an over-

| BOX 13-1 | Advantages and Disadvantages of Using Free Weights and Machines Weights |

ADVANTAGES OF FREE WEIGHTS
1. Incorporates either multi- and single-joint exercises
2. Wide versatility of exercise selection
3. Effectively mimics athletic and ergonomic tasks
4. Greater mechanical specificity and variation of exercises
5. Greater specificity to muscular activation patterns of a specific task
6. Greater metabolic contribution (use more muscle groups per exercise)
7. Greater contribution to proprioception because of three-dimensional movement
8. Greater contribution to training intensity because of multi-joint muscle involvement
9. Greater sensitivity to manipulate loads (1.25-kg plate increments)

ADVANTAGES OF MACHINE WEIGHTS
1. Safe and ease of use for novice trainers
2. Guided through range of motion reducing technique learning
3. Limited coordination or experience required to use (less supervision)
4. Isolation of muscle groups

DISADVANTAGES OF FREE WEIGHTS
1. Greater technique learning component for the novice trainer
2. Safety concerns: require spotters and proper instruction
3. Need to develop coordination to successfully use

DISADVANTAGES OF MACHINE WEIGHTS
1. Machines do not readily accommodate all sized individuals
2. Movement pattern limited
3. Exercise selection limited per machine
4. Limited mechanical exercise variation
5. Single movement plane
6. Some machines restrict normal acceleration and velocity patterns
7. Machines lack the ability to provide smaller incremental weight changes
8. Machines are not portable

estimation stemming from cross-sectional studies, the unwillingness of subjects to provide a maximal effort when performing strength measures, and the contraction type and velocity of movement of the muscles tested (also see Chapter 4). Resistance training is a relatively safe method of training, and the assessment of maximal muscular strength and strength endurance can be achieved safely and with no more injuries than those experienced by younger individuals[39–41]. To ensure safe strength testing in elderly populations, preparticipation screening procedures are critically important. Guidelines for screening subjects should follow recognized standards from professional organizations such as the American College of Sports Medicine (ACSM)[42], the American Heart Association (AHA)[43], or the U.S. Surgeon General's Report (see Chapter 6 and GETP7 Chapter 2)[44]. When screening subjects, particular attention should be directed to medical contraindications to intense exercise such as high blood pressure (BP>160/95 mmHg), musculoskeletal or joint injury, neuromuscular injury, or heart conditions that may be problematic. In addition, the tester should focus on instructing correct lifting technique, maintain sufficient rest between lifts, consider lifts in which the body is supported, use safety precautions (collars, roll bars, spotters) during lifts, and communicate with participants being tested to determine their health status during testing.

CARDIOVASCULAR DISEASE

Cardiovascular disease (CVD) is a term used to describe a number of pathological conditions that can affect the heart and blood vessels (see Chapter 29). These conditions include heart attack and angina, cerebrovascular disease, stroke, high BP, blood clotting, and other heart or blood vessel diseases[41]. The presence of these conditions can be linked to the gradual clogging of blood vessels by fatty or fibrous material that narrow and harden the arteries, thereby reducing oxygen transport to the cells. The arteries associated with the heart, brain, and kidneys appear to be most commonly affected. When assessing maximal muscular strength and muscular endurance in individuals with CVD, it is important to consider that a load that is heavy and sustained for long periods of time, such as a maximal isometric contraction, can compress small arteries and result in substantial increases in total peripheral resistance[45]. Caution is required when assessing CVD patients; however, high-intensity resistance training has been shown to be beneficial for this population (see Chapters 25 and GETP7 Chapter 8)[42,43]. When screening CVD patients, the tester should be aware of contraindications to individual medications, physical activity habits, and the severity of the disease and any comorbidities.

ARTHRITIS

Arthritis simply means inflammation of the joint. There are over 150 forms of arthritis that affect the joints and sometimes affect the muscles or soft tissue of the body[41]. Osteoarthritis (OA) and rheumatoid arthritis are the two most common forms of arthritis. Normally, the two bones of a joint are cushioned with cartilage. In OA, the cartilage deteriorates, causing joint pain and stiffness. Because the joint cartilage lacks a sufficient blood supply, it relies on synovial fluid to lubricate and remove wastes from the joint. Exercise helps improves cartilage health by facilitating these two processes and reducing some of the symp-

toms of arthritis[41]. Although inflammation is common, pain and stiffness can also hinder joint motion. Arthritis is not a condition linked exclusively with aging; the most common and serious forms are often found in young adults and children.

Exercise is vital in the management of arthritis because it increases lubrication of the joints and strengthens the surrounding muscles, resulting in less stress on joints (see Chapter 36)[41,42]. Strengthening exercises are a key aspect of arthritis care, with the intention of building up strength and endurance of the muscles that help move and support the affected joints. Flexibility exercise is also strongly advocated for arthritis care, with the aim of improving the ROM of muscles and joints, which can become stiff, particularly as a result of pain and swelling[43]. When assessing maximal muscular strength and muscular endurance in this population, it is important to consider any joint replacements or movements that may cause damage to the painful joint. It is also important to warm up thoroughly, progress gradually into testing, do not force the joint beyond a comfortable range (use safety stops or spotters), and stop if joint pain increases. Additionally, a constant testing environment should be maintained because extreme changes in temperature caused by air conditioning or environmental conditions can cause pain and discomfort to arthritic sufferers.

DIABETES

Diabetes is a disorder of the endocrine system that is characterized by the body's inability to use blood sugar (glucose). The two main types of diabetes are type I (or juvenile-onset) diabetes and type II (or mature-onset) diabetes. Type I can affect anyone of any age, but is more common in people younger than age 30 years, and it is an insulin-dependent form of diabetes mellitus (IDDM). Type II diabetes usually develops slowly, later in life, after the age of 35 years, and is a non–insulin-dependent form of diabetes mellitus (NIDDM). However, the incidence of type II diabetes is becoming more prevalent in children, especially teenagers, but cases have been reported in children younger than age 4 years. The alarming increase in cases reported in children has been linked to rising levels of inactivity, poor diet, and obesity.

The health-related problems that arise from diabetes include, but are not limited to, CVDs, reduced circulation, kidney disorders, and blindness[36,40]. Weight loss, regular exercise, and a healthy low-fat diet are typically recommended in order to control the symptoms of diabetes. The effectiveness of resistance training, as an integral component of the treatment plan for diabetic patients, continues to be an important area of research (see Chapter 33)[41,45].

Diabetics' physical condition should be assessed before any strength assessment or strength training program. Blood glucose levels should be carefully monitored because hypoglycemic symptoms appear when blood glucose levels fall below 60 mg·dL^{-1}, and emergency carbohydrates need to be kept on hand. Eccentric contractions and high-intensity resistance training have been linked to increased BP, which may damage sensitive blood vessels. Individuals with extreme retinopathy (damage to retina) or increased micro- (small blood vessels) and macrovascular complications should avoid this type of training[45]. The greater the time under tension or load, the greater the potential for damage.

Another condition that should be considered when testing a diabetic individual would be hypoglycemia which can lead to dizziness, fatigue, confusion, sweating, hunger, headache and change in mood. Also the hydration status of these individuals is a concern given the potential for dehydration. Subjects should be carefully monitored and safety precautions in place prior to any testing.

OSTEOPOROSIS

Osteoporosis is a condition in which the bones become less dense, lose strength, become fragile and brittle, and can fracture more easily because of calcium loss. Most people show no signs of reduced bone mineral density (BMD) or developing osteoporosis until a fracture occurs. This is a condition that afflicts almost one in two women and one in three men after the age of 60 years.

Sufficient exercise during childhood and adolescence, particularly the prepubertal years, is more effective for increasing bone mass and strength than exercise in adulthood. To influence BMD, physical activities undertaken two or three times per week at training intensities between 70% and 80% of functional capacity may influence the maintenance of BMD[40]. Maximal strength testing and heavy-percentage RM training has been performed safely on elderly populations[40]. The primary benefit of resistance exercise for adult bones is conservation, not acquisition (see Chapter 35).

When assessing this population, it is important to eliminate movements that create high-impact loads during activities that involve twisting and bending, explosive movements, and staccato (high impacts) movements because they may cause bone damage. Proper screening and bone scans may provide information as to the loading capabilities of this population. Individuals with osteoporosis can perform maximal and muscular endurance assessments after preparticipation screening procedures have been implemented and when the proper precautions have been implemented.

MULTIPLE SCLEROSIS

Multiple sclerosis (MS) is an inflammatory disease of the central nervous system (CNS) in which the myelin covering of the nerve fibers gradually disintegrates. The gradual elimination of the protein and lipid covering of the axons influences the ability of the nerve fibers to conduct signals that may affect motor pathways and cause muscle weakness[46,47]. MS includes symptoms such as excessive fatigue, muscular weakness, spasticity, tremors, balance and gait disturbances, and a decrement in physical mobility[46]. The symptoms of MS are extremely variable, depending on the area of the CNS that has been affected. Sufferers often have multiple episodes or attacks of the condition. MS is very common among the 20- to 40-year-old age group and appears more frequently in women than men.

When assessing and training this population, it is important to consider their mobility (see Chapter 37). The most debilitating aspect of this condition is the lack of muscular control or precision. There appears only one major contraindication with MS, and that is the heat intolerance that accompanies this condition. A consideration when testing and training this population is to perform all exercise in a cool (air-conditioned) environment, incorporating long rest periods so as not to raise core body temperature. Caution and care also include testing and training on machines to improve strength and coordination before progressing to free-weight exercises.

STROKE

Stroke is also referred to as *cerebrovascular accident* (CVA) and occurs when there is a sudden loss of function caused by restricted blood supply (ischemia) or through bleeding (hemorrhage) affecting brain cells. Strokes are most frequent after the age of 60 years and result in muscle weakness, abnormal muscle activation patterns, and impaired postural control[48]. When testing and training this population, care and caution should be used because stroke sufferers usually have poor muscular endurance and functional ability. Testing should incorporate long rest periods between trials and tests, and training should progress based on rest periods.

Flexibility

Joint flexibility or **range of movement (ROM)** is an important component of muscular fitness. ROM describes the movement associated with a joint or series of joints and provides an important indication of joint function[41]. The ROM is measured from the joint axis and is joint specific, thus, each type of joint may have a different "normal" ROM. The ball-and-socket (triaxial = 3 degrees of freedom [df]) joint at the hip and shoulder allows for a greater degree of flexibility than either the gliding (biaxial = 2 df) joint at the wrist or the hinge (uniaxial = 1 df) joint at the knee, elbow, and ankle. When measuring the ROM of the various joints throughout the human body, it is very clear that a person can be highly flexible in one joint and have limited ROM in another.

The ROM that a joint can move through from an anatomical position to the extreme limits of that joint depends on the type of flexibility (see Chapters 1 and 2). Joint flexibility can be subdivided into either static and dynamic flexibility. Whereas a **static flexibility** measure or movement requires the joint to be passively moved by another individual, **dynamic flexibility** requires the active movement of the joint in response to the contraction of its surrounding muscles[49]. The ROM about the joint is partly related to the laxity of the muscles and connective tissues surrounding the joint. As the muscle and connective tissue around a joint are stretched, two important neuromuscular responses occur[8,9,13]. When muscle fibers are stretched, the muscle spindles—specialized muscle fibers that are very sensitive to the changes in length and rate of length change of muscle fibers—send impulses to the nervous system. The nervous system responds by sending an almost immediate response, resulting in tension development in the muscle to resist the stretch. The second neuromuscular response occurs within the sensory receptors known as golgi tendon organs (GTO)[8,9,13]. These specialized organs, located in the muscle–tendon junction, respond after the muscle spindles and only if a stretch has been sustained for a period of 5 seconds or longer. As such, the location of muscle spindles is better suited to "monitor" length changes, and GTOs are better suited to "monitor" tension because they are in parallel and series, respectively, with the muscle fibers. The impulse sent to the CNS by the GTO overrides those from the muscle spindles, thereby allowing the muscle to relax. This is why long, slow stretching (held for a minimum of 6 to 10 seconds) is recommended to enhance flexibility.

Joint ROM results from a combination of factors and is primarily influenced by the shape and structure of the articulating bones and surrounding connective tissues. The factors that limit joint flexibility can be classed as internal, relating to the physical structures of body materials and tissue. The internal structures influencing joint flexibility include:

1. **The type of joint:** Ball and socket, condyloid, gliding, hinge, pivot, and saddle
2. **The internal bony structures:** The articulating bony surfaces of joints limits the ROM. Examples of this can be seen in the ball-and-socket joint of the shoulder and the hinge joint of the elbow. The loose fit between the head of the humerus and the glenoid fossa of the scapula offers very little restrictions to movement. In contrast to the shoulder, the elbow joint is restricted by the olecranon of the ulna and the olecranon fossa of the humerus as the elbow moves into an extended position.
3. **The elasticity of muscle tissue:** The extensibility (ability to stretch beyond resting length) of muscle tissue limits the ROM at the joint. The extensibility of muscle is maintained with stretching and activity of the muscles and is diminished with inactivity.
4. **The elasticity of tendons, ligaments, and skin:** The extensibility of these tissues is another important factor in ROM at the joint. The elastic nature of the tendons and ligaments about the joint can be lost because of disuse, injury, and overextending these tissues. Also, as a consequence of aging, there is a change in the cell structure and fluid content of cells, resulting in a reduction of elasticity of the tendons, ligaments, and skin.
5. **The ability of a muscle to relax and contract:** Joint ROM is also dependent on the sensory receptors of the muscle spindles and GTOs.
6. **The temperature of the joint and associated tissues:** Increasing the temperature of muscles and collagenous tissue around the joint has been reported to increase the ROM of the joint[50].

The external factors that limit joint flexibility are nonstructural. These include environmental temperature, gender, age, excess fatty tissue or hypertrophied muscles, and restrictions of any clothing or equipment. Published normative data on ROM for joint movements are not related to age, gender, or body type (Table 13-3).

Types of Stretching

The ROM of joints throughout the human body can be assisted by exercise programs that involve stretching. Like most aspects of physical training there are many variations of stretching. The different types of stretching include but are not limited to the following:

1. **Active stretching** involves holding a stretch at or near the extreme of the ROM. This can be accomplished by actively contracting antagonistic muscle groups. An example is to stretch the hamstrings muscle group requires the contraction of the quadriceps muscle group.
2. **Passive stretching** involves the use of gravity or the assistance of another person to assist in moving the joint to the limits of its range.
3. **Static stretching** involves a slow, deliberate movement that can be sustained for a period of 10 to 30 seconds to train the neuromuscular responses of the sensory receptors within the muscle.
4. **Ballistic stretching**, sometimes referred to as bounce stretching, attempts to use the momentum of a moving body or a limb to force the joint beyond its normal ROM.
5. **Prioceptive neuromuscular facilitation (PNF) stretching** usually involves a partner. This style of stretching involves a passive static stretch that can be initiated with a partner and is immediately followed by an active contraction against resistance, which is followed by a further passive stretch.

There are no set training guides for flexibility except to say that stretching may benefit the ROM of the stretched joint (or joints)[51,52]. Likewise, there is no evidence to suggest that stretching will reduce the incidence of injury or

TABLE 13-3. Range of Motion of the Major Joints

Joint	Motion	Average Range (degrees)	Joint	Motion	Average Range (degrees)
Spinal			**Upper Extremity**		
Cervical	Flexion	0–60	Shoulder	Flexion	0–180
	Extension	0–75		Extension	0–50
	Lateral flexion	0–45		Abduction	0–180
	Rotation	0–80		Adduction	0–50
Thoracic	Flexion	0–50		Internal rotation	0–90
	Rotation	0–30		External rotation	0–90
Lumbar	Flexion	0–60	Elbow	Flexion	0–140
	Extension	0–25	Forearm	Supination	0–80
	Lateral flexion	0–25		Pronation	0–80
			Wrist	Flexion	0–60
				Extension	0–60
Lower Extremity				Ulnar deviation	0–30
Hip	Flexion	0–100		Radial deviation	0–20
	Extension	0–30	Thumb	Abduction	0–60
	Abduction	0–40	Flexion	Carpal—metacarpal	0–15
	Adduction	0–20		Metacarpal—phalangeal	0–50
	Internal rotation	0–40		Interphalangeal	0–50
	External rotation	0–50	Extension	Carpal—metacarpal	0–20
Knee	Flexion	0–150		Metacarpal—phalangeal	0–5
Ankle	Dorsiflexion	0–20		Interphalangeal	0–20
	Plantarflexion	0–40	Fingers		
Subtalar	Inversion	0–30	Flexion	Metacarpal—phalangeal	0–90
	Eversion	0–20		Proximal interphalangeal	0–100
				Distal interphalangeal	0–80
			Extension	Metacarpal—phalangeal	0–45

Also see GETP7 Table 4-14.

improve performance[51,52]. What is known is that gains from stretching can diminish relatively quickly, within 3 to 4 weeks, without regular training. A stretching program performed three times a week for 10 to 20 minutes each time incorporating static and sport specific dynamic stretching appears beneficial to increasing or maintaining ROM and movement suppleness. (see GETP7 Table 7-2)

Flexibility Evaluation

The two common methods that are available for the assessment of joint ROM are subjective visual estimates and measurements that involve instrumentation. The accuracy of the assessment of ROM depends on which method of assessment is used. Regardless of the assessment method implemented, it is important to follow standard procedures to ensure the accuracy and reliability of these measures. Attention to the following standards help improve the accuracy of joint ROM assessments. The accurate identification and use of bony landmarks[49,53], correct positioning of subjects so the proximal segment is stable and a full ROM is attained in the distal segment[49,53], performing repeat trials of the measurement, and the placement and stabilization of the instruments to measure joint ROM[49,54] are all essential. In addition, it is important to

report warm-up procedures, test time, injuries, joint deterioration, and training background.

Measurement of Flexibility

The measurement of joint ROM can involve indirect assessment techniques such as the sit-and-reach box, goniometers, inclinometers, dynamometers and video analyses, and subjective visual assessment techniques.

SIT AND REACH

The sit-and-reach box is fixed with a ruler and moveable slide so that when the feet are positioned flush on the box, the ruler is at a neutral position. Movement that extends past this point is incremented and results in a positive flexibility score; movement that falls short of this point scores a negative flexibility value. The setup for the sit-and-reach test requires subjects to sit comfortably and relaxed with their feet positioned against a measuring box with the toes pointing up and the legs straight (see GETP7 Box 4-7). The subject bends forward slowly from the waist, reaching forward with the fingertips as far as possible, and holds this position momentarily. The fingertips should be overlapped and be in contact with the moveable slide. The score is recorded as the most distant point reached by the fingertips. (see GETP7 Tables 4-15 and 4-16)

A modified version of the sit-and-reach test follows an identical setup as above with the subject positioned so that subjects sit up against a wall with their legs straight out in front and the soles of their feet touching the sit and reach box. However, the sit-and-reach test results in only moderate reliability (ICC: r = 0.53)[54]. An inherent limitation associated with this test is that it does not allow for proportional differences in leg and arm length and torso height. When these measures are considered in the measurement using a modified sit-and-reach test, then the reliability increases substantially (ICC: r = 0.90)[54,55].

GONIOMETER

Goniometers are the most commonly used measuring device for ROM. Measures are reported in degrees of motion. The goniometer is a large protractor that consists of two arms that are joined at a central axis point. The center of the goniometer is placed at the axis of rotation of the joint, and the arms of the goniometer are aligned along the long axis of the bones of the adjacent segments. The reliability of goniometers ranges between moderate and high, with values (ICC: r = 0.63 to 0.98) expressing up to 10° to 15° error[56–58]. The main limitations of using a goniometer arise when measuring triaxial joints and in positioning and secur-

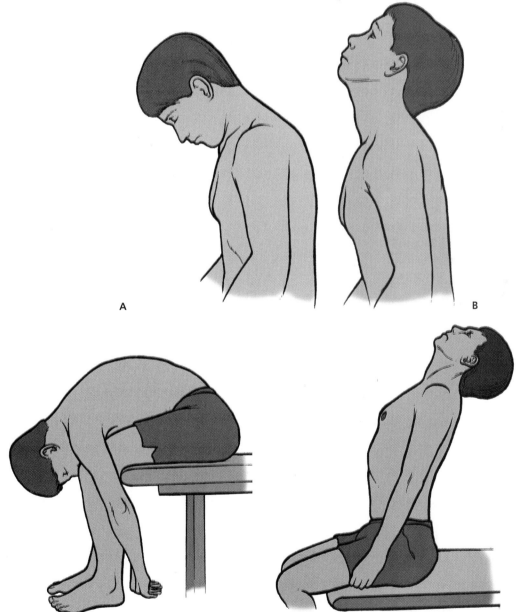

FIGURE 13-2. Neck and trunk flexibility screening. **A.** Cervical flexion (chin to chest). **B.** Cervical extension (move head posteriorly). **C.** Vertebral flexion (trunk to thighs). **D.** Vertebral extension (move trunk posteriorly).

ing the goniometer arms along the long axis of the bone. Electronic goniometers that incorporate position sensors and computer software are also used to measure ROM about the joint. The electronic goniometer is positioned over the joint axis and fastened to the long bones to track motion. The advantages of the electronic goniometer include continual monitoring of the joint, accuracy of measurement, and hands-free action; however, it is only as accurate as the instructor aligning the joint axis and long bones.

INCLINOMETERS

Inclinometers are handheld electronic or mechanical devices that measure motion against a constant vertical component using gravity as a reference. Most inclinometers are fastened to the joint via a mounting strap and incorporate a self-zeroing protractor and indicator, a locking device for both protractor and indicator, and oscillation-reduction devices to increase the sensitivity of measures. Similar to the goniometer, reliability has been reported to be moderate to high (ICC: r = 0.63–0.71)[58]. Inclinometers are acceptable for measuring complex movements associated with the head or trunk and are reported to provide greater accuracy for extremity measures than do goniometers.

ISOKINETIC DYNAMOMETER

The isokinetic dynamometer has an inbuilt protractor that allows the measurement of joint ROM. This device is not traditionally used for this purpose, but it does have a limited capability to measure single joint movements. Another limitation of the device is that the resistance from the lever arm of the machine may influence joint ROM. In

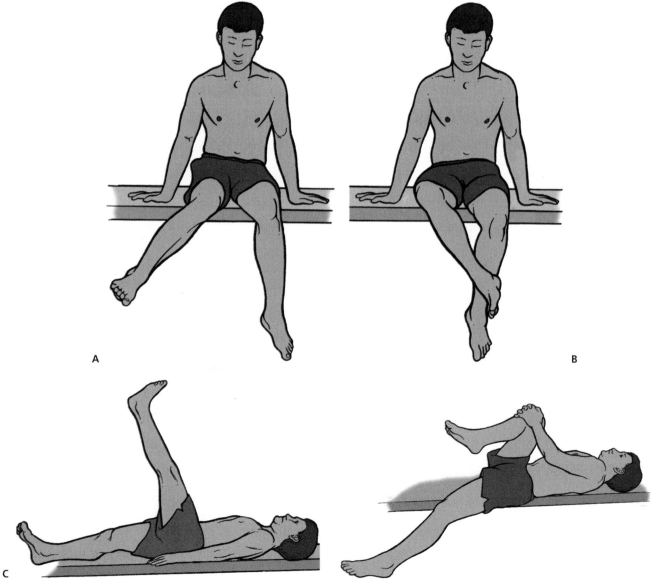

FIGURE 13-3. Hip flexibility screening. **A.** Internal rotation (move thigh laterally). **B.** External rotation (move thigh medially). **C.** Straight-leg raising (opposite leg in full extension). **D.** Combined test (bent knee to chest).

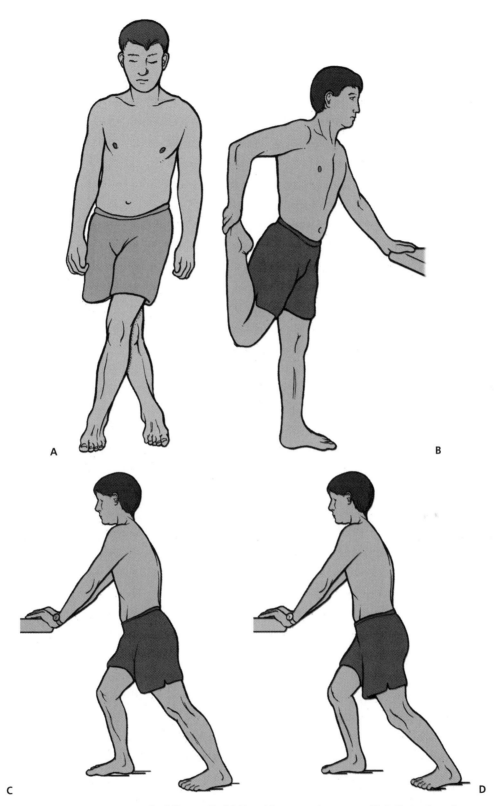

FIGURE 13-4. Lower extremity flexibility. **A.** Illiotibial band (cross over leg to stretch). **B.** Rectus femoris length (maintain upright posture). **C.** Gastrocnemius (knee straight, foot flat). **D.** Soleus (bent knee).

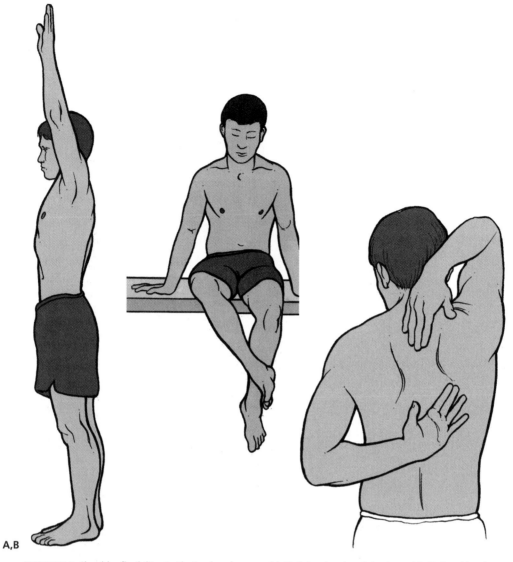

FIGURE 13-5. Shoulder flexibility. **A.** Flexion (reach upwards). **B.** Extension (reach backwards). **C.** Combined (attempt grasp hands).

addition, no reliability measures have been reported on the use of isokinetic dynamometers to assess joint ROM.

VIDEO ANALYSIS

The use of video analysis allows for multiple joint movements to be accurately tracked in three dimensions. The main limitations of this analysis technique are that it requires expensive equipment and software to calculate in three or two dimensions, is time consuming to place multiple markers, requires postprocessing, and requires subjects to wear limited clothing.

SUBJECTIVE VISUAL ASSESSMENT

When highly accurate measurements of ROM are not desired, this form of field testing allows for the observation of postural alignment by comparing ranges of movement between opposing body segments. The most common field tests are shown in Figures 13-2 to 13-5. These measures are best suited to situations in which the left and right sides of the body are compared or when an individual is tested placed on an intervention and then retested. There are no physical qualitative measurements or recordings for this style of assessment. The observed information is recorded in written or diagrammatical reports.

Acknowledgments
The authors wish to acknowledge the authors of this content from previous editions of this text. Their efforts greatly assisted our compilation of information for the current chapter.

REFERENCES

1. Atha J: Strengthening muscle. In Miller D, ed. Exercise and Sport Science Reviews, vol. 9, pp. 1–73. Philadelphia: Franklin Institute Press; 1981.

2. Komi P, ed: Strength and Power in Sport, vol 3. Oxford: IOC Medical Commission Publication; 1992.

3. Abernethy P, Wilson G, Logan P: Strength and power assessment. Issues, controversies and challenges. Sports Med 19:401–417, 1995.

4. Sale D: Testing strength and power (pp. 21–106). In MacDougall J, Wenger H, Green H, eds. Physiological Testing of the High Performance Athlete, 2nd ed. Champaign, IL: Human Kinetics Publishers; 1991.

5. Knuttgen HG, Kraemer WJ: Terminology and measurement in exercise performance. J Strength and Cond Res 1:1–10, 1987.

6. Perrin DH: Isokinetic exercise and assessment. Champaign, IL: Human Kinetics; 1993.

7. Sale D: Neural adaptation to resistance training. Med Sci Sports Exerc 20:S135–S145, 1988.

8. Enoka R: Neural adaptations with chronic physical activity. J Biomech 30:447–455, 1997.

9. Komi PV: Training of muscle strength and power: Interaction of neuromotoric, hypertrophic, and mechanical factors. Int J Sports Med 7:10–15, 1986.

10. Hakkinen K: Neuromuscular and hormonal adaptations during strength and power training. A review. J Sports Med Phys Fit 29:9–26, 1989.

11. Kraemer WJ: Endocrine responses to resistance exercise. Med Sci Sports Exerc 20:S152–S157, 1988.

12. Brooke MH, Kaiser KK: Muscle fiber types: how many and what kind? Arch Neurol 23 69–79, 1970.

13. Åstrand PO, Rodahl K: Textbook of Work Physiology: Physiological Bases of Exercise, 2nd ed. New York: McGraw-Hill; 1977.

14. Pette D, Staron RS: Myosin isoforms, muscle fiber types, and transitions. Micro Res Tech 50: 00–509, 2000.

15. Sale DG, MacDougall JD, Alway SE, et al: Voluntary strength and muscle characteristics in untrained men and women and male bodybuilders. J Appl Physiol. 62:1786–1793, 1987.

16. Tesch PA, Komi PV, Hakkinen K: Enzymatic adaptations consequent to long-term strength training. Int J Sports Med 8(suppl 1):66–69, 1987.

17. Kraemer WJ, Patton JF, Gordon SE, et al: Compatibility of high-intensity strength and endurance training on hormonal and skeletal muscle adaptations. J Appl Physiol 78:976–989, 1995.

18. Abernethy PJ, Jurimae J, Logan PA, et al: Acute and chronic response of skeletal muscle to resistance exercise. Sports Med 17:22–38, 1994.

19. Hay JG: Biomechanics of Sports Techniques, 4th ed. Englewood Cliffs, NJ: Prentice-Hall; 1993.

20. Kraemer WJ, Ratamess NA: Fundamentals of resistance training: progression and exercise prescription. Med Sci Sports Exerc 36:674–688, 2004.

21. Fleck SJ, Kraemer WJ: Designing Resistance Training Programs. Champaign, IL: Human Kinetics; 1987.

22. Grimsby O: More on 1RM testing. J Ortho Sports Phys Ther 31:264–265, 2001.

23. Fernandez R: One repetition maximum clarified. J Ortho Sports Phys Ther 31:264, 2001.

24. Hoeger WWK, Hopkins DR, Barette SL, et al: Relationship between repetitions and selected percentages of one repetition maximum: A comparison between untrained and trained males and females. J Appl Sport Sci Res 4:47–54, 1990.

25. Mayhew JL, Ball TE, Arnold MD, et al: Relative muscular endurance performance as a predictor of bench press strength in college men and women. J Appl Sport Sci Res 6:200–206, 1992.

26. Anderson T, Kearney JT: Effects of three resistance training programs on muscular strength and absolute and relative endurance. Res Q Exerc Sport 53:1–7, 1982.

27. Keating JL, Matyas TA: The influence of subject and test design on dynamometric measurements of extremity muscles. Phys Ther 76:866–869, 1996.

28. Snow CJ, Blacklin K: Reliability of knee flexor peak torque measurements from a standardized test protocol on a Kin-Com Dynamometer. Arch Phys Med Rehab 73:15–22, 1992.

29. Steiner LA, Harris BA, Krebs DE: Reliability of eccentric isokinetic knee flexion and extension measurements. Arch Phys Med Rehab 74:1327–1335, 1993.

30. Frisiello S, Gazaille A, O'Halloran J, et al: Test-retest reliability of eccentric peak torque values for shoulder medial and lateral rotation using the Biodex isokinetic dynamometer. J Ortho Sports Phys Ther 19:341–344, 1994.

31. Emery CA, Maitland ME, Meeuwisse WH: Test-retest reliability of isokinetic hip adductor and flexor muscle strength. Clin J Sport Med 9:79–85, 1999.

32. Li RC, Wu Y, Maffulli N, et al: Eccentric and concentric isokinetic knee flexion and extension: a reliability study using the Cybex 6000 dynamometer. Br J Sports Med 30:156–160, 1996.

33. Requa RK, DeAvilla LN, Garrick JG: Injuries in recreational adult fitness activities. Am J Sports Med 21:461–467, 1993.

34. Knutzen KM, Brilla L, Caine D, et al: Absolute vs. relative machine strength as predictors of function in older adults. J Strength Cond Res 16:628–640, 2002.

35. Frontera WR, Bigard X: The benefits of strength training in the elderly. Sci Sports 17:109–116, 2002.

36. Stone MH, Fleck SJ, Triplett NT, et al: Health- and performance-related potential of resistance training. Sports Med 11:210–231, 1991.

37. Skelton DA, Greig CA, Davies JM, et al: Strength, power and related functional ability of healthy people aged 65–89 years. Age Ageing 23:371–377, 1994.

38. Larsson L, Sjödin B, Karlsson J: Histochemical and biochemical changes in human skeletal muscle with age in sedentary males, age 22–65 years. Acta Physiol Scand 103:31–39, 1978.

39. Faigenbaum AD, Milliken LA, Westcott WL: Maximal strength testing in healthy children. J Strength Cond Res 17:162–166, 2003.

40. Humphries B, Newton RU, Bronks R, et al: The effect of exercise intensity on bone density, strength and calcium turnover in older women. Med Sci Sports Exerc 32:1043–1050, 2000.

41. Winett RA, Carpinelli RN: Potential health-related benefits of resistance training. Prev Med 33:503–513, 2001.

42. American College of Sports Medicine Position Stand: The recommended quantity and quality of exercise fro developing and maintaining cardiorespiratory and muscular fitness, and flexibility in healthy adults. Med Sci Sports Exerc 30:975–991, 1998.

43. Fletcher GF, Balady GJ, Amsterdam EA, et al: Exercise standards for testing and training: a statement for healthcare professionals from the American Heart Association. Circulation 104:1694–1740, 2001.

44. U.S. Department of Health and Human Services. Physical Activity and Health: a report of the Surgeon General. Atlanta: U.S. Department of Health and Human Services, the Center for Disease Control and Prevention, National Center for Chronic Disease Prevention and Health, 1996.

45. Albright A, Franz M, Hornsby G, et al: American College of Sports Medicine position stand. Exercise and type 2 diabetes. Med Sci Sports Exerc 32:1345–1360, 2000.

46. DeBolt LS, McCubbin JA: The Effects of Home-Based Resistance Exercise on Balance, Power, and Mobility in Adults With Multiple Sclerosis. Arch Phys Med Rehabil 85:290–297, 2004.

47. Rik Gosselink R, Kovacs L, Ketelaer P, et al: Respiratory muscle weakness and respiratory muscle training in severely disabled multiple sclerosis patients. Arch Phys Med Rehabil 81:747–751, 2000.

48. Teixeira-Salmela LF, Olney SJ, Nadeau S, et al: Muscle strengthening and physical conditioning to reduce impairment and disability in chronic stroke survivors. Arch Phys Med Rehabil 80:1211–1218, 1999.

49. Lea RD: Current concepts review: range of motion measurements. J Bone Joint Surg 77A:78A, 1995.

50. Wiemann K, Hahn K: Influences of strength, stretching and circulatory exercises on flexibility parameters of the human hamstrings. Int J Sports Med 18:340–346, 1997.

51. Thacker SB, Gilchrist J, Stroup D, et al: The impact of stretching on sports injury risk: A systematic review of the literature. Med Sci Sports Exerc 36:371–378, 2004.

52. Gleim GW, McHugh MP: Flexibility and its effects on sports injury and performance. Sports Med 24:289–299, 1997.

53. Greene, WR Heckman JD, eds: The clinical measurement of joint motion. Rosemount, IL; American Academy of Orthopeadic Surgeons; 1994.

54. Hopkins DR, Hoeger WWK: A comparison of sit and reach test and the modified sit and reach test in the measurement of flexibility for males. J Appl Sport Sci Res 6:7–10, 1992.

55. Fernandez JE, Stubbs NB: Mathematical modeling and testing of the sit and reach test. Int J Indust Ergo 3:201–205, 1989.

56. Rothstein JM, Miller PJ, Roettger RF: Goniometric reliability in a clinical setting. Elbow and knee measurements. Phys Ther 63:1611–1615, 1983.

57. Waddell G, Somerville D, Henderson I, et al: Objective clinical evaluation of physical impairment in chronic low back pain. Spine 17:617–628, 1992.

58. Awan R, Smith J, Boon AJ: Measuring shoulder internal rotation range of motion: A comparison of 3 techniques. Arch Phys Med Rehabil 83:1229–1234, 2002.

SELECTED REFERENCES FOR FURTHER READING

Abernethy PJ, Jurimae J, Logan PA, et al: Acute and chronic response of skeletal muscle to resistance exercise. Sports Med 17:22–38, 1994.

Gleim GW, McHugh MP: Flexibility and its effects on sports injury and performance. Sports Med 24:289–299, 1997.

Kraemer WJ, Ratamess NA: Fundamentals of resistance training: progression and exercise prescription. Med Sci Sports Exerc 36: 674–688, 2004.

Stone MH, Fleck SJ, Triplett NT, Kraemer WJ: Health- and performance-related potential of resistance training. Sports Med 11: 210–231, 1991.

Thacker SB, Gilchrist J, Stroup D, et al: The impact of stretching on sports injury risk: A systematic review of the literature. Med Sci Sports Exerc 36:371–378, 2004.

Winett RA, Carpinelli RN: Potential health-related benefits of resistance training. Prev Med 33:503–513, 2001.

INTERNET RESOURCES

American College of Sports Medicine: http://www.acsm.org

American Council on Exercise: http://www.acefitness.org/

Biomechanics World Wide: http://www.per.ualberta.ca/biomechanics

ExRx.net: http://www.exrx.net

International Fitness Association
http://www.ifafitness.com/stretch/index.html

Medem Medical Library: http://www.medem.com/MedLB/medlib_entry.cfm?sid=103AF635-C640-11D4-8C0100508BF1C1F1&site_name=Medem

NSCA: National Strength & Conditioning Association: http://www.nsca-lift.org

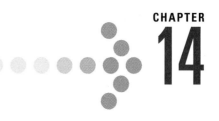

Clinical Exercise Testing Related to Cardiovascular Disease

CARL FOSTER AND JOHN P. PORCARI

This chapter addresses KSAs from the following content areas:

1 **Exercise Physiology and Related Exercise Science**
2 Pathophysiology and Risk Factors
3 **Health Appraisal, Fitness, and Clinical Exercise Testing**
4 **Electrocardiography and Diagnostic Techniques**
5 Patient Management and Medications
6 **Medical and Surgical Management**
7 Exercise Prescription and Programming
8 Nutrition and Weight Management
9 Human Behavior and Counseling
10 Safety, Injury Prevention, and Emergency Procedures
11 Program Administration, Quality Assurance, and Outcome Assessment

Exercise testing is an extension of the history and physical examination that has been of widespread clinical value for at least the past 50 years. Traditionally, exercise testing has been a preliminary step in the **diagnosis** of hemodynamically significant coronary artery disease (CAD). The primary diagnostic criteria have been ST-segment changes on the electrocardiogram (ECG) and their correlation with symptoms (e.g., angina pectoris, shortness of breath) consistent with exertional myocardial ischemia. Within this context, exercise tests have been of established value in the evaluation of patients with an intermediate likelihood of CAD and of lesser value in patients at either very low or very high pretest likelihood of CAD. In view of the limited sensitivity and specificity of ST-segment changes during exercise and the likelihood that the reported sensitivity and specificity (60% to 70%) of exercise testing is influenced by workup bias, the true sensitivity and specificity of exercise testing may be as low as 40% to 50%[1]. Beyond this, the limitation of coronary angiography as the gold standard, particularly with reference to detecting unstable plaques, the traditional view of exercise testing must be reconsidered. Within the past several years, the application of exercise testing has been broadened in response to a better understanding of the considerable prognostic information to be derived from the exercise test[1–9].

Why Do an Exercise Test?

There are several reasons for conducting a clinical exercise test (see GETP7 Chapter 5). These indications are enumerated in Box 14-1. Before assuming the risk of conducting an exercise test, one must always be certain that the indications for the test are adequate. Beyond this, an understanding of the indications for the test will dictate how the relative criteria for terminating the test are judged and how the test results are evaluated. For example, the attitude taken when conducting a test on an otherwise healthy individual at risk for occult cardiovascular disease (CVD) will be somewhat different than in a patient who presents clinically with a history consistent with stable angina pectoris. Likewise, the interpretative approach will be quite different when one is trying to make a new diagnosis of exertional myocardial ischemia versus trying to define **prognosis** in a patient with known CAD.

Preliminary Decisions

Before conducting an exercise test, several things must be considered that will greatly affect the type of information to be derived from the test. These include the indications and contraindications to exercise testing, the type of ergometer, the endpoint of the exercise test, the protocol, and safety considerations.

The indications for exercise testing are listed in Box 14-1. In the most general sense, the overriding concept is that exercise testing is an extension of the history and physical designed to allow the physician to evaluate the patient in circumstances likely to be provocative of the signs or symptoms consistent with exertional myocardial ischemia or other manifestations of CVD. There are both absolute and relative contraindications to exercise testing, which are presented in GETP7 Box 3-5. For the most part, contraindications are relatively commonsense decisions designed to avoid unstable **ischemic** or hemodynamic situations and other situations in which the risk of exercise

KEY TERMS

Chronotropic: Affecting the heart rate

Diagnosis: The determination of the presence of a disease

Ischemic: Inadequate circulation of blood to a tissue

Prognosis: The probable outcome of a disease

testing might exceed the additional information to be gained from the exercise test. It is remarkable that the number of conditions considered to be absolute contraindications have decreased over the past 50 years while at the same time, the general practice of exercise testing has become safer[10]. Given that there is a discrete risk of untoward events during exercise testing[10], subjects should provide informed consent before undergoing testing (see GETP7 Fig. 3-1). As a general principle, the person actually conducting the test should go over the informed con-

sent with the patient immediately before the test even if the patient has already signed the form. It is particularly important to tell the patient what he or she is likely to feel during the test (e.g., "I'm going to try to make you have that chest discomfort you were telling your doctor about. If you don't get the pain, I'm still going to make your legs get very tired and make you get sweaty and out of breath"). At the same time, it is probably worth going over the history and indications for the test just to make sure that the goals of the test are well understood by both the patient and laboratory personnel. Lastly, the resting ECG should be examined before beginning the test, first to identify contraindications for testing and second to make sure that the resting ECG is normal enough to allow for interpretation of changes that might occur during the exercise test.

The exercise protocol represents a convenient way to conduct the exercise examination for both the patient and the physician. There are several general principles that can be applied to the selection of the exercise protocol. The initial level of exertion should be clearly submaximal, the increments between stages should be comparatively small and of consistent size, the protocol should allow easy estimation of the exercise capacity, and the test should be efficient of patient and physician time. The classic Bruce treadmill protocol is the most widely used exercise protocol in the United States[11,12]. From the standpoint of physician familiarity, availability of equations to predict functional capacity[13-15], and efficiency of physician and patient time, the Bruce treadmill protocol is very good. However, this protocol is ideal only for younger individuals with a fairly normal exercise capacity and a good ability to communicate with the physician conducting the test. For older and more debilitated patients, the relatively high starting aerobic requirements and the large increases between stages make the Bruce protocol less than optimal and encourage extensive handrail support, which compromises accurate evaluation of exercise capacity[14,16]. A variety of modifications of the Bruce treadmill protocol and many other treadmill and cycle protocols have been developed. Most recently, patient-specific ramping protocols have gained popularity[15-19] (see GETP7 Figure 5-3).

Termination criteria for exercise testing are well established (see GETP7 Box 5-2). In general, it is safe to say that the test should be continued until the clinical question that prompted the exercise test to be ordered has been answered. Arbitrary termination criteria based on a predetermined workload or percent of the age-predicted heart rate (HR) are difficult to justify, primarily in that they heav-

BOX 14-1   **Clinically Accepted Reasons for Performing an Exercise Test, Including the Level of Evidence Supporting the Indication[a]**

Extension of the history and physical (allowing the physician to examine the patient during symptoms) (I)

Evaluate exertional discomfort (I)

    Chest discomfort
    Dyspnea
    Leg discomfort
    Palpitations
    Cerebral symptoms

Evaluate the presence of occult coronary artery disease (Ia, IIb)

Risk stratification in patients with known cardiovascular disease (I)

Follow-up of therapy (IIa)

Exercise prescription (IIb)

[a] **Class I:** Conditions for which there is evidence and/or general agreement that a given procedure or treatment is useful and effective.

Class II: Conditions for which there is conflicting evidence and/or a divergence of opinion about the usefulness/efficacy of a procedure or treatment.

    IIa: Weight of evidence/opinion is in favor of usefulness/efficacy.

    IIb: Usefulness/efficacy is less well established by evidence/opinion.

Class III: Conditions for which there is evidence and/or general agreement that the procedure/treatment is not useful/effective and in some cases may be harmful.

Adapted from the American College of Cardiology/American Heart Association: ACC/AHA 2002 Guideline Update for Exercise Testing. A Report of the American College of Cardiology/American Heart Association Task Force on Practice Guidelines Circulation 106:1883–1892, 2002.

ily stress the most debilitated patients and fail to challenge more hardy patients (see GETP7 Figure 7-3). Particularly considering the recent recognition of the importance of exercise capacity as a prognostic marker[8], failure to take the patient to either a fatigue or symptom or sign limitation is hard to defend. However, after clearly abnormal findings have been documented, there is little justification for continuation of the test. Some clinicians view the achievement of 85% of the age-predicted maximal HR as adequate stress for revealing exertional ischemia. This practice is based on older observations that 50% of ischemic abnormalities were observed by the time 85% of age-predicted maximal HR was achieved. Although it is true that the sensitivity of exercise testing is increased in tests in which more than 85% of the age-predicted HR is achieved, it makes more sense to argue that achievement of a particular threshold HR is primarily a "security blanket" in an otherwise normal test. In the setting of interpreting a clinically indicated test with no abnormal findings, the clinician is compelled to ask themselves if they have really ruled out exertional ischemia, or if they have missed something. Given that severe exercise in a previously sedentary person is an established trigger of acute myocardial infarction[20,21], and the likelihood that patients receiving reassurance after a normal exercise test result might be willing to engage in severe exercise without proper buildup, the risk of missing an abnormal finding by inadequately stressing the patient is both real and clinically relevant. Accordingly, it seems reasonable to argue that the best place to provoke abnormal findings is in the exercise laboratory, where complications can be responded to appropriately.

A decision needs to be made concerning procedures immediately after the exercise test. Some studies support the concept that the sensitivity of ST-segment changes can be maximized by placing the patient in a sitting or supine position immediately after exercise[22–24]. However, other data have demonstrated that important data derived from the pattern of HR and blood pressure (BP) recovery during the postexercise period[1,2,3,5,7,25,26] suggest that the gain in ECG sensitivity from passive postexercise recovery is less than the information that can be gained by choosing to continue light exercise during the recovery period. These data suggest that it is probably best to perform a short period of low-intensity exercise during the postexercise period to promote hemodynamic stability. It is also important to recognize that the moments immediately after the exercise test are uniquely "teachable moments" during which the clinician conducting the exercise test can effectively communicate with the patient (e.g., the value of habitual exercise, weight loss, stopping smoking, or the safety of resuming normal activities that the patient might fear).

Interpretative Strategy

Interpreting exercise test results can only be accomplished within the clinical context of the exercise test.

Within the context of the reason for performing the test in the first place, at least five factors must be considered during the interpretation of the exercise test, including clinical responses; ECG responses; exercise capacity; hemodynamic responses; and the integrated response, as reflected by exercise test scores.

The *clinical response* to the exercise test must be evaluated in terms of the clinical context of the test. The clinical context is well reflected by the pretest likelihood of ischemic CVD that might have been the indication for the exercise test (see Chapter 19 and GETP7 Table 5-1). This concept is well expressed in terms of Bayes theorem of conditional probability. For CAD, well-accepted quantitative guidelines have been established. *Symptoms* observed during the exercise test must be interpreted in terms of their correspondence to the patients' presenting symptoms. In the case of chest discomfort that is potentially angina pectoris, the timing and character of the chest discomfort must be carefully considered. It is also important to recognize that in older patients, dyspnea is often an anginal equivalent. Ideally, the appearance of symptoms will be correlated with either ECG or hemodynamic abnormalities. There is a tendency for fewer symptoms to be observed during exercise testing than during spontaneous exercise, perhaps because of the influence of warm-up during exercise testing[27].

Changes in the *ST segment* of the ECG are the traditional interpretative benchmark related to the presence of exercise-induced ischemia (see Chapter 21). Traditionally, greater than 1 mm of horizontal or downsloping ST depression is considered the minimal diagnostic threshold to support evidence of myocardial ischemia. In the case of ST-segment depression (or elevation), there is usually a lead with the greatest degree of ST change, surrounded by leads with progressively less ST change. Although it is common to refer to ST-segment changes relative to an area of the heart that might be ischemic or even to a particular coronary artery that might have an obstructive lesion, the fact is that ischemic abnormalities map onto the surface of the chest fairly poorly. Using the traditional criteria of a 70% narrowing of at least one epicardial artery, the sensitivity and specificity of ECG exercise testing is on the order of 70% and 80%, respectively. However, there is likely a significant workup bias, and the true sensitivity may be as low as 40%[1]. Beyond this, high-grade angiographic lesions are probably not an ideal criterion against which to measure exertional ischemia. Given the minimal diagnostic criteria of 1 mm of horizontal or downsloping ST-segment depression, ST-segment changes that occur particularly early during an exercise test, are evident in multiple leads, and persist into recovery are predictive of either severe CAD or multivessel disease.

Dysrhythmias, especially ventricular dysrhythmias, are particularly disturbing during exercise testing because they are widely thought to portend a catastrophic hemodynamic collapse (see Chapter 20). In general, dysrhythmias that increase in frequency or complexity with progressive exercise, are associated with ischemia, or are associated with hemodynamic instability are thought to be more malignant than isolated dysrhythmias. Recent evidence indicating that high-grade dysrhythmias occurring during exercise or recovery are associated with a poor long-term prognosis have served to reinforce the traditional concern about the ominous nature of dysrhythmias[4].

Exercise capacity has always been viewed as an important aspect of exercise testing. Within the context of our understanding of central oxygen transport, a relatively high maximal oxygen uptake ($\dot{V}O_{2max}$) can be inferred to predict a relatively high cardiac output and likewise infers the absence of serious limitations of left ventricular function. Within the past decade, a number of studies have been published demonstrating the profound importance of exercise capacity relative to the prognosis of patients with CVD[8,28]. Either absolute exercise capacity or age and gender normalized exercise capacity is highly related to survival. A significant issue relative to exercise capacity is the imprecision of estimating exercise capacity from exercise performance. The error in estimating exercise capacity from various published prediction equations is about ± 1 MET (metabolic equivalent)[13–16,18,29]. This is comparatively unimportant (< 10% error) in young, healthy individuals with 13 to 15 MET exercise capacities but is much more significant (15% to 25% error) in individuals with reduced exercise capacities typical of those observed in patients with CVD (4 to 8 METs). In view of the prognostic importance of exercise capacity, the frequent custom of stopping the exercise test early because the subject has reached an arbitrary HR seems hard to justify. More importantly, the spurious elevation of the estimated functional capacity resulting from the frequent practice of allowing patients to use handrail support causes an inaccurately favorable prognosis. Although some equations for predicting functional capacity from exercise performance account for handrail support, their relative predictive error is larger than for predictive equations in which the patient is not allowed to use handrail support[14].

Exercise capacity is best understood in terms of the age- and gender-predicted norms. Historically, this has been difficult because age and gender average values in a sedentary population in a species that is not designed to be sedentary are hardly appropriate. Normative data are widely available. Morris et al.[29] present data based on physically active individuals, which probably should be the interpretative norm. Although these data are for men, other data can be used to estimate appropriate age-related values for women (see GETP7 Table 4-8). Historically, exercise capacity has been reported in terms of functional aerobic impairment[11]. However, because physically fit patients have a negative functional aerobic impairment and because negative numbers are intuitively difficult to understand, the concept of functional aerobic impairment is

becoming less popular, and simple percentages of the age- and gender-predicted norm is now most widely reported.

Hemodynamic responses have long been used to evaluate momentary safety issues during exercise testing. Abnormalities in either the pattern or magnitude of the systolic BP response have long been recognized for their prognostic significance[25,26]. The most interesting recent developments in our understanding of exercise testing has been in the recent data regarding the prognostic significance of hemodynamic responses during and immediately after exercise testing[1,2,3,5,7,9,25,26]. Lauer[1] has presented evidence that patients who cannot achieve an adequate HR response to exercise have an unfavorable prognosis beyond that accounted for by symptoms or ECG changes. The most widely accepted cutpoint is a failure to achieve 80% of the predicted HR reserve in patients with no pharmacologic reason to have a limitation in the HR response. The magnitude of the prognostic value of a poor HR response is as powerful as is an exercise-induced myocardial perfusion deficit. An abnormal **chronotropic** response apparently provides information that is independent of myocardial perfusion because the combination of perfusion deficit and an abnormal chronotropic index provides a worse prognosis than either abnormality alone[1]. In a similar, but apparently unrelated, fashion, the failure of the HR to recover promptly after exercise provides independent information related to prognosis[1]. Logistic regression analysis suggests that a failure to decrease HR by 12 bpm during the first minute of recovery is strongly associated with death during the follow-up period[1]. The unfavorable prognosis conveyed by the failure of HR to recover is apparently related to the inability to reassert vagal control over HR, which is independently known to predispose to arrhythmias[1].

Within the past decade, the use of exercise test scores that combine both favorable and unfavorable exercise test results into a single prognostically useful term has gained popularity[6,30]. Although the concept of exercise test scores has been around for a generation, the first widely accepted and most widely used is the Duke Index[6]. The Duke Index (see GETP7 Fig. 6-2) balances a favorable result (exercise capacity) against two unfavorable results (the magnitude of ST-segment depression and the presence and severity of angina pectoris). The calculated score has been shown to be related to a well-defined 5-year survival rate and allows the categorization of patients into low-, moderate-, and high-risk subgroups that may be treated conservatively or aggressively depending on classification.

The Duke Index can also be used in combination with other simple hemodynamic findings such as an abnormal pattern of recovery of HR or the combination of an abnormal chronotropic index or an abnormal HR recovery[1]. Each of these abnormalities of exercise testing contributes independent prognostic information to the result of exercise testing. Although there is a general belief that physicians informally integrate much of this information without the specific calculation of the various prognostically useful results of exercise testing, recent data suggest that estimates of the presence of CAD provided by scores are superior to physician estimates and analysis of ST-segment changes alone[30].

Although not as well tested relative to prognostic risk, there is apparently independent information to be gained from the pattern of increase in HR during exercise. In the majority of healthy individuals, the rate of increase in HR is negatively accelerated at exercise intensities above the second ventilatory threshold[31]. In about 5% of healthy individuals and a high percentage of individuals with CVD, the HR performance curve is positively accelerated[30]. Independent data suggest that this increase in the rate of increase in HR is a method of defending the cardiac output in individuals who have large decreases in stroke volume at high exercise intensities[32].

BLOOD PRESSURE

Systolic BP normally increases in a negatively accelerated manner during incremental exercise. The magnitude of increase is normally in the range of 5 to 10 mm Hg per MET, with a minimal increase of 10 mm Hg from rest to maximal exercise being considered normal (see GETP7 Box 6-1). A peak systolic pressure of more than 250 mm Hg or an increase by more than 140 mm Hg is considered a hypertensive response and is somewhat predictive of future resting hypertension[33]. In patients with limitations of cardiac output, there is either an inappropriately slow increase in BP or a decrease in systolic BP midway through the exercise test. A decrease of systolic BP to below the resting value or by more than 10 mm Hg after a preliminary increase, particularly in the presence of other indices of ischemia, is grossly abnormal and sufficient reason to stop the test immediately (see GETP7 Box 5-2). Diastolic BP is difficult to measure with accuracy during exercise testing. An increase by more than 10 mm Hg is generally considered to be an abnormal finding and consistent with exertional ischemia, as is an increase to more than 115 mm Hg[33].

During the postexercise period, systolic BP normally decreases promptly[25,26]. Over the past 2 decades, a number of investigators have demonstrated that a delay in the recovery of systolic BP is highly related both to ischemic abnormalities and to a poor prognosis[25,26]. As a general principle, the 3-minute postexercise systolic BP should be less than 90% of the systolic BP at peak exercise or if peak exercise pressure cannot be measured accurately, the 3-minute postexercise systolic BP should be less than the systolic BP measured 1 minute after exercise. Although not yet as well documented, abnormalities of the systolic BP recovery ratio may be more prognostically discriminative than abnormalities of the HR recovery pattern.

GAS EXCHANGE

Although the majority of exercise testing is performed without direct measurements of respiratory gas exchange, such measurements have recently been shown to be clinically useful. A major advantage of measuring gas exchange is the more accurate measurement of functional capacity. As indicated earlier, the practice of stopping exercise tests at predetermined workload or HR endpoints may cause clinicians to miss important information about exercise capacity. When exercise capacity is directly measured, values for $\dot{V}O_{2max}$ collected over periods of less than 30 seconds may significantly overestimate exercise capacity. In addition to a more accurate measurement of exercise capacity, gas exchange exercise testing may be particularly useful in defining prognosis (and thus helping to define the timing of transplantation) in patients with heart failure[28,34–36] and may help to guide the differential diagnosis in patients with possible cardiovascular or respiratory disease[37,38]. Gas exchange measurements also allow the determination of ventilatory threshold.

Summary

Recent evidence suggests that there is much more information in the simple incremental exercise test that formerly believed. However, these data are much more important in terms of defining prognosis than in making a specific diagnosis of obstructive CAD. Somewhat surprisingly, changes in the ST segment of the ECG are not particularly central features of this contemporary approach to evaluating exercise test results. The central feature appears to be the functional exercise capacity, which is probably because this serves as a surrogate of cardiac output. The prognostic impression gained from the exercise capacity is typically balanced by either ECG or symptomatic evidence of exertional myocardial ischemia. This relationship is well expressed in exercise test scores such as the Duke Index. Lastly, hemodynamic responses have been shown to be very powerful prognostic markers. It is probably not unreasonable to suggest that if all of the components of the exercise test are put together that exercise testing may be more powerful than myocardial perfusion scans or ventricular function measurements, which have been the *sine qua non* of non-invasive diagnostics for a decade.

Acknowledgments
The authors wish to acknowledge the contributors of this content area from previous editions of this text. Their efforts greatly assisted our compilation of information for the current chapter.

REFERENCES

1. Lauer MS: Exercise electrocardiogram testing and prognosis: Novel markers and predictive instruments. In Balady GJ, ed. Cardiol Clin 19:401–414, 2001.
2. Cole CR, Blackstone EH, Pashkow FJ: Heart rate recovery immediately after exercise as a predictor of mortality. N Engl J Med 341:1351–1357, 1999.
3. Cole CR, Foody JM, Blackstone EH, Lauer MS: Heart rate recovery after submaximal exercise testing as a predictor of mortality in a cardiovascularly healthy cohort. Ann Intern Med 132: 552–555, 2000.

4. Frolkis JP, Pothier CE, Blackstone EH, Lauer MS: Frequent ventricular ectopy after exercise as a predictor of death. N Engl J Med 348:781–790, 2003.

5. Lauer MS, Francis GS, Okin PM: Impaired chronotropic response during exercise stress testing as a predictor of mortality. JAMA 281:524–529, 1999.

6. Mark DB, Shaw L, Harrell FE, et al: Prognostic value of a treadmill exercise score in outpatients with suspected coronary artery disease. N Engl J Med 325:849, 853, 1991.

7. Morshedi-Meibodi A, Larson MG, Levy D, et al: Heart rate recovery after treadmill exercise testing and risk of cardiovascular disease events (The Framingham Heart Study). Am J Cardiol 90:848–852, 2002.

8. Myers J, Prakash M, Froelicher V, et al: Exercise capacity and mortality among men referred for exercise testing. N Engl J Med 346:793–801, 2002.

9. Nissines SI, Makikallio TH, Seppanen T, et al: Heart rate recovery after exercise as a predictor of mortality among survivors of acute myocardial infarction. Am J Cardiol 91:711–714, 2003.

10. Foster C, Porcari JP: The risks of exercise training. J Cardiopulm Rehabil 21:347–352, 2001.

11. Bruce RA, Hosmer F, Kusumi K: Maximal oxygen intake and nomographic assessment of functional aerobic impairment in cardiovascular disease. Am Heart J 85:546–562, 1973.

12. Myers, JN, Voodi, L, Froelicher VF: A survey of exercise testing: methods, utilization, interpretation, and safety in the VAHCS. Med Sci Sports Exerc 32:S143, 2000.

13. Foster C, Jackson AS, Pollock ML, et al: Generalized equations for prediction of functional capacity from treadmill performance. Am Heart J 107:1229–1237, 1984.

14. McConnell TR, Foster C, Conlin NC, Thompson NN: Prediction of functional capacity during treadmill testing: Effect of handrail support. J Cardiopulm Rehabil 11:255–260, 1991.

15. Myers J, Bellin D: Ramp exercise protocols for clinical and cardiopulmonary exercise testing. Sports Med 30:23–29, 2000.

16. Haskell WL, Savin W, Oldridge N, DeBusk R: Factors influencing estimated oxygen uptake during exercise testing soon after myocardial infarction. Am J Cardiol 50:299–304, 1982.

17. Foster C, Crowe AJ, Daines E, et al: Predicting functional capacity during treadmill testing independent of exercise protocol. Med Sci Sports Exerc 28:752–756, 1996.

18. Kaminsky LA, Whaley MH: Evaluation of a new standardized ramp protocol: The BSU/Bruce Ramp protocol. J Cardiopulm Rehabil 18:438–444, 1998.

19. Peterson MJ, Pieper CF, Morey MC: Accuracy of VO_2max prediction equations in older adults. Med Sci Sports Exerc 35:145–149, 2003.

20. Mittleman MA, Maclure M, Tofler GH: Triggering of acute myocardial infarction by heavy physical exertion: protection against triggering by regular exertion. N Engl J Med 329:1677–1683, 1993.

21. Willich SN, Lewis M, Lowell H: Physical exertion as a trigger of acute myocardial infarction. N Engl J Med 329:1684–1690, 1993.

22. Gutman RA, Alexander ER, Li YB, et al: Delay of ST depression after maximal exercise by walking for 2 minutes. Circulation 42:229–235, 1970.

23. Lachterman B, Lehmann KG, Abrahamson D, Forelicher VF: Recovery only ST-segment depression and the predictive accuracy of the exercise test. Ann Intern Med 112:11–16, 1990.

24. Bigi R, Cortigiani L, Gregori D, et al: Exercise versus recovery electrocardiography in predicting mortality in patients with uncomplicated myocardial infarction. Eur Heart J 25:558–564, 2004.

25. Amon KW, Richards KL, Crawford MH: Usefulness of the postexercise response of systolic blood pressure in the diagnosis of coronary artery disease. Circulation 70:951–956, 1984.

26. McHam SA, Marwick TH, Pashkow FJ, Lauer MS: Delayed systolic blood pressure recovery after graded exercise: An independent correlate of angiographic coronary disease. J Am Coll Cardiol 34:754–759, 1999.

27. Maybaum S, Ilan M, Mogilevsky J, Tzivoni D: Improvement in ischemic parameters during repeated exercise testing: A possible model for myocardial preconditioning. Am J Cardiol 78:1087–1091, 1996.

28. Mancini DM, Eisen H, Kussmaul W, et al: Value of peak exercise oxygen consumption for optimal timing of cardiac transplantation in ambulatory patients with heart failure. Circulation 83:778–786, 1991.

29. Morris CK, Myers J, Froelicher VF, et al;: Nomogram based on metabolic equivalents and age for assessing aerobic exercise capacity in men. J Am Coll Cardiol 22:175–182, 1993.

30. Lipinski M, Froelicher V, Atwood E, et al: Comparison of treadmill scores with physician estimates of diagnosis and prognosis in patients with coronary artery disease. Am Heart J 143:650–658, 2002.

31. Pokan R, Hofmann P, von Duvillard SP: The heart rate performance curve and left ventricular function during exercise in patients after myocardial infarction. Med Sci Sports Exerc 30:1475–1480, 1998.

32. Foster C, Spatz P, Georgakopoulos N: Left ventricular function in relation to the heart rate performance curve. Clin Exerc Physiol 1:29–32, 1999.

33. American College of Sports Medicine: Position stand: Exercise and hypertension. Med Sci Sports Exerc 36:533–553, 2004.

34. Myers J: Effect of exercise training on abnormal ventilatory responses to exercise in patients with chronic heart failure. Congest Heart Fail 6:243–249, 2000.

35. Myers J, Madhavan R: Exercise testing with gas exchange analysis. In Balady GJ, ed. Cardiol Clin 19:433–446, 2001.

36. Ramos-Barbon D, Fitchett D, Gibbons WJ, et al: Maximal exercise testing for the selection of heart transplantation candidates: Limitation of peak oxygen consumption. Chest 115:410–417, 1999.

37. Eschenbacher WL, Mannina A: An algorithm for the interpretation of cardiopulmonary exercise tests. Chest 97:263–267, 1990.

38. Wasserman K: Diagnosing cardiovascular and lung pathophysiology from exercise gas exchange. Chest 112:1091–1101, 1997.

SELECTED REFERENCES FOR FURTHER READING

Myers, J.N. Essentials of Cardiopulmonary Exercise Testing. Champaign, IL: Human Kinetics; 1996.

Wassermann K, Hansen JE, Sue DY, et al: Principles of Exercise Testing and Interpretation, 2nd ed. Baltimore: Lippincott, Williams & Wilkins; 1994.

Froelicher VF, Myers J, Follansbee WP, Labovitz AJ: Exercise and the Heart, 3rd ed. St. Louis: Mosby; 1993.

INTERNET RESOURCES

ACC/AHA 2002 Guideline Update for Exercise Testing:
http://www.americanheart.org/presenter.jhtml?identifier=3005237

American College of Cardiology/American Heart Association Clinical Competence Statement on Stress Testing, 2000:
http://circ.ahajournals.org/cgi/content/full/102/14/1726

American Heart Association: Scientific Statement: Exercise Standards for testing and training. 2001:
http://circ.ahajournals.org/cgi/content/full/104/14/1694

Assessment and Limitations Associated with Pulmonary Disease

BRIAN W. CARLIN AND KHALEELUR SALAHUDEEN

Patients with lung disease typically present with shortness of breath precipitated by exercise or strenuous conditions. Lung diseases are generally classified into one of three categories: obstructive, restrictive, and vascular. Although the presenting symptom behind each of these disease types is the same, the pathophysiology associated with the limitations is varied. This chapter addresses the pathophysiology of each of these disease processes, their associated limitations, and the clinical assessment of patients with these diseases. See Chapter 32 for information related to exercise training for patients with lung disease.

Normal Ventilatory Mechanics

During inspiration, the diaphragm contracts and moves downward, and the rib cage moves upward and outward. A negative pressure within the thorax develops and causes air to move into the lungs from the mouth. During expiration, the diaphragm relaxes and moves upward, and the rib cage moves inward, moving air from the lungs to the mouth. Such expiration is aided by the lung parenchyma's intrinsic elastic recoil, which allows air to leave the lungs.

The large airways are supported by cartilage in their walls, allowing them to remain open. The amount of cartilage present is reduced as the size of the airways decreases, thus leaving the smallest airways with no cartilage. These smaller airways are tethered open by the surrounding meshwork involving the alveoli. They are pulled open during inspiration by the development of negative intrathoracic pressure. During expiration, a positive intrathoracic pressure is generated, causing a reduction in the lung volume and traction over the smaller airways. Resulting in smaller airway caliber (Fig. 15-1). The smaller airways are affected more so because there is no cartilage to help support them to remain open.

Obstructive Airway Diseases

Chronic obstructive pulmonary disease (COPD) is a common disorder characterized by progressive expiratory airflow obstruction. Symptoms develop insidiously over years or decades and include **dyspnea** (at rest and with exertion), cough, and sputum production. The obstructive airway diseases include emphysema, chronic bronchitis, and asthma. Although these are often considered to be distinct entities, their physiological and clinical features often overlap in individual patients.

Chronic obstructive pulmonary disease is characterized by nonuniform narrowing of airways. Such airway narrowing increases resistance to airflow and results in uneven distribution of ventilation and expiratory flow limitation (Fig. 15-2). Loss of elastic recoil of the lung occurs, causing the small airways to close at an abnormally high lung volume, resulting in an increase in residual volume (RV) at the end of a forced expiration (also known as air trapping). Air trapping places the diaphragm at a mechanical disadvantage for contraction (Fig. 15-3). All of these mechanisms lead to an increase in the work of breathing, resulting in dyspnea.

EMPHYSEMA

Emphysema is a disease of the lung parenchyma that secondarily affects the smaller airways. Destruction of lung tissue occurs secondary to a variety of mechanisms involving the inflammatory and the protease–antiprotease

KEY TERMS

Asthma: A continuum of disease processes characterized by inflammation of the airway wall

Chronic bronchitis: A clinical diagnosis for patients who have chronic cough and sputum production

Chronic obstructive pulmonary disease (COPD): A group of lung diseases (e.g., emphysema, chronic bronchitis, asthma) that result in airflow obstruction

Dyspnea: The perception of shortness of breath

Emphysema: A pathological or anatomical description marked by abnormal permanent enlargement of the respiratory bronchioles and alveoli accompanied by destruction of the lung parenchyma

Hypercapnia: Excess carbon dioxide in the blood

Hypoxemia: Deficient oxygenation of the blood

Pulmonary hypertension: An elevation in the blood pressure within the arteries of the lung

Restrictive lung disease: A group of diseases characterized by the inability to normally inflate the lungs

Timed walk test: One of a variety of tests (e.g., 6-minute walk test, shuttle walk test, endurance shuttle walk test) used to assess functional status. The distance walked over a certain period of time is measured during these tests.

Vascular lung disease: A group of diseases that affect the vascular supply (pulmonary arteries, capillaries, and veins) of the lung

---

systems. Chronic inflammation throughout the airways, parenchyma, and pulmonary vasculature is mediated by a variety of cell types (macrophages, lymphocytes, and neutrophils). This inflammation often results after exposure to cigarette smoke[1–4]. Destruction of the lung parenchyma (respiratory bronchioles and alveolar walls), also occurs as a result of the imbalance between enzymes (e.g., proteinases and antiproteinases) within the lung[5–7]. Changes in the pulmonary vascular bed (e.g.,

vessel wall thickening and smooth muscle proliferation) also occur as a result of the inflammation and lung destruction[8].

As a result of these processes, the lung loses its elasticity and its elastic recoil pressure. Small airways lose traction with the surrounding alveolar walls and become easily collapsible during expiration. Distribution of ventilation is nonuniform, and alterations in perfusion occur. Some ventilation reaches areas that are not well perfused because of destruction of the capillary bed, and an increase in dead space ventilation occurs.

To overcome this elevation in dead space ventilation and alteration of the normal ventilation–perfusion balance, a patient with emphysema must maintain a high minute ventilation (by increasing the tidal volume [V_T] for each breath and, after it is maximized, increasing the respiratory rate). An increase in the amount of work of breathing occurs, and a larger than normal supply of oxygen is needed by the respiratory muscles to maintain a stable ventilatory process. Oxygen supply is then diverted from the gut toward the respiratory muscles. Coupled with an overall increase in metabolism, malnutrition results. Functional skeletal muscle (in terms of strength and endurance) is lost, and severe muscular deconditioning occurs.

Patients with emphysema alter their pattern of breathing in an attempt to place the ventilatory muscles in a greater position to perform the work necessary to breathe. For example, patients with emphysema can minimize air trapping by breathing through pursed lips. This causes external resistance to flow and maintains a more positive intra-airway pressure during exhalation, minimizing compression of the small airways. This results in a decrease in the overall work of breathing.

Patients with pure emphysema are known as "pink puffers." They complain of significant dyspnea, are barrel

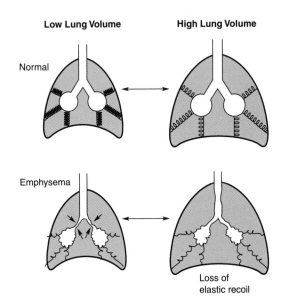

FIGURE 15-1. Small airways are tethered open by radial traction of lung tissue. Airway caliber depends on recoil of the lung, which is greater at high lung volume; hence, airway caliber is also greater at a high lung volume. In diseases in which elastic recoil is lost, small airways are prone to dynamic collapse when pressure outside the airway becomes more positive, as during forced expiration.

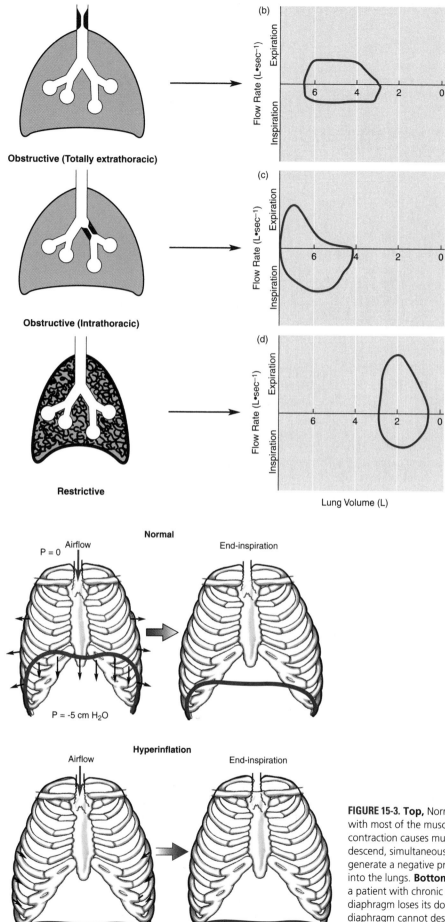

Obstructive (Totally extrathoracic)

Obstructive (Intrathoracic)

Restrictive

(b)

(c)

(d)

Lung Volume (L)

FIGURE 15-2. Maximal flow–volume curves in a normal subject, a patient with obstructive airways disease, and a patient with restrictive lung disease.

Normal

Airflow

P = 0

End-inspiration

P = -5 cm H₂O

Hyperinflation

Airflow

End-inspiration

FIGURE 15-3. Top, Normally, the diaphragm is dome shaped, with most of the muscle fibers nearly vertical. Diaphragm contraction causes muscle fibers to shorten and the dome to descend, simultaneously expanding the rib cage. These actions generate a negative pressure inside the thorax causing airflow into the lungs. **Bottom,** In the lung that is hyperinflated (as in a patient with chronic obstructive pulmonary disease), the diaphragm loses its dome shape. With contraction, the diaphragm cannot descend normally, which can create a paradoxical inward movement of the lower rib cage.

chested because of the marked lung hyperinflation, and have little cough or sputum production. They are typically thin with general muscle wasting. In moderate disease, the arterial oxygen and carbon dioxide tensions are relatively normal. As progressive inflammation and destruction of the alveolar–capillary units occurs, worsening arterial oxygen desaturation and progressive elevation in pulmonary artery pressure may develop followed by right heart failure (Fig. 15-4)[9].

CHRONIC BRONCHITIS

Chronic bronchitis is characterized by a chronic cough and mucus production. Unlike emphysema, which primarily involves abnormalities within the lung parenchyma and smaller airways, chronic bronchitis primarily involves the large airways. Airway wall injury occurs because of the effects of infiltration of inflammatory cells and mucus gland enlargement. As the body attempts to repair the inflamed areas, structural remodeling occurs, with an increase in the deposition of collagen in the airway walls[5]. Such bronchial and peribronchiolar inflammation results in further airway narrowing and an increase in airway resistance[10,11]. Lung areas with an elevation in airway resistance receive little ventilation, and the blood flow to this area remains unchanged or decreases, causing the lung to become underventilated and overperfused. This ventilation–perfusion imbalance leads to arterial **hypoxemia**, which, in turn, may lead to increased pulmonary vascular resistance and pulmonary arterial hypertension. Eventually, right ventricular failure (cor pulmonale) may develop (Fig. 15-5). Unlike in patients with emphysema, the intrathoracic pressure generated by muscular effort and lung elastic recoil is normal in patients with chronic bronchitis.

Hypoxemia stimulates the production of erythropoietin, resulting in excess blood volume, hemoglobin concentration, and hematocrit level (also known as secondary polycythemia). Polycythemia may lead to a high blood viscosity, increasing flow resistance in blood vessels and further compromising blood flow. Typical patients with severe chronic bronchitis are known as "blue bloaters" because they exhibit a stocky habitus with central and peripheral cyanosis. Reduced airflow rate is associated with only mildly increased lung volumes and a relatively normal rate of oxygen transfer across the alveolar–capillary membrane (normal diffusing capacity for carbon monoxide). Secondary derangements in ventilatory control may develop. Patients with chronic bronchitis tend to maintain low minute ventilation, which may further decrease during sleep and may result in nocturnal hypoxemia. Daytime hypoxemia and hypercapnia may develop in some patients.

ASTHMA

Asthma is characterized by increased airway reactivity to a variety of stimuli, resulting in widespread reversible narrowing of the airways. Its episodic nature and reversibility

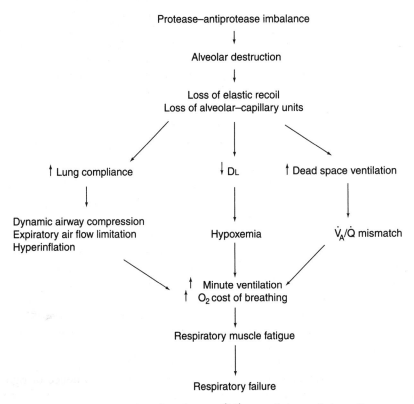

FIGURE 15-4. Progression of emphysema. $\dot{V}_A/\dot{Q}$ = ventilation-perfusion ratio.

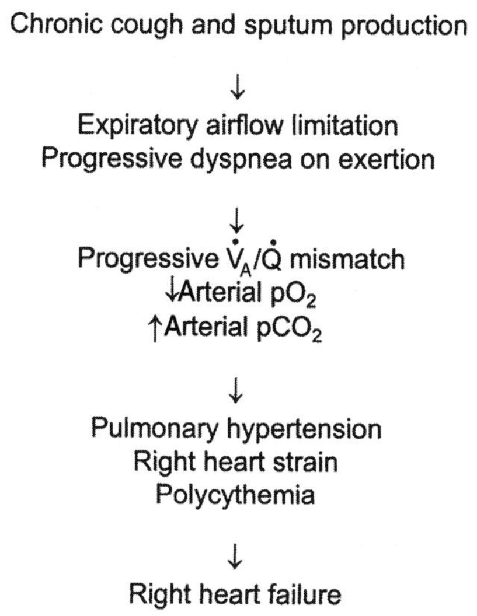

Chronic cough and sputum production

↓

Expiratory airflow limitation
Progressive dyspnea on exertion

↓

Progressive $\dot{V}_A/\dot{Q}$ mismatch
↓Arterial pO_2
↑Arterial pCO_2

↓

Pulmonary hypertension
Right heart strain
Polycythemia

↓

Right heart failure

FIGURE 15-5. Progression of chronic bronchitis.

are important features separating it from the two other major types of obstructive airways disease (i.e., emphysema and chronic bronchitis) Although a precipitating factor often cannot be identified, it is possible in some instances to identify a specific agent (e.g., pollens, dust mites, chemical, animal dander, drugs, exposure to the cold) in these instances, appropriate avoidance of the precipitating agent can be recommended.

As with the other obstructive lung diseases, the pathophysiology of asthma is related to inflammation. Asthma is often initiated by an antigen presented to the airway. An antibody response results in the release of various chemical mediators from mast cells and eosinophils, which promotes inflammation of the airway walls and airway smooth muscle[12,13]. The airway lumen is structurally changed, becoming occluded by a combination of mucus and denuded epithelium. Abnormal collagen deposition in the airways and subepithelial fibrosis result in airway narrowing[14].

The clinical symptoms of a patient with asthma are similar to that of the other obstructive lung diseases. Shortness of breath and wheezing are commonly present. A diagnosis is made by using a combination of the patient's history, clinical examination, and pulmonary function tests. Reduced maximal expiratory flow rates, increased expiratory airway resistance, and elevated RV and total lung capacity (TLC), which are abolished by the administration of a bronchodilator, are hallmarks of this disease. Bronchial hyperresponsiveness to methacholine (a medication that causes airway irritation) is seen in patients with asthma. In some, asthma is only present during or after exercise[15].

During an acute asthma exacerbation, the lung units distal to the areas of airway narrowing are underventilated, and ventilation perfusion imbalance occurs. A patient initially hyperventilates maintaining a normal arterial oxygen tension and a decreased arterial carbon dioxide tension. As

the exacerbation worsens, the distribution of ventilation and perfusion becomes more imbalanced, the arterial oxygen tension decreases, and the arterial carbon dioxide tension increases. This ultimately leads to respiratory failure (hypoxemia and **hypercapnia**).

CLINICAL FEATURES AND LABORATORY ASSESSMENT OF PATIENTS WITH CHRONIC OBSTRUCTIVE PULMONARY DISEASE

Common presenting symptoms of COPD include a shortness of breath or cough developing in the fourth to fifth decades of life. Sputum production occurs only in the morning; throughout this time course, the patient often has dyspnea that worsens with exercise. Exacerbations, characterized by an increase in dyspnea, purulent sputum, wheezing, and fever, may also develop and become more frequent as the disease progresses. Hypoxemia may develop and eventually lead to cor pulmonale. All of these factors result in the development of exercise intolerance, leading to deconditioning and worsening of exercise tolerance.

The patient's history is a very important part of the assessment. Most patients with COPD are current or former smokers, and the amount of cigarettes smoked, characterized by pack years (e.g., one pack year equals one pack of cigarettes smoked per day per year), should be noted. The development of symptoms may lag up to 20 years after the initiation of cigarette smoking. The time course of cigarette smoking and duration of abstinence is also important. A family history of lung disease is pertinent because several diseases processes (e.g., alpha-1 antitrypsin deficiency) are known to be genetically transmitted. A history of childhood illnesses such as asthma and allergies is helpful. A complete work history (including all work performed by the patient dating back to his or her first work experience) is important (e.g., exposures to coal dust, secondhand smoke, molds). Finally, the patient's gender appears to play an important role in the development of lung disease: women may be prone to developing lung disease at an earlier age than men[16,17].

Early in the course of the disease, the patient has normal physical examination findings. As the disease progresses, wheezing may be noted only on a forced expiration maneuver, and hyperinflation of the lung and chest wall occurs. A decrease in breath sounds with a decrease in movement of the diaphragm and a decrease in heart sounds become noticeable. A prolongation of the time for a forced expiration (greater than 3 seconds) is seen. With further progression, the patient may use techniques that are more effective to relieve dyspnea such as leaning forward with the arms outstretched and weight supported by the palms or breathing using pursed lips. When cor pulmonale develops, evidence of right-sided heart failure (neck vein distention, enlarged liver, peripheral edema) may then be seen.

Routine laboratory testing supplements the patient's history and physical examination and is helpful in the evaluation and management process. A chest radiograph is an essential part of this assessment to not only confirm the presence of COPD (e.g., lung hyperinflation, retrosternal airspace increase, diaphragmatic flattening, enlarged pulmonary artery size) but also to determine whether or not there are other causes for dyspnea (e.g., pleural effusion, lung cancer, congestive heart failure).

An electrocardiogram (ECG) is helpful to determine whether a cardiac disease may be present. Measurement of oxyhemoglobin saturation by cutaneous pulse oximetry or arterial oxygen tension/carbon dioxide tension by arterial blood gas analysis help in the assessment of the patient. Measurements of hemoglobin may help to determine the duration of hypoxemia (e.g., a significant elevation in hematocrit level above 50 $g \cdot dL^{-1}$ may indicate long-standing arterial oxyhemoglobin desaturation) or the presence of anemia (e.g., a significant decrease in hematocrit level may be responsible for a patient's symptoms of shortness of breath). Computed tomography (CT) scanning of the chest is helpful to assess the lung parenchyma and to evaluate for intrathoracic masses.

Measurement of lung volumes and flow rates should be performed on all patients suspected of having lung disease. This includes the measurement of TLC, RV, vital capacity (VC), inspiratory capacity (IC), forced expiratory volume in 1 second (FEV_1) and in 6 seconds (FEV_6), forced vital capacity (FVC), peak flow rate (PEFR), and diffusing capacity for carbon monoxide (Dl_{CO}). These measures can be easily and reliably reproduced[17] and help in the determination of the type of disease process present (Table 15-1). Although some of the measures (e.g., TLC, VC, RV, Dl_{CO}) require the use of sophisticated equipment, other measures (e.g., FEV_1, FEV_6, FVC) can be performed using very simple equipment. To promote the early detection of COPD, the National Lung Health Education Program recommends simply spirometry testing for all smokers over the age of 45 years and for any smoker who has respiratory symptoms (e.g., cough, sputum production, dyspnea), regardless of age[18–20].

Pulmonary function testing is helpful not only with the diagnosis of the disease but also with staging of the disease. The FEV_1 is the best correlate with morbidity and mortality in these patients, and several proposals for staging have been developed using the FEV_1. The American Thoracic Society suggests a staging on the basis of the severity of airflow obstruction: stage I is an FEV_1 of more than 50% predicted, stage II is an FEV_1 of 35% to 49% predicted, and stage III is an FEV_1 of less than 35% predicted[21]. In general, patients with stage I disease have little impairment in their quality of life. Patients with stage II disease have significant impairments in their quality of life, and patients with stage III disease are significantly impaired, often requiring many hospitalizations for severe exacerbations (also see GETP7 Table 3-4).

More recently, another staging system has been proposed. This system is part of the Global Initiative for Lung Disease (GOLD Guidelines) and although it is similar to the American Thoracic Society system, differences exist[22]. Stage 0 (at risk) is characterized by a patient who has chronic cough and sputum production with normal lung function. Stage I (mild COPD) is characterized by a patient who has mild airflow limitation (FEV_1/FVC < 70% but FEV_1 > 80% predicted) and usually, but not always, has symptoms. Stage II (moderate COPD) is characterized by a patient who has worsening airflow limitation (FEV_1 between 30% and 80% predicted) and who usually has progression of symptoms to include dyspnea with exertion. Stage III (severe COPD) is characterized by a patient who has severe airflow limitation (FEV_1 < 30% predicted) or the presence of respiratory failure or clinical signs of right heart failure.

The important difference between these two staging systems is that in the latter, the patient's symptoms are a part of the classification system. This may allow patients who have minimal or no symptoms to be staged and potentially make them aware that they may have or may be developing COPD. The latter staging system is the becoming the more widely accepted severity staging system for patients with COPD.

EXERCISE LIMITATIONS IN CHRONIC OBSTRUCTIVE PULMONARY DISEASE

A variety of factors interact to cause exercise intolerance in patients with COPD. Such intolerance is often initially manifested as increase in shortness of breath or easy fatigability with exercise. As COPD progresses, dyspnea and fatigability at even minimal levels of exercise occurs. The factors involved in exercise intolerance for patients with COPD include ventilatory abnormalities (impaired respiratory system mechanics and ventilatory muscle dysfunc-

TABLE 15-1. Pulmonary Function Testing: Interpretation for Various Disease States

	Obstructive	Restrictive	Vascular
FEV_1 (L)	↓	↓	↔
FVC (L)	↓	↓	↔
FEV_1/FVC (FEV_1/FEV_6)	↓	↔ or ↑	↔
TLC (L)	↑	↓	↔
VC (L)	↓	↓	↔
FRC (L)	↑	↓	↔
RV (L)	↑	↓	↔
Dl_{CO}	↔ or ↓	↔ or ↓	↓

↔ = no change; ↑ = increased; ↓ = decreased. ↔ or ↑ = no change early in disease process, increase late in disease; ↔ or ↓ = no change early in disease process, decrease late in disease; Dl_{CO} = diffusing capacity for carbon monoxide; FEV_1 = forced expiratory volume in one second; FRC = functional residual capacity; FVC = forced vital capacity; RV = residual volume; TLC = total lung capacity; VC = vital capacity.

No change early in disease process, decrease late in disease

<table>
<tr><td>

BOX 15-1

</td><td>

Abnormalities Noted During Exercise in Patients with Chronic Obstructive Pulmonary Disease

</td></tr>
</table>

Dyspnea

Leg discomfort

Reduced maximal oxygen consumption

Reduced work rate

High dead space ventilation (V_D/V_T)

Decreased V_T response with increased respiratory rate

Reduced inspiratory capacity with exercise (i.e., dynamic hyperinflation)

Variable arterial oxyhemoglobin desaturation

V_D = dead space; V_T = tidal volume.

tion), metabolic and gas exchange abnormalities, peripheral muscle dysfunction, cardiovascular limitations, and intolerable dyspnea. The typical abnormalities and limitations noted during exercise for patients with COPD are listed in Box 15-1.

Ventilatory limitations constitute the primary cause for exercise limitation in patients with COPD. Airflow limitation, prominent on maximal expiratory efforts, is the hallmark of COPD and results from a variety of mechanisms, including loss of elastic lung tissue, airway inflammation, and airway collapse. As effort increases (e.g., during exercise), expiratory flow increases to a point beyond which further effort does not produce any further increase in expiratory flow (Fig. 15-6). In patients with normal ventilatory systems, only a small fraction of the expiratory flow is used during tidal breathing, and airflow limitation is not reached. But in patients with COPD, the anatomic and physiologic processes already mentioned cause expiratory flow limitation (noted as scalloping of the expiratory portion of the flow volume curve). This expiratory airflow limitation may be so severe in some patients that it can be reached even during tidal breathing. Patients with expiratory airflow limitation cannot reach the increased demands placed on the ventilatory system during exercise by increasing their expiratory flow as would occur in normal individuals.

As expiratory flow limitation occurs, the lung cannot fully empty during resting breathing. End-expiratory lung volume remains elevated compared with that of normal individuals and is termed *dynamic hyperinflation*. Dynamic hyperinflation causes a limitation to be placed on each inspiratory effort and causes a decrease in the inspiratory capacity[23]. Severe mechanical constraints on V_T expansion during exercise occur despite an increase in the respiratory drive. The reduced resting inspiratory capacity and resting expiratory flow limitation

in such patients result in poorer exercise performance compared with patients who have a better preserved inspiratory capacity and no evidence of expiratory flow limitation at rest[23,24].

Dynamic hyperinflation also causes increased elastic loading of the inspiratory muscles, resulting in an increase in muscle oxygen utilization and muscle work. Alterations of the normal length–tension relationship of the inspiratory muscles (e.g., the diaphragm, sternomastoids, and scalenes) compromise the ability of these muscle groups to function efficiently. As exercise increases, dynamic hyperinflation causes progressive limitation of the normal increase in V_T despite maximal inspiratory efforts. Dyspnea may well be more linked to dynamic hyperinflation, even more so than to airflow obstruction.

Gas exchange abnormalities are commonly seen in patients with COPD. A variety of mechanisms are responsible for the development of hypoxemia and hypercapnia. Airflow limitation is not uniformly distributed within the lung and results in an uneven distribution of ventilation with blood perfusion. Destruction of the lung parenchyma (e.g., as might occur in patients with emphysema), alveolar hypoventilation (e.g., as might occur in patients with chronic bronchitis), and an elevation in the resting physiologic dead space that does not decrease with exercise also play roles in the gas exchange abnormalities. As patients exercise, the gas exchange abnormalities become more prominent, resulting in worsening hypoxemia.

Ventilatory and peripheral muscle dysfunction (both structural and functional) is present with patients who have COPD[25,26]. Strength and endurance (the primary characteristics of muscle performance) are significantly reduced for the muscle groups used to effect ventilation. The work of breathing increase significantly for a given level of ventilation as the disease progresses (Fig. 15-7). The ventilatory and peripheral muscle groups are affected

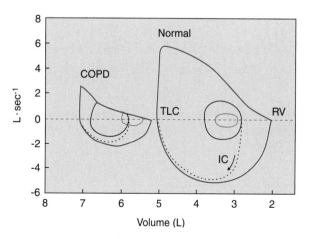

FIGURE 15-6. Flow volume curve for a patient with chronic obstructive pulmonary disease (COPD) (rest and exercise). IC = inspiratory capacity; RV = residual volume; TLC = total lung capacity.

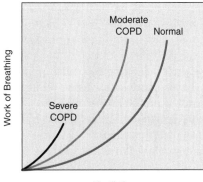

FIGURE 15-7. Work of the respiratory muscles increases as ventilation increases. As chronic obstructive pulmonary disease (COPD) progresses, the work of breathing is higher than normal at any given level of ventilation. In addition, the maximum work that can be generated by the respiratory muscles is diminished as the disease progresses.

differently however: whereas endurance limitation (fatigue) is noted with the peripheral muscles, strength limitation is noted with the ventilatory muscles. Muscle biopsies of the peripheral muscles in patients with COPD show a consistent reduction in type I (slow-twitch, low-tension, fatigue-resistant) fibers and an increase in type II (fast-twitch, high-tension) fibers. Few studies have evaluated the ventilatory muscle, but it appears that there is an opposite effect on these muscle fibers (replacement of the type II fibers with the type I fibers). Current evidence also suggests an alteration of the oxidative capacity (reduction in citrate synthase and hydroxyacyl-CoA dehydrogenase activities and increase in glycolytic activities) of both the peripheral skeletal muscles and the ventilatory muscles along with a reduction in the capillary density[27]. The early production of lactic acid is related to this skeletal muscle dysfunction.

Various factors have been implicated as potential mechanisms for such muscle dysfunction. Hypoxia and oxidative stress (caused by reactive oxygen species, oxygen free radicals), disuse atrophy (deconditioning), malnutrition, skeletal muscle myopathy, and weight loss with altered substrate (e.g., amino acid, anabolic steroids, leptin) metabolism have all been shown to be associated with muscle dysfunction in patients with COPD. Ongoing research is looking into each of these areas because the relative contribution of each of these mechanisms to the resultant skeletal muscle dysfunction needs to be more fully defined.

Restrictive Lung Diseases

Restrictive lung diseases reduce lung volume through the involvement of the thorax or the lung parenchyma. They include more than 200 disorders affecting either the pleural space (e.g., hemothorax, pleural effusion), alveoli (e.g., pulmonary alveolar proteinosis, pneumonia), inter-

stitial space (e.g., interstitial lung disease), neuromuscular system (e.g., myasthenia gravis, spinal cord injury), and thoracic cage (e.g., kyphoscoliosis, ankylosing spondylitis). The cause for the patient's primary symptom of dyspnea is related to the reduction in lung volume caused by the underlying disease process.

CLINICAL EVALUATION AND LABORATORY ASSESSMENT OF PATIENTS WITH RESTRICTIVE LUNG DISEASE

The initial evaluation of the patient should include a complete history and physical examination. The patient often seeks medical attention because of progressive shortness of breath (particularly with exertion) or a nonproductive cough. The history is a vital part of such an evaluation because it often elicits clues to the diagnosis, particularly when interstitial lung disease is being considered as part of the differential (Box 15-2). Attention should be paid to the patient's occupational history, environmental exposure history, medication history, family history, and smoking history.

The shortness of breath progresses insidiously because patients often decrease their level of activity to compensate for the worsening impairment. As the shortness of breath progresses and interferes with the patient's activities of daily living, medical attention is sought. The duration of shortness of breath is helpful in the evaluation process. A short, rapid onset of symptoms is suggestive of hypersensitivity pneumonitis, eosinophilic pneumonia, or alveolar hemorrhage syndromes. A more prolonged course, with the development of symptoms over years or longer, is more characteristic of the interstitial lung diseases (particularly idiopathic pulmonary fibrosis).

The physical examination may be helpful but often not until the patient has developed significant symptoms. A thorough examination of the patient with particular atten-

---

BOX 15-2 | **Causes of Interstitial Lung Disease**

1. Occupational and Environmental Exposures
   Inorganic dusts (silica, asbestos, tin, coal, hard metals)
   Organic (hypersensitivity pneumonitis caused by bacteria, fungi, animal proteins)
2. Drugs or medications (chemotherapy agents, radiation exposure, oxygen)
3. Collagen vascular diseases (scleroderma, systemic lupus erythematosis, rheumatoid arthritis, polymyositis)
4. Neoplasm (bronchoalveolar carcinoma, lymphoma)
5. Unknown causes (interstitial pulmonary fibrosis, sarcoidosis, lymphangioleiomyomatosis, eosinophilic granuloma, nonspecific interstitial pneumonia, bronchiolitis obliterans organizing pneumonia)

tion to the chest and neuromuscular systems is important. A decrease in excursion of the chest with an increase in respiratory rate at rest is often present. A decrease in breath sounds over one side of the chest is seen in patients with pleural disease; an anatomic deformity of the chest and thoracic cage is seen in patients with kyphoscoliosis; and fine-end inspiratory rales (Velcro crackles) are seen in patients with interstitial fibrosis. Weakness of the extremities is present in patients with neuromuscular disease (e.g., myasthenia gravis). Arthritis occurs in those with collagen vascular diseases and sarcoid. Integration of the history and physical findings should then prompt further diagnostic testing.

The diagnostic tests should initially include a chest radiograph. This helps to assess the volume of the lungs, presence of a pleural effusion, structure of the chest wall and thorax, and presence or absence of interstitial or alveolar infiltrates. CT scanning (particularly high-resolution scanning) can assess for the presence of interstitial fibrosis and may help in the differentiation of the various types of interstitial fibrosis (e.g., usual interstitial pneumonia, nonspecific interstitial pneumonia). Pulse oximetry and arterial blood gases are helpful to assess the degree of gas exchange abnormalities that may be present. If neuromuscular disease is suspected, a comprehensive neurologic evaluation, possibly including nerve conduction studies, should be performed. Pulmonary function tests reveal a decrease in the FEV_1, FVC, and TLC with maintenance (or an increase) in the FEV_1/FVC ratio. A low diffusing capacity may be seen late in the disease course, particularly for patients with interstitial fibrosis. A reduction in the maximal expiratory and inspiratory pressures may be seen in patients with neuromuscular diseases. Results of routine pulmonary function testing alone cannot be meaningfully used in the prediction of responses to exercise. It has been shown that many patients with interstitial lung disease have abnormal exercise responses[28].

EXERCISE LIMITATIONS ASSOCIATED WITH PATIENTS WITH RESTRICTIVE LUNG DISEASE

The abnormality common to all of the restrictive lung diseases is a reduction in the TLC and FVC. This reduction in lung volume may lead to collapse of the smaller airway units with subsequent decrease in the functional alveolar–capillary interface and may lead to impaired gas exchange. A decrease in the diffusing capacity of the lungs may result in patients who have disruption of this alveolar–capillary unit.

Interstitial lung disease is the most well studied of the restrictive lung processes, and although a variety of causes for interstitial lung disease have been found, the clinical and pathophysiological characteristics for these diseases are similar. Chronic inflammation of the interstitium and alveoli results in fibrosis of these structures. These changes reduce lung compliance and increase lung stiff-

ness[28]. A stiff lung requires more energy to stretch, with a requirement of having an increased transpulmonary pressure to achieve a given V_T. Not only is the lung capacity decreased and the lung stiffness increased, but the alveolar–capillary units can be replaced with fibrous tissue.

Gas exchange is often disrupted as a result of these processes and is the major factor in exercise limitation. In the early stages of the disease process, the resting arterial oxygen tension is normal but decreases during exercise, and the alveolar–arterial oxygen gradient increases (Box 15-3). As the disease progresses, resting hypoxemia and widening of the alveolar–arterial oxygen gradient occurs because of imbalance of ventilation and perfusion, shunting, and impaired oxygen diffusion[28].

A characteristic ventilatory response to exercise occurs in these patients[29]. An increase in minute ventilation occurs through an increase in the respiratory rate rather than an increase in V_T (because the V_T is functionally limited because of the interstitial process). With such constraints, the patient breathes with very rapid, shallow breaths in an attempt to reduce the work of breathing. This type of breathing results in an increase in dead space ventilation (V_D/V_T) because of the decrease in V_T. Normally during exercise, V_D/V_T decreases because of the increase in V_T, but in patients with interstitial lung disease, the V_D/V_T remains constant or increases.

An increase in elastic recoil of the lung at functional residual capacity is present in patients who have interstitial lung disease. In combination with the reduction in lung volumes, this results in an adverse impact on the ability of the respiratory system to adapt to the increasing ventilatory demands required during exercise.

Pulmonary hypertension develops because of hypoxic vasoconstriction and obliteration of the pulmonary vascular bed by the underlying interstitial process. Most patients with interstitial lung disease develop significant pulmonary hypertension with exercise[30], and nearly all patients with interstitial lung disease have right ventricular hypertrophy.

BOX 15-3 | **Abnormalities Noted During Exercise in Patients with Interstitial Lung Disease**

Dyspnea

Reduced maximal oxygen consumption

Reduced work rate

Reduced V_T with increased respiratory rate at submaximal work rates

Increased dead space ventilation (V_D/V_T)

Arterial oxyhemoglobin desaturation during exercise

Unchanged $PaCO_2$ during exercise

V_D = dead space; V_T = tidal volume.

Pulmonary hypertension has been shown to significantly correlate with hypoxemia during exercise. Hypoxemia plays a more important role than does the abnormal ventilatory mechanics in the exercise limitation found in these patients. In fact, it has been suggested that the gas exchange abnormalities (secondary to this circulatory pathophysiology) are perhaps the most important factors in exercise limitation in patients with interstitial lung disease[28].

Vascular Lung Disease

As with the restrictive lung diseases, a variety of diseases result in **vascular lung disease**. These include diseases that involve the pulmonary veins and arteries and are generally characterized by obstruction of the pulmonary circulation and disruption of the alveolar–capillary membrane. This results in a decrease of the effective vascular bed for gas exchange and impairment of diffusion and gas exchange. Pulmonary hypertension and right ventricular failure ultimately develop.

Pulmonary hypertension is a mean pulmonary artery pressure at rest of more than 25 mm Hg or more than 30 mm Hg with exercise. Pulmonary hypertension can occur because of increased cardiac output or increased pulmonary vascular resistance. It is often characterized as either primary or secondary pulmonary hypertension . Primary pulmonary hypertension is a disease, by definition, of uncertain etiology[31]. Other causes of pulmonary hypertension must not be present in order for a patient to be classified as having primary pulmonary hypertension. Secondary pulmonary hypertension is a disease that is also characterized by elevation in pulmonary artery pressure attributable a known cause, including severe COPD, interstitial lung disease, left ventricular (LV) dysfunction, mitral valvular stenosis, chronic thromboembolic disease[32], HIV infection[33], sleep-disordered breathing, connective tissue disease, medications, and portopulmonary hypertension.

CLINICAL ASSESSMENT AND LABORATORY EVALUATION OF PATIENTS WITH VASCULAR LUNG DISEASE

Patients with vascular lung disease present with symptoms of shortness of breath often first noted during exercise. Patients may have had exposure to certain diet medications (as associated with primary pulmonary hypertension) or a history of venous thromboembolism (as associated with chronic thromboembolic pulmonary hypertension). Typically, very few historical clues are present as to the cause of the patient's pulmonary hypertension. The clinical examination of the patient is often normal, with clear lung fields and normal mechanical movement of the chest and abdominal walls during inspiration and expiration. A cardiac murmur heard best at the base of the heart may suggest mitral stenosis. A gallop is suggestive of LV systolic dysfunction. A loud second heart sound, heard best over the second left intercostal space, is noted and is secondary to the accentuated closure of the pulmonary valve. With long-standing disease, evidence of right-sided heart failure (hepatomegaly, peripheral edema, jugular venous distention) may become apparent. Clubbing of the fingers is also seen.

The laboratory evaluation of a patient with pulmonary hypertension should include a chest radiograph and ECG. The radiograph will show clear lung fields and an enlargement of the cardiac silhouette. An ECG will show a right ventricular strain pattern. Pulse oximetry determination of oxyhemoglobin saturation and arterial blood gas analysis are helpful to determine the presence of gas exchange abnormalities. The diagnosis is often afforded by an echocardiogram. This study can help determine the presence of valvular heart disease or LV systolic dysfunction. The presence (and degree) of right ventricular dysfunction can also be noted, and an estimation of the pulmonary artery pressures can be made using this technique. Ventilation perfusion scanning is helpful to determine the presence of chronic thromboembolic pulmonary hypertension. CT scanning and pulmonary angiography can help to assess the pulmonary parenchyma and the pulmonary vascularity. A right heart catheterization with measurement of the right atrial, right ventricular, pulmonary artery, and left atrial pressures is necessary to confirm the diagnosis and to help direct therapy. It must be remembered that pulmonary vascular disease is associated with cardiac dysfunction and that a comprehensive cardiac evaluation must be a primary consideration in the evaluation of such patients.

EXERCISE LIMITATION OF PATIENTS WITH VASCULAR LUNG DISEASE

The normal pulmonary circulation is able to receive a five- to sixfold increase in blood flow with only a minimal resultant increase in pressure. Although pulmonary artery pressure increases during exercise, the right atrial pressure increases only minimally. The pressure gradient increase across the pulmonary vascular occurring during

BOX 15-4	Abnormalities Noted During Exercise in Patients with Pulmonary Vascular Disease (Pulmonary Hypertension)

Reduced maximal oxygen consumption

Reduced work rate

Decreased anaerobic threshold

Arterial oxyhemoglobin desaturation

Elevation in pulmonary artery wedge pressure (>30 mm Hg)

Elevation in right atrial pressure (>14 mm Hg)

exercise is actually less than the increase in cardiac output. This results in a decrease in the pulmonary vascular resistance. It is believed that this occurs because of recruitment and distention of pulmonary capillaries. At peak exercise, improved efficiency of ventilation and perfusion and a decrease in the alveolar dead space occur (resulting in an increase in the V_D/V_T ratio).

The exercise limitation associated with pulmonary hypertension is primarily associated with cardiac dysfunction (Box 15-4). Pulmonary vasoconstriction and remodeling of the vascular bed increase right ventricle afterload and limit stroke volume in response to exercise[34]. As the right ventricle dilates over the course of the disease, a decrease in LV compliance and diastolic filling occurs. With exercise, an abnormal increase in right atrial and mean pulmonary artery pressure with a relatively normal pulmonary capillary wedge pressure occurs[35].

Maximal oxygen consumption is significantly reduced in patients presenting with pulmonary hypertension. This is related to a decrease in the maximal cardiac output and arterial oxyhemoglobin desaturation. Low oxygen delivery occurs with the production of lactic acidosis at a lower level of exercise (reduced anaerobic threshold) [see Chapter 3].

Underperfused, well-ventilated lung units are present secondary to the lack of the normally seen increase in pulmonary distention and recruitment during exercise. This increases the V_D/V_T and the ventilatory requirements for exercise. A normal breathing reserve is usually found because the ventilatory mechanisms themselves are usually intact.

Exercise Assessment

Exercise testing is an important component of the evaluation and management of most patients with pulmonary disease (Box 15-5). It is important to determine the patient's ability to undergo exercise testing. Contraindications to exercise testing (also see GETP7 Box 3-5) include an unstable cardiac condition (e.g., unstable angina), severe hypoxemia, orthopedic impairment, neurologic impairment, psychiatric disorders, inability to perform the test, or poor motivation. Neither carbon dioxide retention nor age are contraindications to the performance of exercise testing.

MODE OF EXERCISE TESTING

The assessment of exercise capacity is an important component of the overall evaluation and management of patients with lung disease (also see GETP7 Chapter 9). A variety of types of exercise tests are available. The selection of the exercise testing modality depends on the clinical question being asked, available equipment, and having a facility that is able to manage the testing protocols (Box 15-6). Exercise testing should be performed when further questions need answered beyond the information obtained from the history and physical examination, chest radiograph, pulmonary function tests, and ECG.

Stair Climbing

This very simple and inexpensive test has been primarily used to assess postoperative risk for patients undergoing thoracic or upper abdominal surgery and is currently being used to evaluate the functional capacity in patients with COPD[36]. Although there is no standardized procedure for the performance of this test, the patient is asked to climb as many stairs as possible until needing to stop for symptoms (e.g., dizziness, shortness of breath, fatigue, chest pain). Measurements to be made during the test include the number of stairs walked, oxyhemoglobin saturation, level of dyspnea, and heart rate (HR). Variable reporting of the pace of the stair climbing and the actual number of stairs climbed (often referred to as "flights of stairs") adds to the nonuniform nature of the testing procedure.

A good correlation ($r = 0.7$) has been reported between the number of steps climbed and the maximal oxygen consumption (measured during cycle ergometry) in a study of 31 patients with COPD[37]. In several studies, the inability to walk two flights of stairs resulted in a significant increase in the number of postoperative complications[36,38]. This test can provide one with a general idea of the postoperative risk for patients with lung disease in a simple and low-cost manner.

BOX 15-5	**Indications For Exercise Testing in Patients with Lung Disease**

Evaluation of exercise tolerance

Evaluation of undiagnosed exercise intolerance

Evaluation of patients with respiratory symptoms

Exercise evaluation and prescription for pulmonary rehabilitation

Evaluation of impairment or disability

Evaluation for lung transplantation

Evaluation for oxyhemoglobin desaturation

BOX 15-6	**Modalities of Clinical Exercise Testing for Patients with Lung Disease**

Stair climbing

Timed walk tests (6- or 12-minute walk)

Shuttle walk tests

Graded exercise tests

Cardiopulmonary exercise test

Timed Walk Tests

The **timed walk tests** (6-minute walk [MWT], shuttle walks) are practical and simple to perform[39]. They do not require advanced training or advanced equipment, and they provide an objective assessment of exercise tolerance or functional capacity in a manner that is comfortable for most patients to perform. The 6 MWT is the most commonly used because it allows for most patients with lung disease to complete the test with accommodation for their degree of lung impairment.

Standardized protocols exist for the performance of the 6 MWT[40]. Guidelines have been recently developed and include a track for the 6 MWT, patient preparation, monitoring, protocol, measurements, and practice test. The track should be 30 m in length and clearly marked every 3 m. The patient should wear comfortable shoes, and the test should be performed each time at the same time of day with the patient taking his or her usual medication regimen. Monitoring equipment should include a stopwatch, a pulse oximeter, and a sphygmomanometer. The number of laps should be counted. Before beginning the test, baseline HR and blood pressure (BP) measurements should be made as well as a measure of the patient's level of dyspnea (e.g., using a Borg scale)[41] [see GETP7 Table 4-7] and oxyhemoglobin saturation. Standardized instructions should be read to the patient, and the words for encouragement and notification of time elapsed should be consistent for all patients. At the end of the testing, immediate measurements of oxyhemoglobin saturation, pulse, BP, level of dyspnea, and length of walk should be made. Because there may be a training effect noted with such testing, it is important to perform several tests (up to three) on the same day (with 1 hour of rest in between tests) with reporting of the highest distance walked. Studies have reported reference values in healthy adults[42].

The 6 MWT has good reproducibility and has good correlation with other measures of functional capacity and, thus, has been used in lieu of cardiopulmonary exercise test (CPET) when this testing modality is not available. A good correlation between the 6 MWT and maximal oxygen consumption ($r = 0.73$) has been shown in patients with COPD[43]. The 6 MWT test represents a submaximal and motivational alternative compared with the CPET. It also represents a test for which patients are familiar with the testing modality (i.e., walking).

The 6 MWT test has been usefully applied to the evaluation of functional capacity for patients with lung disease (e.g., COPD, interstitial lung disease)[44], evaluation of medical interventions[45], evaluation of response to pulmonary rehabilitation[46], and prediction of morbidity[47]. It has also been used successfully in the evaluation and management of patients with congestive heart failure[48].

There are some concerns about the actual performance of the test and the comparisons that are made from one testing site to another, but the 6 MWT has been used in large multicenter trials[49]. There is a statistically significant improvement (averaging 7%) in distance walked when the test is repeated on a second day. The shape of the walking course (continuous versus straight) appears to be more a determinant of the distance walked than does the length of a straight course[50].

Shuttle Walk Tests

The incremental shuttle walk test (ISWT) is a symptom-limited, maximal exercise test[51]. Subjects are instructed to walk around a 10-m course at a speed indicated by beeps played from a CD player. The speed increases incrementally until the patient is unable to continue or maintain the required speed. The total time walked is recorded. Performance in the ISWT is predictive of peak oxygen consumption, and the test is reproducible after a single practice walk.

The endurance shuttle walk test (ESWT) is a constant work rate exercise test. After a 2-minute warm up period, the subject is asked to walk around a 10-m course. The speed is constant and is set at an equivalent of 85% of the predicted peak maximal oxygen consumption achieved during the ISWT. The total time walked is recorded[52]. These tests are externally paced tests of maximal and submaximal exercise performance, respectively. Each may be used to compare the distance walked before and after an intervention (e.g., response to pulmonary rehabilitation).

Cardiopulmonary Exercise Test

Cardiopulmonary exercise testing (CPET) assesses the integration of the systems (e.g., heart, lung, muscular) involved with the performance of exercise. This type of testing allows an evaluation of the patient's ability to perform exercise and of the system responsible for the exercise impairment. CPET involves a continuous ramped increase in workload continuing until the patient develops symptoms (e.g., fatigue or dyspnea). The test can be performed on either a treadmill or a cycle ergometer. Expired gases from the patient are collected using a metabolic cart that has the capability to determine the V_T, respiratory rate, rate of oxygen consumption, and rate of carbon dioxide elimination. Measurement of HR and oxyhemoglobin saturation (via pulse oximetry) are also made. All measurements are made on a continuous basis, thus allowing for interpretation at various levels of exercise.

Interpretation of CPET can be daunting given the significant amount of information obtained with each study[53,54]. Several questions should be evaluated sequentially when interpreting the data. These include is the exercise capacity normal (as assessed by maximal oxygen consumption, work rate maximum), is cardiovascular function normal (as assessed by oxygen pulse, anaerobic threshold), is ventilatory function normal (as assessed by ventilatory reserve, maximum respiratory rate), and is gas exchange normal (as assessed by dead space ventilation, oxyhemoglobin saturation)?

The various disease states discussed in this chapter have major distinguishing features in regard to the measurements obtained during CPET. Patients with COPD have a reduced exercise capacity (reduced maximal oxygen consumption), ventilatory limitation (reduced or absent ventilatory reserve, hypercapnia), and a normal cardiovascular response (normal oxygen pulse) with exercise. Patients with interstitial lung disease have a reduced exercise capacity (reduced maximal oxygen consumption), ventilatory limitation (high maximum respiratory rate and low TV at end exercise, elevated dead space ventilation with an abnormal reduction during exercise), and a normal cardiovascular response with exercise. Patients with vascular lung disease have a reduced exercise capacity (reduced maximal oxygen consumption), no ventilatory limitation, and an abnormal cardiovascular response (early onset of anaerobic threshold, early plateau of the oxygen pulse with a low maximum value) with exercise.

Summary

Shortness of breath is a common presenting symptom for patients with lung disease. There are three general types of lung disease: obstructive, restrictive, and vascular. Patients with obstructive lung disease have airflow limitation, primarily during expiration. Those with restrictive lung disease have reduction in lung volumes, and those with vascular lung disease have alterations of the pulmonary vascular bed. Each disease process has a specific pathophysiology, both at rest and during exercise. Appropriate assessment of patients with lung disease includes performance of a thorough history and physical examination, laboratory studies (including chest radiograph, ECG, arterial blood gas, pulse oximetry, complete blood count, and pulmonary function tests), and, in some instances a CT scan of the chest or a ventilation–perfusion scan. Exercise testing is helpful to confirm the disease's pathophysiology and to help direct treatment.

Acknowledgments
The authors wish to acknowledge the contributors of this content area from previous editions of the text. Their efforts greatly assisted our compilation of information for the current chapter.

REFERENCES

1. Hill AT, Bayley D, Stockley RA: The interrelationship of sputum inflammatory markers in patients with chronic bronchitis. Am J Respir Crit Care Med 160:893–898, 1999.
2. Keatings VM, Collins PD, Scott DM, Barnes PJ: Differences in interleukin-8 and tumor necrosis factor-alpha in induced sputum from patients with chronic obstructive pulmonary disease or asthma. Am J Respir Crit Care Med 153:530–534, 1996.
3. Vernoy JH, Kucukaycan M, Jacobs JA, et al: Local and system inflammation in patients with chronic obstructive pulmonary disease: Soluble tumor necrosis factor receptors are increased in sputum. Am J Respir Crit Care Med 166:1240–1247, 2002.
4. Niewoehner DE, Kleinerman J, Rice DB: Pathologic changes in the peripheral airways of young cigarette smokers. N Engl J Med 291:755–758, 1974.
5. Saetta M, Di Stefano A, Turato G, et al: CD8+ T-lymphocytes in peripheral airways of smokers with chronic obstructive pulmonary disease. Am J Respir Crit Care Med 157:822–826, 1998.
6. Repine JE, Bast A, Lankhorst I: Oxidative stress in chronic obstructive pulmonary disease. Oxidative Stress Study Group. Am J Respir Crit Care Med 156:341–357, 1997.
7. McLean KA: Pathogenesis of pulmonary emphysema. Am J Med 25:62–74, 1958.
8. Peinado VI, Barbera JA, Abate P, et al: Inflammatory reaction in pulmonary muscular arteries of patients with mild chronic obstructive pulmonary disease. Am J Respir Crit Care Med 159:1605–1611, 1999.
9. MacNee W: Pathophysiology of cor pulmonale in chronic obstructive pulmonary disease. Part two. Am J Respir Crit Care Med 150:1158–1168, 1994.
10. Mullen JB, Wright JL, Wiggs BR, et al: Reassessment of inflammation of airways in chronic bronchitis. BMJ 291:1235–1239, 1985.
11. Mueller R, Changez P, Campbell AM, et al: Different cytokine patterns in bronchial biopsies in asthma and chronic bronchitis. Respir Med 90:79–85, 1996.
12. Barnes PJ, Chung KF, Page CP: Inflammatory mediators of asthma: An update. Pharmacol Rev 50:515–596, 1998.
13. Holgate ST: The cellular and mediator basis of asthma in relation to natural history. Lancet 350(suppl II):5–9, 1997.
14. Roche WR, Beasley R, Williams JH, Holgate ST: Subepithelial fibrosis in the bronchi of asthmatics. Lancet 1(7965):882–884, 1989.
15. McFadden ER Jr, Gilbert FA: Exercise induced asthma. N Engl J Med 330:1362–1367, 1994.
16. Chen Y, Horne SL, Dosman JA: Increased susceptibility to lung dysfunction in female smokers. Am Rev Respir Dis 143:1224–1230, 1991.
17. Gold DR, Wang X, Wypij D, et al: Effects of cigarette smoking on pulmonary function in adolescent boys and girls. N Engl J Med 335:931–937, 1996.
18. Ferguson GT, Enright PL, Buist AS, Higgins MW: Office spirometry for lung health assessment in adults. Chest 117:1146–1161, 2000.
19. Petty TL, Weinmann GG: Building a national strategy for the prevention and management of and research in chronic obstructive pulmonary disease. National Heart, Lung, and Blood Institute Workshop Summary. JAMA 277:246–253, 1997.
20. Petty TL, ed: Strategies in preserving lung health and preventing COPD and associated diseases. The National Lung Health Education Program Chest 117:1146–1161, 2000.
21. American Thoracic Society: Standards for the diagnosis and care of patients with chronic obstructive pulmonary disease. Am J Respir Crit Care Med 152:S77–S152, 1995.
22. Pauwels RA, Buist SA, Calverley PMA, et al: Global strategy for the diagnosis, management, and prevention of chronic obstructive pulmonary disease. Am J Respir Crit Care Med 163:1256–1276, 2001.
23. O'Donnell DE, Revill S, Webb KA: Dynamic hyperinflation and exercise intolerance in COPD. Am J Respir Crit Care Med 164:770–777, 2001.
24. Diaz O, Villanfranco C, Ghezzo H, et al: Exercise tolerance in COPD patients with and without tidal expiratory flow limitation at rest. Eur Respir J 16:269–275, 2000.
25. Casaburi R: Skeletal muscle dysfunction in chronic obstructive pulmonary disease. Med Sci Sports Exerc 33:662–670, 2001.
26. Debigare R, Cote CH, Maltais F: Peripheral muscle wasting in chronic obstructive pulmonary disease. Am J Respir Crit Care Med 164:1712–1717, 2001.
27. Maltais FA, Simard A, Simard C, et al: Oxidative capacity of the skeletal muscle and lactic acid kinetics during exercise in normal subjects and in patients with COPD. Am J Respir Crit Care Med 154:442–447, 1996.
28. Hansen JE, Wasserman K: Pathophysiology of activity limitation in patients with interstitial lung disease. Chest 109:1566–1576, 1996.
29. Markovitz GH, Cooper CB: Exercise and interstitial lung disease. Curr Opin Pulm Med 4:272–280, 1998.

30. Widimsky J, Riedel M, Stanek V: Central haemodynamics during exercise in patients with restrictive pulmonary disease. Bull Eur Physiopathol Respir 13:369–379, 1997.

31. Rubin LJ: Primary pulmonary hypertension. N Engl J Med 336: 111–117, 1997.

32. Fedullo P, Auger W, Channick R, et al: Chronic thromboembolic pulmonary hypertension. Clin Chest Med 22:561–581, 2001.

33. Mehta JN, Khan IA, Mehta RN, Sepkowitz DA: HIV-related pulmonary hypertension. Chest 118:1133–1141, 2000.

34. Sun XG, Hansen JE, Oudiz RJ, Wasserman K: Exercise pathophysiology in patients with primary pulmonary hypertension. Circulation 104:429–435, 2001.

35. Raeside DA, Smith A, Brown A, et al: Pulmonary artery pressure measurement during exercise testing in patients with suspected pulmonary hypertension. Eur Respir J 16:282–287, 2000.

36. Girish M, Trayner E Jr, Dammann O, et al: Symptom-limited stair climbing as a predictor of postoperative cardiopulmonary complications after high-risk surgery. Chest 120:1147–1151, 2001.

37. Pollock M, Roa J, Benditt J, Celli B: Estimation of ventilatory reserve by stair climbing. A study in patients with chronic airflow obstruction. Chest 104:1378–1383, 1993.

38. Holden DA, Rice TW, Stelmach K, Meeker DP: Exercise testing, 6-minute walk, and stair climb in the evaluation of patients at high risk for pulmonary resection. Chest 102:1774–1779, 1992.

39. Montes de Oca M, Ortega Balza M, Lezama J, Lopez JM: Chronic obstructive pulmonary disease: evaluation of exercise tolerance using three different exercise tests. Arch Bronchopneumol 37:69–74, 2001.

40. American Thoracic Society: Guidelines for the six minute walk test. Am J Respir Crit Care Med 166:111–117, 2002.

41. Borg GAV: Psychophysical bases of perceived exertion. Med Sci Sports Exerc 14:377–381, 1982.

42. Enright PL, Sherrill DL: Reference equations for the six-minute walk in healthy adults. Am J Respir Crit Care Med 158:1384–1387, 1998.

43. Cahalin L, Pappagionopolous P, Prevost S, et al: The relationship of the 6-minute walk test to maximal oxygen consumption in transplant candidates with end-stage lung disease. Chest 108:452–459, 1995.

44. Chang JA, Curtis JR, Patrick DL, Raghu G: Assessment of health-related quality of life in patients with interstitial lung disease. Chest 105:163–167, 1994.

45. Oga T, Nishimura K, Tsukino M, et al: The effects of oxitropium bromide on exercise performance in patients with stable chronic obstructive pulmonary disease. A comparison of three different exercise tests. Am J Respir Crit Care Med 161:1897–1901, 2000.

46. DeTorres JP, Pinto-Plata V, Ingenito E, et al: Power of outcome measurements to detect clinically significant changes in pulmonary rehabilitation of patients with COPD. Chest 121:1091–1098, 2002.

47. Kessler R, Faller M, Fourgaut G, et al: Predictive factors of hospitalizations for acute exacerbations in a series of 64 patients with chronic obstructive pulmonary disease. Am J Respir Crit Care Med 159: 158–164, 1999.

48. Cahalin L, Mathier MA, Semigran MJ, et al: The six-minute walk test predicts peak oxygen uptake and survival in patients with advanced heart failure. Chest 110:325–332, 1996.

49. National Emphysema Treatment Trial: A randomized trial comparing lung-volume-reduction surgery with medical therapy for severe emphysema. N Engl J Med 348:2059–2073, 2003.

50. Sciurba F, Criner GJ, Lee SM, et al: Six-minute walk distance in chronic obstructive pulmonary disease. Am J Respir Crit Care Med 167:1522–1527, 2003.

51. Singh SJ, Morgan MD, Hardman AE, et al: Comparison of oxygen uptake during a conventional treadmill test and the shuttle walking test in chronic airflow limitation. Eur Respir J 7:2016–2020, 1994.

52. Revill SM, Morgan MD, Singh SJ, et al: The endurance shuttle walk: A new field test for the assessment of endurance capacity in chronic obstructive pulmonary disease. Thorax 54:213–222, 1999.

53. Weisman IM, Zeballos RJ, eds: Clinical exercise testing. Clin Chest Med 15:173–451, 1994.

54. Younes M: Interpretation of clinical exercise testing in respiratory disease. Clin Chest Med 5:189–206, 1984.

SELECTED REFERENCES FOR FURTHER READING

American Thoracic Society/American College of Chest Physicians: ATS/ACCP Statement on Cardiopulmonary Exercise Testing. Am J Respir Crit Care Med 167:211–217, 2003.

Berry MJ, Woodard CM: Chronic obstructive pulmonary disease (pp. 339–365). In JK Ehrman, PM Gordon, PS Visich, SJ Keteyian, eds. Clinical Exercise Physiology. Champaign, IL: Human Kinetics; 2003.

Cherniak NS, Altose MD, Homma I: Rehabilitation of the Patient with Respiratory Disease. New York: McGraw Hill; 1999.

Myers JM: Essentials of Cardiopulmonary Exercise Testing. Champaign, IL: Human Kinetics; 1996.

Tobin MJ: Year in Review: Chronic obstructive pulmonary disease, pollution, pulmonary vascular disease, transplantation, pleural disease, and lung cancer in AJRCCM 2002. Am J Respir Crit Care Med 167:356–370, 2003.

Weisman IM, Zeballos RJ: Clinical Exercise Testing. Basel, Switzerland: Karger; 2002.

INTERNET RESOURCES

AACVPR: American Association of Cardiovascular and Pulmonary Rehabilitation:
http://www.aacvpr.org

American College of Chest Physicians:
http://www.chestnet.org

American Thoracic Society:
http://www.thoracic.org

National Lung Health Education Program:
http://www.nlhep.org

US COPD Coalition:
http://www.uscopd.org

Exercise Testing in Patients with Diabetes

RICHARD M. LAMPMAN AND BARBARA N. CAMPAIGNE

This chapter addresses KSAs from the following content areas:

1 **Exercise Physiology and Related Exercise Science**
2 Pathophysiology and Risk Factors
3 **Health Appraisal, Fitness, and Clinical Exercise Testing**
4 **Electrocardiography and Diagnostic Techniques**
5 **Patient Management and Medications**
6 Medical and Surgical Management
7 Exercise Prescription and Programming
8 Nutrition and Weight Management
9 Human Behavior and Counseling
10 Safety, Injury Prevention, and Emergency Procedures
11 Program Administration, Quality Assurance, and Outcome Assessment

Individuals with diabetes have a higher incidence and prevalence of symptomatic as well as asymptomatic coronary artery disease (CAD), placing them at a higher risk than nondiabetic individuals for an adverse exercise-induced cardiovascular event[1–15]. Compared with woman without diabetes, women with diabetes are at high risk for adverse cardiovascular events[6,16], especially if other risk factors are present[17]. Individuals with diabetes who are asymptomatic for CAD have a higher prevalence of **silent myocardial ischemia** and associated **autonomic nerve dysfunction** than those without diabetes[8]. A high-risk group for having silent myocardial ischemia is asymptomatic men having type 2 diabetes for more than 10 years and presenting with **peripheral macroangiopathy**[14] or with peripheral vascular disease[18]. Patients with diabetes have more than a twofold higher prevalence of exercise-induced silent myocardial ischemia than those without diabetes. Additionally, patients on insulin therapy or who have retinopathy have nearly a threefold higher prevalence of silent myocardial ischemia compared with those not taking insulin or without retinopathy[19].

Routine exercise is an important treatment component for individuals with diabetes[20,21], but strenuous exercise can precipitate cardiac events in these individuals, resulting in sudden death if undetected cardiac disease is present[22]. Because of the risk of exercise-related sudden death[22,23], it is recommended that adults with a long history of diabetes and those with one or more cardiovascular risk factors other than diabetes undergo exercise testing before embarking on vigorous exercise programs[24–27].

For the purpose of this chapter, exercise testing involves a graded progressive workload using a treadmill or cycle ergometer to provide a cardiovascular stress while monitoring an individual's electrocardiogram (ECG), heart rate (HR), and blood pressure (BP) responses to exercise. Detailed guidelines for exercise stress ECG testing can be found Chapter 14 and elsewhere[28–30]. Exercise testing may identify individuals with diabetes who have advanced coronary disease and are possibly at high risk for a cardiac event. Exercise testing can provide other useful information such as: appropriate cardiovascular interventional therapies, long-term prognosis in those with chronic stable CAD, and the efficacy of treatment modalities. In addition, exercise test results can provide important parameters for generating safe and specific exercise training guidelines for those with diabetes[31,32]. Information on exercise training for individuals with diabetes is revised in Chapter 33.

Clinical Evaluation

Patients with diabetes should undergo both a detailed history and thorough physical examination, especially with a focus on determining the presence of macro- and microvascular disease and, if appropriate, diagnostic studies, before embarking on strenuous exercise programs[32,33]. A resting 12-lead ECG may demonstrate evidence of asymptomatic ischemic heart disease or a previous silent myocardial infarction (MI)[6], but a resting ECG is insufficient for predicting a potential ischemic cardiac response induced by high myocardial workloads resulting from exercise stress or pharmaceutical methods[34,35]. Treadmill or cycle ergometer exercise testing is cost effective for private office practices, clinics, and hospital settings. Absolute and relative contraindications to exercise testing should be considered before a patient with diabetes undergoes an exercise test[30,32,36].

Other more expensive myocardial tests exist for diagnosing underlying CAD (see Chapter 19) such as stress echocardiography, stress single-photon emission computed tomography (SPECT) myocardial perfusion imaging, or positron emission tomography (PET); and potentially, an invasive coronary arteriogram if silent exertional ischemia exists[37,38]. Pharmacologic agents, rather than exercise, may be used to increase myocardial work followed by radionuclide imaging studies if a patient is unable to exercise.

Practical Considerations of Routine Exercise Testing

The sensitivity and specificity of exercise testing in an asymptomatic individual may result in minimal diagnostic value depending on many variables, including the type and severity of diabetes, as well as the duration that a patient has had diabetes (see GETP7 Box 6-2). One major concern is that exercise testing can be costly for routine screening and with the large number of individuals with type 2 diabetes, exercise testing so many individuals would place a large financial burden on the health care system. Furthermore, in an asymptomatic population, exercise testing may result in a false-positive diagnosis and may be a poor predictive for major cardiac events[38]. When embarking on a very light-intensity ($<20\%$ $\dot{V}O_{2max}$; 35% max. HR) or light (20% to 39% $\dot{V}O_{2max}$; 35% to 54% of max HR) exercise program, it may not be necessary to have a younger or even a healthy older individuals undergo exercise tests if they are asymptomatic and do not traditional coronary artery risk factors. Testing older diabetics with a long history of di-

abetes and with multiple known risk factors for ischemic heart disease has clinical merit and can be cost effective.

Box 16-1 summarizes clinical guidelines to help determine if an individual with diabetes should undergo a graded exercise test to evaluate his or her cardiac health status before beginning a moderate- to high-intensity exercise program[11,27,32]. A patient may require an additional exercise test when gathering information necessary for devising an individualized exercise prescription because they need to taking their routine medications.

Very Light to Light Exercise Training: Consideration for Exercise Testing

If a patient plans to participate in exercise that is very light ($<20\%$ $\dot{V}O_{2max}$; 35% max HR) or light (20% to 39% $\dot{V}O_{2max}$; 35% to 54% of max HR) based on exercise of 60

BOX 16-1 | **Clinical Characteristics of Individuals with Diabetes: Guidelines for Exercise Testing**

1. Previously sedentary individual with diabetes aged >35 years; or sedentary at any age and having diabetes >10 years

2. Having type 1 diabetes >15 years or type 2 diabetes >10 years[14]

3. Having additional major risk factors for coronary artery disease such as the presence of smoking, hyperlipidemia, obesity, and being sedentary[5]

4. Displaying clinically advanced peripheral vascular or renal disease, microvascular disease, cardiomegaly, or congestive heart failure[5,39–41]

5. Presence of advanced autonomic, renal, or cerebrovascular disease[42–44]

6. Patients with known advanced coronary artery or carotid occlusive disease

1. Anticipating exercise activity level approximately equal to his or her walking pace (<40% $\dot{V}O_{2max}$; <54% max HR)
2. Under age 35 years
3. Without additional major risk factors for coronary artery disease
4. Without additional risk factors for sudden death
5. Normal resting electrocardiogram

[a] It is highly recommend that diabetics, especially those having diabetes fore more than 10 years, have their physicians thoroughly evaluate them before embarking on exercise training programs even if at a low intensity of effort. Those planning a moderate- to high-intensity exercise programs should be evaluated by exercise testing.

HR = heart rate.

minutes[32], and especially if he or she does not have medical conditions that are contraindicative to regular exercise, he or she may not need an exercise test before starting a very light or light exercise program[27,32]. Even when beginning light exercise, it is recommended that an individual with typical or atypical cardiac symptoms or an abnormal resting ECG result have a diagnostic exercise test[32]. Whether or not a patient should undergo an exercise test when beginning a light-intensity exercise program should be left up to the clinical judgment of the individual's physician (Box 16-2).

Moderate- to Hard-intensity Exercise Training: Exercise Testing

It is recommended that an individual with diabetes undergo an exercise test before engaging in moderate-intensity exercise (40% to 59 % $\dot{V}O_{2max}$; 55% to 69% of max HR) to hard (60% to 85 % $\dot{V}O_{2max}$; 70% max HR; exercise based on 60 minutes)[32]. Individuals with diabetes and having advanced disease states, even though these diseases may not commonly be associated with risks for CAD, should undergo exercise testing, because these patients seem to have a high prevalence of sudden death. Typically, these individuals have microvascular complications (e.g., **diabetic neuropathy**).

Cardiac Complications Specific to Individuals with Diabetes

Silent myocardial ischemia in asymptomatic men with diabetes occurs frequently[3,5], especially in those on long-term insulin treatment because they often have autonomic neuropathy[43], which is associated with an increased risk of sudden death[44]. Individuals with diabetes often show an early loss of parasympathetic function with

progression to sympathetic nerve dysfunction. Cardiac autonomic control is frequently altered with diabetes, resulting in reduced HR variability[20], a condition related to chronic hyperglycemia[45].

Using the criteria that a 1-minute post-exercise HR recovery (decrease ≤ 12 bpm) is abnormal, it has been reported that this attenuated HR recovery after exercise is a predictor of mortality[46,47]. Patients with diabetes show an increased likelihood of an abnormal HR recovery (decrease ≤ 12 bpm), and hyperglycemia is inversely associated with a post-exercise attenuated HR recovery[48]. This fact emphasize the clinical value of monitoring post-exercise testing HR and BP recovery rates in those with diabetes. Individuals with autonomic neuropathy may display unusual ECG, hemodynamic, and physiological responses to exercise testing (Table 16-1).

Other Exercise Testing Considerations

Ideally, the time of day individuals with diabetes undergo an exercise test should coincide with the time they would normally exercise if they plan to begin an exercise program, and the time should be coordinated with meals and insulin and oral antihyperglycemic agent doses. Also, these individuals should be tested while taking their usual medications if test results are to be used for planning a systematic, individualized exercise program. Testing should be avoided if the patient's glucose levels are above 250 mg·dL^{-1} and ketosis is present or if glucose levels are above 300 mg·dL^{-1} and ketosis is not present. If glucose

TABLE 16-1. Abnormal Exercise-induced Cardiovascular Parameters in Patients with Diabetes Having Autonomic Neuropathy

Parameters	Abnormalities or Possible Etiologies
Nervous system	Impaired sympathetic Impaired parasympathetic
Electrocardiogram	Resting tachycardia (>100 bpm) Decreased resting beat-to-beat variation Prolonged QT intervals Attenuated chronotropic response Ischemia: ST-T depression
Arrhythmia	Ischemia potentially secondary to exercise-induced hypoglycemic and its stimulation of the sympathetic nervous system
Diastolic function	Abnormal
Left ventricular ejection fraction	Impaired, both at rest and with exercise
Rate-pressure product	Higher resting; lower at exercise maximum
Blood pressure	Hypertension with exercise Hypotension with exercise
Orthostasis (↓ SBP >20 mm Hg upon standing)	Decreased release of catecholamines with increased vasoconstrictive effect
Silent ischemia	Advanced coronary artery disease

levels are below 100 mg·dL^{-1}, then glucose could be ingested before exercise testing to prevent a hypoglycemic response. It is helpful to have patients monitor their blood glucose levels before and after exercise tests, especially patients taking insulin or oral antihyperglycemic agents so they can appreciate any exercise-induced effects on glycemic control. This can be beneficial information to the patients for maintaining their glycemic control when they are balancing their medications, meals, and exercise training programs. Having patients self-monitor their blood glucose also provides their health care team the opportunity to ensure that patients are correct in their glucose monitoring methods.

If the primary intent of the exercise test is to be diagnostic, then medications that have potential antianginal effects by reducing myocardial oxygen demands such as beta-blockers and calcium channel blockers should be removed 2 days and 1 to 3 days, respectively, before exercise testing. Ideally, it is best to have agents discontinued at least 48 hours before the exercise test because they will attenuate exercise-induced HR and BP responses, thus reducing the diagnostic accuracy for detecting cardiac abnormalities or CAD. Antianginal, long-acting nitrates should be discontinued 12 hours before testing, if feasible, because they may influence perfusion imaging[28,30,36].

After exercise testing, patients taking vasodilation medications may experience post-exercise hypotension requiring an extended cool-down period during which they should be closely monitored. Because of low serum potassium levels, arrhythmias are common in patients taking chronic diuretic therapy. For this reason, serum potassium levels should be checked for normalcy before exercise testing (see GETP7 Table 3-3). Those being exercise tested while using an insulin pump should be advised to reduce their insulinization during and after the stress test to prevent exercise-induced hypoglycemia.

Good, supportive shoes should be used for stability and for protection, especially in those with peripheral neuropathy and lost sensations in their feet[49]. The room should be kept at a comfortably cool temperature, and adequate hydration should be given after the test. Patients should be informed of the potential for post-exercise, immediate or late, hypoglycemia. Before testing, vision and neurological problems should be assessed because these complications may interfere with exercise testing protocols.

Persons with Diabetes Requiring Insulin

Several insulin analogs (i.e., modified insulin) have been introduced in the past 10 years. These include rapid-acting insulin with a short duration of activity and, more recently, long-acting, basal-type insulin. The type of insulin and its pharmacodynamic activity (peak and duration of action) need to be considered when insulin-requiring individuals undergo exercise testing or participate in regular exercise programs.

Oral Antihyperglycemic Agents in Type 2 Diabetes

Many oral antihyperglycemic agents, including, sulfonylureas, metformin, and thiazolidinediones (TZDs), are currently available. TZDs may have beneficial effects on lipid profiles (e.g., increase high-density lipoprotein cholesterol and decrease triglyceride levels and improve insulin sensitivity).

Managing Hypertension

The preferred line of treatment for individuals with diabetes is an angiotensi-converting enzyme inhibitor. Beta-blockers can also be used, but loop diuretics may worsen blood glucose control. Managing BP is of critical importance because BP control can result in fewer microvascular complications in patients with type 2 diabetes.

Exercise Testing Modalities

Individuals with diabetes can undergo different modalities of testing for detecting underlying CAD. Certain exercise testing modalities (see Chapters 14 and 19) may be suited for persons with diabetes who may have peripheral artery disease or peripheral neuropathy. These myocardial stress tests are discussed below. Table 16-2 shows the sensitivity and specificity values reported for different stress testing modalities involving individuals with diabetes.

Exercise Testing with Electrocardiography

A standard method to evaluate diabetic patients' cardiac status in response to exercise is through observation of their ECGs during and after progressive stages of treadmill or cycle ergometry exercise testing (see Chapter 14 and GETP7 Chapter 5). This type of exercise testing is relatively easy to administer and less costly than other stress testing modalities such as echocardiography and radionuclide imaging.

A submaximal exercise electrocardiography test (often defined as a peak HR = 120 bpm or 70% of age-predicted HR) may be used when clinical symptoms are present in severely deconditioned individuals or shortly after a patient sustains an MI. Making it one that is symptom-limited rather than one using a set HR response can improve the prognostic value of an exercise test, although test administrators should be aware of the increased possibility of **chronotropic incompetence** in this patient population. If a submaximal test demonstrate the presence of exercise-induced silent myocardial ischemia or cardiac arrhythmias, there exists an increased risk of exercise-related acute cardiac events. The diagnostic sensitivity of the exercise stress ECG test is enhanced if the individual reaches 85% or more of his or her age-predicted maximum HR and the rate pressure product (systolic HR × BP / 100) is above 300.

Although exercise stress ECG testing is the most common stress testing modality for diagnosing underlying

TABLE 16-2. Sensitivity and Specificity of Exercise or Pharmacologic Stress Tests for Diagnosing Coronary Artery Disease[a]

Myocardial Stress Test	Sensitivity (%)	Specificity (%)	Patient Population/Reference
Stress electrocardiogram	68	77	Pooled data[36]
	71	84	Type 2 diabetes[18]
	75	77	Diabetes[58]
Stress echocardiogram	85	77	Pooled data[51]
	84	87	Pooled data[56]
Exercise stress radionuclide			
Thallium-201 or technetium-99m sestamibi	87	64	Pooled data[51]
Planar thallium 201 scintigraphy—Qualitative analysis/quantitative analysis	83/90	88/80	Pooled data[53]
Thallium-201 SPECT—Qualitative analysis/quantitative analysis	89/90	76/70	Pooled data[53]
Thallium-201	97	Unpublished	Diabetes[57]
Technetium-99m pertechnetate	50	67	Diabetes[60]
Pharmacological stress agents			
Dipyridamole + thallium-201	80	87	Diabetes[58]
Dipyridamole + thallium-201	86	72	Type 1[59]
Dipyridamole or adenosine + thallium-201	62	76	Diabetes[60]
Dipyridamole + tetrofosmin	85	55	Study group[55]
PET using dipyridamole	87–97	70–100	Pooled data[53]

[a] Shown are studies involving pooled data, single laboratory data or results for patients with diabetes along with the reference.

SPECT = single-photon emission computed tomography

PET = positron emission tomography

See Chapter 19 and GETP7 Box 6-2 for how to determine sensitivity and specificity.

CAD, it may not be an adequate diagnostic testing method for women with diabetes[16]. Women with diabetes may need to undergo radionuclide imaging because the treadmill ECG exercise test is less accurate for diagnosing myocardial ischemia because of these patients' generally lower pretest likelihood of having advanced CAD compared with men[50]. The diagnostic accuracy obtained from meta-analysis using exercise stress ECG testing results from patients without a prior MI showed the mean sensitivity to be 68% and the mean specificity of 77% for detecting underlying CAD[30]. Sensitivity and specificity values for different patient populations have been reported[30].

Stress Echocardiographic Testing

Stress echocardiography is used to evaluate regional wall motion before and after myocardial stress assessing for adequate myocardial perfusion. If a patient is disabled or otherwise unable to exercise, dobutamine is used most often with echocardiography.

A meta-analysis showed exercise echocardiography to be slightly better than exercise SPECT imaging with thallium-201 or technetium-99m-sestamibi for diagnosing CAD with respect to a mean specificity (77% for echocardiography and 64% for SPECT), with both tests having similar sensitivity of 85% for echocardiography and 87% for SPECT[51]. Dobutamine stress echocardiography has been shown to be equivalent to thallium-201 SPECT in detecting asymptomatic CAD in patients with diabetes, making it a good testing modality for facilities without nu-

clear scanning equipment[52] (see Chapter 19 for more information on diagnostic testing).

Radionuclide Stress Imaging in Combination with Exercise Stress

RADIONUCLIDE VENTRICULOGRAPHY

Patients with diabetes who have an abnormal resting ECG result or a slightly positive ECG response to exercise stress (1.0 to 1.5 mm ST-T depression at a moderate to high exercise-induced HR) and who are asymptomatic for CAD may be further evaluated using other tests such as stress echocardiography or stress SPECT myocardial perfusion imaging. Those with resting ECG nonspecific ST- and T-wave changes or who have exercise-induced nonspecific ECG wave changes may need to be furthered tested using radionuclide imaging. **Radionuclide ventriculography** studies are also useful in patients needing an evaluation for exercise-induced ischemia that have abnormalities such as resting ST-segment depression greater than 1 mm, left bundle branch block (LBBB), or electronically paced rhythm. In the case of LBBB, a pharmacologic agent that causes myocardial vasodilatation can also be used to induce ischemia[53].

A myocardial perfusion image showing a small fixed defect[12,14] should not restrict an individual with diabetes from exercising, but imaging suggesting a large perfusion abnormality area in a patient with diabetes with symptomatic or silent ischemia places him or her at risk for an adverse cardiac event[54].

Along with evaluating for exercise-induced myocardial ischemia, radionuclide imaging can be useful for assessing left ventricular dysfunction, arrhythmias, abnormal BP responses, and inappropriate orthostatic responses during or after exercise testing. Radionuclide scanning may improve the ability of an exercise test to detect cardiac ischemia or infarction, as well as to localize areas of myocardial disorders. Myocardial perfusion imaging can also document any improvement in perfusion to ischemic areas of the myocardium and functional improvements after a therapy such as an exercise training program.

Myocardial perfusion imaging can be performed using planar scintigraphy or SPECT imaging techniques in which gamma cameras are rotated around the patient's body. In most cases, SPECT is generally more accurate than planar imaging for diagnosing CAD[53]. Planar scintigraphy perfusion imaging has average values for sensitivity and specificity of 83% and 88%, respectively, by visual analysis; and for quantitative analysis, it has a sensitivity of 90% and a specificity of 80%[53]. A practical concern with type 2 diabetes is that very obese individuals may be too heavy for most imaging tables used for SPECT because these tables usually have a weight-bearing limit of 300 pounds. Planar scintigraphy could still be used to image. Because surrounding soft tissue my cause photon attenuation, perfusing imaging may provide better quality images with Tc-99m sestamibi rather than with thallium-201 in those with a large body habitus.

Positron emission tomography is a tomographic nuclear imaging procedure using positrons such as fluorodeoxyglucose (FDG), O-15 water, and N-13 ammonia as radiolabels for assessing cardiac perfusion. Myocardial contractile reserve can be demonstrated, after administration of 13-N ammonia and 18-FDG, showing a contrasting under perfusion with 13-N ammonia but viable myocardium with 18-FDG. Using dipyridamole with rubidium-82 or N-13 ammonia has resulted in sensitivity from 87% to 97% and specificities from 78% to 100% with PET scanning[53].

RADIONUCLIDE IMAGING IN COMBINATION WITH PHARMACOLOGIC STRESS

Individuals who are unable to undergo exercise testing can have an assessment for underlying CAD through a pharmacologic stress test using dobutamine, persantine, adenosine, dipyridamole, or guanidine to cause myocardial hyperemia when performing thallium-201 myocardial perfusing imaging. Dobutamine administration results in increased myocardial blood flow because of its action of causing an increase in myocardial oxygen demand secondary to an increase in HR, systolic BP, and myocardial contractility. Dipyridamole, adenosine, and dobutamine cause coronary vasodilatation, resulting in markedly increased coronary blood flow. Sometimes these agents can cause bronchospasm, so they are usually used only with caution in those with asthma or chronic obstruction lung disease[53].

Although pharmacologic agents can stimulate myocardial blood flow in tests for detecting CAD, this testing method dose not provide exercise-induced cardiovascular parameters that can be used to prescribe an individualized exercise program. The sensitivity and specificity of a nuclear scan test depends on the patient population studied, the radioisotopes used, and whether exercise stress or a pharmacologic stress was used. In a population of those with known CAD, the sensitivity and specificity of diagnosis CAD using 99mTc-tetrofosmin myocardial SPECT with vasodilatation accomplished with dipyridamole were 81% and 55%, respectively[55].

Sensitivity and Specificity of Myocardial Stress Tests

The value of stress testing for detecting underlying CAD depends on good clinical judgment as to the best method of testing. One consideration for an appropriate diagnostic testing modality depends on the patient's pretest probability of CAD, which is influenced by factors such as age, gender, symptoms, and medical history. A few examples regarding the sensitivity and specificity values for diagnosing CAD using different myocardial testing modalities are shown in Table 16-2. Pooled data of different patient populations or single laboratory studies are provided[18,36,51,53,56] and when indicated, reports for individuals with diabetes[18,57–60] are reported.

Prognostic Assessment with Exercise Testing

Both the resting and exercise test ECG can help predict mortality in individuals with diabetes. A prolonged QT interval (corrected for HR [QT_c] and calculated as QT/QT_c) can show a lengthening over time in those with diabetes[61]. Those with both type 1 and type 2 diabetes have been shown to have a high prevalence of QT prolongation, and this abnormality is associated with ischemic heart disease in population-based studies[62–64]. Along with associated cardiac ischemia, those with type 2 diabetes and a prolonged QT dispersion have been shown to have other cardiac complications such as left ventricular hypertrophy and autonomic dysfunction[65]. This abnormal electrophysiological condition of the heart is an independent predictor of mortality in those with type I diabetes[66,67].

The presence of poor prognostic signs during exercise testing can also be helpful in evaluating the risk stratification of the patient, influencing medical therapy, and providing valuable guidelines for an exercise prescription. A predictor of mortality associated with exercise testing includes frequent ventricular ectopy during and immediately after exercise[68]. Two other independent predictors of death for older patients (patients studied included those with diabetes) are impaired functional capacity and an abnormal post-exercise HR recovery over the first minute after exercise[69]. In another study, patients without a history of heart failure or valvular disease and showing an attenuated immediate post-exercise HR recovery (1 minute decrease ≤ 18 bpm) in the absence of a post-exercise cool-down period had a 9% prediction of mortality whether or not systolic dysfunction, as assessed by exercise echocardiography, was present[70]. Using HR recovery after exercise testing as an all-cause predictor of mortality has also been examined in those with diabetes, and an attenuated HR recovery was shown to be an independent predictor of cardiovascular and all-cause death[71].

When either exercise or dobutamine stress echocardiograms were used to assess for cardiac ischemia to predict mortality in predominantly type 2 patients with known or suspected CAD, abnormal stress echocardiography results were independent predictors of death, and myocardial ischemia proved to be an independent predictor of mortality, incremental to the clinical risks for CAD and left ventricle dysfunction[72]. Even with a negative stress echocardiogram result, patients with diabetes, compared with without diabetes, have been shown to be at higher risk for major cardiac events secondary to a higher prevalence of CAD[73].

A normal or low-risk myocardial perfusion tomographic study using adenosine-99m tetrofosmin SPECT imaging in patients with suspected cardiac ischemia or for the evaluation of known CAD has been reported to be associated with a low annualized cardiac death rate of 0.6%

TABLE 16-3. One-Year Follow-up Rates for Cardiac Death or Nonfatal Myocardial Infarction for Patients with Diabetes[15]

Nuclide Scan Results	Myocardial Event Rates
Normal	1% to 2%
Mildly abnormal	3% to 4%
Moderate to abnormal	> 7%

in a multicenter study[74]. Major cardiac event rates of 1271 patients with diabetes undergoing rest thallium-201/stress technetium-99m or sestamibi scanning dual-isotope myocardial perfusion SPECT with exercise or adenosine pharmacologic testing have been reported by Kang et al[15] (Table 16-3). Results of this study show higher myocardial events in those with diabetes as compared with those without diabetes.

When comparing treadmill exercise score (derived from the exercise duration, degree of ST-segment depression, and exercise-induced angina) with the results of thallium imaging, only thallium (size of the perfusion defect) uptake and CAD were found to be independent predictors of prognosis[75]. The prognostic value of nuclear testing when studying myocardial perfusion in diabetic patients showed that, over an average 2-year follow-up, a linear relationship existed between the level of cardiac abnormality and adverse cardiac events. These findings

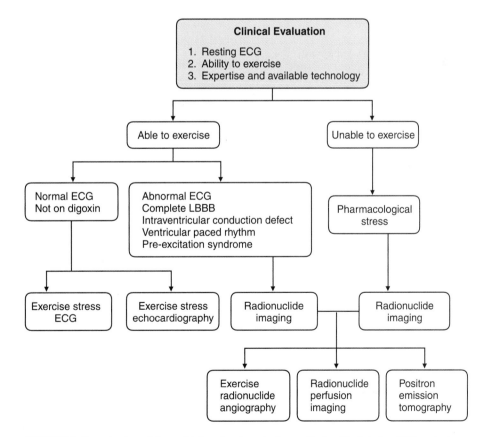

FIGURE 16-1. Flow chart providing guidelines for stress testing patients with diabetes. ECG = electrocardiogram; LBBB = left bundle branch block.

demonstrated that the test results added an incremental prognostic value over clinical risks for cardiac events alone[15]. In a study by Pancholy et al.[54], it was reported that a perfusion abnormality, as diagnosed by thallium-201 defects, and a history of diabetes were the most important predictors of future myocardial events. These authors concluded that the extent of myocardium at risk was more important than the presence or absence of exercise-induced angina pectoris.

Summary

The use of exercise testing for the diagnosis of underlying CAD is clinically important for individuals with diabetes. Because routine exercise is an important component of the management of diabetes, exercise testing can diagnose potential ischemic response to increased myocardial workloads, as caused by exercise training. Exercise test results can be used for diagnostic and predictive purposes, but importantly, test results can be used to prescribe a systematic individualized exercise prescription. Figure 16-1 outlines guidelines for deciding appropriate stress testing modalities for persons with diabetes.

Acknowledgments

The authors wish to acknowledge the contributors of this content area from previous editions of this text. Their efforts greatly assisted our compilation of information for the current chapter.

REFERENCES

1. Chiariello M, Indolfi C, Cotecchia MR, et al: Asymptomatic transient ST changes during ambulatory ECG monitoring in diabetic patients. Am Heart J 110:529–534, 1985.
2. Fazzini PF, Prati PL, Rovelli F, et al: Epidemiology of silent myocardial ischemia in asymptomatic middle-aged men (the ECCIS Project). Am J Cardiol 72:1383–1388, 1993.
3. Nesto RW, Phillips RT, Kett KG, et al: Angina and exertional myocardial ischemia in diabetic and nondiabetic patients: assessment by exercise thallium scintigraphy. Ann Intern Med 108:170–175, 1988.
4. Lane SE, Lewis SM, Pippin JJ, et al: Predictive value of quantitative dipyridamole-thallium scintigraphy in assessing cardiovascular risk after vascular surgery in diabetes mellitus. Am J Cardiol 64: 1275–1279, 1989.
5. Nesto RW, Watson FS, Kowalchuk GJ, et al: Silent myocardial ischemia and infarction in diabetics with peripheral vascular disease: assessment by dipyridamole thallium-201 scintigraphy. Am Heart J 120:1073–1077, 1990.
6. Scheidt-Nave C, Barrett-Connor E, Wingard DL: Resting electrocardiographic abnormalities suggestive of asymptomatic ischemic heart disease associated with non-insulin-dependent diabetes mellitus in a defined population. Circulation 81:899–906, 1990.
7. Koistinen MJ: Prevalence of asymptomatic myocardial ischaemia in diabetic subjects. BMJ 301:92–95, 1990.
8. Langer A, Freeman MR, Josse RG, et al: Detection of silent myocardial ischemia in diabetes mellitus. Am J Cardiol 67:1073–1078, 1991.
9. Paillole C, Passa P, Paycha F, et al: Non-invasive identification of severe coronary artery disease in patients with long-standing diabetes mellitus. Eur J Med 1:464–468, 1992.
10. Valensi P, Sachs RN, Lormeau B, et al: Silent myocardial ischaemia and left ventricle hypertrophy in diabetic patients. Diabetes Metab 23:409–416, 1997.
11. American Diabetes Association: Consensus development conference on the diagnosis of coronary heart disease in people with diabetes. Diabetes Care 21:1551–1559, 1998.
12. Milan Study on Atherosclerosis and Diabetes (MiSAD) Group: Prevalence of unrecognized silent myocardial ischemia and its association with atherosclerotic risk factors in noninsulin-dependent diabetes mellitus. Am J Cardiol 79:134–139, 1997.
13. May O, Arilsen H, Damsgaard EM, et al: Prevalence and prediction of silent ischemia in diabetes mellitus: A population based study. Cardiovasc Res 34:241–247, 1997.
14. Janand-Delenne B, Savin B, Habib G, et al: Silent myocardial ischemia in patients with diabetes: Who to screen. Diabetes Care 22:1396–1400, 1999.
15. Kang X, Berman DS, Lewin HC, et al: Incremental prognostic value of myocardial perfusion single photon emission computed tomography in patients with diabetes mellitus. Am Heart J 138(6 Pt 1):1025–1032, 1999.
16. Manson JE, Colditz GA, Stampfer MJ, et al: A prospective study of maturity-onset diabetes mellitus and risk of coronary heart disease and stroke in women. Arch Intern Med 151:1141–1147, 1991.
17. De S, Searles G, Haddad H: The prevalence of cardiac risk factors in women 45 years of age or younger undergoing angiography for evaluation of undiagnosed chest pain. Can J Cardiol 18:945–948, 2002.
18. Bacci S, Villella M, Villella A, et al: Screening for silent myocardial ischaemia in type 2 diabetic patients with additional atherogenic risk factors: Applicability and accuracy of the exercise stress test. Eur J Endocrinol 147:649–654, 2002.
19. Naka M, Hiramatsu K, Aizawa T, et al: Silent myocardial ischemia in patients with non-insulin-dependent diabetes mellitus as judged by treadmill exercise testing and coronary angiography. Am Heart J 123:46–53, 1992.
20. Schneider SH, Khachadurian AK, Amorosa LF, et al: Ten-year experience with an exercise-based outpatient life-style modification program in the treatment of diabetes mellitus. Diabetes Care 15: 1800–1810, 1992.
21. Smith SC, Blair SN, Bonow RO, et al: AHA/ACC Guidelines for Preventing Heart attack and death in patients with atherosclerotic cardiovascular disease: 2001 Update. A Statement for healthcare professionals from the American Heart Association and the American College of Cardiology. Circulation 104:1577–1579, 2001.
22. Kohl HW 3rd, Powell KE, Gordon NF, et al: Physical activity, physical fitness, and sudden cardiac death. Epidemiol Rev 14:37–58, 1992.
23. Thompson PD, Klocke FJ, Levine BD, et al: 26th Bethesda conference: Recommendations for determining eligibility for competition in athletes with cardiovascular abnormalities. Task Force 5: Coronary artery disease. Med Sci Sports Exerc 26:271–275, 1994.
24. Nesto RW: Screening for asymptomatic coronary artery disease in diabetes. Diabetes Care 9:1393–1395, 1999.
25. Viviani V, Valensi P, Paycha F, et al: The stress test should be the first test performed when assessing silent myocardial ischemia in diabetic subjects. Diabetes 47:119A, 1998.
26. Cosson E, Paycha F, Paries J, et al: Detecting silent coronary stenoses and stratifying cardiac risk in patients with diabetes: ECG stress test or exercise myocardial scintigraphy? Diabet Med 21: 342–348, 2004.
27. American Diabetes Association: Diabetes mellitus and exercise (position statement). Diabetes Care 24(suppl 1):S51–S55, 2001.
28. Fletcher GF, Balady G, Froelicher VF, et al: Exercise standards. A statement for healthcare professionals from the American Heart Association. Writing Group. Circulation 91:580–615, 1995.
29. Gibbons RJ, Balady GJ, Bricker TJ, et al: ACC/AHA 2002 guideline update for exercise testing: Summary article. A report of the American College of Cardiology/American Heart Association Task Force on Practice Guidelines. Circulation 106:1883–1892, 2002

30. Gibbons RJ, Smith SC Jr, Antman E: American College of Cardiology/American Heart Association clinical practice guidelines: Part II (evolutionary changes in a continuous quality improvement project. Circulation 107:3101–3107, 2003.

31. Campaigne B, Lampman R: The clinical application of exercise in type I diabetes (pp. 139–168). In Exercise in the Clinical Management of Diabetes. Champaign, IL: Human Kinetics; 1994.

32. American Diabetes Association: Physical activity/exercise and diabetes. Diabetes Care 27:S58–S62, 2004.

33. Devlin JT, Ruderman N: Diabetes and exercise: The risk-benefit profile revisited. In Ruderman N, Devlin JT, Schneider SH, Kriska A, eds. Handbook of Exercise in Diabetes. Alexandria, VA: American Diabetes Association; 2002.

34. Nabel EG, Rocco MB, Selwyn AB: Characteristics and significance of ischemia detected by ambulatory electrocardiographic monitoring. Circulation.75(6 Pt 2):V74–V83, 1987.

35. Siscovick DS, Ekelund LG, Johnson JL, et al: Sensitivity of exercise electrocardiography for acute cardiac events during moderate and strenuous physical activity. The Lipid Research Clinics Coronary Primary Prevention Trial. Arch Intern Med 151:325–330, 1991.

36. Gibbons RJ, Balady GJ, Beasley JW, et al: ACC/AHH guidelines for exercise testing: A report of the American College of Cardiology/American Heart Association Task Force on Practice Guidelines (Committee on Exercise Testing). J Am Coll Cardiol 30:260–315, 1997.

37. Ambepityia G, Kopelman PG, Ingram D, et al: Exertional myocardial ischemia in diabetes: A quantitative analysis of anginal perceptual threshold and the influence of autonomic function. J Am Coll Cardiol 15:72–77, 1990.

38. Schneider SH, Shindler D: Application of the American Diabetes Association's guidelines for the evaluation of the diabetic patient before recommending an exercise program (pp. 253–268). In Devlin JT, Schneider SH, eds. Handbook of Exercise in Diabetes. Alexandria, VA: American Diabetes Association; 2001.

39. Criqui MH, Langer RD, Fronek A, et al: Mortality over a period of 10 years in patients with peripheral arterial disease. N Engl J Med 326:381–386, 1992.

40. Katzel LI, Sorkin J, Bradham D, et al: Comorbidities and the entry of patients with peripheral arterial disease into an exercise rehabilitation program. J Cardiopulm Rehabil 20:165–171, 2000.

41. Nicolaides AN: The diagnosis and assessment of coronary artery disease in vascular patients. J Vasc Surg 2:501–504, 1985.

42. Giral P, Bruckert E, Dairou F, et al: Usefulness in predicting coronary artery disease by ultrasonic evaluation of the carotid arteries in asymptomatic hypercholesterolemic patients with positive exercise stress tests. Am J Cardiol 84:14–17, 1999.

43. May O, Arildsen H, Damsgaard EM, et al: Cardiovascular autonomic neuropathy in insulin-dependent diabetes mellitus: Prevalence and estimated risk of coronary heart disease in the general population. J Intern Med 248:483–491, 2000.

44. Ewing DJ, Campbell IW, Clarke BF: The natural history of diabetic autonomic neuropathy. Q J Med 49:95–108, 1980.

45. Singh JP, Larson MG, O'Donnell CJ, et al: Association of hyperglycemia with reduced heart rate variability (The Framingham Heart Study). Am J Cardiol 86:309–312, 2000.

46. Cole CR, Blackstone EH, Pashkow FJ, et al: Heart-rate recovery immediately after exercise as a predictor of mortality. N Engl J Med 341:1351–1357, 1999.

47. Nishime EO, Cole CR, Blackstone EH: Heart rate recovery and treadmill exercise score as predictors of mortality in patients referred for exercise ECG. JAMA 284:1392–1398, 2000.

48. Seshadri N, Acharya N, Lauer MS: Association of diabetes mellitus with abnormal heart rate recovery in patients without known coronary artery disease. Am J Cardiol 91:108–111, 2003.

49. Lampman RM: Musculoskeletal disorders and sports injuries (pp. 497–507). In Ruderman N, ed. Handbook of Exercise in Diabetes. Alexandria, VA: American Diabetes Association; 2001.

50. Vanzetto G, Halimi S, Hammoud T, et al: Prediction of cardiovascular events in clinically selected high-risk NIDDM patients. Diabetes Care 22:19–26, 1999.

51. Fleischmann KE, Hunink MG, Kuntz KM: Exercise echocardiography or exercise SPECT imaging? A meta-analysis of diagnostic test performance. JAMA 280:913–920, 1998.

52. Penfornis A, Zimmermann C, Boumal B, et al: Use of dobutamine stress echocardiography in detecting silent myocardial ischaemia in asymptomatic diabetic patients: A comparison with thallium scintigraphy and exercise testing. Diabet Med 18:900–905, 2001.

53. Ritchie JL, Bateman TM, Bonow RO, et al: Guidelines for clinical use of cardiac radionuclide imaging. Report of the American College of Cardiology/American Heart Association Task Force on Assessment of Diagnostic and Therapeutic Cardiovascular Procedures (Committee on Radionuclide Imaging). Developed in collaboration with the American Society of Nuclear Cardiology. J Am Coll Cardiol 25:521–547, 1995.

54. Pancholy SB, Schalet B, Kuhlmeier V, et al: Prognostic significance of silent ischemia. J Nucl Cardiol 1:434–440, 1994.

55. He ZX, Iskandrian AS, Gupta NC, et al: Assessing coronary artery disease with dipyridamole technetium-99m-tetroforsmin SPECT: A multicenter trial. J Nucl Med 38:44–48, 1997.

56. Cheitlin MD, Alpert JS, Armstrong WF, et al: ACC/AHA Guidelines for the Clinical Application of Echocardiography. A report of the American College of Cardiology/American Heart Association Task Force on Practice Guidelines (Committee on Clinical Application of Echocardiography). Developed in collaboration with the American Society of Echocardiography. Circulation 95:1686–1744, 1997.

57. Bell DS, Yumuk VD: Low incidence of false-positive exercise thallium 201 scintigraphy in a diabetic population. Diabetes Care 19:185–186, 1996.

58. Paillole C, Ruiz J, Juliard JM, et al: Detection of coronary artery disease in diabetic patients. Diabetologia 38:726–731, 1995.

59. Boudreau RJ, Strony JT, DuCret RP, et al: Perfusion thallium imaging of type I diabetes patients with end stage renal disease: Comparison of oral and intravenous dipyridamole administration. Radiology 175:103–105, 1990.

60. Vandenberg BF, Rossen JD, Grover-McKay M, et al: Evaluation of diabetic patients for renal and pancreas transplantation: noninvasive screening for coronary artery disease using radionuclide methods. Transplantation 62:1230–1235, 1996.

61. Elming H, Brendorp B, Kober L, et al: QTc interval in the assessment of cardiac risk. Card Electrophysiol Rev 6:289–294, 2002.

62. Veglio M, Chinaglia A, Cavallo-Perin P: The clinical utility of QT interval assessment in diabetes. Diabet Nutr Metab 13:356–365, 2000.

63. Veglio M, Bruno G, Borra M, et al: Prevalence of increased QT interval duration and dispersion in type 2 diabetic patients and its relationship with coronary heart disease: A population-based cohort. J Intern Med 251:317–324, 2002.

64. Linnemann B, Janka HU: Prolonged QTc interval and elevated heart rate identify the type 2 diabetic patient at high risk for cardiovascular death. The Bremen Diabetes Study. Exp Clin Endocrinol Diabetes 111:215–222, 2003.

65. Rana BS, Band MM, Ogston S, et al: Relation of OT interval dispersion to the number of different cardiac abnormalities in diabetes mellitus. Am J Cardiol 90:483–487, 2002.

66. Veglio M, Sivieri R, Chinaglia A, et al: QT interval prolongation and mortality in type 1 diabetic patients: A 5-year cohort prospective study. Neuropathy Study Group of the Italian Society of the Study of Diabetes, Piemonte Affiliate. Diabetes Care 23:1381–1383, 2000.

67. Rossing P, Breum L, Major-Pedersen A, et al: Prolonged QTc interval predicts mortality in patients with Type 1 diabetes mellitus. Diabet Med 18:199–205, 2001.

68. Frolkis JP, Pothier CE, Blackstone EH, et al: Frequent ventricular ectopy after exercise as a predictor of death. N Engl J Med 348:781–790, 2003.

69. Messinger-Rapport B, Pothier Snader CE, Blackstone EH: Value of exercise capacity and heart rate recovery in older people. J Am Geriatr Soc 51:63–68, 2003.

70. Watanabe J, Thamilarasan M, Blackstone EH, et al: Heart rate recovery immediately after treadmill exercise and left ventricular systolic dysfunction as predictors of mortality. The case of stress echocardiology. Circulation 104:1911–1916–2001.

71. Cheng YJ, Lauer MS, Earnest CP, et al: Heart rate recovery following maximal exercise testing as a predictor of cardiovascular disease and all-cause mortality in men with diabetes. Diabetes Care 26:2052–2057, 2003.

72. Marwick TH, Case C, Sawada S, et al: Use of stress echocardiography to predict mortality in patients with diabetes and known or suspected coronary artery disease. Diabetes Care 25:1042–1048, 2002.

73. Kamalesh M, Matorin R, Sawada S: Prognostic value of a negative stress echocardiographic study in diabetic patients. Am Heart J 143:163–168, 2002.

74. Shaw LJ, Hendel R, Borges-Neto S, et al: Prognostic value of normal exercise and adenosine (99m)Tc-tetrofosmin SPECT imaging: results from the multicenter registry of 4,728 patients. J Nucl Med 44:134–139, 2003.

75. Iskandrian AS, Johnson J, Le TT, et al: Comparison of the treadmill exercise score and single-photon emission computed tomographic thallium imaging in risk assessment. J Nucl Cardiol 1:144–149, 1994.

SELECTED REFERENCE FOR FURTHER READING

American Diabetes Association: Standards of medical care in diabetes. Diabetes Care 28:S4-S36, 2005.

American Heart Association Conference Proceedings: Prevention Conference VI: Diabetes and Cardiovascular Disease. Writing Group III: Risk assessment in persons with diabetes. Circulation 105:e144, 2002.

Ruderman N, Devlin JT, Schneider SH, Kriska A, eds: Handbook of Exercise in Diabetes. Alexandria, VA: American Diabetes Association; 2002.

INTERNET RESOURCES

American Diabetes Association: http://www.diabetes.org

CDC Diabetes Public Health Resource: http://www.cdc.gov/diabetes

National Diabetes Education Program: http://ndep.nih.gov

National Institute of Diabetes & Digestive & Kidney Diseases: http://www.niddk.nih.gov

Treadmill and Pharmacologic Stress Testing: http://www.emedicine.com/med/topic2961.htm

Clinical Exercise Testing in Individuals with Disabilities Caused by Neuromuscular Disorders

SUZANNE GROAH

Advances in medical treatment, rehabilitation, and technology have contributed to improved life expectancies for many people with disabilities of neurologic origin. But with this increase in lifespan comes a heightened risk of certain medical conditions, namely chronic diseases such as cardiovascular disease (CVD) and cancer. Thus, medical problems that historically may have been only infrequently seen in certain disabled subpopulations are now being seen with increasing regularity.

This chapter focuses on the specific needs of more severe neurologically impaired individuals with regards to clinical exercise testing, specifically, testing of aerobic capacity. Given the nature of severe neurologic impairment, it is unusual to have other testing, such as strength and flexibility testing, performed outside the rehabilitation setting; hence, these types of testing are not covered in this chapter. The diagnoses of spinal cord injury (SCI),

multiple sclerosis (MS), stroke, and brain injury (BI) are specifically addressed.

Safety of Exercise in Those Disabled Because of Neurologic Impairment

Until recently, it was challenging for individuals with disabilities to participate in a physical activity, an exercise program, or even exercise testing. This is because of multiple barriers to exercise, including limitations imposed by the neuromuscular impairment, geographic barriers, and equipment issues, among others. Furthermore, lack of knowledge and awareness by the health care community and society "discouraged" physical activity and exercise for those with physical disabilities because of a perceived heightened risk of injuries. This pervading perception contributed to the "disability mindset," which is characterized by low self-esteem and low expectations in those who are physically challenged. Now, with improved equipment, the slow elimination of barriers, and the Americans with Disabilities Act (ADA), there is greater opportunity for disabled individuals to acquire and maintain physical fitness.

Furthermore, with the disabled population aging and more often encountering chronic diseases seen in the able-bodied population, disability-specific and -appropriate exercise prescription and assessment are now increasingly essential. Additionally, physical activity, exercise, and exercise testing should be considered safe for individuals with disability, within the confines of the impairment and resultant disability.

Epidemiology

SPINAL CORD INJURY

Spinal cord injury is most often caused by trauma (motor vehicle crashes, falls, violence, and sports-related injuries), although infection, tumor, surgical complications,

KEY TERMS

Dysautonomia: Any disease or malfunction of the autonomic nervous system

Hemiplegia: Weakness of one side of the body caused by damage to one side of the brain

Paraplegia: Weakness of the lower extremities caused by an injury or damage to the spinal cord in the thoracic, lumbar, or sacral region.

Tetraplegia: Weakness of the upper extremities and lower extremities caused by an injury or damage to the spinal cord in the cervical region

and demyelinating disease are being seen with increasing frequency. Males more commonly incur SCIs, and most happen in the third and fourth decades of life. Those injured in falls tend to be older at the time of injury. There are approximately 11,000 people newly injured because of SCIs in a given year, and approximately 200,000 people are currently living in the United States with SCIs[1].

Spinal cord injury is classified primarily by the level and completeness of the injury. An injury that is associated with neurologic impairment between C1 and T1 is termed **tetraplegia** (this is now the accepted terminology so that Greek roots are uniformly used as opposed to the Latin-derived *quadriplegia*) and results in some degree of motor or sensory loss (or both) in the upper and lower extremities as well as the trunk and pelvis. An injury that occurs caudal to (below) T1 is termed **paraplegia** and is associated with motor or sensory loss (or both) in the trunk, pelvis, and lower extremities (Fig. 17-1).

Both often have some degree of autonomic and major organ dysfunction, depending on the level of the injury associated. Function of the major organ systems, such as the autonomic nervous system, respiratory, cardiovascular, gastrointestinal, and genitourinary systems, may be altered and is shown according to injury level in Figure 17-2.

As already stated, SCIs are also classified based on the completeness of injury. The American Spinal Injury Association International (ASIA) Standards for Neurological and Functional Classification of Spinal Cord Injury[2] is an internationally accepted standard for neurologic classification of individuals with SCIs. Components of this classification scheme include measurement of motor strength in 20 key muscles (five in each upper extremity and five in

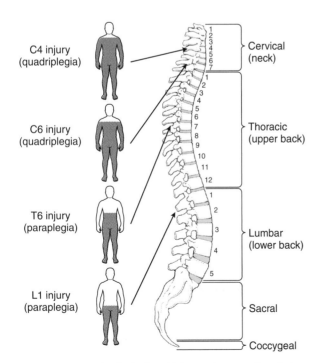

FIGURE 17-1. Levels of spinal cord injury and extent of paralysis.

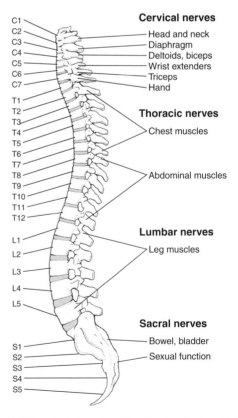

FIGURE 17-2. Neurological level and function in spinal cord injury.

each lower extremity) and assessment of sensation to light touch and pain (via pin stick) sensation in all of the dermatomes, bilaterally. Figure 17-3 shows the ASIA worksheet for neurologic examination.

Finally, the ASIA classification system includes a five-point scale of completeness based on the presence or absence of sacral sensation and the amount of motor and sensory preservation, if any, below the level of injury. A complete injury is defined as no residual motor or sensory function below the level of injury. There are three levels of incomplete injury with increasing amounts of sensory and motor preservation below the level of injury (see Table 17-1).

Thus, an individual's impairment and disability are associated with *both* the level *and* the completeness of the injury, as well as other factors such as age, body habitus, medical comorbidities, and motivation. For example, whereas an individual with a relatively high cervical, or neck, injury resulting in incomplete (ASIA D) tetraplegia may be able to ambulate without assistive devices and may have normal control of his bowel and bladder, an individual with a lower back lesions resulting in thoracic or lumbar complete (ASIA A) paraplegia likely will be mobile using a wheelchair and may have more profound dysfunction of the autonomic, genitourinary, and gastrointestinal systems. Therefore, during the pre-assessment screening, it is important to query the individual specifically about the level *and* completeness of the SCI, as well as other pertinent comorbidities, which are described later.

MULTIPLE SCLEROSIS

Multiple sclerosis is a chronic inflammatory disorder of the brain, spinal cord, or both that is characterized by multifocal demyelination of the central nervous system (CNS) white matter[3]. Grey matter and nerve axons are generally spared, although recent reports indicate there may be some axonal injury. Women are more commonly affected, and disease onset typically occurs between 20 and 40 years old. The etiology of MS is unclear, although most investigators agree that there is an immune component (Box 17-1).

Symptoms vary according to the size and location of the MS plaques, and they might include sensory disturbances in the extremities, optic nerve dysfunction, weakness of the extremities, bladder or bowel dysfunction, sexual dysfunction, incoordination, impaired balance, fatigue, cardiovascular **dysautonomia**, tremor, heat sensitivity, and double vision. Thus, if the spinal cord is solely affected, the impairments and resultant disability seen in MS may be very similar to those seen in SCIs, and they can result in paraplegia or tetraplegia. But if plaques occur in the brain, additional visual, motor, sensory, cognitive, language, or other dysfunction consistent with their location will likely be present. It is important to be aware that some medications used to treat MS may have cardiopulmonary

adverse effects such as hypertension, chest pain, dyspnea, dizziness, syncope, and fatigue, among others.

STROKE AND BRAIN INJURY

A cerebrovascular accident (CVA), or stroke, is a neurologic injury caused by compromised blood flow and characterized by a variety of combinations of loss of motor control, altered sensation, cognitive impairment, and language impairment, among others. It is a significant cause of morbidity and mortality in the United States, with approximately 700,000 people affected per year, and it is the third leading cause of death, exceeded only by CVD and cancer[4]. Stroke usually occurs in individuals older than 65 years of age, men, and African Americans. Risk factors for stroke are listed in Box 17-2.

The majority of strokes (88%) are caused by an ischemic vascular event, and the remaining 9% of strokes are caused by intracerebral hemorrhage and subarachnoid hemorrhage (3%).

Stroke is the leading cause of serious, long-term disability in the United States, with more than 1.1 million Americans reporting functional limitations caused by stroke. Of those who survive the first 3 weeks after stroke, 30–50% report being dependent on others for their activities of daily living (ADLs), 15–30% are permanently disabled, and 20% require institutional care.

Approximately 200,000 Americans incur a BI each year, and another 52,000 Americans die each year because of BIs. Traumatic BIs resulting in disability affect an estimated 2.5 to 6.5 million Americans, with approximately 80,000 experiencing disability caused by BIs each year[5]. The epidemiology of BIs is difficult to elucidate because many people who incur a concussion with mild deficits may not seek medical attention. Conversely, many people die at the scene of an accident because of BIs. Therefore, these subgroups of individuals with BIs are not adequately quantified.

Traumatic BI is most commonly caused by motor vehicle crashes, followed by falls, violence, and sports-related injuries. Risk factors for traumatic BI include youth, male gender, low-income status, being unmarried, ethnic minority, inner-city residence, and history of substance abuse or traumatic BI.

Stroke and BI result in various combinations of cognitive, physical, and psychosocial dysfunction, depending on the location of the injury, and may include but not be limited to those listed in Box 17-3.

Pretest Considerations

During the pretest assessment, it is important to obtain a detailed history, especially of the functional abilities of the individual, because these are critical in the decision of what assessment tools and tests are appropriate. For example, whereas individuals with SCIs or MS resulting in paraplegia may use an arm-crank ergometer, wheelchair

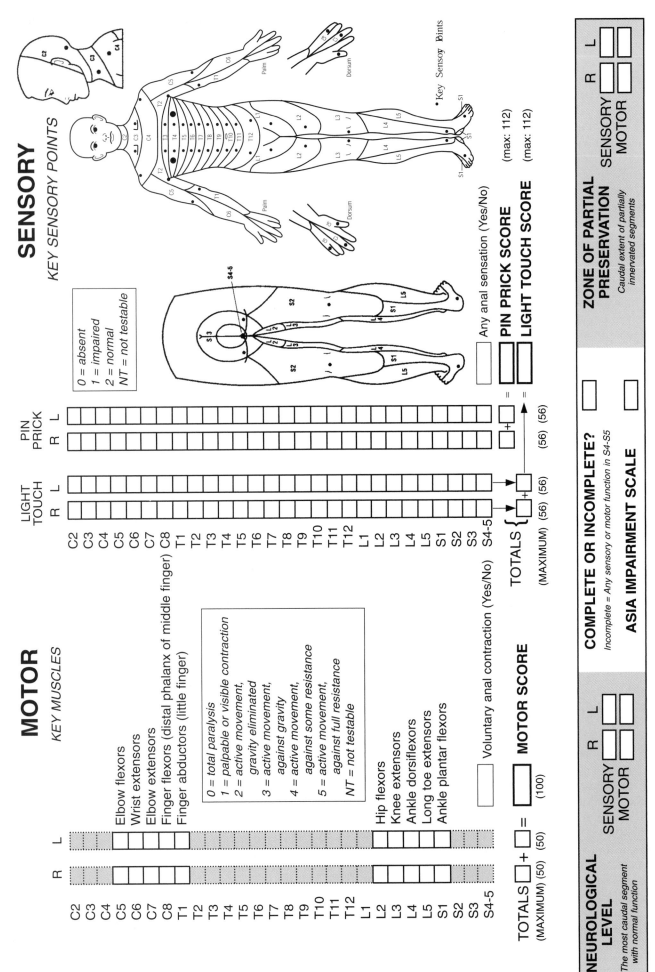

FIGURE 17-3. American Spinal Injury Association spinal cord injury classification system. (Reprinted with permission from the American Spinal Injury Association.)

TABLE 17-1. Description of the American Spinal Injury Association's Classification System for Spinal Cord Injuries

ASIA Classification	Definition
A = Complete	No motor or sensory function in the sacral segments
B = Incomplete	Sensory function only is preserved below the level of injury and through the sacral segments
C = Incomplete	Motor function is preserved and more than half of the muscles below the level of injury have a muscle grade of less than 3
D = Incomplete	Motor function is preserved and at least half of the muscles below the level of injury have a muscle grade of greater than 3
E = Normal	Normal motor and sensory function

ASIA = American Spinal Injury Association.

ergometer, wheelchair treadmill, or wheeling on a track or treadmill for exercise testing, certain individuals with incomplete tetraplegia may actually be able to use a treadmill safely. Likewise, because of balance and coordination problems more so than weakness, individuals with stroke or BIs may be best tested on a bicycle because treadmill testing is unsafe. Often with a severe neurologic impairment, such as with high complete tetraplegia, the functional limitations are severe enough that neither treadmill testing nor arm-crank ergometry are suitable for the client, and pharmacologic testing is necessary.

In addition to the usual pretest history, for safety, planning, and time management, it is important to determine the details of the neuromuscular impairment before exercise testing. Depending on the impairment and functional limitations, extra time might be set aside for mobility issues and additional history attainment. Pertinent questions might include:

Question	Significance
• What is the cause of your disability? Were you born with this condition?	• Tester will be knowledgeble of other areas of concern associated with a paticular condition • Certain birth abnormalities (i.e., spina bifida) have other associated comorbidities, such as latex allergy, implanted cerebral shunts, etc.
• Do you use any devices such as a wheelchair, walker, crutches, cane, or braces to help with mobility?	• Aids with planning the appropriate testing and time management
• Will you be bringing anyone that could help you with any needs you may have?	• Aids with time and staff management
• Will you need assistance with transfers or any other mobility issues?	• Aids with time and staff management

BOX 17-1 | **The Four Clinical Courses of Multiple Sclerosis**

- Relapsing/remitting MS (RRMS)
- Secondary progressive MS (SPMS)
- Primary progressive MS (PPMS)
- Progressive/relapsing MS (PRMS)

Removing Barriers

For any clinician working with an individual with a disability, it is important to note that deficiencies exist between the delivery of health care services to disabled versus able-bodied individuals. Up to one third of women with a disability have reported being refused health care, and nearly one half reported not being spoken to directly by a health care professional.

Clinical tip: Speak directly to the individual with the disability, not necessarily to a friend, family member, or caregiver "about" the individual.

Furthermore, a frequent problem reported by individuals with disabilities is health care providers' unfamiliarity with their disability-related needs.

Another barrier to the attainment of health-related services for the disabled is physical barriers. It should be ensured that the testing facility is free of major geographic barriers to the individual with a disability and should comply with the ADA's general accessibility requirements. Basic recommendations include but are not be limited to those listed in Box 17-4.

Detailed explanations and dimensions to allow adequate space to allow someone to manipulate a wheelchair can be obtained through the Department of Justice[6].

Determinants of Exercise Capacity

Exercise capacity is often limited in individuals with severe neurologic impairments, although data in this area are limited. In individuals with SCIs, maximal values of power output, oxygen consumption, and cardiac output are limited to roughly one third to one half that observed in individuals without SCIs. These limitations are

BOX 17-2 | **Risk Factors for Stroke**

- Hypertension
- Diabetes mellitus
- Carotid or other artery disease
- Atrial fibrillation
- Heart disease
- High cholesterol
- Smoking
- Obesity
- Excessive alcohol use
- Sickle cell disease
- Physical inactivity

BOX 17-3	Dysfunction Resulting from Stroke and Brain Injury

- Weakness, **hemiplegia**
- Loss of trunk control and stability
- Altered balance
- Incoordination
- Anesthesia, hemianesthesia
- Spasticity
- Altered taste, vision, smell, hearing
- Altered speech and language
- Apraxia (disorder of skilled movement)
- Neglect syndrome
- Visual impairments including visuospatial deficit, hemianopia
- Memory deficits
- Behavior/emotional problems
- Seizures

accentuated with higher levels of SCIs because in tetraplegia, the pathologic process involves more extensive muscle paralysis than that seen in paraplegia *and* there is a disruption in the control of the sympathetic nervous system.

The amount of metabolically active tissue is correlated with the amount of physiologic work an individual with an SCI is capable of performing. Although in paraplegics, the percent of lean tissue increases with higher activity level, in tetraplegic individuals, there is no significant relationship between percentage of lean tissue and activity level. Thus, because of the neurologic impairment, there is a reduced ability to stimulate the cardiovascular system to support higher rates of aerobic metabolism; hence, the resting metabolic rate is 12% to 54% lower in patients with SCIs, and this is thought to be attributable to the decrease in muscle mass.

Clinical tip: Anticipate 20% to 36% less work from upper extremity activity compared with lower extremity activity.

BOX 17-4	Americans with Disabilities Act Recommendations

- Accessible parking places for individuals with disabilities
- Ramps or elevators to allow wheelchair access
- If door hardware is not lever or U-shaped, then alternatives must be in place for entry
- An unobstructed path of travel for individuals using wheelchairs or other assistive devices
- Adequate space within the facility to allow wheelchairs to turn
- A wheelchair-accessible changing room (if necessary)
- A wheelchair-accessible bathroom with hand rails and grab bars

There is a reduced association between maximal ventilation and $\dot{V}O_{2peak}$ in individuals with tetraplegia. This is attributed to decreased or absent innervation of muscles of respiration in individuals with tetraplegia versus those with paraplegia.

Compared with active individuals, those who are inactive have decreased left ventricular diastolic dimensions. In contrast, those who are active may maximize physiologic mechanisms to increase preload to the left ventricle, thus increasing left ventricular diameter during diastole. Additionally, individuals with paraplegia above T6 have an attenuated catecholamine release at rest and response to exercise compared with subjects with injuries below T6, which might prevent a better exercise performance in the former group. This may explain, in part, the increase in cardiac output that occurs with exercise in tetraplegics is mainly elicited by an increase in stroke volume; in individuals with paraplegia, it is by heart rate (HR).

Clinical tip: Peak HR is limited, primarily in tetraplegia, and may not exceed 130 bpm.

Similarly, in individuals with MS, $\dot{V}O_{2peak}$ can vary significantly and is related to the degree of lower extremity impairment. Individuals with minimal weakness and little to no dysautonomia have the capability to reach 85% to 90% of age-predicted maximal HR.

After stroke, the ability to exercise depends on the extent of the neurologic involvement and on any other medical comorbidities that might be present. For example, muscle weakness, spasticity, impaired sensation, impaired balance, and impaired vision may all contribute to the inability to ambulate safely. Furthermore, many with a history of a stroke also have comorbidities such as diabetes mellitus, obesity, coronary heart disease, arthritis, or orthopedic problems, further limiting exercise testing. Because of these and other issues, only 20% to 34% of individuals poststroke are able to achieve 85% of age-predicted maximal HR.

Because individuals with BIs are typically younger and have overall fewer physical impairments than the other groups, exercise capacity is better, with most being able to achieve 67% to 74% predicted levels based on height and age. Not surprisingly, submaximal HRs are higher than age-matched control subjects without physical impairments on cycle ergometry.

In summary, it is important to remember that although we use HR, blood pressure (BP), and $\dot{V}O_{2max}$ norms from the general population, because of autonomic and other changes associated with certain neurologic injuries, these may not apply to subpopulations of individuals with neurologic impairment. Unfortunately, for the most part, normal ranges for these subpopulations do not exist. Thus, it is critical to carefully monitor these individuals, especially for signs and symptoms of fatigue, dyspnea, and hypotension, as well as for clinical signs and symptoms of deterioration that are specific to the impairment.

Impairment- and Disability-Specific Guidelines for Exercise Testing and Assessment

Individuals with severe neurologic impairment and disability who present for exercise testing provide an additional challenge to the clinician. Not only is an understanding of the impairment and resultant functional limitations critical, but creativity to allow for safe and adequate testing, as well an understanding of current equipment availability and limitations, is necessary.

Often, because of the disability, treadmill testing is not feasible. Types of testing in the non-ambulatory disabled population include arm-crank testing and wheelchair ergometry. Although arm-crank ergometry is low cost and portable, it is not specific, and its primary limitation is that arm muscle fatigue occurs before a true cardiopulmonary maximum is elicited. Wheelchair ergometry has the advantage of being mobility specific, but it can be difficult to use, and the validity has not been established. Individuals with some motor function in the lower extremities may be able to tolerate treadmill testing with or without body-weight support (through use of a harness).

Recommendations for Exercise Testing

One of the most important factors in determining the type of exercise testing to be performed depends on the functional assessment of the individual. Upper extremity exercise does not necessarily predict lower extremity exercise capacity and vice versa. Thus, upper extremity testing via an arm ergometer or wheelchair testing in the laboratory or outside is often the method of choice used for individuals with SCIs or MS who primarily use their upper extremities for mobility. It is important to be aware, however, that a significant number of individuals with SCIs ambulate in the home and community and have the ability to use their lower extremities for exercise testing. In these cases, bicycle or treadmill testing is appropriate.

Because of the wide range of other conditions associated with SCIs, MS, stroke, and BIs, the degree to which exercise testing can be conducted and monitored is highly variable. The choice of exercise testing depends on symptoms such as weakness, spasticity, impaired balance, sensory disturbance, and visual problems. Because of the potential for dysautonomia, it is important to monitor HR and BP closely. Additionally, some may have cognitive deficits, requiring cueing and additional instructions during testing.

It is important to note that often individuals with MS experience heat sensitivity that may be associated with transient worsening of clinical signs and symptoms of disease. Although physical activity may be beneficial for those with MS, induced thermal loads may preclude participation in exercise and other daily activities. Thus, because of this attenuated or absent sudomotor (sweating) response, the testing room should be kept cool or room temperature (72° to 76°). Furthermore, fluid intake is encouraged during testing. There is some evidence that "precooling" before aerobic exercise may have a beneficial effect on performance by preventing increases in the core body temperature associated with physical work, thereby allowing heat-sensitive individuals with MS to exercise longer with greater physical comfort (also see Chapter 37).

Clinical tip: When testing individuals with MS or SCI higher than T8, make sure to keep the testing room at a temperature to avoid overheating and fatigue (Box 17-5).

The presence of neurological deficits in gait and balance has discouraged systematic application of exercise testing and prescription in the stroke population. It has been shown that a simple floor-walking test using graded velocities similar to a treadmill can be performed to predict adequate neurologic function to perform a treadmill exercise test safely. Additionally, treadmill testing may be possible in individuals who are able to ambulate *without* external assistive devices (the patient may use a lower extremity orthotic such as an ankle foot orthosis or knee brace) such as a walker, cane, or crutch. Body-weight–supported treadmill testing is possible and offers the advantages of being able to partially support the person's weight while allowing lower extremity testing as well as being a safety measure to prevent falls. Also, this kind of testing is well tolerated by individuals poststroke who have cardiovascular problems. The limiting factor is availability of equipment.

Hemiplegia, spasticity, and associated musculoskeletal disorders of the knee, hip, and shoulder are common after stroke and BI and may preclude treadmill testing, thereby necessitating use of the uninvolved extremity for exercise testing with a bicycle ergometer. If possible, consider the use of combined arm/leg ergometry, using the unaffected lower extremity and the upper extremities to assist. A recumbent device might be considered for individuals with impaired torso control and sitting balance. Functional electrical stimulation (FES) has been used in exercise training in those with SCI and has been shown to elicit similar exercise capacity (similar $\dot{V}O_{2peak}$) as arm cranking.

Clinical tip: Consider using toe clips, chest straps, hand mitts, or bicycle racing or lifting gloves in addition to close

---

BOX 17-5	Other Important Issues to Consider in Those with Multiple Sclerosis

- Fatigue may reduce exercise tolerance.
- Because of fatigue, morning is the optimal time for testing.
- Flu-like symptoms may reduce exercise tolerance.
- Avoid testing a person with MS during an exacerbation.

TABLE 17-2. Components of Arm Ergometer Exercise Testing

	Options for Exercise Testing	Protocol	Measures	Endpoints
Aerobic	Arm ergometry	Individually determine initial workload (0–200 kpm·min⁻¹)	Peak HR	Angina
	Wheelchair ergometry	Increase workload by 100–150 kpm·min⁻¹ per stage	METs	ECG changes
		2–4 minute stages	Peak $\dot{V}O_2$	Dyspnea
		Cranking rate 40–60 rpm	BP	Fatigue (RPE scale)
	Wheelchair treadmill		RPE	Muscle discomfort
	Wheeling on track			Dysrhythmia
Flexibility	Goniometer	Test ROM of shoulders, elbows, wrists, fingers, hips, knees, ankles, spine	ROM	Pain
	Stretching tests		Ashworth scale	

BP = blood pressure; ECG = electrocardiogram; HR = heart rate; MET = metabolic equivalents; RPE = rating of perceived exertion ROM = range of motion.

supervision in individuals with weakness caused by a CNS disorder.

It is also important to remember that cognitive and behavioral changes may influence compliance with and retention of information during exercise testing of individuals with stroke or BI. Thus, confirm that the client is able to communicate adequately, especially if there is pain or dyspnea or if the client wants the test terminated. Seizure risk is an important consideration in this subpopulation, and the tester should inquire about any seizure history and medication use.

A variety of arm ergometer exercise testing protocols has been proposed. For aerobic testing, a discontinuous protocol, although more time intensive, is advised to allow for greater monitoring of BP and electrocardiogram (ECG). Table 17-2 summarizes components of an arm ergometer exercise test based on the available protocols.

Common Associated Conditions

Those administering exercise testing should be familiar with the conditions commonly seen in association with SCI, MS, stroke, and BI. Common associated conditions pertinent to exercise testing are summarized in Table 17-3.

CARDIOVASCULAR

The cardiovascular effects of SCI are variable, and there is a correlation with level and completeness of injury. One of the most apparent functions affected is that of BP control. Whereas paraplegics tend to be normotensive or even hypertensive, tetraplegics often have symptomatic or asymptomatic hypotension, with resting BP ranging from 80 to 100/40 to 70 mm Hg.

Clinical tip: Check pretest BP, monitoring BP frequently or continually, and observe for signs of hypotension when testing individuals with CNS impairments.

Individuals with an SCI at the level of T6 or cephalic are at risk of experiencing autonomic dysreflexia (AD).

AD is a relatively unopposed sympathetic response to a noxious stimulus below the level of the SCI. This massive sympathetic surge causes widespread vasoconstriction, leading to peripheral arterial hypertension. Intact baroreceptors detect the hypertensive crisis, but inhibitory impulses are relatively blocked because of the spinal cord lesion. The intact vagus nerve sends impulses, which results in bradycardia, yet this is an inadequate compensatory mechanism. Thus, AD is characterized by systemic hypertension followed by reflex bradycardia. Symptoms include a pounding headache, flushing, sweating, nasal congestion, and pupillary dilatation above the level of the SCI and pallor, piloerection, and penile erection below the level of the SCI. It is critical to be aware of AD because, if left untreated, it can rapidly lead to retinal hemorrhage, subarachnoid hemorrhage, intracerebral hemorrhage, seizure, stroke, myocardial infarction (MI), and potentially death.

The most common causes of AD include noxious stimuli from the bladder (overdistention caused by a clogged urinary catheter or delay in catheterization, urinary tract infection, or urinary stone), bowel (distention caused by constipation), skin (cutaneous stimulation or pressure sore), other (ingrown toenails, fracture, position change, range of motion exercises), or during surgical procedures. An individual with spinal MS may also experience AD, but this is more infrequent.

Clinical tip: If an individual experiences AD during testing, stop the test immediately, ELEVATE the person's head, and then attempt to determine the cause.

Cardiovascular disease is more prevalent in individuals with SCI compared with the general population. Within the SCI population, tetraplegics are at greater risk of cerebrovascular disease and arrhythmias, and hypertension and coronary artery disease tend to be more common in paraplegics. Additionally, hypertriglyceridemia and low high-density lipoprotein cholesterol are prevalent, which can contribute to the development of atherosclerotic heart disease. Another significant issue in the population with SCI is that of silent ischemia and MI in those with injuries

TABLE 17-3. Pertinent Clinical Issues to be Considered During Exercise Testing for Individuals with Spinal Cord Injuries, Multiple Sclerosis, Stroke, and Brain Injuries

System	Spinal Cord Injury	Multiple Sclerosis	Stroke	Brain Injury
Cardiovascular	Hypotension	Hypotension	Hypertension but may be susceptible to hypotension.	
	Silent angina or MI Dysautonomia Autonomic dysreflexia	Dysautonomia	High CVD risk	
Pulmonary	Respiratory insufficiency dependent on level of injury FVC decreased Dyspnea	Respiratory insufficiency dependent on severity of MS	Higher COPD risk	Deficits only caused by deconditioning
Thermal	Thermal instability in those T8 and above	Thermal instability, so avoid overheating; may benefit from "precooling"	Usually unchanged	Usually unchanged
Bowel	Incontinence possible with Valsalva in some	Incontinence possible	May be continent or incontinent	Usually continent
Bladder	Incontinence or overdistention possible	Incontinence or overdistention possible	May be continent or incontinent	Usually continent
Endocrine	Elevated risk of glucose intolerance and diabetes mellitus	No significant endocrine abnormalities	Consider diabetes mellitus	No significant endocrine abnormalities
Skin	High risk of skin breakdown caused by insensate areas	Same as SCI in those insensate	Higher risk of breakdown over insensate areas affected by stroke	At risk for skin breakdown if immobilized or hemiplegic
Musculoskeletal	Spasticity	May have spasticity	May have increased tone, even contractures	Spasticity or contractures
	Heterotopic ossification (usually affects the lower extremities) Osteoporosis: Tend to fracture below the level of injury, typically around the knee	Elevated fracture risk if prolonged immobility	Osteoporosis: Tend to fracture the hip, wrist and spine	Heterotopic ossification (usually affects the upper extremities)
Neurologic	Syringomyelia	Neurologic status may worsen with heat	May have difficulty following and understanding directions and may have problems with memory	May have difficulty following and understanding directions and may have problems with memory
Other concerns		Fatigue	May have deficits in perception, balance, and so on	Seizure risk; may have impaired balance, visual deficits, and so on

COPD = chronic obstructive pulmonary disease; CVD = cardiovascular disease; FVC = forced vital capacity; MI = myocardial infarction; MS = multiple sclerosis; SCI = spinal cord injury.

cephalic to T4 because these individuals may have disrupted the cardiac pain fibers that travel with the sympathetic afferent fibers; therefore, the sensation of ischemic cardiac pain may be eliminated or modified. The risk of CVD is well established in individuals with stroke, as well.

Clinical tip: Consider frequent or continuous ECG monitoring and physician supervision of individuals with severe neurologic impairment because of silent ischemia and the greater risk of CVD.

ENDOCRINE

Individuals with SCI are generally more insulin resistant than are able-bodied individuals. As a result, individuals with SCI are more susceptible to developing non–insulin-dependent diabetes mellitus and impaired glucose tolerance. Similarly, individuals with stroke tend to have more associated medical conditions such as diabetes mellitus.

FATIGUE

Fatigue is a frequent problem encountered by those with MS, with 75% to 95% of people with MS reporting fatigue, and most reporting it as their worst problem[7]. Although chronic fatigue is common, it is also associated with acute bouts of disease, intercurrent illness, and weather changes.

Clinical tip: Before testing, query the individual with MS about fatigue levels and optimal times during the day that testing can be performed.

BOX 17-6 | Additional Cautionary Notes

CONDITION	RECOMMENDATION
• Hypotension (SCI)	• Maintain hydration and monitor BP closely
• Autonomic dysreflexia (SCI)	• Monitor closely for pounding headache flushing, sweating, nasal congestion, and pupillary dilatation above the level of the SCI and for pallor, piloerection, and penile erection below the level of the SCI
• Arrhythmia (SCI, MS, stroke)	• Continuous or frequent ECG monitoring
• Silent ischemia (SCI)	• Continuous or frequent ECG monitoring
• Baseline dyspnea (SCI-T)	• Use RPE scale
• Bladder incontinence (SCI, MS)	• Empty bladder immediately before testing
• Bowel incontinence (SCI, MS)	• Bowel care the evening before or morning of exercise testing
• Poikilothermy, heat sensitivity (SCI, MS)	• Maintain temperature at approximately 72 to 74°
• Skin breakdown (SCI)	• Allow time for pressure reliefs during exercise testing
• Spasticity (SCI, MS, stroke, BI)	• May require strapping
• Shoulder pain (SCI, MS, stroke)	• Discontinue exercise testing if shoulder pain is present
• Nerve impingement (SCI)	• Discontinue exercise testing if there are signs of nerve impingement
• Fracture risk caused by osteoporosis (SCI)	• Avoid standing unless individual is a community ambulator
• Heterotopic ossification (SCI, MS, stroke, BI)	• Do not forcefully position a joint or extremity beyond end of range
• Contracture (SCI, stroke, BI)	• Do not forcefully position a joint or extremity beyond end of range
• Spinal cord syrinx (cyst) characterized by motor or sensory loss, increased spasticity, pain, AD, or visual changes	• Avoid increased abdominal pressure or Valsalva

AD = autonomic dysreflexia; BI = brain injury; ECG = electrocardiogram; MS = multiple sclerosis; RPE = rating of perceived exertion; SCI = spinal cord injury.

PULMONARY

The pulmonary system is often notably affected by SCI and spinal MS. The diaphragm, scalene, and sternocleidomastoid muscles are the major muscles of inspiration, which are all innervated by the upper cervical segments. The major muscles of expiration are the abdominal muscles, innervated by nerves arising from the thoracic and lumbar spinal cord. A complete injury to the spinal cord above C3 causes paralysis of all muscles of inspiration and expiration, thereby necessitating mechanical ventilation for respiratory support. As the level of injury descends, more inspiratory and expiratory function is preserved. Likewise, with motor incomplete injuries, additional inspiratory and expiratory function may be preserved.

Forced vital capacity (FVC) is commonly used to quantify pulmonary insufficiency in patients with SCI. Whereas individuals with C4 SCI have an FVC only 45% of expected, individuals with injuries at the T5 level have an FVC approximately 81% predicted, and those with T12 SCI still have minor FVC deficits (95% predicted)[8]. Clearly, the majority of individuals with SCI and spinal MS have some degree of respiratory insufficiency that is highly related to their level and completeness of injury. Furthermore, pulmonary function declines with age and time since injury, putting individuals with SCI at even greater risk of complications. Therefore, it is important to be aware of these limitations, as well of the associated dyspnea that is a frequent complaint of individuals with SCI. Likewise, people who have had a stroke are more likely to have chronic obstructive pulmonary disease.

Clinical tip: Consider querying individuals with high paraplegia or tetraplegia as to their baseline level of dyspnea before exercise testing (Box 17-6).

REFERENCES

1. Spinal cord injury: Facts & figures at a glance. J Spinal Cord Med 23:153–155, 2000.
2. American Spinal Injury Association/International Medical Society of Paraplegia (ASIA/IMSOP): International Standards for Neurological and Functional Classification of Spinal Cord Injury Patients (Rev). Atlanta; 2000.
3. Paralyzed Veterans of America: Multiple Sclerosis Clinical Practice guidelines. Disease Modifying Therapies In Multiple Sclerosis: Evidence-Based Management Strategies for Disease Modifying Therapies in Multiple Sclerosis.Washington, DC; 2001.
4. American Heart Association: Heart and Stroke Facts: 2005 Statistical Supplement. Dallas: American Heart Association; 2005.
5. Rehabilitation of Persons with Traumatic Brain Injury. NIH Consensus Statement 16(1):1–41, Oct. 26–28, 1998.
6. The ADAAG Standards for Accessible Design were published in the Federal Register. Available at http://www.usdoj.gov/crt/ada
7. Paralyzed Veterans of America: Fatigue and Multiple Sclerosis. Evidence-Based Management Strategies for Fatigue in Multiple Sclerosis. Washington, DC; 1998.
8. Linn WS, Spungen AM, Gong H Jr, et al: Forced vital capacity in two large outpatient populations with chronic spinal cord injury. Spinal Cord 39:263–268, 2001.

SELECTED REFERENCES FOR FURTHER READING

Bauman WA: Carbohydrate and lipid metabolism in individuals after spinal cord injury . In Topics in Spinal Cord Injury Rehabilitation. 2:11–22; 1997.

Figoni SF: Spinal cord disabilities: Paraplegia and tetraplegia (pp. 2457–253). In ACSM's Exercise Management for Persons with Chronic Diseases and Disabilities, 2nd ed. Durstine JL, Moore GE, eds. Philadelphia: Lippincott Williams & Wilkins; 2003.

Mulcare JA: Multiple sclerosis (pp. 267–272). In ACSM's Exercise Management for Persons with Chronic Diseases and Disabilities, 2nd ed. Durstine JL, Moore GE, eds. Philadelphia: Lippincott Williams & Wilkins; 2003.

Palmer-McLean K, Harbst KB: Stroke and brain injury (pp. 238–246). In ACSM's Exercise Management for Persons with Chronic Diseases and Disabilities, 2nd ed. Durstine JL, Moore GE, eds. Philadelphia: Lippincott Williams & Wilkins; 2003.

Phillips WT, Kiratli BJ, Sarkarati M, Weraarchakul G: Effect of spinal cord injury on the heart and cardiovascular fitness. Curr Prob Cardiol 23:641–716, 1998.

Schmid A, Huonker M, Barturen J, et al: Catecholamines, heart rate, and oxygen uptake during exercise in persons with spinal cord injury. J Appl Physiol 85:635–641, 1998.

INTERNET RESOURCES

ADA Home Page: Information and Technical Assistance on the Americans with Disabilities Act: http://www.usdoj.gov/crt/ada/

NSCIA: The National Spinal Cord Injury Association: http://www.spinalcord.org/

Occupational and Functional Assessments

LOIS SHELDAHL

Health care professionals can play an important role in optimizing vocational and nonvocational activity-related decisions for many patients, especially during the early recovery period after a major cardiopulmonary event. The focus of this chapter is on assessment and rehabilitative procedures that may promote optimal short-term as well as long-term activity decisions for those with known heart disease. Many of the same procedures are applicable to those with pulmonary disease.

Occupational Assessment

Employment-related decisions in patients with cardiopulmonary disease can be complex. In addition to the patient and employer, work-related decisions involve various professional agencies, including medical, **disability**, insurance, or legal[1,2]. Several factors may influence the return-to-work process, including the patient's desire to return to work, job satisfaction, perception of disability, previous employment record, age, education level, work tolerance in relation to job demands, disease severity, family concerns, employer or supervisor attitudes or restrictions, support mechanisms, psychological variables, available fi-

nancial resources (e.g., disability income, insurance, savings), or other work incentives/disincentives[1–11]. For those who resume work, employment can produce positive psychosocial, physical, and material benefits.

Because of the variety of factors that can influence work-related decisions, a significant percentage of patients do not resume work after a cardiac event or do not remain employed until a normal retirement age[2,5,10,11]. Some of these individuals are granted disability benefits despite relatively good functional work reserve. In a study of 175 men who were receiving **Social Security Disability Insurance (SSDI)** secondary to ischemic heart disease, 65% were found to have a work capacity $\geq$ 5 METs and 12% a work capacity $\geq$ 7 METs[9]. In this study, peak MET levels were determined with measurement of oxygen uptake. Based on their responses to an activity questionnaire, these men were fairly active with home or leisure-time physical activities. About 20% to 30% of them reported performing relatively demanding home tasks such as gardening, mowing (walking), and snow removal (blowing or shoveling). It is possible that greater reliance on functional work reserve in relation to expected job demands may lead to more optimal decisions regarding granting of disability benefits.

Premature loss of employment has significant societal economic implications and may also impact the social well being of patients. In the United States, coronary heart disease (CHD) is a leading cause of disability under the Social Security Administration (SSA) program[4]. Procedures that may help to optimize work resumption are reviewed in this chapter. Primary topics include clinical assessment, early intervention, **job analysis**, work tolerance testing, counseling, and early rehabilitation.

CLINICAL ASSESSMENT

Information gathered from several sources can be used to assess patients' current medical status and future prognosis in terms of morbidity and mortality secondary to heart disease. Risk stratification of cardiac patients into low-, moderate-, and high-risk categories for future events can be helpful in counseling patients on resuming physical activities[12] (see GETP7 Boxes 2-1 and 2-2). Most jobs today are not physically demanding, so unnecessary delays in

KEY TERMS

Americans with Disabilities Act (ADA): A comprehensive civil rights law that makes it unlawful to discriminate against qualified individuals with disabilities

Disability: The definition varies with how it is being used. Government agencies generally define disability in relation to a particular program or service (refer to http://www.dol.gov/odep/faqs/federal.htm). Disability typically represents an impairment that limits a person's ability to perform a "major life activity'"

Job analysis: Assessment of key job requirements and work conditions

METs (metabolic equivalents): Unit used to estimate the metabolic cost or energy requirements of physical activity, with 1 MET defined as an oxygen uptake of 3.5 mL of oxygen per kilogram body weight per minute.

Simulated work testing: An evaluation of an individual undertaking a test that is designed to represent a specific type of work task or work condition work

Social Security Disability Insurance (SSDI): Benefits provided to disabled or blind individuals who are considered "insured" through contributions to the Social Security trust fund.

work resumption beyond the normal convalescent period should be avoided. This includes avoiding delays specifically to permit completion of a cardiac rehabilitation program or waiting for results from nonessential diagnostic tests before providing medical clearance for work resumption. Patients who have physically demanding jobs, especially those in moderate and high clinical risk categories, may require further diagnostic evaluation or intervention before work resumption. Identification of signs of mental depression and other psychological disorders may be beneficial because psychological issues can have a negative influence work-related decisions in some patients[4,6]. Various methods can be used to help identify and treat psychological disorders[13,14] (also see Chapter 43).

EARLY INTERVENTION AND COUNSELING

For stable patients hospitalized for a cardiac event, an important step is for the clinical staff to discuss work resumption, preferably before discharge[2,5,15]. Some possible factors to consider in approaching hospitalized patients for work-related issues are listed in Box 18-1. Ignoring work-related matters early in the recovery process may cause patients to inappropriately perceive their event as leading to an inability to resume work. Patients can generally be given a positive message regarding work resumption along with a tentative timetable for resuming work before discharge. The actual timing for return to work can vary with several factors such as the cardiac event, disease severity, prognosis, job requirements, safety regulations, and employer attitudes or concerns. Most individuals can resume their jobs within 1 to 12 weeks after a major cardiac event. Some, especially those who work in jobs that may place the public at risk such as commercial truckers and airline pilots, may have greater delays or restrictions on returning to work, including meeting specific medical criteria in order to maintain a license to work[16–18].

JOB ANALYSIS

A job analysis performed soon after a major cardiac event (preferably before discharge) can serve as a basis for (a) delineating expected physical and psychological demands of the patient's job, (b) identifying the patient's concerns regarding work resumption, (c) establishing a tentative timeline for work resumption, and (d) individualizing assessment or rehabilitation procedures that may be undertaken during the early recovery period to optimize return-to-work decisions and capability[2,15,19]. Some of the factors that can be assessed in a job analysis include

BOX 18-1	Checklist for Possible Inpatient Work Resumption Interventions

- Assess disease severity and prognosis of patient after event.
- Ask the patient about pre-admission employment status.
- Discuss expected recovery course with the patient, including work resumption.
- Establish a tentative time table for work resumption, when appropriate.
- Ask the patient about any work resumption concerns.
- Be prepared to discuss qualifying criteria for disability benefits.
- Determine if an inpatient job analysis should be performed.
- Suggest that the patient contact his or her employer after discharge to discuss work resumption.
- Encourage participation in a progressive exercise program to enhance work resumption potential.
- Consider outpatient referrals for procedures or treatments that may represent key elements in getting patients back to work.

determination of specific job tasks from which expected energy cost requirements can be estimated; weight lifting, carrying, pushing, and pulling requirements; environmental conditions, including exposure to potentially hazardous materials; and psychological stressors. Inclusion of employer-related issues that may influence the return-to-work process can be helpful; these issues include the availability of medical staff at the patient's work site, the employer's expectations, a flexible return-to-work policy, sick leave, worker's compensation, light duty options, possibility for job accommodations, and specific job regulations[2,11,19–23]. This information can be obtained with an interview or questionnaire (Box 18-2).

In estimating the average and peak physical demands of work for patients, various resources can be used. The *Dictionary of Occupational Titles*[20] and *Occupational Outlook Handbook*[21] provide general information regarding work requirements under specific job titles. Some employers may be able to provide more specific work requirements that relate directly to their work sites. Metabolic equivalent (MET) tables (See Appendix A) provide approximations for average energy demands of various job and other activity tasks in units of multiples of resting energy expenditure[24,25]. It should be emphasized that the values listed in MET tables are only approximations and that expected energy demands listed for some activities are estimated based on their similarity to other types of activities. The actual MET demands can vary with pace of work, worker efficiency, orthopedic disabilities, automation, assistive devices, protective equipment, body size, terrain, and work. A study on lawn mowing, for example, showed that the mean MET levels for lawn mowing using a walk-behind mower varied from 3 to 10 METs depending on the type of mower (push, power push, or self-propelled), walking speed, lawn terrain, and subject characteristics[26]. In using MET energy cost tables, it should be noted that most on-the-job energy expenditure studies were completed before 1960[27,28]. At our institution, we performed several energy expenditure studies in work simulation settings and at occupational work sites in the past 2 decades[26,29–41]. Table 18-1 shows mean MET data obtained on patients with documented heart disease with our work simulation studies. In our job site studies[41], oxygen uptake was measured for 20 min with a portable device in workers at a variety of physical labor work settings. The mean MET data obtained for selected job categories are shown in Table 18-2. The on-the-job studies indicated that the average energy expenditure of most jobs requiring physical labor correspond to <4 METs. Some job tasks resulted in higher demands such as chain sawing or chipping, power push mowing, barn cleaning, air hammering, drywall and masonry, and weight carrying and repetitive lifting tasks.

In addition to the influence of energy expenditure on myocardial oxygen requirements, it is important to assess whether other work-related conditions (e.g., adverse temperature stress, psychological stress, awkward body positioning, static work) may increase myocardial oxygen demands[2]. The influence of selected environmental factors on myocardial oxygen requirements is discussed later in the chapter.

TRADITIONAL EXERCISE TESTING

The traditional symptom-limited graded exercise test on a treadmill or cycle ergometer can be very helpful in providing realistic vocational recommendations[2,25,42]. Information on work tolerance along with submaximal and maximal exercise-induced hemodynamic responses, electrocardiographic responses, and possible symptoms can help health care professionals and disability agencies assess the ability of patients to resume work within a reasonable level of stress and identify areas that need better management or further assessment. Exercise testing may also reassure the patient, patient's family, and employer regarding the patient's ability to safely resume work[43] (see Chapter 14 and GETP7 Chapters 4 and 5).

An important exercise test measurement is determination of functional MET capacity. In the clinical setting, functional MET capacity is typically estimated based on the peak workload achieved (see GETP7 Appendix D), although oxygen uptake can also be measured with open-circuit spirometry. After functional MET capacity is determined, it can be compared with the estimated average and peak METs of the individual's job. In general, work requirements should not be expected to induce myocardial ischemia or produce excessive fatigue. Over an 8-hour day, fatigue is more likely to occur when the average energy expenditure rate exceeds 50% of the individual's peak aerobic capacity. The appropriate upper intensity level to recommend for short-term (e.g., <60 min) occupational work tasks should be individualized based on patient characteristics (e.g., severity of disease, serious arrhythmias), tolerance for physical work, type of work performed, duration and frequency of work tasks, and work environment. In general, most patients should be able to use the same physical activity guidelines that are individualized for them for home and leisure-time physical activities or for an unsupervised exercise program.

SIMULATED WORK TESTING

For most people with heart disease, the only exercise test needed to assess functional tolerance for work resumption is the traditional graded exercise test. However, there are limitations in advising some on work resumption based only on graded dynamic exercise testing. One limitation is that although the traditional graded exercise test evaluates dynamic exercise tolerance, certain jobs may require a significant static workload (e.g., lift, carry, push, pull). This can result in questions regarding the patient's ability to tolerate the greater myocardial afterload stress expected with static work along with potential questions regarding the appropriate upper static load to recommend. A second

BOX 18-2 | Job Analysis Questionnaire

Patient name_____ Age_____ Date _____

Most recent medical event _____ Date _____

Medical history _____

Major health risk factors _____

Most recent job title_____ DOT#_____ Date last worked _____

Most recent employer _____ Contact person (if available) _____

Employment experience _____

Description of current or last job:

     Physical demands:

         Estimated hours/shift: sitting _____ standing _____ walking _____

         Lifting: maximal weight _____ frequency _____ position _____

                common weight _____ frequency _____ position _____

         Carrying: maximal weight _____ frequency _____ position _____

                common weight _____ frequency _____ position _____

         Pushing: object _____ Pulling: object _____

         Assistive devices/help with heavy static load _____

         Climbing: task _____ height _____ static load _____

         Job tasks:

Name	Estimated METs	Work time	Environment
_____	_____	_____	_____
_____	_____	_____	_____
_____	_____	_____	_____
_____	_____	_____	_____
_____	_____	_____	_____
_____	_____	_____	_____
_____	_____	_____	_____
_____	_____	_____	_____

         Estimated MET requirement of job: peak _____ average _____

         Work conditions: heat _____ cold _____ time pressure _____ fumes _____ other _____

            Work pace: acceptable _____ excessive _____

            Outdoors (%) _____ indoors (%)_____

         DOT class: sedentary _____ light _____ medium _____ heavy _____ very heavy _____

         Work hours: shift _____ hours/week _____ overtime/week _____ breaks _____

         Supervisory responsibilities: _____

         Perceived job stress: _____

         Job satisfaction: strongly dislike 1 2 3 4 5 6 7 8 9 10 strongly like job

         Patient's perception of ability to return to work: _____

         Financial assistance during recovery period (e.g., sick leave, disability, insurance) _____

         Financial or other reason (if any) for not planning on returning to work: _____

     Employer information

         Job site medical staff yes _____ no _____ If yes, contact name _____

         Specific established job criteria for work resumption? Yes____ No _____ If yes, what? _____

DOT = Dictionary of Occupational Title; METs = metabolic equivalents with 1 MET = oxygen uptake of $3.5 \text{ mL} \cdot \text{kg}^{-1} \cdot \text{min}^{-1}$.

Adapted with permission from Sheldahl LM, Wilke NA, Tristani FE: Evaluation and training for resumption of occupational and leisure-time physical activities in patients after a major cardiac event. Med Exerc Nutr Health 4:273–289, 1995.

TABLE 18-1. Mean Metabolic Equivalent Levels of Self-paced Common Home Physical Activities as Determined in Patients with Coronary Artery Disease Using Work Simulation Testing

Activity	METs (mean)	Reference
Auto wash/wax	4.0	
Carpentry tasks performed in different postures		U.S. Department of Labor[22], Wyman[23]
Hammering, manual	2.2–3.8	
Sanding, manual	1.9–2.5	
Sanding, power	1.6	
Sawing lumber, manual	2.7–4.4	
Drill press, power	1.6	
Wrench work, manual	1.7–2.4	
Screwdriver use, manual	1.9–2.5	
Drywall installation, manual	3.3–4.3	
Gardening		U.S. Department of Labor[19]
Hoe	4.2	
Spade	5.3	
Rototill	5.3	
Weed	4.6	
Housework		see Appendix B
Wash dishes, iron, iron, unpack groceries	1.9–2.5	
Vacuum, sweep, mop, change bed linens	2.3–3.4	
Lawn care		U.S. Department of Labor[19]
Power push mower	4.0–4.9	
Self-propelled (three speeds)	2.7–3.9	
Push (no motor)	6.3	
Trim grass, manual	3.0	
Trim grass, power	2.5	
Rake	4.6	
Snow removal		Haskell et al.[25], Passmore and Durnin[27]
Snow shoveling	5.3 (men)	
	5.1 (women)	
Snow blowing	4.9 (men)	
Shovel gravel (cold, neutral, hot environment)	5.7	Sheldahl et al.[26]
Wood splitting	7.1	Sheldahl et al.[29]
Wood stacking	5.6	Sheldahl et al.[29]

METs = metabolic equivalents with 1 MET = oxygen uptake of 3.5 mL·kg^{-1}·min^{-1}.

limitation is that, in contrast to the traditional exercise test, work sites may have less-than-ideal work conditions (e.g., hot or cold climates, air pollution, intermittent heavy work tasks).

It is impractical and unnecessary to evaluate workers under all the various stressors encountered in the course of a typical work routine, although some of the more demanding work tasks can be evaluated in select patients using work simulation testing. Patients most likely to benefit from **simulated work testing** are those whose ability to return to work remain in question despite traditional exercise testing, perhaps because of lower aerobic capacity, left ventricular dysfunction, ischemia at submaximal levels, significant arrhythmias, or the patient's apprehension about resuming a physically demanding job[2,25,44]. Simple, inexpensive work simulation tests can be set up. Use of a limited number of established protocols can help to minimize the expense of this type of testing. In terms of protocols, a weight-carrying test protocol and a repetitive weight-lifting test protocol have been published for evaluating tolerance for static work combined with light to moderate dynamic work[2]. Both of these test protocols are

graded and designed to be applicable to several types of work tasks requiring a static component. Both protocols can be easily modified to evaluate specific patient's job requirements.

The weight-carrying test protocol (Table 18-3) is designed to evaluate tolerance for light to heavy static effort combined with light dynamic work. In the standard protocol, the patient walks on a treadmill at a slow pace while carrying specified weight loads (e.g., dumbbell weights) in one or both hands (Fig. 18-1). The repetitive weight-lift-

TABLE 18-2. Mean Metabolic Equivalent Levels Determined from Oxygen Uptake Measured at Job Sites

Type of Work	Patients (n)	METs (mean)
Factory work	102	2.4
Building construction	85	3.7
Lawn care, landscaping, forestry	41	3.6
Farm work	36	3.5
Auto mechanic	29	2.3
Kitchen or cafeteria work	26	2.4
Laundry service	16	2.6

METs = metabolic equivalents with 1 MET = oxygen uptake of 3.5 mL·kg^{-1}·min^{-1}.

TABLE 18-3. Static-Dynamic Work
Simulation Test Protocols

Stage[b]	Weight-carrying Test Example[a] Protocol			
	Duration (min)	Speed (mph)	Load[c] (lb)	Predicted METs[e]
1	3	2.0	0	2.4
2	3	2.0	20	3.0
3	3	2.0	30	4.2
4	3	2.0	40	5.0
5	2	2.0	50	4.8[d]

Stage[b]	Repetitive Lifting Test Example[a] Protocol			
	Duration (min)	Lift Rate	Load[c] (lb)	Predicted METs[e]
1	6	Self-paced	30	3.8
2	6	Self-paced	40	4.2
3	6	Self-paced	50	4.5
4	6	Self-paced	30,40,50	4.2

[a] Test protocols can be modified to meet specific work conditions.

[b] A seated rest period of 1 to 3 minutes follows each stage.

[c] Weight load in weight-carrying test (e.g., dumbbell) can be carried in one or both hands; weight load in repetitive test can be lifted from floor or pallet to work bench.

[d] The slightly lower MET level for carrying 50 lbs versus 40 lbs is likely because of the shorter walk time and the inability to achieve steady-state conditions.

[e] METs are based on tests using the specific protocol listed.

METs = metabolic equivalents with 1 MET = oxygen uptake of 3.5 mL·kg^{-1}·min^{-1}.

Adapted with permission from American College of Sports Medicine: Guidelines for Exercise Testing and Prescription, 6th ed. Philadelphia: Lippincott Williams & Wilkins; 2000.

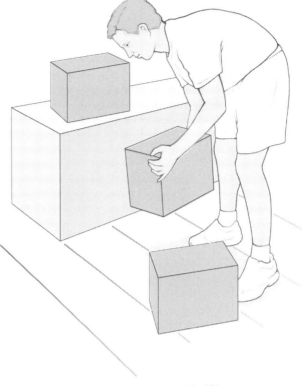

FIGURE 18-2. The repetitive weight-lifting test

ing test protocol (Table 18-3) is designed to evaluate tolerance for intermittent static work combined with a dynamic work component. In this protocol, the patient repetitively lifts specified weight loads, typically from the floor or pallet to a table or bench for a set time period (Fig. 18-2). Patients can be instructed lift at a set pace or select a rate that simulates or somewhat exceeds their job requirement. In assessing blood pressure (BP) responses to static or static–dynamic work, it is important to take BP while handling the static load as BP decreases rapidly

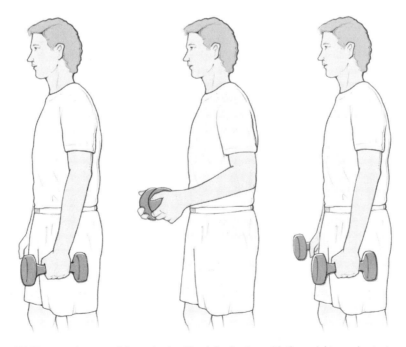

FIGURE 18-1. Three possible methods of load distribution with the weight-carrying test.

upon release of the static load. Electrocardiographic monitoring can be the same as for the traditional exercise test, or telemetry can be used if electrocardiographic ischemia is not expected based on prior traditional exercise testing. In addition to setting up work simulation tests, specialized work simulators (e.g., Baltimore Therapeutic and Valpar work simulators) are available for simulating various tasks, although the energy cost with some stations may be less than when performing tasks in the work setting[30].

ON-THE-JOB MONITORING

Ambulatory electrocardiographic monitoring can be considered for patients in whom concerns exist regarding potential for serious arrhythmias or ischemia on the job despite laboratory testing (see Chapters 20 and 21). Heart rate (HR) responses to work can also be evaluated with this procedure, although inexpensive heart rate monitors can be used or patients can be instructed to check their pulse rates during their more demanding work tasks. Some of the HR monitors can be programmed to emit a sound when a preprogrammed HR is exceeded or to provide average and peak HR information over a period of time. An advantage of on-the-job heart rate monitoring is that it helps evaluate the combined effects of physical work component and other potential work-related factors that can increase myocardial demands such as less-than-ideal environmental or work conditions. Patients may also be assured that their jobs are not causing an excessive myocardial demand by checking their pulse rate.

EARLY REHABILITATION

Participation in cardiac rehabilitation supervised exercise programs after a cardiac event (see GETP7 Chapter 8) has shown mixed results in terms of enhancing work resumption outcomes[4]. Failure to find a positive impact in several studies may stem from the complexity of factors reported to influence work-related decisions. It may be possible that improved tailoring of cardiac rehabilitation programs in the early phase of recovery to address the concerns of patients about resuming work may enhance work resumption potential[2,45]. This may involve providing early intervention for enhancing psychological parameters, as previously discussed, or encouraging use of exercise modes designed to enhance resumption of specific types of work (e.g., arm exercise, resistive exercise). For patients who will need to resume work combined with environmental heat stress, a gradual exposure to outdoor exercise in a warm environment may be more beneficial than restricting exercise to an air-conditioned facility.

DISABILITY

A small percentage of patients with cardiac disease will not be able to resume occupational work because of their disease severity. These patients may qualify for disability income through programs such as the SSDI, private long-term disability insurance, or Veteran's Administration service- and non-service–related pensions. Other patients may inappropriately think they will qualify for disability income. If they are not informed about the stringent qualifying criteria, some of them may unnecessarily go through the long process of applying for SSDI only to be rejected. In discussing return-to-work matters with patients, it is helpful to have a good understanding of the rules and regulations regarding common disability plans such as SSDI[46,47].

In the SSDI program, SSA maintains a list of medical conditions related to the cardiac system and other major body systems that are considered so severe as to automatically qualify an applicant younger than 65 years of age for disability income. In applicants whose condition is severe, but not included in the list, SSA evaluates whether their medical condition hinders the individual's ability to return to previously performed work. If deemed unable to return to this work, applicants will be further evaluated regarding their ability to adjust to other work. From the SSA's viewpoint, the primary issue is whether an applicant is able to engage in substantial gainful employment. In 2004, substantial gainful employment was considered $810 or more a month. To qualify for disability benefits under SSA program, the disability must last or be expected to last for at least 1 year or result in death (i.e., short-term disability is not available through Social Security). For those granted SSDI, the SSA must periodically review continued eligibility. For SSDI beneficiaries who subsequently would like to try returning to work without immediately losing disability benefits, "work incentive" programs (e.g., trial work program, ticket-to-work program) are available[46–48].

In some states, uniformed police officers or firefighters are covered under "accidental disability" (often referred to as "Heart Laws")[1,2,49]. Under these programs, workers may be able to establish the existence of a disabling cardiac disease or hypertension without proving that the job caused the disabling condition. Considerably variability exists among states in terms of the coverage provided under "accidental disability." Contacting the public employee state retirement agency may provide the best source of information to help advise patients.

NEW EMPLOYMENT

Some patients may need to find employment after a cardiac event because they are unemployed or cannot return to their previous employment. Importantly, the **Americans with Disability Act (ADA)** prohibits unlawful discrimination in employment of qualified individuals with disabilities[50]. The ADA applies to private sector employers with 15 or more employees as well as to state and local government. Before making a job offer, an employer may not make any health inquiry or conduct any health examination. The employer may ask applicants about their ability to perform essential job tasks and may condition a job offer based on the outcomes of a medical examination provided the examination is required for all new employees with similar jobs. Employers are also required by the ADA to provide reasonable accommodations. State vocational services may be considered for individuals who need to develop new work skills for employment. The extent of vocational services available varies among states.

NONVOCATIONAL ACTIVITIES

An important goal after a cardiac event is for patients to maintain as active a lifestyle as possible considering the magnitude of the disease, which includes encouraging patients to participate in appropriate home and leisure-time activities. Maintaining an active daily routine with home and leisure-time activities can help those with heart disease achieve the national activity goal of accumulating a moderate amount of physical activity (e.g., 150 kcal) on most, preferably all, days of the week[51]. Leisure-time activities that raise the HR into an aerobic zone can also provide some individuals with an enjoyable way to participate in a regular aerobic-type exercise program. Importantly, regular exercise and good physical fitness provide many benefits in terms of prevention of disease progression and quality of life[52]. Maintaining good physical fitness may also help provide a safety advantage with strenuous activity. Investigators[53,54] have shown that the risk of an acute myocardial infarction (MI) is temporarily increased during high-intensity physical activity, especially in those who are habitually sedentary. People who exercise regularly have a much lower relative risk associated with strenuous exercise plus they have the protective preventive effect associated with a regular program of exercise (also see Chapter 7).

Most of the same procedures used for optimizing occupational work decisions are also applicable to advising patients on resumption of home and leisure-time activities, including medical assessment, early intervention, activity analysis, counseling, work tolerance testing, and exercise conditioning.

A major risk factor for CHD is age and, subsequently, CHD is more common in elderly persons than within other age groups. Just as resumption of occupational work can have important individual and societal ramifications, so can resumption of independent living in the elderly population. In addition to the economic cost associated with assisted living, maintenance of an independent lifestyle impacts on the quality of life in elderly individuals. In a study of CHD people older than 65 years of age, peak aerobic capacity and depression were shown to be predictors of physical functioning in elderly individuals[55]. Encouraging elderly patients to participate in supervised exercise programs as well as resuming their home and leisure-time activities after a cardiac event may promote greater tolerance and confidence among the elderly in performing activities

important for independence. Because of the many comorbidities common in elderly individuals, exercise programs for them may need special tailoring to meet specific needs. Psychological counseling may also help those with depression maintain a more positive outlook on life. This, in turn, may result in a more active lifestyle.

Influence of Environmental Conditions

Many home, leisure-time, and job activities are performed in less-than-ideal environmental conditions, which can alter myocardial oxygen uptake requirements and work tolerance.

HEAT STRESS

During sustained work in a hot environment, circulatory demand typically is increased to meet the dual blood flow demands for metabolism (muscle) and thermoregulation (skin)[56,57]. A common characteristic of work combined with heat stress is a more progressive drift upward in heart rate and drift downward in stroke volume with work time compared with the same type of work performed in a thermoneutral environment. The addition of a humid environment produces an even greater drift. This cardiovascular drift represents an increase in myocardial oxygen requirements.

Most studies involving exercise in a hot environment have been performed on healthy individuals. In a study of asymptomatic men with heart disease, a similar cardiovascular drift response was seen with sustained moderate-intensity work[56]. Left ventricular ejection fraction (LVEF) and cardiac output were maintained, and the incidence of arrhythmias was not increased with heat stress. The effect of work or exercise combined with heat stress in symptomatic patients or those at high risk is not known.

Encouraging individuals to monitor their pulse rate during work in a hot environment provides a useful means for adjusting work rate downward to avoid excessive myocardial demand. Individuals should also be informed about the importance of gradual exposure to exercise combined with heat stress after a period of cool or cold weather exposure to permit heat acclimation. Heat acclimation results in improved capacity to dissipate heat, which, in turn, reduces the magnitude of the cardiovascular drift and thereby myocardial oxygen demands. Heat acclimation can occur within a few days (3 to 10 days) of undertaking mild, sustained (up to 90 min) physical activity in a warm environment (see Chapters 3 and 28 and GETP7 Appendix E for more information).

COLD STRESS

Work in a cold environment may also increase myocardial oxygen requirements by increasing myocardial afterload (e.g., BP, vascular resistance) or by increasing energy expenditure with wearing heavier clothing, walking through snow, and perhaps shivering[33–35]. Some CHD patients report angina at a lower work level in a cold environment[2]. Mortality is increased in the winter months, but it remains uncertain how much of this is related to physical activity performed in a cold environment.

One of the more demanding winter-time physical activities is snow removal[33–36,58]. Anecdotal reports of death from MI during or after snow removal has raised questions regarding the ability of CHD patients to safely perform static–dynamic work tasks in a cold environment. In a work simulation study in our facility, three groups of men (asymptomatic CHD, age-matched without known CHD, young healthy men) were evaluated during self-paced snow shoveling[33]. The mean MET rates varied from 5.3 to 7.3 METs among the three groups. The groups paced their work rate at similar mean relative intensities (75% to 78% of peak treadmill heart rate and 60% to 68% of peak treadmill oxygen uptake in the three groups). With self-paced snow blowing, mean MET levels (4.9. to 5.1) were similar among comparable groups of men[35]. Arrhythmias with snow removal and treadmill testing were comparable. In a subgroup of men with CHD, LVEF did not differ between treadmill testing and snow shoveling. Clearly, snow removal can represent strenuous work and may result in increased risk of MI, especially in those who are sedentary, have low work capacity, or do not pace themselves appropriately. It is important to note that the CHD men included in the snow removal studies had uncomplicated heart disease and relatively good work tolerances. Also, conditions of snow removal were likely not psychologically (e.g., time pressure) and physiologically (e.g., heavy snow, extreme cold) as challenging as happens in some real-life situations.

In a study[58] of younger men shoveling wet snow, mean relative work intensity corresponded to 97% of peak heart rate. In view of the anecdotal reports and work requirements of snow removal, it seems prudent to advise moderate- and high-risk CHD patients and those with a work capacity < 6.5 METs not to remove snow, especially with more physically demanding snow removal conditions (e.g., > 2 inches or wet snow). Some patients, however, continue to remove snow despite being advised not to because factors such as the cost of hiring someone to do the work. For those who plan to remove snow, precautions should be emphasized such as the importance of regular exercise (including resistive training) before and during the winter season, working within appropriate limits, avoiding heavy static loads, dressing appropriately, limiting sustained work time to less than 30 to 45 minutes, stopping at onset of any symptoms, avoiding time pressure conditions, performing warm-up and cool-down exercises, and avoiding taking a hot shower immediately after removing snow. Actually, individuals with unknown significant CHD may be potentially at greatest risk with snow shoveling because they may not realize the importance of some of these precautions.

ALTITUDE

Those traveling to the mountains for skiing or other physical activities should understand that hypoxia at altitude can significantly lower their work tolerance[59,60]. The impact on work tolerance is greatest during the first few of days of going to a high altitude. Over a few days (up to 5 to 10) of altitude exposure, tolerance for physical activities improves through acclimatization. Wyss et al.[60] recently reported that patients with coronary artery disease (CAD) showed a significant decrease in coronary flow reserve (CFR) when evaluated immediately after supine cycle exercise under acute hypoxic conditions comparable to 2500 m altitude. These patients also showed greater electrocardiographic and symptomatic evidence of exercise-induced ischemia with simulated altitude. In contrast, healthy control subjects did not show an exercise-induced decrease in CFR with hypoxic conditions at altitude simulations of 2500 and 4500 m. The investigators concluded that CAD patients with reduced CFR should be cautioned about performing physical activity at moderate or higher altitudes. Another environment factor that needs to be considered at altitude is exposure to less-than-ideal temperature conditions[2,59] (see Chapters 3 and 28 and GETP7 Appendix E for more information).

POLLUTANTS

Air pollutants should be taken into consideration in advising those on resuming work in certain affected communities or work sites, especially in those who have cardiopulmonary disease or are expected to work at relatively high work intensities. Recent reports indicate that both short- and long-term exposure to air pollutants results in an increased risk for cardiopulmonary events[57,61–63] (see Chapters 3 and 28 for more information).

Summary

Enabling patients with cardiopulmonary disease to resume as active and productive a lifestyle as possible for their disease state is an important goal. This includes helping patients resume employment, when appropriate, as well as home and leisure-time activities. Various techniques can be used to help optimize work and activity resumption for patients, including a job or activity analysis, exercise testing, simulated work testing, and activity monitoring. Exercise training programs can also be tailored to enhance the potential of patients to resume specific types of work. To help optimize the return-to-work process for patients, health care professionals should have a basic understanding of job requirements and governmental policies and procedures that can influence work resumption and work conditions for patients.

REFERENCES

1. Sagall EL, Nash IS: Cardiac evaluations for legal purposes (pp. 2519–2532). In Fuster V, Alexander RW, O'Rourke RA, et al, eds. Hurst's The Heart, 10th ed. New York: McGraw-Hill; 2001.

2. Sheldahl LM, Wilke NA, Tristani FE: Evaluation and training for resumption of occupational and leisure-time physical activities in patients after a major cardiac event. Med Exerc Nutr Health 4: 273–289, 1995.

3. Gutmann MC, Sheldahl LM, Tristani FE, Wilke NA: Returning the patient to work. In Pollock M, Schmidt D, eds. Heart Disease and Rehabilitation, 3rd ed. Champaign IL: Human Kinetics Publishers, 405–422, 1994.

4. Agency for Health Care Policy and Research: Cardiac Rehabilitation. Clinical Practice Guideline, Number 17. AHCPR Publication No. 96-0672. Rockville, MD: U.S. Department of Health & Human Services; 1995.

5. Boudrez H, De Backer G: Recent findings on return to work after an acute myocardial infarction or coronary artery bypass grafting. Acta Cardiol 55:341–349, 2000.

6. Soderman E, Lisspers J, Sundin O: Depression as a predictor of return to work in patients with coronary artery disease. Soc Sci Med (England) 56:193–202, 2003.

7. Dougherty CM: The natural history of recovery following sudden cardiac arrest and internal cardioverter-defibrillator implantation. Prog Cardiovasc Nurs 16:163–168, 2001.

8. Kushnir T, Luria O: Supervisors' attitudes toward return to work after myocardial infarction or coronary artery bypass graft. J Occup Environ Med 44:331–337, 2002.

9. Sheldahl LM, Wilke NA, Dougherty SA, et al: Work capacity of men on disability for heart disease [abstract]. Circulation 86(suppl I):400, 1992.

10. Ryan TJ, Antman EM, Brooks NH, et al: ACC/AHA Guidelines for the Management of Patients with Acute Myocardial Infarction: 1999 Update: A Report of the American College of Cardiology/American Heart Association Task Force on Practice Guidelines (Committee on Management of Acute Myocardial Infarction). Available at http://www.acc.org.

11. Leopold RS: A Year in the Life of a Million American Workers. New York: Metlife Group Disability; 2003.

12. American Association of Cardiovascular and Pulmonary Rehabilitation: Guidelines for Cardiac Rehabilitation and Secondary Prevention Programs, 4th ed. Champaign, IL: Human Kinetics; 2004.

13. Valentine D, Byers JF, Peterson JZ: Depression as a risk factor for coronary heart disease: Implications for Advanced Practice Nurses. Topics in Advanced Practice Nursing eJournal 1, 2001. Available at http://www.medscape.com/viewarticle/408416.

14. Blumenthal JA, Babyak MA, Carney RM, et al: Exercise, depression, and mortality after myocardial infarction in the ENRICHD Trial. Med Sci Sports Exerc 36:746–755, 2004.

15. Dennis C, Houston-Miller N, Schwartz RG, Ahn DK, Kraemer HC, Gossard D, Juneau M, Taylor CB, DeBusk RF. Early return to work after uncomplicated myocardial infarction: results of a randomized trial. JAMA 260:214–220, 1988.

16. Blumenthal R, Braunstein J, Connolly H, et al: Cardiovascular advisory panel guidelines for the medical examination of commercial motor vehicle drivers. Available at: http://www.fmcsa.dot.gov/rulesregs/cardio.htm, last updated 10/2002.

17. Aerospace Medical Certification Division. Available at http://www.cami.jccbi.gov/AAM-300/amcdfaq.html, last updated 4/23/2004.

18. Smith TW: Driving after ventricular arrhythmias [editorial]. N Engl J Med 345:451–452, 2001.

19. U.S. Department of Labor, Office of Disability Employment Policy. Available at http://www.dol.gov/odep/pubs/fact/analysis.htm.

20. U.S. Department of Labor. Dictionary of Occupational Titles, 4th ed, revised. Indianapolis: JIST Works Inc; 1991.

21. U.S. Department of Labor, Bureau of Labor Statistics. Occupational Outlook Handbook, 2004–05 Edition. Available at http://www.bls.gov/oco/home.htm. Accessed 6/2004.

22. U.S. Department of Labor, Office of Disability Employment Policy. Available at http://www.dol.gov/odep/search/siteindex.htm.

23. Wyman DO: Evaluating patients for return to work. Am Fam Physician 59:844–848, 1999.

24. Ainsworth BE, Haskell WL, Leon AS, et al: Compendium of physical activities: classification of energy costs of human physical activities. Med Sci Sports Exer 25:71–80, 1993.

25. Haskell WL, Bradfeld N, Bruce RA, et al: Task Force II: Determination of occupational working capacity in patients with ischemic heart disease. J Am Coll Cardiol 14:1025–1034, 1989.

26. Sheldahl LM, Wilke NA, Hanna RD, et al: Responses of people with coronary artery disease to common lawn-care tasks. Eur J Appl Physiol 72:357–364, 1996.

27. Passmore R, Durnin JVGA: Human energy expenditure. Physiol Rev 35:801–840, 1955.

28. Durham JVGA, Passmore R: Energy, Work and Leisure. London: Heinemann Educational Books Ltd; 1967:47–95.

29. Sheldahl LM, Levandoski SG, Wilke NA, et al: Responses of patients with coronary artery disease to common carpentry tasks. J Cardiopul Rehabil 13:283–290, 1993.

30. Wilke NA, Sheldahl LM, Dougherty SM, et al: Baltimore Therapeutic Equipment work simulator: Energy expenditure of work activities in cardiac patients. Arch Phys Med 74:419–424, 1993.

31. Dougherty S, Sheldahl L, Wilke N, et al: Metabolic and hemodynamic responses to gardening in men with and without ischemic heart disease [abstract]. J Cardiopul Rehabil 11:321, 1991.

32. Wilke NA, Sheldahl LM, Dougherty SM, et al: Energy expenditure during household tasks in women with coronary artery disease. Am J Cardiol 75:670–674, 1995.

33. Sheldahl LM, Wilke NA, Dougherty SM, et al: Effect of age and coronary artery disease on response to snow shoveling. J Am Coll Cardiol 20:1111–1117, 1992.

34. Dougherty SM, Sheldahl LM, Wilke NA, et al: Physiologic responses to shoveling and thermal stress in men with cardiac disease. Med Sci Sports Exerc 25:790–795, 1993.

35. Sheldahl LM, Wilke NA, Dougherty S, Tristani FE: Snow blowing and shoveling in normal and asymptomatic coronary artery diseased men. Int J Cardiol 43:233–238. 1994.

36. Sheldahl LM, Wilke NA, Dougherty SM, Tristani FE: Responses of women to snow shoveling and snow blowing [abstract]. Circulation 88:I–612, 1993.

37. Wilke NA, Sheldahl LM, Dougherty SM, et al: Metabolic cost of wood splitting in men with and without ischemic heart disease [abstract]. J Cardiopul Rehabil 10:382, 1990.

38. Sheldahl LM, Wilke NA, Tristani FE, Kalbfleisch JH: Response of patients after myocardial infarction to carrying a graded series of weight loads. Am J Cardiol 52:698–703, 1983.

39. Foss-Campbell B, Sheldahl L, Wilke N, et al: Effects of upper extremity load distribution on weight-carrying in men with ischemic heart disease. J Cardiopul Rehabil 13:37–42, 1993.

40. Sheldahl LM, Wilke NA, Tristani FE, Kalbfleisch JH: Response to repetitive static-dynamic exercise in patients with coronary artery disease. J Cardiac Rehabil 5:139–145, 1985.

41. Sheldahl LM, Wilke NA, Dougherty SM, Tristani FE. Energy cost of occupational work [abstract]. J Am Coll Cardiol 25:173A, 1995.

42. Fletcher GF, Balady G, Froelicher VF, et al: Exercise standards. A statement for healthcare professionals from the American Heart Association. Circulation 91:580–615, 1995.

43. Ewart CK, Taylor CB, Reese LB, DeBusk RF: Effects of early post-myocardial infarction exercise testing on self-perception and subsequent physical activity. Am J Cardiol 51:1076–1080, 1983.

44. Vona M, Capodaglio P, Iannessa A, et al: The role of work simulation tests in a comprehensive cardiac rehabilitation program. Monaldi Arch Chest Dis 58:26–34, 2002.

45. Mital A, Shrey DE, Govindaraju M, et al: Accelerating the return to work (RTW) chances of coronary heart disease (CHD) patients: Part 1—development and validation of a training programe. Disabil Rehabil 22:604–620, 2000.

46. Social Security Administration: Disability evaluation under Social Security. SSA Pub. No. 64-039, 1/2003.

47. Social Security Administration. What's new. Available at http://www.ssa.gov/work/whatsnew.html.

48. Social Security Administration Employment Support For People with Disabilities. Available at http://www.ssa.gov/work/index.html.

49. Massachusetts Public Employee Retirement Administration Commission. Available at: http://www.mass.gov/perac/disguide/disabilityguide16.htm.

50. U.S. Department of Labor. Office of Disability Employment Policy. Available at http://www.dol.gov/odep/archives/adahealt/health.htm.

51. U.S. Department of Health and Human Services. Physical Activity And Health: A Report of the Surgeon General. Atlanta: U.S. Department of Health and Human Services, Centers for Disease Control and Prevention, National Center for Chronic Disease Prevention and Health Promotion; 1996.

52. Lakka TA, Venalainen JM, Raurama R, et al: Relation of leisure-time physical activity and cardiorespiratory fitness to the risk of acute myocardial infarction in men. N Engl J Med 330:1549–1554, 1994.

53. Willich SN, Lewis M, Lowel H, et al: Physical exertion as a trigger of acute myocardial infarction. N Engl J Med 329:1684–1690, 1993.

54. Mittleman MA, Maclure M, Tofler GH, et al: Triggering of acute myocardial infarction by heavy physical exertion. Protection against triggering by regular exertion. N Engl J Med 329:1677– 1683, 1993.

55. Ades PA, Savage PD, Tischler MD, et al: Determinants of disability in older coronary patients. Am Heart J 143:151–156, 2002.

56. Sheldahl LM, Wilke NA, Dougherty S, Tristani FE: Cardiac response to combined moderate heat and exercise in men with coronary artery disease. Am J Cardiol 70:186–191, 1992.

57. Folinsbee LJ: Heat and air pollution (pp. 327–342). In Pollock MLL, Schmidt DH, eds. Heart Disease and Rehabilitation, 3rd ed. Champaign, IL: Human Kinetics; 1995.

58. Franklin BA, Hogan P, Bonzheim K, et al: Cardiac demands of heavy snow shoveling. JAMA 273:880–882, 1995.

59. Pandolf KB, Young AJ: Altitude and cold (pp. 309–326). In Pollock MLL, Schmidt DH, eds. Heart Disease and Rehabilitation, 3rd ed. Champaign, IL: Human Kinetics; 1995.

60. Wyss CA, Koepfli P, Fretz G, et al: Influence of altitude exposure on coronary flow reserve. Circulation 108:1202–1207, 2003.

61. Pope III CA, Burnett RT, Thurston GD, et al: Cardiovascular mortality and long-term exposure to particulate air pollution. Epidemiological evidence of general pathophysiological pathways of disease. Circulation 109:71–77, 2004.

62. Johnson RL Jr: Relative effects of air pollution on lungs and heart. Circulation 109:5–7, 2004.

63. Brook RD, Franklin B, Cascio W, et al: Air pollution and cardiovascular disease. A statement for healthcare professionals from the Expert Panel on Population and Prevention Science of the American Heart Association. Circulation 109:2655–2671, 2004.

SELECTED REFERENCES FOR FURTHER READING

Leopold RS: A Year in the Life of a Million American Workers. New York: Metlife Group Disability; 2003.

Ranavaya MI, LeFevre P, Denniston PL Jr: Evidence-based disability duration guidelines. Disabil Med 2:75–78, 2002.

Sagall EL, Nash IS: Cardiac evaluations for legal purposes (pp. 2519–2532). In Fuster V, Alexander RW, O'Rourke RA, et al, eds. Hurst's The Heart, 10th ed, New York: McGraw-Hill; 2001.

Sheldahl LM, Wilke NA, Tristani FE: Evaluation and training for resumption of occupational and leisure-time physical activities in patients after a major cardiac event. Med Exerc Nutr Health 4:273–289, 1995.

Wyman DO: Evaluating patients for return to work. Am Fam Physician 59:844–848, 1999.

INTERNET RESOURCES

Social Security Online: Employment Support for People with Disabilities: http://www.ssa.gov/work

Social Security Online: Medical/Professional Relations: http://www.socialsecurity.gov/disability/professionals/bluebook

Social Security Online: 2004 Red Book: http://www.ssa.gov/work/ResourcesToolkit/redbook.html

U.S. Department of Labor: Occupational Outlook Handbook, 2004–05 Edition: http://www.bls.gov/oco

U.S. Department of Labor, Office of Disability Employment Policy: http://www.dol.gov/odep

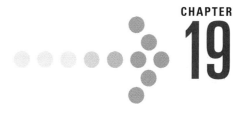

Diagnostic Procedures for Cardiovascular Disease

JONATHAN K. EHRMAN AND JOHN R. SCHAIRER

This chapter addresses KSAs from the following content areas:

1 Exercise Physiology and Related Exercise Science
2 **Pathophysiology and Risk Factors**
3 **Health Appraisal, Fitness, and Clinical Exercise Testing**
4 **Electrocardiography and Diagnostic Techniques**
5 Patient Management and Medications
6 **Medical and Surgical Management**
7 Exercise Prescription and Programming
8 Nutrition and Weight Management
9 Human Behavior and Counseling
10 Safety, Injury Prevention, and Emergency Procedures
11 Program Administration, Quality Assurance, and Outcome Assessment

Today, the diagnosis of heart disease is made using a medical history and physical examination as well as a variety of non-invasive and invasive tests. These tests are ordered by physicians (typically internists and cardiologists), and the order in which they are performed is based on recommendations made by the American College of Cardiology (ACC) and the American Heart Association (AHA) Task Forces[1,2].

The review of the literature and weighting of the significance of a scientific paper to make these recommendations is referred to as the practice of **evidence-based medicine**. The weighting system used by the ACC/AHA Task Force applies an A, B, or C weighting system involving data derived from multiple randomized clinical trials that involved large numbers of patients (level A); derived from a limited number of randomized trials with fewer patients or analysis of nonrandomized studies or observational registries (level B); and derived from an expert consensus (level C). From this evidence, three levels of recommendations for performing a certain diagnostic test or treatment are made. Level I includes recommendations made using a strong level of evidence; level II includes recommendations made using conflicting evidence; and Level III includes recommendations made using contrary evidence. An example of this type of guideline is the ACC/AHA 2002 guideline update for the management of patients with chronic stable angina[1].

Clinical exercise professionals should be familiar with both the general decision-making process of heart disease diagnosis and the specific diagnostic procedures used to make the diagnosis. Often in the cardiac rehabilitation setting, for instance, patients ask about diagnostic procedures and why a diagnostic assessment was, or was not, performed. Even though clinical exercise professionals would not be expected to provide a definitive answer to these types of questions, they can provide some insight during a teaching moment with the patient, provided they have the requested knowledge. Specific questions should be referred to the patient's physician.

Additionally, there is an increasing role for the clinical exercise professional in the administration and preliminary interpretation of some cardiac diagnostic procedures. Often, non-invasive cardiology laboratories use these individuals to perform the technical duties and, possibly, even the supervisory role in exercise testing. Recently, clinical exercise professionals can also find technical opportunities in the cardiac catheterization laboratory.

This chapter focuses on the process of determining which diagnostic tests should be performed, and in which order, to assist in the diagnosis of cardiac disease. The primary focus is on coronary artery disease (CAD), which is the most prevalent cardiac disease (see Chapter 29).

History and Physical Examination

The cornerstone of the evaluation and clinical work-up of the patient with suspected heart disease is the history and physical examination. This is the basis of any subsequent

KEY TERMS

Akinesis: Absence of movement

Augmentation: Enhancement of movement

Bruits: A harsh or musical intermittent auscultatory sound, especially an abnormal one

Cine: Movement, usually relating to motion pictures

Clubbing: A condition affecting the fingers and toes in which proliferation of distal soft tissues, especially the nail beds, results in thickening and widening of the extremities of the digits; the nails are abnormally curved nail beds that are excessively compressible, and the skin over them is red and shiny.

Cyanosis: A dark bluish or purplish discoloration of the skin and mucous membrane caused by deficient oxygenation of the blood, evident when reduced hemoglobin in the blood exceeds 5 g/100 mL

Differential diagnosis: The determination of which of two or more diseases with similar symptoms is the one from which the patient is suffering, by a systematic comparison and contrasting of the clinical findings

Dyskinesis: Reduction in normal movement

Edema: An accumulation of an excessive amount of watery fluid in cells or intercellular tissues

Evidence based medicine: Medical care that is based on the rigorous and expert analysis of the available data documenting relative benefits and risks of those procedures and therapies to produce helpful guidelines that improve the effectiveness of care, optimize patient outcomes, and have a favorable impact on the overall cost of care

False-negative: An initial negative diagnostic assessment that is ultimately untrue

False-positive: An initial positive diagnostic assessment that is ultimately untrue

Gold standard: The diagnostic test that serves as the comparison for all other tests evaluating the same condition, disease, or physiologic response

Hypokinesis: Diminished or slow movement

Predictive value: Calculated as number of true-positive tests divided by the number of true-positives plus the number of false-positives; provides the percentage of tests that effectively identified disease in a population with the disease

Pretest likelihood: The probability that an individual has a given disease, based on physical and history findings before the performance of a diagnostic test

Prevalence: The number of cases of a disease existing in a given population at a specific period of time (*period prevalence*) or at a particular moment in time (*point prevalence*)

Sensitivity: The proportion of affected individuals who give a positive test result for the disease that the test is intended to reveal

Specificity: The proportion of individuals with negative test results for the disease that the test is intended to reveal

True-negative: Denoting an initial negative diagnostic assessment that is ultimately true

True-positive: Denoting an initial positive diagnostic assessment that is ultimately true

diagnostic testing that may performed. The history and physical examination should be performed by a physician, a physician assistant, or a clinical nurse specialist and available to any personnel (e.g., exercise physiologist) who are working with a patient during a diagnostic test or treatment protocol such as an exercise program or behavioral management session. GETP7 Boxes 3-1 and 3-2 provide a comprehensive list of the components of a medical history and physical examination.

When evaluating a patient for the first time, it is always best to perform a complete history and physical and obtain as many of the previous medical records as possible. It is only with a complete knowledge of all of the patient's health and medical information that an accurate diagnosis and effective treatment plan can be designed. The eight symptoms most common to patients with heart disease are listed in Box 19-1.

Each patient should be questioned regarding the presence of these symptoms at each visit. For each symptom, additional information needs to be obtained such as how long ago it began, the duration of the symptom with each occurrence, any precipitating event, and how the patient relieves the discomfort. The most common symptom in those with cardiac disease is chest discomfort. With chest discomfort, the key components to assess include (a) location and type of sensation, (b) if it occurs with myocardial stress such as exertion or mental stress, and (c) if it is relieved by using nitroglycerin or rest and relaxation. If a patient has only one of these components, then it is considered "non-angina" pain; if he or she has two components, then it is "atypical" angina; and if the patient has all three components, then it is considered "typical" angina[1]. It should be noted that women typically have more atypical chest pain that is angina than do men.

BOX 19-1	Eight Symptoms of Heart Disease

1. Chest discomfort
2. Dyspnea (shortness of breath with exertion)
3. Orthopnea (shortness of breath with lying down)
4. Paroxysmal nocturnal dyspnea (waking at night short of breath)
5. Peripheral edema
6. Cardiac palpitations
7. Syncope (fainting)
8. Cough

Also see GETP7 Table 2-3.

BOX 19-2	Four Steps of the Physical Examination

1. Inspection
2. Palpation
3. Percussion
4. Auscultation

Inspection includes assessment of the patient's general condition such as the appearance of distress; the color and texture of the skin; the presence of **cyanosis**, **clubbing**, or **edema** of the extremities; the presence of skin lesions or jugular venous distention. Palpation involves feeling the major arteries, including the abdominal aorta, femoral, pedal, radial, and carotid arteries, to determine the presence and magnitude of the pulse, and in the case of the abdominal aorta, to estimate its size. The apex of the left ventricle (LV; point of maximum intensity [PMI]) can be palpated to determine if cardiac enlargement is present. Peripheral edema is assessed by palpation, first to determine its presence and second to grade its severity. Percussion of vital organs is performed next but is of little value in the assessment for cardiac disease. The final step of the physical examination is auscultation. Each of the major arteries should be evaluated for **bruits**. The lungs are auscultated for signs of pneumonia, emphysema, or heart failure, and the heart is auscultated for regularity of rhythm, murmurs, and extra sounds.

For patients with symptoms that are potentially related to myocardial ischemia, a resting electrocardiogram (ECG) should be performed. In the majority of patients who are asymptomatic at the time of the resting ECG recording, the tracing will be normal. However, it is useful as a baseline for future reference and as a screen for previous or current cardiac problems, including infarction, arrhythmia, and left ventricular hypertrophy (LVH). It is also an important aid for determining the type of diagnostic test to next perform. For instance, any preexisting abnormality may suggest the need to add an imaging study to a graded exercise test to evaluate the patient with ischemic symptoms.

Finally, after the examination, it may be useful to obtain a chest radiograph if there is suspicion of congestive heart failure, valvular or pericardial disease, aortic dissection or aneurysm, or pulmonary disease. However, its use in those presenting with an initial suspicion of ischemic heart disease (i.e., angina) is limited.

Angina typically presents as a dull pressure or burning type (also, gripping, heavy, suffocating, tightness, burning, or aching are used to describe the sensation) discomfort in the chest, jaw, shoulder, back, or arm. It usually occurs with physical exertion or emotional stress and is relieved with rest or nitroglycerine use. It is incorrect to ask about chest pain. Most patients do not experience pain in their chest as a symptom of heart disease. Rather, they may describe the discomfort as "bothersome" rather than painful. By asking about chest pain, many patients with heart disease may be missed. Discomfort that persists for hours or days, is localized to a small area defined by a fingertip, or is sharp in nature is less likely to be angina. The other symptoms listed in Box 19-1 may occur in association with angina or with other types of cardiac disease (e.g., valvular, non-ischemic heart failure).

The history intake should also include an evaluation of the risk factors associated with cardiac disease, including hypertension[3], dyslipidemia[4], smoking, obesity, impaired fasting glucose, lack of exercise, and a family history heart disease in a parent or sibling before age 55 years for men and 65 years for women (GETP7 Table 2-2). Any previous history of cardiac disease should also be assessed. All patients identified with risk factors, whether cardiac disease is present or not, should be counseled about the risk factors, educated about how lifestyle plays a role in risk factor and disease development, and treated accordingly. The physician may also consider ordering clinical laboratory tests for fasting blood lipids (total cholesterol, high- and low-density lipoproteins, and triglycerides), hemoglobin (anemia evaluation), and fasting blood glucose (diabetes evaluation) [see GETP7 Box 3-3]. In some instances, blood lipids and glucose may be assessed at the time of the clinic visit using point-of-care testing procedures.

The physical examination should include blood pressure; pulse; respiratory rate; and body weight, including the body mass index (BMI). The person who places the patient in the exam room typically determines the vital signs. The general physical examination performed by the physician is best described by dividing it into four steps (Box 19-2).

Determining Cardiac Disease Likelihood and Further Evaluation

After the history and physical examination are completed and the previous records obtained and reviewed, a list of symptoms and abnormal findings can be compiled. A second list of possible diseases causing each symptom, called a **differential diagnosis**, can also be compiled (Box 19-3). This is a very important step in the process of determining the necessity and type of diagnostic testing to

BOX 19-3	Differential Diagnosis of Chest Discomfort

- Cardiac
  - Angina
  - Myocardial infarction
  - Mitral valve prolapse
  - Pericarditis
  - Aortic stenosis
  - Aortic dissection
- Gastrointestinal
  - Peptic ulcer disease
  - Esophageal spasm or reflux disease
  - Cholecystitis or cholelithiasis
- Pulmonary
  - Pneumonia
  - Pleurisy
  - Pulmonary embolism
- Musculoskeletal
  - Costochondritis
  - Trauma
  - Cervical and thoracic spine disorders

be performed. It is possible that the origin of symptoms is noncardiac in nature.

The clinician should estimate the **pretest likelihood** of the patient's having heart disease. This is a rating of the probability of cardiac disease in an individual patient. There are a variety of sources that can be used to make this determination[5–7]. The Diamond and Forrester model uses age, gender, and discomfort type (see previous discussion of typical, atypical and noncardiac chest discomfort in this chapter) to determine the probability of CAD[5]. Their scheme stratifies the patient's risk into a low-, intermediate-, or high-risk group which is used to determine the next step in the evaluation process (see GETP7 Table 5-1). In general, those in whom a low probability of CAD is suspected based on the history and physical examination should be considered for treatment of cardiac disease risk factors and assessed for a noncardiac cause of their symptoms (e.g., referrals for gastrointestinal testing, pulmonary function testing, musculoskeletal assessment). However, patients with risk stratified into the intermediate- or high-risk groups should be assessed using diagnostic tests for cardiac disease. Intermediate-risk patients, who are appropriate candidates for a graded exercise test, should undergo an ECG or an ECG plus imaging (radionuclide or echocardiography) stress test. Pharmacologic stress assessment is considered when a patient cannot perform exercise on a treadmill. Patients who are in the high-risk group may begin with an exercise test or directly undergo cardiac catheterization, depending on their individual clinical situation. Cardiac catheterization is also appropriate for those who are initially categorized as intermediate risk and move into the high-risk group after stress testing.

ACCURACY OF DIAGNOSTIC TESTS

The ability of a diagnostic test to accurately identify individuals with heart disease is dependent on the sensitivity and specificity of the test as well as the prevalence of the disease in the population being tested. The Bayes theorem (see Chapter 14) clarifies the importance these variables play in the selection of the appropriate test in the work-up of patients for heart disease. Depending on the specific test and patient and on the pretest likelihood (low, intermediate, or high) of the patient's having heart disease, physicians have a variety of clinical tests at their disposal that can be performed. The following paragraphs define the terms used in the process of determining and understanding about the accuracy of these diagnostic tests.

A positive test result is considered one in which the clinical judgment is that the patient evaluated has an abnormality that was identified by the test. Likewise, a negative test result is one that did not find an abnormality—or in others words, the finding was normal. It must be understood that any clinical test, even if considered the "**gold standard**," will not always correctly identify whether a person has or does not have an abnormality. When the test result is considered positive and the patient is later found to not have the abnormality, the test result is then considered a **false-positive** result. On the other hand, if a test result is determined to be negative and later the patient is found to have the abnormality or disease, the initial test is considered a **false-negative** result. And likewise, tests that accurately assess a patient as positive or negative for an abnormality or disease are considered **true-positive** and **true-negative** results, respectively.

Based on this knowledge, the **sensitivity** and **specificity** of a type of clinical test can be determined (see GETP7 Box 6-2 to determine how to calculate sensitivity and specificity). Sensitivity refers to how often the test uncovers an abnormality or disease in a population with the abnormality or disease. Specificity is the percentage of tests that are negative or normal in a population without the abnormality or disease. For any type of clinical test, the success of a test to uncover an abnormality, if it is present, is only as good as the technical performance of the test, the appropriateness of the test for the person being evaluated, and the interpretation or clinical judgment of the clinician who evaluates the test results.

The **predictive value** of a clinical test provides us with an insight to the ability of a test to accurately determine the presence or absence of an abnormality or disease in a person. The predictive value relies on the test sensitivity and specificity and the **prevalence** or rate of the abnormality or disease in the population being tested. Thus the predictive value of a test speaks to how likely a test finding is accurate for an individual. As such, it is important that the proper population, techniques, and interpretation be applied to any clinical test to enhance the predictive value or accuracy. It is this criteria

TABLE 19-1. Comparison of Tests for Sensitivity, Specificity, and Predictive Accuracy

Grouping	Studies, n	Total Patients, n	Sensitivity, %	Specificity, %	Predictive Accuracy, %
Standard exercise test	147	24,047	68	77	73
Thallium scintigraphy	59	6038	85	85	85
SPECT	30	5272	88	72	80
Adenosine SPECT	14	2137	89	80	85
Exercise echocardiography	58	5000	84	75	80
Dobutamine echocardiography	5	<1000	88	84	86
Dobutamine scintigraphy	20	1014	88	74	81
Coronary calcium score	16	3683	60	70	65

SPECT = single-photon emission computed tomography.

Adapted from http://www.cardiology.palo-alto.med.va.gov/slides/ExerciseTest.ppt.

on which studies in the literature are evaluated and recommendations made for diagnostic testing. Table 19-1 provides an overview of the sensitivity, specificity, and predictive accuracy of various cardiac tests that are presented in the next several sections.

HOW TO DECIDE WHICH DIAGNOSTIC TEST TO SELECT

As mentioned in the previous section, it is important to select the appropriate test for the person being evaluated. This requires the initial evaluation of the patient, determining the pretest likelihood of an abnormality or disease, and applying evidence-based decision making to determine the best clinical test to order. In addition, the scenario in which the patient presents is also important to consider. For instance, is the patient presenting to his internist for a routine physical examination? Or is she presenting to the emergency room to be evaluated in a chest pain clinic for ongoing symptoms? Or maybe he has been referred to a cardiologist for further evaluation? Or is she experiencing chest pain in a cardiac rehabilitation program and further evaluation is being considered? Each of these situations requires a different sequence of decisions to be made, with subsequent decisions based on the previous decisions and test or evaluation results. The "decision tree" in Figure 19-1 was developed by the ACC and the AHA[2]. It can be used to illustrate to clinical exercise physiologists and specialists how decisions are made during the diagnosis of CAD.

The next several sections review the common diagnostic methods for detecting CAD. These techniques are from the ACC/AHA guidelines for stable angina[1].

GRADED EXERCISE TESTING WITH ELECTROCARDIOGRAPHY

In-depth information regarding the performance and interpretation of graded exercise tests can be found in Chapter 14 and in GETP7 Chapters 5 and 6. This section discusses only the decision-making process with respect to the entire process of patient evaluation for ischemia. The decision to perform a graded exercise test should be made based on several criteria, including the pretest likelihood that the patient has CAD (see GETP7 Table 5-1), whether the patient can adequately exercise to symptom-limited maximum, and whether the ECG will be interpretable at peak exercise for possible ischemia.

It is generally accepted that patients who are initially considered to be at intermediate risk for CAD during the history and physical examination will benefit most from having a graded exercise test using ECG for ischemic assessment[1]. Those with a low or high pretest probability of CAD will not generally move to another category based solely on a graded exercise test with ECG assessment. After the graded exercise test, patients are reassigned to either the low- or high-risk categories based on the test results. Patients restratified to the low-risk category generally do not require further diagnostic assessment. Those in the high-risk category may be referred for coronary angiography. If a patient remains in the intermediate-risk category he or she should be assessed using graded exercise with imaging.

Patients with repolarization abnormalities (left bundle branch block [LBBB], LVH, using digoxin) are not appropriate candidates for graded exercise testing without imaging. However, those with right bundle branch block or less than 1 mm ST-segment depression (not including V1–3) can be tested. Box 19-4 lists the types of patients who are appropriate and inappropriate candidates for diagnostic testing using graded exercise testing without imaging. Those in the inappropriate category should be considered for stress testing with imaging, for angiography if considered at an intermediate or high risk, or for noncardiac testing or risk factor treatment if considered low risk. Depending on the interpretation of the graded exercise test (see Chapter 14 and GETP7 Chapter 6), a recommendation for no further testing (negative test result) or for further testing (equivocal or positive test result) is made.

There is a clinical work-up "gap" between what is recommended by the ACC/AHA Guidelines for Exercise Testing and what is commonly practiced by the medical community when faced with making a decision about a patient requiring assessment for heart disease[2]. The

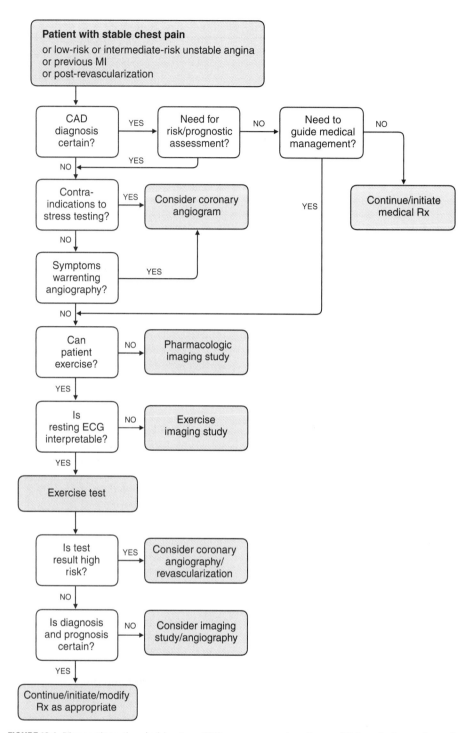

FIGURE 19-1. Diagnostic testing decision tree. CAD = coronary artery disease; ECG = electrocardiography.

guidelines recommend that patients with chest pain, a normal resting ECG, and who are able to ambulate be scheduled for an exercise test with ECG monitoring alone. In clinical practice, many physicians faced with this scenario begin with an imaging test. Instead, an exercise test with imaging is recommended by the guidelines as an initial diagnostic test for patients with an abnormal resting ECG, those who are unable to walk, and those with a history of coronary bypass surgery. Although this strategy provides a slight improvement in predictive accuracy over

the stress ECG combined with the Duke Treadmill Score[8] (see GETP7 Figure 6-2), it does so at a significantly increased cost[9].

Imaging Methods

Imaging techniques for the diagnosis of CAD provide slightly higher sensitivity and specificity than exercise testing with ECG analysis. Candidates for imaging studies, versus stress ECG, are those with an uninterpretable ECG,

---

BOX 19-4   Candidates for Exercise Electrocardio-graphic Assessment

APPROPRIATE CANDIDATES

Intermediate-risk patients based on age, gender, and symptoms

If repolarization abnormality is either right bundle branch block or <1 mm ST-segment depression not caused by digoxin use

INAPPROPRIATE CANDIDATES

Low or high risk of ischemic heart disease, including asymptomatic patients with possible ischemia during ambulatory electrocardiographic monitoring and asymptomatic patients with severe coronary calcification

Preexisting repolarization abnormality (left bundle branch block, left ventricular hypertrophy with strain, digoxin, ventricular pacing, nonspecific ST-segment depression >1 mm)

Pre-excitation syndrome (Wolff-Parkinson-White)

Patients unable to exercise to an adequate myocardial stress level (i.e., <85% of predicted peak heart rate or double product < ~240 × 10^{-2})

Patients with angina who have undergone a previous revascularization procedure in whom localization and other characterization of ischemia is important

---

and those unable to exercise to a level high enough to produce an adequate myocardial stress. In general, imaging studies allow for the patient to be further risk stratified to either a low- or high-risk group. If the test is equivocal, then either a different imaging test or coronary angiography may be suggested as a next step in the diagnostic process. These imaging techniques are categorized as echocardiography or myocardial perfusion imaging and are reviewed in the next several sections (also see GETP7 Chapter 5).

ECHOCARDIOGRAPHY

Over the past 25 years, echocardiography has become the second most frequently ordered test in the evaluation of cardiac patients after the resting ECG. With its high resolution, echocardiography provides a very accurate anatomic view of the heart. Doppler allows the evaluation of the physiology (e.g., blood flow) of the heart. The two procedures are almost always used in combination and provide an assessment of pathophysiology of cardiac disease processes. The principle of cardiac ultrasound is that high-frequency sound waves bouncing off cardiac structures and returning to the transducer provide information regarding that structure. The time it takes for the sound wave to return to the transducer is twice the time (which

can be converted to distance) that it takes to travel from the transducer to the structure, such as a wall of the LV or a valve. By analyzing all of the returning sound waves with computers, it is possible to identify multiple structures and their relationships to each other. This allows the measurement of chamber size and wall motion, as well as identifying valvular structures and pericardial effusions.

Cardiac Doppler assessment uses the principle of Doppler shift to evaluate intracardiac blood flow. The frequency of the returning sound wave varies depending on whether the object is moving toward or away from the transducer. For example, whereas objects moving toward the transducer reflect a sound wave with a higher frequency than the emitted sound wave, objects traveling away from the transducer have a lower frequency. Therefore, blood flow toward the transducer can be distinguished from blood flow away from the transducer. Using Doppler, blood velocity and volumetric flow can be measured to determine intracardiac gradients, valve areas, valvular regurgitation, and intracardiac pressures.

The transesophageal echocardiogram is performed using a transducer mounted on the end of a flexible tube that is swallowed. The attainment of the echocardiographic images is performed in the mid-esophagus. Being closer to the heart than a surface transthoracic transducer, this technique allows for better visualization of the left and right atrium as well as the interatrial septum, mitral valve, aorta, and atrial appendages.

Exercise echocardiography combines surface echocardiography and graded exercise testing. The echocardiographic images are obtained at rest and within 1 to 2 minutes after exercise. These images are then viewed using a side-by-side digital display format that allows the visualization of cardiac function both at rest and during exercise. Similar to radionuclide ventriculography (i.e., multiple-gated acquisition [MUGA]), exercise echocardiography allows assessment of wall motion abnormalities, ejection fraction, and systolic and diastolic function. The normal response to exercise is for the LV to decrease in size, the ejection fraction to increase, and **augmentation** of LV wall motion to occur. Patients with ischemia have normal wall motion at rest and during exercise develop **hypokinesis** or **akinesis** of the LV wall(s) being supplied by an artery with 70% or more stenosis. Patients with a previous myocardial infarction (MI) have akinesis, or possibly **dyskinesis**, of the infarcted wall at rest as well as with exercise. Dilatation of the LV with exercise is a sign of triple-vessel disease.

It is always best to use exercise to deliver the increased myocardial oxygen demand because this best replicates the physiologic processes leading to ischemia. However, some patients may not be able to perform exercise. Intravenous dobutamine, a beta-adrenergic–stimulating agent, offers a pharmacologic alternative for patients who are unable to exercise. Infusion of an incremental dose of dobutamine evokes a positive inotropic and chronotropic response. Unlike dipyridamole and adenosine, dobutamine closely parallels the exercise response by creating an oxygen supply and demand imbalance. In cases in which a patient who is scheduled for a "non-exercise" stress test is actually able to perform an adequate amount of exercise, an alternate plan using graded exercise testing should be discussed.

When to Use Echocardiography

Echocardiography is useful at *rest* in patients who present with symptoms suggestive of valvular disorders, pericardial disease, or LV dysfunction. *Exercise* echocardiography is useful for those with suspected ischemic heart disease and improves the predictive accuracy of the graded exercise test from about 75% to 80%–85%. This improved predictive accuracy remains even after excluding normal submaximal stress tests and nondiagnostic exercise ECGs[10]. An increased test predictive accuracy, compared with exercise ECG assessment alone, has also been observed in a population with a high prevalence of symptomatic CAD[11]. Specificity is also enhanced by exercise echocardiography[12].

Box 19-5 lists candidates for resting or exercise echocardiographic testing and those who are inappropriate candidates. In addition, stress echocardiography is useful in patients with a high likelihood of false-positive test results such as women and in patients with concurrent valvular or primary myocardial disease. Stress echocardiography is less useful in patients with multiple MIs, complex wall motion abnormalities, or a poor imaging window (e.g. obese individuals, individuals with chronic obstructive pulmonary disease).

MYOCARDIAL PERFUSION IMAGING

Radionuclide imaging in combination with exercise or pharmacologic stress is a commonly applied means of diagnosis of coronary disease. Use of radionuclide imaging is indicated in follow-up of patients with abnormal ECG test findings and in the diagnostic evaluation of women, patients taking digitalis, and those with an abnormal resting ECG (i.e., LBBB, LVH, Wolff-Parkinson-White syndrome, intraventricular conduction defects and resting ST-T wave abnormalities). It is also useful for the assessment of myocardial perfusion in patients with angiographically documented CAD and to study myocardial viability.

Thallium 201 ($_{201}$Th) and technetium 99m ($_{99m}$TC) injected at peak exercise and at rest are proportionally distributed within the myocardium in relation to regional myocardial blood flow and muscle viability. Newer $_{99m}$TC-based radiopharmaceutical flow tracers, such as sestambi, provide diagnostic benefits over $_{201}$Th on the basis of their physical and biological attributes. $_{99m}$TC sestambi has a higher energy output and a shorter half-life than $_{201}$Th. This allows administration of a larger dose, providing superior images. Also, the traditional stress–rest $_{201}$Th scan can be replaced with a protocol in which the rest images are acquired before stress, reducing the time required for the study and allowing acquisition of ECG-gated functional images.

In a normal myocardium, rest and stress images show accumulation of the isotope throughout the LV, reflecting integrity of regional blood supply. In areas of decreased perfusion, there is delayed uptake and slower washout. The presence of a perfusion defect on the stress images not present on the rest images suggests ischemia. Areas of scar from previous infarction characteristically show no uptake, either at rest or with stress. In addition to uniformity of isotopic uptake, ventricular size, wall motion, ejection fraction, and wall thickness can be assessed.

The diagnostic accuracy of $_{201}$Th and $_{99m}$TC are similar[13]. Recent advances in radionuclide imaging, such as quantification of radionuclide data, tomographic imaging, and single-photon emission computed tomography (SPECT) have enhanced the sensitivity and specificity beyond that provided by planar imaging. A review of studies using SPECT analysis indicated an overall sensitivity of 89% and a specificity of 70%[14].

As stated previously, it is always best to use exercise to deliver the myocardial stress in patients. However, some patients may not be able to exercise. In these cases,

---

BOX 19-5	**Candidates for Rest or Exercise Echocardiography Assessment**

APPROPRIATE CANDIDATES

Rest

Suspected valvular disease

Suspected ventricular dysfunction

Patients with systolic murmur suggestive of aortic stenosis

Exercise

Intermediate pretest probability of coronary artery disease and uninterpretable rest electrocardiogram; high- and low-risk patients may also be considered but may be more appropriate for myocardial perfusion imaging studies

Previous revascularization (percutaneous coronary intervention or coronary artery bypass surgery)

INAPPROPRIATE CANDIDATES

Patients with multiple myocardial infarctions

Those with complex wall motion abnormalities

Those with a poor imaging window (e.g., obese patients and patients with chronic obstructive pulmonary disease)

Those who cannot adequately ambulate (may be able to perform a pharmacologic test)

pharmacologic techniques, including the use of dipyridamole or adenosine, which are coronary artery selective vasodilators, can be used. With exercise, the myocardial oxygen demand is increased and after it exceeds the ability of oxygen delivery by the blood, ischemia can be detected, if present. Use of the coronary artery vasodilators results in a mismatch of blood flow increase between the normal and diseased coronary arteries that can be detected on the perfusion imaging studies.

When to Use Myocardial Perfusion Imaging

Myocardial perfusion imaging is most useful in patients who are intermediate- (or high-) risk patients for CAD, have abnormal ECG findings, have a history of bypass surgery, or have poor echocardiographic images (Box 19-6). Additionally, those who cannot exercise are candidates for pharmacologic imaging studies using dipyridamole or adenosine. However, these agents cannot be used in patients with reactive airway disease because severe bronchospasm may occur.

CORONARY ANGIOGRAPHY

Coronary angiography using the cardiac catheterization technique is considered the gold standard for assessing the presence of CAD[12]. Despite this, angiography frequently underestimates the size of the plaque and cannot determine whether the plaque is stable or unstable and at risk of rupture.

The technique requires the placement of a catheter through an incision in the groin or arm area. The catheter is then guided through the femoral or brachial artery and to the location of the coronary arteries. A contrast medium or dye is injected during radiographic fluoroscopy that allows for its visualization while flowing through the coronary tree. An area of narrowing can then be identified, located with respect to the coronary artery anatomy, and quantified for the amount of stenosis within a given artery. Although angiography cannot determine if a coronary artery lesion is flow limiting and causing ischemia during stress, and, therefore, most patients undergoing this test are previously symptomatic, the assumption that an identified lesion is causing ischemia can be made. Generally, coronary artery stenosis of 70% or more is required to cause ischemia. Those lesions between 50% and 70% of lumen diameter are considered borderline significant and are only considered clinically important if they corresponded to abnormalities seen on the stress imaging test or the patient is experiencing typical angina. Lesions 50% or smaller of lumen diameter are not generally thought to cause ischemia.

When to Use Angiography

Referral for angiography is appropriate when non-invasive assessment cannot be made because of contraindications or inadequacy or in symptomatic patients who are considered to be at high risk for CAD either before or after non-invasive testing. Additionally, patients who have an equivocal non-invasive test and thus an uncertain diagnosis are also potential candidates for referral for coronary angiography. Box 19-7 presents appropriate and inappropriate patients for angiography referral.

Over the past few years, there has been a rapid increase in the development of imaging techniques that may be useful in the detection of CAD. Although many of these have not yet been incorporated into standardized algorithms for the detection of heart disease, many cardiologists commonly use them as a diagnostic tool. The next several sections review some of these imaging methods.

BOX 19-6 | **Candidates for Myocardial Perfusion Imaging**

APPROPRIATE CANDIDATES

Those who have an uninterpretable resting electrocardiogram (i.e., left bundle branch block, left ventricular hypertrophy, digoxin, >1 mm ST-segment depression)

Use in conjunction with pharmacologic modes if patient cannot exercise

Those unable to achieve a high heart rate or systolic blood pressure

Intermediate- and high-risk symptomatic patients

INAPPROPRIATE CANDIDATES

Contraindications to testing

History of bronchospasm if adenosine or use of Persantine

BOX 19-7 | **Candidates for Coronary Angiography**

APPROPRIATE CANDIDATES

High risk for coronary artery disease, either at initial history and physical or after a non-invasive test

Unstable angina

Non–ST-segment elevation myocardial infarction

INAPPROPRIATE CANDIDATES

Those stratified to low risk of heart disease

Those at intermediate risk who are candidates for additional non-invasive testing

Medically unstable patients (non-cardiac medical problems)

INTRAVASCULAR ULTRASOUND

In addition to the standard cardiac catheterization assessments commonly performed, many laboratories also offer intracoronary diagnostic procedures to evaluate the severity of coronary artery stenosis. Atherosclerotic plaque development in the wall of the coronary artery results in a remodeling process of the entire blood vessel, which helps to maintain the lumen diameter. Traditional coronary angiography allows only for the visualization of the lumen of the coronary artery and thus may underestimate the size of a plaque in a remodeled artery. Also, coronary angiographic evaluation of coronary artery stenosis frequently identifies a lesion that appears "borderline significant" (i.e., stenoses of 50% to 70%). Further evaluation of these lesions using intravascular ultrasound (IVUS), intravascular Doppler (coronary flow velocity), and fractional flow reserve helps to determine which of these stenoses requires revascularization with either percutaneous transluminal intervention (PCI) and stenting or coronary bypass surgery.

During diagnostic evaluation IVUS provides the visualization of the lumen and wall of the vessel, and provides the size of the plaque. During interventional angiography, IVUS can be used after angioplasty to evaluate vessel patency and to look for complications such as coronary artery dissection. Additionally, IVUS is used in coronary stenting to provide information about the deployment of the stent.

Intravascular Doppler techniques provide information about the amount of obstruction to blood flow from an individual plaque within a coronary artery. By measuring the velocity of blood flow at the level of the lesion and determining the vessel's cross-sectional area, an estimate of coronary blood flow distal to the coronary stenosis can be made. Adenosine, a vasodilator that is infused into the coronary artery, is used to assess coronary artery vasodilatation. Normal coronary arteries increase blood flow by 250% or more in response to the adenosine challenge. Increases of less than 250% suggest that the distal vasculature is maximally dilated and that the coronary stenosis is limiting vasodilatation and thus negatively affecting blood flow.

Fractional flow reserve is a measure of the pressure across a section of a coronary artery. It is performed using small guidewires capable of measuring pressure. A decrease in pressure across a coronary artery stenosis indicates a reduction in blood flow. Fractional flow reserve of less than 0.75 suggests the lesion is significantly affecting blood flow and likely resulting in ischemia.

POSITRON EMISSION TOMOGRAPHY

Positron emission tomography (PET) scanning, a newer and significantly more costly and labor-intensive image acquisition technology, is one of the most accurate methods for non-invasively identifying and assessing the severity of CAD. There are two specific clinical applications for PET scanning in patients with suspected CAD. The first is the non-invasive detection of coronary artery stenosis. This is performed using a PET perfusion agent at rest and during pharmacologic vasodilatation and measuring coronary artery flow reserve. Limited coronary flow reserve is consistent with coronary artery stenosis. Radionuclide tracers used to diagnose coronary artery stenosis are nitrogen-13, ammonia, and rubidium-82. A review of the literature[13] reveals 10 studies, totaling 915 patients, that have evaluated the ability of PET scanning to diagnose CAD. Both the sensitivity and specificity were reported to be 93%. In institutions with both SPECT and PET scanning, PET scanning is reserved for patients with equivocal SPECT scans. The second and more frequent clinical application of PET is the assessment of myocardial viability in patients with CAD and LV impairment, which is useful in determining if revascularization would be beneficial. Hibernating myocardium can be differentiated from scar using fluorine-18 fluorodeoxyglucose. In a summary of three studies that included 313 patients, if PET scanning demonstrated myocardial viability, mortality was reduced from 41% in medically treated population to 8% in the surgically revascularized group[13].

CARDIAC MAGNETIC RESONANCE IMAGING

Magnetic resonance imaging (MRI) provides an anatomic view of the heart by measuring the emitted electromagnetic waves from resonating nuclei and locating these nuclei in space. Because of a natural high contrast that exists between blood and cardiac tissue, no contrast agent is needed to identify the blood pool. In cardiology, MRI is used primarily to evaluate the patient for anatomic pathology. The most frequent uses are to (a) assess the extent of damage to the LV as a complication of ischemic heart disease; (b) assess the type of cardiomyopathy and quantify physiologic parameters such as wall stress and LV volume; (c) visualize the pericardium and assess its thickness in pericardial disease; (d) evaluate intracardiac and pericardial neoplastic disease; (e) provide information regarding morphology, size of shunts, and valvular function in congenital heart disease; and (f) evaluate the thoracic aorta for dissection, false lumens, periaortic disease, and abnormalities of the thoracic aortic arch.

Recent advances in MRI have allowed the visualization of the coronary arteries. This is known as magnetic resonance angiography (MRA). One report suggested a 90% correlation between MRA and conventional coronary angiography[15]. MRA has been used to evaluate saphenous vein graft patency with 80% to 90% accuracy[16]. Acquisition of magnetic resonance images during various phases of the cardiac cycle have allowed the development of **cine** MRI, which allows for the assessment of the cardiac cycle. This allows for LV global and regional function to be assessed.

CORONARY CALCIUM SCORING

Two technologies are currently used to assess coronary artery calcium. These are electron beam computed tomography (EBCT) and spiral computed tomography (CT). Each of these techniques requires only a few minutes to complete. Simplified, the patient is prescanned to determine the length of the scanning field (i.e., the length of the heart). Patients slide feet first through the scanner. Electrodes placed on chest to allow imaging to be gated, or coordinated with the cardiac cycle. The scan takes approximately 30 seconds and requires a breath hold to minimize thoracic movement. During this time, 20 to 30 slices are scanned during the diastolic phase of the cardiac cycle. Each separate scan takes 50 msec per slice, and each slice is about 3 mm thick. This may vary slightly based on the type of scanner used.

The idea for this type of assessment came from work in the 1950s that found calcium deposits in the radiographs of coronary atheromas. These appeared as whitened areas. Using current technology, the whitened areas can be quantified (i.e., scored) based on their intensity (i.e., Hounsfield unit). The scanned slices are reviewed to visualize the major coronary arteries; a higher score indicates a greater amount of calcium. Calcium detected in the coronary arteries is always indicative of disease. However, this technique cannot quantify the stenosis. A limited number of data sets are currently available that allow a calcium score, along with age and gender, to be rated as minimal or severe[17].

Although still controversial and not a standard technique for the diagnosis of CAD, this technique provides the promise of uncovering preclinical disease before it leads to myocardial ischemia or MI. The argument is that after the preclinical disease is found, the treatment of risk factors should be no different than if the coronary calcium score were not known. The potential likely lies in discovering the preclinical lesion that is susceptible to rupture and subsequent MI.

Box 19-8 lists potential appropriate and inappropriate candidates for coronary calcium scoring assessment. Nallamothu et al.[18] performed a meta-analysis that stated coronary artery calcium testing has a sensitivity of 92% and a specificity of 51% for occlusive disease. The low specificity is related to the fact that coronary calcium scoring is effective for identifying preclinical, non-occlusive disease. Wong et al.[19] reported the calcium score to be a modest predictor of future cardiovascular events, and Arad et al.[20] reported that calcium scoring predicts coronary death, nonfatal MI, and the need for revascularization procedures in asymptomatic adults. To date, the sensitivity of calcium scoring to detect occlusive disease is similar to that of stress testing, suggesting no advantage. However, in addition to its possible role of detecting preocclusive disease, coronary calcium scoring may be useful in predicting those who will do poorly during or after a stent procedure[21] and

---

BOX 19-8 | **Candidates for Calcium Score Testing[a]**

APPROPRIATE CANDIDATES

Asymptomatic patients with increased risk of coronary artery disease

INAPPROPRIATE CANDIDATES

Patients with established coronary artery disease

Patients younger than age 40 years (men) or 50 years (women)

Patients older than 75 years

[a] Note that the recommendations in Box 19-8 are not based on a practice guideline or clinical statements.

---

in assisting the diagnosis of a suspected false-positive exercise test result[22])

Summary

The diagnosis of cardiac disease relies on an adequate history and physical examination and subsequent adherence to evidence-based principles to determine the appropriate diagnostic test to perform. Graded exercise testing, with or without imaging (echocardiography or radionuclide methods), and cardiac angiography remains the primary method to detect disease. Cardiac MRI, MRA, and PET scanning are increasing in use and may be incorporated into practice guidelines for detecting heart disease in the future. In the future, tests that are able to identify preclinical disease or the status of existing disease composition and structure may become mainstream. Coronary calcium scoring and IVUS, respectively, may be able to detect these timepoints of the CAD progression.

REFERENCES

1. Gibbons RJ, Abrams J, Chatterjee K, et al: ACC/AHA 2002 guideline update for the management of patients with chronic stable angina: A report of the American College of Cardiology/American Heart Association Task Force on Practice Guidelines (Committee to Update the 1999 Guidelines for the management of Patients with Chronic Stable Angina); 2002. Available at http://ww.acc.org/clinical/guidelines/stable/stable.pdf

2. Gibbons RJ, Balady GJ, Bricker JT, et al: ACC/AHA 2002 guideline update for exercise testing: A report of the American College of Cardiology/American Heart Association Task Force on Practice Guidelines (Committee on Exercise Testing); 2002. Available at: http://www.acc.org/clinical/guidelines/exercise/dirIndex.htm

3. Joint National Committee on Prevention, Detection, Evaluation, and Treatment of High Blood Pressure: The seventh report of the Joint National Committee on Prevention, Detection, Evaluation, and Treatment of High Blood Pressure. JAMA 209:2560–2572, 2003.

4. Executive Summary of the Third Report of the National Cholesterol Education Program (NCEP) Expert Panel on Detection, Evaluation, and Treatment of High Blood Cholesterol in Adults (Adult Treatment Panel III). JAMA 285:2486–2497, 2001.

5. Diamond GA, Forrester JS: Analysis of probability as an aid in the clinical diagnosis of coronary-artery disease. N Engl J Med 300:1350–1358, 1979.

6. Pryor DB, Harrell FE, Lee KL, et al: Estimating the likelihood of significant coronary artery disease. Am J Med 75:771–780, 1983.

7. Sox HC, Hickam DH, Marton KI, et al: Using the patient's history to estimate the probability of coronary artery disease: a comparison of primary care and referral practices [published erratum appears in Am J Med 89:550, 1990]. Am J Med 89:7–14, 1990.

8. Mark DB, Shaw, L, Harrell FE, et al: Prognostic value of a treadmill exercise score in outpatients with suspected coronary artery disease. N Engl J Med 325:849–853, 1991.

9. Ladenheim ML, Kotler TS, Pollack BH, et al: Incremental prognostic power of clinical history, exercise electrocardiography, and myocardial perfusion scintography in suspected coronary artery disease. Am J Cardiol 59:270–277, 1987.

10. Marwick TH, Nemec JJ, Paskow FJ, et al: Accuracy and limitations of exercise echocardiography in a routine clinical setting. J Am Coll Cardiol 19:74–81, 1992.

11. Orlandi A, Picano E, Lattanzi F, et al: Stress echocardiography and the human factor: Importance of being an expert. Am J Cardiol 15:52a, 1990.

12. O'Rourke RA, Schlant RC, Douglas JS: Diagnostic and management of patients with chronic ischemic heart disease. In Hurst's The Heart, 10th ed. New York: McGraw Hill; 2001.

13. Wackers FJT, Soufer R, Zaret BL: Nuclear cardiology (pp. 306–307). In Braunwald E, ed. Heart Disease: A Textbook of Cardiovascular Medicine. Philadelphia: Saunders; 1997.

14. Maddahi J, Rodrigues E, Berman DS, et al: State of the art myocardial perfusion imaging (pp. 199–202). In Verani MS, ed Nuclear Cardiology: State of the Art. Philadelphia: WB Saunders; 1994.

15. Manning WJ, Lil W, Enderman RR: A preliminary report comparing magnetic resonance angiography with conventional angiography. N Engl J Med 328:828–832, 1993.

16. White RD, Caputo CR, Mark AS, et al: Non-invasive evaluation of coronary artery bypass graft patency using magnetic resonance imaging. Radiology 164:681–686, 1987.

17. Rumberger JA, et al: Electron beam computed tomography coronary calcium scanning: A review and guidelines for use in asymptomatic persons. Mayo Clin Proc 74:243–252, 1999.

18. Nallamothu BK, Saint S, Bielak LF, et al: Electron-beam computed tomography in the diagnosis of coronary artery disease: A meta-analysis. Arch Intern Med 161:833–838, 2001.

19. Wong ND, Hsu JC, Detrano RC, et al: Coronary artery calcium evaluation by electron beam computed tomography and its relation to new cardiovascular events. Am J Cardiol 86:495–498, 2000.

20. Arad Y, Spadaro LA, Goodman K, et al: Prediction of coronary events with electron beam computed tomography. J Am Coll Cardiol 36:1253–1260, 2000.

21. Sinitsyn V, Belkind M, Matchin Y, et al: Relationships between coronary calcification detected at electron beam computed tomography and percutaneous transluminal coronary angioplasty results in coronary artery disease patients. Eur Radiol 13:62–67, 2003.

22. LaMont DH, Budoff MJ, Shavelle DM, et al: Coronary calcium scanning adds incremental value to patients with positive stress tests. Am Heart J 143:861–867, 2002.

SELECTED REFERENCES FOR FURTHER READING

Cheitlin MD, Armstrong WF, Aurigemma GP, et al: ACC/AHA/ASE 2003 guideline update for the clinical application of echocardiography: a report of the American College of Cardiology/American Heart Association Task Force on Practice Guidelines (ACC/AHA/ASE Committee to Update the 1997 Guidelines for the Clinical Application of Echocardiography); 2003. Available at: http://www.acc.org/clinical/guidelines/echo/index.pdf

Ehrman JK, Gordon PM, Visich PS, Keteyian SJ: Clinical Exercise Physiology. Champaign, IL: Human Kinetics; 2003.

Klocke FJ, Baird MG, Bateman TM, et al: ACC/AHA/ASNC guidelines for the clinical use of cardiac radionuclide imaging: A report of the American College of Cardiology/American Heart Association Task Force on Practice Guidelines (ACC/AHA/ASNC Committee to Revise the 1995 Guidelines for the Clinical Use of Radionuclide Imaging); 2003. Available at: http://www.acc.org/clinical/guidelines/radio/rni_fulltext.pdf

INTERNET RESOURCES

American College of Cardiology: http://www.acc.org

American Heart Association: Scientific statements and practice guidelines topic list: http://www.americanheart.org/presenter.jhtml?identifier=2158

International Atherosclerosis Society: http://www.athero.org

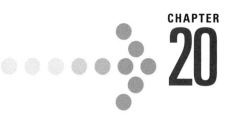

Dysrhythmias and Selected Conduction Defects

JOHN A. LARRY AND STEPHEN F. SCHAAL

Anatomy of the Conduction System

The anatomy of the conduction system is depicted in Figure 20-1. The impulse that drives electrical depolarization of the heart originates in the sinoatrial (SA), or sinus node. This area is located in the right atrium near the superior vena cava. The wave of activity initially spreads in a radial fashion through the right atrium and subsequently the left atrium. The impulse reaches the atrioventricular (AV) node, an ovoid structure that lies at the base of the intra-atrial septum. The impulse takes approximately 100 ms to traverse the AV node and depolarize the bundle of His. In the normal heart, the AV node and the His bundle are the

---

Editor's Note: The information in Chapters 20 and 21 is limited to electrocardiographic (ECG) abnormalities frequently associated with exercise testing or training. For basic information regarding normal ECGs and additional types of abnormalities, readers are directed to the ECG reference texts listed at the end of this chapter.

---

only point of connection between the atria and ventricles. The bundle of His extends through the fibrous skeleton of the heart into the superior portion of the intraventricular septum and divides into right and left bundles. The right bundle is quite discrete and travels down the right side of the interventricular septum and through the moderator band, beyond which it branches into the right ventricle (RV). The left bundle divides into anterior and posterior divisions; in reality, these divisions are more complex and diffuse as they fan out into the left ventricle (LV). The bundle branches terminate in Purkinje fibers (specialized cells that spread the electrical activity rapidly through the myocardium). The depolarization wave stimulates myocardial cells to contract by initiating a series of events referred to as excitation–contraction coupling (also see Chapter 1).

The sinus node is typically responsible for initiating depolarization of the myocardium. The impulse generated then travels through the atria, AV node, His–bundle branch–Purkinje system, and finally the ventricular myocardium. However, in patients with structural heart disease, as well as those with normal hearts, deviations from the normal depolarization sequence occur. These abnormalities in heart rhythm are called dysrhythmias. Dysrhythmias may be fast (tachydysrhythmia) or slow (bradydysrhythmia). Apart from abnormal rhythms, the AV node or bundle branches may be impaired, leading to conduction defects (i.e., AV blocks or bundle branch blocks). This chapter examines the most common dysrhythmias and selected conduction defects as well as the mechanisms responsible for their generation (also see GETP7 Appendix C).

Premature Complexes

It is fairly common for patients to exhibit either premature atrial complexes (PACs) or premature ventricular complexes (PVCs), especially during exercise testing when catecholamine levels are increased. PACs occur when a site in the atrium other than the sinus node depo-

---

KEY TERMS

Atrioventricular block: An obstruction or delay in electrical conduction that occurs in the normal conduction pathways between the sinus node and the Purkinje fibers

Automaticity: The ability of specialized cells in the heart (normally in the sinus node) to spontaneously depolarize and initiate a new electrical impulse

Bigeminy: A conduction pattern in which a premature beat (either supraventricular or ventricular) follows every normal sinus beat

Bundle branch block: A block in electrical conduction that occurs in one or both of the ventricular bundle branches

Dysrhythmia: Any cardiac rhythm that is not a regular sinus rhythm; it may be a single beat or a sustained rhythm

Fascicular block: A conduction block that occurs in one or more of the fascicles of the intraventricular purkinje system

---

larizes prematurely (Fig. 20-2). The resulting impulse traverses the AV node, bundle of His, bundle branches, and Purkinje system and, in the absence of bundle branch block or myocardial disease, generates a narrow QRS complex.

Occasionally, the premature atrial complex occurs early enough that a portion of the conduction system may be refractory. If the impulse finds the AV node not recovered, the impulse extinguishes at that point, and no QRS complex results. These are *blocked PACs*. The block at the AV node is physiological if the PAC occurs quite early. If the AV node conducts the impulse but one of the bundle branches is refractory, the QRS complex exhibits features of a bundle branch block (discussed later in this chapter), a phenomenon termed *bundle branch aberration*. If one of the fascicles of the left bundle is refractory when the premature beat arrives, the QRS complex may exhibit features of left anterior fascicular or left posterior fascicular block aberration. A normal sinus beat alternating with a premature atrial contraction is atrial **bigeminy**.

Premature ventricular complexes occur when a site in the ventricle fires before the next wave of depolarization from the sinus node reaches the ventricle (Fig. 20-3). These QRS complexes have bizarre, wide morphologies. Unlike PACs, these beats may not reset the periodicity of the sinus node; that is, the next sinus beat is often two cycle lengths (referred to as a *full compensatory pause*) from the beat before the PVC. A pattern of a sinus beat alternating with a PVC is ventricular bigeminy, and every third beat, is ventricular trigeminy. PACs and PVCs may occur in patients with normal hearts during rest or exercise, or they may be markers of underlying cardiac disease.

Mechanisms of Tachydysrhythmias

Electrophysiological mechanisms responsible for the generation of most cardiac dysrhythmias have been iden-

tified as circus re-entry, enhanced **automaticity**, and triggered activity. The substrate for re-entry requires two pathways for current to travel. The first pathway depolarizes rapidly and recovers slowly, and the second depolarizes slowly but recovers rapidly (Fig. 20-4). Re-entry occurs when an area of altered conduction exists and unidirectional block occurs. If an impulse arrives prematurely at a time when the slow pathway has recovered but the fast pathway is refractory (not recovered from the previous depolarization), the impulse conducts over the slow pathway. If conduction over the slow pathway reaches the fast pathway when recovered, the impulse may travel retrograde over the fast pathway. If the slow pathway has recovered, depolarization of the slow path occurs and a re-entrant loop is established.

Enhanced automaticity is another mechanism responsible for the generation of dysrhythmias. In this situation, an increased rate of depolarization of a myocardial cell occurs, thereby reaching the threshold potential more rapidly than usual. The cell depolarizes, and the impulse generated depolarizes the remainder of the myocardium.

A third mechanism of dysrhythmias is called triggered activity, which exhibits features of both re-entry and automaticity. Myocardial cells may exhibit after-depolarization or increases in the membrane potential that occur during the repolarization phase of the action potential. These depolarizations can be characterized as early (occurring during phase 3) and late (occurring after phase 3). If the magnitude of these after-depolarizations is great enough, depolarization may be triggered. Early afterdepolarizations are related to conditions that prolong the action potential, such as antiarrhythmic agents (type IA and III drugs) and electrolyte disorders (e.g., hypokalemia and hypomagenesemia). Generally, the tachycardia develops after a pause. Delayed after-depolarizations occur in the setting of myocardial ischemia, digitalis toxicity, and congenital long-QT syndromes. These after-depolarizations are tachycardia dependent. and high catecholamine states contribute to the development of the tachycardia.

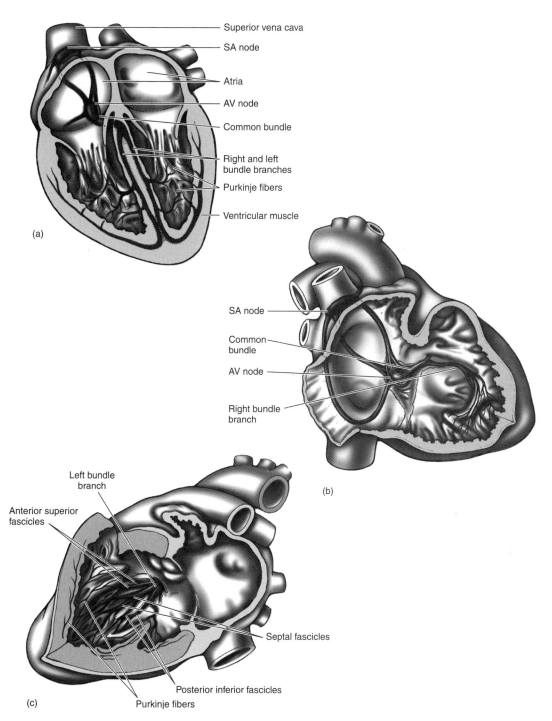

Figure 20-1. The anatomy of the conduction system from three different views: (a) arterior; (b) right; (c) left. AV = atrioventricular; SA = sinoatrial. Also see figure 1-10.

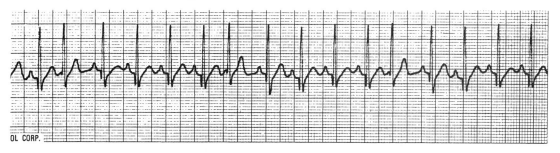

Figure 20-2. Sinus tachycardia with frequent premature atrial complexes.

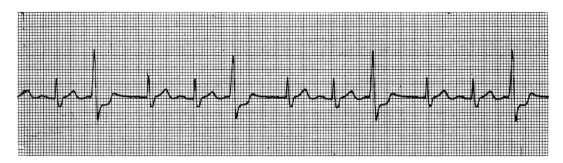

Figure 20-3. Normal sinus rhythm with premature ventricular complexes.

Circus re-entry, enhanced automaticity, and triggered activity may occur in any portion of the myocardium or specialized conducting tissue. The atrial myocardium, ventricular myocardium, SA node, AV node, and the His–Purkinje system all may be susceptible to variations in conduction. The location of the abnormality and the underlying cardiac substrate govern the type of dysrhythmia and its properties.

Types of Tachydysrhythmias

SINUS TACHYCARDIA

Sinus tachycardia (Fig. 20-5) is a sinus rhythm beating greater than 100 bpm, and it is the result of enhancement of the rate of firing of the sinus node. The sinus node is under the control of the parasympathetic and sympathetic nervous systems and, therefore, accelerates or decelerates depending on the physiological requirements. Sinus tachycardia results when increased activity of the sympathetic nervous system is present. These include situations such as fear, exercise, fever, hypovolemia, bleeding, thyrotoxicosis, hypoxia, and other acute illness. Decreased stroke volume in severe LV dysfunction may also result in sinus tachycardia because the sympathetic nervous system is activated in an attempt to preserve adequate cardiac output.

Three key features of sinus tachycardia are important. First, patients typically exhibit a gradual increase in heart rate (i.e., sudden acceleration from 80 to 150 bpm does not occur). Second, although exceptions occur, the sinus

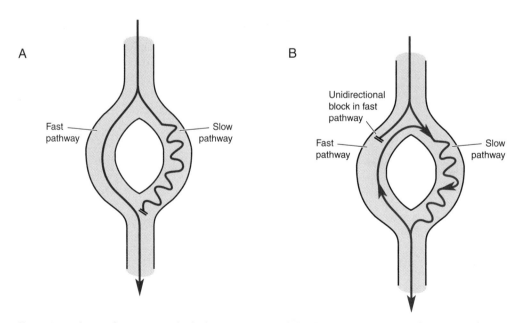

Figure 20-4. Substrate for re-entrant dysrhythmias. **A.** A normal depolarization wave arrives, finding both fast and slow pathways recovered from previous depolarization. An impulse travels via the fast pathway to distal conducting tissue. **B.** A premature beat blocks in the fast pathway but is able to travel over the slow pathway, which has a short refractory period. The impulse travels to the distal conducting tissue and retrograde over the fast pathway, which has recovered by this time. If the slow pathway is recovered, a re-entrant loop is generated, resulting in tachycardia.

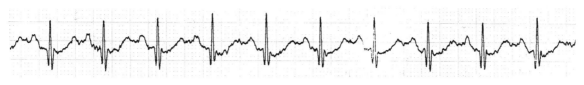

Figure 20-5. Sinus tachycardia.

rate typically does not exceed the maximum rate (see GETP7 Figure 7-3) as estimated by this formula:

$$\text{Maximum heart rate} = 220 - \text{age}.$$

Finally, the P-wave vector must be normal.

ATRIAL FIBRILLATION

Atrial fibrillation (Fig. 20-6), a relatively common **dysrhythmia**, is the result of multiple re-entrant waves of electrical activity in the atria. These depolarization waves do not result in organized atrial contraction, and the appearance of the atria has been described as a bag of worms when in fibrillation. The AV node is stimulated at frequent and irregular intervals by the very rapid atrial activity, resulting in an irregular ventricular rate (R-R response). The rate of the ventricular response is governed by the AV node's refractory period. The hallmarks of atrial fibrillation are the absence of organized P-wave activity and an irregular ventricular response. This rhythm has important consequences for the patient: the absence of a properly timed atrial contraction results in decline of the cardiac output (as much as 20% in those with relatively normal ventricles). In patients with cardiac disease, the cardiac output may decline by up to 40%. Atrial fibrillation may compromise ability to perform physical activities.

In addition, patients with atrial fibrillation are at increased risk for developing atrial thrombus, which may embolize to the brain, kidneys, a peripheral artery, and so on. The incidence of embolic stroke in patients with atrial fibrillation is fivefold the incidence among age-matched patients in normal sinus rhythm.

Treatment of atrial fibrillation focuses initially on decreasing the ventricular response with agents such as digitalis, calcium channel blockers (specifically diltiazem and

verapamil), and beta-blockers, which prolong the refractory period of the AV node. Anticoagulation is necessary before the restoration of normal sinus rhythm, which is usually attempted with types IA, IC, or III antiarrythmic agents, namely quinidine, propafenone, sotalol, or amiodarone. Electrical cardioversion is required if the rhythm does not convert to normal sinus rhythm with the use of an antiarrhythmic drug.

Most patients with atrial fibrillation have underlying cardiac disease. A list of the common causes is presented in Box 20-1. Rarely, a patient has lone atrial fibrillation, in which the dysrhythmia exists in the absence of structural heart disease or another definable trigger. Because of the presence of underlying cardiac disease, even when sinus rhythm has been restored, almost 50% of patients have reverted to atrial fibrillation 1 year later.

ATRIAL FLUTTER

Atrial flutter (Fig. 20-7) classically results from a macro–re-entrant circuit in the atria, generating flutter waves at a rate of 250 to 350 atrial depolarizations per minute. The atrial waves are typically best seen in the inferior leads (II, III, aVF) and lead V1. As in atrial fibrillation, the ventricular rate depends on the refractory period of the AV node, and the QRS complexes may be regular or irregular depending on whether a fixed or variable relationship exists between the atria and ventricles. The classic appearance of this rhythm is the sawtooth shape of the flutter waves in the inferior leads at a rate of 250 to 350 per minute. In the absence of medications or disease of the AV node, 2:1 block exists, so that one of every two atrial flutter waves is conducted to the ventricle. Consequently, whenever a ventricular rate near 150 bpm is detected, the tracing must be scrutinized for atrial flutter waves. The same underlying

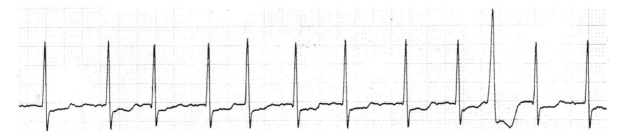

Figure 20-6. Atrial fibrillation with rapid ventricular response. The wide QRS complex likely represents aberrant ventricular conduction, although a premature ventricular complex cannot be excluded.

BOX 20-1	**Cardiac and Noncardiac Conditions Predisposing to Atrial Dysrhythmias**

Hypertensive heart disease

Valvular heart disease

Ischemic heart disease

Cardiomyopathy

Congenital heart disease

Conduction system disease

Pericarditis

Thyrotoxicosis

Pulmonary embolus

Hypoxia

Holiday heart syndrome

Sepsis

causes listed in Box 20-1 for atrial fibrillation apply to atrial flutter. In general, this rhythm may not persist for extended periods but often converts to sinus rhythm or more commonly degenerates into atrial fibrillation.

Patients with hypoxemia, hypokalemia, and other metabolic abnormalities, as occasionally seen in those with chronic obstructive lung disease or congestive heart failure, may exhibit a rhythm known as multifocal atrial tachycardia (Fig. 20-8). This rhythm is likely attributable to multiple sites within the atrium functioning as the pacemaker of the heart, thereby generating multiple P-wave morphologies. The AV node is stimulated at variable intervals by the atrial impulses, leading to irregular, narrow QRS complexes. Recognition of this rhythm depends on defining at least three different P-wave morphologies in the same lead with an irregular and usually rapid ventricular response.

ATRIOVENTRICULAR NODAL RE-ENTRANT TACHYCARDIA

Atrioventricular nodal re-entrant tachycardia (AVNRT) is a narrow complex tachycardia that occurs when a patient has two functional pathways in the AV node region. The pathways exhibit the classic characteristics that promote re-entry: a fast pathway that depolarizes rapidly but recovers slowly and a slow pathway that depolarizes slowly but recovers quickly. The initiation of this rhythm is usually a premature atrial contraction timed so that it finds the fast pathway refractory and the slow pathway recovered. The PAC blocks in the fast pathway and conducts down the slow pathway. After the slow pathway depolarizes, the fast pathway has recovered, allowing the impulse to conduct in a retrograde fashion to the atria and again arrive at the slow pathway. This results in a re-entrant loop of depolarization traveling down the slow pathway and up the fast pathway. The atria and ventricles are depolarized nearly simultaneously. The P waves are typically inverted in the inferior leads (the atria are depolarized in a retrograde fashion from the AV node with the vector going superiorly) and may occur shortly after the QRS complex or even simultaneously with the QRS complex, so that the P wave cannot be visualized on the surface electrocardiogram (ECG; Fig. 20-9).

ATRIOVENTRICULAR RE-ENTRANT TACHYCARDIA

Atrioventricular re-entrant tachycardia (AVRT) occurs in the setting of the substrate of an accessory pathway (AP). The AP is a muscle bridge of connection between the atria and ventricles. The onset of the tachycardia occurs when a PAC conducts over the AV node and returns to the atrium via retrograde conduction over the AP. Alternatively, depolarization from a PVC may travel retrograde over the AP, stimulating the atrium, and return antegrade down the AV node. The P waves are typically at some interval after the QRS complex, usually greater than 100 ms (Fig. 20-10).

ATRIAL TACHYCARDIA

Atrial tachycardia (Fig. 20-11) may be the result of rapid firing of an automatic or triggered atrial focus or re-entry within the atrium. The ventricular rate depends on the atrial rate and the refractory period of the AV node. The P wave has altered morphology (exhibits a different vector from sinus rhythm), and the PR interval is often short.

SUPRAVENTRICULAR TACHYCARDIA

The term *supraventricular tachycardia* is often used to describe tachydysrhythmias that present with a narrow

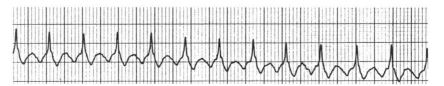

Figure 20-7. Atrial flutter with 2:1 atrioventricular conduction. Note the "sawtooth" pattern of the atrial flutter waves.

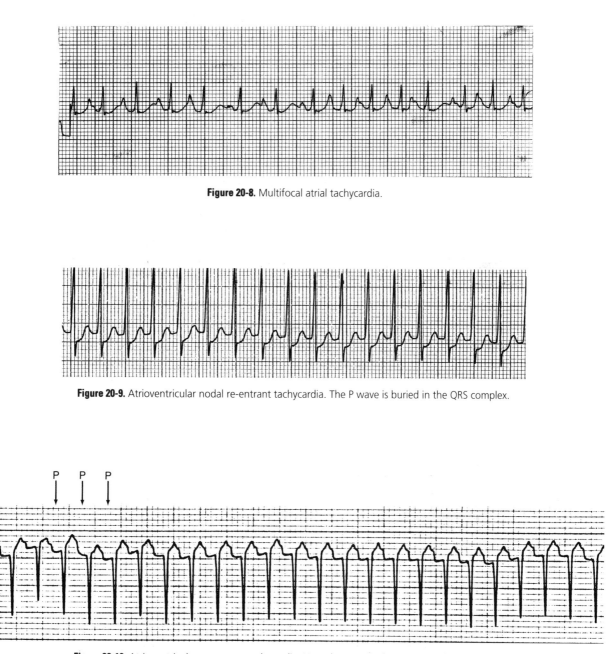

Figure 20-8. Multifocal atrial tachycardia.

Figure 20-9. Atrioventricular nodal re-entrant tachycardia. The P wave is buried in the QRS complex.

Figure 20-10. Atrioventricular re-entrant tachycardia. Note the retrograde P waves within the T wave.

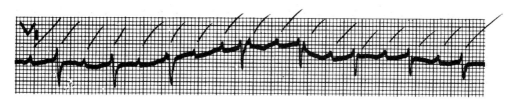

Figure 20-11. Atrial tachycardia with variable atrioventricular block. Markers label the atrial activity.

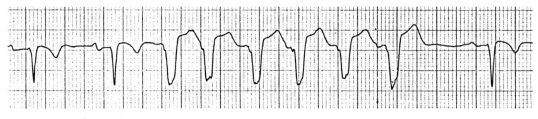

Figure 20-12. Normal sinus rhythm with a run of nonsustained ventricular tachycardia.

QRS morphology that do not originate in the sinus node. These include the AVNRT, AVRT, and atrial tachycardia rhythms already described.

VENTRICULAR TACHYCARDIA

Ventricular tachycardia (Figs. 20-12 and 20-13) is typically seen in patients with underlying heart disease, most commonly coronary artery disease with previous myocardial infarction or cardiomyopathy. Three or more consecutive ventricular beats at 100 bpm or faster defines ventricular tachycardia. Nonsustained ventricular tachycardia is a run of tachycardia lasting less than 30 seconds. Sustained ventricular tachycardia is tachycardia lasting longer than 30 seconds or terminated because of hemodynamic consequences before 30 seconds. Ventricular tachycardia is usually recognized by the presence of a wide QRS complex ($\geq$ 120 ms), AV dissociation (the P waves and QRS complexes have no relationship), and a QRS complex that does not have the morphology of typical bundle branch block. Re-entry is the most common mechanism of ventricular tachycardia; however, abnormal automaticity or triggered activity caused by after-depolarizations may be responsible. Depending on the cardiac and hemodynamic status of the patient and the rate of the tachycardia, the patient may have normal blood pressure with minimal to no symptoms or be in cardiac arrest and require immediate cardioversion.

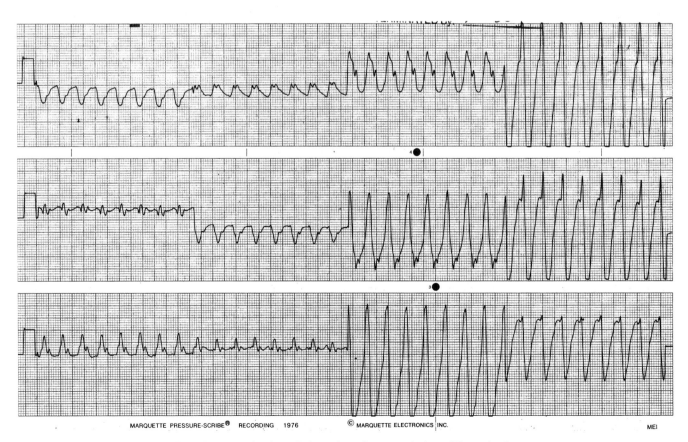

MARQUETTE PRESSURE-SCRIBE® RECORDING 1976   © MARQUETTE ELECTRONICS INC.   MEI

Figure 20-13. Sustained ventricular tachycardia as seen in three different leads.

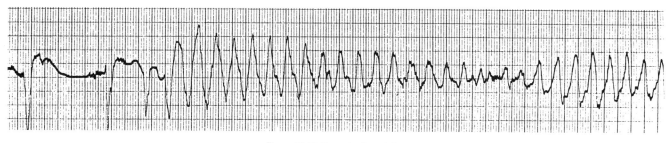

Figure 20-14. Torsade de pointes.

TORSADE DE POINTES

Torsade de pointes is a type of ventricular tachycardia named because the morphology of the ventricular tachycardia exhibits a twisting of the points. An example of this rhythm is shown in Figure 20-14.

VENTRICULAR DEFIBRILLATION

Ventricular fibrillation (Fig. 20-15) is a life-threatening rhythm that must be treated with immediate electrical defibrillation per advanced cardiac life support protocol (see Chapter 28 and GETP7 Appendix B).

Bradydysrhythmias and Disorders of the Conduction System

SINUS NODE DYSFUNCTION

Sinus bradycardia (Fig. 20-16) occurs when the impulse originates from the sinus node at a rate less than 60 bpm. This may be seen in individuals who are well trained and exhibit high parasympathetic (vagal) tone, in patients who are receiving drugs that slow the heart rate (e.g., beta-blockers) or in individuals who have disease of the sinus node (e.g., sick sinus syndrome).

Sinus pauses may be attributable to high vagal tone or disease of the sinus node. If the pause interval is a multiple of the intrinsic sinus rate, one may suspect sinus exit block. In this instance, the sinus node fires but the impulse does not conduct through the perisinus nodal tissue,

and the atrium is not depolarized. Sinus dysrhythmia, a variation of the rate of firing of the sinus node, is commonly seen in younger persons and does not reflect disease of the sinus node.

If the sinus node fails and none of the atrial cell take over the pacemaker role, the AV junction (His bundle region) may assume the role of pacemaker, resulting in a junctional rhythm (Fig. 20-17). This rhythm is typified by narrow QRS complexes at regular intervals; the P waves are often generated by retrograde atrial conduction. P waves may occur during or after the transcription of the QRS complex. Typically, the AV junction has a much slower depolarization than the sinus node. Therefore, the normal junctional rate ranges between 40 and 60 bpm. Occasionally, the rate is more than 60 bpm; the rhythm is called junctional tachycardia or accelerated junctional rhythm.

If the sinus and AV junction pacemaker cells fail, cells within the ventricles may initiate pacemaker activity. This rhythm is typified by wide QRS complexes in regular, slow rhythm (typically 15 to 40 bpm). This rhythm is referred to as a ventricular rhythm or idioventricular rhythm. This rhythm may be observed in the setting of third-degree AV block (described below) or in isolation (i.e., no P-wave activity).

DISORDERS OF THE ATRIOVENTRICULAR NODE AND HIS–PURKINJE SYSTEM

Atrioventricular nodal disease may be attributable to a number of causes; infarction, ischemia, primary conduction system disease, and medication effect are the most com-

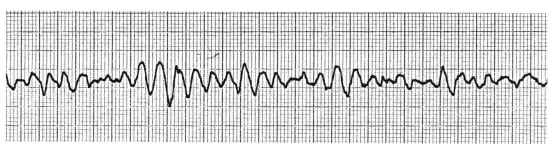

Figure 20-15. Ventricular fibrillation (coarse).

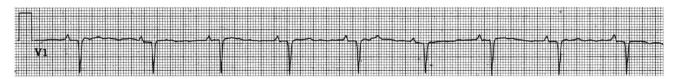

Figure 20-16. Sinus bradycardia.

mon. The types of AV block are classified as follows:

- First-degree **atrioventricular block** is simply prolongation of the PR interval. This may be the result of intra-atrial or interatrial conduction delay, delayed conduction through the AV node, impaired conduction through the His–Purkinje system, or a combination of these.
- Second-degree AV block may be divided into two types: Mobitz type I and Mobitz type II. In type I, also known as Wenckebach, the disease process is usually in the AV node. In Mobitz type I, the PR interval progressively lengthens with each beat until a P wave is not conducted to the ventricles (Fig. 20-18). In type II block, the disease usually is below the AV node in the His bundle branch region. The PR interval is fixed until a P wave is not conducted to the ventricles (Fig. 20-19). Type II block is often associated with a wide QRS complex. A rhythm disorder that may cause confusion is called *2:1 AV block* (Fig. 20-20). The confusion arises with the semantics used to describe *dysrhythmias*. Constant 2:1 AV block may indicate second-degree type I or second-degree type II. Although the width of the QRS complex may be helpful, it is impossible to distinguish whether a progressively prolonging PR interval with a dropped beat or a fixed PR interval with every other beat dropped is present unless the onset or offset of 2:1 AV block is recorded. Further confusion results in the setting in which atrial flutter is present with 2:1 AV block. In this setting, no disease of the AV nodal–His bundle system exists; the refractory period of the normal AV node prevents the atrial impulses from reaching the ventricle in a one-to-one relationship. Therefore, depending on the clinical setting, 2:1 AV block may indicate disease below the AV node, disease in the AV node, or no disease.
- Third-degree or complete heart block occurs when the atrial activity is unable to traverse the AV junction to generate a QRS complex (Fig. 20-21). The atrial rate is faster than the ventricular rate, and the P waves have no influence on the QRS complexes. Depending on the site of origin of the QRS complexes, the QRS complexes may be narrow or wide.

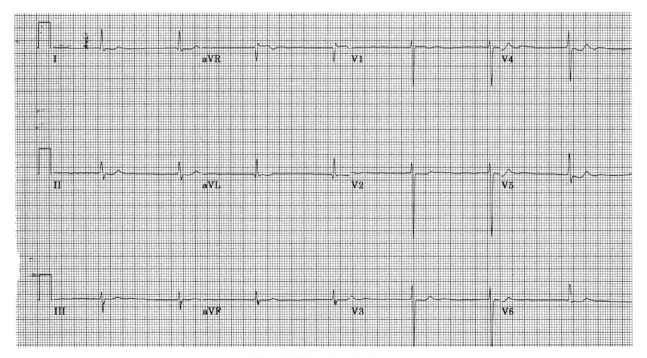

Figure 20-17. Junctional rhythm.

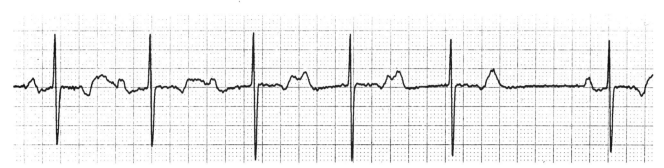

Figure 20-18. Second-degree type I atrioventricular block (Wenckebach).

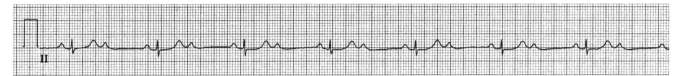

Figure 20-19. Second-degree atrioventricular block, type II.

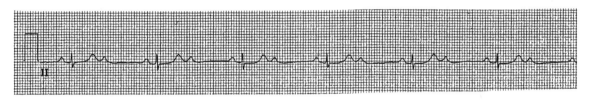

Figure 20-20. 2:1 Atrioventricular block.

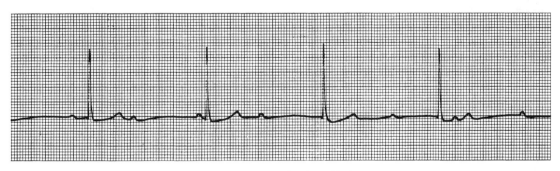

Figure 20-21. Complete heart block.

Disorders of the Bundle Branches and Fasicles

BUNDLE BRANCH BLOCKS

When one of the bundle branches is diseased, the QRS complex is wide (≥ 120 ms). Wide QRS complexes may result from disease in the bundle branches; abnormalities of the ventricular myocardium; or the effects of drugs, electrolyte, or metabolic disorders on the ventricular myocardium. Depending on the morphology of the QRS complex, these may be characterized as right bundle branch block (RBBB), left bundle branch block (LBBB), or nonspecific intraventricular conduction defects (IVCDs).

In right **bundle branch block** (Fig. 20-22), activation of the LV occurs before that of the RV. The initial force caused by left-to-right activation of the septum is normal. Consequently, the small Q waves seen in the inferior and lateral leads and the small R waves seen in leads V1 and V2 are unchanged. After the septum is depolarized, the impulse travels through the mass of the LV, generating the initial portion of the QRS complex. After the LV has been partially depolarized, the RV depolarizes, resulting in a terminal vector that is directed anteriorly and rightward. This results in a triphasic complex in lead V1, often described as a rabbit ears configuration or an RSR complex. The abnormal depolarization results in abnormal repolarization

with ST- and T-wave vectors directed away from the QRS complex in leads V1, V2, and sometimes V3. RBBB does not prohibit ECG interpretation of ST changes in leads other than V1, V2, and V3 during an exercise test.

In LBBB (Fig. 20-23), the initial force travels across the septum from right to left, altering the initial QRS deflection. This results in an initial negative deflection in lead VI and an initial upright deflection in lead V6. As the remainder of the LV is depolarized, the QRS vector continues to be toward V6. The depolarization of the RV is mainly obscured by that of the LV; therefore, little effect of RV depolarization on the vector forces is noted. The repolarization pattern is altered in LBBB, with the ST and T vector directed rightward and anteriorly. Consequently, the ECG may not be used to ascertain ischemic changes during an exercise study.

A QRS ≥ 120 ms without the morphology of RBBB or LBBB is best termed a nonspecific IVCD.

FASCICULAR BLOCKS

Disease in the fasicles of the left bundle branch results in minimal prolongation of the QRS complex. Fascicular block (hemiblocks) are recognized by their effects on the frontal plane axis. Left anterior **fascicular block** causes significant left axis deviation (> approximately 30 degrees), resulting in small Q waves in lead I and aVL and small R

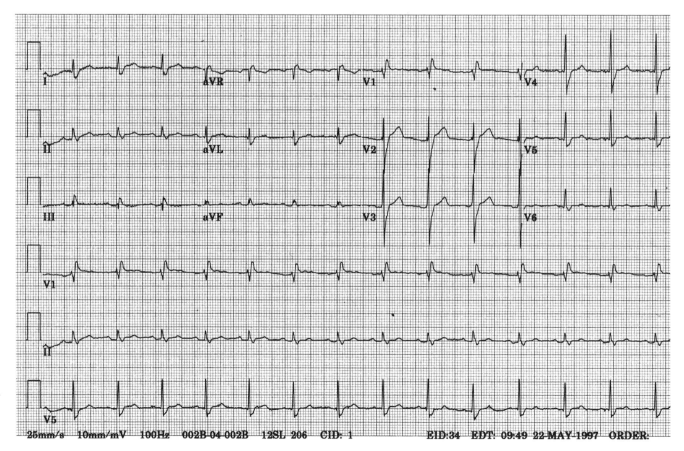

Figure 20-22. Normal sinus rhythm with right bundle branch block.

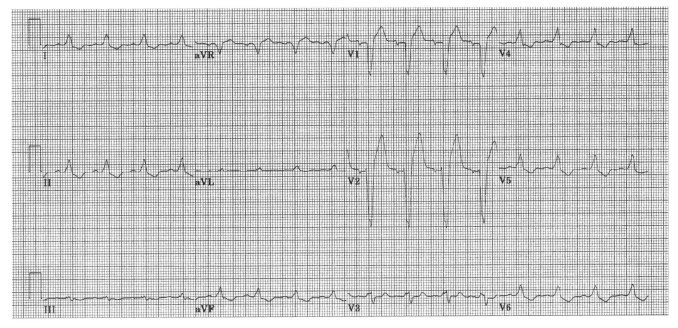

Figure 20-23. Normal sinus rhythm with left bundle branch block.

waves in leads II, III, and aVF. Left posterior fascicular block (Fig. 20-24) produces right axis deviation, (usually 90 to 110 degrees) with small Q waves in leads II, III, and aVF and a small R waves in leads I and aVL. Unlike left bundle branch, these entities have no adverse effect on the ability to interpret ECG changes during exercise tests.

Summary

Many derangements in the normal depolarization sequence may occur. Three mechanisms for dysrhythmia genesis have been described. By careful interpretation of the relationship between the P waves and QRS complexes

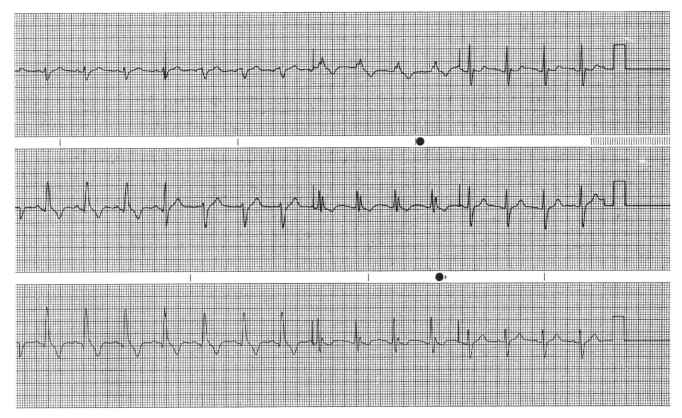

Figure 20-24. Normal sinus rhythm with right bundle branch block and left posterior fascicular block.

and the effect on other aspects of the ECG (i.e., axis, intervals, complex width, and P-wave and QRS vectors), one may readily ascertain the causes of tachydysrhythmias, bradydysrhythmias, AV-blocks and IVCDs.

SELECTED REFERENCES FOR FURTHER READING

Atwood S, Stanton C, Storey-Davenport J: Introduction to Basic Dysrhythmias, 3rd ed. St. Louis: Mosby; 2003

Huff J: ECG Workout: Exercises in Arrhythmia Interpretation, 4th ed. Philadelphia: JB Lippincott, 2002

Huzar RJ. Basic Dysrhythmias: Interpretation and Management, 3rd ed. St. Louis: Mosby; 2002

Lip GYH, Godtfredsen J: Cardiac Arrhythmias. St. Louis: Mosby; 2003.

INTERNET RESOURCES

The Alan E. Lindsay ECG Learning Center: http://medstat.med.utah. edu/kw/ecg

ECG Library: http://www.ecglibrary.com

EKG World Encyclopedia: http://sprojects.mmi.mcgill.ca/heart/egcyhome.html

Myocardial Ischemia and Infarction

JOHN A. LARRY AND STEPHEN F. SCHAAL

Myocardial ischemia is typically the result of the myocardium not receiving an adequate supply of oxygen to meet the current metabolic needs and is a reversible phenomenon. Myocardial infarction (MI) occurs when a portion of the myocardium receives an inadequate oxygen supply for several minutes or longer and results in the death of myocardial cells in the affected area. Certain changes are typically noted in the electrocardiogram (ECG) when either of these events occurs.

Myocardial Ischemia

Myocardial ischemia is best interpreted within the milieu of the entire clinical picture because the patient typically has chest pain or other signs or symptoms of ischemia (see Chapter 24). ECG changes associated with

Editor's Note: The information in Chapters 20 and 21 is limited to electrocardiographic (ECG) abnormalities frequently associated with exercise testing or training. For basic information regarding normal ECGs and additional types of abnormalities, readers are directed to the ECG reference texts listed at the end of this chapter.

ischemia include **ST-segment** depression or inversion of the **T waves** (Fig. 21-1 and GETP7 Fig. 6-1). Alteration in the ST segments and T waves is, in most cases, nonspecific, as numerous factors may contribute to similar appearing ST-segment and T-wave changes. Although symmetrically inverted T waves suggest ischemia, other disorders typically cause asymmetrical inversion. Although many ECGs are interpreted as nonspecific ST- and T-wave changes, some of these changes may actually be the result of myocardial ischemia. The location of the ischemia may be determined by noting, which leads exhibit the ST-segment or T-wave changes, as summarized in Table 21-1.

Exercise Electrocardiographic Testing

Monitoring the ECG during exercise testing affords the opportunity to detect *dysrhythmias* and to ascertain ischemic changes. Dysrhythmias, discussed in Chapter 20, may be provoked during or after exercise. It is important for individuals performing exercise testing to be comfortable with the interpretation of these rhythm disorders and the advanced cardiac life support (ACLS) protocols to treat them (see Chapter 28 and Appendix B).

The lead placement for an exercise ECG deviates slightly from the standard 12-lead ECG. The leads typically placed on the right and left wrists are moved proximally to the upper chest near the shoulders. The lower extremity leads are moved to the lower abdomen. These recording sites reduce the motion artifact that occurs with movement of the extremities during exercise.

A history and examination are necessary to rule out contraindications to exercise testing (see Box 3-5). ECG monitoring is continuous throughout the test and during the recovery. After exercise is initiated, a 12-lead ECG is recorded according to protocol and during any symptoms or change in heart rhythm. Monitoring should continue for 4 to 6 minutes during recovery or until changes on the ECG have resolved. Ischemia may induce several changes on the ECG; the most common change is ST-segment depression. When baseline ST abnormalities exist, the test becomes less specific. In addition to the magnitude of change, the character of the ST depression is important. Upsloping ST depression has less specificity for significant

KEY TERMS

Acute pericarditis: Infected or inflamed pericardium

Bundle branch blocks: Conduction block in either the left or right bundle branch; results in a wider (>0.12 sec) than normal QRS and a QRS configuration that is different for a left versus a right bundle branch block

Digitalis: A class of drugs called cardiac glycosides that increase the force of myocardial contraction and decreases heart rate

False-positive: A test result that indicates the presence of disease when no disease is present

Intrinsicoid deflection: The duration in seconds as measured from the start of the QRS complex to the peak of the R wave in that same QRS complex

Left ventricular hypertrophy: An increase in thickness of the left ventricular wall that results in increased amplitude of the R wave in leads over the left ventricle (V5, V6)

and increased amplitude in the S wave in leads over the right ventricle (V1, V2)

Pathological Q waves: Q waves that have a longer duration (>0.04 sec) than normal and greater amplitude (≥ one third the amplitude of the R wave in the same QRS complex

R waves: The first upward deflection in the QRS complex

ST segment: The line in the electrocardiogram connecting the end of the QRS to the beginning of the T wave; a measure of time from the end of ventricular depolarization to the start of ventricular repolarization

T waves: The wave or deflection on the electrocardiogram that reflects repolarization of the ventricles

Ventricular aneurysm: Thinning of the ventricular wall, resulting in a paradoxical bulging in that area during ventricular contraction

---

coronary disease than does horizontal or downsloping ST depression. Several clinical and ECG criteria exist for termination of the exercise test (see GETP7 Box 5-2).

Because the subendocardial area of the left ventricular apex region is most often rendered ischemic during exercise, the ST segment shifts in V4, V5, and V6 are the most sensitive for detection of ischemia.

Factors Affecting Interpretation of the ST Segment

Digitalis is a medication that interferes with the accurate interpretation of ST segment changes for myocardial ischemia. Digitalis is often used to treat patients with congestive heart failure or atrial dysrhythmias. In addition to its effect of prolonging the refractory period of the

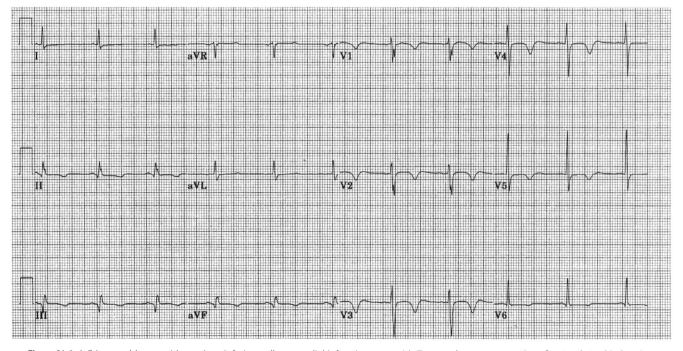

Figure 21-1. A 54-year-old man with previous inferior wall myocardial infarction now with T-wave changes suggestive of anterolateral ischemia.

TABLE 21-1. Locations of Myocardial Infarction and Ischemia

Location	Leads Affected
Anteroseptal	V1, V2
Anterior	V1–V4
Extensive anterior	V1–V6, I, aVL
Anterolateral	V3–V6, I, aVL
High lateral	I, aVL
Inferior	II, III, aVF
Posterior	V1, V2 (ST depression, tall R waves noted)

atrioventricular (AV) node, digitalis affects the ST segment and T wave. Figure 21-2 demonstrates these changes. The ST segment appears scooped out and depressed. These changes typically occur in the inferior and lateral leads. Digitalis may cause **false-positive** stress ECG findings, and additional imaging modalities may be required to increase the specificity of the study.

Left ventricular hypertrophy (LVH) or enlargement (Fig. 21-3), as detected by ECG, can also be a cause of ST-segment changes without the presence of ischemia. LVH is associated with two mechanisms: hypertrophy of the walls and dilatation of the chamber. LVH is an important ECG finding because it has been associated with increased morbidity and mortality. Increased voltage on the ECG tracing is the result of a greater mass of myocardium, which must be depolarized. Repolarization changes that develop with LVH classically are described as a strain pattern. The ST segments are depressed but ex-

hibit an upward convexity and blend into a biphasic or inverted T wave. This pattern is most commonly seen in the inferior and lateral leads. Often, left atrial enlargement can be found in association with LVH. The QRS width may increase, and the time from the R wave to the S wave, the **intrinsicoid deflection**, may also increase.

The presence of LVH on the baseline tracing may result in an indeterminate or false-positive stress ECG result. Because of this, evaluation for chest pain requires supplemental radionuclide imaging to confirm or exclude ischemia.

Myocardial Infarction

Myocardial infarction results when blood flow to a region of heart muscle is interrupted by total occlusion of a coronary artery (see Chapter 29). ECG changes occur as a result of the impairment of flow to the myocardium. The initial manifestation is elevation of the ST segment and peaking of the T waves. The ST-segment change is termed an *injury current*. The ST segments exhibit an upward convex shape, as shown in Figure 21-4, an example of anterior myocardial injury. Within hours or days, the T waves invert and the ST segment gradually returns to baseline. **Pathological Q waves** or loss of R waves may develop in the involved leads, depending on the location and extent of myocardial damage. These may develop soon after the occlusion or take several days to evolve. Q waves or loss of **R waves** are caused by the loss of electrical activity that normally results from the depolarization of that region of myocardium. MIs that do not develop Q

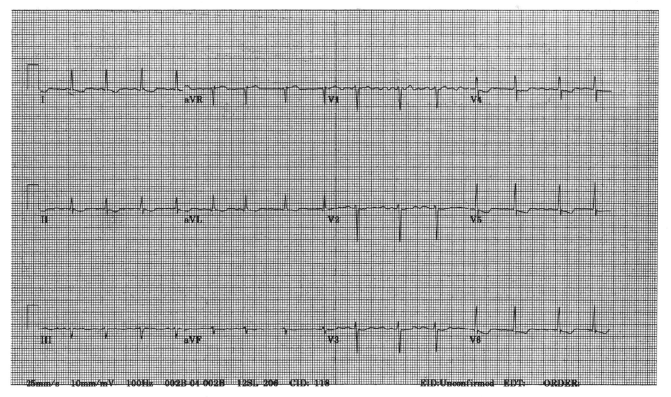

Figure 21-2. ST depression caused by digitalis. The rhythm is atrial fibrillation.

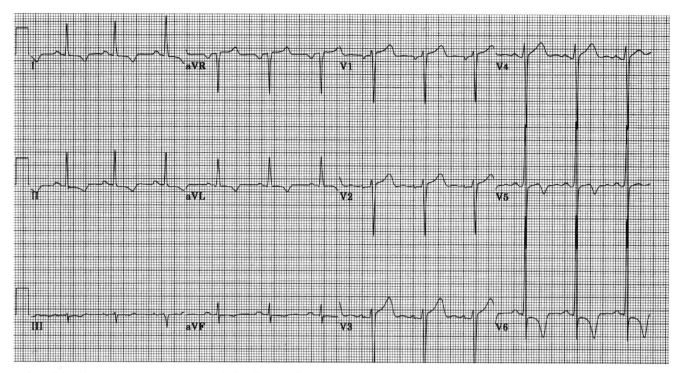

Figure 21-3. Left ventricular hypertrophy and left atrial enlargement.

waves are termed non–Q-wave infarcts. Patients with non–Q-wave infarcts have a better short-term but a worse long-term prognosis than patients with Q-wave infarcts.

The age of the infarct may be determined in relative terms. When ST elevation or hyperacute T waves are identified, acute injury is present. When Q waves are present, the ST segments have returned to baseline, and the T waves remain inverted, the infarct is recent, between 2 weeks and 1 year old. These are often read as in-

farcts of indeterminate age. When the only manifestation is the presence of Q waves and no ST or T-wave changes are present, the infarct is considered to be remote.

The ECG leads that exhibit changes permit determination of the region of MI (Table 21-1). Figure 21-5 is an ECG from a patient with acute inferior wall injury. Note the ST segment elevation in leads II, III, and aVF. Inspection of Figure 21-6 shows loss of R wave in the precordial leads consistent with an anterior wall MI. The ST changes have

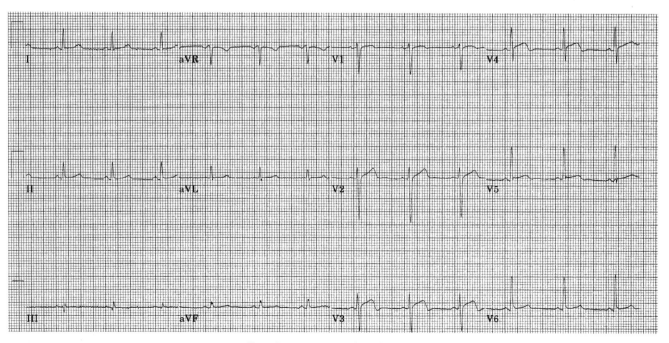

Figure 21-4. Acute anterolateral injury.

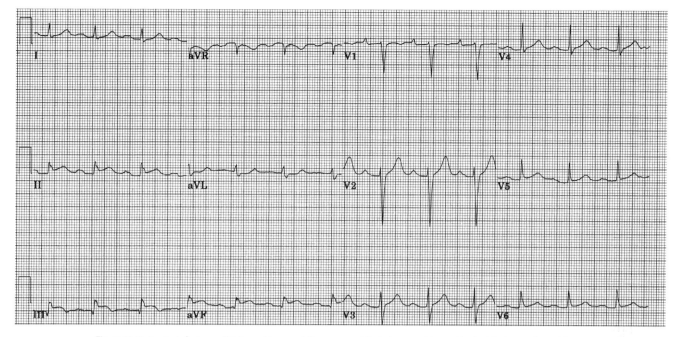

Figure 21-5. Acute inferior wall injury. Abnormal P waves and first-degree atrioventricular block are also evident.

resolved, but T-wave inversions persist in leads V6, I, and aVL, suggesting that this is a recent but not acute infarction.

A common difficulty is differentiation of pathological Q waves from those resulting from the normal depolarization sequence of the myocardium. The location, depth, and width of the Q waves may be useful in this determination. As previously stated, the normal vector loop of depolarization results in small Q waves in leads I, II, III, aVL, aVF, V5, and V6. These deflections are typically quite small in

amplitude and narrow in width (<30 ms). Significant Q waves are typically greater than 30 ms, often at least one third the height of the R wave, and occur in contiguous leads that reflect a particular region of the heart.

Myocardial infarction is not the only entity affecting ST segments. Causes of ST-segment elevation other than myocardial injury are common. Whereas pericardial inflammation present in **acute pericarditis** (Fig. 21-7) causes generalized ST-segment elevation (all ECG leads), acute injury

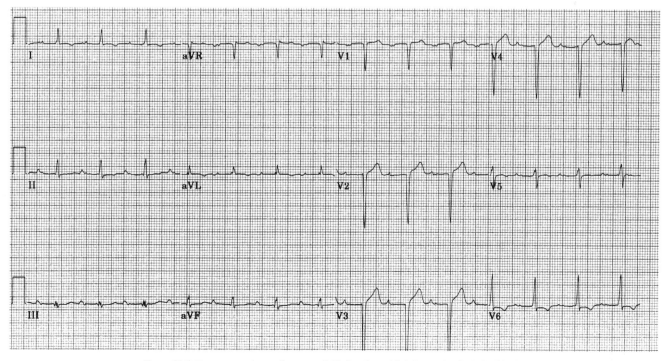

Figure 21-6. Recent anterior wall myocardial infarction with left anterior fasicular block.

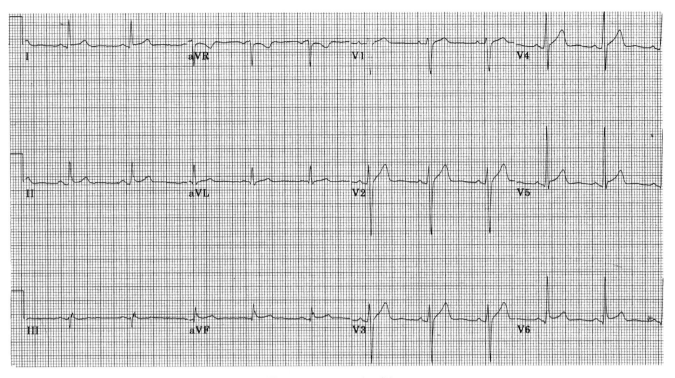

Figure 21-7. Acute pericarditis.

caused by an occluded coronary artery affects contiguous leads. In general, whereas the ST segment typically has an upward concave appearance in pericarditis, the appearance is convex upward in the setting of myocardial injury.

Benign repolarization variants (also called early repolarization) are another common cause of ST-segment elevation. These variants are most commonly seen in young African American men but may be seen in other patients as well. Elevation of the J point from the baseline is present. The ST segments are elevated but exhibit a concave upward appearance; this helps in the differentiation from myocardial injury (Fig. 21-8).

Bundle branch blocks (see Figs. 20-22 and 20-23) also exert influence on the ST segment. In a left bundle branch, the ST vector is directed away from the QRS vector, resulting in elevated ST segments in the right precordial leads,

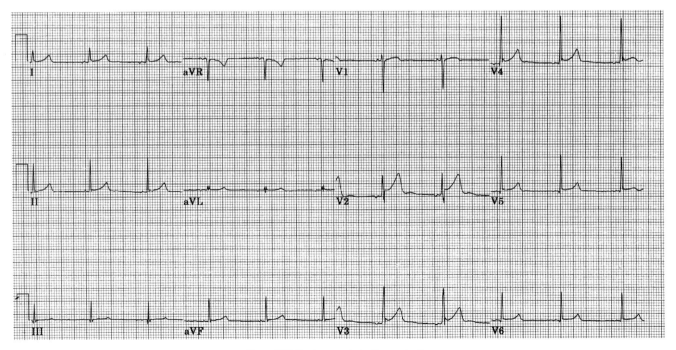

Figure 21-8. Benign repolarization variant.

which makes any changes in the ST segment during exercise uninterpretable for ischemia (see Fig. 20-23).

Persistent ST-segment elevation after an infarction may suggest **ventricular aneurysm** formation. This typically involves the anterior wall of the left ventricle and occurs after large infarcts. The presence of Q waves in the involved leads in a patient after MI suggests this diagnosis.

Summary

Electrocardiography is useful in determining the presence of acute or remote infarctions and may detect resting ischemia. Combining exercise testing with ECG recording is a useful strategy for evaluating patients for exertional angina.

SELECTED REFERENCES FOR FURTHER READING

Dubin D: Rapid Interpretation of EKG's: An Interactive Course. Tampa: Cover Publishing Company; 2001.

Huzar RJ: Basic Dysrhythmias: Interpretation and Management, 3rd ed. St. Louis: Mosby; 2002.

Thaler MS: The Only EKG Book You'll Ever Need, 4th ed. Philadelphia: Lippincott, Williams & Wilkins; 2003.

Wagner GS: Marriott's Practical Electrocardiography, 10th ed. Philadelphia: Lippincott, Williams & Wilkins;, 2001.

INTERNET RESOURCES

The Alan E. Lindsay ECG Learning Center: http://medstat.med.utah. edu/kw/ecg

ECG Library: http://www.ecglibrary.com

EKG World Encyclopedia: http://sprojects.mmi.mcgill.ca/heart/egcyhome.html

Exercise Prescription, Exercise Programming, and Adaptations to Exercise Training

SECTION EDITOR: STEPHEN C. GLASS, PhD, FACSM

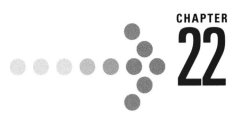

Cardiopulmonary Adaptations to Exercise

STEVEN J. KETEYIAN AND CLINTON A. BRAWNER

This chapter addresses KSAs from the following content areas:

1 Exercise Physiology and Related Exercise Science
2 Pathophysiology and Risk Factors
3 Health Appraisal, Fitness, and Clinical Exercise Testing
4 Electrocardiography and Diagnostic Techniques
5 Patient Management and Medications
6 Medical and Surgical Management
7 Exercise Prescription and Programming
8 Nutrition and Weight Management
9 Human Behavior and Counseling
10 Safety, Injury Prevention, and Emergency Procedures
11 Program Administration, Quality Assurance, and Outcome Assessment

---

Every day, we engage in some type of physical activity. It may be carrying a load of laundry up one flight of stairs, washing a car, playing soccer, or running an 800-m race. In each case, however, the heart and pulmonary systems must alter their function in a manner that allows them to complete the activity. Additionally, repeated and regular exposure to physical activity or sports stimulates the body to acquire permanent adaptations, and it does so in a manner that is usually quite favorable in terms of both performance and health. Exercise training principles and exercise prescription recommendations are reviewed in GETP7 Chapter 7 and in Chapter 24 of this Resource Manual.

This chapter summarizes the chronic adaptations (training effects) that develop in the cardiac and pulmonary systems (cardiopulmonary system) when an individual repeatedly performs exercise. Acute responses to exercise were reviewed in Chapter 3. It also describes the loss of these training adaptations that occurs when an individual stops training. Whenever possible, the chapter provides examples and data comparing healthy, unconditioned individuals with well-trained athletes because doing so helps exemplify how the cardiac and pulmonary systems adjust to chronic exercise.

Chronic Adaptations to Exercise

MAXIMAL OXYGEN CONSUMPTION

Physical inactivity is a major contributing risk factor for heart disease, with an overall risk that is similar to elevated blood cholesterol, cigarette smoking, and hypertension[1]. Moreover, longitudinal studies show that higher levels of aerobic or **cardiorespiratory fitness** ($\dot{V}O_{2max}$) are associated with a lower mortality rate from heart disease, even after statistical adjustments for other disease-related risk factors[2]. It is important to note that cardiorespiratory fitness relies greatly on the effective integration of the cardiac and pulmonary systems, as it pertains to the movement, exchange, and circulation of gases (e.g., O_2 and CO_2) into and through the body. To better appreciate the effect of exercise training on $\dot{V}O_{2max}$, it is appropriate to physiologically define it by rearranging the classic Fick equation (Adolph Fick, circa 1870):

$$\dot{V}O_2 = \text{Heart rate (HR)} \times \text{Stroke volume} \times \text{a-}\bar{V}O_2 \text{ diff}$$

Where:

$\dot{V}O_2$ = oxygen consumption ($mL \cdot kg^{-1} \cdot min^{-1}$)

HR = number of times per minute that the heart contracts (bpm).

Stroke volume = volume of blood ejected from the left ventricle per heart beat ($mL \cdot min^{-1}$).

a-$\bar{V}O_2$ diff = Arteriovenous oxygen difference (i.e., arterio = mixed venous O_2 difference, mL of O_2 per liter of blood.)

Based on this equation, it should be clear that cardiorespiratory fitness (i.e., $\dot{V}O_{2max}$) is defined as the ability of the body to transport (i.e., central transport or cardiac output) and use (i.e., a-$\bar{V}O_{2\text{ diff}}$) oxygen. Both of these components can impact the magnitude of the measure and both can be influenced by age, gender, regular exercise training, detraining, bed rest, different environments (e.g., hypobaria, microgravity), use of certain medications, and illness. For example, a person with chronic heart failure may experience increased breathlessness during exertion because of a reduced ability to circulate blood to the metabolically active skeletal muscles.

KEY TERMS

Cardiac hypertrophy: Increase in the size of the heart; among athletes, the increase may be caused by an increase in the size of the ventricles or an increase in the ventricular wall thickness, but the observed increase should not exceed the upper limit for a normal-sized heart.

Cardiorespiratory fitness: The ability of the body to transport and use oxygen

Detraining: Changes in body structure or function caused by reduction or cessation of regular physical training

Dyspnea: Labored breathing; shortness of breath disproportionate to the work being performed

Myocardial oxygen consumption: The amount of oxygen used by the heart; expressed as milliliters of O_2 per 100 g of muscle per minute

Ultimately, improving exercise performance for most people is dependent, in part, on the ability of the cardiopulmonary system to adapt. Generally, most exercise studies involving healthy people demonstrate 10% to 30% increases in $\dot{V}O_{2max}$, with the greatest relative improvements among the least fit[3]. Among national- or Olympic-level Nordic skiers or runners, $\dot{V}O_{2max}$ may exceed 80 $mL \cdot kg^{-1} \cdot min^{-1}$ in men and approach 70 $mL \cdot kg^{-1} \cdot min^{-1}$ in women[4].

Because an absolute submaximal work rate (e.g., walking at 2 mph) requires a fixed aerobic or oxygen requirement, physically trained individuals work at a lower percentage of their $\dot{V}O_{2max}$, especially during tasks of daily living. Enhanced oxygen transport, particularly increased maximal stroke volume and cardiac output, is traditionally regarded as the primary mechanism underlying the increase in $\dot{V}O_{2max}$ with training. Other favorable changes during submaximal or peak exercise that reflect improved cardiorespiratory fitness include changes in HR, arteriovenous oxygen difference (a-$\bar{V}O_{2\ diff}$), blood lactate, and ventilation. Table 22-1 summarizes the cardiopulmonary adaptations to exercise training in previously unconditioned persons.

It is important to point out that the above-mentioned increases in $\dot{V}O_{2max}$ are usually associated with participation in an aerobic or large motor activity such as walking, swimming, running, in-line skating, or Nordic skiing. Resistance training, both isotonic (concentric) and isometric, may have a small effect, if any, on improving cardiopulmonary health or fitness (see Chapter 23). However, a balanced conditioning program that incorporates both aerobic training and dynamic resistance training is preferred, which helps clients and patients improve both their health and performance.

CARDIAC PERFORMANCE

Regular endurance exercise training in previously sedentary, apparently healthy people is associated with improved stamina, an improved ability to tolerate routine

TABLE 22-1. Physiologic Responses to Regular Aerobic Conditioning in Untrained Individuals

Variable[a]	Unit of Measure	Response
$\dot{V}O_{2max}$	$mL \cdot kg^{-1} \cdot min^{-1}$ or $mL \cdot min^{-1}$	↑
Resting HR	bpm	↓
Exercise HR (submax)	bpm	↓
Maximum HR	bpm	↔ (or slight ↓)
a-$\bar{V}O_{2diff}$	$mL\ O_2$/100 mL blood	↑
Maximum minute ventilation	$L \cdot min^{-1}$	↑
Stroke volume	$mL \cdot beat^{-1}$	↑
Cardiac output	$L \cdot min^{-1}$	↑
Blood volume (resting)	Liters	↑
Systolic BP	mm Hg	↔ (or slight ↑)
Blood lactate	mL/100 mL blood	↑
Oxidative capacity skeletal muscle	Multiple variables[b]	↑

[a]At maximum exercise unless otherwise specified.

[b]Increases in skeletal muscle mitochondrial number and size, capillary density, or oxidative enzymes.

↑ = increase; ↓ = decrease; ↔ = no change; BP = blood pressure; HR = heart rate.

activities of daily living, and less fatigue during the day, often occurring within just weeks after starting a program. These changes in healthy people are partly caused by an improved cardiac or central response to exercise.

Patients with coronary artery disease (CAD) who undergo aerobic training also experience improved function and often experience a decrease in angina symptoms. In fact, until the late 1980s, when evidence was presented that regular exercise in these patients improved clinical outcome (i.e., mortality), a primary reason for referring these patients to cardiac rehabilitation programs was symptom management. These reasons, along with the fact that most patients with clinically manifest CAD have below normal cardiorespiratory fitness (50% to 70% of age, gender-predicted), support the use of cardiac rehabilitation among eligible individuals. However, unlike untrained healthy people who experience an exercise training–related improvement in exercise capacity that is partly caused by improved central or cardiac function, improvement in exercise function in patients with CAD appears to be primarily mediated by improved peripheral oxygen utilization (see Chapter 30).

HEART RATE

Heart rate and stroke volume both contribute to increases in cardiac output during a single bout of acute exercise. However, among unconditioned persons, exercise causes a proportionally greater increase in HR at any fixed submaximal work rate compared with better-conditioned persons. Therefore, in untrained persons, HR plays a greater role in increasing cardiac output (than stroke volume) during graded exercise[5].

Chronic exercise training induces a reduction in myocardial oxygen demand at rest and during exercise and a reduction in resting HR (~10 bpm decrease) that may be caused by altered autonomic function or a direct effect within the myocardium. Maximal HR is unchanged or slightly decreased (3 to 10 bpm) after aerobic conditioning[4]. The latter is probably attributed to two training adaptations: **cardiac hypertrophy** via an increase in the size of the ventricular cavity and decreased sympathetic drive.

STROKE VOLUME

Stroke volume, the second factor used in determining cardiac output, increases during an exercise bout secondary to (a) increased venous return (Frank-Starling mechanism), which allows left ventricular end-diastolic volume to remain unchanged or increase slightly and (b) increased contractile state (perhaps by neurohormonal influences)[6–8]. Chronic aerobic exercise training leads to cardiac hypertrophy, usually characterized by normal wall thicknesses and an enlarged ventricular chamber that does not usually exceed the upper limits of normal (normal < 56 mm). For example, left ventricular end-diastolic

diameter may approach 55 mm in highly trained endurance athletes versus less than 45 mm in non-active, age-matched unconditioned people[4]. One important factor contributing to this adaptation of the left ventricle is the 10–15% increase in blood volume that develops soon (days) after starting an exercise training program[9]. Finally, another contributing factor induced by chronic training is that it likely strengthens myocardial tissue and enables more forceful contractions[10–13]. The result is an augmented ejection of end-diastolic volume (i.e., increased ejection fraction).

Comparatively, cardiorespiratory training allows conditioned individuals to increase ejection fraction to a greater degree than their sedentary counterparts; hence, stroke volume is higher in conditioned individuals at any fixed or relative submaximal work rate. The increased stroke volume caused by training allows conditioned individuals to exercise at similar absolute work rates but with a lower HR, thus decreasing the myocardial oxygen demand of submaximal exercise[7,8]. The increase in ejection fraction is generally quite modest, if at all, approximating 5% to 10% during maximal exercise.

The above-mentioned cardiovascular morphological characteristics, along with increases in central blood volume and total hemoglobin, are closely correlated with the $\dot{V}O_{2max}$.

CARDIAC OUTPUT

Maximum cardiac output is significantly higher in trained than in untrained individuals, primarily because of the ability to increase stroke volume[4,10]. Among endurance-trained male subjects, maximal cardiac output can easily exceed 30 L·min^{-1}, which represents a five- to sixfold increase over resting values. In fact, in elite class endurance athletes, it is common to observe maximal cardiac outputs near 40 L·min^{-1}. Generally, the higher the maximal cardiac output, the higher the maximal aerobic power or $\dot{V}O_{2max}$. However, cardiac output is essentially the same at any fixed submaximal work rate, in both conditioned and unconditioned individuals[10].

ARTERIOVENOUS OXYGEN DIFFERENCE

A final major contributor to the training-induced increase in $\dot{V}O_2$ is an improved a-$\bar{V}O_{2diff}$ during exercise. The difference between arterial and venous content of oxygen in blood reflects the ability of skeletal muscle tissue to extract and use oxygen[10,14]. Chronic endurance-type training increases the number of capillaries surrounding each muscle fiber[4] and enhances the activity of the mitochondrial enzymes used in aerobic metabolism, thereby enhancing the ability to extract and use the oxygen that is transported in circulating blood. This increased ability to transport oxygen to the working skeletal muscle and to remove and use it for generating energy is a hallmark of aerobic training.

a-$\bar{V}O_{2diff}$ is similar in trained and untrained persons at submaximal levels of exercise. However, at $\dot{V}O_{2max}$, a-vDO₂ is greater in trained than untrained persons (e.g., 135 mL·L^{-1} vs. 155 mL·L^{-1} in untrained versus trained athletes, respectively).

BLOOD PRESSURE AND BLOOD FLOW

Systolic blood pressure (BP) increases in a relatively linear fashion with cardiac output (and $\dot{V}O_2$) during exercise. Mean arterial BP can be expressed as follows:

$$BP_{mean} \sim CO \times T_SP_R$$

Where:

BP_{mean} = mean arterial blood pressure

CO = cardiac output

T_SP_R = total systemic peripheral resistance

Primary control of BP is regulated by adjusting T_SP_R, which is accomplished by (a) neural mechanisms affecting peripheral arterioles, (b) locally released substances called *endothelial-derived relaxing factors* (the most studied is nitric oxide), and (c) changes in local chemistry (temperature and hydrogen ion, adenosine, and potassium ion concentrations) within the metabolically more active skeletal muscles[15–17]. There is vasoconstriction in some areas (e.g., splanchnic areas) during exercise and vasodilation in others (e.g., skeletal muscle and myocardium). The net or overall effect is a decreased T_SP_R[4,18]. These changes in vasomotor tone allows for a 15-fold or more increase in blood flow to the metabolically active skeletal muscles, a reduction of blood flow to the splanchnic areas, an increase in blood flow to the heart, and no change in blood flow to the brain.

Systolic BP increases during progressive exercise in healthy individuals because the magnitude of the increase in cardiac output is greater than the decrease in T_SP_R. Diastolic BP remains constant or may decrease slightly in both conditioned and unconditioned individuals. At any fixed submaximal workload, conditioned individuals demonstrate a comparable or lower change in systolic BP than untrained individuals. Relative to $\dot{V}O_{2max}$, systolic BP is lower in trained than untrained people. In individuals with known mild or moderate high BP (i.e., hypertension), regular exercise training lowers both systolic and diastolic pressures approximately 6 to 8 mm Hg at rest (see Chapter 31 and GETP7 Chapter 9). The proposed mechanisms responsible for this decrease include neurohumoral, vascular, and structural adaptations. A decrease in plasma catecholamines, improved insulin sensitivity, and favorable changes in endogenous vasoconstricting and vasodilating agents are also postulated as being responsible for the antihypertensive effects of regular exercise. It is important to point out that after completing a bout of endurance exercise, BPs can remain below pre-exercise values for up to 22 hours.

RATE–PRESSURE PRODUCT

At rest, the heart consumes about 70% of the oxygen brought to it in the blood flowing through the coronary arteries, which is almost three times more than what is consumed by the skeletal muscles at rest. As a result, the heart responds to increased demand for oxygen by increasing blood flow. In fact, coronary blood flow can increase some fourfold during exercise, from 250 mL·min^{-1} to approximately 1000 mL·min^{-1}.

The main factors that influence **myocardial oxygen demand or consumption** are HR, left ventricular size, and myocardial oxygen contractility. However, except for HR, it is difficult to gather these measures in most exercise physiology laboratories. Instead, prior studies have shown that the product of HR and systolic BP provides a reasonable estimate of myocardial oxygen demand, called the *rate–pressure product*.

During exercise, the rate–pressure product increases in direct proportion to increases in HR and systolic BP. After several weeks or more of exercise training, the rate–pressure product during exercise still increases; however, the magnitude of the increase is less compared with pretraining values. This attenuated increase is attributable to the previously mentioned chronic adaptations in HR and BP, both of which increase less after training and translate to a lesser increase in rate–pressure product and myocardial oxygen demand. Chapter 30 provides a detailed summary of how rate–pressure product is used to assess the effects of exercise training in patients with myocardial ischemia.

PULMONARY FUNCTION

Because of the pulmonary system's ability to respond quickly to acute exercise and the fact that it does not limit maximal exercise, the demand on it to adapt to exercise training is less than other systems (e.g., cardiovascular, skeletal muscle). However, there are several pulmonary-related adaptations that are worth mentioning that result from a physical conditioning regimen.

Before discussing these adaptations, it is important to point out that among patients with pulmonary diseases, such as those with chronic bronchitis, emphysema, or asthma, limitations in pulmonary function caused by the disease often minimizes expected physiological gains attributable to exercise training (see Chapter 32 and GETP7 Chapter 9). Also, the **dyspnea** or labored breathing that is associated with so many pulmonary disorders often causes individuals to avoid being active, which leads to a vicious circle of further self-imposed restriction of activity. This does not mean that these patients do not improve exercise tolerance as a result of participating in an exercise or pulmonary rehabilitation program. Both submaximal endurance and total walking time are usually improved, but typically with little change in $\dot{V}O_{2max}$.

MINUTE VENTILATION

Minute ventilation during exercise is augmented by increasing tidal volume and breathing frequency, and it is controlled by neural and chemical factors and by sensory mechanisms within the lungs and breathing muscles. Although ventilation generally does not limit exercise performance in apparently healthy individuals, the limits of ventilation may be reached at $\dot{V}O_{2max}$ in elite athletes[4].

After a program of structured, regular exercise, minute ventilation is unchanged at rest, at approximately 6 $L \cdot min^{-1}$ (tidal volume ~500 mL·breath^{-1}; breathing frequency ~12/min). However; minute ventilation at maximal exercise is increased after training, with the increase attributable to increases in both maximal tidal volume and breathing frequency. Tidal volume and breathing frequency may approach 3000 mL·breath^{-1} and 55 breaths/min, respectively.

Whereas untrained college-aged individuals may achieve a peak ventilation of 120 $L \cdot min^{-1}$, a 60 year-old patient with heart disease may achieve a peak value of 60 to 80 $L \cdot min^{-1}$. In both cases, it is reasonable to assume that a regular exercise training program will increase maximal minute ventilation by 15% to 25%. In contrast, well-conditioned male and female athletes may achieve maximal ventilation that approaches 200 $L \cdot min^{-1}$ and 150 $L \cdot min^{-1}$, respectively. Although exercise training may increase maximal ventilatory capacity, it is unclear that this provides any advantage other than increased buffering capacity for lactate.

Minute ventilation at a standardized submaximal work rate might not change with training, or it may decrease. One likely reason for the latter is the decreased production of lactate attributable to training, which coincides with a decreased need to buffer this metabolic byproduct and, therefore, decreased ventilation. Keep in mind that changes in ventilation during exercise are in response to neural and chemical feedback mechanisms (see Chapter 3). There is also increased ventilatory efficiency, as evidenced by a reduced ventilatory equivalent for oxygen ($\dot{V}_E/\dot{V}O_2$) in trained, compared with untrained, individuals.

PULMONARY DIFFUSION CAPACITY

Diffusion capacity is defined as the volume of gas that diffuses through a membrane each minute for a pressure difference of 1 mm Hg. During exercise, diffusion capacity increases in a near-linear manner, before leveling off near peak exercise. This pattern is observed in trained and untrained individuals, regardless of gender.

At rest and during submaximal and peak exercise, diffusion capacity is greater in endurance-trained individuals. Among untrained and trained individuals, maximal diffusion capacity may approach 54 and 74 mL O_2/min/mm Hg, respectively[4]. Interestingly, it is common to note that the resting diffusion of well-trained runners may approach the peak values observed at maximal exercise in unconditioned individuals. The precise mechanism responsible for the increase in diffusion capacity with training is not known.

BLOOD LACTATE, ANAEROBIC THRESHOLD, AND VENTILATORY THRESHOLD

Unlike $\dot{V}O_2$, which progressively increases during incremental exercise to exhaustion, blood lactate is essentially unchanged until $\dot{V}O_2$ exceeds approximately 50% of maximum. The point at which blood lactate demonstrates a nonlinear increase is called the *lactate threshold* or *onset of blood lactate accumulation*, and it occurs among most people at a blood concentration approximating 4 mmol·L^{-1}. At rest, blood lactate is approximately 0.5 mmol·L^{-1} to 1.0 mmol·L^{-1}; during or after exercise, it may exceed 10 to 12 mmol·L^{-1}. In fact, among elite and well-motivated athletes, it may approach 16 mmol·L^{-1} during exhaustive exercise[4].

Some exercise scientists suggest that the lactate threshold is directly related to an event called anaerobic threshold, with the lactate threshold representing that point during exercise at which anaerobic glycolysis markedly increases to supplement energy production in metabolically more active skeletal muscle because demand for oxygen within cellular mitochondria outpaces supply (see Chapter 3). We are quick to point out; however, that a direct connection between blood lactate threshold and anaerobic threshold is not appreciated by all scientists. One reason for this is that several factors can contribute to the blood lactate threshold, including increased anaerobic glycolysis in the metabolically active skeletal muscles (i.e., increased production of lactic acid), increased recruitment of type II muscle fibers, and decreased blood flow to tissues responsible to remove lactate from the blood (e.g., liver, kidneys).

Blood lactate concentrations throughout submaximal exercise are all reduced as a result of exercise training (Fig. 22-1). This means that at any fixed submaximal work rate, blood lactate concentration is lower. Conversely, with training, the velocity (e.g., running, swimming, cycling) at the onset of lactate threshold is increased, reflecting improved performance. In fact, among athletes, it is common to guide training intensity using lactate threshold. For example, elite male rowers and swimmers often periodically have HR at lactate threshold identified, then use HR alone to train at, just below or just above lactate threshold. As these athletes adapt physiologically, they notice a decrease in HR at a certain pace, forcing them to increase their pace in order to again achieve the training level initially specified.

Although the precise physiological adaptations responsible for the above-mentioned decrease in blood lactate during submaximal exercise are not known, there are several possibilities. These include a smaller oxygen deficit incurred at the beginning of exercise attributable to a faster adjustment of oxygen uptake relative to energy demand; a greater use of the lactate produced during exercise as a fuel source for energy (via the Cori cycle in the liver); and

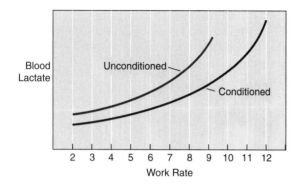

Figure 22-1. Blood lactate concentration during progressive exercise in conditioned versus unconditioned persons. The conditioned response typically exhibits lower lactate concentrations at any given work rate than unconditioned but has higher maximum lactate at $\dot{V}O_{2}max$.

exercise training-induced increases in the size of skeletal muscle mitochondria and in the concentration of enzymes involved in fatty acid oxidation. Concerning the latter, the net result is an improved ability of the skeletal muscle to use fatty acids and to operate aerobically during prolonged exercise versus having to rely sooner on anaerobic glycolysis to generate adenosine trisphosphate (ATP).

From a practical point of view, measuring blood lactate during exercise is not common. It requires willing participants and some additional equipment that is not routinely available in most health and medical fitness centers. Fortunately, lactate threshold can be relatively easily identified using one or a combination of several non-invasive respiratory parameters, most all of which rely on measuring expired air during exercise (so-called ventilatory-derived anaerobic threshold). One common method is the V-slope method, which involves plotting the volume of carbon dioxide exhaled as a function of $\dot{V}O_{2}$ through incremental exercise to maximum. Ventilatory threshold usually occurs somewhere between 60% and 80% of $\dot{V}O_{2max}$; with training, the $\dot{V}O_{2}$ at ventilatory threshold increases 10% to 25%.

Detraining and Bed Rest

Although exercise training promotes a variety of physiological adaptations, long periods of inactivity (i.e., detraining) are associated with a reversal of many of these favorable chronic changes. This detraining concept implies that when physical training is stopped or reduced, the bodily systems readjust in accordance with the diminished physiological stimuli. Because endurance exercise training generally improves cardiovascular function and promotes metabolic adaptations within the exercising skeletal musculature, the reversibility of these specific adaptations is now considered.

Before describing the changes that occur with detraining, we ask that you not limit your thinking to just those times when an active person stops exercising but also consider the magnitude of loss in cardiac and peripheral muscle aerobic function that occurs when an individual is confined to bed for several days or more. An example of

this is a person who suffers a myocardial infarction (MI) and is then confined to bed while in the hospital. In the 1970s, such a person may have been ordered to bed for 7 to 10 days out of a 3-week hospital stay. Upon arriving home from the hospital, these people often complained of being easily fatigued and having a loss of stamina throughout the day, much of it caused by the marked detraining effect that occurred within just 1 week of bed rest.

Conversely, patients who now suffer an uncomplicated MI are allowed to ambulate up and down the hospital's hallway within 48 to 72 hours of their event and find themselves discharged for home within 4 days or so (see Chapter 31 and GETP7 Chapter 8). The direct connection here is that much less time is spent in bed, which means much less detraining and preserved exercise tolerance and $\dot{V}O_{2max}$.

MAXIMAL OXYGEN CONSUMPTION

Mild to moderate endurance training increases $\dot{V}O_{2max}$ by 10% to 30%, mostly attributable to increases in cardiac output and stroke volume[5,18]. Conversely, prolonged detraining (8 to 10 weeks or more) has been reported to result in a complete return of $\dot{V}O_{2max}$ to pretraining levels[19]. Generally, $\dot{V}O_{2max}$ values decline rapidly during the first month of inactivity, with a slower decline to untrained levels occurring during the second and third months of detraining[4,20–22]. Therefore, the available evidence suggests that increases in $\dot{V}O_{2max}$ produced by endurance training involving exercise of low to moderate intensities and durations are totally reversed after several months of detraining and adoption of a more sedentary lifestyle.

Whether years of intensive endurance training result in a more persistent maintenance of $\dot{V}O_{2max}$ after subsequent inactivity than do shorter periods of less intensive training has also been studied[23]. Figure 22-2 illustrates

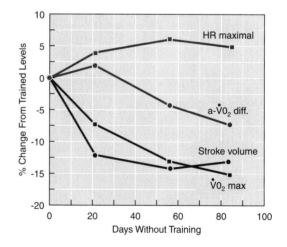

Figure 22-2. Effects of detraining on percent changes in stroke volume during exercise, maximal oxygen uptake ($\dot{V}O_{2max}$), maximal heart rate (HR), and maximal arteriovenous oxygen difference (a-$\dot{V}O_{2diff}$). (Adapted with permission from Coyle EF, Martin WH 3rd, Sinacore DR, et al: Time course of loss adaptations after stopping prolonged intense endurance training. J Appl Physiol 57:1857–1864, 1984.)

the time course of the decline in $\dot{V}O_{2max}$ and related variables (maximal stroke volume, HR, and a-$\bar{V}O_{2diff}$) when subjects become sedentary after training intensively for approximately 10 years. Note the rapid 7% decline in $\dot{V}O_{2max}$ in the first 12 to 21 days and its association with a marked decline in maximal stroke volume. Table 22-2 summarizes the changes associated with detraining at the central and peripheral levels[23–25].

STROKE VOLUME AND HEART SIZE

As already mentioned, whereas prolonged and intensive endurance training promotes increased heart mass (i.e., cardiac hypertrophy), detraining results in decreased heart mass[18,26,27]. However, it is not clear whether training-induced increases in left ventricular dimension and myocardial contractility regress totally with inactivity. Athletes who become sedentary have larger hearts and higher $\dot{V}O_{2max}$ than those of people who have never trained[28].

One of the most striking effects of detraining in endurance-trained individuals is the rapid decline in stroke volume. To gain information regarding the cause of this large marked and rapid decline, Martin et al.[29] measured stroke volume during exercise in trained subjects in both the upright and supine positions and again after 21 and 56 days of inactivity (Fig. 22-3). Simultaneous measurements of the diameter of the left ventricle were obtained using echocardiography. The large decline in stroke volume during upright cycling was associated with parallel reductions in the diameter of the left ventricle at end-diastole (LVEDD). However, when the subjects exercised in the supine position, which usually augments ventricular filling because of increased venous return from elevated lower extremities, reduction in LVEDD was minimal. As a result, stroke volume during exercise in the supine position was maintained within a few percent of trained levels during the 56-day detrain-

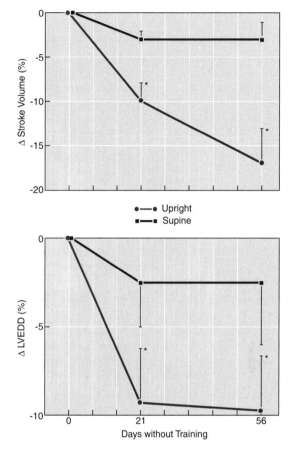

Figure 22-3. Percent decline in exercise stroke volume (**A**) and left ventricle at end-diastole (LVEDD), measured by echocardiography (**B**) during exercise in upright and supine postures when trained and after 21 and 56 days of inactivity.* Responses in upright position are significantly ($P < 0.05$) lower than in supine position and lower than when trained (i.e., day 0). (Reprinted with permission from Costill DL, Fink WJ, Hargreaves M, et al: Metabolic characteristics of skeletal muscle during detraining from competitive swimming. Med Sci Sports Exerc17:339–343, 1985.)

TABLE 22-2. Data for Control Subjects Compared with Highly Trained Athletes and After 3 Months of Detraining

	Sedentary Control	% Difference from Control	
		Trained	**Detrained**
$\dot{V}O_{2max}$ (mL·kg^{-1}·min^{-1})	43.3	143[a]	117[ab]
Stroke volume (mL)	128.0	120[a]	101[a]
Maximum a-vDO$_2$ (mL/100 mL blood)	12.6	122	116[ab]
Citrate synthase activity (mol·kg^{-1}·hr^{-1})	4.1	243[a]	149[ab]
Whole muscle fibers			
Type I fibers	4.8	140[a]	108[ab]
Type II fibers	2.6	246[a]	180[ab]
Capillary density (cap/mm$_2$)	318.0	146[a]	150[a]

[a]Higher ($P \geq 0.05$) than sedentary control.

[b]Detrained lower ($P \geq 0.05$) than trained.

Adapted from Coyle et al.[23], Coyle et al.[24], and Costill et al.[25].

ing period (see Fig. 22-3). These observations indicate that cardiac filling is an important factor in establishing stroke volume during exercise and that when it declines, perhaps as a result of reductions in blood volume, stroke volume also declines.

Not all studies report a decline in left ventricular mass or $\dot{V}O_{2max}$ when endurance-trained subjects stop training. Cullinane et al.[30] found that 10 days of detraining in runners did not alter $\dot{V}O_{2max}$ or echocardiographically determined left ventricular mass. Furthermore, Pavlik et al.[31] reported that 60 days of detraining resulted in no reduction in LVEDD while at rest. Houmard et al.[32] found $\dot{V}O_{2max}$ to decline 4% when a runner stopped training for 14 days and endurance performance declined 9%.

BLOOD VOLUME

It appears that rapid detraining-induced reduction of stroke volume during exercise in the upright position is related to decreased blood volume (Fig. 22-4)[33]. Intensive exercise training usually results in the blood volume's increasing by approximately 500 mL through the expansion of plasma volume[9,34]. This adaptation is gained after only a few bouts of exercise but quickly reverses when training ceases. Therefore, the decline in stroke volume and the increase in HR during submaximal exercise, which normally accompany several weeks of detraining, can be reversed, returning to near-trained levels when the blood volume expands to a level similar to that of trained subjects (Fig. 22-4)[33].

Because stroke volume during exercise is maintained near-trained levels when blood volume is high, the ability

of the heart to fill with blood is not significantly altered by detraining. If ventricular mass does decrease, then thinning of ventricular walls, not decreased LVEDD, may be responsible[29]. Thus, decreased intrinsic cardiovascular function, at least during submaximal exercise, is apparently minimal after several weeks of inactivity in men who had been training intensively for several years[33]. The large reduction in stroke volume during exercise in the upright position is largely a result of reduced blood volume, not deterioration of heart function.

HEART RATE DURING MAXIMAL AND SUBMAXIMAL EXERCISE

Maximal HR may increase with detraining, reflecting an attempt (cardiovascular compensation) to offset the large reductions in blood volume and stroke volume. Coyle et al.[23] observed 4% and 6% increases in maximal HR after 3 and 12 weeks of inactivity, respectively (see Fig. 22-2). These results agree with the findings of others[30,35]. During the course of detraining, HR also increases significantly at a given submaximal work rate. For example, 12 days of inactivity was shown to increase HR from 158 to 170 bpm, then to 184 bpm after 84 days of detraining[24].

CARDIAC OUTPUT

Despite the detraining-related increase in HR that occurs at rest and during submaximal exercise, there is no appreciable change in cardiac output because of the above-described and offsetting decrease in stroke volume that occurs both at rest and during exercise. At peak exercise; however, cardiac output is lower, because of the decrease in peak stroke volume.

RETRAINING

No discussion of detraining would be complete without at least mentioning the concept of retraining. Popular belief once held that the training effects one achieved via endurance training could be increased if the athlete had previously undergone a training and detraining period[4]. However, the scientific evidence does not support this concept. We now know that prior endurance training does not, in itself, positively influence the gains made through a subsequent retraining period. What is more important to remember is that a relatively brief layoff can significantly decrease exercise capacity.

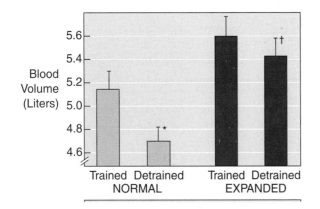

Figure 22-4. Responses to upright exercise with normal and expanded blood volume when trained and detrained. Significantly different from trained normal (*$P < 0.05$). Detrained with expanded blood volume significantly different from detrained with normal blood volume (†$P < 0.05$). (Reprinted with permission Pavlik G, Bachl N, Wollein W, et al: Resting echocardiographic parameters after cessation of regular endurance training. Int J Sports Med 7:226–231, 1986.)

Arm and Leg Exercise

Arm aerobic training for persons with and without heart disease is widely accepted as an integral component of a comprehensive physical conditioning program. Until recently, however, few data regarding the relative trainability of the upper extremities were available. Franklin et al.[36] reported the effects of a 6-week aerobic circuit training program in 13 patients who previously suffered a MI, a trial that involved alternating upper and lower extremity exercise devices for 15 minutes each at an intensity of 70% to 85% of peak HR. The postconditioning rate–pressure products during submaximal arm and leg ergometry were similarly decreased, and arm and leg $\dot{V}O_{2max}$ increased 13% and 11%, respectively (Fig. 22-5). These findings indicated that the upper extremities respond to aerobic exercise conditioning in the same qualitative and quantitative manner as the lower extremities.

Gender-specific Improvement and Trainability

The salutary effects of chronic endurance training in men are well documented. However, numerous studies now also provide ample data on $\dot{V}O_{2max}$, cardiovascular hemodynamics, body composition, and serum lipids in younger, middle-aged, and older women who undergo exercise training. The results demonstrate that women with and without CAD respond to aerobic training in much the same way as men when subjected to compara-

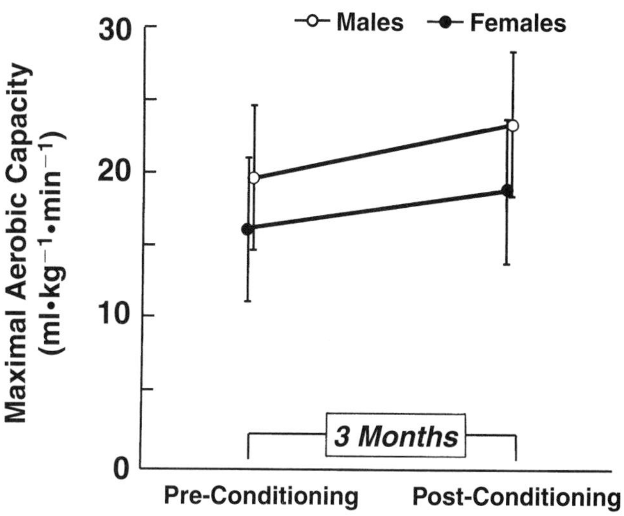

Figure 22-6. Aerobic capacity before and after physical conditioning in older ($\geq$ 62 years) men and women with coronary heart disease. Maximal $\dot{V}O_2$ increased by 19% and 17% in the men and women, respectively (both $P < 0.001$) [36].

ble programs in terms of frequency, intensity, and duration of exercise (Fig. 22-6)[37,38]. Improvement in cardiorespiratory fitness is negatively correlated with age, habitual physical activity, and initial $\dot{V}O_{2max}$ (which is generally lower in women than men) and is positively correlated with conditioning frequency, intensity, and duration[39]. Please note that $\dot{V}O_{2max}$ in women, when expressed in $mL \cdot kg^{-1} \cdot min^{-1}$, is approximately 15% to 25% below that of men. This difference is caused by a slightly greater amount of essential body fat (15% vs. 6%), a smaller peak stroke volume attributable to smaller left ventricular dimension, and a lower hemoglobin concentration (about 10% lower).

There are, however, large interindividual differences among women in the effects of a physical conditioning program, independent of age, initial exercise capacity, or type of conditioning program. These individual variations in response to aerobic exercise training may be attributable to childhood patterns of activity, state of conditioning at the initiation of the program, or degree of physiological aging. Body compositional differences in trainability may also play an important role with respect to the results of physical conditioning. Obese women demonstrate lower aerobic capacity, altered cardiovascular hemodynamics, and elevated serum lipids compared with leaner women[40]. This initial varied profile may serve to modify the outcome of an aerobic conditioning program with respect to the magnitude of quantitative changes.

In general, an average increase in $\dot{V}O_{2max}$ of between 10% and 25% is anticipated for college-age men and

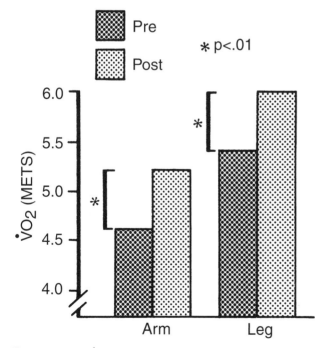

Figure 22-5. Mean $\dot{V}O_{2max}$ values, expressed as metabolic equivalents (METs; 1 MET $\sim$ 3.5 $mL \cdot kg^{-1} \cdot min^{-1}$), during arm and leg exercise testing before and after training in men with previous myocardial infarction[35].

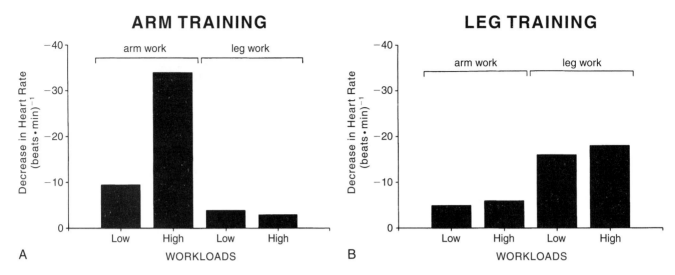

Figure 22-7. A. Whereas exercise training using an arm ergometer markedly decreased the heart rate (HR) response during arm exercise at low and high work loads, the HR reduction during leg work was small. **B.** Similarly, whereas leg training markedly decreased the HR during leg work, the HR reduction during arm work was minimal[40].

women after an 8- to 12-week endurance training program. When gain in $\dot{V}O_{2max}$ is expressed in mL of oxygen per kg of body weight per minute, the values achieved for men and women are similar. However, because the initial $\dot{V}O_{2max}$ of women is generally lower than men, the percent increase is generally greater among women (e.g., 15% vs. 10%, for similar absolute increases in $\dot{V}O_{2max}$).

Specificity of Training

To improve one's ability to perform a certain task or exercise, regardless of whether or not it is walking up two flights of stairs or swimming 100 m, involves working specific muscles or organ systems at an increased resistance. This concept emphasizes both the specificity of training and progressive overload. For purposes of this discussion, we wish to address the former and can do so because numerous studies of normal subjects and patients with heart disease have investigated the cardiorespiratory adaptations of trained versus untrained muscle to physical conditioning. Results generally demonstrate little or no crossover of arm and leg training. After endurance training of one limb or set of limbs, several investigators report increased $\dot{V}O_{2max}$ and anaerobic (ventilatory) threshold or decreased HR (Fig. 22-7), blood lactate, pulmonary ventilation, ventilatory equivalent for $\dot{V}O_2$, BP, and perceived exertion during submaximal exercise in trained but not untrained limbs[41,42]. These limb-specific training effects imply that a substantial portion of the conditioning response is attributed to

extracardiac or peripheral factors such as alterations in blood flow and cellular and enzymatic adaptations in the trained limbs alone[43–45].

On the other hand, studies in both normal subjects and patients with heart disease indicate some transfer effects (i.e., increased $\dot{V}O_{2max}$ or reduced submaximal exercise HR in untrained limbs), providing evidence for central circulatory adaptations to endurance training[46,47]. Although the conditions under which the crossover of arm and leg training may vary, some evidence suggests that the initial fitness, as well as the intensity, frequency, and duration of training, may be important variables in determining the extent of cross-training benefits from arms to legs and vice versa.

The limited degree of cardiorespiratory and metabolic crossover from one set of limbs to another appears to discount the general practice of restricting aerobic conditioning to the lower extremities alone. Many recreational and occupational activities require sustained arm work to a greater extent than leg work. Consequently, individuals who rely on their upper extremities for vocational or leisure-time pursuits should train their arms as well as their legs, with the expectation of improved cardiorespiratory, hemodynamic, and perceived exertion responses to both forms of effort. Specially designed arm ergometers or combined arm–leg ergometers are particularly beneficial for upper extremity training. Several exercise modalities that include upper body exercise are now available, including rowing machines, wall pulleys, vertical climbing devices, and cross-country skiing simulators. Other various factors affecting the training response are summarized in Table 22-3.

TABLE 22-3. Factors Influencing Cardiopulmonary Adaptations

Variable(s)	Comments
Prolonged bed rest	Results in physiological deconditioning, including a significant reduction in VO_2max.
Intensity, frequency, and duration of training	Improvement in aerobic capacity generally demonstrates a positive correlation to these variables.
Age, habitual physical activity, and initial VO_2max	Improvement generally demonstrates an inverse relationship with these variables; however, recent studies suggest that older and younger adults demonstrate comparable exercise trainability.
Adherence to the exercise prescription	Parallels the magnitude of improvement in cardiorespiratory function.
Detraining	When physical conditioning is stopped or reduced, training-induced cardiorespiratory and metabolic adaptations are reversed to varying degrees over time.
Coronary artery disease	Exercise training is generally safe and effective in improving cardiorespiratory function; however, the severity or progression of disease may present an obstacle to improvement.
Left ventricular dysfunction (ejection fraction ≤35%)	Exercise training appears to be generally safe and effective in improving cardiorespiratory function.
Beta-blockade	Patients may derive considerable physiological benefit from exercise training in the presence of both cardioselective and nonselective beta-blockers, despite a reduced training heart rate.
Calcium antagonists	No adverse effect on exercise trainability.

Summary

When exposed to repeated bouts of exercise, both the cardiac and pulmonary systems adapt in a manner consistent with what is referred to as a training effect. Generally, these changes are associated with improved health and performance. The adaptations that take place are somewhat organ system or tissue specific and occur generally the same in men and women. Consistent with the above, periods of detraining, lesser training, and bed rest are associated with loss of exercise tolerance, and many, if not all, of the accompanying training effects.

Acknowledgments
Much of the writing in this chapter was adapted from the 4th edition of ACSM'S Resource Manual. As a result, we wish to gratefully acknowledge and thank the previous efforts of Edward F. Coyle, PhD; Barry A. Franklin, PhD; and Jeffery L. Roitman, EdD.

REFERENCES

1. Fletcher GF, Balady G, Blair SN, et al: Statement on exercise: benefits and recommendations for physical activity programs for all Americans. A statement for health professionals by the Committee on Exercise and Cardiac Rehabilitation of the Council on Clinical Cardiology, American Heart Association. Circulation 94:857–862, 1996.

2. Blair SN, Kohl HW III, Paffenbarger RS, et al: Physical fitness and all-cause mortality. A prospective study of healthy men and women. JAMA 262:2395–2401, 1989.

3. Pate RR, Pratt M, Blair SN, et al. Physical activity and public health. A recommendation from the Centers for Disease Control and Prevention and the American College of Sports Medicine. JAMA 273:402–407, 1995.

4. Foss ML, Keteyian SJ: Fox's Physiological Basis for Exercise and Sport, 6th ed. New York: WCB McGraw-Hill; 1998.

5. Rowell LB: Human cardiovascular adjustments to exercise and thermal stress. Physiol Rev 54:75–159, 1974.

6. Bevegard BS, Shepherd JT: Regulation of the circulation during exercise in man. Physiol Rev 47:178–213, 1967.

7. Longhurst JC, Kelly AR, Gonyea WJ, Mitchell JH. Chronic training with static and dynamic exercise: cardiovascular adaptation, and response to exercise. Circ Res 48(6 Pt 2):I171–I178, 1981.

8. Levine BD, Lane LD, Buckey JC, et al: Left ventricular pressure-volume and Frank-Starling relations in endurance athletes. Implications for orthostatic tolerance and exercise performance. Circulation 84:1016–1023, 1991.

9. Green HJ, Thomson JA, Ball ME, et al: Alterations in blood volume following short-term supramaximal exercise. J Appl Physiol 56:145–149, 1984.

10. Rerych SK, Scholz PM, Sabiston DC Jr, Jones RH: Effects of exercise training on left ventricular function in normal subjects: a longitudinal study by radionuclide angiography. Am J Cardiol 45:244–252, 1980.

11. Ehsani AA, Hagberg JM, Hickson RC: Rapid changes in left ventricular dimensions and mass in response to physical conditioning and deconditioning. Am J Cardiol 42:52–56, 1978.

12. Michielli DW, Stein RA, Krasnow N, et al: Effects of exercise training on ventricular dimensions at rest and during exercise. Med Sci Sports 11:82, 1979.

13. Schairer JR, Stein PD, Keteyian S, et al: Left ventricular response to submaximal exercise in endurance-trained athletes and sedentary adults. Am J Cardiol 70:930–933, 1992.

14. Oscai LB, Williams BT, Hertig BA: Effect of exercise on blood volume. J Appl Physiol 24:622–624, 1968.

15. Holloszy JO: Adaptations of skeletal muscle to endurance exercise. Med Sci Sports 7:155–164, 1975.

16. Johnson PC, Wagner PD, Wilson DF: Regulation of oxidative metabolism and blood flow in skeletal muscle. Summary report of the first ACSM Basic Science Specialty Conference, Indianapolis, IN, September 28–30, 1995. Med Sci Sports Exerc 28:305–314, 1996.

17. McAllister RM: Endothelial-mediated control of coronary and skeletal muscle blood flow during exercise: introduction. Med Sci Sports Exerc 27:1122–1124, 1995.

18. Blomqvist CG, Saltin B: Cardiovascular adaptations to physical training. Annu Rev Physiol 45:169–189, 1983.

19. Orlander J, Kiessling KH, Karlsson J, Ekblom B: Low intensity training, inactivity and resumed training in sedentary men. Acta Physiol Scand 101:351–362, 1977.

20. Fringer MN, Stull GA: Changes in cardiorespiratory parameters during periods of training and detraining in young adult females. Med Sci Sports 6:20–25, 1974.

21. Klausen K, Andersen LB, Pelle I: Adaptive changes in work capacity, skeletal muscle capillarization and enzyme levels during training and detraining. Acta Physiol Scand 113:9–16, 1981.

22. Drinkwater BL, Horvath SM: Detraining effects on young women. Med Sci Sports 4:91–95, 1972.

23. Coyle EF, Martin WH 3rd, Sinacore DR, et al: Time course of loss adaptations after stopping prolonged intense endurance training. J Appl Physiol 57:1857–1864, 1984.

24. Coyle EF, Martin WH 3rd, Bloomfield SA, et al: Effects of detraining on responses to submaximal exercise. J Appl Physiol 59:853–859, 1985.

25. Costill DL, Fink WJ, Hargreaves M, et al: Metabolic characteristics of skeletal muscle during detraining from competitive swimming. Med Sci Sports Exerc 17: 339–343, 1985.

26. Ehsani AA, Hagberg JM, Hickson RC: Rapid changes in left ventricular dimensions and mass in response to physical conditioning and deconditioning. Am J Cardiol 42:52–56, 1978.

27. Hickson RC, Hammons GT, Holloszy JO: Development and regression of exercise-induced cardiac hypertrophy in rats. Am J Physiol 236:H268–H272, 1979.

28. Saltin B, Grimby G: Physiological analysis of middle-aged and old former athletes. Comparison with still active athletes of the same ages. Circulation 38:1104–1115, 1968.

29. Martin WH 3rd, Coyle EF, Bloomfield SA, Ehsani AA: Effects of physical deconditioning after intense endurance training on left ventricular dimensions and stroke volume. J Am Coll Cardiol 7:982–989, 1986.

30. Cullinane EM, Sady SP, Vadeboncoeur L, et al: Cardiac size and VO_2max do not decrease after short-term exercise cessation. Med Sci Sports Exerc 18:420–424, 1986.

31. Pavlik G, Bachl N, Wollein W, et al: Resting echocardiographic parameters after cessation of regular endurance training. Int J Sports Med 7:226–231, 1986.

32. Houmard JA, Hortobagyi T, Johns RA: Effect of short-term training cessation on performance measures in distance runners. Int J Sports Med 13:572–576, 1992.

33. Coyle EF, Hemmert MK, Coggan AR: Effects of detraining on cardiovascular responses to exercise: Role of blood volume. J Appl Physiol 60:95–99, 1986.

34. Convertino VA, Brock PJ, Keil LC, et al: Exercise training-induced hypervolemia: Role of plasma albumin, renin, and vasopressin. J Appl Physiol 48:665–669, 1980.

35. Houston ME, Bentzen H, Larsen H: Interrelationships between skeletal muscle adaptations and performance as studied by detraining and retraining. Acta Physiol Scand 105:163–170, 1979.

36. Franklin BA, Vander L, Wrisley D, Rubenfire M: Trainability of arms versus legs in men with previous myocardial infarction. Chest 105:262–264, 1994.

37. Ades PA, Waldmann ML, Polk DM, Coflesky JT: Referral patterns and exercise response in the rehabilitation of female coronary patients aged greater than or equal to 62 years. Am J Cardiol 69:1422–1425, 1992.

38. Getchell LH, Moore JC: Physical training: comparative responses of middle-aged adults. Arch Phys Med Rehabil 56:250–254, 1975.

39. Franklin BA, Bonzheim K, Berg T: Gender differences in rehabilitation (pp. 151–171). In Julian DG, Wenger NK, eds. Women and Heart Disease. London: Martin Dunitz; 1997.

40. Franklin B, Buskirk E, Hodgson J, et al: Effects of physical conditioning on cardiorespiratory function, body composition and serum lipids in relatively normal-weight and obese middle-aged women. Int J Obes 3:97–109, 1979.

41. Clausen JP, Trap-Jensen J, Lassen NA: The effects of training on the heart rate during arm and leg exercise. Scand J Clin Lab Invest 26:295–301, 1970.

42. Rasmussen B, Klausen K, Clausen JP, Trap-Jensen J: Pulmonary ventilation, blood gases, and blood pH after training of the arms or the legs. J Appl Physiol 38:250–256, 1975.

43. Davies CT, Sargeant AJ: Effects of training on the physiological responses to one- and two-leg work. J Appl Physiol 38:377–385, 1975.

44. Henriksson J, Reitman JS: Time course of changes in human skeletal muscle succinate dehydrogenase and cytochrome oxidase activities and maximal oxygen uptake with physical activity and inactivity. Acta Physiol Scand 99:91–97, 1977.

45. Saltin B, Nazar K, Costill DL, et al: The nature of the training response; peripheral and central adaptations of one-legged exercise. Acta Physiol Scand 96:289–305, 1976.

46. Clausen JP, Klausen K, Rasmussen B, Trap-Jensen J: Central and peripheral circulatory changes after training of the arms or legs. Am J Physiol 225:675–682, 1973.

47. Thompson PD, Cullinane E, Lazarus B, Carleton RA: Effect of exercise training on the untrained limb exercise performance of men with angina pectoris. Am J Cardiol 48:844–850, 1981.

SELECTED REFERENCES FOR FURTHER READING

ATS/ACCP Statement on cardiopulmonary exercise testing. Am J Respir Crit Care Med 167:211–277, 2003.

Robergs RA, Keteyian SJ: Fundamentals of Exercise Physiology for Fitness, Performance, and Health, 2nd ed. New York: McGraw-Hill; 2003

Rowell LB, Shephard JT: Handbook of Physiology. Exercise: Regulation and Integration of Multiple Organ Systems. New York: Oxford University Press; 1996.

Wasserman K, Hansen JE, Sue DY, et al: Principles of Exercise Testing & Interpretation: Including Pathophysiology and Clinical Applications, 3rd ed. Baltimore, MD: Lippincott Williams & Wilkins; 1999.

INTERNET RESOURCES

Athletes Heart: http://www.hopkinsmedicine.org/cardiomyopathy/athlete's_heart.htm

Medicine & Science in Sports & Exercise: http:/www.studioorlando.com/News/position_statement_exercise_elderly.htm

Myocardial Adaptations to Training: http://home.hia.no/~stephens/hrttrn.htm

Promoting and Prescribing Exercise for the Elderly: http://www.aafp.org/afp/20020201/419.html

Adaptations to Resistance Training

TAMMY EVETOVICH AND KYLE EBERSOLE

Neuromuscular Adaptations

The interaction between the nervous and muscular systems during acute or chronic periods of resistance training results in several neuromuscular adaptations that, in part, determine the effectiveness of a resistance training program (Table 23-1). The neural component generally includes such factors as changes in motor unit activation strategies and modifications to the function of neural structures such as the neuromuscular junction (NMJ). Muscle-based adaptations include hypertrophy, hyperplasia, fiber-type modifications, and architectural changes. Collectively, the neural and muscular adaptations provide for the increase in strength, improved performance, and enhanced fitness level typical of a scientifically designed resistance training protocol. It is believed that increases in strength during the initial weeks (0 to 4 weeks) of resistance training are partly caused by **neural adaptations.** Subsequent increases in strength during the later stages of a resistance program are attributed to the morphological changes that occur in muscle. The specific time course for the neuromuscular changes and contribution of each factor continues to be investigated by researchers in an at-tempt to elucidate a greater understanding of the science that supports resistance training program design. This section addresses each of these as well as other factors associated with neuromuscular adaptations that occur after resistance training.

Neural Adaptations

The acute physiological responses to resistance training are discussed in Chapter 3. This chapter focuses on the chronic adaptations to resistance training.

MOTOR UNIT RECRUITMENT AND FIRING RATE

The motor unit is the operational unit for modulation of force by the neuromuscular system and has two functional characteristics for regulation of force output: motor unit recruitment and motor unit firing rate. The functional characteristics of the motor unit are driven, in part, by motor neuron contractile properties such as neuron size and type of muscle fiber innervated. Based on the size-ordered recruitment principles, motor neurons are recruited from smallest to largest for any given muscle action. Whereas smaller motor neurons innervate slow-contracting, fatigue-resistant muscle fibers, larger motor neurons innervate fast-contracting, highly fatigable muscle fibers.

Individual motor units also differ in recruitment threshold. Larger motor neurons have a higher recruitment threshold and are associated with fast-twitch muscle fibers. Slow-twitch muscle fibers, however, have smaller motor neurons and a lower recruitment threshold. Because a motor unit is trained in direct proportion to its recruitment, the intensity of the strength training program has significant influence on the motor unit–based neural adaptations[1]. That is, if the training intensity is below that which is required for recruitment of the larger motor neurons, there will be less neural influence on any increased expression of strength. The motor unit training intensity relationship differs between trained and untrained populations so that an untrained person is generally unable to recruit high-threshold motor units to the same extent as a trained athlete. Furthermore, the principles of orderly motor unit recruitment suggest that the larger motor neurons are not recruited un-

KEY TERMS:

Morphological adaptations: Physical changes in the structure of the muscle fiber and connective tissue as a result of training

Muscle soreness: Pain, either acute or of delayed onset, associated with muscular exertion

Neural adaptations: Adaptations within the nervous system resulting in enhance force production (strength)

Neuroendocrine system: Pertaining to the nervous and endocrine systems as an integrated, functioning mechanism

til force outputs reach higher or near maximal levels. Thus, the training intensity would have to be quite high in a trained athlete to attribute strength increases to the recruitment of the additional larger motor neurons.

EVALUATION OF NEURAL CHANGES WITH ELECTROMYOGRAPHY

Electromyography (EMG) has been widely used to quantify the potential neural adaptations. EMG uses either surface or needle electrodes, with surface EMG dominat-

ing the recent human movement science studies. Surface EMG provides a gross representation of whole-muscle electrical activity. Scientists have attempted to use EMG to measure the change in whole-muscle activation after periods of resistance training. Many studies have hypothesized that increases in strength are associated with an increase in recruitment and, thus, an increase in the EMG signal. The current body of literature, however, presents mixed results with regard to the presence or absence of a strength-related increase in EMG. Evidence suggests that compared with pretraining values, a reduction in total

TABLE 23-1. Neuromuscular Adaptations to Resistance Training

Adaptation	Significance
Neural	
↑ Motor unit recruitment (primarily large, high-threshold motor units)	↑ Rate of force development
↑ Inhibition of the Golgi tendon organs	↑ Force production capability
↑ Inhibition of antagonistic muscles (reduced coactivation)	↑ Force production capability and efficiency of force application
↑ Motor unit synchronization	↑ Force production capability and efficiency of force application
Morphological	
↑ Fat-free muscle mass	↑ Muscle strength
↑ CSA through ↑ myofibril size and ↑ quantity of myofilaments	↑ Contractile capacity and ↑ force production capability
↑ Type IIa MHC	↑ Force production capability
↑ Angle of pennation	↑ Amount of contractile tissue attached to tendon
↓ Or no change in capillary volume density	↓ Or no change in diffusion capacity
↓ Mitochondrial volume density	↓ Oxidative capacity
Neuroendocrine	
↑ Or no change in testosterone levels	↑ Protein synthesis, muscle growth, and influence of the nervous system
↑ Or no change in IGF	↑ Amino acid uptake, protein synthesis
↓ Or no change in cortisol	↓ Protein synthesis
Metabolic	
↑ Store adenosine triphosphate	Improves force-producing capability
↑ Creatine phosphate	Improves force-producing capability
↑ Stored glycogen	↑ Glycolytic capacity
Cardiovascular	
↓ Or no change in resting BP	Improved cardiovascular disease profile
↓ Or no change in resting HR	↓ Work for the heart at rest
↑ Or no change in maximal oxygen consumption	↑ Cardiovascular endurance and functionality and reduced relative workload
↑ Or no change in HDL levels	Improved CVD profile
↓ Or no change in LDL levels	Improved CVD profile
Improved glucose tolerance and insulin sensitivity	Improved CVD profile

BP = blood pressure; CSA = cross-sectional area; CVD = cardiovascular disease; HDL = high-density lipoprotein; HR = heart rate; IGF = insulinlike growth factor; LDL = low-density lipoprotein; MHC = myosin heavy chain.

muscle activation is required to perform a given exercise after a resistance training program. Cannon and Cafarelli[2] have suggested that if a maximal muscle action truly represents maximal recruitment of all available motor units, then any increase in EMG must be attributed to a change in the motor unit firing frequency. The contributions of increased motor unit recruitment or firing rate to increased strength are specific to muscle fiber type and may not occur in all muscles. Training-induced neural adaptations may occur in neural mechanisms other than, or at least in addition to, recruitment or firing rate[2,3].

IMPROVED COORDINATION OF ACTIVATION PATTERNS

In addition to alterations in motor unit recruitment or firing rate, other mechanisms of neural adaptations that may contribute to increase strength are associated with an improved coordination of muscle activation strategies. The Golgi tendon organ is a protective proprioceptive organ system located in the muscle tendon. The Golgi tendon organs respond to excessive changes in muscle tension or length by reflexively inhibiting muscle contraction. Excessive increases in muscle tension increase the activity of the Golgi tendon, thereby depressing motor neuron activity and reducing force output. The Golgi tendon remains relatively inactive if a muscle action produces little tension. Progressive resistance training is thought to increase inhibition of the Golgi tendon, allowing more forceful muscle contractions.

Contraction of the agonists is often associated with concurrent activation of the antagonist muscle group. Coactivation is most often evident during strong and rapid types of muscle actions or dynamic movements. The primary physiologic function of coactivation is to provide protection through joint stabilization during rapid agonist contractions or ballistic types of movements. This protective mechanism, however, occurs by impairing the ability of the agonist to maximize its force-producing capabilities. Through reciprocal inhibition pathways, coactivation limits the ability of the agonist to fully activate. Resistance training has been shown to increase inhibition of antagonist muscle (i.e., reducing coactivation), thereby allowing for a greater expression of strength[4]. This training-induced change in coactivation could be a learned adaptation that may or may not result in increased neural drive to the agonist muscle. The protective role of the antagonist, however, suggests that it may be advantageous to retain a certain degree of antagonist activation during rapid alternating movements. The most significant change in coactivation is likely to be an improved coordination of antagonist muscle groups, especially during gross motor movements.

Motor units fire in an asynchronous pattern. Evidence suggests that there is an increase in motor unit synchronization after a period of resistance training[4,5]. The extent to which synchronization occurs is likely to be related to high-force activities such as those requiring rapid production of maximal or near-maximal force. Resistance training–related increases in synchronization, however, do not directly increase muscle strength. Instead, synchronization facilitates the initiation of a muscle action through increasing the rate of force development. The benefits of increased motor unit synchronization intuitively point to ballistic-type activities involving large fluctuations in force in which improved timing in the activation patterns of a muscle (or of muscles) positively impacts performance.

CHANGES IN THE NEUROMUSCULAR JUNCTION

The NMJ is critical to the function of skeletal muscle. Electrical impulses that originate in the central nervous system are propagated from the terminal end of the axon across the NMJ to the postsynaptic membrane of the sarcolemma. The impulse subsequently depolarizes the sarcolemma and initiates an action potential to complete the excitation–contraction process of a muscle fiber. The effect of endurance training on the NMJ has long been the subject of investigation, mostly in animal-based models because of the invasiveness and difficulties of the research methods. The current body of literature suggests that within animals, the NMJ is able to undergo physiological and morphological changes in response to endurance training[6]. Heavy resistance training has been hypothesized to induce morphological changes in the NMJ such as a greater dispersion of electrical impulses and increases in the length of NMJ branching. Resistance training–induced changes in the NMJ may be specific to fiber type and, thus, differ across types and intensity of training. Given the significant role of NMJ to mediate the excitation–contraction process, the results of future studies could have a significant impact on the scientific design of strength training protocols.

Muscular Adaptations

HYPERTROPHY VERSUS HYPERPLASIA

An increase in cross-sectional area (CSA) of a muscle is a common response to a progressive strength training protocol. The increase in muscle size may result from an increase in the CSA of individual muscle fibers (hypertrophy), an increase in the number of muscle fibers (hyperplasia), or a combination of both. The relative contribution of hypertrophy and hyperplasia to the training-induced increase in muscle CSA remains controversial. Muscle hypertrophy, however, accounts for 90% to 95% of the training-induced enlargement of muscle fibers.

The mechanical stress of resistance exercise results in disruptions or damage to the muscle fibers that initiate modifications to the quantity and quality of the muscle and contractile proteins[7,8]. Repeated exposure to the progressive overload of resistance training induces muscle hypertrophy as a result of the chronic repair and remodeling of involved muscle fibers. The resulting increase in muscle fiber diameter and number of contractile protein myofilaments (actin and myosin) is coupled to the enhanced protein synthesis and associated decrease in protein breakdown, which forms additional sarcomeres[7,8]. Because of the enhanced contractile structures, hypertrophy allows the muscle or muscle groups to generate higher levels of force and power. The magnitude of these changes, however, varies across the type of muscle action performed so that eccentric muscle actions appear to provide the greatest degree of disruption to the muscle fiber. Furthermore, the degree to which hypertrophy occurs is specific to the muscle fibers active during the training process and, thus, emphasizes the importance of well-designed training protocols.

Chronic overload of skeletal muscle in some animals has resulted in hyperplasia or an increase in number of muscle fibers[9,10]. The mechanism for hyperplasia appears to be a function of either satellite cells that develop new muscle cells or by longitudinal splitting of the existing muscle fibers[4]. Hyperplasia remains controversial primarily because of the difficulties in generalizing the animal-based evidence of hyperplasia to humans. Hyperplasia may be an explanation for the greater number of muscle fibers in athletes with extremely well-developed muscles (e.g., bodybuilders) compared with their untrained counterparts. Hyperplasia adaptations to resistance training likely occur when fibers reach a theoretical upper limit in cell size. Furthermore, genetics and the number of years of that an athlete has trained in a particular sport or event likely contribute to the presence of hyperplasia. It is also possible that hyperplasia may be more prevalent in type II fibers because of the assumed high intensity of training necessary to stimulate hyperplasia. Regardless of the degree to which hyperplasia may or may not occur, it is widely accepted that hypertrophy is the dominant mechanism for an increase in muscle CSA.

MODIFICATIONS TO MUSCLE FIBER TYPE

Adaptations in the muscle fiber protein content (quantity and quality) may facilitate the onset of fiber-type transitions. The advancement in technology has resulted in improved methods for identifying changes in the myosin heavy chain (MHC) isoforms, which support the suggestion of fiber-type transitions. Most current human-based resistance training literature has examined a continuum of six muscle fiber types of I, IC, IIAC, IIA, IIAB, and IIB[8,11,12]. This continuum goes from most (type I) oxidative to least (type IIB) oxidative (see Chapter 1 for more information on fiber types). The process of fiber-type transformation begins with the activation of type IIB fibers and is associated with changes in myosin ATPase and MHC proteins. Resistance training accounts for the modification of type IIB fibers to IIA if the training intensity is high enough to activate the type IIB fibers. Modification of fibers from IIA to IIC and IIC to I requires an oxidative stimulus. It is less probable that type IIC fibers are transformed to IC fibers because of the distinctly different physiological characteristics. Current evidence suggests that the transitions follow the energetic requirements of the stimulus, and, therefore, the energetic potential of the muscle fiber[8]. Hostler et al.[11] have suggested that the conversion of fast fiber types is related to an increase in the capillary to muscle fiber ratio that is independent of the change in CSA. Independent of the specific physiological changes, the quality and quantity of the training stimuli are critical factors that influence the fiber-type transformation process. When coupled with the neurological adaptations and other **morphological adaptations,** gradual transformation of type IIB fibers may be an integral component for the ability of a muscle to have a greater expression of strength after a resistance training program.

CHANGES IN MUSCLE ARCHITECTURE

The architecture of skeletal muscle is characterized by the geometric arrangement of the muscle fibers. For example, when comparing a pennate muscle (i.e. vastus lateralis) with a fusiform muscle (i.e., biceps brachii), the pennate structure allows for more contractile tissue to attach to the tendon, thereby contributing to its greater force-producing capabilities. The advancement of technology and availability of magnetic resonance imaging (MRI) and ultrasound instrumentation have provided methods to examine the influence of resistance training on muscle architecture. It has been reported that muscle hypertrophy results in an increase in the physiological cross-sectional area (PCSA; the total CSA of all muscle fibers cut at right angles to their long axes) and is coupled with an increase in pennation angle[1,13]. The concurrent changes in PCSA and pennation angle suggest that the muscle should be able to generate more force. As the angle of pennation angle increases, however, force is displaced away from the tendons and, thus, the increased angle of pennation becomes a disadvantage to a muscle. The loss of force associated with an increased angle of pennation (up to 30°) is compensated for by the increased packing of contractile tissue[1]. Thus, the point at which muscle hypertrophy–induced changes in PCSA and pennation angle become disadvantageous varies across muscles as well as within muscles or muscle groups. The continued advancement of technology and improved imaging methods promise to provide outlets for future research to address this issue.

Methods of Strength Training

There are three fundamental muscle actions that can stimulate the contractile elements and result in increased force production after periods of resistance training. They are isometric training, isotonic training, and isokinetic training. The quality and quantity of strength gains differs across each type of muscle action. Furthermore, a number of strength training programs incorporate exercises using multiple types of muscle actions as well as plyometric and concurrent endurance training. Refer to Chapter 25 for further details on the various types of training methods and to GETP7 Chapter 7 for exericse prescription recommendations.

ISOMETRIC TRAINING

Isometric training is simple to administer and requires little to no equipment. Optimal results are generally achieved when using maximal or near-maximal contractions, held for 6 seconds, and repeated five to 10 times daily. However, based on the principles of joint angle specificity, the realized strength gains only occur at the angle that the resistance training was performed. In order to obtain strength across the entire range of motion (ROM) for a given muscle, training would need to occur at multiple angles. This would ultimately nullify the simplistic benefits of isometric training. Furthermore, there is considerable question about the transfer of isometric strength to functional activities. However, isometric training is extremely beneficial in the early stages of rehabilitation during which joint motion may be limited because of the injury.

A well-defined effect of isometric muscle actions is an elevation of arterial blood pressure (BP). This is effect is caused by the expiratory effort that is made against a closed glottis. Intrathoracic pressure is raised from 80 to 200 mm Hg or more, and this increased pressure is transmitted through the thin walls of the great veins. Consequently, venous return is decreased, placing significant strain on the cardiovascular system. The increased pressure that the heart must work against is related to muscle mass. The deleterious effects of isometric muscle actions are an obvious concern to cardiac patients because significant increases in BP are undesirable.

ISOTONIC TRAINING

Isotonic muscle actions involve moving a given resistance through a ROM such as that experienced with free weight or dumbbell types of training. Although the movement across an entire ROM is a clear advantage over isometric muscle actions, joint angle specificity influences the isotonic strength gains. That is, the strength gains only occur at the weakest angle in the ROM. The effectiveness of isotonic resistance training programs is associated with factors such as the number of repetitions, weight of resistance, and the ability to exercise through the entire ROM, both in the muscle shortening and lengthening phases.

ISOKINETIC TRAINING

Isokinetic muscle actions involve movement under a constant angular velocity. Isokinetic training is popular within the clinical setting for rehabilitation after injury or surgery. Isokinetic testing is often used to determine baseline strength values of athletes at the onset of training for a competitive season. The clear advantage of isokinetic training is the ability to train and test muscle strength across a wide range of velocities. A number of research studies have demonstrated a high correlation between isokinetic strength and athletic performance. Another advantage of isokinetic dynamometer equipment is the ability to train and evaluate muscle function under concentric and eccentric modes of muscle actions.

Physiology of Muscle Soreness

It is a common experience that high-intensity exercise may result in muscular pain and discomfort. In general, there are two forms pain and discomfort that are differentiated by their onset: (a) pain experienced during and immediately after exercise and (b) localized discomfort and soreness that appears 24 to 48 hours after activity. The first type of pain is likely caused by increased sensitivity of pain receptors to metabolic byproducts. This is generally not a limiting condition because it is of short duration and is commonly relieved after the exercise session ceases. The second type of pain is commonly referred to as exercise-induced muscle damage or its clinical correlate, delayed-onset **muscle soreness** (DOMS), and it is commonly associated with eccentric-based exercise. DOMS is associated with localized pain that is sensitive to palpation, reduced ROM, loss of strength, muscle stiffness, and swelling. DOMS generally lasts for about 96 hours and rarely develops into a chronic condition requiring medical attention.

A number of mechanisms have been proposed to explain the cause of DOMS, including mechanical trauma to contractile structures and tissues, acute inflammation, local ischemia, muscle spasm, and the proliferation of free radicals. At this time, however, the specific causative factor and associated mechanisms are unknown. It is likely that DOMS is a multifactorial condition that is influenced by each of the identified factors. It is generally accepted that the mechanical stress associated with eccentric muscle actions initiates damage to the sarcolemma and sarcomere and possibly the sarcoplasmic reticulum[14,15]. Thus, the integrity of the contractile structures as well as a possible disturbance in calcium homeostasis are likely contributors to the decrease in muscle function. In response to this mechanical trauma, a cascade of interrelated events occurs. The swelling associated with DOMS is the result of an increased inflammatory response that leads to the release of prostaglandin E_2 and leukotriene synthesis[15]. These inflammatory mediators take advantage of the increased vascular permeability and promote the movement of fluid into the interstitium and increase the sensation of pain by acting on muscle afferents III and IV. It has also been suggested that the respiratory functions of neutrophils (activated by the leukotrienes) generates free radicals, which further compound the damage to the muscle.

It is likely that no single mechanism is entirely responsible for the exercise-induced muscle damage and DOMS that may occur subsequent to eccentric-based exercise. Recent research has attempted to better understand the cause by examining the muscle repair and regeneration process. In the days after the onset of muscle damage, stress proteins are synthesized. It appears that the stress proteins contribute to the maintenance of cellular homeostasis and function in the repair process of the damaged muscle and may limit the magnitude of DOMS[14]. Other research has examined treatment interventions for DOMS such as stretching, hyperbaric oxygen therapy, nonsteroidal antiinflammatory agents, cryotherapy, and nutritional supplementation (i.e., vitamin E, vitamin C, ubiquinone, and L-carnitine). The efficacy of these treatments remains questionable because a number of studies demonstrate therapeutic effects as well as no effects from the various interventions.

Neuroendocrine Response

The endocrine system includes all tissues or glands that secrete hormones, act as chemical signalers, and bind to specific target cells to exert control over the target tissue. The nervous system typically provides the signal that stimulates the endocrine glands to release the hormones; thus, the close association between the endocrine and nervous systems has resulted in a relatively new term called the **neuroendocrine system**. This system plays a vital role in the acute and chronic neuromuscular adaptations that occur as a result of exercise activities. Of particular interest to those involved in high-intensity activities such as resistance training is the neuroendocrine system's effect on protein synthesis (anabolism) or degradation (catabolism). Knowledge of the acute and chronic responses of important neurohormones with regard to their anabolic nature, such as human growth hormone (HGH), testosterone, and insulinlike growth factors (IGFs) as well as a catabolic hormone of interest, cortisol, is vital to understanding the neuromuscular adaptations to resistance training.

TESTOSTERONE

Testosterone is a steroid hormone produced by the testes that functions to stimulate growth, increase protein synthesis and controls the development and maintenance of the secondary sex characteristics. With regard to the neuromuscular system, testosterone is the primary hormone that mediates tissue responses with resistance training of skeletal muscle in both a direct and indirect manner. In-

direct muscular effects of this steroidal hormone are related to its influence on the nervous system (increasing neurotransmitters and interacting with receptors on neurons) and other hormones (promotion of the HGH response and inhibition of the affect of cortisol). In addition, testosterone can interact with skeletal muscle directly in that binding of this hormone to receptors in the sarcoplasm or on the nucleus increases the rate of protein synthesis and inhibits protein breakdown.

Resistance exercise has been shown to elicit an acute postexercise increase in the concentration of testosterone in the blood in men with no change or increases in women. The degree of acute change in testosterone levels can be affected by many factors, including the intensity and volume of training, nutritional supplementation, size of muscle, age, and training experience. In general, greater responses have been shown for heavy resistance and higher volumes of exercise using muscles of larger mass. The chronic effects of resistance exercise have been equivocal in that resting concentrations of testosterone have shown no change or increases over time in men and in women[16,17]. For studies reporting no change in resting blood levels of testosterone with training, it is possible that there are other cellular adaptations (e.g., up or down-regulation of receptors) without changes in testosterone levels that may explain the anabolic nature of testosterone's positively impacting the adaptation to training[18].

HUMAN GROWTH HORMONE

Human growth hormone is a protein hormone with many molecular variants produced in the anterior pituitary gland that stimulates IGF and increases protein synthesis, growth, and metabolism. It has been reported that acute HGH responses may be dependent on the resistance training protocol in that moderate- to high-intensity, high-volume training with short rest periods and using large muscle groups have resulted in the greatest postexercise levels of HGH in both men and women. In addition, an intriguing new study has indicated that, unlike other hormones, acute HGH changes are linked to the type of muscle action (concentric vs. eccentric) performed[19]. Chronic adaptations in resting HGH levels have not been shown in most studies as a result of resistance training. Similar to testosterone, there may be other cellular adaptations (number and sensitivity of receptors) or factors that have not been thoroughly studied (other molecular variants of HGH) that may play a positive role in HGH-related adaptations to resistance training.

INSULINLIKE GROWTH FACTOR

Insulinlike growth factor is a polypeptide hormone that is structurally similar to insulin that is primarily produced by the liver. IGF functions to regulate many of the actions of HGH and facilitate amino acid uptake, glucose transport, protein synthesis, and bone and cartilage synthesis as well as inhibit protein degradation. Studies have reported both an increase and no change in acute levels of IGF after resistance-training bouts[18]. The acute response of IGF may not be evident, however, by measuring changes in circulating levels of this hormone immediately after exercise in that there is some evidence that release of IGF may occur many hours later. Most studies have indicated no change in resting levels of IGF as a result of a resistance training program. It is important to note, however, that more recent long-term studies in men and women have reported a chronic increase in IGF resting concentrations for a single and multiple set training program[19] and in response to tennis practice and conditioning and resistance training (4 to 6 and 8 to 10 repetition maximum [RM] loads) over a 9-month period[17].

CORTISOL

Cortisol is a catabolic hormone released from the adrenal cortex that not only inhibits protein synthesis but also stimulates amino acid release (protein degradation) from muscles in order to maintain blood glucose homeostasis. Similar to HGH and testosterone, there are specific program variables in a resistance training program (high-volume, moderate- to high-intensity with short rest periods) that elicit an acute increase in cortisol levels in response to the "stress" for both men and women. With regard to the chronic adaptations to a resistance training program, it is reasonable to theorize that decreases in basal levels of cortisol over the course of a training program provide an environment that is conducive to building proteins and muscle mass. Studies examining the chronic adaptation in resting cortisol levels, however, have not provided conclusive evidence that this positive adaptation occurs. In fact, the results of a recent investigation has indicated that a high-volume, high-intensity periodized program coupled with sport, specific training may elicit an increase in resting cortisol levels[17].

OVERTRAINING AND THE NEUROENDOCRINE SYSTEM

Overtraining occurs when physical performance decreases despite continued training[20]. The underlying causes of overtraining are difficult to identify, but a few possible markers related to the neuroendocrine system have been proposed. For example, when athletes undergo a large increase in training, blood levels of testosterone have been shown to decrease while cortisol levels increase. A decrease in the ratio of testosterone to cortisol may lead to protein catabolism and account for the body mass decrease seen in overtrained individuals. In addition, other hormones such as epinephrine and norepinephrine are elevated during periods of intense training, which can lead to an increased sympathetic response evidenced by an elevated resting heart rate (HR) and BP in

overtrained individuals. Finally, although it has been theorized that overtraining may affect neural function and ultimately alter motor unit recruitment, motor coordination, and excitation–contraction coupling, this theory remains to be examined. Because of the close association between hormones and the nervous system, a continuation of studies examining hormones that have been purported to be neurohormones may help in understanding changes to neural function that may perpetuate the overtraining syndrome.

It is evident that the neuroendocrine system is an essential part of the neuromuscular adaptations that occur as a result of resistance training. There are many other neurohormones (and their molecular variants as well as other factors related to the neuroendocrine system not discussed here) that synergistically act to positively impact the development of muscular strength. A complete understanding of this system aids strength and conditioning professionals to design programs, paying attention to specific program variables that will result in optimal neuromuscular adaptations for enhanced performance.

Metabolic Response

The bioenergetic adaptations that occur as a result of resistance training revolve around changes in fuel sources or changes in the quantity and activity levels of metabolic enzymes (see Chapter 3 for more information on metabolism). The acute and chronic adaptations of these metabolic factors must be considered when discussing adaptations that may lead to enhanced performance as a result of resistance training.

SUBSTRATES

Fuel sources that may be available to muscle fibers during resistance training come from phosphagen stores (phosphocreatine and adenosine triphosphate), carbohydrates (glucose and glycogen), lipids (free fatty acids, triglycerides), and protein. Intramuscular levels of adenosine triphosphate (ATP), phosphocreatine (PC), and glycogen have been shown to be lower after an acute bout of resistance exercise. In addition, most studies suggest that the ATP and PC concentrations are unchanged by long-term resistance training; however, it appears that muscle glycogen concentration increases in response to resistance training. The degree of change in these energy sources with resistance training may be a function of training status, programming variables, nutritional status, and the muscle group (or groups) being trained.

Although it is generally thought that PC, ATP, and glycogen are the primary energy substrates during acute bouts of resistance training, some evidence suggests that lipid stores are mobilized and that lipolysis may provide energy during resistance training[21]. For the most part, however, intramuscular levels of lipids do not increase with chronic resistance training and, in some instances, have been shown to decrease. With regard to protein as an energy substrate, recent studies have noted that protein metabolism after an acute resistance exercise activity is elevated for 24 to 48 hours[22,23]. This observation may have implications with regard to the timing of protein consumption after a resistance training bout in that a recent study has reported that protein intake immediately after exercise may be more anabolic than when ingested later[24]. It is well known that chronic resistance exercises can have a profound effect on muscle growth but only if muscle protein synthesis exceeds muscle protein catabolism.

ENZYMES

Typically, the adaptations that may occur to metabolic enzymes have revolved around increased concentrations or increased activity of the enzyme of interest. Those enzymes involved in the breakdown of ATP or the ATP-PC system such as creatine phosphokinase, myokinase, or myosin ATPase have shown little or no change in concentration or activity in response to resistance training, and any increases that were observed were purportedly not sufficient enough to enhance performance. Furthermore, glycolytic enzymes (phosphofructokinase [PFK], low-density lipoprotein [LDH], phosphorylase) as well as oxidative enzymes concentration (whether the substrate is of carbohydrate or lipid origin) have been shown to be unaffected by heavy resistance exercises.

CAPILLARY ADAPTATIONS

With regard to capillary adaptations that occur in a muscle, it is important to distinguish between the adaptations that are reported in terms of per muscle fiber and density (capillaries per unit area). Changes in the density depend on whether muscle hypertrophy occurred in response to a particular training program because of the dilution effect. The dilution effect is evident when assessing the pre- to postnumber of capillaries identified per unit area with hypertrophy. When hypertrophy is elicited with resistance training, fewer fibers and, therefore, fewer capillaries occupy the same area as before training. For strength training involving high load and low repetitions (power and weight lifters), the number of capillaries per muscle fiber does not change; however, the density may actually decrease because of hypertrophy of the muscle fibers. With moderate loads using high numbers of repetitions (body builders), capillaries may proliferate (a greater number per muscle fiber) in order to increase the blood supply and remove wastes for a muscle that consistently is exposed to large increases in blood lactate (because of short rest intervals). Capillary density, however, would not change or may decrease in response to this type of training program because of the masking of this adaptation by an increase in the size of the muscle.

MITOCHONDRIAL ADAPTATIONS

Capillary density has been more thoroughly studied than mitochondrial density. Although the number of mitochondria remains constant, mitochondrial density has been shown to decrease because of the dilution effects of muscle fiber hypertrophy with long-term heavy weight training[25,26]. Theoretically, this may have implications with regard to the distribution of energy from the mitochondria to the sites of energy utilization within muscle fibers[25]. It is not clear whether modification of specific program variables would affect the number of mitochondria per muscle fiber, and further study of this issue is necessary

Cardiorespiratory and Health-related Adaptations

Resistance training has been shown to benefit the cardiorespiratory system because of small volumes of blood pumped at a very high pressures. The high pressures observed result in improved heart, lung, and circulatory function, which can expand the physiological capabilities of an individual. In a recent issue of *The President's Council on Physical Fitness and Sports Research Digest*, Pollock and Vincent[27] reviewed the effect of resistance training on cardiovascular adaptations related to health. They concluded that several positive adaptations to resistance training may decrease the risk of chronic disease and improve quality of life. Some important cardiorespiratory or metabolic responses and adaptations that result from resistance training that are linked to an individual's health status include changes in BP, HR, lipid profiles, oxygen consumption rate, and glucose tolerance.

BLOOD PRESSURE AND HEART RATE

Blood pressure increases dramatically (on average >300/180 mm Hg) with acute dynamic resistance exercises (particularly when the Valsalva maneuver is used), has been shown to be higher during the concentric phase than eccentric phase of a repetition, and increases as a set progresses. A common misconception is that resistance-trained individuals have a higher incidence of chronic hypertension. No evidence exists suggesting that this type of training negatively impacts resting BP because most studies indicate that resistance-trained individuals have normal or slightly lower than normal resting BPs. In fact, a recent meta-analysis[28] concluded that resistance training results in decreases of 2% and 4% for resting systolic and diastolic BP, respectively.

Heart rate increases substantially during an acute bout of resistance exercise, with a peak HR response during the last several repetitions of a set and no phase (concentric vs. eccentric) dependent difference in the degree of increase in HR. In addition, resistance-trained athletes show either lower or average resting HRs.

Rate pressure product (RPP) has been purported to be a good measure of myocardial oxygen consumption and is, therefore, an indication of how hard the heart is working. Based on the HR and BP responses discussed previously, it follows that during an acute bout of resistance exercises, RPP (HR × systolic BP) increases dramatically. Similarly, if chronic training results in decreases in resting HR and BP, RPP changes accordingly and is viewed as a positive adaptation to training.

$\dot{V}O_2$

The acute response of oxygen uptake to an exercise session may vary depending on the muscle group being used (more oxygen for bigger muscles), the type of muscle action (more oxygen consumed for concentric vs. eccentric muscle), and the joint action (more oxygen for a multijoint versus single-joint lift). Depending on the type of resistance training program and the training status of the individual, maximal oxygen consumption values have been shown to either not change (conventional programs) or improve slightly (circuit training or untrained individuals). Although these changes may seem insignificant, it is important to note that weight training may have an indirect impact on cardiovascular endurance in that improvements in muscular strength and endurance can increase functionality and mobility and reduce the relative workload (as a percentage of one-repetition maximum [1RM]), which may then lead to improvements in fitness levels.

BLOOD LIPIDS

The effect of resistance training on serum lipid profiles has provided conflicting results and has been shown to either have no effect or resulted in a more positive blood lipid profile. Pollock and Vincent[27] indicated that for studies showing positive adaptations, high-density lipoproteins (HDLs) increased with heavy resistance exercises and LDLs decreased with high-volume, short-rest interval programs. This suggests that high-volume, high-intensity programs may be necessary to elicit the positive adaptations to the blood lipid profile. Because of the conflicting reports, it is not surprising to find results of a recent meta-analysis that indicated that the effect of resistance training on lipid profiles is inconclusive. It should be noted that only three studies were included in Halbert et al.'s[29], meta-analysis because of the low number of studies that met the inclusion criteria. Thus, it appears that more research on the effect of resistance training on blood lipid profiles is warranted.

GLUCOSE TOLERANCE

It has been reported that resistance training can improve the mechanisms involved in glucose metabolism, particularly in elderly individuals and those with high blood glucose levels as well as in nondiabetic subjects[31] (see

Chapter 33 and GETP7 Chapter 9). A recent position stand[31] reported that the direct results of resistance training such as improved muscle strength and endurance, improved body composition, and a decrease in risk factors for coronary artery disease (BP and lipid changes) can result in improved glucose tolerance and insulin sensitivity. It was concluded that resistive exercises should be included as a therapeutic modality for treating diabetics and possibly preventing diabetes as well.

Resistance training has become an integral part of physical activity programs designed to promote health and wellness (see GETP7 Chapter 7). Resistance training has been shown to have a positive impact on many health measures and the collective impact may significantly improve functionality, well-being, and quality of life.

Aging and Neuromuscular Adaptations

Muscular strength reaches its peak between the ages of 25 and 30 years for most muscle groups, decreases very slowly with maturity, and then decreases at a somewhat greater rate after age 60 years. In addition, it has been shown that there is a decrease in explosive strength (muscle power) with the aging process. Box 23-1 provides a list of reasons that have been proposed for the age-related decrease in strength and power as it relates to the neuromuscular system.

It should be noted that these factors do not interact in a linear fashion but are actually interrelated. Thus, it can be theorized that if an older individual has the ability to slow the rate of decay of just a few of these age-related changes by incorporating a resistance training program into his or her exercise routine, a "domino effect" may occur and result in dramatic improvements in strength, power, health, and quality of life.

BOX 23-1	**Neuromuscular Factors Associated with Age-related Decreases in Strength and Power**

- Change in resting hormone levels
- Blunted acute hormonal response to exercise
- Decrease in muscular energy substrate content
- Decrease in anaerobic enzyme concentration and activity
- Decrease in mitochondrial mass
- Dennervation or death of muscle cells
- Decreased muscle mass (atrophy of muscle fibers particularly of type II)
- Decreased ability to develop force rapidly
- Antagonistic coactivation
- Changes in ability to maximally activate a muscle
- Changes at the neuromuscular junction
- Decreased firing rate of motor units
- Decreased insulin sensitivity and tolerance

NEUROMUSCULAR ADAPTATIONS TO TRAINING

From the earliest study[32] to the most recent[33], researchers have shown that the older neuromuscular system is trainable and can display remarkable adaptations. Strength gains of 16% to 174% and increases in muscle size of 7% to 62% (for both types I and II fibers) have been demonstrated in older men and women (age range = 60 to 98 years) as a result of various types of strength training programs[18]. In addition to strength gains, resistance training involving higher velocities and more powerful movements has been shown to increase the maximal rate of force production in older men and women[34,35]. In fact, from a practical outlook, power training was more effective than strength training for improving physical function in older adults[35].

The primary adaptations that allow for strength and power gains in an older population in response to resistance training are related to neural, endocrine, and hypertrophic factors. The neural adaptations that have been shown to accompany a chronic resistance training program include greater activation of agonistic, increased coordination of synergistic, and reduced coactivation of antagonistic muscle groups. The acute and chronic responses of various hormones (HGH, free testosterone, cortisol, IGF) to a resistance training program have been studied as well. In general, depending on which hormone and the duration of the training, hormonal adaptations of aged populations to resistance training occur but are not of the magnitude nor the rate of change as in younger persons. Finally, although originally thought that older muscles were not capable of hypertrophy, more recent studies with more sensitive techniques have reported significant hypertrophic adaptations of both types I (range = 8% to 46%) and II (range = 5% to 43%) muscle fibers for older men and women. In addition, it has been shown that hypertrophy of type II fibers occurs in the subtypes (IIa, IIb) and that the transformation of type IIb to IIa that is observed in younger individuals has been shown in older subjects as well[36,37].

Research, therefore, has demonstrated that resistance training can promote muscular strength and power gains in older individuals and, in some respects, slows the decay for certain neuromuscular factors. Given this information, it becomes evident that inclusion of resistance training in the exercise programming of aging men and women is vitally important to their well being and functionality (see GETP7 Chapter 10). Pollock and Vincent[27] have indicated that although the best program recommendations for older adults remain to be confirmed, it was suggested that a 10- to 15-repetition guideline may result in less stress and injury for the joints. Furthermore, because of the importance of strength and power in the performance of activities of daily life, when designing resistance training activities for an older population, the inclusion of powerful movements should be considered as a program variable.

REFERENCES

1. Brooks GA, Fahey TD, White TP, et al: Muscle strength, power, and flexibility (pp. 424–457). In Exercise Physiology Human Bioenergetics and Its Applications, 3rd ed. New York: McGraw-Hill; 2000.
2. Cannon RJ, Cafarelli E: Neuromuscular adaptations to training. J Appl Physiol 63:2396–402, 1987.
3. Gardiner P: Strength training (pp. 143–170). In Neuromuscular Aspects of Physical Activity. Champaign, IL: Human Kinetics; 2001.
4. Sale DG, Martin JE, Moroz DE: Hypertrophy without increased isometric strength after weight training. Eur J Appl Physiol 64: 51–55, 1992.
5. Semmler JG: Motor unit synchronization and neuromuscular performance. Exer Sci Sport Rev 30:8–14, 2002.
6. Deschenes MR, Maresh CM, Kraemer WJ: The neuromuscular junction: Structure, function, and its role in the excitation of muscle. J Strength Cond Res 8:103–109, 1994.
7. Kraemer WJ, Fleck SJ, Evans WJ: Strength and power training: physiological mechanisms of adaptation. Exer Sci Sport Rev 24: 363–398, 1996.
8. Pette D: Training effects on the contractile apparatus. Acta Physiol Scand 162:367–376, 1998.
9. Kelley G: Mechanical overload and skeletal muscle fiber hyperplasia: A meta-analysis. J Appl Physiol 81:1584–1588, 1996.
10. McCall GE, Byrnes WC, Dickinson A, et al: Muscle fiber hypertrophy, hyperplasia, and capillary density in college men after resistance training. J Appl Physiol 81:2004–2012, 1996.
11. Hostler D, Schwirian CI, Campos G, et al: Skeletal muscle adaptations in elastic resistance-trained young men and women. Eur J Appl Physiol 86:112–118, 2001.
12. Kraemer WJ, Dudley GA, Tesch PA, et al: The influence of muscle action on the acute growth hormone response to resistance exercise and short-term detraining. Growth Hormone and IFG Research 11:2, 75–83, 2001.
13. Kawakami Y, Abe T, Kuno SY, et al: Training-induced changes in muscle architecture and specific tension. Eur J Appl Physiol 74: 2740–2744, 1995.
14. Clarkson PM, Sayers SP: Etiology of exercise induced muscle damage. Can J Appl Physiol 24:234–248, 1999.
15. Connolly DA, Sayers SP, McHugh MP: Treatment and prevention of delayed onset muscle soreness. J Strength Cond Res 17:197–208, 2003.
16. Kraemer WJ, Staron RS, Hagerman FC, et al: The effects of short-term resistance training on endocrine function in men and women. Eur J Appl Physiol 78:69–76, 1998.
17. Kraemer WJ, Hakkinen K, Triplett-Mcbride NT et al: Physiological changes with periodized resistance training in women tennis players. Med Sci Sports Exerc 35:157–168, 2003.
18. Komi PV, ed: Strength and Power in Sport: The Encyclopedia of Sports Medicine. Oxford, UK: Blackwell Scientific; 2003.
19. Borst SE, De Hoyos DV, Garzarella L, et al. Effects of resistance training on insulin-like growth factor-I and IGF binding. Med Sci Sports Exerc 33:648–53, 2001.
20. Fry AC, Kraemer WJ: Resistance exercise overtraining and overreaching. Sports Med 23:106–129, 1997.
21. Essen-Gustavsson B, Tesch PA: Glycogen and triglyceride utilization in relation to muscle metabolic characteristics in men performing heavy-resistance exercise. Eur J Appl Physiol 61:5–10, 1990.
22. MacDougall JD, Gibala MJ, Tarnopolsky MA, et al: The time course for elevated muscle protein synthesis following heavy resistance exercise. Can J Appl Physiol 20:480–486, 1995.
23. Tipton KD, Wolfe R: Exercise, protein metabolism, and muscle growth. Int J Sport Nutr Exerc Metab 11:109–132, 2001.
24. Biolo G, Tipton KD, Klein, S, et al: An abundant supply of amino acids enhances the metabolic effect of exercise on muscle protein. Am J Physiol 273(1 Pt 1):E122–129, 1997.
25. Chilibeck PD, Syrotuik DG, Bell GJ: The effect of strength training on estimates of mitochondrial density and distribution throughout muscle fibres. Eur J Appl Physiol 80:604–609, 1999.

26. MacDougall JD, Sale DG, Moroz JR, et al: Mitochondrial volume density in human skeletal muscle following heavy resistance training. Med Sci Sports Exerc 11:164–166, 1979.

27. Pollock ML Vincent KR: Resistance training for health. PCPFS Research Digest Series 2 No. 8 1996.

28. Kelley GA, Kelley KS: Progressive resistance exercise and resting blood pressure: A meta-analysis of randomized controlled trials. Hypertension 35:838–843, 2000.

29. Halbert JA, Silagy CA, Finucane, P, et al: Exercise training and blood lipids in hyperlipidemia and normolipidemic adults: A meta-analysis of randomized, controlled trials. Eur J Clin Nutr 53:514–522, 1999.

30. Hurley BF, Roth SM: Strength training in the elderly: Effects on risk factors for age-related diseases. Sports Med 30:249–268, 2000.

31. ACSM Position Stand on Exercise and Type II Diabetes. Med Sci Sports Exerc 32:1345–1360, 2000.

32. Moritani T, DeVries HA: Potential for gross muscle hypertrophy in older men. J Gerontol 35:672–682, 1980.

33. Izquierdo M, Hakkinen K, Ibanez J, et al: Effects of strength training on submaximal and maximal endurance performance capacity in middle-aged and older men. J Strength Cond Res 17:129–139, 2003.

34. Hakkinen K, Kallinen M, Izquierdo, et al: Changes in agonist-antagonist EMG, muscle CSA, and force during strength training in middle-aged and older people. J Appl Physiol 84:1341–1349, 1998.

35. Miszko TA, Cress ME, Slade JM, et al. Effect of strength and power training on physical function in community-dwelling older adults. J Gerontol A Biol Sci Med Sci Feb;58(2):171–5 2003.

36. Hakkinen K, Newton RU, Gordon SE, et al: Changes in muscle morphology, electromyographic activity, and force production characteristics during progressive strength training in young and older men. J Gerontol A Biol Sci Med Sci 53:B415–B423, 1998.

37. Hikida RS, Staron RS, Hagerman FC, et al: Effects of high-intensity resistance training on untrained older men. II. Muscle fiber characteristics and nucleo-cytoplasmic relationships. J Gerontol A Biol Sci Med Sci 55:B347–B354, 2000

SELECTED REFERENCES FOR FURTHER READING

Deschenes MR, Kraemer WJ: Performance and physiologic adaptations to resistance training. Am J Phys Med Rehabil 81(suppl):S3–S16, 2002

Graves JE, Franklin BA (eds): Resistance Training for Health and Rehabilitation. Champaign, IL: Human Kinetics, 2001.

Komi PV, ed: Strength and Power in Sport: The Encyclopedia of Sports Medicine. Oxford, UK: Blackwell Scientific; 2003

Kraemer WJ, Fleck SJ, Evans WJ: Strength and power training: Physiological mechanisms of adaptation. Exer Sci Sport Rev 24:363–398, 1996.

INTERNET RESOURCES

American College of Sports Medicine Current Comments
www.acsm.org/health&fitness/pdf/currentcomments/resisttrain-injuryprev071702.pdf

24
Principles of Cardiorespiratory Endurance Programming

JAN WALLACE

Cardiorespiratory endurance is the ability to perform large muscle, dynamic, moderate- to high-intensity exercise for prolonged periods of time. Cardiorespiratory endurance, along with muscle strength, muscle endurance, and flexibility, is one of the components of physical fitness. Both physical activity[1,2] and cardiorespiratory endurance[3] have been found to produce significant health benefits. **Physical activity** is defined as any bodily movement produced by skeletal muscles that results in energy expenditure[2]. The health benefits from physical activity and exercise are summarized in GETP7 Chapter 1. This chapter addresses cardiorespiratory endurance programming designed to achieve health and physical fitness benefits and to treat or rehabilitate modern chronic disease and associated comorbidities (also see GETP7 Chapter 7).

Principles of Training

Exercise training is defined as planned, structured, and repetitive bodily movement done to improve or maintain one or more components of physical fitness. The principles of training apply to exercise training and exercise treatment more so than to physical activity. A basic assumption in exercise programming is that something useful or beneficial occurs as a result of repeated bouts of exercise. This assumption is predicated on a number of physiological principles. The most central of these is the *principle of adaptation*, which states that if a specific physiological capacity is taxed by a physical training stimulus within a certain range and on a regular basis, this physiological capacity usually expands. Adaptation also depends on two correlated physiological principles, *threshold* and *overload*. To elicit an adaptation, the physiological capacity must be challenged beyond a certain minimal intensity called the *training threshold*. If training stimulus exceeds this threshold, it is a training *overload*, and the process of physiological adaptation usually occurs. As the physiological capacities of the body expand, the initial training stimulus may be rendered subthreshold, and the workload must increase (*progression*) to maintain overload. The concept of progression also encompasses the practice of using very modest intensities of work during the initial sessions of an exercise program. *Regression*, or de-adaptation, refers to the transience of physiological enhancement from training that occurs when training ceases and the physiological capacities regress toward pretraining. *Retrogression* is excessive taxing of physiological capacities leading to their diminution. Retrogression can refer to either acute or chronic periods of excessive overload. That is, either a single bout or chronic bouts of excessive overload can cause retrogression.

A final principle of central importance in exercise programming is the concept of *specificity*. Specific physiological capacities expand only if they are stressed in the course of an exercise program. For example, swimmers have an 11% increase in swim ergometry performance over the course of a training season but show no change in run time to exhaustion on a treadmill[4].

Each of these principles guides the design of an exercise program. In exercise training, the mode of exercise, as well as the frequency, duration, and intensity of training are critical in achieving fitness, athletic, or health outcomes. The mode must be specific to the targeted component of fitness, and the frequency, duration, and intensity must be combined in a systematic overload that will result in physiologic adaptations.

Exercise Prescription for Training

The process of **exercise prescription** can be divided into three steps, which are illustrated in Figure 24-1. The first step is assessing health and fitness information. The second step is to interpret that information. The third step is to use the information with the interpretation as well as the goals of the client or patient to formulate an exercise prescription.

Exercise training spans a broad continuum from improving and maintaining physical fitness, including athletic performance, to disease prevention, treatment, and rehabilitation. Exercise prescription is a means of using the principles of training along with assessment to provide an effective exercise training regime. The extent of the assessment often depends on the setting. The nature of the assessments may vary by setting (clinical vs. health or fitness) program goals (weight loss vs. athletic performance) and clientele (low fit vs. high fit)

An example of exercise prescription in the commercial health and fitness industry is when an exercise professional use information from a health and medical history,

anthropometric estimation of body fat, one-repetition maximum, and submaximal cycle ergometer test with heart rate (HR) monitoring to develop an exercise program for a client. On the opposite end of the spectrum, in exercise prescription in the clinical setting, medical records, blood reports, pulmonary functions, and symptom limited maximal exercise testing with the analysis of expired gases and electrocardiography (ECG) may be incorporated to develop an exercise prescription to treat a patient with chronic obstructive pulmonary disease.

One of the most common uses of exercise training in the health and fitness setting has been to improve physical fitness. As stated earlier, the mode is selected specific to the targeted fitness component, whether it is muscle strength, muscle endurance, cardiorespiratory endurance, or flexibility. Intensity, duration, and frequency combine to create the overload. After fitness is achieved, exercise training can be modified to maintain physical fitness. Most often, the overload intensity, duration, or frequency can be reduced to maintain the physical fitness. Athletic performance requires similar but more intensive exercise training. In addition to the higher levels of physical fitness, skill practice and strategic development combine to develop athletic performance. Exercise treatment is the use of exercise training to treat modern chronic diseases and associated comorbidities. The principles of mode, frequency, duration, and intensity may appear to be similar in exercise training and exercise treatment. However, it may be the precautions for exercise, which are included in the exercise prescription for chronic disease, that become the most important element of the exercise treatment. More recently, physical activity has been used for health benefits such as reduced morbidity and mortality[2]. Physical activity has not been considered to be exercise training because it does not improve any aspect of fitness.

Elements of the Exercise Prescription

Whether the purpose is athletic training or treatment of disease, the exercise prescription must include mode, frequency, duration, and intensity. *Mode*, the type of exercise, uses the specificity of exercise principle to choose a

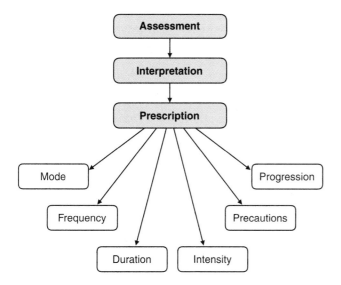

Figure 24-1. The process of developing an exercise prescription.

type of exercise that will stimulate the desired outcome. *Frequency* is number of sessions per week or the number of sessions per day. *Duration* is the total time, measured in minutes, for each exercise session. *Intensity*, measured as percent of capacity, is the effort. As stated earlier, frequency, duration, and intensity combine to produce an overload. In exercise prescription, the recommended frequency, duration, or intensity is called the *target*.

Additional aspects of the exercise prescription include progression and precautions, when appropriate. Guidelines for the progression of exercise become a factor in the success of individuals who are beginning exercise programs or who are engaging in specific types of exercise programs. An example of exercise progression for beginning exercisers is provided in GETP7 Table 7-1.

Precautions for exercise are the modifications in the prescription or the additional concerns that must be addressed for each disease process, comorbidity, or disability to make exercise safe (see Section IV). For example, individuals with diabetes who exercise should be given several precautions for the timing of meals, insulin injections, and glucose monitoring that are not given to apparently healthy individuals without diabetes who exercise (see Chapter 33 and GETP7 Chapter 9). Precautions given to individuals with angina are not the same as those given to individuals with low back pain. Each chronic disease and disability has a specific set of precautions. These precautions are discussed later in this chapter.

Cardiorespiratory Endurance

In 1998, The ACSM updated its position stand on the recommended quantity and quality of exercise for developing and maintaining cardiorespiratory fitness in healthy adults[5]. The recommendations for cardiorespiratory endurance exercise are:

- **Mode:** Using large muscle groups
- **Frequency:** 3 to 5 days per week
- **Duration:** 20 to 60 min
- **Intensity:** 40% to 50% to 85% of $\dot{V}O_2R$

For older and extremely deconditioned individuals, an exercise intensity of 40% can be effective in improving cardiorespiratory endurance.

Within the breadth of these variables, an exercise prescription of 3 days a week for 20 minutes at 50% of $\dot{V}O_2R$ may be more effective for some individuals, but an exercise prescription of 5 days a week for 60 minutes at 85% of $\dot{V}O_2R$ may be more effective for others. How do exercise professional determines what will be most effective for each individual?

DETERMINING THE MODE

Cardiorespiratory exercise should be used to improve cardiorespiratory endurance. Cardiorespiratory exercises are continuous, dynamic exercises that use large muscle masses and require aerobic metabolic pathways to sustain the activity. Examples of these exercises include walking, jogging, cycling, swimming, dancing, rollerblading, and cross-country skiing. Cardiorespiratory exercise can improve cardiorespiratory endurance as well as prevent and treat modern chronic disease[6]. Even though physical activity has a similar effect on the prevention of disease, the role of physical activity in the treatment of modern chronic disease has yet to be established. When physical activity is programmed for health, activities that produce an energy expenditure beyond the intensity of activities of daily living (i.e., greater than 2.5 METs) should be recommended. Examples of physical activities can be found in the Appendix A, Compendium of Physical Activities.

Cardiorespiratory activities can be classified in different ways. One way is to classify by skill and energy expenditure, and another is to classify by the dependence of body weight. Categories for skill and energy expenditure groupings are listed in Table 24-1.

Group 1 activities are recommended for exercise programs and prescriptions in which the intensity is important to regulate and maintain. For example, control of exercise intensity to prevent overuse injuries in novice exercisers who are overweight may limit the mode of exercise to those in group 1. Similarly, more group 1

TABLE 24-1. Grouping of Cardiorespiratory Exercise and Activities

	Group 1	Group 2	Group 3
Definition	• Ease of maintaining constant intensity • Low interindividual variation in energy expenditure	• Ease of maintaining constant intensity • Energy expenditure is related to skill	• Skill highly variable • Energy expenditure highly variable
Use	Desirable for more precise control of exercise intensity: • Beginning an exercise program • Rehabilitation	Not contraindicated for the early stages of conditioning, but skill must be considered.	Good for group interactions, but caution must be taken for • High risk-low fit • Symptomatic patients
Examples	• Treadmill walking • Cycle ergometry	• Swimming • Cross-country skiing	• Racquet sports • Basketball • Soccer

Modified from GETP7 Box 7-1.

exercises are used in rehabilitation programs in which the control of exercise intensity is vital to the safety of the exercise program. However, as individuals progress to higher fitness progression, exercises from groups 2 and 3 may provide more variation in the types of activities.

Classifying cardiovascular exercise by body weight dependency is a different classification system than by skill and energy expenditure. Weight-dependent exercises, or weight-bearing activities, are those in which the body weight is moved throughout the exercise. Examples of weight-bearing exercise are walking, jogging, running, and hiking. On the other hand, in weight-independent exercise, or non–weight-bearing activity, the body weight is supported by the implement or media and does not contribute to the energy expenditure. Examples of non–weight-bearing exercise are cycling and swimming. Non–weight-bearing exercise may be more effective in preventing lower limb overuse injuries associated with exercise.

The mode of exercise that is effective in producing the desired outcome must be the first consideration in choosing the mode of exercise. However, modifications and variations can be made in mode to promote adherence if needed. Varying the mode of exercise among the weekly workouts and substituting recreational activities may be strategies that promote a higher adherence to the exercise.

DETERMINING THE FREQUENCY AND DURATION

Frequency is prescribed in sessions per day and in days per week. To improve cardiorespiratory fitness for apparently healthy adults, the range of frequency is between 3 to 5 days per week. For sedentary individuals, the minimum overload is the 3 days per week; for higher fit individuals, the overload must be increased to 4 to 5 days per week. In patients with some chronic conditions or diseases, such as obesity or hypertension, the most effective frequency may be a higher frequency per week. In these cases, the initial exercise prescription for sedentary individuals with obesity or hypertension may have higher frequencies than for apparently healthy adults. Recommendations for exercise progression are essential for injury prevention when high-frequency prescriptions are given to sedentary individuals. In the inpatient setting, frequency is prescribed in sessions per day for 3 to 5 days per week. These sessions may be as high as 3 to 5 per day. When programming for physical activity, most, if not all, days of the week should be recommended.

Exercise durations range from 5 to 60 minutes. Prescribed exercise duration rarely exceeds 60 minutes. Most individuals do not receive significantly more benefit by working more than 60 minutes. In fact, the risk of overuse injury increases the risk-to-benefit ratio of exceeding 60 minutes of cardiorespiratory exercise for apparently

healthy adults. The lower exercise duration, between 5 to 10 minutes, is used in the clinical setting for chronic disease and disabilities. The minimum duration to achieve an improvement in cardiorespiratory fitness in apparently healthy adults is 20 minutes[6]; the range is 20 to 60 minutes. The range of prescribed duration, similar to frequency, is broad. Similar to the principles of prescribing frequency, duration is prescribed in shorter, 10- to 20-minute ranges depending on the fitness and health of the individual. For apparently healthy individuals who are sedentary, the shorter durations from 20 to 30 or 30 to 40 minutes are adequate to improve cardiorespiratory fitness. For more fit individuals, 40 to 60 minutes may be the required overload to achieve further improvements in cardiorespiratory fitness. When programming for physical activity, a duration of at least 30 minutes should be recommended.

The combination of exercise frequency and duration should be viewed with caution. Pollock, in a 1977 classic study, exercised six groups of men within the range frequency and duration for the exercise prescription for apparently healthy adults to improve cardiorespiratory fitness[8]. Intensity was the same for all groups of men. Three groups exercised for 15, 30, and 45 minutes per session for 3 days a week. Three other groups of men exercised at varying frequencies of one time per week, three times per week, and five times per week for 30 minutes per session. As expected, the improvements in fitness were related to the overload (Fig. 24-2). However, high overloads were also related to high injury rates. The highest duration and the highest frequency resulted in the highest injury rates. Therefore, caution should be taken in determining the optimal duration and frequency to improve fitness without causing overuse injuries.

DETERMINING THE INTENSITY

Intensity of cardiorespiratory exercise is measured as a percent of maximal capacity, or more specifically, as a percent of $\dot{V}O_2$ reserve ($\%\dot{V}O_2R$). Table 24-2 summarizes the

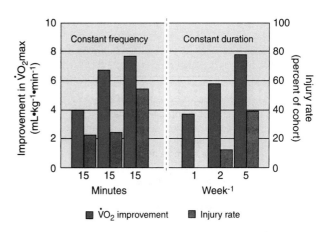

Figure 24-2. The influence of overload on improvement in $\dot{V}O_{2max}$ and subsequent injury rates[9].

TABLE 24-2. Classification of Exercise Intensity for Cardiorespiratory Endurance[5]

Intensity	Percent of HRR or $\dot{V}O_2R$	Percent of HR_{max}%	RPE
Very light	< 20	< 35	< 10
Light	20–39	35–54	10–11
Moderate	40–59	55–69	12–13
Hard	60–84	70–89	14–16
Very hard	> 85	> 90	17–19
Maximal	100	100	20

HRR = heart rate reserve; $\dot{V}O_2R$ = oxygen uptake reserve; HR_{max} = maximum heart rate; RPE = rating of perceived exertion

ACSM classification system for exercise intensity[5]. The three steps in prescribing exercise intensity for cardiorespiratory exercise are:

- Determine the target intensity
- Provide the client or patient with a means of monitoring intensity
- Translate the prescribed intensity to actual work rates for the exercise session

Determining the Cardiorespiratory Intensity

Cardiorespiratory exercise intensity is based on a measured or estimated maximal $\dot{V}O_2$ or heart rate. The ACSM recommends an intensity of exercise corresponding to between 55% and 65% to 90% of maximum HR (HR_{max}), or between 40% and 50% to 85% of oxygen uptake reserve ($\dot{V}O_2R$) or HR reserve (HRR). Whereas the $\dot{V}O_2R$ is the difference between $\dot{V}O_{2max}$ and resting $\dot{V}O_2$, the HRR is the difference between HR_{max} and resting HR. When exercise intensities are set according to $\dot{V}O_2R$, the percent values are approximately equal to the percent values for the HRR[7].

The range to improve cardiorespiratory fitness is 50% to 85% of $\dot{V}O_2R$, with some more sedentary populations being as low as 40%. Individuals with lower cardiorespiratory fitness can improve their fitness with lower exercise intensities, but individuals with higher cardiorespiratory fitness require higher exercise intensities to make improvements. For most individuals, intensities within the range of 70% to 85% HR_{max} or 60% to 80% HRR are sufficient to achieve improvements in cardiorespiratory fitness when combined with an appropriate frequency and duration of training[5].

EXERCISE INTENSITY PRESCRIPTION

Choosing the Prescriptive Range for Exercise Intensity

When prescribing exercise intensity, a range of intensities is recommended rather than a single intensity. When choosing an exercise intensity for your clients, give them a range of target HRs within the 50% to 85% $\dot{V}O_2R$ that best meets their physical condition at that time. A range of exercise intensities can be effective for most health or fitness outcomes. These ranges are often quite broad. An example is the 50% to 85% $\dot{V}O_2R$ intensity range for im-

proving fitness. Even though the range spans 35%, it will be easier for the client or patient to use a 10% range somewhere within the 35% range. For example, the exercise professional could prescribe a range of 60% to 70% $\dot{V}O_2R$, providing a target range to exercise within.

The duration of exercise is measured by minutes, and the frequency of exercise is measured by days. Minutes and days are easy for the client or patient to monitor. Intensity of exercise, on the other hand, is measured by percent of $\dot{V}O_{2max}$ and is much harder for the client or patient to monitor. If a client is instructed to exercise between 60% to 70% of $\dot{V}O_2R$, it may be difficult for him or her to determine how hard to work. Therefore, other variables that reflect the intensity of exercise must be monitored to estimate the intensity of exercise. These variables must exhibit a linear relationship with exercise intensity and be simple for the client or patient to monitor. Figure 24-3 illustrates the model linear relationship that allows these variables to be used for exercise intensity. In the linear model, the resting value of variable A corresponds to the resting value of variable B. Likewise, the maximal value for variable A corresponds to the maximal value of variable B. Because these two variables exhibit a direct linear relationship, 50% of variable A should correspond to 50% of variable B. Therefore, the use of variable B to

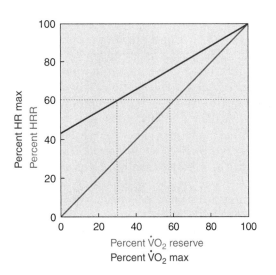

Figure 24-3. A comparison of the relationships between percent heart rate (HR) maximum and HR reserve (HRR).

estimate variable A allows for an accurate estimation. The three most common linear variables used to monitor intensity are:

- $\dot{V}O_{2max}$, metabolic equivalents (METs) or energy expenditure
- HR
- Ratings of perceived exertion (RPE)

As exercise intensity increases, so does HR, perceived exertion, and energy expenditure (METs or $\dot{V}O_2$). These variables can be used alone or in combination to guide exercise intensity. HRs and RPE are most often used in the health and fitness setting, but all three are more often used in exercise treatment.

Exercise Prescription Using $\dot{V}O_2$

ACSM Guidelines suggest exercise intensity prescription be implemented using a percentage of the $\dot{V}O_2R$. To calculate the target $\dot{V}O_2$ based on $\dot{V}O_2R$, the following equation is used:

Target $\dot{V}O_2$ = (exercise intensity) $(\dot{V}O_{2max} - \dot{V}O_{2rest}) + \dot{V}O_{2rest}$

An example of utilizing the equation is given below:

Assessed $\dot{V}O_{2max}$ = 25.0 mL·kg^{-1}·min^{-1}

Assumed Resting $\dot{V}O_2$ = 3.5 mL·kg^{-1}·min^{-1}

If we wish to determine exercise intensity at 55% of $\dot{V}O_2R$:

Target $\dot{V}O_2$ = (exercise intensity) $(\dot{V}O_{2max} - \dot{V}O_{2rest}) + \dot{V}O_{2rest}$

$(0.55) (25.0 - 3.5) + 3.5$

$= (0.55)\qquad (21.5) + 3.5$

$= 11.8 + 3.5$

$= 15.3$ mL·kg^{-1}·min^{-1}

ACSM metabolic equations (see GETP7 appendix D) could then be used to convert the target $\dot{V}O_2$ into a walk speed or cycle watt work rate.

Using Metabolic Equivalents to Guide Exercise Intensity

Using METs is a method of categorizing energy expenditure based on one metabolic unit being resting metabolism. METs and $\dot{V}O_2$ are both measures of energy expenditure and can be converted to each other using the following relationships.

1 MET = 3.5 mL·kg^{-1}·min^{-1}

1 MET = 1.05 kcal·kg^{-1}·hr^{-1}

Metabolic equivalents are often easier for those who are not exercise physiology clinicians to understand because the energy the expenditure is measured in multiples of 1 MET. For example, an exercise that is 10 METs has an energy expenditure 10 times greater than that of rest. Exercise intensities are easier to understand based on METs.

Prescribing exercise intensity with METs is the truest method to guide intensity. Keep in mind the principle of specificity of exercise. The desired outcome of the cardiorespiratory exercise program is an increase in cardiorespiratory energy. METs are energy expenditure. There is no purer form of estimating energy expenditure. Therefore, the formula to determine target METs is:

Target METs = (exercise intensity) (max METs − resting MET) + resting MET

Using the same example as the $\dot{V}O_2R_{max}$ method (55% of max), target METs is computed this way:

Assessed $\dot{V}O_{2max}$ = 25.0 mL·kg^{-1}·min^{-1} = 7.1 METs

Assumed Resting $\dot{V}O_2$ = 3.5 mL·kg^{-1}·min^{-1} = 1.0 MET

Target METs = (exercise intensity) (max METs − resting MET) + resting MET

$(0.55) (7.1 - 1.0) + 1.0$

$= (0.55)\qquad (6.1) + 1.0$

$= 3.4 + 1.0$

$= 4.4$ METS

The energy expenditure of physical activities, exercise, occupational activities, leisure activities, recreational activities, and sports has been determined. See the appendix (compendium of physical activities). for MET expenditures for various activities. Choose the appropriate activities in which the energy expenditure is within the target METs.

Using Heart Rate to Guide Exercise Intensity

There are several ways to choose target heart rates to guide exercise intensity.

- Percent HRmax (%HR$_{max}$)
- HRR
- Direct determination

Which method is best? Before discussing how to use HR to guide exercise intensity, we need to explore the variability of the linear relationship between HR and exercise intensity. The linear relationship between HR and exercise intensity varies with the mode of exercise and the calculation of target HRs. These three relationships can be made more similar to our ideal linear model by plotting them as the %HRmax. The percent HR formula is:

%HRmax = Maximum HR × Percent intensity

A problem with using the %HRmax method is that 50% of HR max does not reflect 50% $\dot{V}O_2R$. Looking at the relationship based on working range rather than a straight percentage may improve the linear relationship for use in guiding exercise intensity. The working range of HR has been termed the HRR. The reserve can be calculated by the following formula, developed by Karvonen et al[9]. The working range or reserve formula is:

Reserve = Maximum value − Resting value

To apply this formula to HR:

$$HRR = HR_{max} - HR_{rest}$$

In a similar fashion as $\%HR_{max}$ was calculated, to calculate a percentage of the reserve:

$$Percentage\ of\ reserve = Reserve \times Percent$$

$$\%HRR = (HR_{max} - HR_{rest}) \times Percent\ (\%)$$

Note that when using this method, the percentage of the reserve is added to the resting heart to calculate the target HR for exercise.

What does all of this mean about using HRs to monitor exercise intensity?

1. HR has a liner relationship with $\dot{V}O_2$. This relationship varies with the:
   a. Mode of exercise
   b. Calculation of target HRs
2. The linear relationship between HR and $\dot{V}O_2$ is best in cardiorespiratory exercise for guiding exercise intensity.
3. Within the spectrum of cardiorespiratory exercise, the more muscle mass involved in the exercise, the better target HRs reflect exercise intensity ($\% \dot{V}O_2R$).
4. A target HR calculated from one test mode may not be as accurate for other modes of exercise because of differences in muscle mass and, therefore, the HR response to the mode of exercise (e.g., exercise test using leg ergometer for walking exercise prescription).

Estimating Maximal Heart Rate

Caution should be taken when using equations to estimate maximal HR[10]. These formulas have large standard deviations; some formulas can be off ± 12 to 15 bpm. If the formula, 220 − age were used to estimate maximal HR, the range of variation for the target HRs for 60% intensity can exhibit a significant variation. For example, what is the target HR at 60% intensity for a 50-year-old man with a resting HR of 70 bpm? To estimated his HR_{max}:

$$Estimated\ HR_{max} = 220 - age$$
$$= 220 - 50$$
$$= 170\ bpm$$

If the standard deviation for this equation is ± 15 bpm, his maximal HR may be anywhere between 155 to 185 bpm. Using all three of these estimated maximal HRs in the formula for HRR, the range of target HRs for 60% intensity is to 121 to 139 bpm:

Using the higher estimated HR_{max} in the Karvonen formula:

$$Target\ HR = [(HR_{max} - HR_{rest})\%] + HR_{rest}$$
$$= [(185 - 70)\ 0.60] + 70$$
$$= [115 \times 0.60] + 70$$
$$= 69 + 70$$
$$= 139\ bpm$$

Using the estimated HR_{max}:

$$Target\ HR = [(HR_{max} - HR_{rest})\%] + HR_{rest}$$
$$= [(170 - 70)\ 0.60] + 70$$
$$= [100 \times 0.60] + 70$$
$$= 60 + 70$$
$$= 130\ bpm$$

Using the lower estimated HRmax (Karvonen equation):

$$Target\ HR = [(HR_{max} - HR_{rest})\%] + HR_{rest}$$
$$= [(155 - 70)\ 0.60] + 70$$
$$= [85 \times 0.60] + 70$$
$$= 51 + 70$$
$$= 121\ bpm$$

Alternative Heart Rate Prescription Methods

In clinical settings, a maximal HR may not be advisable to achieve because of postoperative limitations, recent myocardial infarction, or ischemic conditions. Therefore, target HR intensity can be based on the limiting factor or "threshold" achieved during an exercise test.

At or Below Submaximal Test Endpoint

Whether it is a one mile walk test or a maximal graded exercise test, an assessment of exercise capacity is given before exercise prescription. For safety, exercise intensity should not be prescribed above the intensity used in the exercise assessment. According to the work of Cumming[11], 50% of the individuals who exhibited a positive ECG response to maximal graded exercise testing would have been missed had the test terminated at 80% of HRmax. Had these individuals been tested to 80% HRmax yet prescribed exercise intensity above the 80%, they may have been in danger of an adverse event during exercise. It is prudent to prescribe exercise intensity at or below the intensity of exercise that has been evaluated.

If submaximal graded exercise is used for the exercise testing, choosing the stage below the test endpoint would assure a margin of error between the prescribed intensity and the endpoint intensity. If the exercise assessment involves a one mile walk or 12-minute run, choose a speed below the average speed or a HR below the highest HR exhibited during the assessment.

Exercise Below an Abnormal Cardiovascular Response

Abnormal cardiovascular responses to exercise are often reproducible. That is, an ischemic response to exercise will occur at the same double product for patients who exhibit stable angina. An ischemic response may manifest during an exercise test as a decrease in blood pressure (BP), dysrhythmia, ST-segment depression, or angina.

Prescribing the exercise intensity below the ischemic response decreases the incidence of an abnormal response compromising the exercise or resulting in an adverse event. Often, rate pressure product (RPP; double product), which is calculated as systolic BP multiplied by HR, is a tool used to determine the threshold of abnormality. Subsequent exercise, regardless of mode, can thus be monitored by the HR, BP (and therefore, RPP) response. Further discussion on the RPP is found in Chapters 22 and 31.

Target Heart Rate Summary

In summary, HRs are used to guide intensity because of a direct linear relationship between HR and oxygen consumption. %HRmax and HRR are the two methods to calculate target HRs. The percentage of HRR corresponds to the actual relative intensity as measured by $\dot{V}O_2$ much better than %HRmax. Target HRs must be calculated 10% to 15% higher than the desired intensity when using %HRmax. Caution should be used when estimating maximal HR.

The determination of exercise intensity is more a science than an art. Where the "art" emerges is during the exercise session when any aspect of the exercise program or prescription may be modified in the "art of exercise leadership" to help the client or patient reach his or her goals.

USING RATED PERCEIVED EXERTION TO GUIDE EXERCISE INTENSITY

Rating of perceived exertion (RPE) is a subjective rating system for exercise intensity based on general fatigue. RPE can be used in conjunction with target HRs. RPE is often used as a substitute for target HRs when:

- The ability to monitor HR is compromised.
- No exercise test HRs exist.
- The client is applying effort to physical activities other than cardiorespiratory endurance (e.g., playing tennis or gardening).
- Medications such as beta-blockers alter the HR–oxygen consumption relationship, negating the usefulness of beta-blocker HRs.

Two scales of RPE now exist[12]. Table 4-7 in GETP7 summarizes both scales. The first is called a category scale, in which effort perception has a linear relationship with cardiorespiratory exercise intensity. The scale ranges from 6 to 20, with word description anchors every odd number on the scale. The category-ratio scale has a nonlinear relationship that mimics the blood lactate or minute ventilation response to increasing exercise intensities. The word anchors were improved for better understanding with more common phrases used to describe exercise. Onset of blood lactate is between 4 and 5 on the category-ratio scale and represents 12 to 16 on the category scale.

The target RPE can be chosen in a similar manner as the direct method to determine target HRs. If both target HRs and RPE are to be used to guide intensity, the RPE should be taken from the exercise test that corresponds to the target HR[13]. However, caution must be used with this approach as the relationship between testing RPE and HR may be different in the training setting[14].

The instructions for RPE are important to guide individuals to focus on general fatigue. Reading a standardized script to all clients may be helpful. A recommended version of these instruction is found on page 78 of GETP7.

These instructions should be given before the exercise test as well as when giving the exercise prescription. Additional orientation to the RPE scale during exercise helps the individual focus on the feelings of exertion. After an exercise prescription is given and before the individual begins to exercise, have the individual walk on a treadmill or ride a cycle ergometer at the target exercise intensity. This intensity should also elicit the target RPE. Instruct the individual to remember that this effort is the target RPE. Occasional orientations ensure proper use of the RPE to monitor exercise intensity.

Translating Exercise Intensity from the Prescription to the Workout

Whether you are prescribing exercise intensity by METs or suggesting a work rate for your client to exercise, the exercise intensity needs to be translated from percent intensity, HRs, perceived exertions, and METs to actual work rates for each activity. The metabolic equations can be used to estimate the work rate for group 1 activities recommended in the exercise prescription. The metabolic equations are summarized in GETP7 Table D.1.

Using the prescribed intensity, calculate the $\dot{V}O_2$. Using the in GETP7 Table D.1, calculate approximate work rates for the individual to try on the treadmill, cycle ergometer, arm crank, and stepper. For example, What are the recommended work rates for a 70-kg individual whose physical work capacity is 7 METs and whose prescribed exercise intensity is 60% to 70%? The steps to determine the recommended work rates are:

1. Determine the target $\dot{V}O_2$.

$$1 \text{ MET} = 3.5 \text{ mL·kg}^{-1}\text{·min}^{-1}$$

$$7 \text{ METs} = 3.5 \text{ mL·kg}^{-1}\text{·min}^{-1} \times 6 = 24.5 \text{ mL·kg}^{-1}\text{·min}^{-1}$$

$$\text{Lower range target } \dot{V}O_2 = ([24.5 - 3.5] \text{ mL·kg}^{-1}\text{·min}^{-1}) \times 0.6$$

$$= 12.6 \text{ mL·kg}^{-1}\text{·min}^{-1}$$

$$\text{Higher range target } \dot{V}O_2 = ([24.5 - 3.5] \text{ mL·kg}^{-1}\text{·min}^{-1}) \times .7$$

$$= 14.7 \text{ mL·kg}^{-1}\text{·min}^{-1}$$

2. Calculate a recommended work rate for the target $\dot{V}O_2$ range. These examples will only use the 60% intensity.

a. For treadmill grade of 2.5%:

$$\dot{V}O_2 \,(\text{mL}\cdot\text{kg}^{-1}\cdot\text{min}^{-1}) = [0.1\,(\text{speed})]$$
$$+ [1.8\,(\text{speed})(\text{grade})]$$
$$+ 3.5\,(\text{mL}\cdot\text{kg}^{-1}\cdot\text{min}^{-1})$$

$$12.6\,(\text{mL}\cdot\text{kg}^{-1}\cdot\text{min}^{-1}) = [0.1\,(\text{speed})]$$
$$+ [1.8(\text{speed})(.025)]$$
$$+ 3.5\,(\text{mL}\cdot\text{kg}^{-1}\cdot\text{min}^{-1})$$

$$12.6\,(\text{mL}\cdot\text{kg}^{-1}\cdot\text{min}^{-1}) - 3.5\,(\text{mL}\cdot\text{kg}^{-1}\cdot\text{min}^{-1})$$
$$= [0.1\,(\text{speed})] + [1.8(\text{speed})(0.025)]$$

$$9.1\,(\text{mL}\cdot\text{kg}^{-1}\cdot\text{min}^{-1}) = [0.1\,(\text{speed})]$$
$$+ [1.8(\text{speed})(0.025)]$$

$$9.1\,(\text{mL}\cdot\text{kg}^{-1}\cdot\text{min}^{-1}) = [0.1\,(\text{speed})]$$
$$+ [0.045(\text{speed})]$$

$$9.1\,(\text{mL}\cdot\text{kg}^{-1}\cdot\text{min}^{-1}) = \text{speed}\,[0.1 + 0.045]$$

$$9.1\,(\text{mL}\cdot\text{kg}^{-1}\cdot\text{min}^{-1}) = \text{speed}\,[0.145]$$

$$9.1\,(\text{mL}\cdot\text{kg}^{-1}\cdot\text{min}^{-1})/[0.145] = \text{speed}$$

Speed = 62.8 m/min or 2.3 mph @ 2.5%

b. For the cycle ergometer:

$$\dot{V}O_2\,(\text{mL}\cdot\text{kg}^{-1}\cdot\text{min}^{-1}) = [1.8(\text{work rate})/\text{Mass}]$$
$$+ 7.0\,(\text{mL}\cdot\text{kg}^{-1}\cdot\text{min}^{-1})$$

$$12.6\,(\text{mL}\cdot\text{kg}^{-1}\cdot\text{min}^{-1}) = [1.8(\text{work rate})/70\,\text{kg}]$$
$$+ 7.0\,(\text{mL}\cdot\text{kg}^{-1}\cdot\text{min}^{-1})$$

$$12.6\,(\text{mL}\cdot\text{kg}^{-1}\cdot\text{min}^{-1}) - 7.0\,(\text{mL}\cdot\text{kg}^{-1}\cdot\text{min}^{-1})$$
$$= [1.8(\text{work rate})/70\,\text{kg}]$$

$$5.6\,(\text{mL}\cdot\text{kg}^{-1}\cdot\text{min}^{-1}) = 1.8(\text{work rate})/70\,\text{kg}$$

$$5.6\,(\text{mL}\cdot\text{kg}^{-1}\cdot\text{min}^{-1}) \times 70\,\text{kg} = 1.8(\text{work rate})$$

$$392\,(\text{mL}\cdot\text{min}^{-1}) = 1.8\,(\text{work rate})$$

Work rate = 217 kpm·min$_{-1}$ or 35 watts

These recommended work rates would be used to begin the exercise program. If these work rates elicit the target HRs or RPE, the work rates would be incorporated into the exercise session. If these work rates elicited higher or lower HRs or RPE than the target values, the work rates would be adjusted accordingly.

Intensity Summary

Exercise intensity is programmed or prescribed in three steps. The first is to determine the target exercise intensity that will elicit a training effect. The second is to provide HR, RPE, or MET guides to measure the exercise intensity. The third is to recommend work rates that should produce the exercise intensity.

Exercise Prescription Summary

Exercise training can be used to improve health, improve and maintain physical fitness, and treat and rehabilitate chronic diseases and their associated comorbidities. The elements of the exercise prescription vary for each purpose. Table 24-3 summarizes the variations in mode, frequency, duration, intensity, progression, and precautions used for each purpose. In general, exercise professionals in the health and fitness setting use exercise programming to improve and maintain health and to improve physical fitness. Exercise prescription will be used more in the clinical setting to treat and rehabilitate modern chronic disease and the associated comorbidities.

CONSIDERING THE CALORIC COST OF THE EXERCISE PRESCRIPTION

The interaction of physical activity intensity, duration, and frequency determines net caloric expenditure from the activity. It is generally accepted that many of the health benefits and training adaptations associated with increased physical activity are related to the total amount of work accomplished during training[5,15]. However, the caloric thresholds necessary to elicit significant improvements in $\dot{V}O_{2max}$, weight loss, or a reduced risk of premature chronic disease may not be the same. Therefore, individualized exercise prescriptions should be designed with energy expenditure goals in mind.

The ACSM recommends a target range of 150 to 400 kcal·day^{-1} of energy expenditure in physical activity and exercise[5,15]. The lower end of this range represents a minimal caloric threshold of approximately 1000 kcal·wk^{-1} from physical activity, which is associated with a significant 20%

TABLE 24-3. General Exercise Programming and Prescription Variables in Various Settings

	Physical Activity and Health	Physical Fitness	Exercise Treatment
Mode	Any physical activity	Cardiorespiratory endurance Groups 1 to 3	Cardiorespiratory endurance, primarily group 1 and non–weight bearing or walking
Frequency	Most, if not all days of the week	3–5 days per week	3–5 sessions per day 3–5 days per week
Duration	Accumulation of > 30 min per day	30–60 minutes per session	5–10 minutes per session inpatient 20–60 minutes per day
Progression	Dose response: Increased benefit seen with more activity	Recommended for sedentary individuals Begin with group 1	Recommended per disease or disability
Precautions	Only if contraindication to physical activity exists	Specific to disease or disability	Specific to disease or disability

to 30% reduction in risk of all-cause mortality[16], and this should be the initial goal for previously sedentary individuals. Based on the dose–response relationships between physical activity and health and fitness, individuals should be encouraged to move toward attainment of the upper end of the recommended range (e.g., 300 to 400 kcal·day^{-1} from activity) as their fitness improves during the training program. The application of the 1000-kcal threshold (150 kcal·day^{-1} × 7 days·wk^{-1}) for weight loss and weight loss maintenance may be insufficient for effective control[17]. The Institute of Medicine suggests that 60 min·day^{-1} may be necessary, which is double the current recommendation[18]. Energy expenditure in excess of 2000 kcal·wk^{-1} have been successful for both short- and long-term weight control[19, 20].

Estimating caloric expenditure during exercise has been problematic for exercise professionals, and developing an exercise plan based on caloric thresholds should not be viewed as an exact science. Interindividual differences in skill, coordination, and exercise economy (the $\dot{V}O_2$ at a given submaximal work rate) and the variable intensities within each available activity strongly influence estimation of caloric expenditure during exercise. One useful method to approximate the caloric cost of exercise is by using the following equation based on the MET level of the activity:

$$(\text{METs} \times 3.5 \times \text{body weight in kg})/200 = \text{kcal·min}^{-1}$$

This formula helps an individual understand the components of the exercise prescription and the volume of exercise necessary to achieve the caloric goals of the program.

Consider the following example. The weekly goal of the exercise program has been set at 1000 kcal for an individual who weighs 70 kg, and the MET level of the prescribed activity is 6 METs. In this example, the *net* caloric expenditure from the exercise would be 5 METs because 1 MET of the activity represents resting metabolic rate. Therefore, the *net* caloric expenditure from the exercise is 6 kcal·min^{-1}, which requires 167 minutes per week to attain the 1000 kilocalorie threshold. Given a 4-d·wk^{-1} program, the individual would require approximately 42 minutes per day to achieve the 1000 kcal goal (or 33 minutes per day, 5 d·wk^{-1}). Working backward from the caloric goal to determine the volume of exercise needed to reach the goal is useful in determining the appropriate exercise prescription components. If the goal was a more aggressive 2000 kcal·week^{-1}, the net caloric expenditure of 6 kcal·min^{-1} would require 333 minutes·wk^{-1} or approximately 48 min·day^{-1} on all days of the week (see Appendix A).

Interpreting Fitness and Laboratory Assessments to Develop the Exercise Prescription

Exercise prescription depends on prior assessment. The extent of the assessment is dependent on the environment and cost. Chapter 14 and GETP7 Chapters 4 and 5 discuss methods of assessment. This section presents how the assessment information is used to develop an exercise prescription. It is assumed that the assessment has ruled out individuals with contraindications to exercise, so this discussion is for clients and patients who are appropriate for exercise.

In using exercise tests to develop the exercise prescription, different testing scenarios exist. These include maximal graded exercise testing, submaximal graded exercise testing, field tests, and estimating exercise capacity by questionnaire.

Maximal graded exercise tests are the "ideal" scenario to develop an exercise prescription because maximal HR is determined and the cardiovascular response throughout the whole range of exercise has been observed for normal responses and safety. However, maximal graded exercise testing is rarely used outside of the research setting. Field tests and submaximal tests are more often used in the health and fitness setting. All different forms of testing can be found in the clinical setting. Field tests are often used with pulmonary or cancer patients in which the ECG monitoring of the graded exercise testing is not essential. The following section describes implementing an exercise prescription based on findings from an initial fitness assessment.

Implementing the Exercise Prescription

Several considerations must be made when implementing the exercise prescription. Decisions must be made on the need for exercise supervision. Before exercise can begin, individuals must be taught how to monitor the exercise intensity of their prescription. Instruction on the components of the exercise session is essential to preventing injury and adverse events during exercise. Proper exercise progression is also fundamental to successful outcomes.

SUPERVISION OF EXERCISE

There are several levels of exercise supervision, ranging from none at all to a team consisting of nurses, physical therapists, and exercise physiologists in the inpatient hospital setting. Supervision may only be needed in the initial stages of training in which education and orientation enhances the outcomes. On the other hand, in high-risk patients (e.g., those with risk of sudden death), supervision may be required for as long as the patient exercises (GETP7 Table 7-3).

In the health and fitness setting, supervision is provided for instruction and adherence. Supervision scenarios include orientation to equipment, group exercise, and individual training. Supervision of clients by the health/fitness instructor is limited to a few days during periods of equipment orientation. However, the client can approach the health/fitness instructor whenever advice is needed. In group exercise, one or more exercise leaders lead a group of clients through choreographed routines of different forms of fitness, including mind–body, core stabilization, and aquatic activities. The ratio of clients to leaders is recommended to be 40 to one[21]. In this scenario, the exercise leader may have less opportunity to modify each individual's exercise.

In some setting, the health/fitness instructor may supervise every exercise session early in the initial stages of training. Later, in the improvement and maintenance stages of training, the personal trainer may supervise fewer exercise sessions until the client can exercise on his or her own. Good assessments of fitness, closer focus on exercise outcomes, and improved exercise adherence are advantages of personal training.

In the clinical setting, supervision is provided because of medical status. Supervision levels in the clinical setting include inpatient rehabilitation, outpatient rehabilitation, secondary prevention programs, and the initial stages of exercise training for moderate-risk patients.

The most extensive supervision is found in the inpatient and outpatient hospital settings where the "supervisor" includes a team of nurses, physical therapists, and exercise physiologists. In the inpatient setting, the ratio of supervisors to patients may be four to one; the ratio may be four to 10 in the outpatient setting[21]. Daily monitoring of ECG, BP, and other clinical measures such as oxygen saturations or blood glucose are used in this form of supervision. Even though the exercise habit is well established for patients in secondary prevention exercise programs, supervision is still required to prevent and respond to adverse events. The secondary prevention supervision is less than that of the inpatient and outpatient settings; perhaps two supervisors to 20 patients. Supervision of exercise is essential for initial stages of training to ensure that the patients know how to exercise and how to manage the precautions for exercise. For example, for a patient with diabetes, the exercise specialist will supervise the timing of meals and medications as well as monitor blood glucose to assure the safety for the patient and teach the patient proper monitoring skills.

MONITORING EXERCISE INTENSITY

A critical element of the exercise prescription is exercise intensity. Adherence to the prescribed intensity is important for making the necessary changes in fitness and health as well as for the prevention of injuries and other adverse events. In the exercise prescription, methods of guiding exercise intensity are given. These include the use of HRs, RPE, and METs.

Whether intensity is guided by HRs or RPE, each should be maintained within the target values to assure adherence to the prescribed intensity. For example, the target HRs for an individual are 120 to 130 bpm. The individual walks around a track at 3.5 mph. After 5 minutes, the individual checks his HR to see if he is exercising at the prescribed intensity. If he is not within the prescribed range, he can make appropriate pace adjustments until he is within the prescribed range. The same is true for monitoring RPE. The absolute exercise intensity should be adjusted so that it elicits the target RPE.

Under ideal conditions, the actual walking speed an individual chooses should elicit similar HRs from day to day. However, environmental conditions such as heat, cold, pollution, and altitude add physiological work in addition to the actual work of the exercise. For example, work in the heat is the sum of the work of the activity and the work of cooling the body. Therefore, a workout in a comfortable environment can be more physiologically demanding (e.g., increased cardiac strain) in a hot, humid environment. To adjust to the environmental conditions, the walking speed should be decreased to ensure adherence to the target HRs (see Chapter 28 and GETP7 Appendix E).

If the intensity is guided by METs and the MET range is wide for a specific activity, RPE or HRs should be used to ensure the prescribed intensity within a wide MET range. For example, hiking has a MET range from 3 to 7 METs. Our individual's prescribed intensity is 5 METs. Hiking is an activity that can be chosen to target the 5-MET intensity. On the other hand, hiking also has the possibility of being too intense. If the individual guides the hiking with HRs or RPE, she can be more assured to stay within the target intensity by adjusting their pace.

Monitoring Heart Rates

Heart rates can be monitored by palpation, HR monitors, or ECG. In the health and fitness industry, HRs are most often monitored in the recovery from exercise unless the HR can be palpated during the exercise or if the individual uses a HR monitor. HR monitors can be worn or built into the exercise equipment. In the clinical setting, HRs are monitored more often during exercise through HR monitors, ECG, or palpation.

Whether target HRs are calculated by %HRmax or HRR, the individual is given a range of HRs to maintain during the workout. These HRs are calculated in bpm and in a shorter time frame (10, 12, 15 seconds) that will estimate the minute count because it is unrealistic for the individual to take 1-minute HR counts. If the individual takes the HR in the recovery from the effort, the HR will decrease too fast for an accurate estimation of the exercise HR.

The best HR palpation sites are the peripheral pulses. The radial pulse is the most often monitored site. The temporal pulse is also possible to use. The carotid site is not recommended unless the other sites cannot be palpated. Caution should be used with the carotid site to avoid palpation of the baroreceptors, which can cause a decrease in HR. Using a light touch with two fingers can avoid a baroreflex.

To obtain a pulse rate:

1. Locate a pulse with the index and long fingers of one hand.
2. Count the number of pulsations in the given period.

3. Count the first pulsation as zero.
4. To determine the pulse rate, multiply the number of pulse beats by the number of counting intervals in 1 minute (e.g., take the pulse for 10 seconds and multiply the pulse beats by 6)

The margin of error may be one pulse count within the counting period, which can lead to substantial errors in HR (in bpm) when short counting periods are used. Longer pulse counts during exercise afford greater accuracy and provide more time for detection of some dysrhythmias. However, the HRs of fit persons can decrease quite rapidly after exercise, possibly making long counts less accurate than short ones. The 10-second counting period is most often recommended immediately after exercise unless exceptions are necessary.

Locally telemetered HR monitors (watch style) are commonly available and can be a useful aid in training, particularly for athletes and others desiring frequent, immediate feedback regarding exercise HR. However, the only advantages such monitors have over manual pulse counts are the ability to assess HR without interrupting exercise, the capacity for data storage, and their use for those who have difficulty manually assessing pulse. These devices do not perform any of the functions of a medical ECG monitor such as dysrhythmia or ischemia detection. Manual pulse counts have the advantages of detecting some forms of dysrhythmia and being constantly available to any person who carries a timepiece. Thus, it may be preferable to continue to use manual pulse counts in clinical or older populations. HR monitors usually measure the pulse rate for 5- to 15-second time intervals and correct the pulse rate to a minute. The same margin of error exists for HR monitors as for palpation for short intervals. HR monitors may not detect specific dysrhythmias such as premature ventricular contractions (PVCs). If the HR monitor fails to count PVCs, the HR it reports will be lower than the true HR. It will skip the counting of the PVC. In this case, the individual may increase the intensity of exercise so that his or her HR will meet the target HRs, which may increase the risk of an adverse event.

EXERCISE PROGRESSION

The rate of progression of exercise depends on VO_2 max, health status, age, individual activity preferences and goals as well as the tolerance to training. Exercise progression is essential for sedentary individuals beginning exercise programs. Additional populations that benefit from exercise progression include individuals with chronic disease and disabilities. Most training programs feature three progressive stages: initiation, improvement, and maintenance (see GETP7 Table 7-1).

Initiation Stage

The goal of the initial stage of training allows time to begin the adaptive process. Typically, this is accomplished by working at lower intensity and shorter duration and with careful attention to signs of intolerance, particularly musculoskeletal or cardiopulmonary. The initial stage is the time to develop the habit of exercise with minimal discomfort and soreness. It is also a time to allow the exercise professional to instruct the individual as to proper exercise form.

Suitable initial intensities may range from 40% of VO_2R for beginners to more than 50% of VO_2R for individuals with higher aerobic capacities or experienced exercisers returning from time off regular exercise. Appropriate initial duration of exercise ranges from 15 to 30 minutes per session. Older, obese, and profoundly sedentary individuals may start with as little as 15 to 20 minutes or less of continuous exercise. In such situations, especially if the factor-limiting duration is stable angina or claudication, intermittent exercise or multiple daily sessions may be helpful. If intensity is kept low to moderate, sedentary but otherwise healthy adults may be able to start with sessions of 15 to 20 minutes, and higher fit individuals may begin with 20 to 30 minutes.

The exercise session itself may be modified during the initial stage of training by expanding the warm-up period, using it to inventory possible signs of injury or soreness (e.g., "Let's stretch out our quadriceps now. Is anyone sore here?"), providing information, and answering questions. The initial stage of training generally lasts 4 weeks but may be expanded for those requiring additional time to adapt. Monitoring exercise HRs may also be an indication for progression. If exercise or recovery HRs are lower for the same amount of work, the intensity or duration can be increased.

Improvement Stage

The goal of this stage of training is to provide a gradual increase in the overall exercise stimulus to allow for significant improvements in cardiorespiratory fitness. In the improvement stage, expanding physiological capacities are further challenged. This stage is typified by the phrase *progressive overload*. Small increments in intensity and duration may occur nearly every week. In fact, the challenge of the improvement stage is to increase training at a rate that continues to stimulate further advancement without causing overtraining and retrogression.

Several benchmarks of progression are discussed later in the chapter, but self-observation of subjective and objective responses to training may be the most important. Failure to complete an exercise session, lack of normal interest in training, increased HR or RPE at the same rate of external work, and an increase in minor aches and pains are all signs that progression may be too rapid[22] (see Chapter 28). In an appropriately incremented improvement stage, interest and appetite for exercise normally increase in tandem with the subjective and objective impressions that progress is being made. In general, frequency, intensity, and duration should not be increased together in any single week, and should total weekly training volume should not be advanced by more than 10%[23]. Increasing duration by 5 to 10 minutes per session on a weekly basis is usually well tolerated, as is building intensity gradually through the range of 60% to 85% of aerobic capacity over months. Progression of both intensity and duration in a single session is not recommended.

In this stage, adjusting the training program is commonly accomplished by increasing frequency, duration, or intensity rather than more than one in a saltatory approach toward individual goals. Competitive athletes who train intensively and those encountering musculoskeletal or other physical obstacles impeding progress may benefit from the early incorporation of techniques such as cross-training, which are more typical of the maintenance stage.

The adaptive potential of physiological function is finite, and large increments in fitness, typical in the improvement stage, always taper at some point. Aerobic capacity can be expected to expand by approximately 10% to 30% in the course of a program following ACSM guidelines. Improvements of more than 30% rarely occur unless accompanied by a large reduction in body weight and fat. If training is discontinued, gains in fitness regress by approximately 50% within 4 to 12 weeks[5]. After approximately 6 months of training, most individuals make the transition from improvement to maintenance.

Maintenance Stage

The goal of this stage of training is the long-term maintenance of cardiorespiratory fitness developed in the previous stage. The maintenance stage is typified by diversification of the training program and purposeful attempts to rotate and reduce the stresses of continued training. Diversification may take the form of using several modes of exercise to maintain enjoyment and explore new capabilities. This may be particularly important to lifelong programs with goals such as weight management and general health. For those with a goal of general health, caloric expenditure should exceed 1000 per week and can be obtained through different combinations of frequency, duration, and intensity.

For those using the maintenance phase as a sustained period of performance or competition, diversification may be used as a means of reducing the potential for overuse injuries, particularly in programs with high training volumes or for participants with musculoskeletal limitations. *Cross-training*, as this approach is often called, refers to using a variety of modes of cardiorespiratory endurance exercise (e.g., swimming, running, biking) to maintain a high training stimulus for central aerobic adaptations such as enhanced stroke volume and expanded blood volume. This approach allows rotation of local fatigue and musculoskeletal stresses across a range of muscle groups.

Cognitively, the maintenance stage is a time for enjoyment, surveillance, and reappraisal. It is a time for enjoying the fruits of labor by competing, engaging in new activities, or reducing the demands of weekly training. Surveillance for overuse injury must continue during the maintenance phase. Equipment and footwear should be re-evaluated. Finally, the goals of the program may be re-examined, physiological or performance testing may be repeated, and new goals may be established. Further advancing performance and cardiorespiratory endurance often requires special techniques such as periodization and isolation of performance demands.

Summary

In summary, following the exercise prescription recommendations can provide as safe and effective exercise program or treatment. Combining the principles of exercise training with the principles of exercise leadership can assure adherence to an exercise prescription that can be followed for a lifetime.

REFERENCES

1. Pate RR, Pratt M, Blair SN, et al: Physical activity and public health. A recommendation from the Centers for Disease Control and Prevention and the American College of Sports Medicine. JAMA 273: 402–407, 1995.
2. U.S. Department of Health and Human Services: Physical Activity and Health: A Report of the Surgeon General. U.S. Department of Health and Human Services, Centers for Disease Control and Prevention, National Center for Chronic Disease Prevention and Health Promotion (Ed.) Washington, D.C.; 1996.
3. Blair SN, Kohl HWI, Paffenbarger RS, et al: Physical fitness and all-cause mortality: A prospective study of healthy men and women. JAMA 262:2395–2401, 1989.
4. Magel JR, Foglia GF, McArdle WD: Specificity of swim training on maximum oxygen uptake. J App Physiol 38:151, 1975.
5. American College of Sports Medicine: The recommended quantity and quality of exercise for developing and maintaining cardiorespiratory and muscular fitness, and flexibility in healthy adults. Med Sci Sports Exerc 30:975–991, 1998.
6. MacAlpin RH, Kattus AA: Adaptation to exercise in angina pectoris: The electrocardiogram during treadmill walking and coronary angiographic findings. Circulation 33:183, 1966.
7. Swain DP, Leutholtz BC: Heart rate reserve is equivalent to %VO$_2$ reserve, not to %VO2 max. Med Sci Sports Exerc 29:410–414, 1997.
8. Pollock MJ, Gettman L, Milesis C, et al: Effects of frequency and duration of training on attrition and incidence of injury. Med Sci Sports 9:31–37, 1977.
9. Karvonen M, Kentala K, Musta O: The effects of training on heart rate: A longitudinal study. Ann Med Exp Biol Fenn 35:307–315, 1957.
10. Whaley MH, Kaminsky LA, Dwyer GB, et al: Predictors of over- and underacheivement of age-predicted maximal heart rate. Med Sci Sports Exerc 24:1173–1179, 1992.
11. Cumming G: Yield of ischemic exercise ECG patterns to exercise intensity in a normal population. Br Heart J 34:919, 1972.
12. Borg G: Borg's Perceived Exertion Scales. Champaign, IL: Human Kinetics; 1998
13. Glass SC, Knowlton RG, Becque MD: Accuracy of RPE from graded exercise to establish exercise training intensity. Med Sci Sports Exerc 24:1303–1307, 1992.
14. Glass SC, Whaley MH, Wegner MS: Ratings of perceived exertion among standard treadmill protocols and steady state running. Int J Sports Med 12:77–82, 1991.

15. Haskell WL, Wolffe JB: Memorial lecture. Health consequences of physical activity: Understanding and challenges regarding dose-response. Med Sci Sports Exerc 26:649–660, 1994.

16. Lee IM, Skerrett PJ: Physical activity and all-cause mortality: What is the dose-response relation? Med Sci Sports Exerc 33:S459–S471, S493–S494, 2001.

17. American College of Sports Medicine: Position stand: Appropriate intervention strategies for weight loss and prevention of weight regain for adults. Med Sci Sports Exerc 33:2145–2156, 2001.

18. Saris W, Blair SN, van Baak M, et al: How much physical activity is enough to prevent unhealthy weight gain? Outcome of the IASO 1st Stock Conference and consensus statement. Obesity Reviews 4: 101–114, 2003.

19. Food and Nutrition Board, Institute of Medicine: Dietary Reference Intakes for Energy, Carbohydrates, Fiber, Fat, Protein and Amino Acids (Macronutrients). Washington, D.C.: National Academy Press; 2002.

20. Ross R, Janssen I: Physical activity, total and regional obesity: Dose-response considerations. Med Sci Sports Exerc 33:S521–S529, 2001

21. American College of Medicine: ACSM's Health/Fitness Facility Standards and Guidelines, 2nd ed. Champaign, IL: Human Kinetics; 1997.

22. Lehmann M, Foster C, Keul J: Overtraining in endurance athletes: A brief review. Med Sci Sports Exerc 25:854, 1993.

23. Skinner JS: General principles of exercise prescription. In Skinner JS, ed. Exercise Testing and Exercise Prescription. Philadelphia: Lea & Febiger; 1993.

SELECTED REFERENCES FOR FURTHER READING

ACSM's Metabolic Calculations Tutorial CD-ROM. Philadelphia: Lippincott, Williams & Wilkins; 2000.

Bruce RA, Kusumi F, Hosmer D: Maximal oxygen intake and homographic assessment of functional aerobic impairment in cardiovascular disease. Am Heart J 85:546–562, 1973.

Brubaker PH, Kaminsky LA, Whaley MH: Coronary Artery Disease: Essentials of Prevention and Rehabilitation Programs. Champaign IL: Human Kinetics, 2002.

Cooper KH: A means of assessing maximal oxygen uptake. JAMA 203: 201–204, 1968.

Fletcher GF, Balady G, Amsterdam EA, et al: Exercise standards for testing and training by the American Heart Association Science Advisory and Coordinating Committee. Circulation 104:1694–1740, 2001.

INTERNET RESOURCE

ExRx.net: http://www.exrx.net

Principles of Musculoskeletal Exercise Programming

JOSEPH P. WEIR AND JOEL T. CRAMER

This chapter addresses KSAs from the following content areas:

1   **Exercise Physiology and Related Exercise Science**
2   Pathophysiology and Risk Factors
3   **Health Appraisal, Fitness, and Clinical Exercise Testing**
4   Electrocardiography and Diagnostic Techniques
5   Patient Management and Medications
6   Medical and Surgical Management
7   **Exercise Prescription and Programming**
8   Nutrition and Weight Management
9   Human Behavior and Counseling
10   Safety, Injury Prevention, and Emergency Procedures
11   Program Administration, Quality Assurance, and Outcome Assessment

This chapter focuses on the elements of design for exercise programs geared toward stressing the musculoskeletal system. Specifically, the focus is on resistance exercise and flexibility training. Chapters 3 and 23 explain the physiological responses and adaptations to these types of training programs. But this chapter briefly addresses the broad benefits of this type of exercise, as well as address the possible risks. Emphasis is placed on exercise for improving health and fitness as opposed to training for high-level athletic competition. Nonetheless, the terminology and principles are the same. This chapter also addresses special populations. Resistance exercise, in a variety of forms, is incorporated into activity programs for children, so the unique issues associated with the pediatric population are addressed.

Proper flexibility training elongates the musculotendinous unit and improves range of motion (ROM) about the joints. These improvements may decrease the risk for both acute and chronic injury, although the evidence is equivocal. Resistance exercise is designed to increase muscle strength, size, speed, and power. The health benefits of resistance exercise are becoming increasingly clear. Resistance training has been shown to elicit im-

provements in muscular fitness for a number of populations, including healthy adults[1], older adults[1,2], children and adolescents, and diseased populations[3]. Resistance exercise improves muscle mass, therefore ameliorating aging-induced sarcopenia (i.e., loss of muscle mass). This can translate into improved body composition. Resistance training improves glucose tolerance independent of changes in body composition. Increased strength and muscle power makes activities of daily living easier and decreases the stress of tasks such as carrying groceries and changing a tire. Greater strength may decrease the risk of falling. In addition, the stress on the skeletal system may enhance peak bone density and retard the decline in bone mass with age. Other adaptations to resistance training that may also contribute to increased levels of muscular fitness include increases in balance, stability, coordination, and flexibility. Finally, resistance exercise can enhance appearance and improve self-confidence. Collectively, the health, performance, and aesthetic benefits of resistance exercise improve quality of life.

The American College of Sports Medicine (ACSM) has recognized the importance of resistance training as an integral part of a regular exercise program[4]. Additionally, the U.S. Surgeon General recommends strength developing exercises at least twice per week for all Americans. Recent advances in scientific research have shown the numerous health- and fitness-related benefits of resistance training, which has stimulated the need to establish guidelines for designing resistance training programs. The initial position stand by the ACSM that provided basic guidelines for resistance training was written in 1998: "The recommended quantity and quality of exercise for developing and maintaining cardiorespiratory and muscular fitness, and flexibility in healthy adults"[4]. In 2002, a position stand more specific to resistance training was written: "Progression Models in Resistance Training for Healthy Adults"[1]. Other organizations such as the National Strength and Conditioning Association (NSCA) have also taken an active role in bridging the gap between the science and practice of resistance training principles by publishing position statements not only for athletes[6,7] but for the general population and youths as well.

Despite the many benefits of resistance exercise, as with all exercise, there is risk in participation. Clearly, orthopedic injuries can occur with resistance exercise, and care must be taken to teach proper form and technique. Continued monitoring and supervision minimize injury risk. It has been suggested that the use of free weights poses higher risks than resistance exercise machine and devices such as elastic tubing, but no data support this contention. Furthermore, free weights may challenge balance and posture in positive ways. The ACSM recommends that participants choose a form of resistance training (free weights, bands, or machines) that is comfortable throughout the full pain-free ROM[7].

Resistance exercise poses risks to the cardiovascular system, and individuals with severe cardiovascular conditions such as uncontrolled hypertension and unstable angina should not participate until their conditions are under control. A more detailed list of cardiovascular-associated contraindications is listed in Table 25-1. In general, the contraindications for participation in resistance exercise in those with cardiovascular disease (CVD) are also those for participation in aerobic exercise[3]. Finally, it should be noted that the available evidence indicates that for healthy adults and those with mild CVD, orthopedic injuries are rare, and cardiovascular events have not been reported[3].

TABLE 25-1. Contraindications for Resistance Exercise

Contraindication	Details
Unstable angina	
Uncontrolled hypertension	Systolic BP ≥ 160mm Hg or diastolic BP ≥ 100 mm Hg
Uncontrolled dysrhythmias	
Severe valvular disease	
Hypertrophic cardiomyopathy	
LVOT	
CHF	Until medically treated
Myocardial ischemia or poor LV function	Until fitness > 5 to 6 METs, no angina, and no ischemic ST-segment depression

CHF = congestive heart failure LV = left ventricular; LVOT = left ventricular outflow obstruction; MET = metabolic equivalent.

Adapted from Pollock et al.[3] and GETP7.

Basic Terminology

Strength is defined as the ability to produce a force. As such, the proper unit for strength is Newtons; however, in most settings, actual force production is not measured, and proxies such as the amount of weight that can be lifted is measured. *Work* is defined as the product of force times distance, and *power* is work divided by time. Thus, power is a function of both strength and speed and is exhibited by producing high forces very rapidly. Although strength and power are clearly related, the methods used to develop strength versus power can vary considerably.

Muscle force and power are created by the contraction of skeletal muscles. There are however, different types of muscle contractions. *Concentric contractions* occur when actual shortening of muscle fibers occurs. In this case, the muscle force exceeds the resistance, and the muscle insertion and origin move closer together. Concentric contractions are what are typically thought of as muscle contractions. In contrast, *eccentric contractions* are muscle actions in which active muscle lengthening occurs. That is, the muscle is generating force, but the resistance exceeds the muscle force, and the muscle origin and insertion move farther apart. It is important to note that eccentric contractions occur all the time in normal movements. Examples include the action of the quadriceps muscles when walking down steps or sitting down into a chair and the action of the forearm flexors when setting a cup on a table. Indeed, everyday tasks such as walking involve cyclical coupling of concentric and eccentric contractions. This is referred to as the stretch–shortening cycle. Finally, *isometric* or static contractions occur when muscle force is generated but no movement occurs. In this case, muscle force and the resistance are equal.

Resistance exercise can be performed using a variety of equipment. In general, however, training equipment can be segregated into two broad categories: machines and free weights. Machines have been designed to stress every major muscle group and include machines that use weights for resistance, isokinetic machines, and pneumatic devices. Free weights are typically barbells and dumbbells, and although these are very simple implements, it is a testament to their effectiveness that they have thrived in an era of expensive machines. Most resistance exercise, whether free weights or machines, use gravity to create resistance. This type of resistance is often referred to as *isotonic* resistance. In a strict sense, the term is improper because the derivation means constant ("iso-") tension and the tension actually experienced by the muscle varies throughout the ROM. Other terms have been suggested as a replacement for *isotonic*, and these include isoinertial and **DCER (dynamic constant external resistance)**. Both of these terms reflect the idea that the mass of the object—and, therefore, the influence of gravity—is constant. That said, the term *isotonic* is so well embedded in the literature and is operationally defined as resistance created by moving an object of fixed mass against gravity, so it is unlikely and probably unnecessary to eliminate its usage. *Isokinetic* machines are designed to control speed of motion as opposed to mass moved. Typically, isokinetic devices control the angular velocity about a joint, and the torque (rotary force) and power are measured. The torque-versus-velocity relationship is such that higher torque is generated at slow velocities and lower torque is generated at higher velocities. However, the power-versus-velocity relationship is characterized by an inverted U shape in which the highest power outputs are achieved at intermediate velocities (Fig. 25-1). Isokinetic machines control angular velocity using so-called *accommodating resistance*. That is, the resistance is varied so that the velocity of motion is fixed. No matter how hard the contraction, the angular velocity will not accelerate above the preset value; however, the harder the contraction, the greater the torque that is generated and recorded. Most devices use a servomotor of some sort to achieve accommodating resistance. Most isokinetic machines are limited to single joint motions (open kinetic chain; see below), and angular velocity is controlled. Early isokinetic machines were limited to only concentric contractions (or isometric if the speed was set at

zero), but current machines can involve both concentric and eccentric contractions. An eccentric isokinetic contraction is performed by having the motor actively create motion at some user-defined velocity. The harder the motion is resisted, the greater the torque that is produced. Pneumatic machines typically use pistons in which the exerciser pushes air through an aperture. The size of the aperture is adjustable and dictates the resistance experienced by the participant and the speed of the contraction. These devices are limited to only concentric contractions, and extension/flexion cycles at a joint are accomplished using reciprocal concentric contractions of agonist/antagonist pairs.

The design of resistance exercise programs is based on the manipulation of volume and intensity through factors such as sets, repetitions, and load. A repetition (rep) is one complete cycle of a resistance exercise maneuver. For example, one repetition of the biceps curl exercise consists of concentric contraction of the forearm flexors from full extension to full flexion and the subsequent eccentric contraction from full flexion to full extension. A group of repetitions is called a set. The load simply refers to the amount of resistance (e.g., weight lifted) during each repetition. The volume of training is most easily estimated by the product of the load and the total number of repetitions performed. The number of repetitions performed in a set is primarily determined by the load. That is, high loads can only be performed for a relatively few number of repetitions, and light loads can be performed for relatively high numbers of repetitions. With isotonic resistance exercise, exercise intensity is typically quantified via the load using repetitions maximum. A one-repetition maximum (1RM) is defined as the most amount of weight that can be successfully lifted one time. Similarly, the 5RM and 10RM are the most amount of weight that can be successfully lifted five and ten times, respectively. Training intensities of greater than 80% 1RM are typically required to elicit increases in muscle strength, power, and size in experienced strength trainers (see section titled "Training Load" later in this chapter for specific recommendations). Beginners can improve strength with relative intensity levels of 45% to 50% of 1RM[1].

Motions of the body in general, and resistance exercises in particular, have been described in terms of open versus closed kinetic chain motions. An open kinetic chain motion or exercise occurs when the motion of one joint does not require the motion of an adjacent joint. In this context, the biceps curl is an open kinetic chain exercise because the motion at the elbow does not require motion at the shoulder or the wrist. A closed kinetic chain motion occurs when motion at one joint requires motion at an adjacent joint. As an example, when the feet are on the floor, flexion at the knee also requires motion at the ankle and the hip. Thus, the squat exercise is a closed kinetic chain exercise. The practical distinction here is one between single-joint versus multijoint exercises. So-called "isolation" exercises

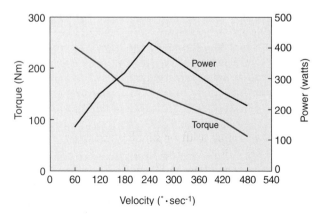

Figure 25-1. Isokinetic torque and power-versus-velocity relationships for knee extension from a representative subject. Data courtesy of the Human Performance Laboratory, University of Nebraska—Lincoln.

such as seated knee extensions and biceps curls are open kinetic chain motions, and compound multijoint exercises such as the bench press and the power clean are closed kinetic chain motions. (In the case of the power clean, both the upper and lower body segments are closed kinetic chain exercises.)

Resistance Training Technique and Equipment Considerations

BREATHING

The pattern of breathing during a set of resistance exercise is important because it influences the cardiovascular response to the exercise bout. Notably, the blood pressure (BP) can increase dramatically during a set of resistance exercise[8,9]. For example, MacDougall et al.[8] reported a mean BP response during the double leg press of 320/250 mm Hg with values as high as 480/350 mm Hg in one subject. Heavy resistance exercise is often accompanied by the **Valsalva maneuver,** which is a forced exhalation against a closed glottis that results in increases in intrathoracic pressure. The Valsalva maneuver most frequently occurs during the sticking point (hardest part) of the concentric phase of a repetition and induces considerable changes in cardiac physiology. It is frequently recommended that the participant inhale during the eccentric phase of a repetition and exhale during the concentric phase. The exhalation prevents the Valsalva maneuver and likely minimizes the BP response to the repetition. In practice, this is difficult to do during a hard repetition. It appears that the precise pattern of inhalation and exhalation in conjunction with the concentric versus eccentric phases of a repetition has little effect on the BP response, as long as the Valsalva maneuver is avoided[10]. Interestingly, avoiding the Valsalva maneuver may actually increase the risk of cerebral hemorrhage because the maneuver also increases the intracranial pressure, which balances the increases in arterial pressure, so that increases in cerebrovascular transmural pressure are minimized[11].

SPOTTING

Spotting refers to the practice of having another person serve as a safety and assist the participant when a repetition cannot be completed. This is particularly important when using free weights because there have been incidents of serious injury and death to individuals who have become trapped by weights without a spotter. Proper spotting requires good communication between the participant and the spotter so that the spotter knows when to intervene. It is good practice to tell the spotter how many repetitions are anticipated and perhaps give a signal for when intervention is needed. In general, the lifter has the responsibility to do most of the work when a spotter intervenes because the spotter is often in a poor mechanical position and may be injured.

WEIGHT BELTS

Weight belts are a popular accouterment for weight training. The logic of the weight belt is that it increases intraabdominal pressure, which serves to stabilize the spine during heavy lifts, and increases in intra-abdominal pressure have been reported with the use of weight belts during the squat lift[12]. In addition, increases in intramuscular pressure of the erector spinae occur with weight belt use, which may increase spinal stiffness (and decrease injury risk) during lifting[13]. During the squat, individuals using weight belts tend to increase repetition speed during both the concentric and eccentric phases relative to repetitions without weight belts, indicating higher power generation[12], an observation consistent with anecdotal evidence of greater 1RM squat values with the use of a weight belt. To date however, it is unclear if weight belt use decreases injury risk during resistance exercise. In addition, weight belt use may increase diastolic BP during lifting tasks[14].

GRIPS AND GRIP WIDTHS

Understanding how to grip a barbell is essential to the safe and effective performance of many resistance training exercises. There are two basic classifications of bar grips: closed and open. Whereas closed grips involve wrapping the thumb around the bar, open grips do not allow the thumb to contain the bar. Because the thumb does not contain the bar like in the closed grip, the open grip is more dangerous and may allow the bar to "fall out." Therefore, in nearly all situations, the open grip is contraindicated. There are, however, several types of closed grips that can be used, including the supinated grip, pronated grip, neutral grip (halfway between supinated and pronated), and alternated grip (one hand supinated and one hand pronated). In addition to the type of grip, the grip width is equally important for safety and effectiveness. A grip width that corresponds with approximately shoulder width is recommended for most applications. An even grip width, however, is the highest priority and is essential before initiating the lift. Most barbells have precisely measured knurled areas and standardized markings to help lifters clearly identify even grip widths.

STANCE

Whether initiating a lift or simply picking up a barbell from the floor, it is essential to begin with a stable body position. Earle and Baechle[15] suggest that when standing erect, the body should be in a stable position when the feet are approximately shoulder width apart, the heels and balls of the feet should be in full contact with the floor, the knees should be slightly bent, and the head and shoulders should be in line with the hips. To remain stable while lying supine on a utility bench, there are five points of the body that must remain in contact with either the bench or the floor throughout the duration of the lift: head, shoulders, low back or buttocks, left foot, and right foot.

IMPORTANCE OF ECCENTRIC PHASE

As noted in Chapters 3 and 23, eccentric contractions are both a normal part of everyday movement and are associated with development of delayed-onset muscle soreness (DOMS). Several studies[16,17] have shown that inclusion of eccentric contractions also facilitates hypertrophy and strength development relative to programs with concentric-only contractions. Therefore, it is recommended that training programs should include both concentric and eccentric actions[1]. This naturally occurs during most isotonic training programs.

STICKING POINTS

The sticking point is the part of the ROM in which a weight is hardest to lift. For example, in the biceps curl exercise, the sticking point usually occurs with the elbows at about 90°. A sticking point exists because of changes in mechanics during a movement. Moment arms change through the ROM, and the changes in muscle and, therefore, sarcomere lengths, contribute to these changes and affect the difficulty of the movement. All isotonic training exercises have sticking points, although attempts have been made to manipulate the shape of cams of resistance training machines to make the difficulty more even throughout the ROM.

Resistance Training Program Design

Specific guidelines exist for designing resistance training programs that safely and effectively optimize the ability to achieve higher levels of muscular fitness. Because training-induced increases in muscular fitness can be multifaceted, a resistance training program must be designed specifically to meet the individual's needs and unique goals. For example, an 18-year-old high school volleyball player participating in a resistance training program to better her playing skills will desire a different training outcome than a 40-year-old obese, sedentary man who has never participated in any kind of exercise program. Therefore, it is essential to understand the principles of resistance training to safely and accurately prescribe effective individualized programs.

According to GETP7, the following guidelines apply for individuals participating in resistance training programs:

- Choose a mode of exercise (free weights, bands, or machines) that is comfortable throughout the full pain-free ROM.
- Perform a minimum of eight to 10 separate exercises that train the major muscles of the hips, thigh, legs, back,

chest, shoulders, arms, and abdomen. A primary goal of the program should be to develop total body strength and endurance in a relatively time-efficient manner. Total exercise training programs lasting longer than 1 hour per session are associated with higher dropout rates.

- Perform one set of each exercise to the point of volitional fatigue for healthy individuals while maintaining good form.
- While the traditional recommendation of eight to 12 repetitions is still appropriate, choose a range of repetitions between three and 20 (e.g., three to five, eight to 10, 12 to 15) that can be performed at a moderate repetition duration (~3 sec concentric, ~3 sec eccentric).
- Exercise each muscle group 2 to 3 nonconsecutive days per week and, if possible, perform a different exercise for the muscle group every two or three sessions.
- Adhere as closely as possible to the specific techniques for performing a given exercise.
- Allow enough time between exercises to perform the next exercise in proper form.
- For people with high cardiovascular risk and those with chronic disease (e.g., hypertension, diabetes), terminate each exercise as the concentric portion of the exercise becomes difficult (rating of perceived exertion [RPE] 15 to 16) while maintaining good form.
- Perform both the lifting (concentric phase) and lowering (eccentric phase) portions of the resistance exercises in a controlled manner.
- Maintain a normal breathing pattern; breathholding can induce excessive increases in BP.
- If possible, exercise with a training partner who can provide feedback, assistance, and motivation.

PROGRAM DESIGN CONSIDERATIONS

Several fundamental considerations must be understood before manipulating the design variables to construct a resistance training program. These considerations can be viewed as "underlying concepts" that exist for all types of resistance training programs; therefore, they can be applied to any scenario. The three primary program design considerations are specificity, variation, and progressive overload[1,18].

Specificity

The body adapts specifically to the unique demands placed upon it; this concept has been termed the *SAID* (specific adaptations to imposed demands) *principle*[18]. Therefore, *specificity* as it relates to resistance exercise can be defined as training in a specifically designed manner to produce a specific training adaptation or outcome. Applying the specificity principle to resistance training helps to ensure that the adaptations will be consistent with the needs and goals of the individual using the program. Despite some carryover of training-induced adaptations, the effects of resistance training are specific to the muscle group, muscle action, muscle action velocity, ROM, metabolic system, intensity, and volume involved in the program. For example, a person engaging in a resistance training program to increase his or her long-distance running performance will most likely need a program that emphasizes muscular endurance for the core and trunk muscle groups at moderate velocities with moderate volume (i.e., low intensity, high repetitions, and short rest periods).

Variation

The principle of *variation* in resistance training can be defined as altering one or more program design variables over time to maintain an optimal training stimulus. Several studies have indicated that variations in training volume and intensity are more effective for eliciting gains in muscular fitness. The most common approach for incorporating structured variation into a resistance training program is called **periodization**, which is defined as a logical, phasic method of manipulating training variables in order to increase the potential for achieving specific performance goals. However, it is not limited to athletic populations. The goals of a periodized resistance training program through structured variation schemes are to optimize the stimulus for increases in muscular fitness to avoid training plateaus, overtraining, and overreaching. A periodized resistance training program typically involves three phases:

- Macrocycle (i.e., long duration; typically 1 year)
- Mesocycle (middle duration; 3 to 4 months)
- Microcycle (i.e., short duration; 2 to 6 weeks).

There are two general forms of periodization: the classic (linear) model and undulating (nonlinear) model. With linear periodization, for example, a mesocycle may contain five basic microcycles:

- **General prepreparation phase (6 to 8 weeks):** The purposes of this phase are to attain basic levels of fitness, master exercise techniques, and establish the number of exercise and initial tolerance. The duration is longer than a typical microcycle.
- **Preparation phase (2 to 4 weeks):** Generally considered to be the first formal phase of the mesocycle, this microcycle is characterized by a high training volume and low intensity.
- **Strength phase (2 to 4 weeks):** This phase progresses toward lower volumes, higher intensities, and longer rest period durations.
- **Power phase (2 to 4 weeks):** This phase typically involves a progression toward velocity-specific training at low volumes and very high intensities with adequate rest periods. This cycle also incorporates additional training modalities such as plyometrics, isokinetic training, and pneumatic devices that can be used safely at high speeds to peak the levels of muscular fitness.

- **Transition phase (several days to 2 weeks):** Also called active recovery, this cycle is incorporated by using endurance (rather than resistance) training to allow time in the mesocycle for recovery.

Figure 25-2 illustrates the theoretical relationship between resistance training volume and intensity throughout a typical macrocycle.

Progressive Overload

The term *progressive overload* was coined from the combination of the principles of overload and progression. The *overload principle* refers to placing greater demands on the body than what it is accustomed to, and the *principle of progression* refers to the constant application of the overload principle throughout a resistance training program. Clearly, these two principles must interact to elicit continual increases in muscular fitness. Therefore, the term **progressive overload** accurately represents this interaction and can be defined as the gradual increase in stress placed on the body throughout a resistance training program[1]. Progressive overload can be applied to a resistance training program by any one or combination of the following methods:

- Increased load
- Increased repetitions (for the current load)
- Altered repetition velocity (with submaximal loads)
- Decreased rest period duration (for increases in muscular endurance)
- Increased rest period duration (for increases in muscular strength or power output)

These methods work well as a short-term model for progressive overload; however, long-term progression is much more complex and must account for the individual's training status. For example, it is likely that general increases in muscular fitness will occur as a result of a general resistance training program for a novice individual. This type of program applied to an advanced, well-trained individual, however, will not yield the same benefits and will require a more specifically designed program to elicit increases in muscular strength, power output, hypertrophy, or endurance. Therefore, for the application of progressive overload over the long-term duration of a resistance training program, the ACSM recommends the general-to-specific model of progression, which states that a resistance training program should progress from simple to complex as the training status of a lifter progresses from novice to advanced[1].

PROGRAM DESIGN VARIABLES

Designing a resistance training program is a complex process that requires an understanding of the principle components as well as how they interact to provide an optimal stimulus for increases in muscular fitness. The previous section discussed the principles of specificity,

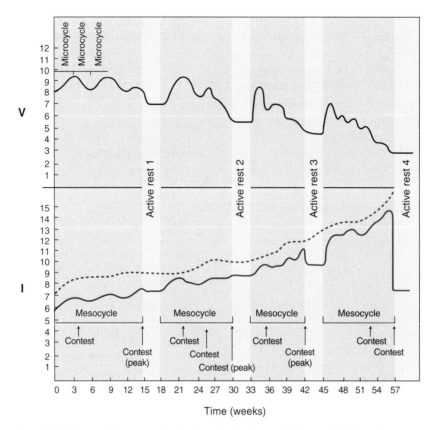

Figure 25-2. A theoretical, macrocycle-length periodization model for an elite shotputter showing microcycle and mesocycle variation. Whereas volume begins relatively high and decreases, training intensity begins relatively low and increases. (Adapted with permission from Stone et al.[58].)

variation, and progressive overload (i.e., program design considerations), but to apply these concepts, it is essential to also understand the program design variables. There are six basic program design variables: exercise selection, training frequency, order of exercises, training load, training volume, and rest period duration. Additional variables include the type and velocity of the muscle actions involved. Before the design variables can be applied and the program is underway, however, the first step should be a needs analysis to assess the safety considerations, needs, and goals of the individual who will be engaging in the resistance training program.

Needs Analysis

Traditionally, a needs analysis is conducted for athletes competing in specific sports and identifies movement patterns, muscle groups, and metabolic demands that are specific to the target athlete. However, a needs analysis can be adapted to other populations that may include steps such as completing a health history questionnaire, risk assessment, and the determination of realistic and attainable goals based on training status.

As with all types of exercise programs, the first steps should include a health history questionnaire; risk assessment; and medical clearance, if necessary. Because resistance training can place an abnormally high amount of stress on the cardiovascular system, there is a clear need for precautionary measures before prescribing a resistance training program (see Chapter 31). For example, if maximal exercise is contraindicated as a result of the health history questionnaire and risk assessment, a submaximal estimation of 1RM loads must be used and the designated training load and volume should be reduced and carefully monitored.

The second component of the needs analysis is the determination of realistic and attainable goals through the use of a resistance training program. During this process, a detailed record of the individual's exercise training history should be obtained. From the individual's experiences with resistance training, a classification should be made regarding his or her training status: novice, intermediate, or advanced. Novice individuals have little or no resistance training experience; intermediate or "trained" lifters typically have approximately 6 months of consistent experience; and advanced lifters often have years of experience and already exhibit high levels of muscular fitness. In general, the higher the training status, the slower the rate of progression will be for training-induced increases in muscular fitness. For example, whereas novice individuals typically exhibit large and rapid increases in muscular fitness parameters, the gains attained by intermediate and advance lifters tend to be smaller in magnitude and slower in progression. Therefore, the combined information of an individual's goals and training status should provide the impetus for designing a relatively general or specific resistance training program based on the general to specific model of progression.

Exercise Selection

Exercise selection is choosing the specific exercises for a resistance training program. Resistance exercises are classified into two primary categories: core and assistance exercises. Core exercises are multijoint exercises that involve large muscle groups such as the chest, shoulder, back, hip, or thigh. Assistance exercises are single-joint exercises that target smaller muscle groups such as the neck, trapezius, biceps, triceps, forearm, abdomen, low back, or anterior and posterior leg muscles. Additional classifications include structural (axial loading) and power exercises (i.e., power clean, snatch). Table 25-2 provides the names, classifications, and targeted muscle groups of selected resistance training exercises. It is recommended that a sufficient number of exercises be chosen to target all of the core muscle groups (as tolerated) as well as various assistance muscle groups as needed. Special attention should be given to choosing exercises that balance the agonist and antagonist muscles that surround a joint. For example, a triceps extension exercise should be chosen in addition to the biceps curl to balance the muscles that flex and extend the forearm. Although both multijoint and single-joint exercises are acceptable, it is recommended that an emphasis be placed on multijoint exercises that optimize muscle strength and closed kinetic chain movement capabilities in novice, intermediate, and advanced individuals.

For the most part, many facilities offer both free-weight and machine exercises as viable forms of resistance training. Machines are generally considered safer than free weights because the patterns of movement and ROMs are controlled and spotters are not required. Free-weight exercises offer the advantage of concurrently training numerous stabilizer muscles, in addition to the primary agonist, and promoting increases in coordination, balance, and kinesthetic awareness. For novice and intermediate individuals, the GETP7 recommends that the resistance training program include either free-weight or machine exercises. For advanced training, emphasis should be placed on free-weight exercises plus the use of machines to complement the overall program[1].

Order of Exercises

The order of resistance exercises within a particular session is important and can influence the strength capabilities of exercises ordered secondarily because of the fatigue that occurs throughout a workout.

For Increases in Muscular Strength, Power Output, Hypertrophy, and Endurance

- When training all of the core muscle groups in a single session, core exercises should come before assistance exercises, and upper and lower body exercises should be alternated (Table 25-3A).
- When training upper and lower body muscle groups during separate sessions, core exercises should be done before assistance exercises, and agonist and antagonist exercises should be alternated (Table 25-3B).
- When training individual muscle groups during separate sessions, core exercises should come before assistance exercises, and higher intensity exercises should come before lower intensity exercises (Table 25-3C).

Training Frequency

Training frequency is the number of resistance training sessions per week. The most important consideration when determining the optimal frequency is the allotted recovery time between sessions. The general guideline is to schedule workouts so that there is at least 1 day of recovery, but not more than 3 days, between consecutive training sessions involving the same muscle groups.

For Increases in Muscular Strength, Power Output, Hypertrophy, and Endurance

- For individuals beginning resistance training, the entire body should be trained during the same session at a frequency of 2 to 3 days per week (see Table 25-3A).
- For intermediate level resistance training, individuals can continue at a frequency of 2 to 3 days per week. Or for variation, a split routine can be adopted with an overall frequency of 3 to 4 days per week, allowing each muscle group to be trained only 1 to 2 days per week (see Table 25-3-B).
- For advanced level resistance training, a frequency of 4 to 6 days per week is recommended so that each core muscle group is trained no more than 2 to 3 days per week (see Table 25-3C).

Training Load

Because the training load is a critical variable that can affect acute and chronic responses to resistance training exercise, it is essential to understand the guidelines for loading. As a general guideline, progressive overload can be applied by using the two-for-two rule[1]. This rule states that the training load should be increased when an individual can perform two additional repetitions (beyond the allotted number of repetitions) with a given load on two consecutive resistance training sessions. For example, if

TABLE 25-2. A List of Popular Resistance Training Exercises with the Exercise Classification, Equipment, and the Targeted Muscle Groups

Exercise Name	Exercise Classification	Equipment	Target Muscle Groups
Back Squat	Core, Structural	Free-weights with barbell	Quadriceps Femoris (extensors of the knee), Hamstrings, and Gluteal Muscles (extensors of the hip)
Leg Press/ Hip Sled	Core	Machine	Quadriceps Femoris (extensors of the knee), Hamstrings, and Gluteal Muscles (extensors of the hip)
Leg Extension	Assistance	Machine	Quadriceps Femoris
Leg Curl	Assistance	Machine	Hamstrings
Calf (heel) Raises	Assistance	Free-weights with dumbbells or machine	Gastrocenemius, Soleus (extensors of the foot)
Bent-Over Row	Assistance	Free-weights with barbell	Latissimus Dorsi, Biceps Brachii, Brachialis, Brachioradialis
Seated Row	Assistance	Machine	Latissimus Dorsi, Biceps Brachii, Brachialis, Brachioradialis
Dumbbell Row	Assistance	Machine	Latissimus Dorsi, Biceps Brachii, Brachialis, Brachioradialis
Lat Pulldown	Assistance	Machine	Latissimus Dorsi, Biceps Brachii, Brachialis, Brachioradialis
Biceps Curl	Assistance	Free-weights with barbell	Biceps Brachii, Brachialis, Brachioradialis
Lying Triceps Extension	Assistance	Free-weights with barbell or dumbbells, or machine	Triceps Brachii
Wrist Curl	Assistance	Free-weights with barbell or dumbbells or machine	Hand Flexors
Wrist Extension	Assistance	Free-weights with barbell or dumbbells or machine	Hand Extensors
Supine Bench Press	Core	Free-weights with barbell or dumbbells or machine	Pectoralis Major, Triceps Brachii, Anterior Deltoid
Vertical Chest Press	Core	Machine	Pectoralis Major, Triceps Brachii, Anterior Deltoid
Incline Press	Core	Free-weights with barbell or dumbbells or machine	Pectoralis Major, Triceps Brachii, Anterior Deltoid
Dumbbell Fly	Assistance	Free-weights with dumbbells	Pectoralis Major
Seated Shoulder Press	Core	Free-weights with barbell or dumbbells or machine	Deltoid, Triceps Brachii
Lateral Raise	Assistance	Free-weights with dumbbells	Deltoid
Trunk Curls	Assistance	Manual exercise	Rectus Abdominus
Power Clean	Core, Power, Structural	Free-weights with barbell	Hamstring and Gluteal Muscles (extensors of the hip), Erectors (extensors of the back) Quadriceps Femoris (extensors of the knee), Trapezius (shoulder elevators)
Power Snatch	Core, Power, Structural	Free-weights with barbell	Hamstring and Gluteal Muscles (extensors of the hip), Erectors (extensors of the back), Quadriceps Femoris (extensors of the knee), Trapezius (shoulder elevators)
Push Jerk	Core, Power, Structural	Free-weights with barbell	Hamstring and Gluteal Muscles (extensors of the hip), Quadriceps Femoris (extensors of the knee), Gastrocenemius and Soleus (extensors of the foot) Deltoid

the resistance training program (Monday, Wednesday, and Friday) calls for 65% of 1RM for three sets of 10 reps, and 12 reps were achieved on both Monday and Wednesday, an increase in the load is warranted. Increases in training load of 2% to 10% are recommended for progression. Decisions regarding specific increases (within the 2% to 10% range) should be based on the size and involvement of the target muscle group (i.e., greater increases for core muscle groups; smaller increases for assistance muscle groups).

For Increasing Muscular Strength and Hypertrophy

- For novice to intermediate level training, 60% to 70% of 1RM for eight to twelve repetitions is recommended for strength and 70% to 85% of 1RM for eight to twelve repetitions is recommended for hypertrophy

TABLE 25-3 Schedules for Three Different Training Frequency Scenarios with the Correct Order of Exercises

A		B		C	
M, W, and F *or* T, R, and Sa		M and R *or* T and F (alternating schedule with LB)		M, W, S, F (alternating schedule with Back/Biceps)	
Exercises for the entire body	Leg Press/Hip Sled Vertical Chest Press Leg Curl Seated Shoulder Press Leg Extension Lat Pulldown	UB exercises	Supine Bench Press Seated Row Seated Shoulder Press Biceps Curl Triceps Extension Low-back Extension	Exercises for the shoulders, chest, and triceps	Supine Bench Press Dumbbell Fly Seated Shoulder Press Lateral Raise Triceps Extension
	Calf (Heel) Raise	T and F or M and R (alternating schedule with UB)		M, W, or F (alternating schedule with Chest/Shoulders/Triceps)	
	Biceps Curl Trunk Curls Triceps Extension Low-back extension	LB exercises	Back Squat Leg Curl Leg Extension Calf (Heel) Raise Trunk Curls	Exercises for the biceps, back, and trunk	Lat Pulldown Seated Row Biceps Curl Low-back extension Trunk Curls
				T and Sa LB exercises	Back Squat Leg Curl Leg Extension Calf (Heel) Raise
Days off: T, R, Sa, and Su or M, W, F, and Su		Days off: W, Sa, and Su		Days off: R and Su	

M = Monday, T = Tuesday, W = Wednesday, R = Thursday, F = Friday, Sa = Saturday, Su = Sunday, UB = upper body, LB = lower body

A. An example of a novice assistance training program for the entire body that can be performed 3 days per week with 4 days of recovery. B. An example of an intermediate resistance training program split into upper body exercises performed 2 days per week, lower body exercises performed on 2 separate days per week, and 3 days of recovery. C. One example of an advanced resistance training program split into separate muscle groups performed on separate days. In this example, exercises for the chest, shoulders, and triceps are grouped together and performed 1-2 days per week, the back and biceps exercises are performed 1–2 days per week, and the lower body exercises are performed 2 days per week with 2 days of recovery.

- For advanced level training, 80% to 100% of 1RM for one to 12 repetitions (in a periodized fashion) with emphasis on 70% to 85% of 1RM for six to 12 repetitions (for hypertrophy)

For Increasing Muscle Power Output[1]

- For novice and intermediate level training, 60% to 80% of 1RM for eight to 12 repetitions (for increases in muscular strength and power output)
- For progression to intermediate level training, incorporate power exercises, 30% to 60% of 1RM for three to six repetitions (not performed to failure) at fast, explosive velocities
- For advanced training, place emphasis on 85% to 100% of 1RM (at slow to moderate velocities) in conjunction with power exercises performed at 30% to 60% of 1RM (at fast, explosive velocities) for one to six repetitions in a periodized fashion using multiple sets (three to six)

For Increasing Muscular Endurance[1]

- For novice and intermediate level training, 50% to 70% of 1RM for 10 to 15 repetitions
- For advanced training, 30% to 80% of 1RM for 10 to 25 repetitions (in a periodized fashion)

Training Volume

Training volume is equal to the sum of the total number of repetitions multiplied by the sum of the resistance used during a single training session. Training volume can be varied by the number of exercises performed, the number of repetitions per set, or the number of sets per exercise. One commonly debated aspect of training volume is the use of multiple- versus single-set programs. As reviewed in both the GETP7 and the ACSM position stand, there is a body of literature that has shown that single-set programs produce similar strength gains as multiple-set program and there are other studies that have shown that multiple-set programs are superior[1]. Given that it is well accepted that single-set programs do produce significant strength gains, the decision about advancing to a multiple set program hinges on the requirement of additional training time for the potential for additional strength gains.

For Increases in Muscular Strength, Hypertrophy, and Endurance

- As reviewed in GETP7 and the ACSM Position Stands, for novice individuals, either multiple- or single-set resistance training programs (one to three sets) can be performed initially, although single set programs may improve exercise compliance.
- For more serious weight lifters (athletes), a regimen of heavier weights (6 to 12RM) of one to three sets using periodization techniques usually provides greater benefits.

For Increases in Muscle Power Output[1]

- For progression to advanced training, multiple-set resistance training programs (three to six sets in a periodized fashion) are recommended to optimize increases in muscle power output.

- To help avoid overtraining and overreaching for all types of resistance training programs, dramatic increases in training volume are contraindicated.

Rest Period Duration

Rest period duration is the amount of rest that is allowed between consecutive sets. The rest period duration can substantially affect the performance of subsequent sets as well as the acute and chronic responses to resistance exercise. As a general rule, whereas longer rest periods are associated with resistance training programs that emphasize increases in muscle strength and power output, shorter rest periods are associated with increases in muscular endurance. Therefore, rest period duration should vary based on the individual exercise (core vs. assistance) and the goals of the program.

For Increases in Muscular Strength, Power Output, and Hypertrophy[1]

- For all levels of training, 2- to 3-minute rest periods for core exercises and 1- to 2-minute rest periods for assistance exercises

For Increases in Muscular Endurance[1]

- For all levels of training, 1- to 2-minute rest periods for high-repetition sets and <1 minute rest periods for 10- to 15-repetition sets

Additional Design Variables

Two additional variables should be considered when designing a resistance training program: the muscle action involved and the muscle action velocity. Two dynamic muscle actions occur during traditional DCER (isotonic) training: the concentric and eccentric phases. Fundamental differences exist between concentric and eccentric muscle actions. For example, eccentric muscle actions require less motor unit activation, produce greater force outputs, and result in more severe DOMS than concentric muscle actions. The ACSM recommends, however, that both concentric and eccentric muscle actions should be included in resistance training programs for novice, intermediate, and advanced individuals[1].

Resistance training can be performed at very slow, slow, moderate, and fast muscle action velocities. During maximal isokinetic muscle actions, resistance training at velocities of 180 to 240 deg·sec^{-1} has been shown to optimize gains in strength[19]. Most studies have suggested that DCER resistance training at moderate or fast velocities produces greater increases in muscular fitness parameters than does slow training[20,21]. A recent study[22] indicated that resistance training at very slow (intentionally slow)

muscle action velocities resulted in significantly lower gains in strength compared with traditionally slow velocities. However, resistance training at slow velocities may be particularly useful for untrained, sedentary individuals. Based on these findings, it is recommended that for novice individuals, resistance training should be performed at slow and moderate velocities. For intermediate individuals, moderate velocities are recommended, and for those who are advanced, a wide range of velocities is warranted, from unintentionally slow to fast, explosive velocities. Training at fast velocities is particularly useful when the emphasis of the program is to increase muscle power output.

Resistance Training for Special Populations

CHILDREN AND ADOLESCENTS

Numerous research studies[23,24] have indicated that children and adolescents can increase strength through resistance training. In addition, several other benefits are associated with resistance training in youths, including injury prevention, improved athletic and motor skill performance, and improved overall health. Most importantly, properly supervised resistance training in youths appears to be quite safe and poses an injury risk comparable to adults[25,26]. This is true for both pre- and as well as postpubescent youths. In prepubescence, gains in muscle strength occur with limited changes in muscle hypertrophy. The minimal hypertrophy is likely attributable to the low levels of anabolic hormones that are present before puberty. The strength increases with minimal levels of hypertrophy suggest that neurological adaptations are the primary mechanism for enhanced strength[25]. After puberty, significant strength and hypertrophy can occur with resistance training. The enhanced hypertrophic capability after puberty is likely caused by the higher concentration of anabolic hormones that are present during this period, which contributes to the accretion of fat-free weight independent of resistance training[27]. This factor likely also explains both the growth-induced as well as training-induced differences in hypertrophy and strength between young men and women after puberty.

The current recommendations for resistance training program design for children include repetitions in the range of 8 to 15 for one to three sets per exercise using both open and closed kinetic chain exercises[5] that target all major muscle groups (8 to 10 different exercises). Training frequency should be limited to two times per week. All types of equipment and devices, including free weights, machines, and body weight resisted calisthenics, are acceptable for use with children and adolescents. Care must be taken to ensure that the equipment fits the size of the youth. When learning new exercises, participants should be encouraged to use a light weight or even a broomstick at the start so that proper form can be learned. Implementation of overload should emphasize increasing repetitions versus increasing load[5].

Case reports exist that indicate a potential risk of testing or training-induced damage to epiphyseal plates of the long bones, which can deform limbs and retard subsequent growth, especially when unsupervised or using improper form[26]. In all cases, resistance training programs should be supervised by qualified personnel. Furthermore, to minimize injury risk, attempts to lift weights that are at or near 1RM have been discouraged[25]. Instead, lighter weights that can allow multiple repetitions are preferred. That said, the limited data that exist indicate that 1RM testing can be safely performed in children[26] and with high reliability[28].

OLDER ADULTS

Resistance training in older adults is an important component of maintaining health and vigor. Sarcopenia is the loss of muscle mass associated with aging, and it is associated with many debilitating conditions linked with aging such as weakness, poor balance, and increased risk of falls[2]. Resistance training has been shown to be a potent stimulus for combating sarcopenia and improving function. Indeed, in the case of frail elderly persons, resistance training may be a prerequisite before individuals are physically capable of starting an aerobic exercise program such as walking[2]. Other potential benefits in elderly individuals include effects on bone density, metabolism and weight control, and insulin resistance[9].

For older adults, the resistance training prescription parameters are similar to those of young adults, with the exception that the intensity is recommended to be lower. Specifically, intensity levels in the range of 8 to 15RM, which roughly corresponds to 60% to 80% of 10RM, have been suggested[2,9]. At the start of a training period, or after a lay off, lower training intensities (< 50% 1RM) may be appropriate. Exercises should target all the major muscle groups (see Table 25-2). When implementing progression, preference may be given to increasing the number of repetitions versus increasing load. It should be noted that higher intensity training is likely to provide a more effective training stimulus, but this must be weighed against compliance and injury risk[29]. Similarly, although one set of each exercise may elicit training effects that are somewhat lower than when using multiple sets, the tradeoff with time constraints, compliance, and injury risk must be weighed[9]. A training frequency of two to three times per week is a reasonable compromise between optimal training response (facilitated by more frequent training) and compliance and dropout considerations. It has been suggested that relative to free weights, isotonic machines decrease injury risk in elderly individuals[9]. However, to date, no studies have tested this, and many individuals may benefit from incorporation of some free-weight activities to simultaneously stress coordination and balance[2].

CARDIOVASCULAR DISEASE

Exercise prescription for CVD has historically emphasized aerobic exercise training. However, it is becoming increasingly clear that resistance exercise can have favorable effects on a variety of factors associated with CVD and in rehabilitation after a cardiovascular event[3]. These include the previously mentioned effects on strength, muscle mass, metabolism, bone health, and glucose tolerance. In addition, improved muscle strength eases the burden of daily activities and decreases the physiological stress associated with various activities[3,29,30].

Resistance exercise is now recommended as part of a comprehensive cardiac rehabilitation program (see Chapter 31). The basic principles underlying the design of resistance exercise programs are the same for individuals with CVD as they are for other groups; however, extra care is required to minimize cardiovascular risk during training. The contraindications for resistance exercise in persons with CVD are presented in Table 25-1. In general, low- to moderate-risk patients are prime candidates for resistance training, and other patients should be considered more carefully because data on safety and efficacy are lacking. All patients should receive physician approval before initiating the training. It may be prudent to delay resistance exercise until after 2 to 4 weeks of aerobic exercise training have been performed[3]. In addition, it is generally recommended that initial training programs incorporate light loads and progress slowly. Indeed, use of elastic bands or extremely light weights (1 to 2 lbs) may be prudent in early phase II cardiac rehabilitation followed by more intense training at a later date[3]. Postsurgical patients may require up to 3 months of recovery before incorporating exercises that specifically apply stress to the sternum[3].

Interestingly, only recently has resistance exercise been examined in patients with chronic heart failure (CHF). CHF is a CVD characterized by fatigue and shortness of breath during physical activity. Although the clinical focus of heart failure is on central hemodynamic function, it is clear that peripheral skeletal muscle abnormalities significantly contribute to exercise intolerance. CHF is associated with a myopathy characterized by atrophy of type I muscle fibers, poor muscle endurance, and exercise intolerance. Recently, Pu et al.[31] found that 10 weeks of high-intensity resistance training (pneumatic machines) significantly improved exercise capacity (6-min walk test), muscle endurance, and muscle strength in women with CHF, with no change in peak VO_2 or indices of central cardiac function. Similarly, Delagardelle et al.[32] reported that combined strength and endurance training elicited improvements in peak VO_2 and left ventricular function than endurance training alone. These results suggest that resistance exercise may be an important adjunct to aerobic exercise in the treatment of patients with CHF.

Flexibility Training

Flexibility is a term that is used to characterize the pain-free ROM of a single joint (i.e., elbow) or a series of joints (i.e., spine). Joint ROM and flexibility are directly proportional and joint specific. For example, stretching exercises that focus on increasing the ROM of the hip augment hip flexibility, but they do not increase shoulder flexibility. Likewise, an individual can have joints that are highly flexible, some of average flexibility, and some that are inflexible. Therefore, it is recommended that flexibility training programs incorporate multiple stretching exercises that target the primary joints of the body to maintain overall flexibility. Adequate flexibility is not only desirable for athletes, but it also contributes to efficient movement in daily activities, such as walking, stair climbing, and lifting objects. The maintenance of good joint ROM through flexibility training may also help prevent the age-related decreases in flexibility that occur in middle-aged[33] and older adults[34]. In fact, a review of the literature indicates that stretching exercises can improve flexibility throughout the life span[35–38].

NEUROMUSCULAR CONSIDERATIONS

There are two primary proprioceptors that provide protective reflex responses to stretching: muscle spindles and Golgi tendon organs. These receptors are activated during strong, tension-producing muscle actions and stretches. After they are stimulated, they send afferent signals to lower control centers in the central nervous system to protect the musculotendonous unit from injuries resulting from overcontraction or overstretch. Muscle spindles, for example, are composed of intrafusal fibers that lie parallel to the regular muscle (extrafusal) fibers, and they respond to stretching-induced muscle tension in two ways. First, when a musculotendonous unit is lengthened, muscle spindles are activated, which sends a very rapid monosynaptic signal that stimulates the stretched muscle to contract. This is called the *myotatic reflex* or *stretch reflex*[39]. Second, the same afferent signal originated by the muscle spindle also triggers a bisynaptic inhibitory response that causes the antagonistic muscle to relax. This is called *reciprocal innervation*[39]. In contrast, however, *Golgi tendon organs* are located in the tendon and myotendonous junctions (in series with the muscle) and respond to lengthening caused by either muscle action or stretching. For example, when the stretching-induced tension becomes great enough, Golgi tendon organs are activated, which sends a bisynaptic inhibitory impulse that overrides the myotatic reflex causing a sudden relaxation of the stretched muscle. This is called the *inverse myotatic reflex, autogenic inhibition*, or the *clasp-knife reflex*[39]. In both cases, the reflex arcs created by muscle spindles and Golgi tendon organs manipulate neural activation of the stretched muscle and its antagonist by either facilitating or inhibiting the motor neuron as a protective mechanism.

MECHANICAL CONSIDERATIONS

Limitations in joint ROM may be caused by any one or combination of the following factors:

- Joint mechanics
- Muscle or fat tissue obstruction
- Soft tissue stiffness

For some joints, the bony structure sets a very definite limit on ROM. For example, extension at the elbow and knee joints is limited by the joint structures, which cannot be modified to any large extent. Individuals who have large muscle mass or a large fat mass (obese) may also have difficulty moving through a full ROM because of the physical obstructions imposed by excessive muscle or fat mass. Probably the most common factor that limits joint ROM, which can be modified through flexibility training, is the stiffness of soft tissues that surround the joint, such as muscle, fasciae sheaths, tendons, ligaments, joint capsules, and the skin. When considering muscle as one of the soft tissue components that limits joint ROM, it is important to note that the limiting factor does not lie in the contractile elements but instead in the connective tissue components of the muscle. Therefore, changes in flexibility are primarily attributed to changes in the connective tissues.

Connective tissue exhibits both elastic and plastic properties. *Elasticity* is defined as the ability to return to resting length after passive stretching (i.e., elastic recoil), and *plasticity* is the tendency to assume a greater length after passive stretching (i.e., plastic deformation)[40]. The goal of a flexibility training program, therefore, is to maximize joint ROM by carefully and repeatedly stretching to surpass the acute elastic recoil properties of the connective tissue and elicit a chronic plastic deformation over time. Several studies have suggested that a slow, sustained stretch for 30 to 60[38] or 90[41] seconds is necessary to get beyond the acute elastic recoil and produce the mild discomfort that will stimulate chronic plastic deformation.

APPROPRIATE TIMES TO STRETCH

Although stretching can be done at any time during the day, the ACSM has traditionally recommended that flexibility training should be incorporated into the warm-up and cool-down phases of workout sessions[5]. Recent studies, however, have provided evidence against the inclusion of flexibility training before exercise sessions. For example, several studies[42–47] have suggested that stretching compromises the force-producing capabilities of muscles. This information may be particularly useful for those who incorporate stretching as a warm-up before resistance training. Recent findings have also shown that applying heat packs for 20 minutes to increase muscle temperature can increase hamstring flexibility more so than 30 seconds of static stretching[44]. This evidence implies that a pre-exercise warm-up consisting of only cardiovascular exercise to increase body temperature may be adequate for increasing flexibility before an exercise session.

BASIC MODES OF STRETCHING

Two basic classifications of stretching can be made independent of the specific mode used: active (unassisted) and passive (assisted) stretching. Whenever there is only one individual involved in the stretching procedure and he is providing his own stretching stimulus without assistance, it is termed *active* or *unassisted stretching*. When another person such as a partner or trainer is supplying the stimulus for stretching, it is referred to as **passive** or **assisted stretching**. Both methods are effective for increasing flexibility and can generally be applied to most stretching modes.

Static Stretching

This is the most common method of stretching and is appropriate and effective for nearly all individuals when using the correct technique. A static stretch is slow, controlled, and constant. The general procedure involves gradually applying tension to a muscle or muscle group toward the end of the joint ROM until the point of mild discomfort is reached. The stretch is then held in this position for at least 10 seconds (preferably 30 to 60 seconds). This process is repeated after a 20- to 30-second rest period for additional repetitions. Studies showing the duration of a static stretch that is necessary to elicit chronic increases in flexibility are conflicting. At least one study[36] has indicated that 10-second stretch durations were sufficient to increase flexibility, but other studies[37,38] indicate that the minimal stretch duration should be at least 30 seconds. In addition, it has been suggested that 30 to 90 seconds of static stretch is necessary to overcome the initial neuroexcitatory response and to elicit the chronic plastic deformation that is necessary for increases in flexibility over time[41,48,49]. It is recommended, therefore, that although novice individuals may experience increases in flexibility with static stretch durations of only 10 seconds, an emphasis should be placed on progressing toward stretch durations of at least 30 seconds.

Ballistic Stretching

A ballistic stretch involves forceful bouncing and ballistic-type movements that quickly exaggerate the joint ROM but do not hold the position for any extended duration. The most recent ACSM position stand[4] recommends that static, ballistic, or proprioceptive neuromuscular facilitation (PNF; see related section in this chapter for details) stretching techniques should be incorporated into the overall fitness program. A study by Lamontagne et al.[50], however, suggested that slow and gradual stretching procedures (e.g., static and PNF techniques) should be used instead of ballistic stretching to reduce the risk of injury

attributable to excessively high tensions created during ballistic stretching maneuvers. Others[40,51] have suggested that ballistic stretching may predispose muscles or joint connective tissues to injury, especially when there has been a previous injury involving the target joint. It should be noted, however, that one study[52] has reported significant elevations in DOMS and creatine kinase (a biochemical marker of muscle damage) in response to both static and ballistic stretching exercises, and the static stretching elicited significantly greater DOMS than the ballistic stretching. Therefore, based on previous suggestions[40,47,51,52] and the recommendations of the ACSM[4], caution should be taken when incorporating ballistic stretching into an overall fitness program, and the comfort level and experience of the client, patient, or subject should be considered. For example, whereas those exhibiting relatively poor flexibility, little experience with flexibility training, or previous musculoskeletal injury may be at lower risk and benefit more from static or PNF stretching[40,50,51], more experienced individuals with no history of musculoskeletal injuries may benefit from using movement- or sport-specific ballistic stretching exercises for increasing joint ROM.

Dynamic Stretching

Dynamic stretching incorporates flexibility training during dynamic, sport- or exercise-specific movements[53]. This form of stretching is similar to ballistic procedures in that there are dynamic movements, but it does not use forceful bouncing. Rather, dynamic stretching involves movements that mimic a specific sport or exercise in an exaggerated but controlled manner. This mode of stretching is often used by athletes in preparation for events and may be preferred over static stretching for inclusion in warm-ups[45,47,53]. For example, a sprinter may use 10 consecutive exaggerated stride lengths performed quickly as a dynamic stretching exercise[53] to improve hip ROM.

Proprioceptive Neuromuscular Facilitation Stretching

Types of **proprioceptive neuromuscular facilitation (PNF)** techniques for stretching include the hold–relax, contract–relax, and hold–relax–contract stretches[40]. For the hold–relax form of PNF stretching, a muscle is contracted isometrically, relaxed, then stretched further into the available ROM during the relaxation phase. The contract–relax PNF technique is identical to the hold–relax procedure, except rather than an isometric muscle action, there is a concentric muscle action through the full ROM before the relaxation phase. A similar procedure is used for contract–relax–contract PNF stretching, except the antagonist muscle is also contracted during the relaxation phase to gain addition increases in ROM. PNF stretching often requires assistance (i.e., passive technique) or at least external equipment, such as a towel or rubber tubing. There is conflicting evidence regarding the superiority of PNF stretching; some studies have found PNF to better than static stretching, but others have not[54,55]. Although recent evidence supports the efficacy of PNF stretching[56], further research is necessary before specific recommendations can be made regarding the use of static or PNF stretching.

Yogic Stretching

Yoga is a form of abstract meditation, mental concentration, and spiritual expression that often involves unique stretching maneuvers[57]. The stretching involved with yoga is largely static and is focused primarily on the trunk musculature.

FLEXIBILITY TRAINING PROGRAM DESIGN

In conjunction with the advantages discussed earlier in this section, the following guidelines for flexibility training are recommended:

- **Mode:** Static, ballistic, or PNF stretching (with static and PNF being the preferred method) should be used.
- **Exercises:** The joint specificity of flexibility training advocates the need for multiple stretching exercises that target the primary joints of the body, including the neck, shoulders, elbows, wrists, trunk, hips, knees, and ankles.
- **Repetitions:** Two to four repetitions of each stretching exercise should be performed.
- **Duration of each repetition:** A minimum of 10 seconds with an emphasis on progression to 30 to 90 seconds should be done.
- **Frequency:** Minimum 2–3 days/week, ideally 5–7 days/week.
- **Intensity:** To the point of tightness or mild discomfort

REFERENCES

1. American College of Sports Medicine Position Stand: Progression models in resistance training for healthy adults. Med Sci Sports Exerc 34:364–380, 2002.
2. American College of Sports Medicine Position Stand: Exercise and physical activity for older adults. Med Sci Sports Exerc 30:992–1008, 1998.
3. Pollock ML, Franklin BA, Balady GJ, et al: AHA Science Advisory. Resistance exercise in individuals with and without cardiovascular disease: Benefits, rationale, safety, and prescription: An advisory from the Committee on Exercise, Rehabilitation, and Prevention, Council on Clinical Cardiology, American Heart Association; Position paper endorsed by the American College of Sports Medicine. Circulation 101:828–833, 2000.
4. American College of Sports Medicine Position Stand: The recommended quantity and quality of exercise for developing and maintaining cardiorespiratory and muscular fitness, and flexibility in healthy adults. Med Sci Sports Exerc 30:975–991, 1998.
5. U.S. Department of Health and Human Services: Physical Activity and Health: A Report of the Surgeon General. Atlanta: U.S. Department of Health and Human Services, Centers for Disease Control and Prevention, National Center for Chronic Disease Prevention and Health Promotion, 1996.
6. Strength training for female athletes: A position paper: Part I. National Strength and Conditioning Association Journal 11:43–51, 1989.
7. Strength training for female athletes: A position paper: Part II. National Strength and Conditioning Association Journal. 11:29–36, 1989.
8. MacDougall JD, Tuxen D, Sale DG, et al: Arterial blood pressure response to heavy resistance exercise. J Appl Physiol 58:785–790, 1985.
9. Mazzeo RS, Tanaka H: Exercise prescription for the elderly: Current recommendations. Sports Med 31:809–818, 2001.
10. Linsenbardt ST, Thomas TR, Madsen RW: Effect of breathing techniques on blood pressure response to resistance exercise. Br J Sports Med 26:97–100, 1992.
11. Haykowsky MJ, Eves ND, Warburton DER, Findlay MJ: Resistance exercise, the Valsalva maneuver, and cerebrovascular transmural pressure. Med Sci Sports Exerc 35:65–68, 2003.
12. Lander JE, Hundley JR, Simonton RL: The effectiveness of weight-belts during multiple repetitions of the squat exercise. Med Sci Sports Exerc 24:603–609, 1992.
13. Miyamoto K, Iinuma N, Maeda M, et al: Effects of abdominal belts on intra-abdominal pressure, intra-muscular pressure in the erector spinae muscles and myoelectrical activities of trunk muscles. Clin Biomech (Bristol, Avon) 14:79–87, 1999.
14. Rafacz W, McGill SM: Wearing an abdominal belt increases diastolic blood pressure. J Occup Environ Med 38:925–927, 1996.
15. Earle RW, Baechle TR: Resistance training and spotting techniques (pp. 343–389). In Baechle R, Earle RW, eds. Essentials of Strength Training and Conditioning. Champaign, IL: Human Kinetics; 2000.
16. Dudley GA, Tesch PA, Miller BJ, Buchanan P: Importance of eccentric actions in performance adaptations to resistance training. Aviat Space Environ Med 62:543–550, 1991.
17. Hather BM, Tesch PA, Buchanan P, Dudley GA: Influence of eccentric actions on skeletal muscle adaptations to resistance training. Acta Physiol Scand 143:177–185, 1991.
18. Baechle TR, Earle RW, and National Strength & Conditioning Association (U.S.): Essentials of strength training and conditioning, 2nd ed. Champaign, Ill.: Human Kinetics; 2000, xiii, 658.
19. Kanehisa H, Miyashita M: Specificity of velocity in strength training. Eur J Appl Physiol Occup Physiol 52:104–106, 1983.
20. Hay JG, Andrews JG, Vaughan CL: Effects of lifting rate on elbow torques exerted during arm curl exercises. Med Sci Sports Exerc 15:63–71, 1983.
21. Morrissey MC, Harman EA, Frykman PN, Han KH: Early phase differential effects of slow and fast barbell squat training. Am J Sports Med 26:221–230, 1998.
22. Keeler LK, Finkelstein LH, Miller W, Fernhall B: Early-phase adaptations of traditional-speed vs. superslow resistance training on strength and aerobic capacity in sedentary individuals. J Strength Cond Res 15:309–314, 2001.
23. Falk B, Tenenbaum G: The effectiveness of resistance training in children. A meta-analysis. Sports Med 22:176–186, 1996.
24. Payne VG, Morrow Jr JR, Johnson L, Dalton SN: Resistance training in children and youth: A meta-analysis. Res Q Exerc Sport 68:80–88, 1997.
25. Bernhardt DT, Gomez J, Johnson MD, et al: Strength training by children and adolescents. Pediatrics 107:1470–1472, 2001.
26. Faigenbaum AD, Milliken LA, Westcott WL: Maximal strength testing in healthy children. J Strength Cond Res 17:162–166, 2003.
27. Kraemer WJ, Fry AC, Frykman PN, et al: Resistance training and youth. Pediatr Exerc Sci 1:336–350, 1989.
28. Faigenbaum AD, Westcott WL, Long C, et al: Relationship between repetitions and selected percentages of the one-repetition maximum in healthy children. Pediatr Phys Ther 10:110–113, 1998.
29. McCartney N, McKelvie RS, Martin J, et al: Weight-training-induced

attenuation of the circulatory response of older males to weight lifting. J Appl Physiol 74:1056–1060, 1993.

30. Goldberg L, Elliot DL, Keuhl KS: Cardiovascular changes at rest and during mixed static and dynamic exercises after weight training. J Appl Sport Sci Res 2:42–45, 1988.

31. Pu CT, Johnson MT, Forman DE, et al: Randomized trial of progressive resistance training to counteract the myopathy of chronic heart failure. J Appl Physiol 90:2341–2350, 2001.

32. Delagardelle C, Feiereisen P, Autier PR, et al: Strength/endurance training versus endurance training in congestive heart failure. Med Sci Sports Exerc 34:1868–1872, 2002.

33. Shephard RJ, Berridge M, Montelpare W: On the generality of the "sit and reach" test: An analysis of flexibility data for an aging population. Res Q Exerc Sport 61:326–330, 1990.

34. Bassey EJ, Morgan K, Dallosso HM, Ebrahim SB: Flexibility of the shoulder joint measured as range of abduction in a large representative sample of men and women over 65 years of age. Eur J Appl Physiol Occup Physiol 58:353–360, 1989.

35. Bandy WD, Irion JM., Briggler M: The effect of time and frequency of static stretching on flexibility of the hamstring muscles. Phys Ther 77:1090–1096, 1997.

36. Borms J, Van Roy P, Santens JP, Haentjens A: Optimal duration of static stretching exercises for improvement of coxo-femoral flexibility. J Sports Sci 5:39–47, 1987.

37. Chan SP, Hong Y, Robinson PD: Flexibility and passive resistance of the hamstrings of young adults using two different static stretching protocols. Scand J Med Sci Sports 11:81–86, 2001.

38. Feland JB, Myrer JW, Schulthies SS, et al: The effect of duration of stretching of the hamstring muscle group for increasing range of motion in people aged 65 years or older. Phys Ther 81:1110–1117, 2001.

39. Ganong WF: Review of Medical Physiology, 20th ed. Stamford, CT: McGraw Hill; 2001; 870.

40. Holcomb WR: Stretching and warm-up (pp. 321–342). In Baechle TR, Earle RW, eds. Essentials of Strength Training and Conditioning. Champaign, IL: Human Kinetics; 2000.

41. Mozam K, Lawrence J, Keagy R: Muscle relationships in functional fascia. Clin Orthop 150:403–409, 1978.

42. Behm DG, Button DC, Butt JC: Factors affecting force loss with prolonged stretching. Can J Appl Physiol 26:261–272, 2001.

43. Cramer JT, Housh TJ, Johnson GO, et al: The acute effects of static stretching on peak torque in women. J Strength Cond Res, in press.

44. Funk D, Swank AM, Adams KJ, Treolo D: Efficacy of moist heat pack application over static stretching on hamstring flexibility. J Strength Cond Res 15:123–126, 2001.

45. Kokkonen J, Nelson AG, Cornwell A: Acute muscle stretching inhibits maximal strength performance. Res Q Exerc Sport 69: 411–415, 1998.

46. Nelson AG, Guillory IK, Cornwell C, Kokkonen J: Inhibition of maximal voluntary isokinetic torque production following stretching is velocity-specific. J Strength Cond Res. 15:241–246, 2001.

47. Nelson AG, Kokkonen J: Acute ballistic muscle stretching inhibits maximal strength performance. Res Q Exerc Sport 72:415–419, 2001.

48. Astrand P-O, Rodahl KA: Textbook of work physiology: Physiological bases of exercise, 3rd ed. New York: McGraw Hill; 1986: xii, 756.

49. Garfin SR, Tipton CM, Mubarak SJ, et al: Role of fascia in maintenance of muscle tension and pressure. J Appl Physiol 51:317–320, 1981.

50. Lamontagne AF, Malouin, Richards CL. Viscoelastic behavior of plantar flexor muscle-tendon unit at rest. J Orthop Sports Phys Ther 26:244–252, 1997.

51. Corbin CB, Dowell LJ, Lindsey R, Tolson H: Concepts in Physical Education. Dubuque, IA: Brown; 1978.

52. Smith LL, Brunetz MH, Chenier TC, et al: The effects of static and ballistic stretching on delayed onset muscle soreness and creatine kinase. Res Q Exerc Sport 64:103–107, 1993.

53. Hedrick A: Dynamic flexibility training. Strength and Conditioning Journal 22:33–38, 2000.

54. Etnyre BR, Lee EJ: Chronic and acute flexibility of men and women using three different stretching techniques. Res Q Exerc Sport 59:222–228, 1988.

55. Hardy L, Jones D: Dynamic flexibility and proprioceptive neuromuscular facilitation. Res Q Exerc Sport 57:150–153, 1986.

56. Funk DC, Swank AM, Mikla BM, et al: Impact of prior exercise on hamstring flexibility: A comparison of proprioceptive neuromuscular facilitation and static stretching. J Strength Cond Res 17:489–492, 2003.

57. Carrico M: Yoga Journal's Yoga Basics: The Essential Beginner's Guide to Yoga for a Lifetime of Health and Fitness. New York: Henry Holt; 1997:xiv, 191.

58. Stone MH, O'Bryant HS, Schilling BK, et al: Periodization: Effects of manipulating volume and intensity (part 2). Strength and Conditioning J 21:54–60, 1999.

SELECTED REFERENCES FOR FURTHER READING

Baechle TR, Earle RW: Essentials of Strength Training and Conditioning, 2nd ed. Champaign, IL: Human Kinetics; 2000.

Fleck SJ, Kraemer WJ: Designing Resistance Training Programs. Champaign, IL: Human Kinetics; 1997.

Faigenbaum AD, et al: Youth resistance training: Position statement paper and literature review. Strength and Conditioning Journal 18: 62–75, 1996.

Graves JE, Franklin BA (eds): Resistance training for health and rehabilitation. Champaign, IL: Human Kinetics; 2001.

INTERNET RESOURCES

Health World: Strength Training: http://www.healthy.net/fitness/training/strength.htm

NSCA: National Strength & Conditioning Association: http://www.nsca-lift.org

NSCA Certification Commission: http://www.nsca-cc.org

Training for Seniors: http://www.burkespencer.com/training_for_seniors.htm

USA Weightlifting: http://www.msbn.tv/usavision/index.aspx

"Today, at the start of the new year, millions of Americans will resolve to lose weight, but by tomorrow or next week, or maybe next month, most of them will give up trying. Few will have lost weight, and even fewer will sustain that weight loss"[1].

Approximately 97 million people in the United States are considered overweight or obese[2], and the World Health Organization (WHO) acknowledges that obesity is a "global epidemic"[3]. The Centers for Disease Control and Prevention has reported that individuals who are obese and overweight comprise about 30% and 70% of the U.S. population, respectively (Fig. 26-1). Obesity has been related to many chronic diseases, such as coronary heart disease, hypertension, stroke, diabetes mellitus, gallbladder disease, and some cancers[4,5], and prevention of obesity would decrease chronic disease, improve quality of life, and decrease health care costs in the United States (also see Chapter 9).

As individuals age, they lose their ability to regulate energy intake based on physiological cues, leading to overeating and weight gain[6]. These cues can be further "ignored" in an environment that promotes overeating by offering large portion sizes in restaurants[7] and in the home. In addition, many of the foods readily available are high-fat foods[7,8], which are high in energy density[8,9] but low in nutrient density. This inability to regulate energy intake, coupled with a sedentary lifestyle, are two major reasons why obesity has become increasingly more prevalent in the United States. Thus, it is imperative that both eating healthily and increased physical activity are promoted and encouraged.

One goal of this chapter is to discuss the impact nutrition has on weight management. This chapter highlights several areas that pertain to nutrition and weight management, including determining energy needs and macronutrients needs, the role of some micronutrients on body weight, and guidelines for proper weight loss.

Establishing a Healthy Body Weight Goal

Several methods can be used to determine his or her "ideal body weight." However, in many cases, especially for athletes, ideal body weight may be unrealistic. Thus, it is better to focus on a "healthy body weight" rather than an "ideal body weight." A healthy body weight is different for each individual, athlete or non-athlete, and is one that is relative to a person's overall health profile (e.g., serum lipid levels, glucose levels, blood pressure). Thus, probably the simplest way to determine a healthy body weight would be for a person to use body mass index (BMI). BMI is defined as a person's height (in kilograms) divided by his or her height in meters squared (m^2). BMI is not perfect because it does not take into account body fat; thus, a muscular athlete may have a BMI that is considered "obese." However, for the average population, BMI typically works well. For an overview of body composition measurement, refer to Chapter 12. Table 4-1 in the GETP7 lists the different BMI levels and how they match to overweight and obesity.

Note that a BMI between 18.5 and 24.9 $kg \cdot m^{-2}$ is considered healthy because individuals within this range are at the lowest risk for developing chronic disease. Nonetheless, although obesity has been shown to increase chronic diseases risk, a BMI of less than 18.5 can place a person at risk for gastrointestinal diseases, immune impairment, and diseases of the heart that are related to electrolyte imbalances and may also be an indication of an eating disorder. Aside from being overweight or obese, other risk factors to consider are hypertension, high levels of low-density lipoprotein cholesterol (LDL-C), low levels of high-density lipoprotein cholesterol (HDL-C), high serum triglyceride levels, high blood glucose levels, family history of heart disease, sedentary lifestyle, and cigarette smoking[10]. Another important point to note is that, although it places a person at a lower risk of chronic disease if he or she is within a healthy BMI range, losing as little as 10% of one's body weight reduces the risk of developing an obesity-related disease[10].

Effects of Diet Only, Exercise Only, and Diet Plus Exercise on Weight Loss

Researchers have assessed the effects of diet alone, exercise alone and a combination of diet plus exercise on weight loss and the prevention of weight gain. In over 100 men and women assessed for 2 years, Skender et

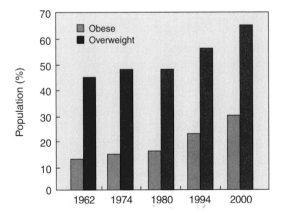

Figure 26-1. "The fattening of America." Note that obesity has increased to about 30% of the U.S. population from 1962 to 2000. The percent of individuals in the United States considered overweight has increased to about 70%. (Adapted from: Centers for Disease Control, 2003) http://www.cdc.gov/nccdphp/dnpa/obesity/trend/ maps/index.htm

al.[11] reported that, although their diet-plus-exercise and diet-only groups had the greatest weight loss at 1 year, the exercise group was able to maintain their weight loss at the 2-year mark, but the other groups gained weight (the diet-only group gained more weight than at baseline). Kraemer et al.[12,13] reported that fat-free mass was better maintained in their groups who included weight training as part of their exercise regimen. Nonetheless, these studies were only 12 weeks in duration and did not include an exercise-only group but did include control groups. Although Utter et al.[14] reported significant weight loss in their diet-only and diet-plus-exercise groups, compared with their control and exercise only groups, their study was also only 12 weeks in duration. Both Kraemer et al.[12,13] and Utter et al.[14] reported cardiorespiratory improvements in their exercise groups.

More recently[15], intensity of exercise was compared in men and women with a BMI of about 41 kg·m^{-2}. Although body weight loss was equal between the low- and high-intensity exercise groups, the authors concluded that the higher intensity exercise program showed greater generalized improvement in muscle performance and physical fitness, as well as a stronger motivation for spontaneous physical activity compared with the low-intensity group[15].

In addition to exercise intensity, some researchers have demonstrated that exercising in multiple bouts throughout the day can be as effective for weight loss and cardiovascular benefits as exercising for one continuous bout[16,17]. Exercising in multiple short bouts throughout the day may provide greater adherence for some individuals who have erratic schedules. Jakicic et al.[17] also reported that weight loss is greatest if energy expended is more than 150 min·wk^{-1}.

Although exercise alone does not provide the greatest weight loss over time, it does appear that exercise prevents weight gain and results in modest levels of weight loss[18]. Nonetheless, with consistent exercise, the weight loss will be maintained. However, combined with a lower energy intake, a greater weight loss will be achieved. Furthermore, with greater intensity exercise, greater improvements in physical fitness are observed. If weight loss or prevention of weight gain is the key, then the intensity of physical activity is not as important. However, if greater spontaneous exercise and, hence, greater energy expenditure will occur with higher intensity exercise (and perhaps with multiple bouts of exercise), then these may be other motivational tools used with some individuals (see also Chapter 24).

So what does this mean for exercise physiologists and other health care professionals working with the public? In the most basic sense, people need to get moving throughout their day, and the more minutes they are active, the more likely they will lose weight or prevent weight gain. The level of intensity and type of exercise need to be individualized based on the goals of particular clients, their likes and dislikes, and their overall health.

Importance of an Adequate Daily Energy Intake for Healthy Weight Management

The basic premise of weight maintenance is that energy intake equals energy expenditure. If weight loss is to be achieved, then energy intake must be less than energy expenditure (or energy expenditure must be greater than energy intake). It is important to maintain adequate energy intake because micronutrients (vitamins and minerals) are required for physiological processes in the body. If micronutrients are not adequately consumed, other problems such as impairment of the immune system may occur.

In general, a weight loss of no more than 2 lbs (~1 kg) per week is best for several reasons: (a) this smaller amount of weight loss better preserves lean body mass; (b) although slower, this lower amount of weight loss results in better adherence and better ability of the person to maintain that weight loss because, typically, the person has made lifestyle changes rather than drastic changes to their dietary intake; and (c) slower weight loss typically means that less water loss and, thus, a "false weight loss," has not occurred.

To lose 1 lb of body fat per week, a person should be in a 500-kcal deficit per day. Because 3500 kcals = 1 lb of fat. It is important to note that not everyone loses 1 lb of fat with a 3500-kcal deficit, but this is an estimate or average. Individuals vary on the amount of weight they lose with this 3-500-kcal deficit. Nonetheless, in general, a person can achieve this deficit by exercising enough to burn 250 kcal and decrease intake by just 250 kcal daily. These would need to be doubled if a 2-lb per week weight loss is desired. This level of deficit is moderate and increases compliance while also decreasing a person's likelihood of regaining the body weight lost. Although a combination of a moderate energy intake deficit and a moderately increased energy expenditure may provide the best method to achieve weight loss, weight loss can be achieved by exercise alone. Donnelly et al.[19] reported that, after 16 months, exercise alone prevented weight gain in women and resulting in a significant weight loss for men (~5.2 kg weight loss, on average) compared with a sedentary control group.

Determining Energy Needs

Energy needs can be determined by a number of ways. One way consists of using the Harris-Benedict equation, then multiplying it by the appropriate factors; however, this may overpredict a person's energy needs. Simply multiplying a person's body weight in pounds by 10 (providing a crude estimate of a person's resting metabolic rate [RMR]), then adding appropriate factors based on energy expenditure, is another way. Determining a person's intake over time and assessing body weight is a more tedious method of assessing energy needs; however, this provides a more accurate estimate. Another more tedious but more accurate method is to assess an individual's RMR (kcal·day^{-1} used at rest), dietary-induced thermogenesis (energy expended after a meal; this must be conducted for up to 4 hours after a meal), and energy expended during exercise, all through indirect calorimetry (either using a metabolic cart or a whole-room calorimetry). These methods measure oxygen consumption and expiration of carbon dioxide, and then energy expenditure is calculated. Doubly labeled water provides the best estimate of a person's energy expenditure each day; however, it is expensive and does not partition how much energy is used for each activity.

Because many of these methods may not be practical, a useful tool for determining energy needs is to refer to the Food and Nutrition Board of the Institute of Medicine, National Academy of Sciences'[20] newest recommendations for energy intake based on energy expenditure. Table 26-1 lists the newest recommendations for moderately active individuals. These energy intake levels can be adjusted based on energy expenditure and amount of weight loss required. Referring to the previous section, a deficit of 500 kcal·day^{-1} is required to lose 1 lb of body fat per week.

The Macronutrients: Carbohydrates, Fat, and Protein

Equally as important as consuming the proper amount of energy is the consumption of a good balance of energy (see Chapter 10). Although proper nutrition should be individualized, it is generally recommended that individuals consume about 45% to 65% of their total energy intake from carbohydrates (which provides 4 kcal·g^{-1})[20]. These carbohydrates should consist mostly of whole grains (e.g., whole wheat products; brown rather than white rice). The consumption of whole grains provides more nutrients (vitamins and minerals) as well as greater amounts of fiber, all of which can help to stave off cardiovascular disease and cancer. Protein is another macronutrient that is often perceived as the "building block" of muscle in the body. Although it is true that protein (which provides 4 kcal·g^{-1}) is required for muscle growth, if protein intake is above what the body requires, much of it is stored as fat in

TABLE 26-1. Criteria and Dietary Reference Intake Values for Energy by Moderately Active Individuals by Life Stage Group[a]

Life Stage Group	Criterion	Active PAL EER (kcals·day^{-1}) Males	Females
0–6 months	Energy expenditure + energy deposition	570	520 (3 months)
7–12 months	Energy expenditure + energy deposition	743	676 (9 months)
1–2 years	Energy expenditure + energy deposition	1046	992 (24 months)
3–8 years	Energy expenditure + energy deposition	1742	1642 (6 years)
9–13 years	Energy expenditure + energy deposition	2279	2071 (11 years)
14–18 years	Energy expenditure + energy deposition	3152	2368 (16 years)
> 18 years[b]	Energy expenditure	3067	2403 (19 years)

[a] Established for healthy, moderately active Americans and Canadians.

[b] Subtract 10 kcals·day^{-1} for men and 7 kcals·day^{-1} for women for each year of age above 19 years.

EER = estimated energy requirement; PAL = physical activity level.

Source: Food and Nutrition Board, Institute of Medicine, National Academy of Sciences (2003).[20]

adipocytes. In general, individuals need about 0.4 to 0.5 g of protein per pound of body weight[20]. For example, a 150-lb person requires, on average, about 75 g of protein per day. Each ounce of a protein food provides about 7 g of protein. A person who exercises strenuously may require slightly more protein per day (e.g., about 0.5 to 0.6 g·lb^{-1} body weight), especially if he or she is novice to the specific exercise program. Fat, which is a nutrient that is often thought of as "bad," is required for proper bodily function. Fat provides 9 kcal·g^{-1} of energy. It is recommended that individuals consume about 20% to 35% of their total energy intake from fat[20]; however, the type of fat consumed is most important. Monounsaturated fats (e.g., olive oil, nuts, avocados) and polyunsaturated fats (e.g., safflower oil, sunflower oil) should be consumed in higher amounts than saturated fats (e.g., butter, lard, fat from meat). The reason is because saturated fats lead to increased risk of heart disease because they increase blood levels of LDL. Finally, although alcohol provides energy (7 kcal·g^{-1}), it should be consumed in moderation because high consumption of alcohol can lead to malnutrition.

The Micronutrients

Vitamins and minerals are required for life, but they are required in much lower values than the macronutrients. Their functions are many, but they do *not* provide energy as do the macronutrients. However, many vitamins and minerals are required for energy metabolism and can affect exercise performance and overall health if they are not consumed in the right balance. It is beyond the scope of this chapter to review all the vitamins and minerals; therefore, only two minerals that relate to weight management are highlighted in this chapter: chromium and calcium.

CHROMIUM

Chromium is a mineral that became popular in the early 1990s as a possible weight loss supplement. It was especially popular with body builders, who thought it would increase muscle mass because some researchers reported improvements in body composition with chromium supplementation[21–23]. However, a number of researchers have reported that chromium intake (either picolinate or nicotinate) does not result in significant reductions in weight loss[24–27]. Thus, the efficacy of chromium as a weight loss supplement is not warranted.

However, more recent work on chromium supplementation as an adjuvant therapy for type 2 diabetes mellitus has shown some positive effects on glucose control[28]. The National Institutes of Health has funded research to further assess the efficacy of chromium as a therapy for type 2 diabetes mellitus; therefore, more research will be available in the next several years to provide more evidence of a possible role for chromium in the management of type 2 diabetes mellitus (see Chapter 33).

CALCIUM

It has been proposed that low calcium intake may lead to lipogenesis and that high calcium intake may lead to up-regulation of lipolysis, thereby increasing thermogenesis, resulting in less fat deposition in the adipocyte (fat cell)[29]. There are several mechanisms that may cause this altered lipid metabolism when calcium intake is low. First, calcium is the primary signal of insulin release in the pancreatic beta cell. Increased insulin results in increased fatty acid synthase (FAS) transcription inside the adipocyte, leading to increased FAS, resulting in greater de novo lipogenesis[30]. A lack of dietary calcium intake upregulates

1,25-dihydroxyvitamin D, the most active form of vitamin D, to increase calcium deposition into the adipocytes, which, in turn, increases FAS transcription activity, leading to increased FAS and de novo lipogenesis[30]. Furthermore, decreased dietary calcium intake leads to a reduction in the number of fatty acids in the small intestine that get bound to calcium; thus, more unbound fat is absorbed, increasing fat deposition directly into the adipocytes[31]. Additionally, calcium may increase thermogenesis, perhaps by expressing uncoupling protein 2 (UCP2); however, this mechanism has not been fully elucidated[43]. Finally, the whey protein in milk is a rich source of bioactive compounds, some of which can partly inhibit the autocrine/paracrine renin-antiogensin system within the adipocytes[43]. Calcium may inhibit the production of angiotensin II in the adiopocytes.

Zemel et al.[29] placed transgenic mice expressing the agouti protein (agouti protein is also found in humans and increases FAS transcription activity, as well as low calcium intake) on four different diets: basal diet (0.4% calcium), 1.2% calcium via supplementation with calcium carbonate (supplemented), 1.2% calcium via supplementation with nonfat dry milk (medium dairy), and 2.4% calcium via supplementation with nonfat dry milk (high dairy). Weight gain and fat pad mass were significantly reduced ($P < 0.001$) in all of the calcium diets compared with the basal diet; however, the high-dairy diet had the greatest reduction[29].

In relation to humans, Davies et al.[32] assessed five clinical studies they had initially conducted to assess the effects of calcium supplementation on bone mineral density. They reported that, in the 780 women studied, ranging from the third to the eighth decade of life, a 1000-mg difference in calcium intake resulted in an 8-kg difference in body weight. Carruth and Skinner[33] conducted a longitudinal study in children, 2 to 5 years of age, and reported that those who consumed higher intakes of calcium, monounsaturated fat, and dairy products had lower body fat than children who consumed lower amounts.

In a 2-year exercise intervention study in young women (18 to 31 years of age), Lin et al.[34] assessed the relationship between dietary calcium and changes in body composition. They reported that, regardless of the exercise group assignment, when calcium was adjusted for energy intake, subjects with higher calcium intake gained less body weight and fat over 2 years than those with low calcium intake. This prediction was stronger when dairy calcium was used in the statistical regression models.

Although compelling evidence suggests that higher calcium intake, particularly low-fat dairy calcium, may result in weight loss or prevention of weight gain, more studies are required that define the dose of calcium needed to elicit this effect, further assess if other sources of calcium elicit an effect, and fully elucidate the mechanism (or mechanisms) involved.

Inappropriate Weight Loss Methods

Fad diets are promoted by television, newspaper, and magazine articles on a daily basis. The weight loss industry is a billion dollar industry, and dieting books are among the top sellers. However, many times, these fad diets are promoted by individuals who are not qualified or trained in any way to provide this information. Furthermore, because the weight loss may be unhealthy, these fad diets may be dangerous.

When assessing diet books, those that restrict certain food groups, especially fruits and vegetables, and state that their diets will cure everything, are not appropriate. Furthermore, exercise books that state that a person only needs to exercise 5 minutes per day to lose weight are usually greatly overstating the truth. A book that provides balance in eating and exercise is one that does not restrict foods and does not state that exercise can be done in 5 minutes per day. These books are usually written by registered dietitians or exercise physiologists.

Other inappropriate weight loss methods that can be dangerous are use of saunas or steam rooms, exercising in the heat with heavy clothing on to "sweat off the pounds," starvation diets, liquid diets that are not supervised by physicians and other health care professionals, diets that require mega dosing of vitamin and mineral supplements (mega-dosing can be dangerous because many minerals compete for one another within the body if they share the same carrier), and diets that are only several weeks long, promising rapid weight loss. As stated before, rapid weight loss can be dangerous and can lead to loss of muscle mass and water. If the claims seem too good to be true, they probably are, and that weight loss regimen should be avoided.

Furthermore, rapid weight loss is not recommended because negative consequences can ensue. These consequences can be as simple as a high water weight loss, to as serious as electrolyte imbalances leading to cardiac dysrhythmias. Individuals who lose weight rapidly also tend to lose more lean muscle mass, which can lead to an overall decline in RMR. This decline in RMR may make it more difficult for weight loss to occur in the future. In addition, most individuals who lose weight rapidly do not change their behavior, so their weight loss may not be maintained over time.

Very low-energy diets (VLEDs) are often used for rapid weight loss for morbidly obese individuals. They are typically associated with hospitals, and individuals undergoing these diets are monitored by physicians, as well as a team of other medical personnel. However, are the risks of consuming VLEDs worth the weight loss? Do individuals maintain this weight loss after they return to regular foods? Leser et al.[35] reported that, 3 years after weight loss using a VLED, the women who were most successful were those who maintained physical activity and low-fat diets. Conversely, Wadden et al.[36] reported that women who were first placed on a VLED (420 kcal·d^{-1} for 16 weeks) and then placed on a balanced deficit diet of 1200 kcal/d lost the same amount of body weight (~11 kg) after 1 year compared with those individuals placed on the balanced deficit diet for the entire year. Thus, an overall balanced energy intake that results in lifestyle changes should be the goal. Many individuals want to see rapid results, which typically leads to their weight's cycling over a lifetime. Although lifestyle changes seem "boring" and too lengthy for people, it is an approach that needs to be taken, and each person will have individual lifestyle changes that will make a difference in their overall health and body weight in the long term.

GUIDELINES FOR PROPER WEIGHT LOSS

The American College of Sports Medicine (ACSM) published its most recent position stand in 2001[18]. In brief, it stated that "the combination of reductions in energy intake and increases in energy expenditure, through structured exercise and other forms of physical activity, [should] be a component of weight loss intervention programs"[18]. An energy deficit of 500 to 1000 kcal·d^{-1} was recommended by a combination of a reduction in energy intake and increases in energy expenditure. Furthermore, and as stated previously, it was reported that, although health benefits can be attained with a minimum of 150 min (2.5 hours) of moderate-intensity exercise per week, overweight and obese individuals may better maintain weight loss if they gradually increase exercise to 200 to 300 minutes (3.3 to 5.0 hours) of exercise per week[18]. The incorporation of resistance training was also encouraged to increase strength and function, but it may not significantly prevent the loss of fat-free mass when incorporated with a weight loss program. Finally, although weight loss via sensible exercise and healthy eating was promoted, "When medically indicated, pharmacotherapy may be used for weight loss, but pharmacotherapy appears to be most effective when used in combination with modifications of both eating and exercise behaviors"[18].

Proper weight loss takes time. People do not gain their excess weight in a short period of time; therefore, they need to be reminded that weight loss will not take a short period of time. As far as dietary intake is concerned, a small deficit in food consumption (e.g., 250 kcal·d^{-1}), coupled with an increase in energy expenditure (e.g., 250 kcal·d^{-1}), can lead to a weight loss of about 1 lb·wk^{-1}. It appears that individuals who are successful at maintaining weight loss consume a moderately lower energy intake, exercise on a daily basis, and have had some behavioral therapy to change their overall lifestyle[10].

Although there has been a great deal of argument over the present Food Guide Pyramid (see Fig. 10-1), much of the confusion to the lay public is that many individuals do not understand what one serving size is. Thus, if better education is given to the public that, for example, a bagel

from a fast food restaurant is typically large enough to be three servings, individuals may better understand the Food Guide Pyramid. Depending on the number of calories a person requires, it is recommended that individuals consume from 6 to 11 servings from the base of the Pyramid (Bread, Cereal, Rice, Pasta Group). Examples of one serving from this group are 1 slice of bread, 1/2 cup of cooked rice, 1 cup of cold cereal, 1/2 of a hotdog or hamburger bun, or 4 small crackers. The next two groups on the Food Guide Pyramid are the Fruit Group and the Vegetable Group; these are two groups from which more Americans should be consuming. Individuals should strive to consume from 3 to 5 servings from the Vegetable Group and 2 to 4 servings from the Fruit Group. Examples of what constitutes one serving from these groups include 1/2 cup of cooked vegetables, 1 cup of raw leafy vegetables, 1/2 to 3/4 cup of 100% vegetable juice, 1 whole medium fruit (about 1 cup), 1/2 cup of canned fruit, and 1/2 to 3/4 cup of 100% fruit juice. The next level of the Food Guide Pyramid consists of the Milk, Yogurt and Cheese Group (2 to 3 servings) and the Meat and Meat Alternatives Group (2 to 3 servings). Examples of one serving for the Milk, Yogurt and Cheese Group include 8 oz of milk or yogurt (skim or low-fat are preferred), 2 slices (or 1.5 ounces) of cheese, and 2 cups of cottage cheese. Examples of what constitutes a serving in the Meat and Meat Alternatives Group are 2 to 3 ounces of cooked lean meat, poultry, or fish; 2 eggs; 7 ounces of tofu; 1 cup of cooked legumes; 4 tablespoons of peanut butter; and 1/2 cup of nuts or seeds. The tip of the Food Guide Pyramid

---

BOX 26-1 | **Dietary Guidelines for Americans**

AIM FOR FITNESS
- Aim for a healthy weight.
- Be physically active every day.

BUILD A HEALTHY BASE
- Let the Food Guide Pyramid guide your food choices.
- Choose a variety of grains daily, especially whole grains.
- Choose a variety of fruits and vegetables daily.
- Keep food safe to eat.

CHOOSE SENSIBLY
- Choose a diet that is low in saturated fat and cholesterol and moderate in total fat.
- Choose beverages and foods to moderate your intake of sugars.
- Choose and prepare foods with less salt.
- If you drink alcoholic beverages, do so in moderation.

Adapted from U.S. Department of Agriculture
http://www.health.gov/dietaryguidelines/dga2000/document/contents.htm

BOX 26-2	Be Leery of Weight Loss Plans That Suggest Any of the Following[39]:

- A diet should be drastically different from the recommendations given in the Dietary Guidelines for Americans and the Food Guide Pyramid.
- The diet plan promotes or stresses dietary supplements or herbal products.
- The diet plan requires purchasing of special foods, especially if they are only available at a certain place.
- The diet plan is heavily endorsed through testimonials by famous people or even "everyday" people.
- The diet plan claims to be a cure-all for a number of different medical conditions.
- The plan includes any catch phrases such as: "Lose weight while you sleep" or "Melt pounds away" are used.
- The plan includes exercise gadgets that require the individual to do nothing (e.g., "If you wear this product, it will exercise your stomach for you").

BOX 26-3	Components of Good Weight Loss Programs

- The program should offers clear, scientific information about the success of their clients.
- The program has qualified individuals (e.g., registered dietitians, exercise physiologists, physicians) running it
- Know about the risk of disease. For example, a very low-fat diet can lead to gallbladder disease in some individuals.
- A realistic approach to the weight goal is important.
- Avoid diets of less than 800 kcal·d^{-1} except under medical supervision.
- A dietary program needs to be coupled with an exercise program. This exercise program needs to be tailored to the individual.

Adapted from Food and Nutrition Board of the Institute of Medicine, National Academy of Sciences[40].

consists of fats and sweets (e.g., butter, margarine, oils, cake, donuts, candy), and these should be consumed sparingly[37]. It is important to note that the Food Guide Pyramid encourages consumption of a variety of foods and that, if weight loss if the goal, a decreased number of servings is encouraged.

The Dietary Guidelines for Americans is also a helpful guide for eating more healthily. If people simply increase their fruit and vegetable intake, their overall energy intake usually decreases, and they are consuming products that provide a good deal of fiber and antioxidants, both of which help stave off some chronic diseases. In 2000, the fifth edition of the Dietary Guidelines were published and

stress the importance of eating well and exercising. The three main premises of these guidelines are "Aim for Fitness," "Build a Healthy Base," and "Choose Sensibly"[38]. Box 26-1 lists the details of how to achieve each of these main guidelines.

Recommendations related to weight loss programs are summarized in Boxes 26-2 to 26-4.

Summary

Although weight loss is a challenge for clients and health care professionals, it can be achieved. People striving to lose weight need to understand that weight loss, done properly, takes time, and involves both healthy eating and exercise. A lifestyle change is the key to successful weight loss. It is important that individuals understand inappropriate weight loss methods to prevent any serious side effects from occurring.

BOX 26-4	Components of Good Weight Loss Programs

- Satisfy all nutritional needs.
- Protect an individual from hunger between meals, provide a sense of well being, and not result in fatigue.
- Be one that, with suitable alterations in energy intake and expenditure, can be conducted throughout a lifetime.
- Be simple to maintain, whether at home or away.
- Parallels normal eating habits and tastes as much as possible.
- Uses foods readily available from the grocery store.
- Includes exercise or physical activities that are enjoyable and do not require a certain instrument to promote increased physical activity.

Adapted from Kantor[39].

REFERENCES

1. Kassirer JP, Angell M: Losing weight—an ill-fated New Year's resolution. N Engl J Med 338:1–7, 1998.
2. U.S. Department of Health and Human Services: Clinical Guidelines on the Identification, Evaluation, and Treatment of Overweight and Obesity in Adults: The Evidence Report. NIH Publication No. 98-4083. Bethesda, MD: National Institutes of Health; 1998.
3. Andersen RE: What can physicians do about obesity? Phys Sportsmed 28:15–16, 2000.
4. Must A, Anderson SE: Effects of obesity on morbidity in children and adolescents. *Nutrition in Clinical Care*, 6(1): 4–12, 2003.
5. U.S. Department of Health and Human Services: Healthy People 2010, vol 1. McLean, VA: International Medical Publishing; 2000:28–29.
6. Birch LL, Davison KK: Family environmental factors influencing the developing behavioral controls of food intake and childhood overweight. Child Adolesc Obesity 48:893–907, 2001.

7. French SA, Jeffery RW, Story M, et al: A pricing strategy to promote low-fat snack choices through vending machines. Am J Public Health 87:849–851, 1997.

8. Hill JO, Peters JC: Environmental contributions to the obesity epidemic. Science 280:1371–1374, 1998.

9. Yao M, Roberts SB: Dietary energy density and weight regulation. Nutr Rev 59:247–258, 2001.

10. National Heart, Lung and Blood Institute: Aim for a healthy weight. Available at http://www.nhlbi.nih.gov/health/public/heart/obesity /lose_wt/risk.htm.

11. Skender ML, Goodrick KG, Del Junco DJ, et al: Comparison of 2-year weight loss trends in behavioral treatments of obesity: Diet, exercise, and combination interventions. J Am Dietetic Assoc 4:342–346, 1996.

12. Kraemer WJ, Volek JS, Clark KL, et al: Influence of exercise training on physiological and performance changes in weight loss in men. Med Sci Sports Exerc 9:1320–1329, 1999.

13. Kraemer WJ, Volek JS, Clark KL, et al: Physiological adaptation to a weight-loss dietary regimen and exercise programs in women. J Appl Physiol 83:270–279, 1997.

14. Utter AC, Nieman DC, Shannonhouse EM, et al: Influence of diet and/or exercise on body composition and cardiorespiratory fitness in obese women. Int J Sport Nutr 8:213–222, 1998.

15. Lafortuna CL, Resnik M, Galvani C, Sartorio A: Effects of non-specific vs individualized exercise training protocols on aerobic, anaerobic and strength performance in severely obese subjects during a short-term body mass reduction program. J Endocrinol Invest 26:197–205, 2003.

16. Jakicic JM, Wing RR, Butler BA, Robertson RJ: Prescribing exercise in multiple short bouts versus one continuous bout: effects on adherence, cardiorespiratory fitness, and weight loss in overweight women. Int J Obes Rel Metab Disord 19:893–901, 1995.

17. Jakicic JM, Winters C, Lang W, Wing RR: Effects of intermittent exercise and use of home exercise equipment on adherence, weight loss and fitness in overweight women: A randomized trial. JAMA 282:1554–1560, 1999.

18. Jakicic JM, Clark K, Coleman E, et al: American College of Sports Medicine position stand: Appropriate intervention strategies for weight loss and prevention of weight regain for adults. Med Sci Sports Exerc 33:2145–2156, 2001.

19. Donnelly JE, Hill JO, Jacobsen DJ, et al: Effects of a 16-month randomized controlled exercise trial on body weight and composition in young overweight men and women: The Midwest exercise trial. Arch Intern Med 163:1343–1350, 2003.

20. Food and Nutrition Board, Institute of Medicine, National Academy of Sciences: Dietary Reference Intakes for Energy, Carbohydrate, Fiber, Fat, Fatty Acids, Cholesterol, Protein, and Amino Acids. Washington, DC: The National Academies Press; 2003.

21. Crawford V, Scheckenbach R, Preuss HG: Effects of niacin-bound chromium supplementation on body composition in overweight African-American women. Diabet Obes Metab1:331–337, 1999.

22. Evans GW: The effect of chromium picolinate on insulin controlled parameters in humans. Int J Biosoc Med Res 11:163–180, 1989.

23. Hasten DL, Rome EP, Franks BD, Hegsted M.: Effects of chromium picolinate on beginning weight training students. Int J Sports Nutr 2:343–350, 1992.

24. Campbell WW, Joseph LJ, Davey SL, et al: Effects of resistance training and chromium picolinate on body composition and skeletal muscle in older men. J Appl Physiol 86:29–39, 1999.

25. Vincent JB: The potential value and toxicity of chromium picolinate as a nutritional supplement, weight loss agent and muscle development agent. Sports Med 33:213–230, 2003.

26. Volpe SL, Huang H-W, Larpadisorn K, Lesser II: Effect of chromium supplementation on body composition, resting metabolic rate, and selected biochemical parameters in moderately obese women following an exercise program. J Am Coll Nutr 20:293–306, 2001.

27. Walker LS, Bemben MG, Bemben DA, Knehans AW: Chromium picolinate effects on body composition and muscular performance in wrestlers. Med Sci Sports Exerc 30:1730–1737, 1998.

28. Anderson RA, Cheng N, Bryden NA, et al: Elevated intakes of supplemental chromium improve glucose and insulin variables in individuals with type 2 diabetes. Diabetes 46:1786–1791, 1997.

29. Zemel MB, Shi H, Greer B, et al: Regulation of adiposity by dietary calcium. FASEB J 14:1132–1138, 2000.

30. Zemel MB: Mechanisms of dairy modulation of adiposity. J Nutr 133:252S–256S, 2003.

31. Parikh SJ, Yanovski JA: Calcium intake and adiposity. Am J Clin Nutr 77:281–287, 2003.

32. Davies KM, Heaney RP, Recker RR, et al: Calcium intake and body weight. J Clin Endocrinol Metab 85:4635–4638, 2000.

33. Carruth BR, Skinner JD: The role of dietary calcium and other nutrients in moderating body fat in preschool children. Int J Obesity 25:559–566, 2001.

34. Lin Y-C, Lyle RM, McCabe LD, et al: Dairy calcium is related to changes in body composition during a two-year exercise intervention in young women. J Am Coll Nutr 19:754–760, 2000.

35. Leser MS, Yanovski SZ, Yanovski JA: A low-fat intake and greater activity level are associated with lower weight regain 3 years after completing a very-low-calorie diet. J Am Dietetic Assoc 102:1052–1056, 2003.

36. Wadden TA, Foster GD, Letizia KA: One-year behavioral treatment of obesity: Comparison of moderate and severe caloric restriction and the effects of weight maintenance therapy. J Consult Clin Psychol 62:165–171, 1994.

37. U.S. Department of Agriculture: Healthy school meals resource system. Available at http://schoolmeals.nal.usda.gov/

38. U.S. Department of Agriculture: Aim. . . Build. . . Choose. . . for Good Health. Available at http://www.health.gov/dietaryguide-lines/dga2000/document/contents.htm

39. Editor 2 Kantor M: Evaluating weight loss programs. Available at http:// www.agnr.umd.edu/MCE/Publications/Publication.cfm? ID=132&cat=11

40. Food and Nutrition Board, Institute of Medicine, National Academy of Sciences: Weighing the Options: Criteria for Evaluating Weight-Management Programs. Washington, DC: National Academies Press; 1995.

SUGGESTED READINGS

Binkley HM, Beckett J, Casa DJ, et al: National Athletic Trainers' Association Position Statement: Exertional heat illnesses. J Athlet Training 37:329–343, 2002.

Casa DJ, Armstrong LE, Hillman SK, et al: National Athletic Trainers' Association position statement: Fluid replacement for athletes. J Athlet Training 35:212–224, 2000.

Hill JO, Peters JC: Environmental contributions to the obesity epidemic. Science 280:1371–1374, 1998.

Hill JO, Wyatt HR, Reed GW, Peters JC: Obesity and the environment: Where do we go from here? Science 299:853–855, 2003.

Insel P, Turner RE, Ross D: Nutrition. Boston: Jones & Bartlett Publishers; 2001.

Jakicic JM, Clark K, Coleman E, et al: American College of Sports Medicine position stand: Appropriate intervention strategies for weight loss and prevention of weight regain for adults. Med Sci Sports Exerc 33:2145–2156, 2001.

Must A, Anderson SE: Effects of obesity on morbidity in children and adolescents. Nutr Clin Care 6 4–12, 2003.

National Institutes of Health: Clinical Guidelines on the Identification, Evaluation, and Treatment of Overweight and Obesity in Adults: The Evidence Report. NIH Publication No. 98–4083; September 1998.

Yao M, Roberts SB: Dietary energy density and weight regulation. Nutr Rev 59:247–258, 2001.

INTERNET RESOURCES

American Dietetic Association: http://www.eatright.org/Public

National Heart, Lung, and Blood Institute: Clinical Guidelines on the Identification, Evaluation, and Treatment of Overweight and Obesity in Adults: http://www.nhlbi.nih.gov/guidelines/obesity/ob_home.htm

NHLBI Health Information Network: Online Continuing Medical Education Programs on Obesity: http://hin.nhlbi.nih.gov/joinhin/news /OEI 0415.htm

North American Association for the Study of Obesity: http://www. naaso.org

United States Department of Health & Human Services: Overweight and Obesity: The Surgeon General's Call to Action to Prevent and Decrease Overweight and Obesity: : http://www.surgeongeneral.gov/topics/obesity

Weight-control Information Network: http://win.niddk.nih.gov/publications/prescription.htm

Applied Exercise Programming

LEN KRAVITZ

The varieties of organized group-led class offerings have grown extensively in the past quarter century. Instructor-led classes in indoor cycling, step training, walking, kickboxing, water exercise, mixed-impact aerobics, yoga, Pilates, and rebounding are just a few of the numerous classes now offered in fitness facilities throughout North American and in countries all over the world. Most group-led exercise courses are founded by design to help improve and sustain the lifetime health and well being of the class participants. In this chapter, exercise class design components are applied from the scientific principles presented in previous chapters. It should be emphasized that the certified health/fitness instructor must always take into account the fitness level of the students, age, skill level, and overall goal of the program when designing a safe and effective exercise class.

Warm-up

Traditionally, the group-led exercise class begins with a warm-up. The warm-up consists of a 5- to 10-minute combination of rhythmic movements, advancing in a logical progression from full-body general movements to more specific muscle–joint isolation exercises. The full-body exercises often mimic the movements that will be performed in the subsequent workout (referred to as "rehearsal moves"), only they are executed at a much lower level of intensity. For instance, in a cardio kickboxing class, the warm-up may include several jabs, punches, and kicks performed at a light intensity. The full-body movements heighten blood flow to the working muscles, increase the speed of nerve impulses, and advance oxygen and energy substrate delivery to working muscles while removing waste products[1]. These physiological responses ready the body for vigorous exercise by accelerating metabolism in muscle fibers and decreasing intramuscular resistance, thus improving movement efficiency[1]. This general warm-up phase also provides the instructor with an opportune time to demonstrate and create awareness of correct execution and posture of many of the workout exercises to ensue.

The muscle–joint isolation segment of the warm-up session consists of limbering movements such as shoulder circles, neck rotation, spinal rotation, spinal lateral flexion, knee flexion and extension, and ankle plantarflexion and dorsiflexion movements. These specific joint movements are rhythmically performed to prepare the movable body joints and attached muscles for the dynamic exercises to follow. Often, the specific joint exercises are performed in similar patterns of motion that they will be completed during the workout. For instance, in a sports conditioning class warm-up, the inclusion of some easy lunges may be a most beneficial preparation for the challenging workout lunges that simulate forward, diagonal, and side exercises completed for ski and soccer sport conditioning skills and drills. This specific warm-up technique, in effect, provides the neuromuscular system with a comparable movement pattern rehearsal of some of the workout exercises.

The incorporation of stretching movements in the warm-up, for purposes of injury reduction, is currently uncertain (see Chapter 25). Presently, there is insufficient evidence to endorse or discontinue stretching in the warm-up as a means of injury prevention[1,2]. However, stretching clearly has been shown to increase flexibility, and for optimal effectiveness, it should be conducted after an appropriate warm-up is performed[1].

Cardiorespiratory Program Design

According to the American College of Sports Medicine (ACSM) guidelines reviewed in Chapter 24 and GETP7 Chapter 7, the cardiorespiratory section should consist of between 20 and 60 minutes of continuous or intermittent (minimum of 10-min bouts) aerobic activity and be at an intensity of exercise corresponding to between 55% and 65% to 90% of maximum heart rate (HR_{max}) or between 40% and 50% to 85% of oxygen uptake reserve ($\dot{V}O_2R$) or HR reserve (HRR). The objective of this phase of the group-led class is to sufficiently challenge the cardiorespiratory system for the improvement or maintenance of cardiovascular function. A second objective may be promoting the positive realization of weight management goals (see Chapter 26). Before discussing the actual cardiorespiratory design, a brief discussion of exercise mode and intensity modification considerations is warranted.

EXERCISE MODE CONSIDERATIONS

Cardiorespiratory fitness is exemplified by being able to do physical activity for a prolonged period of time. Aside from energy expenditure, some factors to consider when selecting a mode of exercise include the personal interests of the students, equipment and facility availability, physical needs, injury risk, and fitness goals.

Because of the great variety of cardiorespiratory modes and types of programs presently available, many exercise enthusiasts now prefer to cross train on a variety of exercise modes, which combines high exercise enjoyment and possible lowered musculoskeletal risk.

VARYING THE INTENSITY OF EXERCISE

With most exercise programs, it is necessary to be able to vary the intensity of the exercise, such as for interval training programs (discussed later), or to adapt the program for special populations (e.g., sedentary, elder, overweight). Therefore, in selecting exercise programs and modes for group-led exercise, it is helpful to evaluate how the particular mode of exercise can be adjusted or graded to vary the stress placed on the cardiorespiratory and musculoskeletal systems. For instance, indoor cycling intensity can easily be made more or less demanding by adjusting the pedaling resistance or cadence. Typically, with indoor cycling classes, when pedaling resistance is increased, there is an accompanying decrease in pedaling cadence. Adding or removing a step riser to stepping height has been conclusively shown to affect the step training workout intensity[3–7]. In addition, the inclusion of propulsive movements while performing traditional step training significantly increases the exercise intensity[8].

When sequencing the cardiovascular segment, always allow for a 3- to 5-minute progressive cardiovascular warm-up to prepare the cardiorespiratory and musculoskeletal systems for the succeeding workout. Just as important, make sure there is a 3- to 5-minute (or longer) recovery period of gradually decreasing exercise intensity at the end of the cardiovascular segment. This recovery phase provides a physiological transition for cardiovascular parameters to return towards a resting state.

It should be pointed out that the addition of light (up to 4 lbs in each hand) handheld weights to a cardiorespiratory exercise program has not been shown to significantly improve **cardiorespiratory endurance** or muscular fitness as compared with not using handheld weights[5,9,10]. In addition, in traditional low-impact[11] and step training[12] classes, it has been found that the larger traveling patterns of movement and choice of exercises involving greater muscle mass[13] are associated with higher oxygen costs and caloric expenditure. Lastly, increasing the speed of movement in many exercise programs (e.g., step training) also increases the exercise intensity[14]. However, caution is always recommended because speed of movement may sometimes lead to a compromise in range of motion (ROM) performed and possible increase the risk of injury.

APPLIED CARDIORESPIRATORY SECTION DESIGN

Group-led exercise classes, which may range in time from 30 to 90 minutes, now offer continuous or intermittent (in 10-min bouts) aerobic segments. Depending on the mode of exercise, such as with indoor cycling programs, the length of the aerobic section may be carefully designed to challenge the participants without consequential musculoskeletal risk. However, in weight-bearing activities, the certified instructor must always be concerned with preventing lower body injuries in students. Group-led instructors are encouraged to vary the type of exercise movements (e.g., avoiding the performance of several consecutive high-impact movements in a sequence) and to gradually increase the intensity of the exercise.

The varieties of group-led exercise programs currently being taught are virtually boundless. The discussions of applied cardiorespiratory designs to follow initially focus on the three major formats of the majority of these classes: continuous training, interval training, and circuit formats.

CONTINUOUS TRAINING

Continuous training endeavors to maintain a specific workout intensity level throughout the entire workout. The types of exercises, as evaluated by the physical exertion needed to perform them and the speed of exercise execution, are carefully chosen to sustain this intensity throughout the workout. Participants are encouraged to attain a target heart rate (HR) or target ratings of perceived exertion (RPE) and maintain this target level throughout the workout. Continuous training classes exemplify "steady state" or "steady rate" workout formats, in which as soon as the target intensity is reached, all physiological variables (e.g., HR, oxygen consumption, and respiratory rate) remain relatively stable.

INTERVAL TRAINING

Interval training is a form of cardiorespiratory training that combines segments of high-intensity work with segments of light- to moderate-intensity work. More recently, interval training is becoming an increasingly popularized training method that can be incorporated with most modes of exercise.

Interval training has been a meaningful part of athletic training programs for many years because a variety of sport and recreational activities demand variation in the bursts of movement intensities. The incorporation of interval training into a group-led exercise class helps to achieve the development or maintenance of cardiorespiratory fitness, as well as the accomplishment of body composition goals[15].

In principle, interval training delivers an exercise method of completing high-intensity work bouts mixed with recovery periods of less intense aerobic work (Table 27-1 provides definitions of terms related to interval training). The specific duration of the work and rest intervals, number of cycles and sets of intervals, and type of recovery (active versus passive) depend on the energy systems in which training adaptations are primarily desired (refer to Chapter 3 for a review of exercise metabolism). It

TABLE 27-1. Terms Related to Interval Training

Term	Definition
Work interval	Time of work effort or work bout
Recovery interval	Time between work intervals; the recovery interval may consist of light activity such as walking (passive recovery) or light to moderate exercise such as jogging (active recovery)
Work/recovery ratio	Time ratio of the work and recovery intervals; a work/recovery ratio of 1 to 3 means the recovery interval is three times that of the work interval
Cycle	One cycle includes a work and recovery interval
Set	Number of cycles completed per workout

should be kept in mind that although a certain combination of training factors may primarily challenge a particular energy system, training adaptations, to some extent, are likely to be seen in all three energy systems with interval training programs

INTERVAL TRAINING FOR GROUP-LED EXERCISE CLASSES

Putting theory into practice, here is an applied example of an interval training design for a group-led exercise program. For this interval aerobic workout, choose any mode of cardiorespiratory activity (i.e., walking, rebounding, cycling, stepping, cardio kickboxing). Always begin the interval training segment gradually with 3 to 5 minutes of light-intensity aerobics to prepare the heart, lungs, and musculoskeletal system for the workout to follow.

Then, with the interval training design, exercise for 4 minutes at a higher intensity followed by 4 minutes at a light to moderate intensity. Alternate these 4-minute intervals for the duration of the workout. This is an example of a one-to-one work/recovery ratio (see Table 27-1). During the 4-minute high-intensity interval, a possible goal with a fit and healthy population is to exercise in the 70% to 80% HRR intensity (or a 15 to 16 on the RPE scale). A likely goal intensity for the light- to moderate-intensity recovery period is 50% to 60% HRR intensity (or 11 to 12 on the RPE scale). Determine the intensity level of the program according to the fitness levels of the particular exercise population. Also, depending on the fitness level, age, health, mode of exercise, and goals of the class, progress into a range of 20 to 60 minutes with this interval training workout.

Modifying for special populations (e.g., obese, senior, injury recovery, entry-level student) is very easy. The key is that all participants work out at a relative exercise intensity of their fitness level.

The diverseness of possible interval training designs is quite extensive, and the ease of design for multilevel abilities is noteworthy. Presented here in text is only one example of an interval training program for use with group-led exercise classes. Feel free to be creative and design other interval training program designs depending on which energy systems you wish to challenge.

CIRCUIT TRAINING

The term *circuit* refers to a number of carefully selected exercises arranged successively in a specific sequence. In its classical format, 9 to 12 stations comprise the circuit. This number may vary according to the design of the program (Table 27-2 provides an example of a basic **circuit training** format that may be performed in a group-led body conditioning class, although equipment availability and choice will determine class size). Each participant moves from one station to the next with little (15 to 30 seconds) or no rest, performing a 15- to 45-second set of eight to 20 repetitions at each station (using a resistance of about 40% to 60% of one-repetition maximum [1RM]). The program may be performed with exercise machines, handheld weights, elastic resistance, or muscle conditioning exercises using the body as the resistance (e.g., squats, push-ups, curl-ups, lunges).

By adding a 30-second to 3-minute (or longer) aerobics station between each station, referred to as *aerobic circuit training*, the method attempts to improve cardiorespiratory endurance, although experimental research reviewed[15] is somewhat equivocal. Applied design variations of this aerobic circuit training model include performing two to four or more exercise stations in series and then performing the aerobics station. For example, Box 27-1 is a functional exercise circuit example of participants completing two functional exercise stations in series then alternating with aerobics. With functional exercise training, movements and muscles are trained to better perform in everyday activities[16].

BOX 27-1	Example of a Functional Exercise Circuit

1. Alternating step forward lunges while holding a medicine ball
2. Standing alternating hip adduction lateral raises
3. 3 minutes of aerobics (walking)
4. Seated overhead press with dumbbells on stability ball
5. Seated (on floor) high row with elastic tube
6. 3 minutes of aerobics (bench stepping)
7. Squats with upright rows using dumbbells
9. Preacher biceps curl on a stability ball
10. 3 minutes of aerobics (jogging)
11. Reverse flys on stability ball
12. Standing unilateral frontal raises with tubing
13. 3 minutes of aerobics (rope skipping)
14. Alternating pull-down with tubes while performing a squat
15. Alternating knee lifts while extending a medicine ball overhead
16. 3-minute aerobics (cardio kickboxing alternating front kicks)
17. Stability ball elbow balance
18. Stability ball rotation crunches

GUIDELINES FOR CONDUCTING CIRCUIT TRAINING PROGRAMS

The various types of circuit training programs that can be developed are only limited by the creativity of the instructor and the space and equipment available. As well, circuit programs can be designed to meet the needs of numerous populations, including sedentary, physically challenged, cardiac rehabilitation, weight management, and team sports. The following are some applied exercise guidelines for administering circuit training programs.

Music, Station Changes, and Timing

Select music that will particularly motivate your students to exercise. Because the participants typically do not have to exercise to the tempo of the music, a number of different types of music and tempos may be used that inspire the class to exercise.

Having students change from station to station can be handled effortlessly. With the availability of a microphone, the instructor can just direct students to change stations. As well, the use of a unique sound, such as a bicycle horn or musical party instrument, works most handily. The use of a stopwatch or large clock helps to maintain the appropriate timing at each station.

Room Size, Traffic Flow, and Station Signs

With a little planning, even small rooms can be made very space effective for station setup and traffic flow of students. For traffic flow of students going from station to

TABLE 27-2. Example of a Basic Circuit Training Format[a]

Exercise	Muscle Groups
Squat or leg press	Hamstrings, quadriceps, gluteals
Chest press	Pectorals, anterior deltoid, triceps, coracobrachialis, subscapularis
Lunge	Hamstrings, quadriceps, gluteals
Seated row pull	Latissimus dorsi, middle and posterior deltoid, rhomboids, infraspinatus, teres minor
Shoulder press	Anterior deltoid, upper trapezius, pectorals-clavicular, coracobrachialis
Lateral pull	Latissimus dorsi, teres major, pectorals—sternal
Triceps extension	Triceps brachii, anconeus
Biceps curl	Biceps brachii, brachialis, brachioradialis
Heel raise	Gastrocnemius, soleus
Supine abdominal curls	Rectus abdominals, internal and external obliques

[a]This circuit can be done with resistance machines, free weights, elastic resistance, or any combination of resistance devices. Adding an aerobics station between one or more stations creates an aerobic circuit training format.

station, a simple clockwise direction is usually most effective and easy to follow. Placing signs (with illustrations or pictures with exercise names) at each station is very useful for students to know what exercises to do.

Equipment

Make sure you maximize the available equipment resources in all possible ways. For instance, a step aerobics bench and risers can be inclined or declined for use for abdominal crunches or chest flies.

Class Size

Most instructors know the attendance range in a particular class which helps with the circuit planning. Plan for the higher number of that range to avoid administration obstacles when starting the class.

Mainstreaming New Students

Frequently, new participants (or newcomers to exercise) may come to class the day a circuit is being taught. Because the teacher is quite involved with managing and supervising the circuit program, there is not always a lot of one-on-one time available for new students. One workable solution is to have new participants buddy up with regularly attending students, who can guide them through the circuit and be good role models for correct exercise performance at each station.

Safety Considerations

One key safety concern is to make sure the exercises are explained and taught well to the students so the exercises can be performed with proper technique. Although the concept of circuit training indicates movement, make sure the circuit does not seem to rush the students through the circuit. Also, with circuits such as a ski conditioning, in which some of the exercises may involve jumping and leaping over objects, teachers are highly encouraged to use "plastic cones" for obstacles to jump over as opposed to heavy objects (e.g., benches), which may cause someone to trip and fall. Lastly, an important concern is to avoid repeating overuse-type exercises in the circuit. For instance, in a cardio kickboxing circuit, use a variety of movements such as jabs, hooks, upper cuts, elbow strikes, front kicks, knee strikes, and sidekicks to challenge the body with a balanced approach to training the total body.

Muscular Fitness Segment

Most group-led exercise classes also incorporate a muscular fitness component. Depending on the goals of the class and time for this segment, this section can be as short as a few sets of abdominal and back exercises up to a full-body, comprehensive muscular fitness workout. Additionally, not all group-led classes have the necessary equipment to provide

an adequate overload stimulus for the attainment of muscular strength (maximal or near-maximal muscle force production). Therefore, in group-led exercise programs, the muscular fitness segment is usually designed with an emphasis on enhancing muscular endurance (sustained, repeated submaximal muscular actions). Equipment often available may include exercise tubes, dumbbells, exercise bands, weighted bars, medicine balls, and barbell sets. It is important to remember that the GETP7 now recommends at least one set (of three to 20 repetitions with eight to 12 usually recommended) of eight to 10 separate exercises for the major muscle groups (arms, shoulders, chest, abdomen, back, hips, and legs) of the body to be performed two to three times per week (see Tables 1-5 and 1-6). For older or more frail persons, 10 to 15 repetitions may be more appropriate. The following are applied exercise design considerations for muscular fitness training that complement the information presented in Chapter 25.

PARTICIPANT CHARACTERISTICS

As mentioned previously in Chapter 5 and GETP7 Chapter 2, it is recommended to have the health and fitness background information as well as the medical history of the students in a class. For example, it would be most useful to know if a student was suffering from arthritis because depending on the severity of this health condition, some exercises may need to be modified or eliminated to avoid discomfort to the student.

EXERCISE SELECTION

When choosing exercises for a particular class or group, factors to consider include the level of fitness of the participants, years of exercise training, average age of participants, any potential risks with the exercise (and possible modifications), and the overall purpose of the exercises.

A new method of exercise design selection and progression is provided in **Functional Exercise Progressions**[16]. This novel design progresses from simple to complex exercises that include an underlying theme in strengthening the core muscles (internal obliques, transverse abdominus, multifidus, quadratus lumborum) of the body. Yoke and Kennedy's[16] six-step exercise design system is described below.

> **Level #1: Isolate and educate:** The student is learning how to focus on the muscle and movement. Exercises in this level are often performed in the supine or prone position.
> **Level #2: Isolate and educate and add resistance:** Resistance is added to the exercise in Level #1.
> **Level #3: Add functional training position:** To better challenge the stabilizing muscles, an exercise in a seated or standing position (for the targeted muscles) is performed.
> **Level #4: Combined increasing function with resistance:** Some type of overload (e.g., weights,

tubing, bands) is added to challenge the body's stabilizers in the functional position.

Level #5: Multi-muscle groups with increasing resistance and core challenge: More complex exercises (e.g., squats and lunge variations) are added that combine muscular fitness, balance, coordination, and stability.

Level #6: Add balance, increased functional challenge, speed, or rotational movements: The use of stability balls, wobble boards, or spinal rotation to exercise movements is added. Yoke and Kennedy[16] note that some individuals may never reach this level because of their fitness level or health history.

MUSCULAR FITNESS MAIN CATEGORIES

Muscular fitness program designs typically fall into three main categories: general training, functional training, and sport-specific training. In the health and fitness field, general training has been traditionally what most individuals fall within. This category fundamentally represents resistance exercise designs that focus on training the major muscles of the body. However, in the past few years, functional training has gained tremendous empirical support and usage for inclusion in muscular fitness designs. The concept of functional exercise may be described as adding "movement that matters" or "purposeful movement" to daily life activities. Yoke and Kennedy[16] propose that training muscles in this deliberate fashion improves people's ability to function independently in the real world. Sport-specific muscular fitness programs include training exercises that are considered to be associated with the improvement of performance of a particular sport.

The muscular fitness program variables (e.g., sets, repetitions, rest periods between sets, progressive overload, and the intensity of resistance) are thoroughly covered in Chapter 25.

Cool-down Segment

The purpose of the final cool-down segment is to return the body toward a resting or pre-exercise state. This segment helps to prevent pooling of the blood in the arms and legs, thus maintaining blood pressure (BP) and aiding the body's return to a pre-exercise state. The cool-down normally consists of slow moving rhythmical bodily movements (similar to those completed in the warm-up) and standing and seated stretches of the muscle groups used during the workout. It may typically last between 4 and 10 minutes. A secondary goal that may be accomplished within the cool-down segment is the improvement of flexibility (or ROM) of the targeted joints. A thorough discussion of flexibility methods is presented in Chapter 25. A third goal of the cool-down segment may be to include a relaxation component to further help to relax the mind from daily stressors.

Popular Group-led Class Programs

A diverse number of group-led class programs has emerged in an effort to meet the retention needs of regular exercisers and to attract new fitness participants. Some of these programs are choreographed to accompanying music, and others use music as a background source of inspiration. Music is customarily arranged in measures of four beats, alternating between emphasized and deemphasized beats, referred to as the downbeat and upbeat, respectively. Some programs, such as step, need to follow a specialized 32-beat phrasing. This necessitates further understanding, training, and practice for instructors to effectively learn how to integrate the movement with the music. Other exercise programs, such as indoor walking with music, more readily incorporate a blend of music phrases, with less demand on movement and music integration. Regardless of the music phrasing, group-led instructors have an obligation to their students to make sure the music loudness does not put any of their students at hearing loss risk. In reference to instructor voice safety, whenever possible, instructors should use a microphone when teaching group-led exercise classes. Some of the popular group-led programs briefly highlighted in this section include mixed-impact aerobics, step training, martial arts exercise, water fitness, indoor cycling, yoga, stability ball workouts, and Pilates.

MIXED-IMPACT AEROBICS

Mixed-impact, or high–low, classes combine high-impact aerobic movements that are associated with greater stresses on the lower extremities (e.g., running, jumping, and hopping) with low-impact movements that provide minimal stress on the lower extremities (e.g., step touches and side lunges). Combinations and routines are choreographed to music approximately 130 to 150 bpm incorporating a variety of arm movements, leg movements, traveling patterns, and directional turns. An advantage of mixed-impact classes is the ability to modify the intensity of the exercise. With all exercise programs, modification involves analyzing the movements or exercises and determining safe ways the programs can be introduced to people of different fitness levels. A review of literature reveals a wide difference in energy cost between the low-impact (4 to 5 kcal·min^{-1}) and the high-impact (10 to 11 kcal·min^{-1}) movement styles[17]. Typically, the most common ways to modify any group-led exercise are to alter the speed of movement, modify the ROM of the movement, vary the amount of traveling completed with a movement, and change the vertical direction of the movement.

With mixed-impact classes, there is no single preferred method of combining the impact styles. Some classes alternate impact styles using the music songs for the style changes. For example, some mixed-impact programs alternate between high- and low-impact movement with every song (3- to 5-min) change on a soundtrack. Other programs combine the impact styles within all sections of the choreography, thus interspersing the low- and high-impact movements throughout the program. The best suggestion to group-led instructors is to evaluate what they think would best minimize injury risks while maximizing health benefits of their participants. General exercise safety recommendations for most group-led exercise classes appropriately apply to mixed-impact classes as well, and are as follows:

1. Always wear exercise shoes designed for the particular class.
2. Regularly monitor the exercise intensity with pulse rate checks or ratings of perceived exertion.
3. Encourage all students to work out at their own preferred intensity.
4. Drink water before, during, and after aerobic exercise workouts.
5. Gradually wind down the aerobic section to a walking pace to ensure safe and proper recovery

Recommendations specific to mixed-impact classes include:

1. Do not hop on one foot more than four times in a row.
2. Stay away from twisting hop variations that may lead to spinal stress.

STEP TRAINING

Step training has become a mainstay cardiorespiratory class format because of its widespread popularity and ease of administration to the multilevel ability levels that are commonly seen in exercise classes. Researchers of step training describe it as being a safe, low-impact exercise program that may potentially provide high-intensity aerobic conditioning for participants[4]. The workouts can be as challenging as a rigorous jogging workout and yet produce impact forces as safe as walking. The cadence of step aerobics classes generally ranges from 118 to 128 bpm[18,19]. To increase workout intensity, many instructors unwisely teach at speeds above 130 bpm. However, the research clearly demonstrates that changing bench height is the most consequential variable to alter step exercise intensity[3–7]. As well, these faster stepping cadences result in greater vertical ground reaction forces on the body in less-experienced step enthusiasts[20]. The most widely used step platforms have adjustable heights from 4 to 12 inches, with a stepping surface 14 inches wide and 42 inches long. Instructors are encouraged to regularly inform and educate their students that the progression of exercise intensity is best accomplished with changes in step height. The typical riser increase allows for a 2-inch change in step height. Students are recommended and encouraged to begin gradually, using a lower step height and then progressively increasing the platform height as they become more capable of performing the instructor-led workouts.

Group-led instructors should be alerted to the fact that some participants will find the unfamiliarity of stepping up onto and off the step to be a challenging motor skill. One suggestion is to introduce many of the step combinations gradually and without musical accompaniment for these learners. The following are other key safety tips to follow when implementing a step training program.[15,18,19,21]:

1. Step entirely on the top part of the platform with each step, not allowing any part of the foot to hang over an edge. Keep participants from adopting a bouncy style of stepping.
2. Most participants find progressing up to a 6-inch step height to provide a satisfactory workout. Discourage flexing the knees more then 90° with the step height. Avoid flexing the knees more than 60° for participants predisposed to patellofemoral pain.
3. Additional handheld weights while step training are not recommended by several certification organizations because of the fact that long-term training effects (12 weeks) have not demonstrated the use of handheld weights (up to 4 lbs) to provide superior physiological benefits.
4. To lower the step intensity quickly, stop stepping and switch to marching in place on the ground.
5. Be careful not to step too far back off the platform. This causes the body to lean slightly forward, placing extra stress on the Achilles tendon and calf. Instruct students to step back about one shoe length away from the step.
6. Use good cross-training shoe or indoor fitness shoes for step workouts. The tread on most running shoes does not provide suitable support for step movements.
7. As the name implies, step training is a stepping motion using the entire foot. Avoid pounding foot movements on the platform and bouncing actions onto and off the floor when step training.
8. Vary choreography but avoid step combinations that travel forward and down off the bench.
9. Be aware of the potential for overuse injury syndrome. Encourage students to participate in a variety of aerobic activities, allowing for different stresses on the lower body.
10. Always look at the step platform when doing step aerobics; however, do not drop the head too far forward.
11. The correct posture in step training involves standing tall and bending at the knees for the ascending and descending movements. Too much hip flexion while stepping may place unwanted stresses on the spine.
12. Change the leading foot when doing the step patterns to avoid overstressing one leg. A good rule of thumb is to change the lead foot every minute or sooner.
13. Step training choreography allows for some moves to be repeating actions. A safe guideline to follow is not to perform more than five consecutive repeating movements on the same leg.
14. Lunges off a step can provide high-intensity challenges but are often performed incorrectly or too

swiftly, with potential trauma to the lower leg from the ground impact. Take the time to teach safe lunges and be careful not to overperform.

15. If any participants complain of knee stress from a step class, they should be advised to seek help from their health practitioners. Step aerobics may not be a suitable exercise mode for all exercise enthusiasts.

16. Include strengthening exercises for both the lower body limb agonist and antagonist muscle groups.

17. Try not to keep the arm movements at or above the shoulder for extended periods of time.

MARTIAL ARTS EXERCISE

Kickboxing aerobics, aerobic kickboxing, cardio boxing, and aerobic boxing are just a few of the many martial arts exercise class workouts that have become a staple component of the group-led fitness industry. Enthusiasts appear to enjoy the power and exhilaration from delivering kicks, punches, elbows, jabs, knee strikes, and combinations used in boxing and martial arts. The athletic drills in these classes are mixed with recovery bouts of basic aerobic movements such as boxer-style rope skipping (with and without a rope), walking, and light jogging in place. Some kickboxing exercise programs involve authentic boxing gloves, punching bags, and martial arts equipment, and other programs incorporate a form of "shadow boxing" that involves no equipment. The majority of these classes are driven by moderately paced music (approximately 120 to 138 bpm), although the music in many instances is more for motivation because the cardio kickboxing choreography is not always performed to a specific tempo. Some of the classes are taught in circuit formats, in which groups of students rotate from station to station, performing different types of kicks, jabs, and punches at each station. Other classes are taught in the more traditional instructor-led format in which a teacher leads the students during the entire class.

A key concern with martial arts exercise classes is the preparation of instructors to properly teach the programs[22]. Instructors need to have proper knowledge of correct punching techniques, as well as the progressive teaching skills in order to evade any joint-related injuries to class participants. Thus, the leadership challenge involves a balance of creating a motivating workout environment while progressively introducing safe, enjoyable, and challenging martial arts exercises. As with all group-led classes, the effectiveness of martial arts instructors highly depends on their ability to modify movement to suit the needs and abilities of the class participants.

The following are some safety guidelines to consider with martial arts exercise classes[22,23].

1. Perform a satisfactory warm-up to properly prepare the muscles and joints for the ensuing challenge of the workout.

2. With all upper body strikes and jabs, make sure the elbow is not taken past its normal extension ROM.

3. Avoid performing complex upper body strike and lower body kick combinations.

4. To protect the supporting leg, execute no more than 10 kicks consecutively. Avoiding high repetitions of any cardio kickboxing move is prudent.

5. Do not do physical contact exercises without proper skill progressions.

6. Be careful not to kick beyond the normal ROM on all lower body kicks. Control for any "snapping" movements during leg extension.

7. Kicking and pivoting may be contraindicated for many learners. Beginners should master the basic moves before progressing to advanced kickboxing movements.

8. Always take the time to slowly break down skills for the proper skill acquisition the students.

9. Make sure the music is not too fast, leading to movements being performed incorrectly and hastily. Safe music speeds are from 120 to 135 bpm. If students are having difficulty with the movements, it is advisable to slow down the music tempo.

10. Be aware that the novelty of martial arts movements may lead to more delayed-onset muscle soreness in those just starting classes.

11. Wear shoes that give ample support to the ankles.

12. To protect ligaments, turn out the toes slightly and flex the knee of the supporting leg when kicking.

13. Make sure each participant has plenty of floor space when using equipment.

14. Deliver punches from the body as opposed to from the shoulders.

15. To progress gradually, start with one cardio kickboxing workout per week and gradually build up. Cross train with other forms of exercise such as indoor cycling, walking, hiking, and step training.

WATER FITNESS

Water fitness classes are steadily growing in popularity with all fitness levels. The surrounding resistance of the water environment provides an effective environment to perform numerous exercise movements. Many recreational athletes use the aquatic environment to complete a greater volume of work with less stress to the body's bones and joints. Key benefits of water exercise have been summarized as the following[24]:

1. Water provides an adequate resistance overload for resistance training as well as for vigorous exercise intensities to improve cardiovascular function.

2. The minimal weight-bearing environment allows for graded exercise intensities without risk to the lower extremities.

3. The aquatic environment medium gives exercisers the ability to explore different types of physical movement that are altogether different than those imposed by gravity.

4. The external pressure of the water medium may be suitably adapted for individuals encumbered with poor blood circulation problems because the external pressure of the water against the body enhances venous return.
5. The external pressure of the water may provide a sufficient challenge for individuals suffering from weakened respiratory muscle function.
6. The aquatic medium provides a unique opportunity for modifying ROM patterns of many exercises and movements.
7. Functional balance and stabilization movement patterns may be improved and practiced in the water.
8. Clients who fear falling on land may find the aquatic environment much less intimidating.
9. The frequent changing movement patterns in the water may translate to improved posture on land because the trunk and abdominal muscles are regularly stimulated to maintain posture in the water.

Generally, the three water depths (in 81 to 84° water) used in water fitness classes are (a) shallow, which is navel to nipple; (b) transitional, which is nipple to neck; and (c) deep, where the feet are not touching the bottom. In deep water exercise, some type of buoyancy gear is required. The choice of water depth may be determined by what is accessible, the available aquatic equipment, the client's fitness level, and the amount of weight-bearing movement desired. For instructors wishing to mimic movements on land, yet with less impact, the shallow water environment is preferred. For some injured exercise enthusiasts, deep water exercise may be preferred because of its completely no-impact environment[25].

Exercises in the water can be graded by the ROM of performance, the speed of motion, and the lower-body load[25]. Lower body load at a shallow water level incorporates more jumping and leaping exercise movements. In deep water exercise, the lower body load can be intensified with the use of aquatic exercise equipment, such as with giant aquatic sandals, which add more resistance to the movement. Finally, for exercise variety, numerous types of aquatic equipment, including webbed gloves, fins, and nonbuoyant bells have been designed to provide multiple training stimulus options to aquatic exercise programs. Some general safety guidelines with water fitness include the following[25]:

1. Design workouts to keep participants warm and comfortable throughout the entire class.
2. If indoors, try to reduce any air currents, which may cause the participants to become chilled, in the room.
3. Format the class to alternate less active work involving smaller muscle groups with more vigorous larger muscle group exercises.
4. Plan to start on time so there is no waiting at the beginning of class.
5. Attempt to keep the students' entire bodies in motion during water fitness classes. Simultaneously combine upper and lower body exercises.

6. Education is important in water fitness classes. Provide the specific cues for the size, speed, and force of the movements being performed.
7. Inform students to move their legs more if they feel themselves getting cold.
8. Communicate with the class regularly. Find out how students feel and if they are warm or cold.
9. Sometimes if participants become too cool in deep water workouts, it is advisable to move them to shallower water where they can move with great force, creating more heat production.
10. Finish the class with full-body movements to help keep participants warm.

INDOOR CYCLING

Indoor or group cycling classes are unique group-led exercise format that have attracted many devoted supporters. Because most people have learned how to ride a bicycle at some time in their lives, indoor cycling classes present a group-led exercise format that many people feel quite comfortable to perform. Because of its non–weight-bearing nature, indoor cycling classes also offer some orthopedic advantages to special populations not able to perform traditional weight-bearing exercise. Also, for seasoned cyclists, indoor cycling offers a viable option to the hazards of wintertime weather cycling.

Indoor cycling classes have singularized themselves from other workouts with the motivational coaching and visual imagery verbalized by instructors[26]. The use of visualization with cycling positions may help some students improve their cycling techniques and body alignment. Whereas traditional group-led exercise formats focus on instructing participants to attain a certain body position, with some indoor cycling classes, the students are instructed to visualize the position and then perform it. Instructors lead exercise enthusiasts through a "virtual" outdoor road ride, complete with valleys, hills, straightaways, and finish lines[26]. Music selection in indoor cycling classes is much more geared toward enhancing the ambient mood of the "ride." No actual bpm guidelines have been established with indoor cycling classes; however, the faster and slower tempos surely can be used to increase or decrease the exercise intensity[27]. It is more apparent that the success of an indoor cycling class depends heavily on the exercise program design knowledge of the instructor as well as the instructor's ability to motivate the fitness enthusiasts[28]. As well, soft-lighting room designs with bikes placed close together creates an atmosphere similar to outdoor riding with a pack of cyclists. Naturally, because of the close nature of the exercisers, good air circulation is a must for indoor cycling classes.

Mainstreaming all fitness levels is easily accomplished with indoor cycling classes. Students can control their own workout intensity with cycling cadence (pedaling speed), cycle workload (wheel resistance), and body position (seated or standing position while cycling)[27]. Successful teaching of indoor cycling requires a fair amount of practice. Indoor cycling instructors are encouraged to attend cycling workshops and courses that provide them with the skills necessary to integrate the physiological goal of the workout segment (endurance, speed, strength) with the imagery (hill, plateau, downhill), music tempo (slow, moderate, fast), and body focus (breathing, body alignment, pedal stroke) into a robust workout for the enthusiasts[27]. The following are some specific safety guidelines to follow with indoor cycling classes[26–29]:

1. Make sure all participants are fitted correctly on their bikes. The upstroke knee should not exceed hip level, and the downstroke knee should be approximately 80% to 85% straight. As well, check the front-to-back seat setting to make sure the knees are over the pedals. Handle bar height should neither be too high nor too low, but students should hold the handlebars with "soft" elbows in a comfortable position on the back.

2. Always review the operation of the emergency brake and the appropriate adjustments of the pedal straps.

3. Have students wear correct cycling apparel. Cycling shorts with padded inserts help to lesson the discomfort of prolonged cycling. Hard-soled cycling shoes are preferred to minimize the pressure on the feet when pedaling and to keep them from slipping off the pedals. Many cycling shoes have a cleat that can snap into the pedal, improving cycling mechanics and power transfer from the body. Shoes that are too tight may cause pain, burning, or numbness in the ball of the foot and toes.

4. Educate students about the relationship in cadence and resistance. High cadence is associated with low resistance, and low cadence is related to high resistance. Both extremes may be stressful on the hips and knees. Encourage students to find a satisfying balance they can maintain and enjoy. Remind students that it is more important to stay in control of their cycling.

5. Regularly instruct students (visually and technically) about proper cycling technique and body alignment. Normally, as students fatigue, their cycling form starts to deteriorate.

6. Because of the multiple fitness levels in a class, always provide resistance or cadence options during the various class segments.

7. Encourage students to bring water bottles to stay hydrated and towels to class wipe off sweat.

8. Create an environment that students can pace themselves individually. Indoor cycling classes, although often marketed for "everyone," may be very challenging on the lower body and cardiorespiratory system.

9. To help students budget their energy throughout the class, give them specific facts about parts of the ride. For instance, share with students how many more seconds may be in a sprint or how many intervals they will be doing. This will help students gauge their exertion more efficiently.

10. The forward riding posture of cycling may become uncomfortable for some participants in the lower back. Strength and flexibility exercises for the lower back may be most helpful to participants. Also, regularly varying the riding position during the class helps to minimize any lower back discomfort.

11. To minimize wrist and upper body tension, educate students not to place too much weight on the handlebars while in a standing position.

12. It is important to keep indoor classes fresh and challenging, but avoid highly repetitive jumping drills (off the seat) because they can lead to knee injury in some participants.

13. Because indoor cycling classes may be quite intensive workouts, instructors should plan enough time to gradually recover the exercise participants appropriately.

YOGA

Although its exact origin in India has yet to be identified, yoga has existed for at least the past 5000 years. **Yoga** means **union**, and it refers to one of the symbolic systems of Hindu philosophy that strives to bring together and develop the body, mind, and spirit[30]. Hindu priests who lived thrifty lifestyles, characterized by discipline and meditation, originally developed yoga. Through observing and mimicking the movement and patterns of animals, the priests hoped to achieve the same balance with nature that animals seem to display. Hatha yoga is the form with which Westerners are most familiar and is defined by a series of exercises (referred to as **asanas**) in physical posture and breathing patterns[31]. Besides balance with nature, ancient Indian philosophers recognized yoga's health benefits, including proper organ functioning and whole well being.

There are several different forms of Hatha yoga that are popularly practiced. Iyengar yoga incorporates traditional Hatha techniques into fluid, dancelike sequences. It uses props such as chairs, pillows, blankets, and belts to accommodate persons with special needs[30,31]. Ashtanga yoga is a fast-paced, athletic style that is the foundation for the power-yoga classes[30,31]. These classes resemble more vigorous workouts as opposed to relaxation sessions. Bikram, or hot yoga, is done in a sauna-style room that is 100°F, so the muscles get very warm for extending and stretching[30]. Kripalu yoga centers on personal growth and self-improvement through the practice of meditation during poses[30,31]. Kundalini merges stretching, breathing, and meditation. Safety guidelines for teaching yoga classes include the following[30,31]:

1. Design classes to the abilities of the students.

2. Incorporate a range of standing, seated, prone, and supine poses in the class.

3. With deconditioned participants, use more stretching and relaxing poses.

4. Be aware of students with muscle or joint problems, and modify poses for these students.

5. Be prudent with the use of advanced poses, such as the headstand, handstand, shoulder stand, and plough.

6. The Kundalini yoga style involves lots of breathing exercises, which may be contraindicated for pregnant women and those with hypertension or glaucoma.

7. Monitor students carefully, but be sensitive and cautious about using any hands-on corrections to some students in an attempt to take them further into a posture.

8. Always teach students how to achieve and maintain the proper postures and alignments for poses.

STABILITY BALL WORKOUTS

Originating in Europe, stability ball training is spreading throughout North America. Although originally used in rehabilitation, stability ball training is now used in group-led exercise classes and by home fitness buffs. These round, beachball-looking exercise devices provide an unstable base for exercises to be performed. The unstable nature of the ball allows more muscles to be challenged when performing exercises on or with the stability ball. Thus, the body's neuromuscular balance-regulating mechanisms have to work harder when performing stability ball exercises, as opposed to the same movements on a solid base of support, such as a bench. Ball size is quite variable; however, a good rule of thumb when selecting a ball is that when the individual is seated on the ball, her or his hips should be level with the knees. The firmness of the ball is another element to consider. Softer balls have larger base or surface areas, making it easier for clients to maintain their balance. Firmer balls provide more balance challenges. With specialized training, a person can learn numerous exercises with stability balls. Because 80% of Americans suffer from some degree of low-back pain, most exercises designed with stability balls have been chosen to strengthen the trunk or "core" musculature. The concept of core training suggests that for the peripheral muscles of the body to act most effectively, the body must be solidly supported at its midpoint[32]. Therefore, a strong core may also help prevent ailments associated with low-back pain. Here are some safety tips for using stability balls.[32,33]:

1. Stability ball training may be intimidating to some persons. Allow them time to become familiar with this new exercise device.

2. The use of stability balls is not recommended for individuals with advanced osteoporosis or vertigo (sensation of spinning) caused by vestibular dysfunction.

3. Initially, have clients just sit on the ball and become aware of their center of gravity on this unstable base of support.

4. Progress with exercises when students can demonstrate the ability to easily maintain a steady position while sitting on the stability ball.

5. For some individuals, it may be safer to place the ball close to the wall, with the student's back facing the

wall. Therefore, if a student loses his or her balance on the ball, it may protect the him or her from a fall.

6. For some learners, placing a chair on either side of the ball provides additional stability.

7. Be aware that stability ball exercises performed on a wood floor provide less surface friction and thus may be more difficult for older and less fit individuals to maintain a stable ball.

8. Individuals with high BP should modify exercises (particularly in the supine position) in which the head drops below the heart. This may lead to lightheadedness and dizziness attributable to lack of blood flow back to the heart and brain.

9. Identify students with ROM limitations and plan modifications for some of their ball exercises.

10. Some instructors have attempted to incorporate bouncing on the ball to train the cardiovascular system. However, with this type of movement, there is potential risk for compromised balance and uneven compression on the vertebral disks; thus, this type of movement cannot be endorsed.

PILATES

The historical roots of Pilates are from World War I, when German expatriate Joseph Pilates (1880–1967), a gymnast turned nurse, created a series of strength and flexibility exercises and equipment for prisoners of war[34]. Pilates eventually opened a training studio in New York, helping professional dancers attain improved strength and endurance. He created more than 500 exercises that emphasize proper breathing and torso strength[34]. Pilates is one of the fastest growing fitness trends in the United States. It uses many different types of equipment such as the Reformer, Trapeze Table (or Cadillac), Combo Chair, as well as exercises on the mat. Pilates programs emphasize the uniform development of all muscle groups while promoting skeletal alignment, circulation, and flexibility[35]. However, the common theme in Pilates programs is the initiation of movement from the core of the body, referring to the deep abdominal and lower back muscles.

Pilates exercises involve rhythmic movements that simultaneously engage many different groups of muscles. It is an integrated mind/body training program involving appropriate breathing techniques and mental concentration. The six basic principles of Pilates training include stabilization (movement is initiated from a stable source), control (all movements are controlled actions), flow (movements flow as opposed to being jerky), concentration (heightened awareness of the body), breathing (optimal uptake of oxygen with improved circulation) and full ROM (for the reduction of possible chronic injuries)[35]. It is proposed (because no scientific studies have been published) that incorporating the six principles of Pilates training results in individuals' optimally developing a healthy spine and torso, which enhances their everyday life activities as well as their exercise and sport pursuits[34,35]. Currently, numerous Pilates programs are available for instructor training and client exercise programs. As may be recommended with any exercise program, before embarking into a Pilates class or program, seek out your options and evaluate the credentials of those presenting the program. Pilates certification courses vary greatly from 15 to 800 hours and depend on the level of certification, the type of program, and the educational background of the instructor[34].

Summary

Group-led exercise is challenging because of the varied nature of the activities and the wide range of clientele fitness and ability. Effective instructors understand that modifications, variations, and individualized intensity monitoring are essential to ensure safe and enjoyable participation by all. Most group-led classes involve some form of cardiovascular conditioning, along with core strengthening exercises, flexibility activities, and proper warm-up and cooldown activities. For specialized group-led classes, it is suggested that instructors obtain additional training specific to the instructional method.

REFERENCES

1. Thacker SB, Gilchrist J, Stroup DF, Kimsey CD: The impact of stretching on sports injury risk: A systematic review of the literature. Med Sci Sports Exerc 36:371–378, 2004.
2. Bracko MR: Can stretching prior to exercise and sports improve performance and prevent injury? ACSM's Health Fit J 6:17–21, 2002.
3. Riker HA, Zabik RM, Dawson ML, Frye PA: The effect of step height and upper body involvement on oxygen consumption and energy expenditure during step aerobics. Med Sci Sports Exerc 30: S945, 1998.
4. Scharff-Olson M Williford HN, Blessing DL, Brown JA: The physiological effects of bench/step exercise. Sports Med 21:164–175, 1996.
5. Wang N, Scharff-Olson M, Williford HN: Energy cost and fuel utilization during step aerobics exercise. Med Sci in Sports Exerc 25:S630, 1993.
6. Woodby-Brown S, Berg K, Latin RW: Oxygen cost of aerobic dance bench stepping at three heights. J Strength Cond Res 7:163–167, 1993.
7. Francis PR, Poliner J, Buono MJ, Francis LL: Effects of choreography, step height, fatigue and gender on metabolic cost of step training. Med Sci Sports Exerc 27:S69, 1992.
8. Greenlaw K, McMillan L, Catalano S, et al: The energy cost of traditional versus power bench step exercise at heights of 4, 6, and 8 inches. Med Sci Sports Exerc 27:S1343, 1995.
9. Kravitz L, Heyward VH, Stolarczyk L,Wilmerding V: Does step exercise with handweights enhance training effects? J Strength Cond Res 11:194–199, 1997.
10. Yoke M, Otto R, Wygand R, Kamimukai C: The metabolic cost of two differing low impact aerobic dance exercise modes. Med Sci Sports Exerc 20:S527, 1988.
11. Otto R, Yoke M, Wygand J, Larsen P: The metabolic cost of multidirectional low impact and high impact aerobic dance. Med Sci Sports Exerc 30:S525, 1988.
12. Calarco L, Otto R, Wygand J, Kramer J, et al: The metabolic cost of six common movement patterns of bench-step aerobic dance. Med Sci Sports Exerc 23:S839, 1991.
13. Scharff-Olson M, Williford HN: The energy cost associated with selected step training exercise techniques. Res Quar Exerc Sport 67:465–468, 1996.
14. Stanforth D, Velasquez K, Stanforth P: The effect of bench height and rate of stepping on the metabolic cost of bench stepping [abstract]. Med Sci Sports Exerc 23:S143, 1991.
15. Kravitz L: The fitness professional's complete guide to circuits and intervals. IDEA Today 14:32–43, 1996.
16. Yoke M, Kennedy C: Functional Exercise Progressions. Monterey, CA: Healthy Learning; 2004.
17. Williford HN, Scharff-Olson M, Blessing DL: The physiological effects of aerobic dance: A review. Sports Med 8:335–345, 1989.
18. Scharff-Olson M, Williford HN, Blessing DL, Greathouse R: The cardiovascular and metabolic effects of bench stepping exercise in females. Med Sci Sports Exerc 23:1311–1318, 1991.
19. Smith J: Injury prevention in step classes. IDEA Health & Fit Source 18:36–45, 2000.
20. Scharff-Olson M, Williford HN, Blessing DL, et al: Vertical impact forces during bench-step aerobics: Exercise rate and experience. Percep Motor Skills 84:267–274, 1997.
21. Kravitz L: Anybody's Guide to Total Fitness, 7th ed. Dubuque, IA: Kendall/Hunt Publishing Company; 2003.
22. Williams A: Injury prevention in kickboxing classes. IDEA Health & Fit Source 18:58–67, 2000.
23. Olson MS, Williford HH: Martial arts exercise: A T.K.O. in studio fitness. ACSM's Health Fit J 3:6–13, 1999.
24. Sanders ME: Cross over to the water. IDEA Health and Fitness Source 17:53–55, 58, 1999.
25. Sanders ME, Curry M: Fundamental skills and exercise design (pp. 102–118). In Sanders ME, ed. YMCA Water Fitness for Health. Champaign, IL: Human Kinetics; 2000.
26. Bryant CX, Wenson J, Peterson JA: Safe and enjoyable group cycling for your members. Fit Man 17:38–42, 2001.
27. Sherman RM: The indoor cycling revolution. IDEA Today 15:30–33, 35–36, 38–39, 1997.
28. Kolovou T: Launching an indoor cycling program. Fit Man 16:40–42, 2000.
29. Vogel AE: Injury prevention in indoor cycling classes. IDEA Health & Fit Source 18:48–57, 2000.
30. Hollingshead S: Yoga for sports performance. IDEA Health and Fit Source 20:30–39, 2002.
31. Carrico M: Contraindications of yoga. IDEA Health and Fit Source 16:34–43, 1998.
32. Schlicht J: Stability balls: An injury risk for older adults. ACSM's Health Fit J 6:14–17, 2002.
33. Eckmann TF: Older adults get on the ball. IDEA Health and Fit Source 16:81–85, 1998.
34. Stott M: How to start a Pilates-based program. Fitness Man 16: 44–48, 2000.
35. Sichel HS: Why Pilates principles work. Personal Fitness Professional 5:17–18, 2003.

SELECTED REFERENCES FOR FURTHER READING

Howley ET, Franks BD: Health Fitness Instructors Handbook. Champaign, IL: Human Kinetics, 2003.
Kennedy CA, Yoke MM: Methods of Group Exercise Instruction. Champaign, IL: Human Kinetics, 2005.

INTERNET RESOURCES

ACSM's Health & Fitness Journal: http://www.acsm-healthfitness.org

Aerobics and Fitness Association of America: http://www.afaa.com

American Council on Exercise: http://www.acefitness.org

IDEA Health and Fitness Association: http://www.ideafit.com

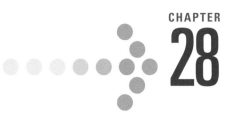

Medical Considerations

JOHN E. KOVALESKI, LARRY R. GURCHIEK, AND ALBERT W. PEARSALL IV

This chapter addresses KSAs from the following content areas:

1   Exercise Physiology and Related Exercise Science
2   Pathophysiology and Risk Factors
3   Health Appraisal, Fitness, and Clinical Exercise Testing
4   Electrocardiography and Diagnostic Techniques
5   Patient Management and Medications
6   Medical and Surgical Management
7   Exercise Prescription and Programming
8   Nutrition and Weight Management
9   Human Behavior and Counseling
10 Safety, Injury Prevention, and Emergency Procedures
11 Program Administration, Quality Assurance, and Outcome Assessment

One of the most important goals of every physical fitness program is to create a safe environment for participation. Regardless of the effort, the nature of exercise participation dictates that accidents can and do occur. An *emergency* is defined as an unexpected event or serious change in one's health status that may lead to injury or illness. Musculoskeletal injuries are common in the physically active population. Cardiovascular, pulmonary, and metabolic abnormalities sometimes arise during exercise testing and participation that result in illness and death. Such challenges and threats to personal health and safety must be met with increased levels of education and training. When such situations arise, prompt care is essential and must be based on effective initial management to ensure the participant's well being. This chapter reviews the medical considerations of exercise and testing related to safety procedures and ongoing safety training. Pertinent information is presented concerning causes, recognition, care, and prevention of injuries and illnesses unique to exercise participation. In addition, environmental influences during exercise and their associated health risks are discussed.

Emergency Plan of Action

Appropriate care and management of emergency situations begin with the development of an emergency plan (see GETP7 Appendix B). A risk management or safety committee is formed to oversee the development of policies and procedures with subsequent audits to assist in the maintenance of all emergency and safety procedures[1]. The plan should address both medical and non-medical (e.g., fire, chemical, weather) emergencies that are likely to occur.

An **emergency action plan** for medical emergencies is defined as a system of policies, procedures, and processes that results in activation of the emergency health care services of the facility and community[2]. Essential elements, strategies, and questions that should be asked in the development of the emergency plan of action are presented in Box 28-1. Staff roles include being assigned very specific and detailed responsibilities, and some staff members are assigned duties at the scene of the incident. Individuals are most effective in responding to emergencies when they are assigned duties as initial responder, team leader, communications staffer, or medical liaison[1]. All individuals must also be familiar with the duties of the other staff members and understand the emergency plan of action protocols for different locations (e.g., testing area, gym, pool, weight room) within the facility. Consideration should be given to both minor (e.g., abrasions, contusions, and strains) and major (life and limb threatening) incidents and events involving bloodborne pathogens[3]. In the event of an emergency, the guidelines presented in Box 28-2 should be followed[1].

Health and fitness facility personnel involved in management or delivery of exercise programs must meet academic and professional standards and have the required experience as established by the American College of Sports Medicine (ACSM)[4]. Specific components of the emergency plan vary because of differences in type of facility, risk stratification of the participant, staff qualifications, and type of emergency equipment available (Box 28-3). Staff members who directly supervise program participants should be trained in basic life support[4]. Training of personnel, periodic practice of the emergency plan, documentation, and the availability of a first aid kit and other equipment (e.g., automated

KEY TERMS

Air quality index: An index for reporting daily air quality that indicates how clean or polluted the air is and what associated health effects might be a concern

Emergency action plan: The actions employees should take to ensure their safety and the safety of their clients if an emergency situation occurs

Overtraining syndrome: A collection of emotional, behavioral, and physical symptoms caused by excess training and inadequate rest

Universal bloodborne pathogen precautions: Policies and procedures implemented to prevent transmission of bloodborne pathogens between patients and workers

---

BOX 28-1 | **Strategies for Developing an Emergency Care Plan[1,2]**

- Is an outline of the entire emergency care plan displayed and accessible at a central staff location?
- Are different emergency procedures developed and posted for various areas within the facility (testing areas, pool, weight room, gymnasium)?
- What care will be provided?
- Who will render care?
- Are all staff and supervisors certified in first aid, CPR, AED, or ACLS?
- Is all staff familiar with OSHA's bloodborne pathogen guidelines and procedures?
- Are the responsibilities of individual staff members identified (e.g., team leader, captain, medical liaison)?
- Who will activate EMS? Are telephone numbers for emergency procedures clearly posted?
- Are all staff members familiar with the information to be provided to EMS over the telephone?
  Type of emergency (injury, illness)
  Current status of involved or injured individuals
  Type of assistance being given
  Exact location of the facility and the afflicted individual within the facility
  Specific point of entry into the facility
  Telephone number being used
- Who will supervise the other activity areas if supervisors must leave to assist at an accident scene?
- Who will help with crowd control?
- Who has access to keys for locked areas or doors?
- Who will direct ambulance or EMS to the emergency scene?
- Have the facility administrators invited representatives from EMS to become familiar with the floor plan and activities of the facility?
- Are emergency response training sessions conducted regularly (at least once every 3 months)?
- Does emergency training consist of both announced and unannounced mock drills?
- Are emergency drills and training documented and evaluated with recommendations for necessary changes?
- Is EMS involved in the training and conduction of drills?
- Do all staff members know the location and have easy access to first aid kits, AED, splints, stretchers, fire extinguishers, and other emergency equipment?
- Is emergency equipment and supplies clearly labeled, routinely checked, and maintenanced?
- Is the facility conducting cardiovascular screening of all new members and prospective users?
- Are persons at high risk directed to seek facilities providing appropriate levels of care and staff supervision?
- Are appropriate documents (health appraisal, physician permission to participate, assumption of risk or waiver, informed consent, and emergency information) completed?
- Have staff members been appropriately informed of orthopedic or other health problems that might affect participation?
- Are emergency notification cards on file for each participant that includes telephone numbers of family members, physician names, telephone numbers with special instructions, and alternative telephone numbers if primary contacts are unavailable?
- Are properly documented injury and accident reports completed and stored in an appropriate secure location for review and follow-up by administration?

CPR = cardiopulmonary resuscitation;

ACLS = advanced cardiac life support; AED = automated external defibrillator; EMS = emergency medical services; OSHA = Occupational Safety and Health Administration.

| BOX 28-2 | Emergency Response Guidelines |

MINOR INCIDENTS

- The initial responder or supervisor assesses and manages injuries and conditions within the facility, if appropriate.
- Supervising staff members should assess the condition of the individual after evaluation and triage within the facility or refer to community medical resource.
- The supervisor arranges for transportation of injured, if necessary.
- Other staff members are responsible for crowd control or site management.

Incident or injury reports are completed and filed.

MAJOR INCIDENTS

- The initial responder is usually defined as the staff member who arrives first or witnesses the accident or event. This individual should render immediate first aid consistent with the protocols for CPR, first aid, or AED of the American Heart Association or the American Red Cross. These protocols include checking the scene for safety, initiating the emergency response system within the facility, and providing immediate care to the injured or ill.
- The team leader directs and controls general care after arriving on the scene.
- The communication staffer contacts the community or facility EMS through 911 or local emergency telephone systems for EMS response or transportation to an emergency room. It is essential to provide the following information to the emergency service: description of the injured or ill, exact location of the facility, location of the individual within the facility, and specific point of entry into the facility. This information should be posted in written form and readily available to cue the communication staffer for each building or area within the facility. Information about the estimated time of arrival of the emergency service is obtained and communicated to the team leader. Medical or emergency records of the injured or ill individual are gathered, and the communication staffer moves to the point of entry to meet the EMS and direct them to the location of the emergency scene.
- The crowd control staffer maintains order and clears the area of individuals to facilitate access and evaluation.
- The incident report is completed and filed by the team leader. Appropriate actions and follow-up documentation are performed.

AED = automated external defibrillator; CPR = cardiopulmonary resuscitation; EMS = emergency medical services.

| BOX 28-3 | Emergency Supplies and Equipment |

- First aid kits should be located within the facility to ensure availability in areas where they are most likely to be needed such as testing and exercise areas, youth and sport activity areas, and central areas such as a control desk.
- Inventory of the first aid kit's contents and documentation of inventory should be completed at least once a month.
- Common items contained within the kit include a first aid manual, disposable latex or vinyl gloves, bandages and dressings of various types and sizes for wound care and musculoskeletal injuries, splints, first aid cream or ointment, hydrogen peroxide, cold packs, ice bags, adhesive tape, eye wash, tongue blades and cotton swabs, CPR mask or barrier, scissors, penlight, safety pins, and bleach solution for blood and body fluids clean up.
- Other first aid and CPR equipment includes the AED, BP cuff, stethoscope, oxygen, and emergency cart.

AED = automated external defibrillator; BP = blood pressure; CPR = cardiopulmonary resuscitation.

external defibrillator [AED], backboard) must also be considered (Table 28-1 and GETP7 Table B-1)[1,5].

Universal bloodborne pathogen precautions were developed by the Centers for Disease Control and Prevention as an aggressive set of guidelines to protect employees from bloodborne pathogens such as HIV and hepatitis B virus. Recommendations include the use of gloves, masks, gowns, and other barriers whenever an individual is likely or potentially likely to come in contact with blood and other body fluids. The Occupational Safety and Health Administration (OSHA) issued a regulation in 1991 requiring the adoption of universal precautions for occupational exposure to bloodborne pathogens[6]. The standard also mandates annual training for all employees who potentially could be exposed to bloodborne pathogens.

Staff members should always use latex gloves and appropriate barriers when treating skin wounds and when handling items such as mouthpieces, resuscitation bags, and equipment that may have been exposed to bloodborne pathogens. Biohazard kits should be available to all employees who may be potentially exposed to blood, cerebrospinal fluid, pleural fluid, saliva, or any body fluid with visible blood. These kits should contain disposable paper towels, a

TABLE 28-1. Emergency Plans and Equipment for Health Fitness Facilities

	Level 1	Level 2	Level 3	Level 4	Level 5
Type of Facility	Unsupervised exercise room (e.g., hotel, commercial building)	Single exercise leader	Fitness center for general membership	Fitness center offering special programs for clinical populations	Medically supervised clinical exercise program (e.g., cardiac rehabilitation)
Personnel[a]	None	Exercise leader; recommended: medical liaison	General manager; H/F instructor; exercise leader; recommended: medical liaison	General manager; exercise specialist; H/F instructor; medical liaison	General manager; exercise specialist; H/F instructor; exercise leader; medical liaison
Emergency Plan	Present	Present	Present	Present	Present
Emergency Equipment	Telephone in room Signs; encouraged: PAD plan with AED as part of the composite PAD plan in the host facility (hotel, commercial building)	Telephone; signs Encouraged: BP kit, stethoscope, PAD plan with AED	Telephone; signs Encouraged: BP kit, stethoscope, PAD plan with AED (the latter are strongly encouraged in facilities with membership > 2500 and those in which EMS response time is expected to be > 5 min from recognition of arrest)	Telephone; signs BP kit stethoscope; strongly encouraged: PAD plan with AED	Telephone; signs BP kit, stethoscope, oxygen, crash cart defibrillator[b]

AED = automated external defibrillator; EMS = emergency medical services; H/F = health and fitness; PAD = public access to defibrillation.

Reprinted with permission from American College of Sports Medicine/American Heart Association Joint Position Statement[5].

[a]Detailed definitions and competencies for personnel positions are outlined in GETP7 Table B-2, B-3, and B-4.

[b]Standard equipment in level 5 facilities includes a defibrillator[4,42].

spray bottle with 10% bleach solution, hydrogen peroxide, assorted sizes of gloves, disposable gauze and towels, red biohazard bags, gowns, masks, and face shields[3].

Legal Implications of Safety

Exercise professionals should have a good understanding of the legal implications pertaining to safety procedures to protect themselves and the institutions that employ them from the risk of lawsuit (see Chapter 50 for an extensive discussion on the legal implications of exercise and testing). Effective policies and procedures, documented safety procedures, use of incident documents, and ongoing safety training help avoid legal liability while improving the quality of services[1,2,4]. Exercise professionals can significantly decrease the risk of *legal wrongs* (torts) involving safety by following several key points, as outlined in Box 28-4.

Health Considerations

MUSCULOSKELETAL CONDITIONS

The risk factors and mechanisms of injury along with recommendations concerning prevention and treatment are

---

BOX 28-4   Prudent Operational Policies for Exercise Professionals

- Maintain qualified supervision of the facility.
- Ensure that proper and safe equipment and facilities are maintained and used at all times.
- Not use or permit the presence of faulty or hazardous equipment.
- Develop and carefully follow an emergency plan.
- Keep all emergency first aid equipment in working order and available to those who will need to use it.
- Keep factually accurate and timely records that document all injuries and set up a record retention policy that allows records to be kept and used in defense of litigation that may be brought against the staff or facility.
- Document hazards and efforts to create a safe exercise environment.
- Ensure that all staff members know and understand the limitations of their expertise as well as the applicable state regulations and restrictions that limit exercise professionals' scope of practice.
- Ensure that all staff members accept and appreciate the responsibility to act within the scope of their practice and training in the event of an emergency.

important concepts for exercise professionals to understand. Most types of physical activities are beneficial because moderate exercise is an important element for general well being[7]. The risk of musculoskeletal injury increases for all levels of participation with increasing physical activity, intensity, and duration of training[8]. Understanding the associated risks, preventive measures, and procedures of immediate care can reduce the incidence and severity of exercise-related musculoskeletal injuries.

Attempts to maintain or improve physical fitness require awareness of injury prevention. Expanded exercise participation by a larger and older population potentiates the incidence of injury as the number of participants and volume of training increases. Exercise professionals are encouraged to perform *health and fitness screenings* before participants begin exercise programs (see Chapter 6). These screenings should be used to detect not only cardiopulmonary and metabolic abnormalities but also musculoskeletal problems that are a contraindication to exercise.

The AHA (American Heart Association)/ACSM Health/ Fitness Screening Questionnaire serves as a useful assessment form (Box 28-5; see GETP7 Table 2.1)[4]. The screening process must document any history of musculoskeletal injury before implementation of the exercise program. A cursory musculoskeletal examination should be performed to identify the ranges of motion of major joints involving both the upper and lower extremities and the cervical and lumbar spines. In addition, muscle strength, motor control, and balance should be assessed using functional activities for the purpose of determining the individual's ability to participate or perform specific activity[9].

Injury Risk Factors

Musculoskeletal injuries are among the most common adverse effects of regular exercise and physical activity for individuals of all ages[10,11]. Musculoskeletal injuries can be attributed to the complex interaction of intrinsic and extrinsic risk factors (Box 28-6) that predispose physically active individuals to specific types of injuries[12–14]. Poor baseline physical fitness, excessive training, improper biomechanics, and improper training techniques also affect the incidence of injury. Helping exercise participants identify modifiable short- and long-term injury risks could assist in developing strategies to decrease injuries.

Requa et al.[15] reported the annual injury rate for recreational adult fitness participants at 2.3 injuries per participant per year. A majority of these injuries (76%) resulted in time lost from physical activity. The risk of musculoskeletal injury associated with various physical activities and cardiorespiratory fitness levels among recreationally active adults has also been reported[16]. The findings indicate that the moderate types and duration of physical activity promoted by the ACSM and national health organizations have lower injury risk than more vigorous

types and longer durations of physical activity[7,17]. The risk of physical activity–related injury among adults increased for runners, sports participants, persons engaging in more than 1.25 hours per week of physical activity, and individuals with moderate to high cardiorespiratory fitness levels. However, walking for exercise was not associated with a significant increased risk of activity-related injuries, even among walkers with the highest duration of activity per week. This low risk of musculoskeletal injury suggests that participation in walking can be safely recommended as a way to improve health and fitness[16,18].

Comparisons of injury rates of athletes and exercise participants provide a perspective for understanding the magnitude of the problem of fitness-related injuries. The annual overall incidence of injury among distance runners is reported to range from 24% to 65% for heterogeneous populations of recreational and competitive runners[19]. The causation of musculoskeletal running injuries is related to the runner, the running activity itself, and the environment[20]. Training errors are reported in 60% to 80% of injuries to runners and are commonly caused by exceeding limits of duration and intensity, high rates of progression, and excessive hill running[21].

High-impact aerobics and dance are also associated with a greater incidence of injury[22]. The incidence of injury in aerobic dance is reported to be approximately 45% of students and 75% of instructors[23]. Eighty percent of these injuries affect the lower legs and are related to frequency of exercise (> three times per week); improper footwear; or exercise on hard, nonresilient surfaces[24]. Low-impact aerobics participation is more common today and is used as an alternative to high-impact aerobics primarily performed in earlier years (see Chapter 27). The injury rate is not known for this type of aerobic dance because no comprehensive study has yet to be published.

The risk of acute injury from weight training and weight equipment is estimated to be from 2.4% to 7.6% of participants per year. A recent study showed a 35% increase in the number of emergency department injuries related to weight training activities[25]. Injuries reported included soft tissue injury, lacerations, concussions, and fractures and dislocations. Most weight training injuries occur from excessive training, improper techniques, and the misuse of weight training equipment[26].

Overtraining is caused by excessive overload precipitated by poorly structured exercise programs. The consequences of overtraining involve complex interactions among biological and psychological factors that may lead to illness, musculoskeletal injury, or dramatic performance decreases in individuals of all training levels[27–29]. The proper design of exercise training programs is essential to avoid overtraining. Proper periodization of training (planned variation), nutrition (glycogen replenishment and rehydration), and sufficient recovery time (recuperation from training) contribute significantly to preventing the overtraining syndrome[29].

BOX 28-5	AHA/ACSM Health/Fitness Facility Preparticipation Screening Questionnaire

Assess your health needs by marking all true statements.

History

You have had:

___ A heart attack

___ Heart surgery

___ Cardiac catheterization

___ Coronary angioplasty (PTCA)

___ Pacemaker, implantable cardiac defibrillator, or rhythm disturbance

___ Heart valve disease

___ Heart failure

___ Heart transplantation

___ Congenital heart disease

If you marked any of the statements in this section, consult your health care provider before engaging in exercise. You may need to use a facility with a **medically qualified staff member** to guide your exercise program.

Symptoms

___ You experience chest discomfort with exertion.

___ You experience unreasonable breathlessness.

___ You experience dizziness, fainting, blackouts.

___ You take heart medications.

Other health issues:

___ You have musculoskeletal problems.

___ You have concerns about the safety of exercise.

___ You take prescription medication(s).

___ You are pregnant.

Cardiovascular risk factors

___ You are a man ≥ 45 years.

___ You are a woman ≥ 55 years, you have had a hysterectomy, or you are postmenopausal.

___ You smoke.

___ Your BP is ≥140/90 mm Hg.

___ You don't know your BP.

___ You take BP medication.

___ Your blood cholesterol level is ≥ 200 mg·dL^{-1}.

___ You don't know your cholesterol level.

___ You have a close blood relative who had a heart attack before age 55 (father or brother) or age 65 (mother or sister).

___ You are diabetic or take medicine to control your blood sugar.

___ You are physically inactive (i.e., you get less than 30 minutes of physical activity on at least 3 days per week).

___ You are more than 20 pounds overweight.

If you marked two or more of the statements in this section, you should consult your healthcare provider before engaging in exercise. You might benefit by using a facility with a **professionally qualified exercise staff member** to guide your exercise program.

___ None of the above is true.

You should be able to exercise safely without consulting your health care provider in almost any facility that meets your exercise program needs.

ACSM = American College of Sports Medicine; AHA = American Heart Association; PTCA = percutaneous transluminal coronary angioplasty.

Reprinted with permission from Balady et al.[4].

BOX 28-6 | Injury Risk Factors

INTRINSIC RISK FACTORS
History of previous injury
Inadequate fitness or conditioning
Body composition
Bony alignment abnormalities
Strength or flexibility imbalances
Joint or ligamentous laxity
Predisposing musculoskeletal disease

EXTRINSIC RISK FACTORS
Excessive load on the body
Type of movement
Speed of movement
Number of repetitions
Footwear
Surface
Training errors
Excessive distances
Fast progression
High intensity
Running on hills
Poor technique
Fatigue
Adverse environmental conditions
Air quality
Darkness
Heat or cold
High humidity
Altitude
Wind
Worn or faulty equipment

Modified with permission from Renstrom and Kannus[13].

Overtraining can occur on a short-term basis, which is defined as overreaching (poor performance in training and competition)[29,30]. **Overtraining syndrome** is untreated overreaching that results in long-term decreased performance, impaired ability to train, chronic fatigue, or other problems that may require medical attention[29,30]. Two clinical types of overtraining syndrome have been described: sympathetic overtraining syndrome (includes elevated sympathetic activity at rest, e.g., increased heart rate [HR] and blood pressure [BP], elevated basal metabolic rate) and parasympathetic overtraining syndrome (includes increased parasympathetic activity at rest, e.g., decreased resting HR and BP, and with exercise an early onset of fatigue or rapid HR recovery after exercise)[28]. The symptoms of overtraining are highly individualized with the presence of one or more of the symptoms of

overtraining syndrome sufficient to identify the individual as over-trained. A review of common anaerobic and aerobic overtraining indicators is presented in Box 28-7.

Disorders of the musculoskeletal system may directly increase the risk of acute or chronic injury by interrupting normal structure and function of bone, joint, and soft tissue. The most common musculoskeletal risk factors include osteoarthritis, osteoporosis, chondromalacia, age-related musculotendinous degeneration, and malalignments of the lower extremities[31]. Excessive body weight has been found to predispose individuals to acute and overuse injuries, including osteoarthritic changes of the hip and knee with weight-bearing recreational activities[32,33]. Weight loss reduces the risk of developing knee osteoarthritis, but its effect on the progression of the disease is unknown[34]. In addition, vigorous physical activity may predispose partic-

BOX 28-7 | Common Signs and Symptoms of the Overtraining Syndrome[27–29]

FUNCTIONAL INDICATORS
- Decline in physical performance and early onset of fatigue
- Decreased desire to train or decreased enjoyment from training or competition
- Loss of muscle strength, coordination, and maximal working capacity
- Increased submaximal HR
- Prolonged recovery from typical training sessions or competitive events
- Presence of tenderness and soreness in muscles and joints
- Overuse injuries

METABOLIC AND PSYCHOLOGIC INDICATORS
- Loss of appetite and body weight loss
- GI disturbances; occasional nausea
- Increased susceptibility to upper respiratory infections (altered immune function)
- Emotional instability characterized by general fatigue, apathy, depression, and irritability
- Sleep disturbances

PHYSIOLOGIC INDICATORS
- Decreased maximal oxygen uptake
- Increased creatine kinase
- Altered cortisol concentration
- Decreased total testosterone concentration
- Decreased ratio of total testosterone to cortisol
- Decreased ratio of total testosterone to sex hormone–binding globulin
- Decreased sympathetic tone (decreased nocturnal and resting catecholamines)
- Increased sympathetic stress response
- Altered resting HR and BP

BP = blood pressure; GI = gastrointestinal; HR = heart rate.

ipants to osteoarthritis by means of mechanical trauma to the joint[32]. For example, an increased risk of osteoarthritis has been shown for competitive sports and running but not recreational running[35].

Obesity, a poor sitting posture that duplicates the fully flexed standing posture, frequent back flexion, loss of back extension, and low physical activity are among proposed causative factors of low back pain[36,37]. Episodes of low back pain are usually related to acute trauma or overuse. However, the individual's age, type of activity, and activity level are also variables. The incidence and recurrence of low back pain are also associated with muscle fatigue and movements such as a poor lifting technique (see Figure 2-11) and failure to correctly position oneself before attempting lifts[36].

Concerns for Exercise Testing and Programming

Musculoskeletal injuries are a health burden because they may lead to permanent reductions in activity, thereby impeding efforts to promote exercise participation. To reduce the incidence and severity of injury, it is important to identify predisposing risk factors through education and clinical intervention. Behavior modifications with regard to early detection of symptoms of overuse are important for preventing injury. Participants should be encouraged to report injuries and symptoms because untreated musculoskeletal injuries are likely to worsen the problem or predispose to future exercise-related injury[38]. Strenuous exercise is contraindicated in the presence of acute joint injury, chronic joint inflammation (osteoarthritis), or uncontrolled systemic joint disease (rheumatoid arthritis). Under medical management, submaximal and symptom-limited fitness testing along with exercise program participation should be possible. The progression and level of physical activity must be pain free, individualized, and otherwise limited by precautions and contraindications associated with specific medical conditions (see Chapter 24). The goal of exercise programs for individuals after musculoskeletal injury or those with orthopedic disease and disability should be to prevent debilitation caused by inactivity and to improve endurance, exercise tolerance, strength, and flexibility[39].

Treatment Considerations

Most activity-related injuries result from either *macrotrauma* (tension, shear, or compression) or *microtrauma* (overuse or repetitive motion). Damage to tissue caused by trauma is defined as the primary injury. With the exception of controlling hemorrhage, initial treatment has little effect on the extent or severity of primary injury. Improper care or delay in treatment may cause additional pain, swelling, and tissue damage of healthy tissues. Secondary hypoxic injury (the death of healthy cells caused by lack of oxygen) is caused by the body's natural response to hemorrhage with a decrease in blood flow to the injured body segment. Secondary hypoxic injury may continue even after bleeding is

controlled, which necessitates that the initial treatment protocol consists of rest, ice, compression, elevation, and stabilization during the 24 to 72 hours after injury.

Exercise professionals are often asked for advice regarding the management of musculoskeletal problems or injuries. This may entail making recommendations about training and modifications in exercise programs, rendering immediate first aid, or referring participants to physicians. To help in decision making, knowledge of common exercise injuries (Table 28-2) and their causative mechanisms (Table 28-3) is important. When injury occurs, the initial evaluation process for musculoskeletal injury should follow a logical sequence (Box 28-8). Evaluation using the HOPS (history, observation, palpation, special tests) procedure is especially important for understanding the cause and severity of the injury[9].

Basic first aid procedures for common exercise-related musculoskeletal injuries are outlined in Table 28-4. The combination of rest, ice, compression, elevation, and stabilization (RICES) is the appropriate treatment for immediate care of patients with acute injuries[40]. When used properly, the RICES treatment regimen reduces the total amount of tissue damage, decreases swelling and pain, and aids in controlling the inflammatory response, which results in quicker rehabilitation and recovery. Rest allows time to control the effects of trauma and to avoid additional tissue damage. Rest is a continuum ranging from complete rest or immobilization to restricted activity (relative rest) of the involved body part. The application of ice or some form of cold application helps lower tissue temperature, thus slowing cell metabolism. Cold applications also are beneficial for reducing pain and muscle spasms that accompany musculoskeletal injuries. Both compression and elevation contribute to swelling control. Stabilization allows musculature around the injury to relax, which, along with the ice, aids in limiting the pain–spasm cycle[40].

Therapeutic treatment and additional exercise procedures that follow initial treatment are designed to promote healing and allow return to activity. Heat modalities and exercise rehabilitation are often prescribed after the initial treatment period. It is recommended that a physician or sports medicine professional direct follow-up treatment.

CARDIOPULMONARY CONDITIONS

In addition to the many musculoskeletal injuries that have been discussed, a variety of additional health-related conditions can potentially affect exercise participants. Occasionally, the stress of physical exertion during exercise, accompanied by pathologic or environmental conditions, can increase the risk for cardiopulmonary or metabolic complications that affect the individual's health.

The AHA/ACSM Health/Fitness Facility Preparticipation Screening Questionnaire uses history, symptoms, and risk factor information to help direct people to either begin an exercise program or contact a physician before

TABLE 28-2. Descriptions of General Exercise Injuries

Condition	Description	Characteristics
Sprain	A stretch or tear to the ligaments and stabilizing connective tissues of a joint	Swelling, pain, joint instability, loss of function
Strain	A stretch or tear in the muscle or adjacent tissue such as the fascia or muscle tendon	Movement pain, local tenderness, loss of strength and ROM.
Contusion	A bruise that occurs from a sudden traumatic blow to soft or bony tissue.	Soft tissue hemorrhage, hematoma, ecchymosis, movement restriction
Acute fracture	A sudden break of a bone	Deformity, bone point tenderness, swelling, ecchymosis
Stress fracture	Microscopic damage to the bone caused by repetitive stress	Insidious onset of pain that persists when attempting activity; tenderness
Bursitis	Inflammation of a bursa between bony prominences and muscle or tendon	Swelling, pain, some loss of function
Tendonitis	Inflammation of a tendon	Gradual onset, diffuse or local pain, tenderness, loss of strength
Plantar fasciitis	Inflammatory condition to the plantar surface of the foot	Inferior heel pain, pain increased with weight bearing
Shin splints	An overuse injury that indicates pain in the anteromedial shin	Pain occurring before, during, or after activity; bone tenderness
Patellar femoral pain syndrome	Knee pain caused by lateral deviation of the patella as it tracks in the femoral groove	Tenderness of the lateral patella, pain, swelling
Low back pain	Condition resulting from trauma or multiple episodes of microtrauma resulting in muscular or joint pain	Pain accentuated by sudden flexion, extension, or rotation; muscle weakness
Rotator cuff tendonitis	Inflammation of the rotator cuff muscles or tendons	Diffuse pain, increased with overhead activities; muscle weakness in external rotation
Tennis elbow	Inflammation of the lateral epicondyle of the humerus	Pain in lateral elbow during and after activity; weakness of the wrist in extension

ROM = range of motion.

starting exercise (Box 28-5)[4]. The AHA and ACSM have jointly published guidelines for classifying exercise participants according to disease risk[4]. The recommendation states that participants should be classified into one of three risk strata: apparently healthy, persons at increased risk, and persons with known cardiovascular disease. After an individual has been stratified, decisions can be made regarding the need for and the types of medical examination and exercise testing. People at higher risk for coronary heart disease are directed to seek exercise facilities providing appropriate levels of staff supervision (see Table 28-1)[41].

With chronic degenerative conditions (atherosclerosis) of the heart, exercise participants may be unaware that disease is present or progressing to where it could cause major health complications. Fewer than 10 of 100,000 men will have a heart attack during exercise[42]. Of the millions of participants in high school, collegiate, and professional sports, fewer than 20 individuals die per year as a result of sudden death syndrome[43]. When death during exercise occurs in people age 30 years or older, it usually results from cardiac arrhythmia caused by cardiovascular disease. Those younger than age 30 years are most likely to die from hypertrophic cardiomyopathy, an aortic aneurysm, or myocarditis. The examination of post-exercise heart attack episodes in 1228 men and women shows that the risk of

heart attack is 5.9 times higher after heavy versus lighter or no physical exertion in those who usually exercise very little. Men may be more susceptible to sudden death because they may participate at higher levels of physical activity and ignore prodromal symptoms compared with women[43,44].

Deaths during exercise in people older than age 35 years usually are caused by a cardiac arrhythmia resulting from atherosclerosis. When blood supply to a part of the heart's myocardium is severely or totally restricted, ischemia can lead to a heart attack, or myocardial infarction (MI). In addition, an irregular heart rhythm or arrhythmia can present as a *tachycardia*. With these arrhythmias, the sinus rhythm itself is usually altered, which can adversely affect circulation. Atrial and ventricular tachycardias are serious arrhythmias that can lead to fibrillation and death[45]. Unstable tachycardia exists when the heart beats too fast, resulting in reduced diastolic filling time and reduced stroke volume. This unstable tachycardia can lead to hemodynamic instability and signs and symptoms such as pain and distress involving non–Q-wave or Q-wave MI, hypotension, or congestive heart failure (Table 28-5).

In untrained individuals, *bradycardia* (decreased resting HR) is usually the result of abnormal cardiac function or a diseased heart. However, a natural consequence of endurance training is a markedly decreased resting HR. The actual mechanisms responsible for this decrease are

TABLE 28-3. Common Acute and Chronic Exercise Injuries and Causes

Body Region	Injury	Mechanism of Injury
Upper Extremities		
Shoulders	Rotator cuff strain	Throwing; swimming
	Rotator cuff tendonitis	Use of arm above horizontal; repetitive overhead activities
	Anterior glenohumeral dislocation	Forced horizontal abduction, external rotation
Upper arms	Bicipital tenosynovitis	Repeated forceful external rotation of the arm
Elbows	Lateral epicondylitis	Repeated forceful extension of the elbow (tennis elbow)
	Medial epicondylitis	Repeated forceful flexion of the elbow
Wrists and hands	Carpal tunnel syndrome	Activities that require repeated wrist flexion
	Strains and sprains	Falling on the wrist or outstretched hand
	Fractures	Falling on the outstretched hand
Lower Extremities		
Feet	Heel bruise	Contusion; sudden stop-and-go movements in running
	Plantar fasciitis	Unequal leg length; inflexible longitudinal arch; tight gastrocnemius– soleus muscle
	Metatarsalgia	Excessive pressure under the forefoot; fallen metatarsal arch
	Metatarsal stress fracture	Training overload; unequal leg length; hyperpronation of foot
Ankle, lower legs	Inversion ankle sprain	Foot forced into inversion-plantar flexion
	Achilles tendon strain	Sudden excessive dorsiflexion of foot
	Achilles tendonitis	Training errors; tight gastrocnemius–soleus muscle
	Anterior, posterior tibial tendonitis	Faulty posture alignment; falling arches; overuse stress
	Stress fracture of the tibia, fibula	Overuse stress; biomechanical foot problems
	Shin splints	Overtraining; running on hard surface; malaligned lower leg
Knees	Patellofemoral pain syndrome	Overuse (e.g., hill running); patellar compression
	Joint sprain	Direct straight-line or rotary forces
	Meniscal lesion	Excessive pressure (squatting); shear forces
	Patellar subluxation, dislocation	Alignment abnormalities; quadriceps weakness
	Chondromalacia patella	Abnormal patellar tracking; anatomical variation
	Degenerative arthritis	Overuse stress; obesity
	Patellar or quadriceps tendonitis	Sudden or repetitive forceful extension of knee
	Iliotibial band friction syndrome	Overuse stress associated with running, cycling
Upper legs	Quadriceps muscle strain	Weak muscles; sudden contraction, as during jumping
	Hamstring muscle strain	Strength imbalance; tightness; explosive movements
Hips	Trochanteric bursitis	Increased Q-angle; unequal leg length; faulty running form
Trunk		
Abdomen	Muscle strain	Sudden twisting of the trunk; reaching overhead
Spine	Lumbar strain and sprain	Poor posture; lumbar lordosis; sudden abrupt extension or contraction, sometimes with trunk rotation
	Low back pain	Acute traumatic event; overuse; poor sitting posture; static or repeated flexion activities

---

BOX 28-8 | **The Injury Recognition Process**

1. Check vital signs and perform immediate first aid, if necessary.
2. Stabilize the individual or the injury.
3. Identify the injury.
   - **History:** Subjective statements by the injured person that include major complaints and injury history (e.g., description of injury mechanism, functional impairments, pain, previous injury, training level and changes, equipment used, and rehabilitation)
   - **Observation:** Inspect or look at the individual and the injured part. Note variations in size, swelling, discoloration, posture, gait, limping, joint ROM, instability or deformity, and atrophy. Compare the injured part with the uninjured part.
   - **Palpation:** Using the fingers, carefully and gently feel the affected part, including soft and bony structures. Examine for edema, skin temperature variations, deformity, and point tenderness.
   - **Special tests:** Detect specific conditions, such as joint ROM and stability, muscle strength, neurological status, and circulation.
4. Decide your course of action.
   - RICES
   - Referral to physician
   - Return to activity
5. Complete administrative procedures.
   - Record injury or incident in file.
   - Inform your immediate supervisor.

RICES = rest, ice, compression, elevation, and stabilization; ROM = range of motion.

TABLE 28-4. Basic First Aid Guidelines for Exercise-related Musculoskeletal and Skin Injuries

Condition	First Aid Procedures
Acute musculoskeletal injuries Contusion Sprain Strain	If no fracture, follow the RICES guidelines: set the area at rest (immobilize), apply an ice bag or cold pack with an elastic wrap for 20 to 30 minutes, and elevate the extremity above the heart. Reevaluate after initial first aid, support the injured area, and apply an elastic wrap to maintain compression keeping the extremity elevated, if possible. Reapply ice or cold packs every 2 hours for 30 minutes and then continue to maintain compression and elevation during periods when cold is not being applied. Repeat these procedures for the first 24 to 72 hours, depending on the severity of injury and symptoms.
Fracture	Keep the individual still with the extremity in the position found without moving the extremity or individual, if possible. Activate EMS or the facility's emergency response system to transport the individual to an ER. Do not apply a commercial or homemade splint unless the individual must be moved. Apply a cold pack. Calm and reassure the individual. Monitor the individual for signs and symptoms of shock, internal bleeding, and other life-threatening conditions. If splinting is warranted, proper splinting technique includes: (a) check distal pulse, skin temperature, color, and sensation for damage to nerves and blood vessels; (b) keep the individual still and immobilize the joints above and below the suspected fracture site along with the broken bone ends with splinting materials, the ground, or other body part; and (c) recheck for circulation and sensation distal to the injury site.
Open skin wounds	With all open wounds, be sure to place a barrier (e.g., disposable latex gloves) between yourself and the individual's blood or body fluids and follow universal precautions to prevent the transfer of bloodborne pathogens. Be sure to wash your hands immediately after providing care. Minor wounds without significant bleeding (e.g., blisters, abrasions, lacerations, and incisions) should be cleaned with soap and water and treated with a germicide cream or solution followed by the application of a sterile dressing such as an adhesive plastic strip, gauze pad, or other commercial wound cover. The individual should be reminded to watch for signs of infection, keep the area clean and dry, and change the dressing as needed. Significant wounds that are bleeding severely should be treated by one or more of the following procedures: (a) apply direct pressure by applying a sterile dressing directly to the wound and applying pressure with the flat of the hand and fingers (if the dressing becomes saturated, apply additional dressings on top of the previous without removing the saturated dressing); (b) elevate the limb (if no fracture is suspected) while maintaining direct pressure elevate the wound above the individual's heart; (c) apply a bandage snugly over the dressing; or (d) if the preceding methods fail to stop the wound from bleeding, apply pressure to the brachial artery in the arm for upper extremity wounds or femoral artery in the groin for lower extremity wounds. Activate EMS or the facility's emergency response system.

EMS = emergency medical services; ER = emergency room; RICES = rest, ice, compression, elevation, and stabilization.

TABLE 28-5. Cardiopulmonary and Metabolic Conditions

Condition or Abnormality	Definition	Description and Etiology
Hypertrophic cardiomyopathy	Hypertrophy of the myocardium	Cardiac palpitations, angina, syncope, vertigo; asymptomatic
Tachycardia	HR ≥ 100 bpm in adults at rest	Chest palpitations; difficulty breathing, severe chest pressure, chest pain, shortness of breath while exercising
Bradycardia	HR < 60 bpm in adults at rest	Chest pain, shortness of breath, fatigue, exercise intolerance, hypotension, decrease in BP when standing;, chest pain
Tachypnea	Abnormal rapidity of respiration	Hyperventilation syndrome
Hypertension	Systolic BP ≥ 140 mm Hg Diastolic BP ≥ 90 mm Hg	Headache; most people are symptom free until complications arise
Hypotension	Decreased systolic and diastolic BP	Syncope and fatigue; occurs in shock, hemorrhage, and dehydration
Fainting	Feeling weak as though about to lose consciousness	Paleness; weakness; dizziness; weak, rapid, irregular pulse
Syncope	Transient loss of consciousness caused by inadequate blood flow to the brain	Peripheral circulatory failure; cardiac arrhythmia; hyperventilation
Hypoglycemia	Abnormal decreased blood glucose level	Headache; shakiness, confusion, faintness, blurred or double vision, tachycardia, pallor, convulsions, unconsciousness
Hyperglycemia	Abnormal increased blood glucose level	Nausea, dizziness when rising, polyuria, blurred vision, weight loss

BP = blood pressure; HR = heart rate.

not entirely known, but training appears to increase parasympathetic activity in the heart while decreasing sympathetic activity. Therefore, it is necessary to distinguish between training-induced bradycardia and pathological bradycardia, which can be a serious cause for concern. Both autonomic influences and the intrinsic pathology of the conducting system can lead to bradycardia. In particular, acute MI can lead to ischemic damage to the conducting system of the heart, producing bradycardias that range from sinus bradycardia to complete third-degree heart block (see Table 28-5)[45].

For individuals with vascular disease, several forms of exercise (i.e., high intensity, resistance training) may prove harmful because of the acute hemodynamic effects caused by the pressor response associated with Valsalva-type maneuvers[46]. Other potential adverse health effects from exercise include cardiac dysfunction, ischemic arrhythmias, excessive hypertensive responses, and post-exercise orthostatic hypotension (see Table 28-5).

Appropriate immediate care must be understood and practiced to avoid deterioration of health status when any adverse health condition occurs. Table 28-6 presents guidelines for the initial management of individuals experiencing hemodynamic and cardiopulmonary conditions. Exercise testing personnel should be trained in cardiopulmonary resuscitation (CPR) and preferably ad-

TABLE 28-6. Basic First Aid Guidelines for Cardiopulmonary and Metabolic Conditions

Condition	First Aid Procedures
Angina	If individual develops new symptomatic chest pain:
	Stop activity; rest or sit in recumbent position.
	Check pulse and BP (and cardiac rhythm if appropriate).
	Activate EMS or evaluate by a physician.
	If patient suffers from chronic stable angina:
	Stop exercise and rest; give medication (if appropriate) and consult primary physician.
Bradycardia	Stop activity, assess vital signs, secure airway, ensure defibrillator is available.
	Activate EMS system.
Tachycardia	Stop activity, assess vital signs, secure airway, ensure defibrillator is available.
	Activate EMS system.
Cardiac Arrest	Assess responsiveness.
	If unresponsive activate EMS and get AED.
	Check ABCs.
	If no pulse or no breathing, perform CPR until defibrillator is attached.
	Operate AED to analyze and attempt defibrillation, if indicated (follow equipment manufacturer instructions).
	After three shocks or after any "no shock indicated": Check for signs of circulation[a]
	If no signs of circulation are present, perform CPR for 1 minute.
	Recheck for signs of circulation[a] If absent, analyze and attempt to defibrillate, if indicated.
	Repeat up to three times.
Dyspnea	Stop activity; maintain open airway.
	Administer bronchodilator, if prescribed.
	If signs and symptoms persist, activate EMS.
Tachypnea	Stop activity; maintain open airway.
	If signs and symptoms persist, activate EMS.
Hyperventilation	Have the individual slow the rate of respiration and concentrate on breathing in through the nose and exhaling through the mouth inhaling and exhaling through one nostril, or breathing slowly into a paper bag.
Asthma or bronchospasm	Preventive: Patient should avoid known irritants, and cold, dry, or polluted air.
	Stop activity; maintain open airway.
	Administer bronchodilator, if prescribed.
	If signs and symptoms persist, activate EMS.
Hypotension or shock	Stop activity and remove patient from exercise area, if possible.
	Position in a supine position.
	Activate EMS.
	Elevate legs unless fracture, head, neck, or back injury is suspected.
	Maintain normal body temperature.
Hypoglycemia	If patient is known diabetic and is symptomatic, stop activity, obtain Accucheck to determine if blood glucose is <70 mg·dL^{-1}.
	If patient remains symptomatic, give glucose (e.g., sugar cube, orange juice, candy, fruit) orally
	Activate EMS if patient is unconscious and cannot be given glucose by mouth.
Hyperglycemia	If patient is known diabetic and is symptomatic, stop activity; obtain Accucheck to determine if blood glucose >250 mg·dL^{-1} or if patient remains symptomatic.
	Administer fluids orally if conscious. Individual should receive insulin.
	Activate EMS.

[a] If pulse is present but no breathing, begin rescue breathing.

ABC = airway, breathing, circulation; AED = automated external defibrillator; BP = blood pressure; EMS = emergency medical services.

TABLE 28-7. Advanced Cardiovascular Life Support Drugs[45,47]

Drug	Mechanism of Action and Indications
ACE Inhibitors Enalapril Captopril Lisinopril Ramipril	Treatment of hypertension
Adenosine	Slows conduction through the AV node, interrupts AV-nodal reentry pathways and can restore normal sinus rhythm in patients with PSVT.
Amiodarone	Potent α- and β-adrenergic blocking properties. Multiple effects on sodium, potassium, and calcium channels in the treatment of atrial and ventricular tachyarrhythmias.
Amrinone	Inotropic vasoactive agent that is a phosphodiesterase inhibitor. Hemodynamic effects include increased cardiac output and diminished peripheral resistance and preload in treatment of severe CHF.
Aspirin	Blocks formation of thromboxane A2, which causes platelets to aggregate and arteries to constrict. Anticoagulant/antiplatelet agent.
Atropine sulfate	A parasympatholytic drug that enhances both sinus node automaticity and AV conduction via its direct vagolytic action. Used to treat symptomatic patients with sinus bradycardia.
β-Adrenergic Blockers Atenolol Esmolol Metoprolol Propranolol Labetalol	Attenuate the effects of circulating catecholamines by blocking their ability to bind to β-adrenergic receptors. Reduction in HR, BP, myocardial contractility, and myocardial oxygen consumption in treatment of patients with MI and unstable angina.
Calcium Channel Blockers Diltiazem verapamil	Inhibit the influx of calcium ions during membrane depolarization of cardiac and vascular smooth muscle; reduce myocardial oxygen consumption; slows conduction and prolong refractoriness in the AV node (treatment of supraventricular tachycardias); antihypertensive effect by relaxation of vascular smooth muscle; anti-ischemic agent.
Calcium chloride	Positive inotropic effect by calcium ions entering the sarcomere units and increasing the force of myocardial contraction.
Digibind	Digoxin-specific antibody therapy for treatment of patients with life-threatening arrhythmias, shock, CHF, hyperkalemia.
Digoxin	Cardiac glycoside that inhibits sodium-potassium ATPase, an enzyme that regulates the quantity of sodium and potassium inside cells; leads to an increase in the intracellular concentration of calcium that results in direct actions on cardiac muscle; treatment of mild to moderate heart failure.
Diltiazem	Inhibits slow channel activity in cardiac and vascular smooth muscle; antihypertensive effect; treatment of angina by its ability to reduce myocardial oxygen demand.
Disopyramide	Decreases the rate of diastolic depolarization in cells with augmented automaticity. Treatment of ventricular arrhythmias.
Dobutamine	Sympathomimetic amine that exerts inotropic effects by stimulating β_1- and α_1-adrenergic receptors in the myocardium; treatment of CHF and pulmonary congestion.
Dopamine	Inotropic vasoactive agent that stimulates β_1-adrenergic receptors and increases cardiac output; treatment of symptomatic bradycardia and hypotension.
Epinephrine	Potent α_1- and α_2- postsynaptic adrenergic agonist effects improve cerebral and coronary blood flow by preventing arterial collapse and increasing peripheral vasoconstriction. For cardiac arrest, symptomatic bradycardia, severe hypotension.
Fibrinolytic agents Alteplase, recombinant tPA Anistreplase APSAC Reteplase, recombinant Streptokinase Tenecteplase	Breakdown fibrin in blood clots, and prevents the polymerization of fibrin into new clots. For acute MI in adults.
Flecainide	Ventricular arrhythmias
Flumazenil	Reverse respiratory depression
Furosemide	Diuretic that inhibits reabsorption of sodium and chloride in the ascending loop of Henle. For hypertensive emergencies.
Glucagon	Adjunctive treatment of toxic effects of calcium channel blocker or ∃-blocker.
GP IIb/IIIa Abciximab Eptifibitide Tirofiban	Inhibit the integrin GP IIb/IIIa receptor in the membrane inhibitors of platelets, inhibiting platelet aggregation.
Heparin (UFH, LMWH) Dalteparin Enoxaparin	Inhibit thrombin generation by factor X_a inhibition and inhibits thrombin indirectly by formation of a complex with antithrombin III.

TABLE 28-7. Advanced Cardiovascular Life Support Drugs[45,47] (*continued*)

Drug	Mechanism of Action and Indications
Ibutilide	Treatment of supraventricular arrhythmias, including atrial fibrillation and flutter.
Isoproterenol	Sympathomimetic amine with potent inotropic and chronotropic properties that frequently result in increased cardiac output despite a reduction in mean BP because of peripheral vasodilation and venous pooling. Treatment of symptomatic bradycardia.
Lidocaine	Suppresses ventricular arrhythmias by decreasing automaticity. Anesthetic properties help to suppress ventricular ectopy after MI.
Magnesium sulfate	Enzymatic cofactor essential for the function of the sodium-potassium ATPase pump. Acts as a physiological channel blocker.
Mannitol	Increased intracranial pressure in management of neurologic emergencies.
Morphine sulfate	Produces analgesic and hemodynamic effects for treating ischemic chest pain by decreasing myocardial oxygen requirements.
Nitroglycerin	Vasodilator; relaxes vascular smooth muscle; treatment of angina or ischemic pain, acute MI, and LV failure.
Nitroprusside (sodium Nntroprusside)	Reduces BP by reducing peripheral arterial resistance by increasing venous capacitance and, thus, preload; increases cardiac output by diminishing vascular impedance and increasing stroke volume.
Norepinephrine	Increases myocardial contractility because of its β_1-adrenergic effects; potent α-adrenergic effects lead to arterial and venous vasoconstriction; treatment of severe cardiogenic shock.
Oxygen	Elevates arterial oxygen tension; increases arterial oxygen content; improves tissue oxygenation.
Procainamide	Suppresses ventricular ectopy and slows intraventricular conduction. Suppresses phase 4 diastolic depolarization and reduces the automaticity of all pacemakers in normal ventricular muscle and Purkinje fibers. Treatment of arrhythmias.
Propafenone	Antiarrhythmic agent with local anesthetic effects and a direct stabilizing action on myocardial membranes; used for treatment of ventricular and supraventricular arrhythmias.
Sodium bicarbonate	Chemical agent that buffers H^+ to prevent acidosis. Indicated for several conditions associated with sudden VF arrest
Sotalol	Treatment of ventricular and atrial arrhythmias.
Vasopressin	Adrenergic agent that is a powerful peripheral vasoconstrictor that increases blood flow to the brain and heart. Treatment of adult shock-refractory VF.

ACE = angiotension-converting enzyme; APSAC = Anisolylated Plasminogen Streptokinase Activator Complex; AV = atrioventricular; BP = blood pressure; CHF = congestive heart failure; GP = glycoprotein; HR = heart rate; LMWH = low molecular weight heparin; LV = left ventricular; MI = myocardial infarction; PSVT = Paroxysmal Supraventricular Tachycardia; tPA = issue plasminogen activator. UFH = unfractionated heparin; VF = ventricular fibrillation. Also see GETP7 Table A-1.

vanced cardiac life support (ACLS). The AHA's approach to cardiovascular and cardiopulmonary emergencies includes the primary ABCD (airway, breathing, circulation, and defibrillation) survey and the secondary ABCD survey[45]. The primary ABCD survey assesses and manages most immediate life-threatening events using CPR and defibrillation. The secondary ABCD survey focuses on assessment and advanced treatment to restore and maintain spontaneous breathing and circulation. Because the secondary survey includes advanced medical interventions, health care providers are required to have advanced skills, which include treating inadequate ventilation with positive-pressure ventilations and administering drugs appropriate for rhythm and condition.

The AHA's *2000 Handbook of Emergency Cardiac Care*[47] presents treatment algorithms for comprehensively managing pre-arrest and cardiac arrest emergencies. The treatment algorithms list interventions and actions, including advanced cardiovascular life support drugs. Knowledge of emergency procedures and the advanced cardiac life support drugs is important for exercise professionals. Table 28-7 presents common advanced cardiovascular life support drugs that should be available for use in physician-supervised exercise testing and training sessions[45,46].

METABOLIC CONDITIONS

Diabetes mellitus (DM) is a chronic metabolic disorder marked by hyperglycemia. Diabetes mellitus results either from failure of the pancreas to produce insulin (type I DM) or from insulin resistance, with inadequate insulin secretion to sustain normal metabolism (type 2 DM). Type 1 DM usually presents as an acute illness with dehydration and often diabetic ketoacidosis. Type 2 DM is frequently asymptomatic in its early years and is, therefore, occult[48]. Diagnosis is based on a fasting plasma glucose level greater than 126 mg·dL^{-1} on more than one occasion or a glucose level exceeding 200 mg·dL^{-1} in a patient with excessive urinary volume (polyuria), excessive thirst (polydipsia), and weight loss[48]. For those individuals experiencing hemodynamic, cardiopulmonary, or metabolic conditions (diabetes), proper immediate care must also be understood and practiced to avoid deterioration of health status (see Table 28-6). If an individual with diabetes has any diabetic complications, consultation with the physician is warranted to determine appropriate exercise guidelines. Some guidelines that may be helpful in avoiding exercise-induced hypoglycemia in the diabetic population include those indicated in Box 28-9[49].

BOX 28-9	Guidelines for Avoiding Exercise-induced Hypoglycemia

- Check blood glucose before exercise.
- If blood glucose <100 mg·dL^{-1}, then eat 15 to 20 g CHO 15 to 30 minutes before training.
- Recheck blood glucose after 30 minutes of training or sooner if symptoms are present
- Exercise 1 to 2 hours after eating.
- Avoid exercise during insulin peak time.
- Inject insulin into less active or nonactive muscle.
- Have fast-acting glucose available at all times (e.g., glucose tablets).
- Check blood glucose immediately after exercise; if blood glucose <60 mg·dL^{-1}, then eat 15 to 20 g CHO (glucose preferred).

Environmental Considerations

The human body experiences unique challenges and occasionally adverse health effects when performing physical activity in extreme environmental conditions (e.g., high temperature, high humidity, high altitude, and pollution).

Environmental stress can adversely affect an individual's ability to exercise and, in some instances, poses a serious health threat. Special precautions and modifications of exercise programming are sometimes needed to reduce health risks related to the exercise environment (Table 28-8). It is vitally important that exercise professionals have knowledge about environmental factors to assist them in planning and conducting safe exercise programs. See Chapter 3 for more information on the physiologic effects of exercise in different environmental conditions.

HEAT

The stress of physical exertion is often complicated by environmental thermal conditions that result in elevated body temperature above the normal range (hyperthermia [see Chapter 3]). Heat stress is not always accurately reflected by air temperature alone. Humidity, air velocity (or wind), and thermal radiation also contribute to the total heat stress when exercising (Box 28-10). Conduction, convection, radiation, and evaporation are thermoregulatory mechanisms that transfer body heat. During exercise, sweat evaporation becomes the most important avenue of heat loss. Because sweat must evaporate to provide cooling, high humidity

TABLE 28-8. Basic First Aid Guidelines for Environmental and Exercise Intolerance Conditions

Condition	Guidelines
Environmental and exercise intolerance	Stop activity; calm and reassure the individual; monitor vital signs; activate EMS, if warranted.
Dizziness	Stop activity; position patient in supine with legs elevated; monitor vital signs and seek medical attention if symptoms persist.
Fainting	Position patient in supine with the legs elevated provided no injury is suspected; monitor vital signs and seek medical attention if symptoms persist. If individual has fallen, check for additional injuries before moving.
Syncope	Position patient in supine with the legs elevated provided no injury is suspected; monitor vital signs; assess for heat stress or other conditions that may predispose syncope; maintain normal body temperature; seek medical attention if symptoms persist or worsen. If individual has fallen, check for additional injuries before moving.
Heat cramps	Stop activity; attempt to reduce muscular cramp by stretching, relaxation, and massage; replace lost fluids with sodium-containing fluids; continue to monitor the individual's hydration status for the next few days.
Heat exhaustion	Stop activity and move the individual to a shaded or air-conditioned area; remove excess clothing and cool individual if body temperature is elevated; place the individual in a reclining position with the legs above the heart; if not nauseated, vomiting, or experiencing any CNS dysfunction rehydrate with chilled water or sports drink; monitor vital signs, core temperature, and CNS status; activate EMS system if rapid improvement is absent.
Heat stroke	Aggressive and immediate whole-body cooling via cold water immersion (35 to 58°F/ or .67 to 14.5°C) if constant monitoring of core temperature is possible; alternative cooling strategies include spraying body with cold water, using fans, placing ice or cold towels over as much of the body as possible, or moving to shaded or air-conditioned facility; activate EMS and monitor ABCs, core temperature, and CNS; cease cooling when core temperature reaches approximately 101°F (38.3°C).
Hyponatremia	Distinguish between hyponatremia, heat exhaustion, and heat stroke; activate EMS and transfer to medical facility; individuals with suspected hyponatremia should not be administered fluids unless directed by a physician.
Systemic hypothermia	Carefully move individual to a warm place; activate EMS; arrange rapid transport to emergency facility; monitor vital signs and provide care for shock; remove wet clothing and cover with blankets to retain body heat; provide external heat; encourage drinking hot liquids.
Local injury (frostbite, chilblain, frostnip)	Remove wet clothing; soak area in warm water (100 to 105°F or 37.8 to 40.5°C); cover the affected area with dry, sterile dressings; check ABCs, monitor vital signs and care for shock; do not rewarm a frostbitten area if there is danger of refreezing; activate EMS or transport individual to an emergency medical facility.

ABC = airway, breathing, circulation; CNS = central nervous system; EMS = emergency medical services.

BOX 28-10 Heat Index

	AIR TEMPERATURE (°F)										
RH	**70**	**75**	**80**	**85**	**90**	**95**	**100**	**105**	**110**	**115**	**120**
30	67	73	78	84	90	96	104	113	123	135	148
35	67	73	79	85	91	98	107	118	130	143	
40	68	74	79	86	93	101	110	123	137	151	
45	68	74	80	87	95	104	115	129	143		
50	69	75	81	88	96	107	120	135	150		
55	69	75	81	89	98	110	126	142			
60	70	76	82	90	100	114	132	149			
65	70	76	83	91	102	119	138				
70	70	77	85	93	106	124	144				
75	70	77	86	95	109	130					
80	71	78	86	97	113	136					
85	71	78	87	99	117						
90	71	79	88	102	122						
95	71	79	89	105							
100	72	80	91	108							

RH = humidity.

HEAT INDEX	EFFECTS ON THE HUMAN BODY
130 or above	Heat stroke highly likely with continued exposure
105–130	Heat stroke likely with prolonged exposure
90–105	Heat stroke possible with prolonged exposure

Adapted from National Oceanic and Atmospheric Administration[55].

limits sweat evaporation and heat loss. Consequently, body temperature can increase to critical levels, seriously jeopardizing health[50,51].

Heat illnesses are more likely in hot, humid weather but can also occur in the absence of hot and humid conditions (Box 28-11). When the exercise session is conducted in hot, humid conditions or if the individual is not acclimated to exercise in the heat, special precautions and modifications of exercise programming for exertional heat illnesses must be undertaken. The most important factors in reducing heat illness are to limit the intensity and duration of activity, wear minimal clothing to allow heat dissipation from the body, increase the number and length of rest breaks, and encourage proper hydration. Several other factors important to preventing heat illnesses are listed in Box 28-12[51,52].

COLD

Increasing year-round participation in such sporting activities as the triathlon, hiking, running, and cycling has created new concerns about exercise in the cold (see Chapter 3). The two major cold stressors, ambient temperature (air) and water, cause a loss of body heat that threatens homeostasis. *Hypothermia* occurs when body temperature falls below 36°C (97°F) and results when a person is exposed to wet or cold conditions or after trauma[50]. Ambient temperature and wind influence the coldness of an environment. The wind-chill index determines the wind's cooling effect on exposed tissue and can be used as a guide to determine suitable outdoor exercise conditions (Box 28-13). When exposed to cold, the body attempts to increase internal heat production by increasing muscular activity, such as shivering, and by increasing the individual's basal metabolic rate. After the body temperature falls below 34.5,dg>C (94°F), the hypothalamus begins to lose its ability to regulate body temperature. This ability is completely lost when the internal temperature falls to about 29.5°C (85°F). Predisposing factors to cold injury include inadequate insulation from wind and cold, restricted circulation because of arterial disease or tight clothing (including footwear), fatigue, and the

| **BOX 28-11** | **Common Exertional Heat Illnesses** |

EXERCISE-ASSOCIATED MUSCLE (HEAT) CRAMPS
- Acute, painful, involuntary muscle contraction
- Present during or after intense exercise sessions
- Caused by fluid deficiencies (dehydration), electrolyte imbalances, neuromuscular fatigue

HEAT SYNCOPE (ORTHOSTATIC DIZZINESS)
- Occurs when exposed to high environmental temperatures or dehydration
- Individuals may be vulnerable during initial exercise sessions in the heat (unacclimated state)
- Caution for individuals with heart disease and those taking diuretics
- Can occur immediately after cessation of activity or after rapid assumption of upright posture after lying or sitting

EXERCISE (HEAT) EXHAUSTION
- The inability to continue exercise associated with any combination of heavy sweating, dehydration, sodium loss, and energy depletion
- Body core temperature generally ranges between 36°C (97°F) and 40°C (104°F); pallor, weakness, headache, dizziness, diarrhea
- Difficult to distinguish from exertional heat stroke without measuring rectal temperature

EXERTIONAL HEAT STROKE
- Elevated core temperature (usually >40°C (104°F) associated with signs of organ system failure caused by hyperthermia
- Tachycardia, hypotension, sweating (skin may be wet or dry at time of collapse), altered mental status, and vomiting
- Can result in death

EXERTIONAL HYPONATREMIA
- Relatively rare condition defined as a blood sodium level $< 130 \ mmol \cdot L^{-1}$, producing intracellular swelling that causes potentially fatal neurologic and physiologic dysfunction
- Disorientation, altered mental status, headache, vomiting, lethargy, swelling of hands and feet, pulmonary and cerebral edema
- Can result in death (Also see Box 3-1)

body's shunting of blood away from the skin when exposed to the cold.

The hazards of excessive cold exposure include potential injury to both peripheral tissues and the life-supporting cardiovascular and respiratory systems. Considerable water loss from the respiratory passages can lead to dehydration during exercise on cold days[28]. Inspired ambient air temperature generally does not pose a danger to the respiratory tract tissues. The early warning signs of peripheral cold injury include tingling and numbness in the fingers and toes

| **BOX 28-12** | **Recommendations for Preventing Heat Illness** |

- Modify activity under high-risk conditions (Wet Bulb Globe Temperature > 28°C (82°F); consider rescheduling or delaying the session until safer conditions prevail.
- Schedule exercise sessions to avoid the hottest time of the day (10 am to 5 PM).
- Avoid radiate heating from direct sun light.
- Progressively increase the intensity and duration of work in the heat over days or weeks (i.e., acclimatization).
- Consume an adequate volume of fluids (water or sports drinks) to maintain hydration.
- Fluid replacement: Maintain proper hydration (educate the individual to match fluid intake with sweat and urine losses).
- Instruct individuals to drink sodium-containing fluids to keep their urine clear to light yellow to improve hydration.
- Individual should weigh themselves before and after exercise to estimate the amount of body water lost during exercise and to ensure a return to pre-exercise weight before the next exercise session.
- Consume approximately 1.00 to 1.25 L (16 to 20 oz) of fluid for each kilogram of body water lost during exercise.
- Wear loose-fitting, absorbent, light-colored clothing, mesh clothing, or new-generation cloth blends specially designed to allow effective cooling.
- Conduct warm-up and stretching sessions in the shade (for outdoor activities).
- Individuals who have lost 2% of body weight should be excluded from participation (as should those who exhibit heat illness symptoms).

BOX 28-13 | Wind Chill Chart

New Wind Chill Chart

Wind (mph)

	Calm	5	10	15	20	25	30	35	40	45	50	55	60
40		36	34	32	30	29	28	28	27	26	26	25	25
35		31	27	25	24	23	22	21	20	19	19	18	17
30		25	21	19	17	16	15	14	13	12	12	11	10
25		19	15	13	11	9	8	7	6	5	4	4	3
20		13	9	6	4	3	1	0	−1	−2	−3	−3	−4
15		7	3	0	−2	−4	−5	−7	−8	−9	−10	−11	−11
10		1	−4	−7	−9	−11	−12	−14	−15	−16	−17	−18	−19
5		−5	−10	−13	−15	−17	−19	−21	−22	−23	−24	−25	−26
0		−11	−16	−19	−22	−24	−26	−27	−29	−30	−31	−32	−33
−5		−16	−22	−26	−29	−31	−33	−34	−36	−37	−38	−39	−40
−10		−22	−28	−32	−35	−37	−39	−41	−43	−44	−45	−46	−48
−15		−28	−35	−39	−42	−44	−46	−48	−50	−51	−52	−54	−55
−20		−34	−41	−45	−48	−51	−53	−55	−57	−58	−60	−61	−62
−25		−40	−47	−51	−55	−58	−60	−62	−64	−65	−67	−68	−69
−30		−46	−53	−58	−61	−64	−67	−69	−71	−72	−74	−75	−76
−35		−52	−59	−64	−68	−71	−73	−76	−78	−79	−81	−82	−84
−40		−57	−66	−71	−74	−78	−80	−82	−84	−86	−88	−89	−91
−45		−63	−72	−77	−81	−84	−87	−89	−91	−93	−95	−97	−98

Temperature (°F)

Frostbite occurs in 15 minutes or less

Wind Chill (°F) = 35.74 + 0.6215T − 35.75($V^{0.16}$) + 0.4275T($V^{0.16}$)

Where, T = Air Temperature (°F)

V = Wind Speed (mph)

Adapted from National Oceanic and Atmospheric Administration[55].

or a burning sensation in the nose and ears[53]. Effects of cold on body function and local injury include:

1. Systemic hypothermia (both core and shell temperatures decrease)
   - Excessive cold exposure
   - Body functions slow down
   - Cardiac arrhythmias, cardiac arrest, and possible death
2. Local injury (core temperature is maintained, but shell [skin] temperature is decreased)
   - Frostnip: Mild cold injury resulting in reversible blanching of the skin
   - Chilblain: Mild cold injury marked by localized redness, burning, and swelling on exposed body parts
   - Frostbite: Severe tissue and cell damage caused by freezing a body part

The principles of care for cold injuries are to prevent further heat loss, rewarm as quickly as possible, and watch for complications. Specific prevention strategies include:

- Prevention through preparation (length of exposure, anticipating weather changes)
- Layer clothing properly.
- Have dry clothing available, if possible.

TABLE 28-9. Air Quality Index[a]

Index Values	Levels of Health Concern	Health Advisory: Ozone	Health Advisory: PM$_{2.5}$	Health Advisory: CO	Health Advisory: SO$_2$	Health Advisory: NO$_2$
0–50	Good	None	None	None	None	None
51–100	Moderate	Unusually sensitive people should limit prolonged outdoor exertion	None	None	None	None
101–150	Unhealthy for sensitive groups	Active children and adults and people with respiratory disease such as asthma	None	People with CVD (e.g., such as angina) should limit heavy exertion and avoid sources of CO (e.g., heavy traffic)	People with asthma should consider limiting outdoor exertion.	None
151–200	Unhealthy	Active children and adults and people with respiratory disease (e.g., asthma; everyone else, especially children, should avoid prolonged outdoor exertion.	People with respiratory or heart disease, the elderly, and children should avoid prolonged exertion; everyone else should limit prolonged exertion.	People with CVD (e.g., angina) should limit moderate exertion and sources of CO, such as heavy traffic.	Children, asthmatics, and people with heart or lung disease should limit outdoor exertion.	None
201–300	Very unhealthy	Active children and adults and people with respiratory disease (e.g., asthma) should avoid all outdoor exertion; everyone else should limit outdoor exertion.	People with respiratory or heart disease, the elderly, and children should avoid any outdoor activity; everyone else should avoid prolonged exertion.	People with CVD (e.g., angina) should avoid exertion and sources of CO (e.g., heavy traffic).	Children, asthmatics, and people with heart or lung disease should avoid outdoor exertion; everyone else should limit outdoor exertion.	Children and people with respiratory disease (e.g., asthma) should limit heavy outdoor exertion.
301–500	Hazardous	Everyone should avoid all outdoor exertion.	Everyone should avoid any outdoor exertion; people with respiratory or heart disease, the elderly, and children should remain indoors.	People with CVD, (e.g., angina) should avoid exertion and sources of CO (e.g., heavy traffic); everyone else should limit heavy exertion.	Children, asthmatics, and people with heart or lung disease should remain indoors; everyone else should avoid outdoor exertion.	Children and people with respiratory disease (e.g., asthma) should limit moderate and heavy outdoor exertion.

CVD = cardiovascular disease.

[a] Pollutants: ground-level ozone, particulate matter (PM$_{2.5}$), carbon monoxide (CO), sulfur dioxide (SO$_2$), and nitrogen dioxide (NO$_2$).

Adapted from the United States Environmental Protection Agency[54].

Also see Table 3-6.

- Avoid overdressing (excessive sweating and poor evaporation of sweat can promote heat loss in the cold).
- Be able to recognize the signs and symptoms of hypothermia,

ALTITUDE

Acute exercise or sports competition at high altitude is associated with performance impairment (see Chapter 3). Hypobaric environments result in lower partial pressures of oxygen, which limits pulmonary diffusion and oxygen transport in the tissues[28]. Hyperventilation and increased submaximal cardiac output via elevated HR are the primary immediate responses to altitude exposure.

Clinical problems associated with exercise at high altitude can include susceptibility to cold-related disorders and dehydration caused by colder and dryer air temperature as altitude increases. In addition, because the atmosphere is thinner and drier, solar radiation is more intense.

Three medical problems resulting from exercising at moderate to high altitudes include[28]:

1. Acute mountain sickness (debilitating headache, dyspnea on exertion, lightheadedness, fatigue, bluish skin color, loss of coordination of trunk muscles, paralysis on one side of the body),
2. High-altitude pulmonary edema (severe fatigue and weakness, dyspnea, and cough)
3. High-altitude cerebral edema (severe headaches, persistent cough with pulmonary infection, impaired mental processing, and ashen skin color)

Exercise considerations when exercising at altitude include:

- The rate of altitude acclimatization depends on the terrestrial elevation.
- Observable improvements occur within several days. Adaptations need about 2 weeks, although acclimatization to relatively high altitudes may require 4 to 6 weeks.
- Aerobic and endurance-related exercise capacity is reduced because acclimatization does not fully compensate for reduced partial pressure of oxygen at altitude.

POLLUTION

The U.S. Environmental Protection Agency (EPA) is responsible for informing and alerting the general population about air quality[54]. The EPA uses the **air quality index (AQI)** for five major pollutants: ground-level ozone, particulate matter, carbon monoxide, sulfur dioxide, and nitrogen dioxide. For each of these pollutants, the EPA has established national air quality standards to protect against harmful health effects. AQI levels can vary depending on the time of day or from one season to the next. Table 28-9 provides a health advisory statement for the major pollutants and guidelines to follow that protect health and prevent unsafe exercise participation[54].

Summary

Musculoskeletal injuries and other adverse health conditions sometimes occur during exercise participation. Adequate screening and evaluation are important to identify and counsel individuals with underlying contraindications before beginning exercise. Health and fitness facility personnel involved in the management or delivery of exercise programs must possess the knowledge to prevent, recognize, and provide treatment for exercise-related injuries and illnesses. When exercise-related emergencies occur, exercise professionals contribute by taking appropriate action to ensure the individual's health and well being.

REFERENCES

1. Peterson JA, Tharrett SJ, eds: American College of Sports Medicine Health/Fitness Facility Standards and Guidelines, 2nd ed. Champaign, IL: Human Kinetics; 1997.
2. Anderson MK, Hall SJ. Fundamentals of Sports Injury Management. Baltimore, MD: Williams & Wilkins; 1997.
3. National Safety Council: Bloodborne Pathogens. Boston: Jones & Bartlett; 1993.
4. Balady GJ, Chaitman B, Driscoll D, et al: American Heart Association/American College of Sports Medicine Joint Scientific Statement: Recommendations for cardiovascular screening, staffing, and emergency policies at health/fitness facilities. Med Sci Sports Exerc 30:1009–1018, 1998.
5. American College of Sports Medicine/American Heart Association Joint Position Statement: Automated external defibrillators in health/fitness facilities. Med Sci Sports Exerc 34:561–564, 2002.
6. OSHA: The OSHA Bloodborne Pathogens Standard. Federal Register 55:64175, 1991.
7. US Department of Health and Human Services: Physical Activity and Health: A Report of the Surgeon General. Atlanta, GA: US DHHS, Centers for Disease Control and Prevention, National Center for Chronic Disease Prevention and Health Promotion; 1996.
8. Powell KE, Heath GW, Kresnow M-J, et al: Injury rates from walking, gardening, weightlifting, outdoor bicycling, and aerobics. Med Sci Sports Exerc 30:1246–1249, 1998.
9. Schenck RC, ed: American Academy of Orthopaedic Surgeons. Athletic Training and Sports Medicine, 3rd ed. Park Ridge, IL: American Academy of Orthopaedic Surgeons; 1999.
10. Arendt EA: Common musculoskeletal injuries in women. Phys Sports Med 7:39–48, 1996.
11. Andrews JR: Overuse syndromes of the lower extremity. Clin Sports Med 2:137–148, 1983.
12. Renstrom P, ed: The Encyclopedia of Sports Medicine: Sports Injuries. Oxford: Blackwell Scientific Publications; 1993.
13. Renstrom P, Kannus P: Prevention of sports injuries In Strauss RH, ed. Sports Medicine. Philadelphia: WB Saunders; 1992.
14. Shephard RJ, Astrand PO, eds: The Encyclopedia of Sports Medicine: Endurance in Sport. Oxford: Blackwell Scientific Publications; 1992.
15. Requa RK, De Avilla LN, Garrick JG: Injuries in recreational adult fitness activities. Am J Sports Med 21:461–467, 1993.
16. Hootman JM, Macera CA, Ainsworth BE, et al: Association among physical activity level, cardiorespiratory fitness, and risk of musculoskeletal injury. Am J Epidemiol 154:251–258, 2001.
17. American College of Sport Medicine: Recommended quantity and quality of exercise for developing and maintaining cardiorespiratory and muscular fitness, and flexibility in healthy adults. Med Sci Sports Exerc 30:975–991, 1998.
18. Colbert LH, Hootman JM, Macera CA: Physical activity-related injuries in walkers and runners in the aerobics center longitudinal study. Clin J Sports Med 10:259–263, 2000.

19. Kaufman KR, Brodine S, Shaffer R: Military training-related injuries: Surveillance, research, and prevention. Am J Prev Med 18:54–63. 2000.

20. Powell KE, Kohl HW, Caspersen CJ, et al: An epidemiologic perspective on the causes of running injuries. Phys Sports Med 14:100–114, 1986.

21. Kopland JP, Rothenberg RB, Jones EL: The natural history of exercise: a 10-yr follow-up of a cohort of runners. Med Sci Sports Exerc 27:1180–1184, 1995.

22. Garrick JG, Gillien DM, Whiteside P: The epidemiology of aerobic dance injuries. Am J Sports Med 14:67–72, 1986.

23. Mutoh Y, Sawai S, Takanashi Y, et al: Aerobic dance injuries among instructors and students. Phys Sports Med 16:81–88, 1988.

24. Richie DH, Kelso SF, Bellucci PA: Aerobic dance injuries: a retrospective study of instructors and participants. Phys Sports Med 13:130–140, 1985.

25. Jones CS, Christensen C, Young M: Weight training injury trends: A 20-year survey. Phys Sports Med 28:61–72, 2000.

26. Reeves RK, Laskowski ER, Smith J: Weight training injuries: Part 2: Diagnosing and managing chronic conditions. Phys Sports Med 26:54–63, 1998.

27. Kreider RB, AC Fry, ML O'Toole, eds: Overtraining in Sport. Champaign, IL: Human Kinetics; 1998.

28. Mcardle WD, Katch FI, Katch VL: Exercise Physiology: Energy, Nutrition, and Human Performance, 5th ed. Philadelphia: Lippincott Williams & Wilkins; 2001.

29. Raglin J, Audrius B, eds: Overtraining In Athletes: The Challenge of Prevention. A Consensus Statement. ACSM's Health & Fitness J 3:27–31, 1999.

30. Fry AC, Kraemer WJ: Resistance exercise overtraining and overreaching. Sports Med 23:106–129, 1997.

31. Nieman DC: Exercise Testing & Prescription, 5th ed. Boston: McGraw Hill; 2003.

32. Felson DT, Zhang Y, Hannan MT, et al: Risk factors for incident radiographic knee osteoarthritis in the elderly: The Framingham Study. Arthritis Rheum 40:728–733, 1997.

33. Ettinger WH, Burns R, Messier SP, et al: A randomized trial comparing aerobic exercise and resistance exercise with a health education program in older adults with knee osteoarthritis: The Fitness Arthritis and Seniors Trial (FAST). JAMA 277:25–31, 1997.

34. Felson DT, Zhang Y, Anthony JM, et al: Weight loss reduces the risk for symptomatic knee osteoarthritis in women. Ann Intern Med 116:535–539, 1992.

35. Lane NE: Physical activity at leisure and risk of osteoarthritis. Ann Rheum Dis 55:682–684, 1996.

36. Heistaro SE, Vartiainen E, Heliovaara M, et al: Trends in back pain in eastern Finland, 1972–1992, in relation to socioeconomic status and behavioral risk factors. Am J Epidemiol 148:671–682, 1998.

37. Carpenter DM, Nelson BW: Low back strengthening for the prevention and treatment of low back pain. Med Sci Sports Exerc 31:18–24, 1999.

38. Almeida SA, Trone DW, Leone DM, et al: Gender differences in musculoskeletal injury rates: A function of symptom reporting? Med Sci Sports Exerc 31:1807–1812, 1999.

39. Durstine JL, Moore GE, eds: ACSM's Exercise Management for Persons with Chronic Diseases and Disabilities, 2nd ed. Champaign IL: Human Kinetics; 2003.

40. Prentice WE: Arnheim's Principles of Athletic Training, 11th ed. Boston: McGraw Hill; 2003.

41. American Association of Cardiovascular & Pulmonary Rehabilitation: Guidelines for Cardiac Rehabilitation and Secondary Prevention Programs, 4th ed. Champaign, IL: Human Kinetics; 2004.

42. Albert CM, Mittleman MA, Chae CU, et al: Triggering of sudden death from cardiac causes by vigorous exertion. N Engl J Med 343:1355–1361, 2000.

43. Marron BJ, Shirani J, Poliac LC, et al: Sudden death in young competitive athletes. JAMA 276:199–204, 1996.

44. Van Camp SP, Bloor CM, Mueller FU, et al: Nontraumatic sports deaths in high school and college athletes. Med Sci Sports Exerc 27:641–647, 1995.

45. Cummins RO, ed: ACLS Provider Manual. Dallas: American Heart Association.; 2001.

46. Soukup JT, Maynard TS, Kovaleski JE: Resistance training guidelines for individuals with diabetes mellitus. Diabetes Educ 20:129–137, 1994.

47. Hazinski MF, Cummins RO, Field JM, eds: 2000 Handbook of Emergency Cardiovascular Care for Healthcare Providers. Dallas: American Heart Association.; 2000.

48. Venes D, ed: Tabers Cyclopedic Medical Dictionary. Philadelphia: FA Davis Company; 2001.

49. American Diabetes Association: Physical Activity/Exercise and Diabetes. Diabetes Care 27:S58–S62, 2004.

50. American College of Sports Medicine: Heat and cold illnesses during distance running. Med Sci Sports Exerc 28:I–X, 1996.

51. Binkley HM, Beckett J, Casa DJ, et al: National Athletic Trainers' Association Position Statement: Exertional heat illnesses. J Athlet Training 37:329–343, 2002.

52. Casa DJ, Armstrong LE, Hillman SK, et al: National Athletic Trainers' Association Position Statement: Fluid replacement for athletes. J Athlet Training 35:212–224, 2000.

53. American Red Cross: Community First Aid and Safety. Manasha, WI: Banta Printing; 2000.

54. United States Environmental Protection Agency: EPA-454/K-03-002, August 2003. Available at: http://www.epa.gov/airnow/agibroch.

55. Adapted from National Oceanic and Atmospheric Administration: Meteorological tables. Available at http://www.erh.noaa.gov/er/iln/tables.htm

SELECTED REFERENCE FOR FURTHER READING

American Association of Cardiovascular & Pulmonary Rehabilitation: Guidelines for Pulmonary Rehabilitation and Programs, 3rd ed. Champaign, IL: Human Kinetics; 2004.

Fletcher GF, Balady GJ, Amsterdam EA, et al: Exercise standards for testing and training. American Heart Association Scientific Statement. Circulation 104:1644–1740, 2001.

INTERNET RESOURCES

American Academy of Orthopaedic Surgeons: http://www.aaos.org

American Heart Association: http://www.americanheart.org

American Red Cross: http://www.redcross.org

National Athletic Trainers' Association: http://www.nata.org

National Safety Council: http://www.nsc.org

Occupational Safety & Health Administration: http://www.osha.gov

Exercise Testing and Training for Individuals with Chronic Disease

SECTION EDITOR: CAROL EWING GARBER, PhD, FACSM

Pathophysiology and Clinical Features of Cardiovascular Diseases

RAY W. SQUIRES

The burden of diseases of the cardiovascular system on our society is horrendous. Since 1900, cardiovascular diseases (CVDs), such as coronary heart disease, stroke, chronic heart failure (CHF), and hypertension have been the leading cause of death in the United States every year with the exception of 1918, the year of the great influenza epidemic[1]. The annual cardiovascular death rate (per 100,000 population) is 320.57. CVDs cause 2600 deaths *every day* in the United States. It is the leading cause of death in men and women and all ethnic groups: whites, African Americans, Hispanics, Asian/Pacific Islanders, and American Indians/Alaskan Natives. Although the overall CVD death rate has decreased 18% from 1992 to 2002, the total number of deaths has increased slightly.

Approximately 150,000 Americans who die each year as a result of CVDs are younger than age 65 years[1]. Distinct regional variations in death rates exist in the United States, with Mississippi having the highest (424.2 of 100,000) and Minnesota the lowest (247.5 of 100,000) death rates. CVDs claim more lives each year than the next five leading causes of death combined: cancer, chronic lower respiratory tract disease, accidents, diabetes mellitus, and influenza and pneumonia. Estimated direct and indirect costs attributed to CVD are $393.5 billion annually[1]. Coronary heart disease claims more than 500,000 lives annually. Approximately 13 million Americans have suffered a myocardial infarction (MI) or have **angina pectoris,** and ≈700,000 new cases will be observed in 2005. Nearly 1 million individuals undergo either percutaneous (coronary angioplasty or stent placement) or surgical (bypass surgery) revascularization annually, and 4.9 million Americans have a diagnosis of CHF, with approximately 550,000 new cases each year. Valvular heart disease and diseases of the arteries (including peripheral arterial disease [PAD]) kill more than 50,000 Americans each year.

This chapter provides information regarding the following topics in the field of CVDs:

1. The disease process of atherosclerosis and thrombosis
2. Myocardial blood flow, metabolism, and ischemia
3. Stable coronary atherosclerosis
4. The clinical features of the acute coronary syndromes (ACS)
5. The basic pathology and clinical characteristics of CHF, cardiomyopathies, valvular heart disease, adult congenital heart disease, and PAD

Atherosclerosis and Thrombosis

Atherosclerosis is a disease process that may result in blood flow–limiting lesions in the epicardial coronary, carotid, iliac, and femoral arteries, as well as the aorta. Some arteries (brachial, internal thoracic, intramyocardial) are resistant to **atherosclerosis** for unknown reasons[2]. The processes of atherosclerosis and thrombosis are interrelated, and the term *atherothrombosis* has been adopted by some investigators to emphasize this point[2]. Atherosclerosis is just one of several types of arteriosclerosis, which is characterized by thickening and hardening of artery walls, but the two terms are often used interchangeably.

Acute coronary syndromes: An umbrella term describing a group of clinical symptoms compatible with acute myocardial ischemia, including unstable angina and myocardial infarction

Acute myocardial infarction: Prolonged myocardial ischemia that results in death (necrosis) of an area of the myocardium

Angina pectoris: Transient pain or discomfort in the chest (or adjacent areas) caused by myocardial ischemia

Atherosclerosis: A process whereby fatty material is deposited along the walls of arteries. This fatty material thickens, hardens, and may eventually block the artery.

Cardiomyopathy: A heart disease characterized by a weakening of the myocardium that usually results in inadequate pumping function of the heart

Chronic heart failure: A heart disease in which the heart loses its ability to pump blood efficiently

Congenital heart disease: A broad term that refers to diseases of the heart that are present at birth

Myocardial ischemia: Insufficient blood supply to the heart muscle (myocardium)

Sudden cardiac death: Sudden, abrupt loss of heart function in a person with or without diagnosed coronary heart disease

Peripheral arterial disease: Arteriosclerosis of the peripheral blood vessels that may result in ischemia of the muscle supplied by the artery

Thrombosis: A blood clot that forms in a blood vessel or heart chamber and remains there

Unstable angina pectoris: Chest pain of new onset or angina pectoris that lasts for a longer duration, at increased frequency, or at a lower level of exertion than usual or that occurs at rest

Valvular regurgitation: A condition characterized by the inability of a heart valve to close completely, leading to regurgitation

Valvular stenosis: A condition characterized by the inability of a heart valve to open completely so that blood is pumped through a reduced passageway

Thrombosis is a blood clot that forms in a blood vessel or heart chamber and remains there. A thrombus that travels from where it was formed to another location in the body is called an *embolus*, and the disorder, an *embolism* (e.g., pulmonary embolism).

THE NORMAL ARTERY

The channel for the flow of blood within the artery is the lumen. The inner, single cell layer of the artery is the endothelium (Fig. 29-1). The endothelium plays a critical role in maintaining vasomotion (the degree of vasoconstriction) and regulating hemostasis (balancing pro- and antithrombotic properties). When intact, the endothelium produces nitric oxide, a vasodilator, and substances such as plasminogen that inhibit thrombosis formation. Various receptors, such as those for low-density lipoprotein (LDL) and growth factors, are located on the endothelial cells[3]. Under normal circumstances, the endothelium protects against the development of atherothrombosis, but when damaged, it plays a central role in the development of the disease[3].

Underneath the endothelial basement membrane is the intima, consisting of a thin layer of connective tissue with an occasional smooth muscle cell (SMC; see Fig. 29-1). The lesions of atherosclerosis form in the intima[3].

The media contains most of the SMCs of the arterial wall, in addition to elastic connective tissue, and is located underneath the intima between the internal and external elastic laminae (see Fig. 29-1). The SMCs maintain arterial tone (partial vasoconstriction). SMCs have receptors for LDL, insulin, and growth factors. When appropriately stimulated, the SMCs are capable of functioning as synthetic tissue, producing connective tissue[4].

The outermost layer of the arterial wall is the adventitia and consists of connective tissue (collagen, elastin), fibroblasts (cells capable of synthesizing connective

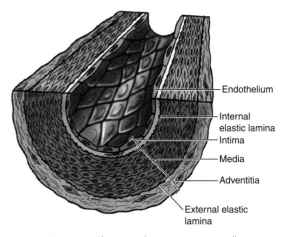

Figure 29-1. The normal coronary artery wall.

tissue), and a few SMCs. This tissue is highly vascularized (i.e., its blood supply is provided by small vessels called the *vasa vasorum*) and provides the media and intima with oxygen and nutrients[3].

ATHEROGENESIS

Our understanding of the development and progression of atherosclerosis (i.e., atherogenesis) is incomplete. However, it is clear that endothelial injury resulting in endothelial dysfunction and a subsequent inflammatory response play critical roles[5]. The disease process may begin in childhood and progress for decades before a clinical event occurs. The rate of progression of atherosclerosis may not be consistent over time and impossible to predict.

Under normal conditions, the endothelium may experience periodic minimal amounts of injury. In these situations, the inherent repair processes of the endothelium are adequate to restore normal function. However, chronic, excessive injury to endothelial cells initiating the process of atherogenesis may result from multiple causes[4–11] (Box 29-1).

Endothelial dysfunction may result from these potentially injurious factors' leading abnormalities characteristic of an inflammatory response (Box 29-2). Platelets adhere to the damaged endothelium (platelet aggregation), form small blood clots on the vessel wall (mural thrombi), and release growth factors and vasoconstrictor substances, such as thromboxane A2[3,4]. These changes indicate a switch in endothelial function favoring a prothrombotic, vasoconstrictive state.

Monocytes, a type of white blood cell, also adhere to the injured endothelium and migrate into the intima. LDL cholesterol (LDL-C) enters the arterial wall and undergoes the process of oxidation. Monocytes accumulate LDL-C, augmenting the oxidation process, and become transformed into a distinctly different type of cell, the macrophage[3,5].

Growth factors expressed by platelets, monocytes, and damaged endothelium result in growth and proliferation

---

BOX 29-1 | **Multiple Causes of Excessive Injury to Endothelial Cells Initiating the Process of Atherogenesis**

- Tobacco smoke and other chemical irritants from tobacco
- Low-density lipoprotein cholesterol
- Hypertension
- Glycated substances resulting from hyperglycemia and diabetes mellitus
- Plasma homocysteine
- Infectious agents (e.g., *Chlamydia pneumoniae*, herpes viruses)

BOX 29-2 | **Abnormalities Characteristic of an Inflammatory Response**

- Increased adhesiveness resulting in platelet deposition and monocyte adhesion
- Increased permeability to lipoproteins and other substances in the blood
- Impaired vasodilation and increased vasospasm

(increase in cell numbers and cell size) of certain types of cells (mitogenic effect), as well as the migration of cells into the area of injury (chemotactic effect)[3,5]. In response to the growth factors, SMCs and fibroblasts (undifferentiated connective tissue cells that can synthesize fibrous tissue) migrate from the media to the intima. Smooth muscle progenitor cells from bone marrow also migrate to the intima[12]. Some of these cells, in addition to monocytes, accumulate cholesterol, forming foam cells that may release their cholesterol into the extracellular space, giving rise to fatty streaks, the earliest visually detectable (yellow macroscopic appearance) lesion of atherosclerosis (Fig. 29-2)[9,13]. Immune system cells, T-lymphocytes, are also present in fatty streaks and are part of the inflammatory state in the arterial wall[14].

With continued migration, proliferation and growth of tissue, the lesion progresses in complexity and size and becomes a fibromuscular plaque (see Fig. 29-2)[13]. The composition of the plaque now includes a fibrous cap, connective tissue extracellular matrix, lipids, inflammatory cells such as macrophages and T-lymphocytes, SMCs, thrombus, and calcium. The typical plaque is firm in texture, pale gray in color, and may contain a yellow cholesterol core.

As the intimal lesions of atherosclerosis progress and thicken the vessel wall, a compensatory outward expansion of the vessel occurs (to a point) and the lumen size remains unchanged. This is called *arterial remodeling* and may be effective in compensating for plaques whose bulk may represent up to 40% of the vessel diameter[15]. With continued progression in plaque bulk, the area of the lumen is reduced and may ultimately result in a reduction in blood flow.

The progression of the size and volume of atherosclerotic lesions is highly variable. Some lesions appear relatively stable over many years, other plaques may slowly progress in size, and other areas of atherosclerosis may enlarge very rapidly[4]. The slowly progressing plaques are thought to gradually internalize monocytes and lipids, and the rapidly progressing lesions incorporate thrombus into the plaque[2]. Local stressors (from turbulent blood flow or vasoconstriction, for example) or chemical factors (enzymes such as metalloproteinases that weaken the fibrous cap) within the lesion may result in plaque rupture or fissuring of the fibrous cap, exposing the internal contents of the plaque to the blood[4,16]. Various amounts of thrombus form in response to this prothrombotic environment and may be incorporated into the plaque. The scenario of plaque rupture, subsequent thrombus formation, and incorporation into the arterial wall may repeatedly occur, giving a layered appearance to the lesion and resulting in rapid progression in the size of the plaque. These lesions, which include organized thrombus, are called *advanced atherosclerotic plaques* (see Fig. 29-2).

Atherosclerosis affects arteries in an extremely diffuse manner with occasional discrete, localized areas of more pronounced narrowing of the vessel lumen[17]. Selective coronary angiography is the gold standard test for determination of the severity of coronary lesions. However, based on comparisons of angiographic and autopsy findings, with the exception of the situation of complete occlusion of the vessel in question (100% stenosis), the degree of stenosis is greatly underestimated by angiography because of the diffuse nature of the disease process[18]. Obstructive coronary lesions (severe enough to reduce blood flow) occur most frequently in the first 4 to 5 cm of the epicardial coronary arteries, although more distal disease may be also seen. Obstructive lesions at the origin (ostial lesions) of the left main and main right coronary arteries may also occur. For reasons not fully understood, women generally lag 5 to 20 years behind men in the extent and severity of coronary atherosclerosis[19].

RISK FACTORS FOR ATHEROSCLEROSIS

Risk factors are associated with an increased likelihood that atherosclerosis will develop over time (see Chapter 5).

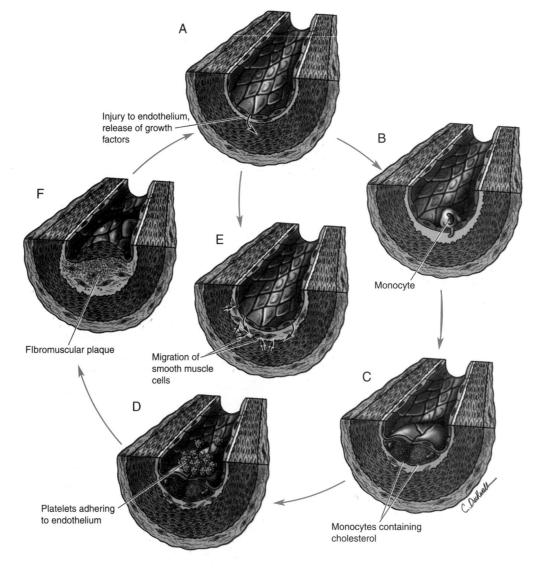

Figure 29-2. The atherosclerotic process: response to injury. **A.** Injury to endothelium with release of growth factors (*small arrow*). **B.** Monocytes attach to endothelium. **C.** Monocytes migrate to the intima, take up cholesterol, form fatty streaks. **D.** Platelets adhere to the endothelium and release growth factors. **F.** The result is a fibromuscular plaque. An alternative pathway is shown with *arrows* from A to E to F, with growth factor–mediated migration of smooth muscle cells from the media to the intima (**E**).

Such factors have been identified on the basis of observational studies evaluating common characteristics of persons with the disease[20,21]. Possible mechanisms of atherogenic effect have been identified for some risk factors. The effects of reducing the severity of some risk factors, especially LDL-C, have been demonstrated to reduce progression of the disease. Predicting whether an individual patient will or will not develop atherosclerosis based on the presence and severity of risk factors is very imprecise, however.

Tobacco usage is a powerful contributor to atherosclerosis, and several atherogenic effects are well established (Box 29-3)[9,22–26].

Dyslipidemia is the term that describes an adverse blood lipid profile. Elevated levels of total cholesterol and LDL-C as well as low levels of high-density lipoprotein (HDL)-C are strongly related to the development of coronary atherosclerosis[27]. Elevated triglycerides are also probably atherogenic. No threshold concentrations for total or LDL-C for atherogenesis have been determined.

Hypertension exerts a direct effect on atherogenesis by causing endothelial dysfunction. It also has detrimental effects on the myocardium by increasing myocyte oxygen requirements and causing left ventricular hypertrophy (LVH)[9,28].

A sedentary lifestyle is a major coronary risk factor with a prevalence of approximately 70% for the U.S. adult population[29]. Poor cardiorespiratory fitness, closely linked to a sedentary existence, is also a prevalent and powerful risk factor[30].

Obesity is closely associated with a lack of regular physical activity but is also an independent major risk factor for the development of coronary atherosclerosis[31]. It is also directly related to several comorbidities related to atherosclerosis: hypertension, glucose intolerance, hypercholesterolemia, hypertriglyceridemia, and reduction in HDL cholesterol[31].

BOX 29-3 Atherogenic Effects of Tobacco Usage[9,22–26]

- Endothelial damage
- Platelet activation and adhesion to the injured endothelium
- Increased release of platelet-derived growth factor
- Carbon monoxide-induced arterial wall proinflammatory state
- Promotion of low-density lipoprotein oxidation
- Increased sympathetic nervous system stimulation; increased blood catecholamines
- Decreased high-density lipoprotein cholesterol (high-density lipoprotein cholesterol)
- Increased thrombosis; increased fibrinogen
- Increased blood viscosity (relative polycythemia)
- Impaired endothelial-mediated vasodilation

BOX 29-4 Potential Mechanisms for Adverse Effects of Diabetes[34]

- Associations of hyperglycemia and hyperinsulinemia with hypertension, low high-density lipoprotein cholesterol, increased triglycerides, and increased obesity
- Increased hemostatic factors (e.g., s fibrinogen)
- Increased inflammatory markers (e. g., C-reactive protein)
- More extensive atherosclerosis in both the proximal and distal coronary arteries
- Diabetic left ventricular diastolic dysfunction
- Dysfunctional autonomic innervation of the heart, resulting in an increased risk of sudden cardiac death

---

A cluster of risk factors, termed the *metabolic syndrome*, is a prevalent (22% of the U.S. adult population) condition closely linked to insulin resistance (impaired normal actions of insulin)[32]. Diabetes mellitus accelerates the development of atherosclerosis and increases the coronary death rate by at least twofold[33]. Potential physiologic mechanisms for these adverse effects of diabetes[34] are shown in Box 29-4 (also see Chapter 33).

A family history of premature coronary events (male first-degree relatives < 55 years; female first-degree relatives < 65 years) is an established risk factor. Although only 2% to 6% of families in the general population have very strong family histories of early coronary disease, they account for nearly 50% of all early coronary deaths in the population[35]. High-risk families share both genetic and environmental factors. Smoking, high saturated fat diet, sedentary lifestyle, depressed HDL-C, and elevated triglycerides cluster in families. With increasing age, cardiovascular risk climbs[21].

Men have a much higher coronary risk than do women, until menopause[26]. After menopause, coronary risk for women increases and coronary atherosclerosis is the leading killer of women, as well as men. The biological basis for these gender differences is not known. Hormonal factors have been proposed, but estrogen replacement therapy has not been demonstrated to lower cardiovascular risk in postmenopausal women. In fact, hormone replacement therapy has been shown to increase the risk of nonfatal MI, stroke, and pulmonary embolus[36].

Some psychosocial factors, such as depression, anxiety, social isolation, lower socioeconomic standing, life dissatisfaction, chronic life stressors, and the coronary-prone behavior pattern, have been established as coronary risk factors[9,26,37]. People with the coronary-prone behavior pattern, also referred to as the type A personality, exhibit specific traits, such as high levels of ambition, aggressiveness, hostility, competitiveness, and a sense of time urgency. This behavior pattern has been shown to be an independent coronary risk factor. Presumably, these psychosocial factors exert their atherogenic potential through neuroendocrine activation mediated by the sympathetic division of the autonomic nervous system[37].

As mentioned previously, prediction of future risk based on the established coronary risk factors is imprecise. Less than half of future cardiovascular events can be predicted using conventional risk factors[38]. Investigators have attempted to discover other "emerging" risk factors that assist in predicting risk, but these factors have not yet become fully established. Plasma homocysteine is an intermediary in the metabolism of the essential amino acid methionine. Elevated concentrations of homocysteine are thought to be atherogenic by damaging the endothelium. Folic acid and B vitamin supplementation lower homocysteine levels but to date have not been demonstrated to lower risk. Fibrinogen, a protein factor in the blood coagulation cascade, is associated with increased cardiovascular risk. Elevated fibrinogen levels are associated with being male, smoking, sedentary lifestyle, diabetes mellitus, and having elevated LDL-C. It is prothrombotic and proinflammatory. Lipoprotein(a) is similar to LDL in lipid composition and in having apo B-100 as a surface lipoprotein. It contains a unique glycoprotein, apo(a) and is associated with elevated cardiovascular risk. This may be because of its LDL-like and prothrombotic properties. LDL particles differ in size and density and may be separated in specialized laboratories. A pattern of having a predominance of small, dense LDL particles is associated with increased coronary risk. Small, dense LDL tends to be associated with elevated triglycerides and low HDL-C. Exercise training and niacin may favorably increase LDL particle size. C-reactive protein (CRP) is a marker for systemic inflammation and is the most well established of the emerging risk factors[39]. It has proinflammatory, proatherogenic, and prothrombotic actions and, in some studies, elevated CRP levels predicted coronary risk better than did LDL-C. Several interventions are known to lower CRP levels: weight loss, exercise, low saturated fat diet, smoking cessation, and use of statin medications and aspirin. It is not known if lowering CRP reduces cardiovascular risk, however.

Myocardial Blood Flow, Metabolism, and Ischemia

Normal contraction and relaxation of cardiac myocytes requires the presence of adequate amounts of adenosine triphosphate (ATP, a high-energy phosphate molecule) in the myocardium. The heart is a highly aerobic organ with an extensive circulatory system and abundant mitochondria[40]. The coronary arterial system includes epicardial arteries (Fig. 29-3) that bifurcate into intramyocardial and endomyocardial branches (Fig. 29-4). At rest, coronary blood flow averages 60 to 90 mL·min^{-1} per 100 g of myocardium and may increase five- to sixfold during exercise[41]. Under usual conditions, the heart regenerates ATP aerobically and myocardial cells are not well adapted to anaerobic energy production. At rest, myocardial oxygen uptake is approximately 8 to 10 mL O_2 per 100 g of tissue per minute. During intense exercise, the oxygen requirement may increase by 200% to 300%[42]. The myocardium

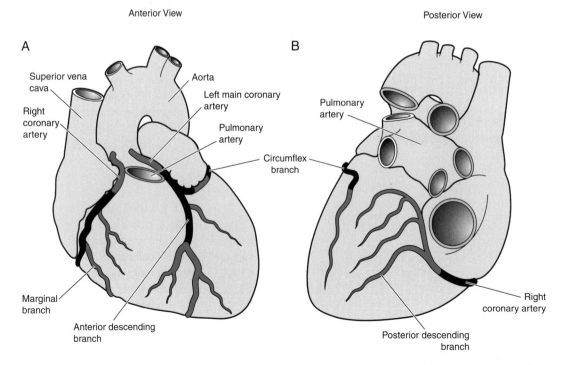

Figure 29-3. The epicardial coronary arteries. **A.** Anterior view. *Black segments* are prime sites for the development of obstructive atherosclerotic plaques. **B.** Posterior view.

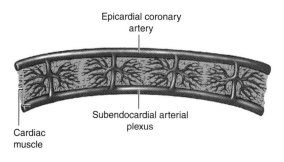

Figure 29-4. Structure of the intramyocardial and subendocardial coronary arteries in relation to the epicardial coronary arteries.

extracts nearly all of the oxygen from the capillary blood flow (unlike skeletal muscle), and coronary blood flow must be closely regulated to the needs of the myocardium for oxygen[43]. With an increase in myocardial work, oxygen demand increases and coronary blood flow must also increase to provide the necessary amount of oxygen (also see Chapter 3).

Blood flow through any regional circulation, including the coronary system, is determined by the blood pressure (BP) and the vascular resistance[43]. During systole, intramyocardial pressure is increased (as is vascular resistance) and the intramural vessels are compressed. Therefore, most coronary blood flow occurs during diastole, when intramyocardial pressure is lower (lower vascular resistance) (Fig. 29-5).

Before a decrease in flow can be measured distal to an atherosclerotic, narrowed coronary artery segment, a substantial reduction in vessel luminal diameter must occur. When plaque bulk reduces the luminal cross-sectional area (CSA) by 75% or more, flow will be reduced under resting conditions (a hemodynamically significant lesion)[41]. Beyond this amount of critical stenosis, further small decreases in CSA of the vessel will result in large

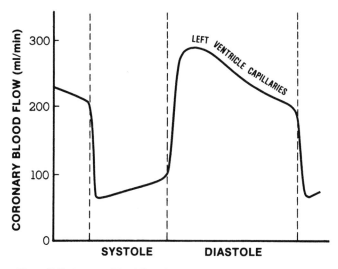

Figure 29-5. Coronary blood flow during systole and diastole. (Reprinted with permission from Guyton AC: Textbook of Medical Physiology, 7th ed. Philadelphia: WB Saunders; 1986.)

BOX 29-5	**Factors Causing Lumen Diameter Reductions**[44,45]

- Significant atherosclerotic plaque
- Vasospasm without underlying plaque
- Vasospasm superimposed over a plaque
- Thrombus associated with plaque rupture

reductions in flow. A reduction in the lumen diameter may be caused by several factors (Box 29-5)[44,45].

Coronary vasospasm may result from several factors, such as endothelial dysfunction, sympathetic nervous system activation (e.g., vasospasm resulting from exposure to very cold ambient temperatures), and bloodborne substances such as epinephrine[46].

Myocardial ischemia results when myocardial blood flow is inadequate to provide the required amounts of oxygen for ATP regeneration (oxygen supply < oxygen demand)[40,41]. Ischemia may result in progressive abnormalities in cardiac function termed the *ischemic cascade*[47]. The first abnormality is stiffening of the left ventricle that impairs diastolic filling of the heart (diastolic dysfunction). Second, systolic emptying of the left ventricle becomes impaired (systolic dysfunction). Localized areas of the myocardium develop abnormal contraction patterns such as hypokinesis (reduced systolic contraction). Left ventricular ejection fraction (LVEF) may decrease. Third, electrocardiographic (ECG) abnormalities associated with altered repolarization (ST-segment changes, T-wave inversion) or arrhythmias may occur. Finally, symptoms of angina pectoris may develop.

Angina pectoris is transient, referred cardiac pain resulting from myocardial ischemia[48]. This chest pain is relieved by rest or nitrate medications within a short period of time (usually less than 15 minutes). A minority of patients with substantial amounts of ischemia do not report pain (silent ischemia). The pain of angina may be located in the substernal region, jaw, neck, or arms, although pain may also occur in the epigastrium and interscapular regions. It is usually described as a feeling of pressure, heaviness, fullness, squeezing, burning, aching, or choking. The pain may vary in intensity and may radiate. The patient may experience dyspnea (anginal equivalent) if the ischemia results in increased left ventricular end-diastolic pressure and increased pulmonary vascular pressure. Typical angina is provoked by exertion, emotions, cold and heat exposure, meals, and sexual intercourse and is relieved by rest or nitroglycerin. Atypical angina refers to similar symptoms but with features that set it apart from typical angina, such as no relationship to exertion. Stable angina is reproducible and predictable in onset, severity, and means of relief. **Unstable angina** is defined as new onset of typical angina, increasing frequency, intensity or duration of previously stable angina, or angina that occurs at rest or in the first few days after **acute myocardial infarction**.

If an episode of ischemia is brief, the contractile abnormalities described above are quickly reversible. Brief, post-ischemic left ventricular dysfunction is called *stunned myocardium*[49]. Chronic, substantial, nonlethal ischemia may result in prolonged but reversible left ventricular dysfunction called *hibernating myocardium*. The myocytes remain viable but exhibit depressed contractile function. Elimination of the chronic ischemia with revascularization results in a gradual return of normal contractile function, although resolution may require up to 1 year[50]. Prolonged, severe ischemia results in myocyte necrosis (irreversible damage, MI).

Stable Coronary Atherosclerosis

Many patients with coronary artery disease have one or more hemodynamically significant lesions that remain anatomically stable over many years. These lesions impair coronary blood flow in a predictable and reproducible manner. Angina pectoris, if present, occurs consistently with various provocative stimuli. The lesions in these patients are thought to be advanced plaques with thick fibrous caps and small amounts of lipid[4].

Medical treatment of patients with stable coronary atherosclerosis includes aspirin, statins, β-blockers, and angiotensin-converting enzyme inhibitors (especially in patients with anterior wall MI or depressed LVEF)[51] Revascularization, percutaneous or surgical, is generally reserved for patients with intractable symptoms or severe ischemia seen with stress testing.

Acute Coronary Syndromes: Unstable Angina Pectoris, Acute Myocardial Infarction, and Sudden Cardiac Death

Unstable angina pectoris, acute MI, and some instances of sudden cardiac death comprise the **acute coronary syndromes (ACS)**[2]. The underlying mechanism resulting in these syndromes is plaque erosion, rupture or other type of plaque disruption resulting in thrombus formation, and possibly vasoconstriction with subsequent vessel occlusion.

The type of ACS that occurs is related to the duration of vessel occlusion. Unstable angina is probably the result of transient vessel occlusion (< 10 minutes) followed by spontaneous thrombolysis (clot dissolution) and vasorelaxation. Vessel occlusion persisting for more than 60 minutes results in acute MI. Ischemia resulting from atherothrombotic vessel occlusion may trigger ventricular tachycardia or ventricular fibrillation and **sudden cardiac death**[2]. Sudden cardiac death is sudden, abrupt loss of heart function in a person with or without diagnosed coronary heart disease. Death occurs immediately or shortly after symptoms appear (within 24 hours). About half of all deaths from coronary heart disease are sudden and unexpected, regardless of the underlying disease, and this disorder is responsible for about 340,000 deaths each year among U.S. adults either before reaching a hospital or emergency room.

Why do some plaques rupture and thrombose? Approximately two thirds of patients with ACS have "high-risk" or "vulnerable" atherosclerotic lesions with thin fibrous caps overlying a lipid-rich core with an abundance of macrophages[2]. Inflammation mediated by various cytokines, including proteases and tumor necrosis factor, erodes the plaque from within. The physical forces assisting with plaque disruption include increased BP or heart rate, local vasoconstriction, and nicotine or immune complexes. After plaque rupture, circulating blood platelets come in direct contact with the thrombogenic internal environment of the plaque, resulting in clot formation[52]. *Angiographic studies have demonstrated that most of these rupture-prone lesions are less than 50% occlusive before they become disrupted*[53]. This explains why many patients who experience an ACS do not have warning symptoms. However, angiographically severe coronary atherosclerosis does increase the likelihood of a coronary event by serving as a marker for the presence of extensive disease, including rupture-prone lesions. Autopsy studies have also demonstrated that many patients have disrupted plaques but no history of an ACS. Thus, not all plaque disruption results in clinical events. In approximately one third of cases, an ACS results from only superficial erosion of a severely stenotic and fibrotic plaque with clot formation caused by a hyperthrombotic state resulting from factors such as smoking, hyperglycemia, or elevated LDL-C levels[2].

ACUTE MYOCARDIAL INFARCTION

Acute MI is the necrosis (death) of cardiac myocytes resulting from prolonged ischemia caused by complete vessel occlusion[54]. The key event in distinguishing reversible from irreversible (infarction) ischemia is disruption of the myocyte membrane, which is a lethal event. The myocyte cannot recover if membrane disruption occurs and cytoplasmic contents spill into the circulation.

In some patients, a precipitating event or "trigger" for the MI may be determined (Box 29-6)[55,56]. Slightly more MIs occur in the early morning hours than at other times, suggesting a role for sympathetic nervous system activation as a trigger[54,56].

Symptoms of MI include chest pain or other anginal sensations, gastrointestinal upset, dyspnea, sweating, anxiety, or syncope. It may be painless (silent MI) in approximately 25% of cases[57]. Pain is often severe, but all intensities of discomfort may be experienced.

The diagnosis of MI is based on the presence of two or more of the following triad: chest pain persisting for 30 minutes or more, ECG ST-segment or T-wave changes, and the presence of blood markers (biomarkers)

BOX 29-6	Potential Events or "Triggers" of Myocardial Infarction[55,56]

- Physical exertion
- Emotional stress or anger
- Surgery associated with substantial loss of blood
- Circadian variation

of myocyte necrosis[57]. The myocardial isoforms (MB) of creatine kinase (CK) and cardiac troponin T are the preferred biomarkers for cardiomyocyte necrosis.

After MI, myocardial cells do not regenerate, and healing occurs via scar formation. Depending on the extent of infarction, scar formation may take days to weeks for completion. The larger the size of the infarction, the larger the size of the scar.

Infarctions are classified as ST segment elevation (STEMI) or non–ST-segment elevation (NSTEMI)[57]. ECG criteria for STEMI and NSTEMI are found in Box 29-7 (also see Chapter 21).

STEMI is the result of an occluded epicardial coronary artery with more extensive myocardial damage and a worse prognosis. NSTEMI have less myocardial damage caused by spontaneous thrombolysis (i.e., clot dissolution). Figure 29-6 shows the evolution of the ECG after STEMI with the formation of a Q wave indicating infarction of all or most of the thickness of the ventricular wall. The STEMI results from ischemic injury, and inverted T waves are caused by ischemia around the outside borders of the infarct. Anatomic localization of MIs is possible if Q waves are formed, as shown in Table 29-1. Several serious complications may arise from acute MI (Box 29-8)[54,56].

Extensive MI, particularly involving the anterior wall, may produce progressive adverse changes in the geometry and contractile function of the ventricle over weeks to months[58]. Left ventricular dilatation involving both the infarcted myocardium (infarct expansion) and the adjacent non-infarcted tissue (ventricular remodeling) may occur. These processes result in progressive thinning of the ventricular wall, enlargement of the cardiac chambers, and the development of CHF.

BOX 29-7	Electrocardiographic Criteria for STEMI and NSTEMI[57]

- STEMI: ST segment elevation of at least 1 mV in two contiguous leads or new left bundle branch block
- NSTEMI: ST segment depression or T-wave inversion persisting at least 24 hours

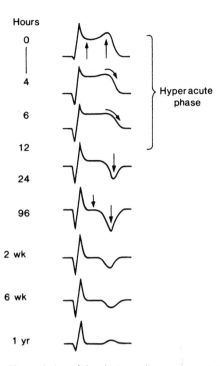

Figure 29-6. The evolution of the electrocardiogram in acute ST segment elevation myocardial infarction resulting in Q-wave formation. (Reprinted with permission from Gau GT: Standard electrocardiography, vectorcardiography and signal-averaged electrocardiography. In Giuliani ER, Fuster V, Gersh BJ, et al, eds. Cardiology: Fundamentals and Practice, 2nd ed. St. Louis: Mosby Year Book; 1991.)

SUDDEN CARDIAC DEATH

Death attributable to cardiovascular causes occurring instantaneously, or within 1 hour of the onset of symptoms, is termed *sudden cardiac death*. This phenomenon accounts for approximately 50% of all cardiac deaths[59]. The vast majority of sudden cardiac deaths are caused by ventricular tachycardia and ventricular fibrillation. The pathophysiology leading to these lethal ventricular arrhythmias may be acute MI, myocardial ischemia, chronic MI (scar-mediated arrhythmia), LVH, or cardiomyopathy. Unfortunately, sudden death may be the first manifestation of cardiac disease for many patients. Additional less common causes of sudden cardiac death include supraventricular tachycardia with an extremely rapid ventricular rate, cardiac rupture (usually in the setting of acute MI), pericardial effusion with cardiac tamponade (i.e., compression of the heart with subsequent rapid decline in cardiac output), and aortic rupture.

Chronic Heart Failure

Chronic heart failure (CHF) is defined as impairment in the ability of the ventricle to eject blood or to fill with blood[60]. CHF is a major public health problem for the United States, accounting for 300,000 deaths every year.

TABLE 29-1. Criteria for Anatomic Localization of Myocardial Infarction by Q-wave Appearance

Inferior wall MI (usually right coronary artery occlusion)	Q-wave (> 40 ms duration; amplitude > 25% of the R-wave) in leads II, III, aVF
Anterior wall MI (left anterior descending coronary artery occlusion)	Q-wave in leads V1–V3 (anteroseptal), QS pattern in leads V1–V3 (anteroseptal), Q wave in leads V2–V4 (anterior), QS pattern in leads V2–V4 (anterior)
Lateral wall MI (usually circumflex coronary artery occlusion)	Q wave in leads V4–V6 or QS pattern in leads V4–V6
Posterior wall MI (usually right coronary artery occlusion)	Prominent R wave in leads V1–V2 with positive T waves
High lateral wall MI (usually circumflex coronary artery occlusion)	Q wave in leads I and aVL or QS pattern in leads I and aVL

MI = myocardial infarction.

Adapted from Gau GT: Standard electrocardiography, vectorcardiography and signal-averaged electrocardiography. In Giuliani ER, Fuster V, Gersh BJ, et al, eds. Cardiology: Fundamentals and Practice, 2nd ed. St. Louis: Mosby Year Book; 1991.

Although patients of all ages may develop CHF, it is primarily a disease of the elderly: 6% to 10% of persons over 65 years of age have the condition, and more Medicare dollars are spent for diagnosis and treatment of CHF than for any other illness.

For the majority of patients with CHF, systolic dysfunction (diagnosed by a below-normal LVEF) is the reason for the inadequate cardiac output. However, for approximately 20% to 40% of patients with CHF, diastolic dysfunction (i.e., impaired ventricular filling with normal systolic function) is the culprit[60]. Some patients have either predominantly systolic or diastolic dysfunction, and others have both conditions concurrently.

For most patients with systolic dysfunction, coronary artery disease is the underlying cause of CHF (ischemic left ventricular dysfunction). Other causes may be identifiable (e.g., hypertension or valvular heart disease) or unidentifiable (e.g., idiopathic dilated cardiomyopathy). Diastolic dysfunction may result from restrictive cardiomyopathy, hypertrophic cardiomyopathy, infiltrative cardiomyopathies, or other unidentifiable conditions[60].

The clinical manifestations of CHF include dyspnea, fatigue, exercise intolerance, and fluid retention that may result in pulmonary or peripheral edema. The natural history of CHF is progressive. It usually begins with a stage of ventricular dysfunction without definite symptoms (asymptomatic left ventricular dysfunction). This progresses to a minimally symptomatic stage and finally to the stage of congestive symptoms of fluid overload. The rate of progression is highly variable. After symptoms of congestion develop, median survival is only 2 to 3 years[60]. Sudden cardiac death is responsible for approximately 40% of deaths in persons with CHF[61]. The classification of CHF is given in Table 29-2 and is based on the progressive nature of the disease and the importance of early treatment for prevention. The progression of CHF is directly related to the process of remodeling, the gradual enlargement of the cardiac chambers and hypertrophy of the walls of the ventricles[60]. Remodeling results in an increase in end-diastolic volume that helps preserve cardiac output in the early stages of the disease. However, with continued remodeling, cardiac size becomes too great, and deterioration in cardiac output occurs, resulting in worsening symptoms in the later stages of CHF[60].

Cardiomyopathies

Cardiomyopathies are a group of diseases of the heart resulting in cardiac dysfunction. They are classified as dilated cardiomyopathy (DCM), hypertrophic cardiomyopathy (HCM), and restrictive cardiomyopathy (RCM).

BOX 29-8	Serious Complications Attributable to Acute Myocardial Infarction[54, 56]

- Life-threatening ventricular arrhythmias (ventricular tachyacardia, ventricular fibrillation)
- Rupture of the ventricular free wall (occurs in < 5% of infarctions)
- Development of a left ventricular aneurysm
- Extension of recurrence of infarction
- Severe left ventricular dysfunction leading to chronic heart failure and cardiogenic shock (a downward cascade of cardiac pump failure resulting in hypotension and reduced coronary blood flow, usually with a lethal outcome)
- Papillary muscle rupture resulting in mitral valve regurgitation
- Pericarditis ("Dressler's syndrome")

TABLE 29-2. Classification of Chronic Heart Failure[60]

Stage	Definition
Stage A	Patients at high risk for developing CHF but have no structural disorder of the heart
Stage B	Patients with structural heart disease but have no symptoms of CHF
Stage C	Patients with past or current symptoms of CHF with underlying structural heart disease
Stage D	Patients with end-stage disease requiring specialized treatment, such as mechanical circulatory support, continuous inotropic infusions, cardiac transplantation, or hospice care

CHF = chronic heart failure.

BOX 29-9	Potential Causes of Idiopathic Dilated Cardiomyopathy

- Genetic predisposition
- Viral or autoimmune processes
- Alcohol abuse
- Chemotherapy (doxorubicin)
- Tachycardia (e.g., atrial fibrillation)
- Peri- or postpartum
- Infiltrative diseases of the myocardium (e.g., hemachromatosis and amyloidosis)

Arrhythmogenic right ventricular dysplasia (ARVD) is a rare form of cardiomyopathy associated with sudden cardiac death in young persons[61].Cardiomyopathy may be caused by viral infections; MI; alcoholism; long-term, severe high BP; or unknown causes.

DILATED CARDIOMYOPATHY

Dilated cardiomyopathy is characterized by dilatation of all four cardiac chambers with depressed systolic function[61]. It is a common cause of CHF. Although the cause of DCM is not apparent in many patients (idiopathic DCM), several causes are responsible in some cases (Box 29-9). In addition, many cases of DCM may be the result of specific diseases (Box 29-10).

Diagnosis of DCM is based on clinical features of heart failure, abnormal ECG findings (left bundle branch block, ventricular tachycardia), and echocardiographic examination.[61]

HYPERTROPHIC CARDIOMYOPATHY

Hypertrophic cardiomyopathy is defined as asymmetric left /or right ventricular hypertrophy involving the interventricular septum with normal or reduced ventricular volume[62]. There are four variants for the location of the sep-

BOX 29-10	Diseases Causing Dilated Cardiomyopathy

- Ischemia cardiomyopathy caused by coronary heart disease
- Valvular cardiomyopathy from severe valvular heart disease
- Hypertensive cardiomyopathy resulting from uncontrolled elevated blood pressure
- Inflammatory cardiomyopathy caused by myocarditis
- Metabolic cardiomyopathy attributable to diseases such as hypothyroidism
- Dilated cardiomyopathy attributable to general system disease (e.g., systemic lupus erythematosus)

tal hypertrophy: subaortic (the most common), apical, mid ventricle, and diffuse. A left ventricular outflow tract (LVOT) gradient may be present at rest or with exercise or may be absent.

Symptoms of HCM include dyspnea on exertion, angina pectoris, syncope or presyncope, heart failure, mitral regurgitation (MR), arrhythmias, and sudden cardiac death. The symptoms are related to the degree of left LVOT obstruction, diastolic dysfunction, and myocardial ischemia (even with completely normal coronary arteries)[62].

Diagnosis is made on the basis of a systolic ejection murmur, abnormal ECG findings (LVH), and echocardiography. Echocardiographic measurement of septal wall thickness greater than 15 mm is the threshold for HCM. HCM is commonly a genetic disorder with transmission to first-degree relatives in half of all cases. The natural history of the disorder is highly variable. Factors associated with a poorer prognosis include a family history of sudden cardiac death, a history of syncope, and severe septal hypertrophy[62].

RESTRICTIVE CARDIOMYOPATHY

Restrictive cardiomyopathy is a rare disorder defined as restrictive filling and reduced end-diastolic volume of either one or both ventricles. Systolic function is normal, as is wall thickness. The primary abnormality is ventricular diastolic dysfunction with a reduced stroke volume[62]. Symptoms include fatigue, dyspnea, and signs of right heart failure. RCM may be idiopathic or associated with other disease processes, such as hemachromatosis, amyloidosis, and eosinophilic endomyocardial disease. Mediastinal radiation therapy may also result in RCM. Doppler echocardiography is helpful in the diagnosis with findings of normal ventricular size and function with marked enlargement of both atria[62].

ARRHYTHMOGENIC RIGHT VENTRICULAR DYSPLASIA

Arrhythmogenic right ventricular dysplasia is a rare genetic form of cardiomyopathy associated with malignant ventricular arrhythmias and sudden cardiac death, often precipitated by exercise. The disease entails progressive fibrous and fatty tissue replacement of the right ventricular myocardium. Patients may present with right heart failure or ventricular arrhythmia. The ECG shows T-wave inversion in the anterior precordial leads. Echocardiographic signs include a dilated, poorly contracting right ventricle[61].

Valvular Heart Disease

The four cardiac valves are shown in Figure 29-7. The leaflets of the valves open and close passively because of transient pressure gradients that occur during the cardiac

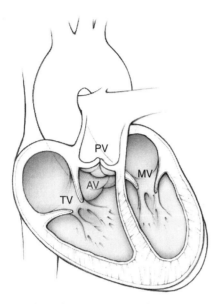

Figure 29-7. The cardiac valves. AV = aortic valve; MV = mitral valve; PV = pulmonic valve; TV = tricuspid valve.

cycle consisting of atrial and ventricular systole and diastole[46]. When functioning properly, the valves maintain the forward flow of blood. The AV valves (mitral valve, tricuspid valve) prevent the backflow of blood from the ventricles into the atria during ventricular systole. The semilunar valves (aortic valve, pulmonic valve) prevent backflow from the aorta and pulmonary artery into the ventricles during ventricular diastole.

Pathology of the cardiac valves includes **valvular stenosis** and **valvular regurgitation**. Stenosis occurs when valve leaflets adhere to each other so that blood flow through the valve orifice (opening) is impeded. Regurgitation is the problem of valve leaflets not closing completely, resulting in a backflow of blood. Stenosis and regurgitation may occur in the same valve at the same time.

AORTIC STENOSIS

Aortic stenosis may result in progressive obstruction of blood flow from the left ventricle, leading to LVH, angina pectoris, dyspnea, syncope, and sudden death[63]. Causes of aortic stenosis include a congenital bicuspid valve (normal aortic valves have three cusps or leaflets), congenital aortic stenosis, rheumatic fever (resulting in thickened, fused valve leaflets), and senile calcific disease. Aortic stenosis is diagnosed by auscultation of the heart (systolic ejection murmur caused by turbulent blood flow through the narrowed valve orifice) and Doppler two-dimensional echocardiography. The severity of stenosis is determined by the valve area and by the mean pressure gradient across the valve measured by echocardiography. This lesion may result in pressure overload of the left ventricle, leading to hypertrophy, dilatation of the chamber, systolic and diastolic dysfunction, ischemia, CHF, and death[63].

MITRAL STENOSIS

The most common cause of mitral stenosis (narrowing of the mitral valve orifice) is rheumatic fever, although this disease is extremely rare today in industrialized countries. Mitral stenosis may lead to increased left atrial and pulmonary vascular pressures and result in significant dyspnea. Echocardiography and auscultation (a "blowing" systolic murmur) are used for diagnosis[63].

AORTIC REGURGITATION

Aortic regurgitation may result from rheumatic fever, a congenital bicuspid valve, infective endocarditis, and senile degeneration of the valve[64]. The regurgitant volume of blood results in an increased left ventricular volume and end-diastolic pressure, leading to pulmonary congestion. Chronic aortic regurgitation results in hypertrophy and reduced systolic function. If severe, the pulse pressure (difference between systolic and diastolic BP) may exceed 100 mm Hg. Doppler echocardiography is helpful in determining the cause and severity of the disease. The auscultatory finding of aortic regurgitation is a "blowing" murmur during diastole. Patients may be asymptomatic for long periods, but after symptoms occur (awareness of overactivity of the heart, exertional dyspnea), prognosis is poor[64].

MITRAL REGURGITATION

The mitral valve is anatomically complex with leaflets and associated structures, chordae tendinae (connective tissue strands from the bottom of the leaflets to the papillary muscles), and papillary muscles (which keep the leaflets from flowing up into the left atrium during ventricular systole). MR results from failure of one or more of these structures. Three mechanisms may cause MR (Box 29-11)[64].

Substantial MR results in a volume overload for the left ventricle and atrium. In severe, acute MR, caused by papillary muscle rupture resulting from MI, pulmonary congestion and dyspnea appear rapidly. Chronic, substantial

---

BOX 29-11 | Mechanisms Causing Mitral Regurgitation[64]

- Abnormal valve leaflets and associated structures, as seen in infective endocarditis, and mitral valve prolapse (billowing of a leaflet into the left atrium during systole)
- Defective chordae tendinea or papillary muscles caused by myocardial ischemia or infarction, degenerative changes in the chordae, and chest trauma
- Increased left ventricular or atrial size, resulting in failure of the valve leaflets to close properly, as observed in severe chronic heart failure

MR may lead to LVH and left atrial dilatation without appreciable symptoms. Eventually, left ventricular function declines and the patient develops symptoms and signs of heart failure. A holosystolic murmur is the characteristic auscultatory finding in MR. The intensity of the murmur does not necessarily correlate with the severity of MR. Doppler echocardiography is performed for assessment of MR severity, as well as for detecting abnormalities of the leaflets, annulus, chordae tendinae, and papillary muscles[64].

TRICUSPID REGURGITATION

The most common cause of tricuspid regurgitation is enlargement of the right ventricle and tricuspid annulus (the valve ring containing the leaflets) because of left-sided valvular disease or CHF[64]. It is rarely an isolated abnormality and is well tolerated in the absence of pulmonary hypertension.

PULMONARY REGURGITATION

In adults, pulmonary regurgitation is usually not clinically important[64]. In fact, Doppler echocardiography frequently demonstrates pulmonary regurgitation in clinically normal patients. The pathology responsible for the lesion is typically pulmonary hypertension or idiopathic dilatation of the pulmonary artery. If it is chronic and severe, it may result in right ventricular overload and right heart failure[64].

Adult Congenital Heart Disease

Congenital heart disease is the general name for any type of congenital (present since birth) malformation of the heart, valves, or great vessels observed in adults. Most severe congenital abnormalities require surgical correction in infancy or childhood[65].

ATRIAL SEPTAL DEFECTS

An atrial septal defect (ASD) is an opening in the atrial septum. If it is large, it results in a left-to-right shunting of blood flow. There are three main types of ASD[65].

- **Secundum ASD:** Most common form in adults. It is a hole in the central portion of the atrial septum. It may result in right ventricular volume overload. Adults with this abnormality are often asymptomatic. If unrepaired, it may result in development of atrial fibrillation with tricuspid valve regurgitation and often right ventricular failure.
- **Primum ASD:** An opening in the lower portion of the atrial septum involving the atrioventricular (AV) septum. The AV valves are abnormal with MR, mitral stenosis and tricuspid regurgitation frequently present.
- **Sinus venosus ASD:** The hole is in the upper portion of the septum. It is usually associated with anomalous pulmonary veins[65].

VENTRICULAR SEPTAL DEFECT

A ventricular septal defect (VSD) is an opening in the ventricular septum. Defects may occur at many different areas of the septum. Small defects often produce a loud murmur but are of little clinical significance. Large defects result in a left-to-right shunt and may produce pulmonary hypertension[65].

COARCTATION OF THE AORTA

This anomaly is a narrowing of the aorta, usually just distal to the left subclavian artery. The narrowing produces systemic hypertension above the coarctation and a reduced BP below the lesion (in the legs). It is more common in men than women and is associated with a congenital bicuspid aortic valve. It is most often diagnosed in childhood and surgically corrected. If not diagnosed earlier, patients may present with systemic hypertension in adulthood[65].

EBSTEIN'S ANOMALY

This abnormality is displacement of the tricuspid valve into the right ventricle, producing an "atrialized" right ventricle above the valve and a small functional right ventricle below. Fifty percent of patients with Ebstein's anomaly have either a patent foramen ovale (a hole in the atrial septum in the fetal heart) or a secundum ASD[65].

CYANOTIC HEART DISEASE

These defects result in deficient oxygen content of the blood of the systemic circulation. These defects usually require surgery early in life, although there are some "natural survivors" who reach adulthood without an operation. Examples of conditions causing cyanotic heart disease are shown in Box 29-12.

Peripheral Arterial Disease

Peripheral arterial disease (PAD), also called peripheral vascular disease, is the highly prevalent condition of progressive atherosclerosis involving the abdominal aorta, iliac, femoral, popliteal, and tibial arteries[66,67]. Ischemia may occur and result in the symptom of intermittent claudication: reproducible aching, cramping, and exercise-induced tightness in one or both legs that is relieved by standing still. Pseudoclaudication, which is caused by lumbar spinal stenosis, is a condition often confused with intermittent claudication and is characterized by bilateral leg pain with standing and walking, which is relieved by sitting and leaning forward. The diagnosis of PAD is made clinically, based on symptoms, or by the ankle–brachial index (ABI) measured supine at rest or before and after treadmill exercise[67,68]. The ABI measurement technique is performed as follows: with the subject in the supine posture, the systolic BPs are recorded in the upper extremities at both brachial arteries and in both lower extremities at the

| BOX 29-12 | Examples of Conditions Causing Cyanotic Heart Disease[65] |

- **Tetralogy of Fallot:** A large subaortic ventricular septal defect (VSD) and obstruction to pulmonary outflow with the aorta overriding the VSD
- **Pulmonary atresia with VSD:** The same intracardiac anatomy as seen in tetralogy of Fallot except that the right left ventricular outflow tract is atretic (severely narrowed or obstructed)
- **Single ventricle:** The most common type in adults is a double inlet left ventricle with associated pulmonary stenosis.
- **Corrected transposition of the great vessels with VSD and pulmonary stenosis:** In this complex abnormality, the right atrium enters into the left ventricle, which ejects blood into the pulmonary artery, and the left atrium enters into the right ventricle, which ejects into the aorta. The circulation flows "correctly" (hence the term "corrected") but flows through the wrong chambers. Although patients with this defect may survive 50 years or more, problems often occur because of the right ventricular support of the systemic circulation.
- **Eisenmenger syndrome:** Defects that begin with a large left-to-right shunt (usually through a VSD) may result in substantial pulmonary hypertension. If the pumonary hypertension is severe, the shunt may reverse itself and become a right-to-left shunt (Eisenmenger physiology).

TABLE 29-4. Fontaine Classification of Peripheral Arterial Disease[66]

Stage	Symptoms
1	Asymptomatic
2	Intermittent claudication
2a	Distance to pain onset > 200 m
2b	Distance to pain onset < 200 m
3	Pain at rest
4	Gangrene, tissue loss

factor in the development of PAD. Additional important risk factors include advancing age, diabetes mellitus, dyslipidemia, hypertension, and elevated plasma homocysteine level[67].

REFERENCES

1. American Heart Association: Heart Disease and Stroke Statistics—2005 Update. Dallas: American Heart Association; 2005.
2. Corti R, Fuster V, Badimon JJ: Pathogenetic concepts of acute coronary syndromes. J Am Coll Cardiol 41:7S–14S, 2003.
3. Ross R: The pathogenesis of atherosclerosis. In Braunwald E, ed. Heart Disease: A Textbook of Cardiovascular Medicine, 5th ed. Philadelphia: WB Saunders; 1997.
4. Fuster V, Chesebro JH: Atherogenesis: Pathogenesis, initiation, progression, acute coronary syndromes, and regression. In Giuliani ER, Gersh BJ, McGoon MD, et al, eds. Mayo Clinic Practice of Cardiology, 3rd ed. St Louis: Mosby; 1996.
5. Ross R: Atherosclerosis—an inflammatory disease. N Engl J Med 340:115–126, 1999.
6. Ross R, Glomset J: Atherosclerosis and the smooth muscle cell. Science 180:1332–1339, 1973.
7. Clowers AW, Reidy MA, Clowers MM: Kinetics of cellular proliferation after arterial injury. I. Smooth muscle growth in the absence of endothelium. Lab Invest 49:327–333, 1983.
8. Faggiotto A, Ross R, Harker L: Studies of hypercholesterolemia in the nonhuman primate. I. Changes that lead to fatty streak formation. Arteriosclerosis 4:323–340, 1984.
9. Fuster V, Gotto AM, Libby P, et al: 27th Bethesda conference: Matching the intensity of risk factor management with the hazard for coronary disease events. J Am Coll Cardiol 27:964–976, 1996.
10. Mayer EL, Jacobsen DW, Robinson K: Homocysteine and coronary atherosclerosis. J Am Coll Cardiol 27:517–527, 1996.
11. Muhlestein JB, Hammond EH, Carlquist JF, et al: Increased incidence of chlamydia species within the coronary arteries of patients with symptomatic atherosclerosis versus other forms of cardiovascular disease. J Am Coll Cardiol 27:1555–1561, 1996.
12. Caplice NM, Bunch TJ, Stalboerger PG, et al: Smooth muscle cells in human coronary atherosclerosis can originate from cells administered at marrow transplant. Proc Natl Acad Sci 100:4754–4759, 2003.
13. Ross R: The pathogenesis of atherosclerosis-an update. N Engl J Med 314:488–500, 1986.
14. Van Furth R: Current view on the mononuclear phagocyte system. Immunobiology 161:178–185, 1982.
15. Libby P: Molecular bases of the acute coronary syndromes. Circulation 91:2844–2850, 1995.
16. Chesebro JH, Zoldelyi P, Fuster V: Plaque disruption and thrombosis in unstable angina pectoris. Am J Cardiol 68:9C–15C, 1991.
17. Lie JT: Pathology of coronary artery disease. In Giuliani ER, Fuster V, Gersh BJ, et al, eds. Cardiology: Fundamentals and Practice, 2nd ed. Chicago: Mosby Yearbook; 1991.

dorsalis pedis and posterior tibial arteries using a Doppler device. The ABI for each leg is calculated by dividing the higher of the two ankle systolic pressures by the higher brachial pressure[68]. Table 29-3 presents a grading system for PAD based on the ABI. The Fontaine Classification System, based on symptom severity, is given in Table 29-4.

Because atherosclerosis tends to affect multiple vascular beds, PAD patients have an extremely poor prognosis with 5-year rates nonfatal MI or stroke of 20% and all-cause mortality of 30%[67]. The ischemia affecting the lower extremities may result in abnormal mitochondrial function and muscle weakness. Walk speed and stride length may decrease, resulting in a further reduction in functional capacity and quality of life. Smoking is the most critical risk

TABLE 29-3. Grading System for Peripheral Arterial Disease Severity[67]

	Supine Resting ABI	Post-exercise ABI
Normal	> 1.0	No change or increase
Mild disease	0.8–0.9	> 0.5
Moderate disease	0.5–0.8	> 0.2
Severe disease	< 0.5	< 0.2

ABI = ahkle-brachial index.

18. Arnett EN, Isner JM, Redwood DR: Coronary artery narrowing in coronary heart disease: Comparison of cineangiography and necropsy findings. Ann Intern Med 91:350–356. 1979.

19. Strong JP, McGill HC Jr. The natural history of coronary atherosclerosis. Ann J Pathol 40:37–49, 1962.

20. Marmot MG: Epidemiologic basis for the prevention of coronary heart disease. Bull WHO 57:331–347, 1979.

21. Kannel WB: Cardiovascular disease: A multifactorial problem (insights from the Framingham study). In Pollock ML, Schmidt DH, eds. Heart Disease and Rehabilitation. Boston: Houghton Mifflin; 1979.

22. Brinson K: Effect of nicotine on human platelet aggregation. Atherosclerosis 20:137–140, 1974.

23. Astrup P: Some physiological and pathological effects of moderate carbon dioxide exposure. BMJ 4:447–452, 1972.

24. Mustard JF, Murphy EA: Effect of smoking on blood coagulation and platelet survival in man. BMJ 1:846–849, 1963.

25. Haft JI. Cardiovascular injury induced by sympathetic catecholamines. Pro Cardiovasc Dis 17:73–86, 1974.

26. Kottke TE, Weidman WH, Nguyen TT: Prevention of coronary heart disease. In Giuliani ER, Gersh BJ, McGoon MD, et al, eds. Mayo Clinic Practice of Cardiology, 3rd ed. St. Louis: Mosby; 1996.

27. Kannel WB: Range of serum cholesterol values in the population developing coronary artery disease Am J Cardiol 76:69C–77C, 1995.

28. Kannel WB, Cuppler LA, D'Agostino RB, Stokes J: Hypertension, antihypertensive treatment, and sudden coronary death: The Framingham study. Hypertension 11(suppl II):II-45–II-50, 1988.

29. U.S. Department of Health and Human Services: Physical Activity and Health: A Report of the Surgeon General. Atlanta: U.S. Department of Health and Human Services, Centers for Disease Control and Prevention, National Center for Chronic Disease Prevention and Health Promotion; 1996.

30. Blair SN, Kohl III HW, Paffenbarger RS, et al: Physical fitness and all-cause mortality: A prospective study of healthy men and women. JAMA 262:2395–2401, 1989.

31. Eckel RH, Krauss RM for the AHA Nutrition Committee, American Heart Association. Call to action: Obesity as a major risk factor for coronary heart disease. Circulation 97:2099–2100, 1998.

32. Ford ES, Giles WH, Dietz WH: Prevalence of the metabolic syndrome among US adults: Findings from the Third National Health and Nutrition Examination Survey. JAMA 287:356–359, 2002.

33. Mokdad AH, Bowman BA, Ford ES, et al: The continuing epidemics of obesity and diabetes in the United States. JAMA 286:1195–1200, 2001.

34. Betteridge DJ: Diabetes and the heart. In Tonkin AW, ed. Atherosclerosis and Heart Disease. New York: Martin Dunitz; 2003.

35. Williams RR, Hopkins PN, Hunt SC, et al: Population-based frequency of dyslipidemia syndromes in coronary-prone families in Utah. Arch Intern Med 150:582–588, 1990.

36. Writing Group for the Women's Health Initiative Investigators: Risks and benefits of estrogen plus progestin in healthy postmenopausal women: Principal results from the Women's Health Initiative controlled trial. JAMA 288:321–333, 2002.

37. Rosenman RH, Brand RJ, Sholtz RI, Friedman M: Multivariate prediction of coronary heart disease during 8.5 year follow-up in the Western Collaborative Study Group. Am J Cardiol 37:903–910, 1976.

38. Kullo IJ, Gau GT, Tajik AJ: Novel risk factors for atherosclerosis. Mayo Clin Proc 75:369–380, 2000.

39. Ridker PM: Clinical application of C-reactive protein for cardiovascular disease detection and prevention. Circulation 107:363–369, 2003.

40. Garratt KN, Morgan JP: Pathophysiology of myocardial ischemia and reperfusion. In Giuliani ER, Fuster V, Gersh BJ, et al, eds. Cardiology: Fundamentals and Practice, 2nd ed. St. Louis: Mosby Year Book; 1991.

41. Braunwald E, Sobel BE: Coronary blood flow and myocardial ischemia. In: Braunwald E, ed. Textbook of Cardiovascular Medicine, 3rd ed. Philadelphia: WB Saunders; 1988.

42. Garratt KN, Morgan JP: Coronary circulation. In Giuliani ER, Fuster V, Gersh BJ, et al, eds. Cardiology: Fundamentals and Practice, 2nd ed. St. Louis: Mosby Year Book; 1991.

43. Guyton AC: Textbook of Medical Physiology, 7th ed. Philadelphia: WB Saunders; 1986.

44. Maseri A: Myocardial ischemia in man: Current concepts, changing views and future investigation. Can J Cardiol July (suppl A): 255A–259A, 1986.

45. Fuster V: Elucidation of the role of plaque instability and rupture in acute coronary events. Am J Cardiol 76:24C–33C, 1995.

46. McGoon MD, Fuster V: Coronary artery spasm and vasotonicity. In Giuliani ER, Fuster V, Gersh BJ, et al, eds. Cardiology: Fundamentals and Practice, 2nd ed. St. Louis: Mosby Year Book; 1991.

47. Nesto RW, Kowalchuk GJ: The ischemic cascade: Temporal sequence of hemodynamic, electrocardiographic and symptomatic expression of ischemia. Am J Cardiol 57:23C–30C, 1987.

48. Shub C: Angina pectoris and coronary heart disease. In Giuliani ER, Fuster V, Gersh BJ, et al, eds. Cardiology: Fundamentals and Practice, 2nd ed. St. Louis: Mosby Year Book; 1991.

49. Ferrari R: Metabolic disturbances during myocardial ischemia and reperfusion. Am J Cardiol 76:17B–24B, 1995.

50. Rahimtoola SH: From coronary artery disease to heart failure: Role of the hibernating myocardium. Am J Cardiol 75:16E–22E, 1995.

51. Smith SC, Blair SN, Bonow RO, et al: AHA/ACC guidelines for preventing heart attack and death in patients with atherosclerotic cardiovascular disease: 2001 update. A statement for healthcare professionals from the American Heart Association and the American College of Cardiology. J Am Cardiol 38:1581–1583, 2001.

52. Frink RJ, Ostrach LH, Rooney PA: Coronary thrombosis, ulcerated plaques and platelet/fibrin microemboli in patients dying with acute coronary disease. A large autopsy study. J Inv Cardiol 2:199–210, 1990.

53. Shah PK, Forrester JJ: Pathophysiology of acute coronary syndromes. Am J Cardiol 68:16C–23C, 1991.

54. Pasternak RC, Braunwald E, Sobel BE: Acute myocardial infarction. In Braunwald E, ed. Textbook of Cardiovascular Medicine, 3rd ed. Philadelphia: WB Saunders; 1988.

55. Mittleman MA, Maclure M, Sherwood JB, et al: Triggering of acute myocardial infarction onset by episodes of anger. Circulation 92:1720–1725, 1995.

56. Gersh BJ, Clements IP: Acute myocardial infarction: Diagnosis and prognosis. In Giuliani ER, Gersh BJ, McGoon MD, et al, eds. Mayo Clinic Practice of Cardiology, 3rd ed. St. Louis: Mosby; 1996.

57. Wright RS, Santrach PJ, Kopecky SL: Diagnosis of acute myocardial infarction. In Murphy JG, ed. Mayo Clinic Cardiology Review, 2nd ed. Philadelphia: Lippincott; 2000.

58. Pfeffer MA, Braunwald E: Ventricular remodeling after myocardial infarction: Experimental observations and clinical implications. Circulation 81:1161–1172, 1990.

59. Osborn MJ: Mechanisms, incidence, and prevention of sudden cardiac death. In Giuliani ER, Gersh BJ, McGoon MD, et al. Mayo Clinic Practice of Cardiology, 3rd ed. St. Louis: Mosby; 1996.

60. Hunt SA, Baker DW, Chin MH, et al: ACC/AHA guidelines for the evaluation and management of chronic heart failure in the adult: Executive summary. J Am Coll Cardiol 38:2101–2113, 2001.

61. Tajik AJ, Murphy JG: Dilated cardiomyopathy. In Murphy JG, ed. Mayo Clinic Cardiology Review, 2nd ed. Philadelphia: Lippincott; 2000.

62. Tajik AJ, Murphy JG: Hypertrophic and restrictive cardiomyopathies. In Murphy JG, ed. Mayo Clinic Cardiology Review, 2nd ed. Philadelphia: Lippincott; 2000.

63. Nishimura RA. Valvular stenosis. In Murphy JG, ed. Mayo Clinic Cardiology Review, 2nd ed. Philadelphia: Lippincott, 2000.

64. Karon BL, Enriquez-Sarano M. Valvular regurgitation. In Murphy JG, ed. Mayo Clinic Cardiology Review, 2nd ed. Philadelphia: Lippincott; 2000.

65. Warnes CA: Adult congenital heart disease. In Murphy JG, ed. Mayo Clinic Cardiology Review, 2nd ed. Philadelphia: Lippincott; 2000.

66. Gardner AW: Exercise training for patients with peripheral artery disease. Phys Sportsmed 29:25–35, 2001.

67. Spittell PC: Peripheral vascular disease. In Murphy JG, ed. Mayo Clinic Cardiology Review, 2nd ed. Philadelphia: Lippincott; 2000.

68. Hirsch AT, Criqui MH, Treat-Jacobson D, et al: Peripheral arterial disease detection, awareness, and treatment in primary care. JAMA 286:1317–1324, 2001.

SELECTED REFERENCES FOR FURTHER READING

Ross R: Atherosclerosis-an inflammatory disease. N Eng J Med 340:115–126, 1999.

INTERNET RESOURCES

American Heart Association: http://www.americanheart.org

Centers for Disease Control and Prevention: Health Topics: Cardiovascular Disease: http://www.cdc.gov/health/cardiov.htm

National Heart, Lung, and Blood Institute: http://www.nhlbi.nih.gov

Treatment of Cardiovascular Disease

NANCY E. O'HARE

Overview and Impact

The economic burden of **cardiovascular diseases (CVDs)** is enormous[1]. In 2004, the indirect (e.g., lost productivity) and direct (e.g., health care) costs of CVD totaled an estimated $351.8 billion dollars in the United States[1]. Appropriate treatment of CVD and risk factor reduction may reduce costs associated with CVD[2–5]. Therapies for the **secondary prevention** of CVD, including smoking cessation; control of hypertension; dyslipidemia; physical activity; cardiac rehabilitation; and treatment with beta blockers, angiotensin-converting enzyme (ACE) inhibitors, and antiplatelet drugs, are believed to be cost effective and are recommended by the American Heart Association (AHA) and the American College of Cardiology (ACC) for nearly all patients with atherosclerosis and related diseases[3,5].

The high cost of CVDs combined with increasing evidence of the cost effectiveness of treatment has led many health care agencies to promote a "disease management" approach to patient care, which consists of a comprehensive plan of care (care map) coordinated among the health care professionals caring for patients[2]. Many experts agree

that future improvements in the **prevalence**, **incidence**, **morbidity**, and **mortality** of CVDs will rely on educating the public to recognize symptoms and obtain prompt medical care; reducing **risk factors** across the life span; and implementing evidenced-based medical, surgical, and emergency treatments promptly and as indicated[2,3,5 6].

Professional organizations, voluntary health care agencies, quality improvement organizations, insurers, and accrediting agencies have identified quality of care indicators to evaluate, promote, and recognize delivery of good health care and adherence to accepted treatment guidelines. The American Medical Association, AHA and the ACC have performance outcome tools available for physicians and health care professionals to assist them in tracking their clinical performance and identifying changes in care over time[7]. The National Committee for Quality Assurance (NCQA) and the Joint Commission on Accreditation of Healthcare Organizations (JCAHO) have both implemented programs for the accreditation and certification of disease management programs in health care settings[2]. The NCQA's Bridges to Excellence Program Cardiac Care Performance Assessment Program recognizes physicians and health care organizations that consistently meet evidence-based treatment guidelines as shown by performance on seven quality of care indicators: hypertension control, blood lipid measurement, control of total and low-density lipoprotein (LDL) cholesterol, aspirin or antithrombotic medication use, and smoking cessation advice[8].

This chapter reviews the treatment of patients with CVDs, including an overview of existing evidence-based treatment guidelines. The first section addresses risk factor management of all CVD diseases (summarized in Table 30-1), and subsequent sections discuss the treatment and secondary prevention specific to several CVD diagnoses (summarized in Table 30-2). Readers will notice that are many similarities in the treatment strategies across the diseases that fall into the category of CVD because of the commonality of the atherosclerosis as the underlying disease process (see Chapter 29 for further disease pathophysiology). Treatment of patients with CVDs is continually being improved as new research is conducted, so readers are encouraged to look at the recommended websites for the most up-to-date information on these topics.

Cardiovascular diseases: Diseases of the circulatory system, including myocardial infarction, coronary artery disease, angina pectoris, valvular heart disease, congestive heart failure, stroke, and peripheral arterial disease

Incidence: How many new cases of a disease have developed in a given population over a particular period of time; usually reported in a 1-year period

Morbidity: The incidence of disease or rate of sickness, usually presented in a specified community or group over a set period of time

Mortality: The number of deaths in a given time or place, usually reported as mortality or death rate, which is

the ratio of deaths to the number of individuals in a population. Mortality rate is usually expressed as number of deaths per hundred or per thousand population for a given period of time

Prevalence: The proportion of a population affected by a disease at a given time, usually a 1-year period

Risk factors: Factors associated with an increased risk or susceptibility for a disease; some examples are cigarette smoking, hypertension, high blood cholesterol, physical inactivity, obesity and overweight, and diabetes

Secondary prevention: Efforts to prevent progression or reoccurrence of disease, performed after the onset of a disease

Education and Risk Factor Management

As discussed in Chapter 5, the primary risk factors for CVD are tobacco smoking, hypertension, high blood cholesterol level, physical inactivity, obesity, and diabetes. Patients with known CVDs have a much greater risk of developing a subsequent CVD event (e.g., myocardial infarction [MI], stroke) compared with persons without disease, so it is extremely important to reduce risk factors in these patients[6,9]. This section emphasizes pharmacologic treatments because lifestyle and behavioral risk reduction methods (e.g., exercise and diet) are discussed in Chapter 31. Secondary prevention guidelines, including risk factor management for all CVDs, are shown in Table 30-1.

SMOKING CESSATION

The risk of CVD morbidity and mortality can be sharply reduced with smoking cessation, with the benefits accruing relatively quickly after smoking is stopped[3,10]. Consider that a person with coronary heart disease (CHD) who quits smoking may reduce risk of death and another MI by as much as 50%[10]. There is also evidence that patients who are advised to quit shortly after a health crisis such as an MI are more likely to stay quit in the long term. Thus, it is particularly important that this risk behavior be addressed by health professionals during the acute phase of the illness[10]. Specific techniques for assisting patients with smoking cessation may be found at the websites of the National Cancer Institute and the American Cancer Society, which are listed at the end of this chapter.

HYPERTENSION

Hypertension is unique in that it is both a CVD (see Chapter 29) and a risk factor for CVD (see Chapter 5). Of con-

cern, hypertension is currently the most common primary medical diagnosis in the United States, affecting more than 50 million people[11]. Elevations in blood pressure (BP), both systolic and diastolic, are an important risk factor for nearly all CVDs[11]. Patients with hypertension have an elevated risk of heart attack and other coronary heart disease events and are more likely to die after an MI. It is also well known that the risk of cerebrovascular disease, such as ischemic stroke, hemorrhagic stroke, and dementia, increases as a direct function of BP levels.

Hypertension is also a major contributory factor to the development of heart failure in more than 90% of all patients with heart failure, with a disproportional effect in African American and elderly persons. Many are not aware that hypertension contributes to renal insufficiency and renal failure as well (see Chapter 33). Hypertension accelerates the decline in renal function that occurs with aging and, thus, increases the risk of development of chronic renal failure and end-stage renal disease. The good news is control of systolic and diastolic hypertension has been found to result in reductions in all-cause and CVD mortality and decrease the morbidities of MI, myocardial ischemia, ischemic and hemorrhagic stroke, and heart failure[11].

The Joint National Committee on Prevention, Detection, Evaluation and Treatment of High Blood Pressure seventh report (JNC-VII) added a striking addition to previous classification and treatment guidelines, with the formal identification of a group of persons who are at high risk of developing hypertension[11]. Prehypertensive individuals include those with systolic BP ranging from 120 to 139 mm Hg or diastolic BP from 80 to 89 mm Hg. Essentially, patients in the prehypertension category are "on watch" and should monitor their BP regularly and modify their risk factors for hypertension and other CVDs. Drug

TABLE 30-1. American Heart Association/American College of Cardiology Secondary Prevention for Patients with Coronary and Other Vascular Disease: 2001 Update

Component	Goal	Intervention Recommendations
Smoking	Complete cessation	Assess tobacco use. Strongly encourage patient and family to stop smoking and to avoid secondhand smoke. Provide counseling, pharmacologic therapy (including nicotine replacement and buproprion), and formal smoking cessation programs, as appropriate.
BP control	< 140/90 mm Hg or < 130/85 mm Hg if heart failure or renal insufficiency < 130/80 mm Hg if diabetes	Initiate lifestyle modification (weight control; physical activity; alcohol moderation; moderate sodium restriction; and emphasis on fruits, vegetables, and low-fat dairy products) in all patients with BP > 130 mm Hg systolic or 80 mm Hg diastolic. Add BP medication, individualized to other patient requirements and characteristics (i.e., age, race, need for drugs with specific benefits) if BP is not < 140 mm Hg systolic or < 90 mm Hg diastolic or if BP is not < 130 mm Hg systolic or 85 mm Hg diastolic for individuals with heart failure or renal insufficiency (< 80 mm Hg diastolic for individuals with diabetes).
Lipid management	Primary Goal: LDL < 100 mg·dL⁻¹	Start dietary therapy in all patients (< 7% saturated fat and < 200 mg/dL cholesterol) and promote physical activity and weight management. Encourage increased consumption of omega-3 fatty acids. Assess fasting lipid profile in all patients and within 24 hours of hospitalization for those with an acute event. If patient is hospitalized, consider adding drug therapy on discharge. Add drug therapy according to the following guide:

$LDL < 100$ mg·dL⁻¹ (baseline or on-treatment) — Further LDL-lowering therapy not required. Consider fibrate or niacin (if low HDL or high TG)

LDL 100–129 mg·dL⁻¹ (baseline or on treatment) — Therapeutic options: Intensify LDL-lowering therapy (statin or resin[a]). Fibrate or niacin (if low HDL or high TG). Consider combined drug therapy (statin, fibrate or niacin) (if low HDL or high TG)

$LDL > 130$ mg·dL⁻¹ (baseline or on treatment) — Intensify LDL-lowering therapy (statin or resin[a]). Add or increase drug therapy with lifestyle therapies

Component	Goal	Intervention Recommendations
Lipid management	Secondary goal If TG ≥ 200 mg·dL⁻¹, then non-HDL[b] should be < 130 mg·dL⁻¹	If TG ≥ 150 mg·dL⁻¹ or HDL < 40 mg·dL⁻¹: Emphasize weight management and physical activity. Advise smoking cessation. If TG 200–499 mg·dL⁻¹: Consider fibrate or niacin after LDL-lowering therapy[a] If TG ≥ 500 mg·dL⁻¹: Consider fibrate or niacin before LDL-lowering therapy[a] Consider omega-3 fatty acids as adjunct for high TG
	Physical activity: Minimum goal 30 minutes 3 to 4 days per week Optimal daily	Assess risk, preferably with exercise test, to guide prescription. Encourage minimum of 30 to 60 minutes of activity (walking, jogging, cycling, or other aerobic activity), preferably daily or at least three or four times weekly, supplemented by an increase in daily lifestyle activities (e.g., walking breaks at work, gardening, household work). Advise medically supervised programs for moderate- to high-risk patients.
Weight management	BMI 18.5–24.9 kg·m⁻²	Calculate BMI and measure waist circumference as part of evaluation. Monitor response of BMI and waist circumference to therapy. Start weight management and physical activity as appropriate. Desirable BMI range is 18.5–24.9 kg·m⁻². When BMI ≥ 25 kg·m⁻², goal for waist circumference is ≤ 40 inches in men and ≤ 35 inches in women.

TABLE 30-1. American Heart Association/American College of Cardiology Secondary Prevention for Patients with Coronary and Other Vascular Disease: 2001 Update *(continued)*

Component	Goal	Intervention Recommendations
Diabetes management	$HbA_{1c} < 7\%$	Provide appropriate hypoglycemic therapy to achieve near-normal fasting plasma glucose level, as indicated by HbA1c.
		Provide treatment of other risks (e.g., physical activity, weight management, BP, and cholesterol management).
	Antiplatelet agents/anticoagulants:	Start and continue indefinitely aspirin 75 to 325 mg·d^{-1} if not contraindicated.
		Consider clopidogrel 75 mg·d^{-1} or warfarin if aspirin is contraindicated.
		Manage warfarin to INR = 2.0 to 3.0 in post-MI patients when clinically indicated or for those not able to take aspirin or clopidogrel.
	ACE inhibitors	Treat all patients indefinitely post-MI; start early in stable high-risk patients (anterior MI, previous MI, Killip class II [S3 gallop, rales, radiographic CHF]). Consider chronic therapy for all other patients with coronary or other vascular disease unless contraindicated.
	Beta-blockers	Start in all post-MI and acute ischemic syndrome patients.
		Continue indefinitely. Observe usual contraindications.
		Use as needed to manage angina, rhythm, or BP in all other patients

aThe use of resin is relatively contraindicated when TG > 200 mg·dL^{-1}.

bNon-HDL cholesterol = total cholesterol minus HDL cholesterol.

ACE = angiotensin-converting enzyme; BMI = body mass index; BP = blood pressure; CHF = congestive heart failure; HbA_{1c} = major fraction of adult hemoglobin; HDL = high-density lipoprotein; INR = international normalized ratio; LDL = low-density lipoprotein; MI = myocardial infarction; TG = triglyceride.

Adapted from Smith SC Jr, Blair SN, Bonow RO, et al: AHA/ACC Guidelines for Preventing Heart Attack and Death in Patients with Atherosclerotic Cardiovascular Disease: 2001 update. A statement for healthcare professionals from the American Heart Association and the American College of Cardiology. J Am Coll Cardiol 38:1581–1583, 2001.

Also see Chapter 5 for more information on risk factor management.

TABLE 30-2. Treatment for Cardiovascular Disease

Diagnosis	Treatments
ACS	Oxygen, IV, ECG, nitroglycerin, aspirin, thrombolysis, primary angioplasty
Chronic CAD	Review and adjust risk factors
	Beta-blocker, ACE inhibitor, antiplatelet therapy
	Angioplasty, stents
	CABG
Hypertension	Review and adjust risk factors
	Weight management
	Reduce salt and alcohol intake
	Antiplatelet therapy, diuretics
	Beta-blockers, ACE inhibitors, CCBs, ARBs
Arrhythmias	Review and adjust risk factors
	Pharmacologic therapy, including anticoagulation
	Cardioversion
	Ablation
	Pacemaker
	Defibrillator
Valvular disease	Pharmacologic therapy, including antibiotic prophylaxis
	Valvuloplasty
	Valve replacement
Heart failure	Review and adjust risk factors
	Diuretic, ACE inhibitor, beta-blocker
	Pacemaker
	Defibrillator
	Biventricular pacing
	CABG
	LVAD
	Cardiac transplant

ACE = angiotensin-converting enzyme; ACS = acute coronary syndromes; ARB = angiotensin receptor blocker; CABG= coronary artery bypass graft; CAD = coronary artery disease; CCB = calcium channel blocker; ECG = electrocardiogram; IV = intravenous; LVAD = left ventricular assist device.

therapy is not indicated for prehypertensive individuals, except in the presence of diabetes or renal failure[11].

The initiation of pharmacologic therapy for hypertension is recommended by the JNC-VII for all people in whom hypertension has been established (systolic BP of ≥ 140 mm Hg or diastolic BP ≥ 90 mm Hg) or for those with diabetes or renal failure who have systolic BP of 130 mm Hg or higher and/or diastolic BP of 80 mm Hg or more[11]. The JNC-VII algorithm for treatment of hypertension is shown in Figure 5-4. Treatment that is more aggressive is recommended for patients with coexisting diseases such as previous MI or stroke. Thiazide diuretics (e.g., hydrochlorothiazide) are the first-line treatment of choice, with beta-blockers, ACE inhibitors, calcium channel blockers, and angiotensin receptor blockers indicated in addition, depending on the presence of other comorbid conditions. Most patients require two antihypertensive agents to gain adequate control of their hypertension (i.e., target systolic BP < 140 mm Hg and diastolic BP ≤ 90 mm Hg with compelling conditions)[11]. Patients with coronary artery disease (CAD) appear to have an increased risk of CVD risk with low diastolic BP (i.e., ≤ 55 mmHg). In the presence of stable angina and silent ischemia, beta blockers are the recommended first-line therapy for hypertension. The JNC-VII recommends that all health care professionals work to enhance BP control by "providing reinforcing messages about the risks of hypertension, the importance of managing both SBP [systolic BP] and DBP [diastolic BP] and achieving goal BP, education about effective lifestyle interventions, pharmacologic therapies, and adherence to treatment"[11].

Exercise training is an important component of treatment for patients with hypertension, whether or not they have overt CVD[11–13] (see Chapter 31). Patients with CVD, multiple risk factors, or older age are at the highest risk of complications during exercise, and it is recommended that all of these patients have a medically supervised peak or symptom-limited exercise test with electrocardiographic (ECG) monitoring before embarking on a program of vigorous exercise[1,12,14]. Moderate exercise is suggested before formal exercise evaluation[12], although there is some controversy about the efficacy of exercise testing before moderate exercise[13]. See Chapter 6 and GETP7 Chapter 2 for further discussion of risk stratification and testing supervision. It is also recommended that ACE inhibitors and calcium channel antagonists be used for recreational athletes and chronic exercisers[12]. The ACSM's position stand on exercise and hypertension recommendations for exercise in patients with hypertension is shown in Box 30-1[12].

DYSLIPIDEMIA

The National Cholesterol Education Program issued its third report (Adult Treatment Panel III; ATP3) in September 2002[15]. The ATP3 address the diagnosis and treatment of dyslipidemia and its treatment algorithm has three risk categories: (a) established CHD and CHD risk equivalents (e.g., noncoronary forms of clinical atherosclerotic disease, diabetes, and two or more CHD risk factors with 10-year risk for CHD greater than 20%), (b) two or more risk factors, and (c) one risk factor or less[15] (see Box 5-2).

Thus, all persons with CHD or CHD risk equivalents are considered by the ATP3 to be at high risk[15]. According to the ATP3 treatment algorithm, the optimal level of LDL cholesterol (LDL-C) for high-risk persons is less than 100 mg·dL^{-1} and high-density lipoprotein (HDL) cholesterol (HDL-C) greater than 40 mg·dL^{-1} in patients with CVD. Triglyceride (TG) levels of 150 mg·dL^{-1} or more also indicate the need for lifestyle or drug treatment. The ATP3 recommends that an LDL-C less than 100 mg·dL^{-1},

whether on baseline or with treatment, needs no further LDL-lowering therapy. Lowering dietary therapy should be initiated for all high-risk patients with LDL-C levels of 100 mg·dL^{-1} or more. When the baseline LDL-C is 130 mg·dL^{-1} or more, an LDL-lowering drug should be started simultaneously with dietary therapy. For LDL cholesterol levels between 100 and 129 mg·dL^{-1}, it is recommended that more intensive dietary therapy be used, and an LDL-lowering drug is optional. In addition, for patients with elevated triglycerides (> 200 mg·dL^{-1}) or low HDL-C (< 40 mg·dL^{-1}), a drug that targets these abnormalities may be added[15].

In 2004, some revised recommendations were added to the ATP3 based on the results of recent randomized clinical trials[16]. The major modification in this report is to add the recommendation for clinicians to consider more aggressive treatment goals for very high- and moderate-risk patients. In very high-risk patients, an LDL-C goal of less than 70 mg·dL^{-1} can be considered, as should combining a fibrate or nicotinic acid with an LDL-lowering drug if the patient has high triglycerides or a low HDL level. In the moderate-risk category, the revised recommendations suggest that an LDL-C goal of less than 100 mg·dL^{-1} is a therapeutic option. This means that lipid-lowering therapy can be considered for persons with a baseline LDL-C of 100 to 129 mg·dL^{-1}. It is also recommended that a reduction in LDL-C levels of at least 30% to 40% is the treatment goal whenever drug therapy is initiated. Finally, this report recommends lifestyle modification for behavioral risk factors (e.g., obesity, physical inactivity, elevated triglyceride level, low HDL-C level, or metabolic syndrome) in all high- and moderate-risk patients with these risk factors, no matter what their LDL-C levels.

PHYSICAL ACTIVITY

The value of regular physical activity and exercise is incontrovertible, with the greatest value is found in moving people from the inactive state to the active state[13,17,18]. The recommendation of the first Surgeon General's Report on Physical Activity and Health[18] applies to patients with CVD as long as there are no contraindications to exercise. Patients with CVD should accumulate of 30 minutes of at least moderate-intensity physical activity, preferably all days of the week. A more detailed discussion of the recommendations for exercise and physical activity may be found in Chapter 31, Chapter 8 of GETP7, and Thompson et al[13].

OVERWEIGHT AND OBESITY

The contribution of obesity to cardiovascular risk is well known[19]. Guidelines for the clinical evaluation and treatment of overweight and obesity have been established based on the classifications of the body mass index (BMI)[20]. The combination of diet and exercise is the most effective to restore a healthy BMI, and readers are referred to Chapter 26 for further details about weight management.

| **BOX 30-1** | **Exercise Prescription for Persons with Hypertension** |

Frequency: on most, preferably all, days of the week

Intensity: moderate-intensity (40–60% of $\dot{V}O_2R$)

Time: 30 min of continuous or accumulated physical activity per day

Type: Primarily endurance physical activity supplemented by resistance exercise

(From Pescatello LS, Franklin BA, Fagard R, Farquhar WB, Kelley GA, Ray CA; American College of Sports Medicine. American College of Sports Medicine position stand. Exercise and hypertension. Med Sci Sports Exerc. 2004 Mar;36(3):533–53.)

DIABETES

The relationship of diabetes to CVD has been described and is of great concern in patients with known CVD. For example, patients with diabetes often encounter greater complications after MI and after revascularization procedures[21]. In all patients with CVD, screening for and identification of diabetes is important. In those with identified hyperglycemia, aggressive management of diabetes is vital, with a target glycosylated hemoglobin level of less than 7%[9]. See Chapter 33 for a more detailed discussion of diagnosis and treatment of patients with diabetes.

Diagnosis and Treatment

ACUTE CORONARY SYNDROME

Acute coronary syndrome (ACS) is an umbrella term encompassing conditions involving myocardial ischemia, including unstable angina, non–Q-wave MI, and Q-wave MI[22]. The most common presentation of ACS in the emergency room is chest pain; however, some patients may have atypical symptoms, which makes it difficult to diagnose ACS by symptoms alone. Misinterpretation of ACS symptoms is thought to produce the greatest number of adverse events in patients presenting to emergency rooms. It is for this reason that many major medical centers have initiated a chest pain center that often includes observation and exercise testing done when the ECG is normal, the first set of enzymes (i.e., creatine kinase-MB and troponin) is normal, and the symptoms are not believed to be angina[22]. Chest pain units may help to more accurately identify low-risk patients who may have coronary artery disease requiring treatment[22].

The treatment algorithms for ACS are aimed at reducing the likelihood of an adverse CVD event; providing symptomatic relief; and after the acute phase, modifying risk factors and secondary prevention.(see Table 30-2[22–24]). The diagnosis of MI is made using patient history and presentation, ECG (non–ST-segment elevation MI and ST-segment elevation MI), and enzyme levels[22,24]. The treatment of patients with acute MI and unstable angina begins out of the hospital with the following[25]:

1. Early recognition of symptoms by the patient or other persons
2. Aspirin (chewed for prompt absorption into the blood)
3. Rapid emergency transport to the hospital
4. Advanced cardiac life support, as needed

In the emergency department, the following steps are taken[23]:

1. Obtain an ECG
2. Determine the presence of cardiac biomarkers of necrosis
3. Administer supplemental oxygen
4. Give sublingual nitroglycerine

5. Provide aspirin (if not administered earlier)
6. Provide opiate analgesia
7. Perform thrombolysis or percutaneous revascularization (i.e., reperfusion therapy)

Early reperfusion (restoring patency) of the infarct-related artery, ideally within 1 to 2 hours of symptom onset with either thrombolytic agents or immediate coronary angioplasty with stent (metal support device) deployment (termed "myocardial salvage") may restore normal blood flow and reduce the size of the area of infarction[23,25]. Thrombolysis may be performed if the infarct is an ST-elevation infarct MI (STEMI) with an age of less than 6 hours. If a cardiac catheterization laboratory is available, angioplasty and the use of stents is the treatment of choice. The speed of application of reperfusion therapy after symptom onset is the critical factor in myocardial salvage. Reperfusion therapy administered more than 12 hours after the onset of infarction is usually of no benefit. Standard treatment during hospitalization includes[23,25]:

1. Continuous ECG monitoring for 24 or more hours
2. Serial ECGs
3. Serial biomarker measurements
4. Intravenous nitroglycerine
5. Beta-blocker medications
6. Aspirin
7. ACE inhibiting drugs with STEMI, left ventricular dysfunction, left bundle branch block
8. Statin medications

CHRONIC TREATMENT FOR POST-MYOCARDIAL INFARCTION PATIENTS

Treatment after MI may include treatment with drugs or revascularization procedures and therapies for secondary prevention (see Table 30-2). Chronic use of beta-blockers, ACE inhibitors, aspirin or its equivalent, and lipid-lowering therapy has been advocated for most post-MI patients[23]. Beta-blockers decrease the work of the heart; ACE inhibitors have the potential to reduce infarct size and remodeling, and aspirin reduces the possibility of the formation of thrombus. Symptomatic relief of angina can be provided by the use of nitroglycerin in the sublingual, spray, or oral form. As mentioned previously, risk factors must be continually reviewed and modified to reduce CVD risk. Regular office visits and scheduled testing, including ECG, exercise or stress testing, and blood work, may be indicated. Patients with positive exercise test results may also be referred for diagnostic cardiac catheterization and revascularization procedures, including percutaneous coronary angioplasty (PTCA) and coronary artery bypass (CABG) surgery[26]. The goal of revascularization is to achieve the largest luminal diameter in a diseased segment of an artery to produce the greatest possible increase in blood flow and to reduce the risk of restenosis. Restenosis is defined as the development of narrowing at a site previously treated by revascularization. Restenosis is considered significant if it occurs in less than 6 months after the procedure and if the site is reduced by 30% or more of previously achieved luminal diameter[26].

The use of devices such as stents (bare metal intracoronary stents and drug-eluting stents), as opposed to angioplasty alone, appear to show the greatest probability of preventing adverse CVD events and restenosis of the vessel[27]. Percutaneous coronary interventions (PCIs) have been used successfully on native coronary arteries, coronary artery grafts, and allografts in cardiac transplant patients. Patients with multivessel disease or lesions that are more complex more often receive CABGs, but recent evidence has supported the efficacy of PTCA in some patients with multivessel disease[28–30]. Other potentially useful interventions include transmyocardial laser revascularization (TMLR) and therapeutic angiogenesis[31].

Coronary artery bypass surgery has been available to patients for several decades. CABG involves the surgical implantation of venous or arterial grafts that are attached to bypass the stenotic coronary artery segment[32]. The procedure can be performed on a single vessel or multiple vessels. CABG can be performed with a cardiopulmonary bypass pump or off pump in selected patients, and promising newer minimally invasive techniques currently are being evaluated (e.g., minimally invasive direct CABG[32,33]). The choice to use PCI rather than CABG depends on the patient characteristics, including the number and complexity of the lesions and concurrent comorbidity[34].

STABLE ANGINA PECTORIS

Initial treatment of stable angina pectoris follows an ABCDE acronym[35]:

A = Aspirin and antianginal therapy
B = Beta-blocker and BP
C = Cigarette smoking and cholesterol
D = Diet and diabetes
E = Education and exercise

Treatment for unstable angina can be divided into two parts: therapy to reduce angina and education and risk factor modification[35]. The goals of treatment of chronic stable angina are to reduce the risk of mortality and morbidity and to reduce symptoms. Antianginal therapy may include beta-blockers, calcium antagonists, long-acting nitrate medications, or a combination[35]. Risk factor modification and secondary prevention strategies previously discussed in this chapter apply to patients with stable angina as well. In addition, every patient with angina pectoris needs to have a prescription for sublingual nitroglycerin and receive education about its use[35]. Revascularization procedures already discussed may also be considered for patients with significant left main or multivessel disease, previous episode of ventricular tachycardia, or chronic stable angina who cannot be adequately treated medically[35]. A summary of treatment for angina pectoris may be found in Table 30-1, and further details about the treatment of angina pectoris may be found in Gibbons et al[35].

SECONDARY PREVENTION RECOMMENDATIONS FOR PATIENTS WITH CARDIOVASCULAR DISEASE

Secondary prevention and risk factor management must be revisited on a regular basis in all patients with CVD[6,36,37]. Guidelines for secondary prevention are shown in Table 30-1[9]. Essentially, the previously discussed risk reduction strategies apply, along with the addition of three pharmacologic therapies: antiplatelet medications (e.g., aspirin), ACE inhibitors, and beta-blockers.

WOMEN AND HEART DISEASE

Cardiovascular disease is the leading cause of death of women in the United States and in most developed areas of the world. In the United States, more than 500,000 women die of CVD each year, with nearly two thirds of women who dying suddenly with no previously recognized symptoms[37]. Since the early 1990s, special attention has been paid to the diagnosis and treatment of women with CVD because there had been few studies that had included women.

The diagnosis of myocardial ischemia and CAD is a challenge in women, partly because of gender differences in pain reporting. It is well recognized that the chest pain is less likely to be associated with significant coronary stenoses in women compared with men[38]. Symptoms in women are generally believed to be less sensitive and specific for the diagnosis of ischemic heart disease compared with men[39]. In addition, standard stress testing methods that evaluate ECG changes, myocardial perfusion defects, and regional wall motion abnormalities often are of limited value in women undergoing evaluation for CAD[38]. The reason for these differences may result from a high prevalence of abnormal endothelial dysfunction, resulting in flow limitations (and probably symptoms), and a lower prevalence of flow limiting large vessel coronary stenoses in women[40]. In 2004, the AHA published an expert panel report on the prevention of CVD in women based on the current evidence from studies of women[37]. This report may be found on the AHA's website (see Internet Resources).

ARRHYTHMIAS

Arrhythmias are disorders of the heart rhythm that include rhythms that originate along the conduction system of the atria and ventricles. Arrhythmias can occur alone or concomitantly with other heart diseases such as acute MI and valvular disorders. Although many potential rhythm disturbances exist, this chapter focuses on the most common arrhythmia, atrial fibrillation (AF; see Chapter 20), and provides an overview of treatments for all arrhythmias. Patients with symptoms of palpitations, syncope, spells of lightheadedness, chest pain, or symptoms of congestive heart failure (CHF) may be suspected of having an arrhythmia[41]. Patients reporting these symptoms should be questioned by their health care providers about the nature of their symptoms. The diagnosis of an arrhythmia includes a 12-lead ECG and possibly an ambulatory ECG[41,42]. There have been many advances in rhythm control, including the use of pharmacologic agents, pacemakers, automatic implantable cardiac defibrillators (AICDs), and tissue ablation. A combination of drugs and medical devices is often used successfully. A summary of treatment for arrhythmias may be found in Table 30-2.

Atrial Fibrillation

Atrial Fibrillation is the most common cardiac arrhythmia, with an estimated 2.2 million Americans having paroxysmal (transient) or chronic (persistent) AF[43]. The number of hospitalizations for AF has increased two- to threefold since 1985, and it is expected that one quarter of all adults over age 40 years will develop AF during their lifetimes[43,44]. AF is associated with an increase in the incidence of ischemic stroke, which is about 5% per year, and approximately 16% of ischemic strokes associated with AF[45,46]. The etiology of atrial fibrillation is frequently unknown, but it is often associated with hypertension, ischemic heart disease, CHD, and diabetes[43]. Longstanding hypertension can result in left atrial enlargement, left ventricular hypertrophy, impaired ventricular filling, and slowing of atrial conduction velocity. These anatomical and physiological changes can initiate sequellae that lead to AF[43].

The three factors that affect hemodynamic stability in AF are the irregular ventricular response, the rapid atrial heart rate, and the loss of synchronous mechanical atrial activity. The three treatment goals for AF are rhythm control, maintenance of sinus rhythm, and prevention of thromboembolism. Although HR control is imperative for all patients, the other treatments should be based on the risk and benefits to the individual patient[43]. The treatment of AF focuses on HR control through the use of cardioversion and drugs[47,48].

Cardioversion is done by use of electrical shocks or pharmacologically. Some new drugs make pharmacologic cardioversion more popular than previously, although these drugs do carry some risk such as drug-induced torsades de pointe ventricular tachycardia and other serious arrhythmias. Electrical cardioversion is more effective than pharmacologic cardioversion, but the need for conscious sedation or anesthesia is a disadvantage of electrical cardioversion[47].

Rhythm control and maintenance of normal sinus rhythm (if cardioversion is successful) is generally achieved by use of drugs, although surgical ablation, pacemakers, and implantable cardioverter/defibrillators (ICDs) may be needed with refractory AF[47]. Beta-block-

ers may be effective in patients with exercise-induced AF and are recommended as a consideration for patients with lone AF (i.e., without CHD). Flecainide, propafenone, and sotalol are very effective drugs for AF, and amiodarone and dofetilide are recommended as alternative therapy[47]. Combinations of antiarrhythmic drugs may be needed if a single drug fails to control AF[43]. Commonly, a beta-blocker with sotalol or amiodarone and a type Ic agent such as flecainide or moricizine are used in combination[44]. In patients with known CHD, sotalol and amiodarone are usually the drugs of choice; amiodarone or and dofetilide are recommended for patients with heart failure. In patients with hypertension, drugs that do not affect the Q-T interval such as propafenone and flecainide are preferred[47] (see GETP7 Appendix A).

Treatment with an anticoagulant, usually warfarin (Coumadin), in appropriate patients can reduce the risk of stroke by about 60% in patients with AF[44]. A balance between stroke prevention and avoiding hemorrhagic complications is the goal of anticoagulant therapy, and the lowest effective intensity of anticoagulation therapy is the target. Most studies support an international normalized ratio (INR) of 2 to 3 are the most effective while minimizing stroke risk. The target intensity of anticoagulation involves a balance between prevention of ischemic stroke and avoidance of hemorrhagic complications. Patients who are older or have greater risk of hemorrhagic complications may need to be monitored more carefully. Aspirin has a modest effect on stroke risk of about 20%, and it can be considered for select patients, particularly those with hypertension or diabetes[45].

Pacemakers and Automated Implantable Cardioverter/Defibrillators

Arrhythmias may be treated with drugs, an implantable pacemaker, or an ICD[49]. Discussion of the specific drug therapy for the wide range of arrhythmias is beyond the scope of this chapter, but readers are referred to the AHA's website for more specific information.

Pacemakers are recommended for some atrioventricular (AV) blocks, chronic bifascicular and trifascicular blocks, sinus node dysfunction, and tachycardias and in certain arrhythmias after MI and some neurologic diseases in adults[49]. There are indications for these devices in some congenital heart diseases in children and adults. Arrhythmias in which pacing is considered to be definitely effective include third-degree or advanced second-degree AV block in the presence of symptomatic bradycardia, asystole lasting at least 3 seconds, after ablation of the AV junction, postoperative AV block that does not resolve, alternating bundle branch block, sinus node dysfunction with documented symptomatic bradycardia (including frequent sinus pauses that produce symptoms), symptomatic chronotropic incompetence, sustained pause-dependent ventricular tachycardia, and high-risk patients with congenital long-QT intervals[49].

Implantable cardioverter/defibrillator devices are recommended in patients after cardiac arrest caused by ventricular fibrillation (VF) or VT that is not caused by a transient or reversible cause, patients with structural heart disease with spontaneous sustained VT, in the presence of known CHD with nonsustained VT, and those with spontaneous sustained VT that is not controlled with other treatments[49]. Pacemakers and ICDs may be effective in other arrhythmias as well, depending on the cause and patient symptoms; readers are referred to the Gregoratos et al[49], available on the AHA's website).

VALVULAR DISEASE

Diseases of the heart valves, or valvular diseases, involve changes in the anatomy or physiology of the aortic, mitral, pulmonic, and tricuspid valves of the heart, and may include stenosis and regurgitation, and result in coronary insufficiency attributable to concomitant changes in neighboring cardiac chambers. Valvular heart disease is diagnosed by clinical evaluation (e.g., auscultation of heart sounds and murmurs), echocardiography, or cardiac catherization. The progression of disease may be evaluated with serial echocardiograms or stress testing in order to evaluate treatment efficacy and the possible need for valvular replacement surgery[50]. Antibiotic prophylaxis is generally recommended in valvular disease to prevent infection of the affected valve. Valve disease is often treated medically with a "watch-and-see" approach until the time when the disease becomes symptomatic and severe, when surgical treatment is often recommended. Valve replacement or percutaneous valvotomy may be indicated in patients with severe aortic or mitral stenosis or aortic or mitral regurgitation[50]. A summary of treatment for valvular disease may be found in Table 30-2.

CONGESTIVE HEART FAILURE

Congestive heart failure is the most rapidly increasing cardiovascular diagnosis in the United States. The number of hospital discharges for CHF increased 165% from 1979 to 2000[1]. The cause to the increased incidence of CHF is believed to be the result of successful treatment and increased survival of patients with CHD. Heart failure is a disease primarily of the elderly, with nearly 5 million patients in the United States having CHF. Approximately 500,000 new patients have their first episode of heart failure each year[51]. Generally, patients with heart failure appear in the health care system because of decreased exercise tolerance, increased dyspnea, edema of the lower extremities, or increased fluid retention, all of which are signs of left ventricular dysfunction. The echocardiogram is the single most important tool for assessing left ventricular function or dysfunction. After left ventricular dysfunction is identified, it may be appropriate for the patient to undergo exercise testing to determine functional capacity.

The treatment of CHF involves pharmacologic therapy and modification of CVD risk factors in accordance with recommended guidelines[51]. A summary of treatment for heart failure may be found in Table 30-2. Pharmacologic therapies include diuretics, ACE inhibitors, beta-blockers, and digoxin[51]. For patients with ischemic left ventricular dysfunction, aspirin and a statin drug are also recommended. Furthermore, it is important to minimize or eliminate behaviors that may worsen the probability of heart failure, including consumption of alcohol. Dietary intervention for weight management and reduction of and salt intake is an important component of treatment. Patients who are not adherent to treatment face a high risk of recurrent heart failure with repeat emergency room visits and hospital stays. Surgical treatment options include the following[52,53]:

- Coronary revascularization (in the setting of coronary artery disease and viable myocardium)
- Biventricular pacing to restore ventricular synchronous contraction in left bundle branch block
- ICDs
- Surgical restoration of left ventricular size and shape
- Left ventricular assist device
- Cardiac transplantation (the treatment of choice for end-stage patients)

PERIPHERAL VASCULAR DISEASES

Peripheral vascular diseases (PVD) are vascular diseases that include cerebrovascular and carotid disease (stroke), peripheral arterial disease (PAD), and abdominal aortic aneurysm[54].

Peripheral arterial disease is an atherosclerotic disease that results in muscular pain or cramping called claudication, which is secondary to ischemia of muscles in the leg. The most common effect of PAD is a reduced ability to walk, which can significantly affect activities of daily living[55].

Peripheral arterial disease is a highly prevalent disease that often goes hand in hand with CHD. Unfortunately, PAD is often overlooked because the symptoms and physical findings may be subtle or atypical. The risk factors are the same as for CVD, and the mechanism of disease is atherosclerosis of the peripheral arteries, causing narrowing or obstruction of the arteries and a limitation of blood flow to local and distal tissues. Screening for PAD is made using the ankle–brachial index (ABI) and Doppler ultrasound, and more specific imaging modalities such as magnetic resonance angiography may be used to identify lesions[55]. Treatment includes intensive risk factor management, and exercise is one of the most effective nonsurgical treatments for patients with PAD[56,57]. Drug therapy includes aspirin (with or without dipyridamole), clopidogrel, cilostazol, and pentoxifylline. Surgical or endovascular revascularization is generally reserved for patients with disabling symptoms, diabetes mellitus, rest pain, ischemic ulceration, or gangrene[58].

STROKE

Stroke is the third leading cause of death after heart disease and cancer[1]. The three types of stroke are ischemic (the most common), intracerebral hemorrhage, and subarachnoid hemorrhage. As with CHD, treatment of cerebrovascular disease includes the medical and surgical treatments and secondary prevention (e.g., management of risk factors)[58]. Medications, specifically, aspirin and the BP-lowering drugs, are essential.

Consideration can be given to angioplasty or the use of devices such as carotid stents and surgical procedures, including carotid endarterectomy in patients with known significant arterial stenoses. Carotid endarterectomy is a well-established surgery that is usually performed with good outcomes[59]. Carotid angioplasty and stenting are relatively new treatments with promising results[60]. Aggressive BP lowering is indicated in patients with a history of stroke, including the hemorrhagic type or transient ischemic attack[61].

Acknowledgments
Thank you to Ray W. Squires, Ph.D., of the Mayo Clinic, Rochester, MN for his assistance with this chapter.

REFERENCES

1. American Heart Association: Heart Disease and Stroke Statistics—2004 Update. Dallas: American Heart Association; 2004.
2. Brown AID, Garber AM: A concise review of the cost effectiveness of coronary Heart disease prevention. Med Clin N Am January 84:279–297, 2000.
3. Probstfield JL. How cost-effective are new preventive strategies for cardiovascular disease? Am J Cardiol 91:22G–27G, 2003.
4. Ofman JJ, Badamgarav E, Henning JM, et al: Does disease management improve clinical and economic outcomes in patients with chronic diseases? A systematic review. Am J Med 117:182–192, 2004.
5. Weintraub WS: Cost-effectiveness in preventive cardiology. Curr Treat Options Cardiovasc Med 6:279–290, 2004.
6. Smith SC Jr, Blair SN, Bonow RO, et al: AHA/ACC guidelines for preventing heart attack and death in patients with atherosclerotic cardiovascular disease: 2001 update. A statement for healthcare professionals from the American Heart Association and the American College of Cardiology. J Am Coll Cardiol 38:1581–1583, 2001.
7. American Heart Association: http://www.americanheart.org/getwiththeguidelines
8. National Committee for Quality Assurance: http://www.bridgestoexcellence.org/bte/physician/cardiacassess.htm#measures
9. Smith SC Jr, Jackson R, Pearson TA, et al: Principles for national and regional guidelines on cardiovascular disease prevention: A scientific statement from the World Heart and Stroke Forum. Circulation 109:3112–3121, 2004.
10. Ockene IS, Miller NH: Cigarette smoking, cardiovascular disease, and stroke: A statement for healthcare professionals from the American Heart Association. American Heart Association Task Force on Risk Reduction. Circulation 96:3243–3247, 1997.
11. National Heart Lung and Blood Institute: Seventh Report of the Joint National Committee on Prevention, Detection, Evaluation and Treatment of High Blood Pressure—JNC VII Bethesda, MD: U.S. Department of Health and Human Services. National Institutes of Health, NIH Pub. No. 04-5230; May 2003.
12. Pescatello LS, Franklin BA, Fagard R, et al, and the American College of Sports Medicine: American College of Sports Medicine position stand. Exercise and hypertension. Med Sci Sports Exerc 36:533–553, 2004.
13. Thompson PD, Buchner D, Pina IL, et al. and the American Heart Association Council on Clinical Cardiology Subcommittee on Exercise, Rehabilitation, and Prevention, American Heart Association Council on Nutrition, Physical Activity, and Metabolism Subcommittee on Physical Activity: Exercise and physical activity in the prevention and treatment of atherosclerotic cardiovascular disease: a statement from the Council on Clinical Cardiology (Subcommittee on Exercise, Rehabilitation, and Prevention) and the Council on Nutrition, Physical Activity, and Metabolism (Subcommittee on Physical Activity). Circulation 107:3109–3116, 2003.
14. Fletcher GF, Balady GJ, Amsterdam EA, et al: Exercise standards for testing and training: A statement for healthcare professionals from the American Heart Association. Circulation 104:1694–1740, 2001.
15. National Heart, Lung, and Blood Institute: Detection, Evaluation and Treatment of High Blood Cholesterol in Adults—Final Report. National Cholesterol Education Program. NIH Publication No 02-5215. September 2002.
16. Grundy SM, Cleeman JI, Merz CN, et al. and the National Heart, Lung, and Blood Institute; American College of Cardiology Foundation, American Heart Association: Implications of recent clinical trials for the National Cholesterol Education Program Adult Treatment Panel III guidelines. Circulation 110:227–239, 2004.
17. Fletcher GF, Balady G, Blair SN, et al: Statement on exercise: Benefits and recommendations for physical activity programs for all Americans. Circulation 94:857–862, 1996.
18. U.S. Department of Health and Human Services: Physical Activity and Health: A Report of the Surgeon General. Atlanta: Department of Health and Human Services, Centers for Disease Control and Prevention, National Center for Chronic Disease Prevention and Health Promotion; 1996.
19. Krauss RM, Winston M, Fletcher BJ, Grundy SM: Obesity—Impact on cardiovascular disease. Circulation 98:1472–1476, 1998.
20. National Heart, Lung, and Blood Institute Clinical Guidelines on the Identification, Evaluation and Treatment of Overweight and Obesity in Adults. U.S. Department of Health and Human Services. National Institutes of Health, Pub. No. 98-4083: September 1998.
21. Grundy SM, Howard B, Smith S, et al: Prevention Conference VI: Diabetes and cardiovascular disease. Circulation 105:2231–2248, 2002.
22. Stein RA, Chaitman BR, Balady GJ, et al: Safety and utility of exercise testing in emergency room chest pain centers: An advisory from the Committee on Exercise, Rehabilitation, and Prevention, Council on Clinical Cardiology, American Heart Association. Circulation 102:1463–1467, 2000.
23. Antman EM, Anbe DT, Armstrong PW, et al: American College of Cardiology, American Heart Association Task Force on Practice Guidelines:ACC/AHA guidelines for the management of patients with ST-elevation myocardial infarction—Executive summary: A report of the American College of Cardiology/American Heart Association Task Force on Practice Guidelines (Writing Committee to Revise the 1999 Guidelines for the Management of Patients With Acute Myocardial Infarction). Circulation 110:588–636, 2004.
24. Braunwald E, Antman EM, Beasley JW, et al: American College of Cardiology/American Heart Association Task Force on Practice Guidelines (Committee on the Management of Patients With Unstable Angina). ACC/AHA guideline update for the management of patients with unstable angina and non-ST-segment elevation myocardial infarction—2002: summary article: a report of the American College of Cardiology/American Heart Association Task Force on Practice Guidelines (Committee on the Management of Patients With Unstable Angina).Circulation 106:1893–1900, 2002.

25. Murphy JG, Wright RS, Kopecky SL, Reeder GS: Management of acute myocardial infarction. In Murphy JG, ed. Mayo Clinic Cardiology Review, 2nd ed. Philadelphia: Lippincott; 2000.

26. Smith SC Jr, Dove JT, Jacobs AK, et al: ACC/AHA guidelines for percutaneous coronary intervention: Executive summary and recommendations: a report of the American College of Cardiology/American Heart Association Task Force on Practice Guidelines (Committee to Revise the 1993 Guidelines for Percutaneous Transluminal Coronary Angioplasty). Circulation 103:3019–3041, 2001.

27. Hill R, Bagust A, Bakhai A, et al: Coronary artery stents: a rapid systematic review and economic evaluation. Health Technol Assess. Sep;8(35):1–256, 2004.

28. Aoki J, Ong AT, Arampatzis CA, et al: Comparison of three-year outcomes after coronary stenting versus coronary artery bypass grafting in patients with multivessel coronary disease, including involvement of the left anterior descending coronary artery proximally (a subanalysis of the arterial revascularization therapies study trial). Am J Cardiol 94:627–631, 2004.

29. Legrand VM, Serruys PW, Unger F, et al: Arterial Revascularization Therapy Study (ARTS) Investigators. Three-year outcome after coronary stenting versus bypass surgery for the treatment of multivessel disease. Circulation 109:1114–1120, 2004.

30. Botman KJ, Pijls NH, Bech JW, et al: Percutaneous coronary intervention or bypass surgery in multivessel disease? A tailored approach based on coronary pressure measurement. Catheter Cardiovasc Intervent 63:184–191, 2004.

31. Kleiman NS, Patel NC, Allen KB, et al: Evolving revascularization approaches for myocardial ischemia. Am J Cardiol 92:9N–17N, 2003.

32. Verma S, Fedak PW, Weisel RD, et al: Off-pump coronary artery bypass surgery: Fundamentals for the clinical cardiologist. Circulation 109:1206–1211, 2004.

33. Detter C, Reichenspurner H, Boehm DH, et al: Minimally invasive direct coronary artery bypass grafting (MIDCAB) and off-pump coronary artery bypass grafting (OPCAB): Two techniques for beating heart surgery. Heart Surg Forum 5:157–162, 2002.

34. Eagle KA, Guyton RA, Davidoff R, et al: ACC/AHA guidelines for coronary artery bypass graft surgery: Executive summary and recommendations: A report of the American College of Cardiology/American Heart Association Task Force on Practice Guidelines (Committee to Revise the 1991 Guidelines for Coronary Artery Bypass Graft Surgery). Circulation 100:1464–1480, 1999.

35. Gibbons RJ, Abrams J, Chatterjee K, et al. and the American College of Cardiology; American Heart Association Task Force on Practice Guidelines. Committee on the Management of Patients with Chronic Stable Angina: ACC/AHA 2002 guideline update for the management of patients with chronic stable angina—Summary article: A report of the American College of Cardiology/American Heart Association Task Force on Practice Guidelines (Committee on the Management of Patients with Chronic Stable Angina). Circulation 107:149–158, 2003.

36. Williams MA, Fleg JL, Ades PA, et al: Secondary prevention of coronary artery diseases in the elderly (with emphasis on patients > 75 years of age). Circulation 105:1735–1754, 2002.

37. Mosca L, Appel LJ, Benjamin EJ, et al: American Heart Association. Evidence-based guidelines for cardiovascular disease prevention in women. Circulation 109:672–693, 2004.

38. Bairey Merz N, Bonow RO, Sopko G, et al: National Heart, Lung and Blood Institute, American College of Cardiology Foundation. Women's Ischemic Syndrome Evaluation: Current status and future research directions: report of the National Heart, Lung and Blood Institute workshop: October 2–4, 2002: Executive summary. Circulation 109:805–807, 2004.

39. Kennedy JW, Killip T, Fisher LD, et al: The clinical spectrum of coronary artery disease and its surgical and medical management, 1974–1979. The Coronary Artery Surgery study. Circulation 66(5 pt 2):III-16–III-23, 1982.

40. Pepine CJ, Balaban RS, Bonow RO, et al. and the National Heart, Lung and Blood Institute, American College of Cardiology Foundation. Women's Ischemic Syndrome Evaluation: Current status and future research directions: Report of the National Heart, Lung and Blood Institute workshop: October 2–4, 2002: Section 1: Diagnosis of stable ischemia and ischemic heart disease. Circulation 109:44–46, 2004.

41. American Heart Association: Evaluating Patients with Arrhythmia. http://www.americanheart.org/presenter.jhtml?identifier=77

42. Crawford MH, Bernstein SJ, Deedwania PC, et al: ACC/AHA guidelines for ambulatory electrocardiography: Executive summary and recommendations. A report of the American College of Cardiology/American Heart Association Task Force on Practice Guidelines (Committee to Revise the Guidelines for Ambulatory Electrocardiography). Circulation 100:886–893, 1999.

43. Wattigney WA, Mensah GA, Croft JB: Increasing trends in hospitalization for atrial fibrillation in the United States, 1985 through 1999: Implications for primary prevention. Circulation 108:711–716, 2003.

44. Lloyd-Jones DM, Wang TJ, Leip EP, et al: Lifetime risk for development of atrial fibrillation: The Framingham Heart Study. Circulation 110:1042–1046, 2004.

45. Hart RG: Stroke prevention in atrial fibrillation. Curr Cardiol Rep 2:51–55, 2000.

46. Hart RG, Sherman DG, Easton JD, Cairns JA: Prevention of stroke in patients with nonvalvular atrial fibrillation. Neurology 51:674–681, 1998.

47. Fuster V, Ryden LE, Asinger RW, et al: American College of Cardiology/American Heart Association Task Force on Practice Guidelines; European Society of Cardiology Committee for Practice Guidelines and Policy Conferences (Committee to Develop Guidelines for the Management of Patients with Atrial Fibrillation); North American Society of Pacing and Electrophysiology. ACC/AHA/ESC Guidelines for the Management of Patients with Atrial Fibrillation: Executive summary: A report of the American College of Cardiology/American Heart Association Task Force on Practice Guidelines and the European Society of Cardiology Committee for Practice Guidelines and Policy Conferences (Committee to Develop Guidelines for the Management of Patients with Atrial Fibrillation). Developed in collaboration with the North American Society of Pacing and Electrophysiology. Circulation 104:2118–2150, 2001.

48. Healey JS, Connolly SJ: Atrial fibrillation: Hypertension as a causative agent, risk factor for complications, and potential therapeutic target. Am J Cardiol 91(suppl):9G–14G, 2003.

49. Gregoratos G, Abrams J, Epstein AE, et al. and the American College of Cardiology/American Heart Association Task Force on Practice Guidelines/North American Society for Pacing and Electrophysiology Committee to Update the 1998 Pacemaker Guidelines. ACC/AHA/NASPE 2002 guideline update for implantation of cardiac pacemakers and antiarrhythmia devices: Summary article: A report of the American College of Cardiology/American Heart Association Task Force on Practice Guidelines (ACC/AHA/NASPE Committee to Update the 1998 Pacemaker Guidelines). Circulation 106:2145–2161, 2002.

50. Bonow RO, Carabello B, de Leon AC Jr, et al: Guidelines for the management of patients with valvular heart disease: executive summary. A report of the American College of Cardiology/American Heart Association Task Force on Practice Guidelines (Committee on Management of Patients with Valvular Heart Disease). Circulation 98:1949–1984, 1998.

51. Hunt SA, Baker DW, Chin MH, et al: ACC/AHA guidelines for the evaluation and management of chronic heart failure in the adult: Executive summary. J Am Coll Cardiol 38:2101–2113, 2001.

52. Young JB, Abraham WT, Smith AL, et al: Combined cardiac resynchronization and implantable cardioversion defibrillation in advanced chronic heart failure: The Miracle ICD Trial. JAMA 289:2685–2694, 2003.

53. Nishimura RA: Valvular stenosis. In: Murphy JG, ed. Mayo Clinic Cardiology Review, 2nd Ed. Philadelphia: Lippincott; 2000.

54. Dillavou E, Kahn MB: Peripheral vascular disease. Diagnosing and treating the 3 most common peripheral vasculopathies. Geriatrics 58:37–42, 2003.

55. Weiner SD, Reis ED, Kerstein MD: Peripheral arterial disease. Medical management in primary care practice. Geriatrics 56:20–22, 25–26, 29–30, 2001.

56. Gardner AW: Exercise training for patients with peripheral artery disease. Phys Sports Med 29:25–35, 2001.

57. deVries SD, Visser K, deVries JA, et al: Intermittent claudication: Cost-effectiveness of revascularization versus exercise therapy. Radiology 222:25, 2002.

58. Spittell PC: Peripheral vascular disease. In Murphy JG, ed. Mayo Clinic Cardiology Review, 2nd ed. Philadelphia: Lippincott; 2000.

59. Biller J, Feinberg WM, Castaldo JE, et al: Guidelines for carotid endarterectomy. Circulation 97:501–509, 1998.

60. Bettman MA, Katzen BT, Whisnant J, et al: Carotid stenting and angioplasty. Circulation 97:121–123, 1998.

61. Chalmers J: Trials on blood pressure-lowering and secondary stroke prevention. Am J Cardiol 91(suppl):3G–8G, 2003.

SELECTED REFERENCES FOR FURTHER READING

American Association of Cardiovascular and Pulmonary Rehabilitation Guidelines for Cardiac Rehabilitation and Secondary Prevention Programs, 4th ed. Champaign, IL: Human Kinetics Publishers; 2003.

Braunwald, E, Zipes DP, Libby P, EDS: Heart Disease: A Textbook of Cardiovascular Medicine. 6th ed. Philadelphia: W.B. Saunders; 2001.

Brubaker P, Kaminsky LA, Whaley, MH: Coronary Artery Disease: Essentials of Prevention and Rehabilitation Programs. Champaign, IL: Human Kinetics Publishers; 2002.

Fuster V, Alexander RW, O'Rourke RA, et al, eds: Hurst's The Heart, 10th ed. Boston: McGraw-Hill Professional; 2000.

Murphy JG, ed: Mayo Clinic Cardiology Review, 2nd ed. Philadelphia: Lippincott, Williams & Wilkins; 1999.

INTERNET RESOURCES

American Cancer Society: Prevention & Early Detection: Quitting Smoking: http://www.cancer.org/docroot/PED/ped_10.asp

American Heart Association:
Scientific Statements and Practice Guidelines Topic List:
http://www.americanheart.com/statements

Clinical Guidelines on the Identification, Evaluation, and Treatment of Overweight and Obesity in Adults:
http://www.nhlbi.nih.gov/guidelines/obesity/ob_home.htm

National Cancer Institute: Tobacco: Quitting and Prevention:
http://www.nci.nih.gov/cancertopics/tobacco/quitting-and-prevention

National Guideline Clearinghouse: Cardiac Rehabilitation: Clinical Guideline Number 17, Bethesda, MD. AHCPR Pub. No. 96-0672.
http://www.guideline.gov/summary/summary.aspx?doc_id=1049&nbr=93&string=exercise+AND+CHD

National Guideline Clearinghouse: http://www.guideline.gov

The Seventh Report of the Joint National Committee on Prevention, Detection, Evaluation, and Treatment of High Blood Pressure (JNC 7):
http://www.nhlbi.nih.gov/guidelines/hypertension/index.htm

Surgeon General's Guide to Quitting Smoking:
http://www.surgeongeneral.gov/tobacco/treating_tobacco_use.pdf

Third Report of the National Cholesterol Education Program Adult Treatment Panel III (NCEP ATP III):
http://www.nhlbi.nih.gov/guidelines/cholesterol/index.htm

Exercise Training in Patients with Cardiovascular Disease

JOHN R. SCHAIRER AND STEVEN J. KETEYIAN

This chapter addresses KSAs from the following content areas:

1 Exercise Physiology and Related Exercise Science
2 Pathophysiology and Risk Factors
3 Health Appraisal, Fitness, and Clinical Exercise Testing
4 Electrocardiography and Diagnostic Techniques
5 Patient Management and Medications
6 Medical and Surgical Management
7 Exercise Prescription and Programming
8 Nutrition and Weight Management
9 Human Behavior and Counseling
10 Safety, Injury Prevention, and Emergency Procedures
11 Program Administration, Quality Assurance, and Outcome Assessment

Physical activity is a behavior with positive effects on physical health and mood. Current public health recommendations state that all people over 2 years of age, including those with disease, should accumulate 30 minutes of moderate-intensity physical activity on most (preferably all) days of the week[1]. Resistance or strength training involving the major muscle groups should be included at least two times per week[2]. Exercise is recommended in patients with heart disease and heart disease risk factors. Similar to other high-risk patients about to embark on an exercise program, it is recommended that a physician or physician extender evaluate individuals with coronary heart disease to determine if they can exercise safely[3].

Disease-specific Effects on Physiologic Responses and Fitness

Patients with coronary artery disease (CAD) may demonstrate a normal or abnormal cardiovascular response during a single bout of exercise, depending on the severity of disease and other factors. Common hemodynamic abnormalities are discussed below.

HEART RATE

A normal response to maximal exercise testing involves the patient achieving a heart rate (HR) that is within 2 standard deviations of an age-predicted maximum value and then decreasing back to baseline fairly quickly during recovery[4,5]. Failure to achieve predicted maximum HR, in the absence of β-adrenergic blocking agents, is called **chronotropic incompetence**. This finding during exercise, even as an isolated anomaly, has been shown to predict the presence of significant CAD and is associated with a higher morbidity and mortality[5,6]. After exercise, increased parasympathetic tone causes the HR to decrease fairly quickly. Measurement of the HR at 1 or 2 minutes into recovery and comparing these rates to peak HR is called HR recovery. Abnormal HR recovery, defined as a delayed decrease in HR of more than 12 bpm at 1 minute and more than 22 bpm at 2 minutes, predicts future cardiac mortality[7].

BLOOD PRESSURE

The normal response of systolic blood pressure (BP) during incremental exercise rises progressively by about 10 ± 2 mm Hg/MET (metabolic equivalents), with a possible plateau at peak exercise. Systolic BP during exercise may respond normally or may increase or decrease abnormally in patients with CAD. Exertional hypertension during an exercise test is defined as a systolic BP of more than 250 mm Hg and is a relative indication to stop the test (see GETP7 Box 4-5). Exertional hypotension is defined as a decrease below resting BP or a failure of systolic BP to increase. A decrease of ≥ 10 mm Hg or more during an exercise stress test is an indication to stop the test[3]. Exertional hypotension may be caused by left ventricular dysfunction, a large area of exercise-induced ischemia, or papillary muscle dysfunction with mitral regurgitation. An abnormal systolic BP response is associated with an increased risk of cardiac events[8,9].

Because of a reduction in systemic vascular resistance in the metabolically active muscles during exercise, diastolic BP usually remains the same or decreases during exercise. Although an increase in diastolic BP of 15 mm Hg or more may be associated with covert CAD, several

KEY TERMS

Angina: Chest discomfort caused by coronary artery stenosis; it occurs with activity and is relieved by rest

Chronotropic incompetence: An attenuated increase in heart rate to exercise; failure to achieve a heart rate that is ≥ 85% or within two standard deviations of the age-predicted maximum

Heart failure: Because of disease or injury, cardiac myocyte function is abnormal to the extent that the heart is no longer able to pump blood at a rate commensurate with the requirement of metabolizing tissues

Ischemic cascade: The temporal sequence of hemodynamic, electrocardiographic, and symptomatic expressions occurring during ischemia

Metabolic syndrome: A syndrome closely linked to insulin resistance that represents a constellation of lipid and nonlipid risk factors of metabolic origin. Risk factors of metabolic syndrome include truncal obesity, hypertriglyceridemia, elevated low-density lipoprotein (LDL) level, hypertension, and elevated fasting blood sugar (FBS)[1]. Prevalent in 24% of the population.

Rate–pressure product: Correlate of myocardial oxygen consumption, computed as the product of heart rate and systolic blood pressure

---

studies have shown that an exaggerated response of the systolic BP (>220 mm Hg) or abnormal diastolic pressure (increase of 10 mm Hg or >90 mmHg) is probably a marker for future hypertension[10–12].

CARDIAC OUTPUT AND OXYGEN UPTAKE

Typically there is an eight- to 10-fold increase in oxygen uptake ($\dot{V}O_2$) at peak exercise in healthy, active individuals. In patients with CAD, however, the increase in peak $\dot{V}O_2$ may be reduced[13]. This reduced ability to transport and use oxygen is primarily caused by diminished cardiac output to and peak blood flow within the peripheral musculature. Cardiac output (HR × stroke volume) during exercise may be reduced because of chronotropic incompetence or left ventricular impairment resulting from myocardial infarction (MI) or transient coronary ischemia that results in a decrease in both ejection fraction and stroke volume[14].

In general, the reduction in cardiac output contributes to a peak $\dot{V}O_2$ in cardiac patients that may be reduced 20% or more when with age-matched, healthy persons. The magnitude of reduction in peak $\dot{V}O_2$ varies in part with the severity of the disease. $\dot{V}O_{2max}$ below the twentieth percentile for age and gender is associated with increased risk of death from all causes. With exercise training, $\dot{V}O_{2max}$ can be increased approximately 15% to 30 %[15–18].

Although progressive dynamic exercise has been shown to be safe in patients with CAD, myocardial oxygen uptake increases while simultaneously shortening diastole and coronary perfusion time, contributing to transient oxygen deficiency or ischemia in some patients. Ischemia can contribute to electrical instability and dysrhythmias.

Scientific Rationale for Exercise Therapy in Patients with Heart Disease

One common symptom of heart disease is **angina** (because of myocardial ischemia that occurs when myocardial oxygen demand exceeds myocardial oxygen supply), which is typically chest discomfort brought on with exertion and relieved by rest. Other symptoms associated with heart disease are shortness of breath, palpitations, dizziness, and syncope. Some patients with CAD do not experience chest discomfort but have shortness of breath as a symptom of myocardial ischemia. Shortness of breath in this instance can be considered an anginal equivalent. Control of symptoms is of paramount importance when treating patients with heart disease.

The development of angina represents the cumulative impact of a sequence of pathophysiologic events, sometimes referred to as the **ischemic cascade**[19,20]. The ischemic cascade has been studied during percutaneous transluminal coronary angioplasty, atrial pacing, and exercise testing. It begins with the imbalance between myocardial oxygen supply and demand and produces an ischemic event that causes initial abnormalities in diastolic function, with subsequent abnormalities of systolic function. Next, electrocardiographic (ECG) changes occur, and, finally, the patient may experience angina. After the myocardial oxygen supply and demand imbalance is corrected, the process is reversed: that is. angina resolves first, then the ECG changes, followed by improvement in systolic function and finally normalization of diastolic dysfunction.

Berger et al.[21] performed bicycle exercise studies in 60 patients with CAD and found that although hemodynamic abnormalities were seen in nearly all patients, radionuclide evidence of global or regional wall motion abnormalities were only noted in 80% of patients and ECG and symptomatic evidence of ischemia occurred in only 50% and 30% of patients, respectively. Thus, although ischemia results in abnormalities of diastolic and systolic function in the majority of patients, ECG changes and angina are seen much less frequently.

MYOCARDIAL OXYGEN DEMAND

Factors that increase myocardial oxygen demand are HR (the more frequently the heart contracts, the more oxygen it requires), left ventricular preload (the greater the stretch on the myocardial muscle fibers, the more energy [oxygen] required), and myocardial contractility (force of contraction). At rest and during exercise, myocardial oxygen consumption can be reliably estimated using a noninvasive method—the simple product of HR and systolic BP called the **rate–pressure product**. The normal exercise response results in a rate–pressure product of 25,000 or higher[22].

During exercise, the rate–pressure product, sometimes called the double product, increases in direct proportion to increases in HR and systolic BP. For patients with CAD and angina symptoms, the rate–pressure product allows us to estimate the myocardial oxygen consumption at which it occurs. This is important when treating patients with CAD. For example, consider a patient undergoing an exercise test who walks for 6 minutes and stops because of angina at an exercise rate pressure product of 19,300 (HR of 140 bpm times systolic BP of 138 mm Hg). After the test, she receives from her doctor a prescription for a common medication called a β-blocker, which attenuates the increase in both HR and BP during exercise. A repeat test 1 month later shows a longer total exercise time of 7.2 minutes, achieving a peak rate pressure product of 15,600, and is now stopped because of fatigue. This means this patient can exercise longer, and she is symptom free. Regular exercise training is similar to a β-adrenergic blocking agent in that it also lowers HR and BP responses during submaximal exercise (Fig. 31-1). This rightward shift in the rate–pressure product curve allows patients to engage in routine and leisure time activities with fewer or no symptoms.

TABLE 31-1. Physiologic Effects of Exercise

Vascular	Acute	Chronic
Vascular stenosis	—	Partial regression (> 2200 kcal·wk^{-1})
Collaterals	—	—
Endothelial dysfunction	—	↓
Capillary flow	—	↑
Autonomic Nervous Symptoms		
Parasympathetic	↓	↑
Sympathetic	↑	↓
Hemostatic		
Fibrinogen	↑	↓
Factor VII	—	—
Platelet aggregation	↑	↓
Fibronolytic	↑	↓
Viscosity	↑	↓

↑ = increase; ↓ = decrease; — = no effect.

MYOCARDIAL OXYGEN SUPPLY

As mentioned, ischemia occurs as a result of an imbalance between myocardial oxygen supply and demand. To better appreciate the pathophysiology leading to angina in patients with stable CAD, also keep in mind four basic pathogenic factors that affect myocardial O_2 supply: coronary artery stenosis with endothelial dysfunction, microvascular dysfunction, abnormalities of the autonomic nervous system, and abnormalities of coagulation and fibrinolytic systems. This discussion focuses on the effects of a chronic exercise program on several of these components (Table 31-1).

Coronary artery stenosis influences myocardial oxygen supply and can be further divided into the components of plaque formation, collateral artery formation, and endothelial dysfunction. To date, three intervention trials addressed the issue of whether exercise, combined with risk factor modification, may be associated with a slowing or regression of obstructive CAD[23–25]. The largest trial, the Stanford Coronary Risk Factor Intervention Project[25], randomized patients with CAD to risk factor modification and exercise ($n = 145$) or usual care ($n = 155$). After 4 years, repeat angiography revealed that the mean rate of lesion progression in the intervention group was half that of patients in the usual care group.

Shuler et al.[26] randomized patients to risk factor modification plus exercise ($n = 56$) or a usual care group ($n = 55$). At 1 year, the intervention group demonstrated no change in the luminal diameter, but the usual care group had a decrease in luminal diameter of 0.13 ± 0.45 mm. Repeat angiography at 6 years also demonstrated significantly less progression in the intervention group. Interesting, a poststudy subgroup analysis[26] of subjects in the intervention group revealed that a weekly caloric

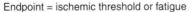

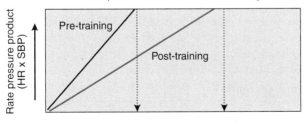

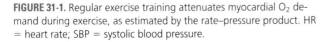

FIGURE 31-1. Regular exercise training attenuates myocardial O_2 demand during exercise, as estimated by the rate–pressure product. HR = heart rate; SBP = systolic blood pressure.

energy expenditure of less than 1000 kcal was associated with progression of disease. Additionally, those with an energy expenditure of more than 1400 kcal per week showed improved cardiopulmonary fitness, and an energy expenditure exceeding 1500 kcal was associated with a slower progression of disease. Partial regression of CAD was associated with an energy expenditure of 2200 kcal or more per week.

Despite data from animal trials, there is no definitive evidence that exercise causes collateral blood vessel formation in humans. Hambrecht et al.[26] and Niebauer et al.[27] assessed the effects of more than 3 hours of exercise per week and a low-fat diet on collateral formation in patients with CAD ($n = 56$) compared with patients receiving usual care ($n = 57$). After 1 year, there was no significant difference between the groups with respect to coronary collateral formation.

Abnormal endothelial function in patients with CAD was first described in 1986 by Ludmer et al[28]. Whereas normal coronary arteries dilate in response to intracoronary acetylcholine, a paradoxical vasoconstriction is observed in patients with coronary disease. Endothelial dysfunction can also be seen in patients with congestive **heart failure**, multiple risk factors for CAD, and sepsis. Endothelial dysfunction is thought to result from a decreased production of nitric oxide within vascular smooth muscle cells. Limited evidence suggests that exercise may help to normalize endothelial dysfunction. Hambrecht et al.[29] randomized 19 patients with CAD and abnormal endothelial function to exercise training or a non-exercising control group. After 4 weeks, endothelial function was again assessed, and the patients in the training group demonstrated less vasoconstriction compared with non-exercise control subjects.

During rest and exercise, the autonomic nervous system, through a complex interplay of the parasympathetic and sympathetic components, mediates changes in HR, BP, and vascular tone (i.e., systemic blood flow). Patients with previous MI[30,31] and chronic congestive heart failure[32,33] often have abnormalities of autonomic function during exercise, as manifested by decreased parasympathetic and increased sympathetic activity. Autonomic nervous system abnormalities are strongly associated with increased cardiac morbidity and mortality.

Beat-to-beat variations in R-R intervals, known as HR variability (HRV), is a surrogate assessment for parasympathetic activity. After an MI, mean values of all measures of HR variability are attenuated by about one third of that of age- and gender-matched healthy control subjects. Mean values of HRV improve with time but never return to normal. The magnitude of the reduction reflects the amount of the myocardial damage. Even after making adjustments for abnormal left ventricular function and ventricular ectopy, patients with attenuated parasympathetic activity manifested as a reduced HRV have a 5.3-fold increase in mortality[34].

Norepinephrine is a surrogate for sympathetic activity. Patients with heart failure have elevated plasma and urinary norepinephrine levels. Among patients with heart failure, an elevated plasma norepinephrine level at rest is associated with worsening heart failure and is a powerful predictor of future mortality.

Chronic exercise training partially reverses autonomic dysfunction in patients with heart disease. Clinical exercise trials on post-MI patients demonstrate significant improvement in HRV[35,36]. One study showed that β-adrenergic blockade therapy and exercise together have a greater impact on parasympathetic activity than either therapy alone[37]. Additionally, exercise training results in decreased resting and exercise plasma norepinephrine levels in both MI patients and patients with heart failure[37–40].

In a review of the literature, Koenig[41] and Imhof and Koenig[42] describe the relationship between hemostatic components, cardiovascular disease (CVD) risk, and exercise. Concentrations of hemostatic elements such as fibrinogen, factor VII, and platelet hyperactivity as well as fibrinolytic elements such as tissue plasminogen activator have been identified as cardiovascular risk factors[41–44]. The viscosity of the blood is also important to coronary blood flow. The major determinants of blood viscosity are hematocrit and fibrinogen levels. Increased fibrinogen levels are associated with a twofold risk for cardiovascular events. Increased factor VII levels, platelet hyperactivity, and decreased tissue plasminogen activator levels have been shown to be predictors of coronary events but to a lesser degree[45,46]. Much, but not all, of the literature describes an inverse relationship for moderate- to high-intensity exercise and fibrinogen levels. Whereas there is no evidence that factor VII levels are affected by exercise, endurance exercise increases activity in the fibrinolytic system. Long-term exercise training trials in patients with a history of a MI have reported reductions in erythrocyte rigidity, platelet aggregability, and adherence. Carroll et al.[46] and others[47,48] have demonstrated an inverse relationship between hematologic parameters such as plasma viscosity and hematocrit and physical activity parameters such as leisure-time physical activity and maximum oxygen consumption in patients with a history of MI. It is important to point out that most of the studies addressing the relationship between exercise and the level of hemostatic components involved individuals without known CAD.

Effects of Exercise on Selected Cardiovascular Risk Factors

Cardiorespiratory exercise training is recommended as an important component of secondary prevention of CVD in patients with CHD(Table 31-2)[49]. A 2000 position paper of the American Heart Association (AHA)[50] endorsed by the American College of Sports Medicine (ACSM)

TABLE 31-2. Summary of Effects of Exercise on Selected Cardiovascular Risk Factors

Risk Factor	Effect
Smoking	By itself: Little or no effect
	Exercise should be part of a comprehensive smoking cessation program
Lipid abnormalities	
Cholesterol	Little or no effect
LDL cholesterol	Little or no effect
HDL cholesterol	Mild to moderate increase
Hypertension	Reduces incidence (especially among white men)
Systolic	Reduced: Average, 6 mm Hg
Diastolic	Reduced: Average, 5 mm Hg
Obesity	By itself: Mild effect
	Exercise should be part of a comprehensive weight management program

HDL = high-density lipoprotein; LDL = low=density lipoprotein.

recommended mild to moderate resistance training for improving muscular strength and endurance, preventing and managing a variety of chronic medical conditions, and modifying risk factors.

In the past 30 to 40 years, there has been a steady decrease in deaths attributable to CVD, with a 24% decline in the past 15 years[51,52]. It might be concluded that the decrease in deaths is the result of new medications and advanced technological treatments for heart disease. However, it is speculated that half of the reduction in CVD deaths is attributable to risk factor modification, including exercise. Thus, the AHA and the American College of Cardiology recommend aggressive risk factor modification for secondary prevention of CVD for patients with CAD (for specifics, see the AHA's website and Chapter 30). It should also be added that although death from CAD is on the decline, the incidence and prevalence of heart failure are increasing, probably because persons with CAD are living longer.

Cardiac rehabilitation programs are more than ever before adopting a comprehensive secondary prevention approach to patient care. This includes management of risk factors in addition to an exercise program. For more information concerning risk factor management in CAD patients, see Chapter 30. Exercise is important for cardiac patients, not only because it independently reduces CVD risk but also because exercise impacts directly on several on risk factors, as described below.

SMOKING CESSATION

Exercise by itself has little or no effect on smoking cessation. However, well-designed education and behavioral interventions have successfully resulted in smoking cessation in 17% to 26% of patients with a history of MI[53–57]. Incorporating multiple treatment components, such as a behavioral intervention with counseling and education

and medical treatment using nicotine and non nicotine products, is recommended for inclusion in a comprehensive cardiac rehabilitation program[49].

Lipid Abnormalities

The National Cholesterol Education Program (NCEP) Adult Treatment Panel III (ATP III)[58] guidelines state that "the appropriate use of physical activity is considered an essential element in the nonpharmacologic therapy of elevated serum cholesterol." However, studies of exercise training have reported no change in total cholesterol and inconsistent effects on LDL cholesterol and triglycerides; therefore, exercise should not be recommended as a sole intervention for lipid management[58,59]. High-density lipoprotein (HDL) cholesterol can be improved by exercise, but a substantial volume of activity is required ($>1,000$ to $1,500$ kcal·wk^{-1}) for 6 months or more[60]. Improvement in lipid profiles can be observed with intensive nutritional education, counseling, and behavioral interventions. The Agency for Health Care Policy and Research (AHCPR) recommends that these types of interventions be included as components of a comprehensive cardiac rehabilitation program[49].

HYPERTENSION

Involvement in physical activity and higher fitness levels is associated with reduced incidence of hypertension in white men without CAD[61]. Aerobic training has also been shown to reduce resting BP in people with hypertension[61–64]. The 2003 Joint National Commission on the Detection Evaluation and Treatment of High Blood Pressure (JNC VII)[65] and the ACSM[61] recommend lifestyle modifications such as weight management, physical activity, and moderation of dietary sodium as definitive or adjunctive treatment for hypertension. There have been no large-scale, multisite randomized controlled studies showing that either exercise only or multi-interventional cardiac rehabilitation programs definitively improve hypertension in patients with coronary heart disease. However, data gathered from trials in individuals without heart disease suggest that patients with a history of heart disease probably also benefit from exercise[49].

The ACSM Position Stand on Exercise and Hypertension[61] states: "Dynamic aerobic training reduces resting blood pressure in individuals with normal blood pressure and in those with hypertension." Higher levels of physical activity and greater fitness levels are associated with reduced incidence of hypertension in white men. The decrease in BP with physical activity is greatest in patients with hypertension and averages 6 mm Hg for systolic BP and 5 mm Hg for diastolic BP[61]. The effectiveness of exercise training as a complement to pharmacologic therapy has been demonstrated in adult African American men with severe hypertension[66].

Patients with hypertension or heart disease should consult their physicians before embarking on exercise programs. In patients with CVD and hypertension, a stress test should be performed before beginning moderate ($\geq 40\%$ $\dot{V}O_{2max}$) or higher intensity exercise training. It is reasonable for the majority of patients to begin with moderate-intensity exercise training (40 to $<60\%$ $\dot{V}O_{2max}$) such as walking. In patients with documented CVD, vigorous training ($\geq 60\%$ $\dot{V}O_{2max}$) is best initiated in dedicated cardiac rehabilitation centers. For patients with high BP, an exercise program that is primarily aerobic based with adjunctive resistance training is recommended[65]. The evidence is limited regarding the optimal frequency, intensity, and duration of exercise for control of hypertension.

OBESITY

For many years, the relationship between CAD and obesity has been controversial. Multivariate analysis of the Framingham data suggests that most of the relationship between obesity and CAD is mediated through cardiovascular risk factors such as hypertension, type II diabetes, and dyslipidemia[67]. However, it is clear that obesity is prevalent in persons with CAD and needs to be addressed as part of a comprehensive program of secondary prevention. The benefits of weight loss for CAD patients are believed to be similar to persons without CAD; however, the urgency of weight loss is greater in CAD patients. The approach to weight loss in CAD patients is generic to all overweight or obese individuals; see Chapter 26 for more specific information.

It should be remembered that optimal body weight does not need to be achieved to receive the health benefits of weight reduction. Modest reductions in body weight of 5% to 10% are associated with health benefits for patients with and without CAD, including decreased BP and improvements in lipid levels and factors related to the onset of type II diabetes mellitus[68,69]. Obesity is associated with increased mortality, but it appears that higher fitness levels may offset some of this increased mortality[70].

Metabolic syndrome, sometimes referred to as syndrome X, is closely linked to insulin resistance and is more common in patients with CAD. It represents a constellation of lipid and nonlipid risk factors of metabolic origin, including truncal obesity, hypertriglyceridemia, elevated LDL level, hypertension, and elevated FBS[58]. Exercise as an intervention is effective alone or as part of a multifactorial risk factor modification program because of its positive impact on many of the components of the metabolic syndrome.

Morbidity, Mortality, and Safety of Cardiac Rehabilitation

The 1995 AHCPR Clinical Practice Guidelines for Cardiac Rehabilitation[49] states that "total and cardiovascular mortality are reduced in patients following myocardial infarction who participate in cardiac rehabilitation exercise training, especially as a component of multifactorial rehabilitation." This statement is based primarily on two meta-analyses of randomized controlled trials of cardiac rehabilitation conducted in the late 1980's[71,72], which showed a 25% reduction in mortality at 3 years among patients participating in multifactorial cardiac rehabilitation. A review of the literature by AHCPR found no difference in the rate of nonfatal MIs between the cardiac rehabilitation group and the control population. A recent meta-analysis of trials conducted over the past decade confirmed that cardiac rehabilitation reduced all-cause mortality by approximately 25% and, again, there was no reduction in nonfatal MI's[73].

The incidence of fatal and nonfatal cardiac events occurring during or shortly after a cardiac rehabilitation exercise session is low. Fatal events occur at a rate of 1 in 900,000 patient hours of participation in supervised exercise training, with most events occurring in patients considered to be at high risk for cardiac events. The rate of nonfatal MIs during cardiac rehabilitation is approximately 1 in 250,000 patient hours[49,73].

Exercise Prescription and Programming

CORONARY ARTERY DISEASE

Individuals with chronic illnesses such as MI, heart failure, and stroke have rates of sedentary behavior of 30% to 40%, exceeding the general population rate of 24%[74,75] (Table 31-3).

The previously cited meta-analyses of secondary prevention in post-MI patients[71-73], combined with data from primary prevention observational studies[74,76,77], provide strong evidence that exercise, whether we measure physical activity or physical fitness levels, reduces all-cause and cardiovascular mortality. Blair et al.[78,79] reported that only a modest level of fitness is necessary to achieve the benefits of reduced mortality from CVD in persons without CAD. In patients who already have CAD higher levels of physical activity may be needed. As cited earlier in this chapter, Shuler et al.[25] found that a weekly caloric expenditure of more than 2200 kcal is necessary to potentially achieve partial regression atherosclerosis in patients with CAD.

The Harvard Alumni Study[76,77] found that 1500 to 2000 kcal per week of exercise is necessary to reduce all-cause mortality and cardiovascular mortality. Two separate groups evaluated the physical activity levels of patients in cardiac rehabilitation to determine whether they were achieving the "threshold" level identified by Paffenbarger et. al. Patients participating in a maintenance program (e.g., phase four cardiac rehabilitation) after a MI or coronary revascularization were found to expend 230 kcal to 270 kcal per 45-minute rehabilitation session[80,81]. A more recent study evaluated total weekly caloric energy expen-

TABLE 31-3. Summary of Unique Exercise Prescription Issues Among Patients with Cardiovascular Disease

Illness	Comments
Coronary artery disease	To impact mortality, frequency, duration, and intensity of training should sum to yield a weekly energy expenditure > 1500 kcal·wk^{-1}.
Myocardial infarction	Achieve 1500 to 2000 kcal of energy expenditure through physical activity each week.
Angina	Consider prophylactic nitroglycerin 15 min before anticipated exertion if symptoms limit routine ADLs or ability to train. Upper HR for training should be set at 10 beats below **angina** or ischemic threshold.
PTCA with or without stent	Achieve 1500 to 2000 kcal of energy expenditure through physical activity each week
CABG	Limited upper body activities to mild intensity and ROM until 10 to 12 weeks after surgery.
Heart failure	If needed, initially guide exercise intensity at 60% of HR reserve and adjust duration to three bouts of 10 min each. Progress to one bout of 30 to 40 min. Titrate using the rating of perceived exertion scale, set at 11 to 14. As patient progresses, maintain upper rate below ventilatory threshold, which approximates a training range between 60% and 70% of HR reserve.
Cardiac transplant	Guide training intensity using RPE (11 to 14).
Pacemaker, ICD, RCT	Restrict all arm activity for 2 months and vigorous arm activity for 1 additional month. Set intensity a 50% to 85% of HR reserve or 10 to 15 beats below ischemic threshold or ICD activation threshold.

ADLs = activities of daily living; CABG = coronary artery bypass graft; HR = heart rate; PTCA = percutaenous transluminal coronary angioplasty; ICD = implantable cardiac defibrillator; RCT = cardiac resynchronization therapy; RPE = rating of perceived exertion.

diture among patients in a maintenance cardiac rehabilitation program and confirmed that the average patient, exercising three times per week, expended 830 kcal per week in cardiac rehabilitation[82]. Cardiac rehabilitation patients were also found to be active outside of the program, expending an additional 675 kcal per week. In contrast to other estimates, 72% of patients exceeded 1000 kcal, and 43% exceeded 1500 kcal in total weekly energy expenditure. Thus, more than one third of patients reached or exceeded a minimum threshold thought to reduce all-cause mortality in a general population. Patients 70 years and older; those with a body mass index (BMI) of 30 or above; and women, regardless of race, were least likely to achieve 1500 kcal per week.

The general principles of exercise prescription apply to cardiac patients as well, and readers are referred to Chapter 24 and Chapters 7 and 8 in *ACSM Guidelines for Exercise Testing and Prescription* for further information[2]. The duration of each exercise session should gradually be increased until the patient is training at least 30 to 40 minutes most days of the week. Exercising large muscle groups through rhythmic activity such as walking, cycling, rowing, or stair climbing is a cornerstone of outpatient cardiac rehabilitation programs. Because training benefits are specific to the activity performed, both the legs and the arms need to be trained[83]. The exercise session should have warm-up and cool-down phases (5 to 10 min), including stretching, range of motion (ROM), and low-intensity aerobic activity. The warm-up phase may reduce the likelihood of developing musculoskeletal injury by increasing connective tissue extensibility, improving joint ROM, and function and enhancing muscular performance. Among patients with CAD low-intensity warmups help them avoid the occurrence of ST-segment depression, threatening arrhythmias, and transient left ventricular dysfunction[84,85]. The cool-down phase permits return of HR and BP to resting values; reduces the likelihood of postexercise hypotension and dizziness; and com-

bats the potential deleterious effects of the postexercise increase in plasma catecholamine levels[86].

Dynamic resistance exercise for the upper and lower body is now commonly recommended as part of a structured cardiac rehabilitation program[50]. Moderate-intensity dynamic resistance exercise (defined as 50% of one-repetition maximum [1RM]) results in improved muscle strength and endurance, both of which are important for the safe return to activities of daily living, vocational and avocational activities, and maintaining independence. However, it remains unclear to what extent, if any, cardiovascular risk factors such as hyperlipidemia and hypertension are favorably modified by resistance training in patients with CVD[88].

A commonly recommended resistance training program involves performing one set of eight to 10 regional exercises, 2 to 3 days per week[2,50]. Typically these programs involve starting at a low weight and progressing to ±10 to 15 repetitions. For more detail about resistance training, see GETP7 Chapters 7 and 8 and the ACSM Position Stands on Exercise Training and Resistance Training[2,88]. The rate–pressure product should not exceed that prescribed for endurance exercise, perceived exertion should range from 11 to 14 on the Borg category scale (see GETP7 Table 4-7) and intensity is set at 50–70% of a 1RM[2,50]. Patients suffering an uncomplicated MI or undergoing a transcatheter procedure (e.g., percutaenous coronary intervention [PCI]) may begin a resistance training program as early as 5 or 3 weeks after the their event, respectively[87]. Patients undergoing coronary artery bypass graft (CABG) surgery should avoid upper limb resistance training until sternal healing has occurred, generally between 4 to 8 weeks after surgery. For many patients, training with the upper limbs might begin with elastic bands and hand weights before progressing to resistance-type exercise machines[87].

When generating an exercise prescription for patients in cardiac rehabilitation, the amount of energy expenditure during both cardiac rehabilitation and leisure time physical activity should to be considered so that the patient achieves at least 1500 kcal per week[82]. Weekly caloric expenditure should be considered as a fifth component of the exercise prescription, in addition to frequency, intensity, duration, and type of activity.

MYOCARDIAL INFARCTION

To prevent deconditioning while in the hospital, patients who suffer a MI should be started in cardiac rehabilitation, as soon as they are stabilized. In-hospital cardiac rehabilitation is often referred to as phase I. The goals of phase I are to minimize the deconditioning that occurs as a result of hospitalization and begin to educate the patient about risk factor modification and the lifestyle changes necessary to reduce future mortality and morbidity. Much of the deterioration in exercise tolerance can be countered through simple exposure to orthostatic or gravitational stress (by intermittent sitting or standing) and ROM exercises[89].

Outpatient cardiac rehabilitation is separated into phases, with each phase differing based on extent of supervision and monitoring, subject independence, and time from the event[3,87]. Outpatient cardiac rehabilitation aims include improving exercise performance and modifying cardiac risk factors, again both meant to reduce future all-cause and cardiac mortality.

Nontraditional exercise programs have been shown to be effective and safe in selected populations[49]. DeBusk et al.[90], as well as others, have reported their experience with medically directed at-home rehabilitation after an uncomplicated MI. A total of 127 male patients were randomized to home training or group training. At 26 weeks, the adherence rate was 72% and 71% for home and group training, respectively. No training complications occurred in either group. When compared with usual care, the patients involved in home training demonstrated a significantly greater functional capacity. These findings support the concept that medically directed at-home rehabilitation has the potential to increase the availability and decrease the cost of rehabilitating low-risk survivors of acute MI.

It is generally recommended that post-MI patients start at the lower end of their training intensity (40% to 60% of $\dot{V}O_2$ or HR reserve or 11 to 13 on the ratings of perceived exertion scale)[87]. Most cardiac rehabilitation programs train patients in a structured environment three nonconsecutive days per week, for 20 to 40 minutes of aerobic exercise, with a 5 to 10 minute warm-up and cooldown period[87]. As patients progress, they should be encouraged to exercise at home as well, so that in the course of a week, they expend more than 1500 kcal[25,76,77,82].

ANGINA

Exercise, lifestyle behavior changes, and medical compliance are beneficial for people with stable angina and help reduce overall cardiac risk and prevent or retard progression of atherosclerotic plaques. It was initially thought that the threshold at which the myocardium becomes ischemic and angina occurs is reproducible and, as mentioned earlier, can be estimated by the rate product pressure product. More recent work by Garber et al.[91] and others[92–94] demonstrated that the angina threshold varies with the type of exercise performed. They found that the ischemic threshold varied depending on whether one was performing a maximal stress test or a longer submaximal exercise session. The ischemic threshold occurred at a lower HR during sustained submaximal exercise and daily activities at home than during a maximal stress test. Circadian rhythm was also thought to play a role. Quyyumi et al.[94] showed that ischemic threshold was found to be lower at 1 pm than 8 am and 9 pm. Forearm vascular resistance was increased at 8 am and 9 pm compared with 1 pm, suggesting that increased vascular resistance may be one of the causes for the variability in anginal threshold. For a given patient performing a specific activity at the same time of the day, there did appear to be reproducibility in the rate–pressure product at which angina occurs[94].

One goal for patients with angina is to increase the amount of work or exercise they can perform at a given pressure–rate product[3,87]. Exercise improves peripheral muscle oxygen extraction and endothelial function and reduces platelet aggregation and vascular tone. As a result, patients perform routine daily activities at a lower rate–pressure product, thus reducing the amount of angina and fatigue. Therefore, more intense activities are subsequently required to reach the rate–pressure product associated with ischemia (i.e., ischemic threshold) (see Fig. 31-1)

Exercise programming for patients with angina requires that they first recognize and understand their symptoms. They need to identify the nature of their angina (e.g., chest, throat, back, arm) and understand that there are no clinical benefits derived from exercising with pain. They also need to identify which activities precipitate their angina and modify the situation accordingly. For example, if walking in the cold causes chest discomfort, then they should exercise indoors or consider wearing a scarf or other protective wear over their mouth to warm or humidify inhaled air. Similarly, if carrying out the garbage or walking the dog frequently causes chest pain, they should talk with their doctor about taking sublingual nitroglycerin beforehand.

The upper HR for exercise should be set 10 beats or more beats below the HR or rate–pressure product at which ischemia was first noticed[3,87,95]. Ischemia may manifest as angina, ST-depression with or without chest pain, ventricular arrhythmias, or abnormal BP response[96].

Medications such as β-blockers, nitrates, and some calcium channel blockers can influence the ischemic threshold. As a result, it is prudent to ensure that patients take their medications before undergoing an exercise test administered for the purpose of establishing the correct exercise training HR range. Ideally, the physician would like to repeat the exercise test if a patient's medication or dose is changed, although this is not always realistic because of reimbursement issues. McLenachan et al.[93] showed whereas that the β-blocker propranolol largely eliminated ischemic events occurring at higher (>100 bpm) and moderate (80 to 100 bpm) HRs, the number of events at low (<80 beats/min) HRs was increased. In contrast, nitrates reduced episodes at low and moderate HRs only.

REVASCULARIZATION (CORONARY ARTERY BYPASS GRAFT AND PERCUTANEOUS CORONARY INTERVENTION)

The three treatment modalities for obstructive coronary arteries, medications, angioplasty with or without stent, and CABG, are discussed in Chapter 30. The effects of anti-ischemic medications are discussed in the previous section on angina. Patients undergoing revascularization by either angioplasty or stent or CABG surgery are expected to demonstrate an improved exercise response. Signs of ischemia during exercise such as angina, ST-segment depression, and hemodynamic abnormalities (i.e., chronotropic incompetence, blunted BP response) are often eliminated after revascularization or occur at higher intensity activities. In short, the benefits and limitations of exercise are the same for patients after revascularization as they are for all patients after an MI.

Recommendations for exercise programming for patients after PCI are generally the same as for other patients with CAD. However, because patients undergoing PCI frequently did not experience myocardial damage or extensive surgery, they can sometimes begin cardiac rehabilitation 24 to 48 hours after the procedure[97]. Patients undergoing CABG surgery often begin rehabilitation as early as 3 to 4 weeks after surgery; however, upper body exercise should be limited to ROM and light repetitive activities such as arm ergometry until 4 to 8 weeks after surgery[95].

HEART FAILURE

A hallmark symptom of patients with chronic heart failure is exercise intolerance or dyspnea on exertion. Compared with age-matched healthy normal individuals, peak exercise capacity is reduced approximately 40% to 50% in patients with heart failure[98,99].

Several mechanisms have been identified to explain the observed exercise intolerance, including a reduction in peak cardiac output (~40%), chronotropic incompetence, and a reduced stroke volume. Also, the ability to increase blood flow to the more metabolically active skeletal muscles during exercise is attenuated, mostly because of both an exaggerated increase in plasma norepinephrine level and an attenuated production of endothelium-derived relaxing factor. There are also abnormalities in the skeletal muscle such as a reduction in myosin heavy chain I isoforms, reduced activity of the enzymes associated aerobic metabolism, and a reduction in fiber size[98].

Current evidence[98,99] indicates that moderate exercise is generally safe and results in improvement in quality of life, autonomic balance (i.e., parasympathetic activity), exercise tolerance (peak $\dot{V}O_2$, ~15% to 35%), endothelial function, chronotropic responsiveness, and skeletal muscle function. However, it is important to point out that other than single-site clinical trial data[39], no definitive multicenter evidence yet addresses the effect of regular exercise on mortality and rehospitalization.

Compared with apparently healthy people and those with ischemic heart disease and normal ventricular function, there are only a few differences relative to prescribing exercise in patients with New York Heart Association Functional class II or III heart failure. Specifically, duration of activity may need to be adjusted to allow these patients more opportunity for rest and to progress at their own pace. In fact, some patients may better tolerate discontinuous training involving short bouts of exercise interspersed with bouts of rest[100,101]. Patients should be encouraged to progressively increase exercise duration, as tolerated, until they are able to tolerate one bout of 30 minutes or more.

Research indicates that different exercise intensities have been used to increase exercise tolerance yet still yield similar relative gains in cardiovascular fitness[98]. Based on these data, for the first few exercise sessions, it seems reasonable to guide exercise intensity at 60% of HR reserve, titrated based on a patient's subjective feelings of fatigue using the rating of perceived exertion scale of 11 to 14. In view of conflicting reports about whether there is a further decrease in left ventricular function when patients with chronic heart failure train above ventilatory threshold (VT)[98,102], it seems prudent to set exercise intensity at 60% to 70% of HR reserve.

Presently, cardiac rehabilitation programs in the United States decide on the use of ECG telemetry monitoring when exercising patients with heart disease, both with and without heart failure, based on a patient's risk for exercise-related events and any limitations imposed by third-party insurance carriers[87]. Although ECG telemetry monitoring during cardiac rehabilitation is common in the United States, it is important to point out that such an approach is not used in either Canada or Europe. Albeit limited, analysis of safety data from the European Heart Failure Training Group[104] and the EXERT (Exercise Prescription trial)[99] suggest that ECG monitoring may not be necessary when exercising patients with stable, chronic heart failure.

CARDIAC TRANSPLANT

Every year, approximately 3000 cardiac transplants are performed worldwide in patients with end-stage heart failure. For adults undergoing this procedure, the 1- and 3-year survival rates are approximately 86% and 80%, respectively[105]. Despite receiving a donor heart with normal systolic function, cardiac transplant recipients continue to experience exercise intolerance after surgery of about 40%

to 50% below that of age-matched normal individuals. This exercise intolerance is believed to be primarily attributable to the absence of efferent sympathetic innervation of the myocardium, residual skeletal muscle abnormalities developed before transplantation due to heart failure, and decreased skeletal muscle strength[105].

After surgery, medical management focuses on preventing rejection of the donor heart by suppressing immune system function while at the same time avoiding complicating side effects such as infections, hyperlipidemia, hypertension, osteoporosis, diabetes, certain cancers, and accelerated graft atherosclerosis of the epicardial and intramural coronary arteries. Except for cyclosporine, which may cause an increase in BP at rest and during submaximal exercise, none of the other medications used to control immune system rejection in cardiac transplant recipients appears to influence the physiologic response of these patients during acute bout of exercises or prevent the development of a safe exercise prescription for aerobic conditioning[105].

Because of the decentralized myocardium, many differences in the cardiopulmonary and neuroendocrine response are evident at rest, during exercise, and in recovery in cardiac transplant recipients. These abnormalities include an elevated resting HR (often >90 bpm), elevated systolic and diastolic BPs at rest attributable to increased plasma norepinephrine and the immunosuppressive medications (i.e., cyclosporine and prednisone), an attenuated increase in HR during submaximal work, a lower peak HR and peak stroke volume, a greater increase in plasma norepinephrine during exercise, and a delayed slowing of HR in recovery[105]. Delayed HR in recovery is thought to be attributable to increased levels of plasma norepinephrine, exerting its positive chronotropic effect in the absence of vagal efferent innervation[106].

To prescribe exercise and guide exercise intensity in cardiac transplant recipients, it is best to simply disregard all rather-based methods because of the abnormal HR control in these patients[107]. For example, it is common to find persons with cardiac transplants achieving an exercise HR during training that not only exceeds 85% of peak but is often equal to or greater than the peak rate attained during their last symptom-limited exercise test. Ratings of perceived exertion between 11 and 14 should be used to guide exercise training intensity[105,107].

Among cardiac transplant patients who undergo exercise training, it has been demonstrated that exercise capacity increases by about 15% to 40%; resting HR is unchanged or decreases slightly; peak HR increases; there is little, if any, change in peak stroke volume or cardiac dimensions; and quality of life is favorably altered[105]. In the most comprehensive prospective, randomized trial to date, Kobashigawa et al.[108] showed a 49% in peak $\dot{V}O_2$ and a 23-bpm increase in peak HR.

In addition, these patients can benefit from a systematic program of resistance training because a leg strength

deficit exists and contributes to the reduced exercise capacity that persists after surgery. Braith and Edwards[109] showed that resistance training improves muscular endurance, but it also partially restores bone mineral density and addresses the skeletal muscle abnormalities (i.e., strength development, lipid content, fiber size) that commonly occur because of long-term corticosteroid therapy. A progressive resistance training program of seven to 10 exercises that focuses on the legs, back, arms, and shoulders; is started at least 12 weeks after surgery; and is performed two times per week should suffice[110].

PACEMAKERS AND DEFIBRILLATORS

Rate-responsive pacemakers respond to exercise by gradually increasing the rate (referred to as the *ramp*) until the upper rate of the pacemaker is reached (referred to as the *upper rate limit*). Both the ramp and the upper rate limit of the pacemaker are adjustable to maximize a patient's exercise performance. As in angina, the pacemaker upper rate limit is usually set so it is 10 or more beats below ischemic threshold. Obviously, patients with pacemakers and an ICD need to have an exercise prescription that takes into account their age, underlying heart disease, functional capacity, and the device being used. Exercise tests performed to evaluate ischemia in patients with pacemakers or ICDs require imaging studies during the test because of the abnormal resting ECG. Generally, exercise HR in these patients should be set at 10% below the ischemic threshold or ICD activation threshold[95,110].

Summary

Over the past 25 years, regular exercise has become increasingly used in patients with a variety of cardiac-related problems. The use of exercise in this manner is because of its beneficial effects on symptoms, functional capacity, physiology, mood, and clinical outcomes.

REFERENCES

1. U.S. Department Of Health And Human Services, Physical Activity and Health: A Report of the Surgeon General. Atlanta: US Department of Health and Human Services, Centers for Disease Control and Prevention, National Center For Chronic Disease Prevention And Health Promotion. Publication no: S/N 017-023-00196-5; 1996.
2. Pollock ML, Gasser GA, Butcher JD, et al: The recommended quantity and quality of exercise for developing and maintaining cardiorespiratory and muscular fitness, and flexibility in adults. Position stand. Med Sci Sports Exerc 30:975–991, 1998.
3. Fletcher GF, Balady GJ, Amsterdam EA, et al: Exercise standards for testing and training: a statement for healthcare professionals from the American Heart Association. Circulation 104:1694–1740, 2001.
4. Ellestad MH, Wan MK: Predictive implications of stress testing: Follow-up of 2700 subjects after maximum treadmill stress testing. Circulation 51:363–369, 1975.

5. Brener SJ, Pashkow FJ, Harvey SA, et al: Chronotropic response to exercise predicts angiographic severity in patients with suspected or stable coronary artery disease. Am J Cardiol 76:1228–1232, 1995.

6. Lauer MS, Okin PM, Larson MG, et al: Impaired heart rate response to graded exercise: Prognostic implications of chronotropic incompetence in the Framingham Heart Study. Circulation 93:1520–1526, 1996.

7. Cole CR, Blackstone EH, Paskow FJ, et al: Heart-rate recovery immediately after exercise as a predictor of mortality. N Engl J Med 341:1351–1357, 1999.

8. Comess KA, Fenster PE: Clinical implications of the blood pressure response to exercise. Cardiology 68:233–244, 1981.

9. Irving JB, Bruce RA, DeRouen TA : Variations in and significance of systolic pressure during maximal exercise (treadmill) testing: Relation to severity of coronary artery disease and cardiac mortality. Am J Cardiol 39:841–848, 1977.

10. Sheps DS, Ernst JC, Briese FW, et al: Exercise-induced increase in diastolic pressure: indicator of severe coronary artery disease. Am J Cardiol 43:708–712, 1979.

11. Wilson N, Meyer E: Early prediction of hypertension using exercise blood pressure. Prev Med 10:62–68,1981.

12. Dlin R, Hanne N, Silverberg DS, et al: Follow-up of normotensive men with exaggerated blood pressure response to exercise. Am Heart J 106:316–320, 1983.

13. American College of Sports Medicine: Exercise for patients with coronary artery disease. Position Stand. Med Sci Sports Exerc 26:i–v, 1994.

14. Clausen JP: Circulatory adjustments to dynamic exercise and effects of physical training in normal subjects and in patients with coronary artery disease (pp. 39–75). In Sonneblick H, Lesch M, eds. Exercise and Heart Disease, New York: Grune and Stratton; 1977.

15. Hartung GH, Rangel R: Exercise training in post-myocardial infarction patients: Comparison of results with high risk coronary and post-bypass patients. Arch Phys Med Rehabil 62:147–150, 1988.

16. Thompson PD: The benefits and risks of exercise training in patients with chronic coronary artery disease. JAMA 259:1537–1540, 1988.

17. Hambrecht R, Niebauer J, Fiehn E: Physical training in patients with stable chronic heart failure: Effects on cardiorespiratory fitness and ultrastructural abnormalities of leg muscles. J Am Coll Cardiol 25:1239–1249,1995.

18. Keteyian SJ, Levine AB, Brawner CA: A randomized controlled trial of exercise training in patients with heart failure. Ann Intern Med 124:1051–1057, 1996.

19. Nesto RW, Kowalchuk GJ: The ischemic cascade: Temporal sequence of hemodynamic, electrocardiograhic, and symptomatic expressions of ischemia. Am J Cardiol 57:23C–30C, 1987.

20. Heller GV, Ahmed I, Tilkemeier PL, et al: Comparison of chest pain, electrocardiographic changes and thallium-201 scintigraphy during varying exercise intensities in men with stable angina pectoris. Am J Cardiol 68:569–574, 1991.

21. Berger HJ, Reduto LA, Johnstone DE, et al: Global and regional left ventricular response to cycle exercise in coronary artery disease: Assessment by quantitative radionuclide angiocardiography. Am J Med 66:13–21, 1979.

22. Wasserman K, Hansen JE, Sue DY, et al: Principles of Exercise Testing and Interpretation, 3rd ed. Baltimore: Lippincott, Williams & Wilkins;1999.

23. Ornish D, Brown SE, Scherwitz LW, et al: Can lifestyle changes reverse coronary heart disease? Lancet 336:129–133, 1990.

24. Haskell WL, Alderman EL, Fair JM, et al: Effects of intensive multiple risk factor reduction on coronary atherosclerosis and clinical cardiac events in men and women with coronary artery disease. Circulation 89:975–990, 1994.

25. Shuler G, Hambrecht R, Schlierf G, et al: Regular exercise and low fat diet-effects on progression of coronary artery disease. Circulation 86:1–11, 1992.

26. Hambrecht R, Niebauer J, Marburger CH, et al: Various intensities of leisure time physical activity in patients with coronary artery disease: Effects of cardiorespiratory fitness and progression of coronary artherosclotic lesions. J Am Coll Cardiol 22:468–477, 1993.

27. Niebauer J, Hambrecht R, Marburger C, et al: Impact of intensive physical exercise and low fat diet on collateral vessel formation in stable angina pectoris and angiographically confirmed coronary artery disease. Am J Cardiol 771–775, 1995.

28. Ludmer PL, Selwyn AP, Shook TL, et al: Paradoxical vasoconstriction induced by acetylcholine in atherosclerotic coronary arteries. N Engl J Med 315:1046–1051, 1986.

29. Hambrecht R, Wolf A, Gielen S, et al: Effect of exercise on coronary endothelial function in patients with coronary artery disease. N Engl J Med 342:454–460, 2000.

30. Bigger JT, Fleiss JL, Steinman RC, et al: Frequency domain measures of heart period variability and mortality after myocardial infarction. Circulation 85:164–171, 1992.

31. Farrell T, Paul V, Cripps T, et al: Baroreflex sensitivity and electrophysiological correlates in patients after acute myocardial infarction. Circulation 83:945–952, 1991.

32. Nolan J, Batin PD, Andrews R, et al: Prospective study of heart rate variability and mortality in chronic heart failure evaluation and assessment of risk trial (UK-heart). Circulation 98:1510–1516, 1998.

33. Nolan J, Flapan AD, Capewell S, et al: Decreased cardiac parasympathetic activity in chronic heart failure. Br Heart J 67:482–485, 1992.

34. Kleiger RE, Miller JP, Bigger JT, et al: Decreased heart rate variability and its association with increased mortality after acute myocardial infarction. Am J Cardiol 59:256–262, 1987.

35. Malfatto G, Facchini M, Bragato R, et al: Short and long term effects of exercise training on the tonic autonomic modulation of heart rate variability after myocardial infarction. Eur Heart J 17:532–538, 1996.

36. Tiukinhoy S, Beohar N, Hsie M: Improvement in heart rate recovery after cardiac rehabilitation. J Cardiopulm Rehabil 23:84–87, 2003.

37. Malfatto G, Facchini M, Sala L, et al: Effects of cardiac rehabilitation and beta-blocker therapy on heart rate variability after first acute myocardial infarction. Am J Cardiol 81:834–840, 1998.

38. Belardinelli R, Georgiou D, Cianci G, et al: Randomized, controlled trial of long-term moderate exercise training in chronic heart failure: Effects on functional capacity, quality of life, and clinical outcome. Circulation 99:1173–1182, 1999.

39. Keteyian SJ, Brawner CA, Schairer JR, et al: Effects of exercise training on chronotropic incompetence in patients with heart failure. Am Heart J 138:2343–2240, 1999.

40. Coats AJS, Adamopoulos, S, Rnadaelli A, et al: Controlled trial of physical training in chronic heart failure. Circulation 85:2119–2131, 1992.

41. Koenig W: Haemostatic risk factors for cardiovascular diseases. Eur Heart J 19(suppl C):C39–C43, 1998.

42. Imhof A, Koenig W: Exercise and thrombosis. Cardiol Clin 19:389–400, 2001.

43. Thallow E, Eriksen J, Sandvik L, et al: Blood platelet count and function are related to total and cardiovascular death in apparently healthy men. Circulation 84:613–616, 1991.

44. Meade TW, Ruddock V, Stirling Y, et al: Fibrinolytic activity, clotting factors and long term incidence of ischemic heart disease in the Northwick Park Heart Study. Lancet 342:1076–1079, 1993.

45. Heinrich J, Balleisen L, Schulte H, et al: Fibrinogen and factor VII in the prediction of coronary risk. Results of PROCAM study in healthy men. Arterioscler Thromb 14:54–59, 1994.

46. Carroll S, Cooke CB, Butterfly RJ: Physical activity, cardiorespiratory fitness, and the primary components of blood viscosity. Med Sci Sports Exerc 32:353–385, 2000.

47. Koenig W, Sund M, Döring A, et al: Leisure-time physical activity but not work-related physical activity is associated with decreased plasma viscosity. Results from a large population sample. Circulation 95:335–341, 1997.

48. Elwood PC, Yarnell JWG, Pickering J, et al: Exercise, fibrinogen and other risk factors for ischaemic heart disease. Caerphilly prospective heart disease study. Br Heart J 69:183–187, 1993.

49. Wenger NK, Froelicher ES, Smith LK, et al: Cardiac rehabilitation clinic practice guidelines no. 17. Rockville, MD: US Department of Health and Human Services, Public Health Service Agency for Health Care Policy and Research and the National Heart, Lung and Blood Institute, Agency for Health Care Policy and Research. Publication no. 96-0672; October 1995.

50. Pollock ML, Franklin BA, Balady GJ, et al: Resistance exercise individuals with and without cardiovascular disease: Benefits, rationale, safety, and prescription: An advisory from the Committee on Exercise, Rehabilitation, and Prevention, Council on Clinical Cardiology, American Heart Association. Circulation 101:828–833, 2000.

51. McGovern PG, Pankow JS. Shahar E, et al: Recent trends in acute coronary heart disease. Mortality, morbidity, medical care, and risk factors. N Engl J Med 334:884–890, 1996.

52. American Heart Association: Heart and Stroke Facts: 2000 Statistical Supplement. Dallas: American Heart Association; 2000.

53. DeBusk RF, Houston-Miller N, Superko HR, et al: A case-management system for coronary risk factor modification after acute myocardial infarction. Ann Intern Med 120:721–729,1994.

54. Sivarajan ES, Newton KM, Almes MJ, et al: Limited effects of outpatient teaching and counseling after myocardial infarction: A controlled study. Heart Lung 6:975–980, 1977.

55. Engblom E, Hietanen EK, Hamalainen H, et al: Exercise habits and physical performance during comprehensive rehabilitation after coronary bypass surgery. Eur Heart J 13:1053–1059,1992.

56. Heller RF, Knapp JC, Valenti LA, et al: Secondary prevention after acute myocardial infarction. Am J Cardiol 72:759–762,1993.

57. Taylor CB, Houston-Miller N, Killen JD, et al: Smoking cessation after acute myocardial infarction: effects of a nurse-managed intervention. Ann Intern Med 113:118–123, 1990.

58. Executive Summary of the Third Report of the National Cholesterol Education Program (NCEP) Expert Panel on Detection, Evaluation, and Treatment of High Blood Cholesterol in Adults (Adult Treatment Panel III). JAMA 285:2486–2497, 2001.

59. Leon AS, Sanchez OA: Response of blood lipids to exercise training alone or combined with dietary intervention. Med Sci Sports Exerc 33:S502–S515, 2001.

60. Williams PT, Wood PD, Haskell WL et al: The effects of running mileage and duration on plasma lipoprotein levels. JAMA 247:2674–2679, 1982.

61. American College of Sports Medicine: Position Stand. Exercise and Hypertension. Med Sci Sports Exerc 36:533–553, 2004.

62. Arroll B, Beaglehole R: Does physical activity lower blood pressure: A critical review of the clinical trials. J Clin Epidemiol 45:439–447, 1992.

63. Kelley G, McClellan P: Antihypertensive effects of aerobic exercise: A brief meta-analytic review of randomized controlled trials. Am J Hypertens 7:115–119, 1994.

64. Hagberg JM: Physical Activity, Physical Fitness, and Blood Pressure. NIH Consensus Development Conference: Physical Activity and Cardiovascular Health. Bethesda MD: National Institutes of Health; 1995:67–71.

65. Chobanian AV, Bakrisg GL, Black NR, et al: The seventh report of the joint national commission (JNC) VII) on detection evaluation and treatment of high blood pressure: The JNC VII report. JAMA 289:2560–2672, 2003.

66. Kokkinos P, Narayan P, Colleran J, et al: Effects of regular exercise on blood pressure and left ventricular hyperthrophy in African-American men with severe hypertension. N Engl J Med 333:1462–1467, 1995.

67. Wilson PWF, D'Agostino RB, Levy D, et al: Prediction of coronary heart disease using risk factor categories. Circulation 97:1837–1847, 1998.

68. Goldstein DJ: Beneficial health effects of modest weight loss. Int J Obes 16:397–415, 1992.

69. Wing RR, Venditti E, Jakicic JM, et al: Lifestyle intervention in overweight individuals with a family history of diabetes. Diabetes Care 21:350–359, 1998.

70. Lee CD, Blair SN, Jackson AS: Cardiorespiratory fitness, body composition, and all-cause mortality in men. Am J Clin Nutr 69:373–380, 1999.

71. O'Conner GT, Burning JE, Yusuf S, et al: An overview of randomized trials of rehabilitation with exercise after myocardial infarction. Circulation 80:234–244, 1989.

72. Oldridge NB, Guyatt GH, Fischer ME, et al: Cardiac rehabilitation after myocardial infarction: combined experience of randomized trials. JAMA 260:945–950, 1988.

73. Jollifee JD, Rees K, Taylor RS, et al: Exercise-Based Rehabilitation for Coronary Heart Disease. Cochrane Database Syst. Rev 2001:(1): CDC01800.

74. Centers for Disease Control and Prevention:. Prevalence of sedentary lifestyle: Behavioral risk factor surveillance system, United States, 1991. Mor Mortal Wkly Rep 42:576–579, 1991.

75. Crespo CJ, Keteyian SJ, Heath GW, et al: Leisure time physical activity among US adults. Arch Intern Med 156:93–98, 1996.

76. Paffenbarger RS, Wing AL, Hyde RT: Physical activity as an index of heart attack risk in college alumni. Am J Epidemiol 108:161–175, 1978.

77. Paffenbarger RS, Hyde RT, Wing AL et al: Physical activity, all-cause mortality, and longevity of college alumni. N Engl J Med 314:605–613, 1986.

78. Blair SN, Kohl HW, Paffenbarger RS, et al: Physical fitness and all cause mortality. JAMA 262:2395–2401, 1989.

79. Blair SN, Kohl HW, Gorgon NF, et al: How much physical activity is good for health? Ann. Rev Public Health 13:99–126, 1992.

80. Schairer JR, Kostelnik T, Proffett SM, et al: Caloric expenditure during cardiac rehabilitation. J Cardiopulm Rehabil 290–294, 1998.

81. Ades H, Savage PD, Brochu M, Scot P, et al: Low caloric expenditure in cardiac rehabilitation. Am Heart J 140:527–533, 2000.

82. Schairer JR, Keteyian SJ, Ehrman JK, et al: Leisure-time physical activity in patients in maintenance cardiac rehabilitation. J Cardiopulm Rehabil 23:260–265, 2003.

83. Clausen JP, Trap-Jensen J, Lassen NA: The effects of training on heart rate during arm and leg exercise. Scand J Clin Lab Invest 26:295–301, 1970.

84. Barnard RJ, Gardner GW, Diaco NV, et al: Cardiovascular responses to sudden strenuous exercise: Heart rate, blood pressure and ECG. J Appl Physiol 34:833–837,1973.

85. Barnard RJ, MacAlpin R, Katus AA, et al: Ischemic response to sudden strenuous exercise in healthy men. Circulation 48:936–942, 1973.

86. Dimsdale JE, Hartly H, Guiney T, et al: Postexercise peril: Plasma catecholamines and exercise. JAMA 251:630–632, 1984.

87. American Association of Cardiovascular and Pulmonary Rehabilitation: Guidelines for Cardiac Rehabilitation and Secondary Prevention, 4th ed. Champaign, IL: Human Kinetics; 2004:65–66, 118–120.

88. Kraemer WJ, Adams K, Cafarelli E, et al: American College of Sports Medicine position stand. Progression models in resistance training for healthy adults. Med Sci Sports Exerc 34:364–380, 2002.

89. Convertino VA: Effect of orthostatic stress on exercise performance after bed rest: Relation to in-hospital rehabilitation. J Cardiac Rehabil 3:660–663, 1983.

90. DeBusk RF, Haskell WL, Miller NH, et al: Medically directed at-home rehabilitation soon after clinically uncomplicated acute myocardial infarction: a new model for patient care. Am J Cardiol 55:251–257, 1985.

91. Garber CE, Carleton RA, Camaione DN, et al: The threshold for myocardial ischemia varies with coronary artery disease depending on the exercise protocol. J Am Coll Cardiol. 17:1256–1262, 1991.

92. Benhorin J, Pinsker G, Moriel M, et al: Ischemic threshold during two exercise testing protocols and during ambulatory electrocardiographic monitoring. J Am Cardiol 22:671–677, 1993.

93. McLenachan JM, Weidinger FF, Barry J, et al: Relations between heart rate, ischemia and drug therapy during daily life in patients with coronary artery disease. Circulation 83:1263–1270, 1991.

94. Quyyumi AA, Panza JA, Diodati JG, et al: Circadian variation in ischemic threshold. Circulation 86:22–28, 1992.

95. American College of Sports Medicine. American College of Sports Medicine's Exercise Management for Persons with Chronic Disease and Disabilities. Champaign, IL: Human Kinetics; 1997.

96. Hoberg E, Schuler G, Kunze B, et al: Silent myocardial ischemia as a potential link between lack of premonitoring symptoms and increased risk of cardiac arrest during physical stress. Am J Cardiol 65:583–589,1990.

97. Schelkum PH: Exercise after angioplasty: How much? How soon?. Phys Sportsmed 20:199–212, 1992.

98. Keteyian SJ, Spring TJ: Chronic heart failure (pp. 261–280). In Clinical Exercise Physiology. Champaign, IL: Human Kinetics; 2003.

99. McKelvie RS, Teo KK, Roberts R, et al: Effects of exercise training in patients with heart failure: The exercise prescription trial (EXERT). Am Heart J 144:23–30, 2002.

100. Meyer K, Samek L, Schwaibold M, et al: Interval training in patients with severe chronic heart failure: Analysis and recommendations for exercise procedures. Med Sci Sports Exerc 29:306–312, 1997.

101. Meyers K, Schwaibold M, Westbrook S, et al: Effects of short-term exercise training and activity restriction on functional capacity in patients with severe chronic heart failure. Am J Cardiol 78:1017–1022, 1996.

102. Normandin EA, Camaione DN, Clark BA III, et al: A comparison of conventional vs anaerobic threshold exercise prescription methods in subjects with left ventricular dysfunction. J Cardiopulm Rehabil 13:110–116, 1993.

103. Strzelczk TA, Quigg RJ, Pfeifer PB: Accuracy of estimating exercise prescription intensity in patients with left ventricular systolic dysfunction. J Cardiopulm Rehabil 21:158–163, 2001.

104. European Heart Failure Training Group: Experience from controlled trials of physical training in chronic heart failure. Eur Heart J 19:466–475, 1998.

105. Keteyian SJ, Brawner C: Cardiac transplant (pp. 70–75). In Durstine JL, Moore GE, eds. ACSM's exercise Management for Persons with Chronic Disease and Disabilities. Champaign, IL: Human Kinetics, 2001.

106. Albrecht AE, Lillis D, Pease MD, et al: Heart rate and catecholamine responses during exercise and recovery in cardiac transplant recipients. J Cardiopulmonary Rehabil 13:182–187, 1993.

107. Keteyian SJ, Ehrman J, Fedel F, Rhoads K: Heart rate-perceived exertion relationship during exercise in orthotopic heart transplant patients. J Cardiopulm Rehabil 10:287–293, 1990.

108. Kobashigawa JA, Leaf DA, Lee N, et al: A controlled trial of exercise rehabilitation after heart transplantation. N Engl J Med 34:272–277, 1999.

109. Braith RW, Edwards DG: Exercise following heart transplantation. Sports Med 30:171–192, 2000.

110. Pashkow FJ: Patients with implanted pacemakers or implanted cardioverter defibrillators (pp. 431–38). In N Wenger and H Hellerstein, eds. Rehabilitation of the Coronary Patient, 3rd ed. New York: Churchill Livingstone; 1992.

SELECTED REFERENCES FOR FURTHER READING

American Association of Cardiovascular and Pulmonary Rehabilitation Guidelines for Cardiac Rehabilitation and Secondary Prevention Programs, 4th ed. Champaign, IL: Human Kinetics; 2004.

Brubaker P, Kaminsky LA, Whaley, MH: Coronary Artery Disease: Essentials of Prevention and Rehabilitation Programs. Champaign, IL: Human Kinetics; 2002.

American College of Sports Medicine: ACSM's Exercise Management for Persons With Chronic Diseases and Disabilities, 2nd ed. Champaign, IL: Human Kinetics; 2003.

Fardy PS, Franklin BA, Pocari JP, Verrill DE: Guidelines for Cardiac Rehabilitation and Secondary Prevention Programs. Champaign, IL: Human Kinetics; 1999.

Graves JE, Franklin BA: Resistance Training for Health and Rehabilitation. Champaign, IL: Human Kinetics; 2001.

Pashkow FJ, Dafoe WA: Clinical Cardiac Rehabilitation: A Cardiologist's Guide, 2nd ed. Philadelphia: Lippincott, Williams & Wilkins; 1999.

INTERNET RESOURCES

AACVPR: American Association of Cardiovascular and pulmonary Rehabilitation: http://www.aacvpr.org

American College of Sports Medicine: Position Stands: http://www.acsm.org/publications/positionStands.htm

American Heart Association: Scientific Statements and Practice Guidelines List: http://www.americanheart.org/presenter.jhtml?identifier=2158

National Clinical Guideline Clearinghouse: http://www.guideline.gov

National Heart Lung and Blood Institute Clinical Guidelines: www.nhlbi.nih.gov/guidelines

Treatment and Rehabilitation of Pulmonary Diseases

LAURA A. PENO-GREEN AND CHRISTOPHER B. COOPER

Successful implementation of any exercise program in individuals with lung disease can be a challenging task. The limited exercise capacity extending from the type and severity of lung disease affects the ability to perform any type of physical activity, including activities of daily living (ADLs). Additionally, the severity of the physiologic aberration can be further amplified by physical activity. The dyspnea and fatigue begins the perpetuating process of anxiety, activity avoidance, and progressive disability.

A basic understanding of disease pathophysiology, particularly in the context of the physiology of exercise, improves the efficacy and success of any exercise program for these patients. The design of the exercise program can be enhanced by recognizing disease features that can be used to individualize the program and optimize the individual exercise response. Through this knowledge base, elements key to the evaluation or assessment of the exercise response become more apparent, providing further direction to modifications that will enhance program design. Acquiring this knowledge base can be a large and complicated task, particularly if the diseases are approached in an individual manner. This task can be simplified by grouping diseases based on physiologic

similarities. Four groups of diseases can be defined and named for their primary limitation: **obstructive pulmonary disease**, **restrictive pulmonary disease**, pulmonary vascular disease, and disturbances in ventilatory control. The physiologic pattern associated with each category can be generally applied to all the diseases within the respective category.

This chapter provides an overview of the key pathophysiologic principles important to exercising individuals with chronic lung disease. A categorical approach is used to convey these concepts. The more prevalent diseases are used to exemplify these concepts. Chapter 15 reviewed assessments and exercise testing of patients with pulmonary disease.

Obstructive Pulmonary Disease

Increased airway resistance is a major physiologic limitation in obstructive pulmonary disease. Generally, a reduced cross-sectional airway diameter attributable to structural or dynamic changes within the airway accounts for the increase in airway resistance[1–3]. Structural airway abnormalities are chronic, specified by disease processes, and are usually related to disease severity. Dynamic changes are variable and precipitated by acute stimuli such as physical activity, stress, or acute illness. Clinically, airway resistance can be attributed to both processes, particularly in exercising individuals. Regardless of the causation, the common endpoint for high airway resistance is air trapping and lung hyperinflation[3,4].

CHRONIC OBSTRUCTIVE PULMONARY DISEASE

The pathologic features for chronic obstructive pulmonary disease (COPD) involve chronic bronchitis, small airway disease, and emphysema[1,5]. The major distinction between **chronic bronchitis** and **emphysema** is anatomic. Conducting airways are primarily affected in chronic bronchitis, and the disease is characterized by sputum production on most days of the week for more than 3 months for at least 2 consecutive years (Medical Research Council definition). On the other hand, the primary abnormality in emphysema involves destruction of alveolar septae and enlargement of the air spaces distal to the terminal bronchi-

KEY TERMS

Asthma: A disease of the lung characterized by airflow obstruction that is usually completely reversible and is usually associated with airway hyperreactivity

Bronchiectasis: A lung disease characterized by irreversible dilatation of the distal bronchi

Chronic bronchitis: A chronic obstructive lung disease that primarily affects the conducting airways

Emphysema: A chronic obstructive lung disease that primarily involves enlargement of the air spaces

Interstitial lung diseases (ILD): A group of restrictive pulmonary diseases involving pathology primarily confined to the lung parenchyma

Obstructive pulmonary disease: A category of diseases of the pulmonary system characterized by increased airway resistance is a major physiologic limitation; also termed chronic obstructive pulmonary disease

Pulmonary hypertension: A category of lung diseases that affect the pulmonary vasculature

Restrictive pulmonary disease: A category of lung diseases in which the underlying pathologic process involved with each disease interferes with ability for normal lung expansion

oles. In this disease, a chronic inflammation occurs, leading to fixed narrowing of small airways and alveolar wall destruction. Increased numbers of alveolar macrophages, neutrophils and cytotoxic T lymphocytes, and the release of multiple inflammatory mediators (e.g., lipids, chemokines, cytokines, growth factors) are characteristic of emphysema[6]. The destruction of the alveolar septae is not associated with fibrosis[1,7,8]. From a practical standpoint, it is usually difficult to separate chronic bronchitis from emphysema, and the majority of individuals manifest a combination of both conditions.

The relationship between COPD and **asthma** has undergone much debate throughout the years[6,9,10]. The classic definition for asthma is airflow obstruction that is completely reversible and usually associated with airway hyperreactivity[8] One perspective considers chronic bronchitis, emphysema, and asthma as mutually exclusive diseases, sometimes manifesting overlapping features (Fig. 32-1)[1]. A recent version of this diagram eloquently pre-

sented by Soriano et. al.[11] proportionally modified the boundaries based on disease incidence both in the United States and United Kingdom.

An alternative perspective claims that asthma, chronic bronchitis, and emphysema are part of a continuum for a single disease process (Fig. 32-2). The latter perspective revisits an older theory proposed in the 1980s, known as

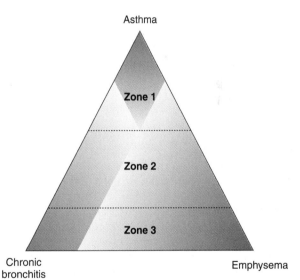

FIGURE 32-2. The Dutch Hypothesis: one disease (i.e., chronic obstructive pulmonary disease [COPD]) with three different manifestations (i.e., asthma, chronic bronchitis, and emphysema). Overlap largely accounts for the variability often seen clinically with COPD, with the degree of variability viewed as a continuum (graded regions) extending from the limits of this spectrum (*darkened corners*). The variable manifestations of COPD are also a function of the degree of airflow obstruction (zones 1, 2, and 3 defined as reversible, partially reversible, and irreversible airflow, respectively). (Adapted from Postma DS, Boezen HM: Rationale for the Dutch Hypothesis. Allergy and airway hyperresponsiveness as genetic factors and their interaction with environment in the development of asthma and COPD. Chest 126:96S–104S, 2004.)

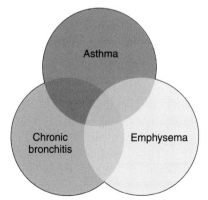

FIGURE 32-1. The interrelationship between asthma, chronic bronchitis, and emphysema depicted as a Venn diagram. (Adapted from Standards for the diagnosis and care of patients with chronic obstructive pulmonary disease. American Thoracic Society. Am J Respir Crit Care Med 152:S77–S121, 1995.)

the Dutch hypothesis[8,12,13]. This hypothesis seems to be driven by the high degree of clinical variability seen in the manner in which these three diseases manifest clinically. This variability is linked to varying degrees of disease overlap, which adds to the difficulty in diagnosing these three diseases clinically. For now, the general consensus is that COPD refers to chronic bronchitis and emphysema alone. Partially reversible airflow obstruction is the primary physiologic abnormality for COPD. The reversible component to the airflow obstruction seen in COPD may sometimes be linked to the coexistence of asthma[1,14].

Chronic obstructive pulmonary disease is a major cause of mortality, morbidity, and disability within the United States. In 2000 the prevalence of COPD was estimated to be at 24.0 million adults[15]. It is the fourth leading cause of death in the United States and worldwide. The socioeconomic implications are huge. A recent report by the Centers for Disease Control and Prevention showed that COPD is responsible for 8 million outpatient medical visits and 1.5 million emergency department visits. During the same year, COPD was responsible for 1.9%, or 726,000, of all hospitalizations, and this diagnosis was listed as a major contributing illness for 25 million additional hospitalizations[15]. Dollars spent on this diagnosis are estimated to be in the billions, with $20 billion linked to direct and $11 billion linked to indirect medical costs[16].

TREATMENT AND EXERCISE CONSIDERATIONS

The vast majority of exercise research in chronic lung disease has been in the area of COPD. The prevalence of this disease facilitates recruitment for clinical research and the severe morbidity and high costs associated with this disease make it a high priority. Many of the exercise principles outlined in this section for COPD are applicable to other diseases classified as in the obstructive lung disease (OLD) category.

Dynamic lung hyperinflation is an important principle to consider when exercising patients with COPD. This process can be a major contributor to the ventilatory impairment seen in OLDs[4]. First, the geometric confines of the thorax define the maximum lung volume. By this principle, lung hyperinflation can induce a restrictive defect[4]. Second, the inspiratory muscles are mechanically disadvantaged by the high load induced by lung hyperinflation[4,7,8]. Thus, the force of muscle contraction is reduced.

Lung hyperinflation also has negative consequences on the exhalation phase, causing significantly higher intrathoracic pressures than seen under normal conditions, both at resting and exercising states[4–7]. Flow-limited conditions are created with pathologic narrowing of the airways. When intrathoracic pressures exceed airway pressures, the patency of these airways can become further compromised, resulting in airway collapse and additional airtrapping[4]. Box 32-1 provides a list of the physiologic effects of dynamic hyperinflation.

BOX 32-1	Negative Effects of Dynamic Hyperinflation During Exercise

Tidal volume restriction during exercise

Mechanical load of inspiratory muscles adversely affected

Incomplete lung emptying during resting tidal breathing

Reduced cardiac output

Dyspnea

Tachypnea

High ventilatory demand

Early exercise termination

Adapted from O'Donnell DE, Revill SM, Webb KA: Dynamic hyperinflation and exercise intolerance in chronic obstructive pulmonary disease. Am J Respir Crit Care Med 164:770–777, 2001.

The work of breathing can also potentially influence ventilatory capacity. Ventilatory work is defined by force, volume, and pressure[17]. With OLD, ventilatory work is raised through an increase in these variables. For inhalation, an increase in ventilatory muscle force is required to overcome the high end-expiratory pressures generated by lung hyperinflation. Furthermore, the negative intrathoracic pressures generated need to be higher to overcome the reduced compliance of the overdistended lungs. For exhalation, lung hyperinflation and high airway resistance impede airflow, requiring a change from passive to active state[17]. Factors increasing ventilatory work also affect energy expenditure and oxygen demand. When work performed exceeds oxygen supply, ventilatory muscle fatigue and early exercise termination result[7].

The stage of COPD influences the severity of illness score, treatment selection, and exercise prescription. Multiple classification schemas have been proposed through the years to describe disease severity. The most recent, known as the GOLD (Global Initiative for Chronic Obstructive Lung Disease) guidelines, was developed through a collaborative effort between National Heart, Lung, and Blood Institute and the World Health Organization (WHO), Global Initiative for Chronic Obstructive Lung Disease[18]. Revisions to these guidelines were published in 2003 (Table 32-1)[19]. A novel feature to the GOLD guidelines is the recognition of individuals having a history of significant risk factors predisposing them to COPD. Individuals within this subgroup often have chronic cough and sputum production but still exhibit normal pulmonary function (stage 0). Beyond this level, stages are determined by the severity of airflow obstruction measured after bronchodilator administration.

A recent article by Celli et al.[20] proposed the use of a new index, the BODE index, to more accurately rate the severity of COPD and predict the risk of death attributa-

TABLE 32-1. Global Initiative for Chronic Obstructive Lung Disease Guidelines for Chronic Obstructive Pulmonary Disease Staging

Stage[a]	FEV1[b]	Symptom	Severity
0	Normal	Chronic cough, sputum	At risk for disease
I	>80%	± Symptoms	Mild
II	50%–80%	± Symptoms	Moderate
III	30%–50%	± Symptoms	Severe
IV	<30% or <50% with chronic respiratory failure	± Symptoms	Very severe

FEV_1 = forced expiratory volume in 1 second; FVC = forced vital capacity.

[a]For stages I through IV, the FEV_1/FVC ratio needs to be < 70%.

[b]FEV_1 values are based on postbronchodilator measurements.

Adapted from: Global Initiative for Chronic Obstructive Lung Disease. Available at: http://www.goldcopd.com

ble respiratory and non-respiratory causes. The BODE index is a 10-point multidimensional scale that assigns points based on the results of four measures: body mass index (B), airflow obstruction (O), dyspnea (D), and exercise capacity (E). Airflow obstruction is measured by use of the FEV_1 (forced expiratory volume in 1 second)[21]; dyspnea with the Medical Research Council (MRC) dyspnea scale[22]; and exercise capacity, measured by the best of two trials on the 6-minute walk test[23] (Table 32-2).

Optimizing lung mechanics before implementing an exercise program is essential for patients with COPD. As detailed earlier in this section, many of the contributing factors possess some degree of reversibility, particularly when dealing with dynamic hyperinflation. Interventions directed toward these factors improve ventilatory function and optimize exercise performance. These interventions are directed toward four primary objectives: (a) control inflammation in the bronchial mucosa, (b) control bronchospasm, (c) control airway mucus, and (d) eliminate any predisposing conditions such as tobacco use[1,19,24].

TABLE 32-2. BODE Index

Variable	Points on BODE Index			
	0	1	2	3
FEV1 (% predicted)	≥56	50–64	36–49	≤35
Distance walked in 6 min (m)	≥350	250–349	150–249	≤149
MMRC dyspnea scale	0–1	2	3	4
BMI	>21	≤21		

BMI = body mass index; FEV_1 = forced expiratory volume in 1 second; MMRC = Medical Research Council.

Adapted from Celli BR, Cote CG, Marin JM, et al: The body-mass index, airflow obstruction, dyspnea, and exercise capacity index in chronic obstructive pulmonary disease. N Engl J Med 350:1005–1012, 2004.

The GOLD guidelines have outlined the list of pharmacologic interventions advocated for COPD but do not provide a clear selection sequence for these agents. A recent review of inhaled therapies in COPD has proposed a three-step approach for mild, moderate, and severe disease[18,25]. Inhaled short-acting anticholinergic agents (e.g., ipatropium) were traditionally advocated as first-line therapy for COPD[17,26]. Short-acting beta-agonist agents (e.g., albuterol) are beneficial before exercise and are useful to relieve dyspnea. More recently, the long-acting anticholinergic bronchodilator tiotropium has become available along with the long-acting beta-adrenoreceptor agonists salmeterol and formoterol. These long-acting drugs will gain acceptance because of their sustained bronchodilator efficacy and convenience (e.g., tiotropium is a once-daily medication). Evidence suggests that inhaled corticosteroids should be prescribed for patients with severe or very severe COPD ($FEV_1 < 50\%$) to reduce the frequency of acute exacerbations. Inhaled agents are usually preferred over oral agents because of their rapid onset and low side effect profile.

After lung mechanics are optimized by bronchodilator therapy, the need for oxygen supplementation should be assessed. The underlying mechanism for hypoxia in COPD involves regional mismatching between ventilation and perfusion[24]. Ventilation is wasted within regions of the lung where emphysema is the dominant pathology. This process is referred to as dead-space ventilation. Under these conditions, ventilatory efforts are wasted because the corresponding capillary bed is destroyed in emphysema. With chronic bronchitis, the capillary perfusion is relatively preserved, but ventilation is altered to the corresponding region because of airway narrowing, resulting in venous admixture of deoxygenated blood into arterial blood. The result is a reduction in the overall oxygen content. Thus, dead-space ventilation and venous admixture can be viewed at opposite ends of the spectrum for the varying degrees of ventilation/perfusion mismatching (V/Q mismatch).

Asthma

Asthma is characterized by reversible airflow obstruction, at least in its earlier stages[27]. This disease is a major health problem that affects 14 to 15 million Americans, one third of whom are children, making it the most common chronic childhood disease. Asthma has been linked to 100 million days missed from work or school and 470,000 hospitalizations annually[28]. Importantly, acute severe asthma accounts for nearly 5000 deaths per year in the United States, many of which might be preventable[28].

Similar to COPD, illness severity is used as the primary determinant for treatment selection. Asthma can be divided into four levels of severity: mild intermittent, mild persistent, moderate, and severe[27]. The frequency and severity of both basal symptoms and exacerbations determine the level of severity. Each severity level corresponds

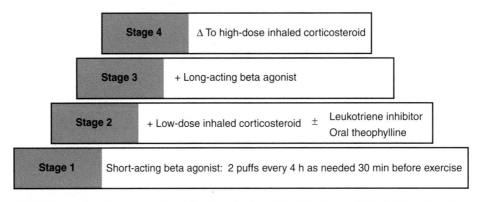

FIGURE 32-3. Systematic approach to adult asthma treatment in stable disease. (Adapted from Expert Panel Report 2. Guidelines for the Diagnosis and Management of Asthma. Bethesda, MD: National Institutes of Health, National Heart, Lung, and Blood Institute. NIH Publication No. 97-4051; 1997.)

to a specific step approach, which define general treatment options (Fig. 32-3).

The chronic nature of asthma has not always been appreciated, but it has gained wide acceptance over the past decade[29]. The chronic pathologic changes seen with asthma primarily extend from bronchial inflammation. This inflammation is the inciting factor responsible for the physiologic aberrations, symptom manifestation, and natural history of this disease. Control of bronchial inflammation is pivotal to asthma treatment. When left unchecked, the inflammation can lead to structural changes within the bronchial wall, which is linked to airway remodeling and basement membrane fibrosis[30,31].

The pathologic consequences of the inflammation in asthma are the changes seen within the bronchial mucosa. Smooth muscle hyperplasia and hypertrophy develop, predisposing to an increase in smooth muscle tone and bronchial spasm. Frequently, there is a diurnal variation in the airway caliber, manifested as nocturnal pulmonary symptoms. Mucus hypersecretion occurs through an increase in goblet cells, and the mucous glands enlarge. The patency of the bronchial lumen is compromised by the excessive mucus production, which compromises the intraluminal bronchial diameter. This development predisposes the individual to distal airway plugging, leading to atelectasis (collapse of alveolar segments). Atelectasis leads to a reduced functional lung volume and hypoxia by V/Q mismatching[32].

Triggers that induce the inflammatory cascade are important to recognize and avoid if possible[27,32]. Triggers can include allergens and inhaled irritants. Common aeroallergen triggers are dust mites, animal dander, pollen, mold spores, and inhaled irritants (e.g., smoke, airborne particulates). Occupational triggers include plastic resin, wood dust mites, animal products, biological enzymes, and certain metals. Non-allergic triggers include the inhalation of noxious fumes; environmental particulate exposure; and hormonal variations, as seen with the menstrual cycle or pregnancy. Some individuals exhibit aspirin sensitivity, frequently in association with nasal polyps. Other sensitiv-

ities that can trigger an inflammatory response include preservatives, sulfites, and latex. Latex sensitivity is increasingly prevalent in health care workers and must be taken into consideration in the rehabilitation environment. Direct contact with latex is not essential for triggering the inflammatory response; aerosolization has been demonstrated. The effect of these triggers is dose dependent and often immediate. However, symptoms that occur after allergen exposure can sometimes manifest a delayed onset that occurs 6 to 8 hours after exposure. Seasonal variations are not uncommon. In sensitive individuals, cool air and humidity can also serve as triggers because of the affect on airway tone. Interventions interrupting the inflammatory pathways will be discussed. Some patients have exercise induced asthma in which the stimulus to bronchoconstriction is thought to be respiratory heat exchange at higher levels of ventilation.

TREATMENT AND EXERCISE CONSIDERATIONS

Asthma is a clinical diagnosis, although direct provocation studies are used by many to confirm or refute the diagnosis[27,32]. The underlying premise to a provocation study is that hypersensitive individuals will develop bronchospasm after inhalation of certain agents, such as methacholine. A significant decrease in FEV_1 and forced vital capacity (FVC) is used as the objective measure for defining bronchospasm during these studies[27,33]. Many question the utility of provocations studies for the diagnosis of asthma. Nevertheless, the concepts underlying these studies convey important principles that can be applied to treatment of patients with asthma[32]. Trigger avoidance and interruption of the inflammatory pathways precipitated by the trigger are essential elements to asthma treatment[27].

The diagnostic cardiopulmonary exercise test (DXT), also known as cardiopulmonary exercise test (CPX), can also be used as a provocation study to identify exercise-induced asthma[34,35]. To meet the criteria for exercise-induced asthma, a 20% decline in the flow volumes (FEV_1 or FVC) must be demonstrated during the 30 minutes after maximum exercise has been achieved[34,35]. The traditional test for exercise-induced asthma recommends an exercise stimulus of greater than 80% of maximum heart rate (HR) for 6 minutes. However, a maximal incremental exercise test usually provides an adequate stimulus and can be used alternatively for this evaluation[34].

Unusual presentations of asthma and should be considered when airflow limitation is suspected during exercise[30]. Cough-variant asthma is an entity described in both children and adults, in whom cough is the only symptom, manifesting reduced bronchial airflow. Postviral hyperreactive airways syndrome has an asthma-like presentation that occurs after a viral illness. However, the distinguishing feature for this syndrome is bronchospastic symptoms that are generally limited to a duration of 3 to 6 months. "Cardiac asthma" is another variant to consider, which can occur in the setting of heart failure. The high-pitched sound generated by this condition results from airway edema; thus, bronchodilators are often not as effective as they are for the bronchial hyperreactivity associated with asthma.

An important asthma mimic is vocal cord dysfunction[36]. This problem is receiving increased attention and can occur with or without the coexistence of asthma. In some individuals, it is only manifested with exertion, making it difficult to differentiate from exercise-induced asthma. Some authors have estimated an incidence of 2% in a series of healthy athletic individuals who complain of exertional dyspnea[27,36]. This disorder is characterized by paradoxical closure of vocal cords during inhalation. The usual manifestation is the sensation of dyspnea, but in more extreme cases, this syndrome can cause alveolar hypoventilation and acute hypercarbia. Often an underlying psychiatric illness is associated with this entity. Stridor auscultated over the larynx, as opposed to wheezing at the thorax, is a common finding with this disorder[36].

Gastroesophageal reflux disease (GERD) is also important to consider. Not only is this condition included in the differential diagnosis of cough, but it is also often seen as a coexisting illness with asthma[37]. The bronchospasm induced by GERD is difficult to control without controlling the reflux. Proposed mechanisms underlying this type of bronchospasm include neuronal pathway and gross aspiration. Exercise can potentially induce gastroesophageal reflux in susceptible individuals, largely by causing changes in the intra-abdominal and intrathoracic pressure[32]. Rigorous exercise does not need to be avoided in individuals manifesting GERD, but measures should be implemented to minimize the severity of reflux. Nonpharmacologic interventions include maintaining head elevation at a minimum of elevation a minimum of 30 degrees while exercising and avoiding stomach overdistention with food or fluids before exercise.

As with COPD, optimizing airflow before exercise cannot be overemphasized for asthmatic individuals[14,38]. Many similarities exist between the pharmacologic interventions for both diseases[39,40], but the reduction and control of airway inflammation is paramount to maintenance care of asthma[8,41]. As mentioned previously, avoiding triggers that induce bronchospasm is considered the first line for inflammation control[27,36,41]. Pharmacologic interventions directed toward this objective primarily include inhaled corticosteroids and leukotriene inhibitors[27,36,41]. Inhaled corticosteroids are available in multiple preparations, each with a different administration route, potency, efficacy, and side effect profile. Leukotriene inhibitors include montelukast sodium (Singulair) and zafirlukast (Accolate). These drugs also provide long-term control of inflammation but are currently considered second line to the inhaled corticosteroids.

Short-acting beta-agonist drugs are the drugs of choice for rapid relief symptoms extending from bronchospasm[27,36,41]. These agents are also useful before exercise. Their mechanism of action is through the innervation of beta-receptors located on the bronchial smooth muscle. A bronchodilator with a short-acting onset of action is ideal. The historically important drug within this category is albuterol. Inhaled administration, either by metered-dose inhaler (MDI) or nebulization renders a significant bronchodilating effect within 15 minutes[29]. However, its duration of action is usually not sustained for longer than 2 to 4 hours, for which reason the long-acting beta-agonists were developed.

Salmeterol (Serevent) and formotalol (Foradil), newer beta-agonist inhalers, are directed toward long-term control of bronchospasm, usually resulting in the maintenance of airflow improvement for up to 12 hours[27,36,41]. These long-acting beta-agonist inhalers are now available in preparations that also contain inhaled corticosteroids to enhance convenience and drug compliance. These agents are not recommended for "rescue" relief from bronchospasm because their onset of control is not comparable to that of the short-acting beta-agonists. The extended duration of action makes these drugs attractive for use in exercise-induced asthma. If used for this purpose, administration optimally needs to be in advance to exercise initiation, at least by 30 minutes.

Additional medications that have been demonstrated to have utility in patients with asthma treatment include theophylline preparations, as well as a newer medication anti-IgE therapy named omalizumab (Xolair)[27,36,41]. Theophylline is administered either orally or parenterally. This drug has direct bronchodilator, with some reports suggesting anti-inflammatory properties. However, theophylline is not considered first line in the maintenance control of asthma, largely because of its cardiovascular and gastrointestinal side effects. The current Food and Drug Administration indication for omalizumab only extends to the atopic or allergic subgroup of asthma. Xolair is a monoclonal antibody that binds directly with the IgE antibody, which is a major inflammatory mediator in allergic asthma. This drug is injected into the subcutaneous tissue and directed toward maintenance therapy.

Side effects extending from beta-agonist drug therapy require some consideration because the cardiovascular side effects such as tachycardia, palpitations, tachyarrhythmias, tremors, and headache could potentially compromise exercise responses[27,36,41]. Many of the beta-agonist preparations are not selective in that beta-receptors outside of bronchial tissue can also be stimulated. After they are stimulated, the end effect to the beta-agonist inhalers seems to be dose responsive. Levalbuterol (Xopenex) was developed as a selective agonist, having little effect on the beta-receptors outside of bronchial tissue, thereby minimizing cardiovascular stimulation. Tachyphylaxis is defined as a reduction in drug efficacy with repeated administration. This development seems to be more common with frequent use of short-acting rather than the longer-acting beta-agonist inhalers, but it can occur with longer acting beta-agonist inhalers as well. To minimize its occurrence, the beta-agonist should be used only when required, either as a rescue agent or before exercise[27,36,41].

To summarize, asthma management, both pharmacologic and nonpharmacologic, requires consideration. Nonpharmacologic interventions include trigger awareness, peak flow monitoring, and control of comorbid conditions that are associated with accentuating the severity of airflow obstruction. Drug selection is largely based on illness severity and is approached in a stepwise manner (see Fig. 32-2). Exercise management of bronchospasm is much more attainable when chronic bronchial inflammation is kept under control. Additional exercise considerations include symptom manifestation and pretreatment with beta-agonists inhalers.

Bronchiectasis

Bronchiectasis is usually an inflammatory condition characterized by irreversible damage and dilatation of the bronchi[42,43]. Regions of bronchiectasis in the lung commonly become chronically infected. The amount of mucus production is variable, influenced largely by the severity and extensiveness of the disease. Acute exacerbations of this disease influence the amount, color, and tenacity of mucus produced. Mucociliary clearance is altered in bronchiectasis, with retained secretions imposing a significant clinical problem. Recurrent lung and bronchial infections are common. Furthermore, the mucus is rich in inflammatory mediators, predisposing affected individuals to a chronic inflammatory bronchitis, which is sometimes associated with bloody sputum referred to as hemoptysis.

Mild cases of bronchiectasis can be asymptomatic and found incidentally by chest radiograph using computerized tomography. This type of bronchiectasis is most often focal, involving only a small portion of the bronchial tree, such as that seen after an episode of pneumonia. The incidence of clinically significant, progressive bronchiectasis is low relative to other OLDs such as asthma or COPD. However, when clinically extensive disease develops, it is often disabling and sometimes requires surgery such as lung resection or lung transplantation[42,43].

Retained secretions cause either partial or complete airway obstruction. This airflow obstruction can lead to atelectasis or post-obstructive bronchial dilatation. Post-obstructive bronchial dilatation can develop through a ball-valve mechanism, allowing air to flow past the obstruction while inspiring but trapped distally while expiring. Bronchiectasis can also develop by the tethering of surrounding uninvolved airways, leading to bronchial distortion[42,43].

Several factors have been linked to the development of bronchiectasis[42,43]. Cystic fibrosis (CF) is an important cause of bronchiectasis in the United States and Europe, and this disorder has a genetic basis. The age of onset for CF is characteristically childhood, but genetic testing has enabled the identification of adult-onset disease, linked to variable gene penetrance. Recurrent lung infection also plays a major role in the pathogenesis and propagation of bronchiectasis. Often, the infections involve resistant bacterial pathogens, particularly gram-negative organisms such as *Pseudomonas* sp. Mycobacterial organisms, including both tuberculous and nontuberculous species, seem to have a higher propensity to induce progressive bronchiectasis.

TREATMENT AND EXERCISE CONSIDERATIONS

Expiratory flow limitations can occur in as much as 50% of individuals with bronchiectasis, depending on the cause of bronchiectasis[44]. In some patients, the airflow limitation is in association with bronchial hyperresponsiveness, as demonstrated by provocation studies. Some authors believe that this observation represents coexisting asthma[45]. Other studies have demonstrated improved airflow after ipratropium bromide inhalation in patients with bronchiectasis after a histamine provocation study[44]. This observation suggests that the bronchospasm in bronchiectasis is different from that seen in asthma, having more of a vagal mediation extending from lung damage and airway irritation[42,43]. Administration of an inhaled bronchodilator should be considered, but should be determined on an individual basis, as outlined by the clinical manifestation.

Bronchopulmonary hygiene, often referred to as pulmonary toilet, is fundamental to bronchiectasis management[42,43]. Pulmonary toilet involves a combination of adequate hydration to reduce mucus tenacity and chest physiotherapy implemented either manually or with the aid of mechanical devices[42,43,46]. From a clinical perspective, exercise quality and endurance could also improve by implementing this intervention before exercise because mucus plugging theoretically impedes the distal lung unit from participation in gas exchange while promoting airtrapping[42,43]. If acute infection exists, antimicrobial therapy is indicated. The decision to exercise during an acute exacerbation is largely dependent on the severity of the disease and the severity of the exacerbation. This principle not only applies to bronchiectasis but also to the other OLDs.

Non-obstructive Lung Diseases

RESTRICTIVE PULMONARY DISEASE

The restrictive pulmonary disease category encompasses a large number of diseases[44]. The overall incidence for these diseases is low compared with that for the OLD. The pathogenesis, pathology, natural history, and treatment are quite variable for the diseases within this group[47]. One commonality exists among this variability: abnormal lung mechanics. The pathologic process involved with each disease interferes with the ability for normal lung expansion[47]. The mechanisms responsible for the abnormal lung mechanics can be divided into the three groups depicted in Figure 32-4, and they include diseases that involve the lung parenchyma, pleura, and thoracic cage.

Relative to the restrictive pulmonary disease category, there has been very little investigation of the exercise physiology of this category, particularly as it applies to the **interstitial lung diseases (ILDs)**[48–51]. Recently, some authors have argued for the usefulness of exercise testing in the evaluation of at least some restrictive pulmonary diseases[52]. This argument probably relates to the low incidence of this group of diseases, particularly when evaluating a specific ILD. Because of the different pathophysiologic features, it is probably not accurate to extrapolate observations on exercise response identified in a specific cohort to all of the lung diseases because there are likely to be multiple disease-specific variances.

Few generalities can be made for this category of diseases. Whether anatomic involvement is intraparenchymal or extraparenchymal, the volume of air entering the lung is restricted[44]. The degree of restriction is usually proportional to disease severity. To meet criteria using pulmonary function testing (PFT), a reduction in the total lung capacity (TLC) must be evident, with severity defined by the vital capacity (VC) measurement[33]. Early disease may show as its only abnormality an isolated reduction in functional

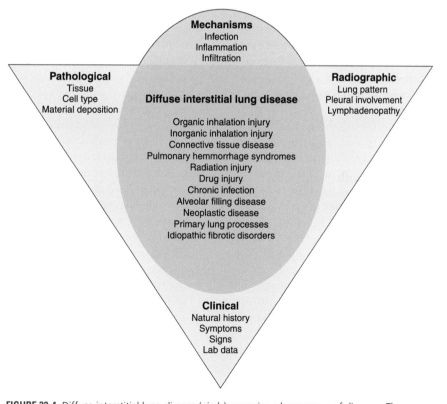

FIGURE 32-4. Diffuse interstitial lung disease (*circle*) comprise a large group of diseases. The etiology for these disease (*lower circle*) can be linked to three basic mechanisms of injury (*upper circle*). Multiple factors are used to characterize each of these diseases. These factors can be simplified by grouping into pathologic, radiographic, and clinical differences (*corners of triangle*). This diagram is used to illustrate the complexity of features to consider when diagnosing diseases+ within this category and the high degree of overlap seen in the characteristics that describe each disease. (Adapted from Nield M, Arora A, Dracup K, et al: Comparison of breathing patterns during exercise in patients with obstructive and restrictive ventilatory abnormalities. J Rehabil Res Dev 40:407–414, 2003.)

residual capacity (FRC) and residual volume (RV). The diffusing capacity is usually low, even with early disease. Investigators have demonstrated that one of the earliest objective pulmonary function measurements for the disease is exercise-induced hypoxemia[48–51].

Flow limitation is usually not a problem with these diseases, unless complicating features develop[44]. Lung fibrosis leading to traction bronchiectasis or the coexistence of COPD extending from tobacco use illustrates complicating features that can occur. Some restrictive lung diseases are classically characterized by a combination of lung restriction and lung obstruction as part of the pathology[44]. The diseases typically associated with both processes include sarcoidosis, hypersensitivity pneumonitis, and eosinophilic granuloma (a disease within the spectrum of histiocytosis X, which involves a proliferation of the Langerhan histiocytes)[44].

The exercise-induced hypoxemia primarily extends from ventilation–perfusion (V/Q) mismatching[48–52]. The V/Q mismatching occurs because of an increase in dead-space ventilation. Increased dead space ventilation extends from a disproportionate rise in the ventilatory rate during exercise, leading to rapid shallow breathing. Respiratory rates will often exceed 50 breaths per minute. The work limitation usually extends from a low breathing reserve. A reduced capillary bed surface area accentuates the dead-space ventilation. This surface area reduction can occur either in the form of pathological disruption of the capillary bed (seen with ILD) or impairment in capillary bed recruitment through the secondary development of pulmonary hypertension (potentially seen with all of the restrictive pulmonary diseases). Even though the diffusing capacity is abnormal, hypoxemia does not usually result from a diffusion defect because of the high oxygen diffusion rates. Only with a high level of exercise or with alveolar proteinosis can a diffusion defect account for the hypoxia.

Relative to the obstructive pulmonary disease category, there has been very little investigation of exercise rehabilitation effects in restrictive pulmonary disease. This phenomenon is largely attributed to the low incidence for all restrictive pulmonary diseases, particularly when comparing them with OLD. Furthermore, it is probably not entirely accurate to extrapolate physiologic responses to exercise rehabilitation observed in one restrictive pulmonary disease and apply it to an unrelated restrictive pulmonary disease that has a different pathologic process.

Interstitial Lung Disease

The first group of restrictive pulmonary diseases involves pathology primarily confined to the lung parenchyma (see Fig. 32-4)[44]. Under normal conditions, the lung interstitium is a potential space that exists between the basement membrane of the alveolar epithelium and capillary epithelium. The matrix or stroma contains collagen and noncollagenous proteins along with a sporadic number of macrophages, fibroblasts, and myofibroblasts. With ILD,

the interstitial stroma consists of a higher percentage of protein material, and the cellularity is often increased. Further magnifying the problem, the pathology is often not limited to the interstitium, and there is involvement of the alveoli and terminal bronchi. The lungs become stiff and noncompliant, lending to the restrictive physiology and diffusion abnormality often seen with this disease. Different natural histories are encountered for each of the ILDs, influencing disease acuity and severity as well as the exercise potential (Box 32-2).

Multiple classifications have been proposed for the ILDs. However, classification schemes are subject to change because the pathogenesis is not clearly understood for many of these diseases and many questions remain unanswered. This phenomenon is largely responsible for the multiple revisions seen with disease nomenclature. The classification scheme used in this chapter (see Fig. 32-4) is structured to enhance clinical practicality. With this approach, the ILDs are grouped into categories based on the most recognized feature causing disease.

Three primary pathologic features are fundamental to this classification schematization. These features include either an infiltrating, inflammatory, or infectious process. Diseases categorized as infiltrating show deposition of a dominant substance within the interstitium, such as amyloid or tumor[44]. Cardiogenic pulmonary edema is arbitrarily included as an infiltrating process because water displaced into the interstitium by hydrostatic forces within the pulmonary vasculature. Diseases categorized as inflammatory include those processes well recognized as having inflammatory mediators propagating the pathogenesis. Noncardiogenic pulmonary edema, or adult respiratory distress syndrome, is arbitrarily assigned to this category because inflammatory mediators are well recognized as the primary mediator of disease. The infectious category includes processes whereby microorganisms are known to be involved disease pathogenesis[44].

Remember, this categorization scheme is used here to simplify the approach to ILD. Not only does it help with disease organization, but it also has clinical utility by simplifying the differential diagnosis for this large and diverse group of diseases. In actuality, most diseases within this group manifest overlapping characteristics and mechanisms of injury, which lends to the inherent complexity of this disease group.

Exercise Considerations

Mechanical limitations directly result from forces generated by the pathology and usually parallel disease severity[44]. Impaired lung expansion translates to a reduced lung volume and lung capacity. The ILDs are characteristically associated with a loss of lung elasticity. PFT criteria for lung restriction require a reduced TLC, with the VC defining the severity[33]. Early disease may only show abnormality after exhalation, including an isolated reduction in the residual capacity and volume measurements (FRC, RV)[44].

BOX 32-2	Diffuse Lung Diseases Outlined by Pathogenesis

ORGANIC INHALATION INJURY
Farmer's lung

Bird fancier's lung

INORGANIC INHALATION INJURY
Asbestosis

Silicosis

Berylliosis

Talc

CONNECTIVE TISSUE DISEASE
Rheumatoid arthritis

Scleraderma

Sjogren's syndrome

Systemic lupus erythematosis

PULMONARY HEMORRHAGE SYNDROMES
Wegener's syndrome

Goodpasture's disease

Vasculitis

PHYSICAL AGENTS
Radiation

Oxygen

Mechanical ventilation

DRUG INJURY
Methotrexate

Bleomycin

Paraquat

Cocaine

CHRONIC INFECTION
Virus

Fungus

Mycobacterial disease

Parasites

ALVEOLAR FILLING DISEASE
Alveolar proteinosis

Amyloidosis

Microlithiasis

NEOPLASTIC DISEASE
Pulmonary lymphoma

Bronchoalveolar cell carcinoma

Lymphangitic carcinomatosis

PRIMARY LUNG PROCESSES
Sarcoidosis

Eosinophilic granuloma

Amyloidosis

Lymphangioleiomyomatosis

IDIOPATHIC FIBROTIC DISEASES, INCLUDING USUAL INTERSTITIAL PNEUMONITIS
Desquamative interstitial pneumonitis

Fibrosing alveolitis

Bronchiolitis obliterans with organizing pneumonia

Lymphocytic interstitial pneumonia

The diffusion capacity measured during the PFT is usually low with restrictive disease[44]. This abnormality reflects impaired gas diffusion through the alveolar and capillary interface. This diffusion abnormality usually does not translate into clinically significant hypoxemia because there is adequate pulmonary capillary transit time to allow complete diffusion equilibrium of the oxygen molecules. The one exception to this rule is exercise[54]. Hypoxemia extending directly from an impaired diffusion rate can be seen when individuals with ILD exercise[48–52].

The restrictive pulmonary diseases extrinsic to the lung parenchyma can be viewed either as an intrapleural or extrapleural process[44]. Intrapleural processes can be viewed by physical properties creating the abnormal pleural characteristics. Pneumothorax occurs when there is a collection of air within the pleural space. When liquid accumulates within the pleural space, it is referred to as a pleural effusion. There are many causes of pleural effusions, including renal disease, heart failure, pneumonia, and malignancy. Infiltration of a solid substance into the pleural space occurs with certain fibrotic processes and malignancy. The last group of restrictive pulmonary diseases includes extrapleural pleural processes that impact muscle strength or function of the diaphragm or thoracic cage[44]. Any process that results in an increase in the intrabdominal pressure will inhibit diaphragmatic function. Exercises performed with a recumbent body position will have the same impact on diaphragmatic excursion. Neuromuscular diseases affect the ventilatory muscle strength. Thoracic deformities and poor posture interfere with the proper function of thoracic cage to operate as a bellows[44].

Physiologic responses to exercise directly extend from the impaired lung inhalation[48–53]. Ventilatory rate increases to compensate for the low lung volume. The rate can exceed 50 breaths per minute, frequently approaching the ventilatory threshold or maximum ventilatory volume (MVV) for that individual. MVV is determined by the lung disease severity regardless of the disease category. The result is reduced work efficiency and reduced exercise endurance[53].

Pulmonary vascular abnormalities are often found with restrictive pulmonary disease[44]. These vascular abnormalities are usually a secondary effect, from advanced lung disease. Secondary **pulmonary hypertension** can result from either vascular bed destruction, seen with many fibrotic lung processes, or from a high pulmonary vascular tone, which can occur with chronic hypoxic states. Exercise limitations associated with pulmonary hypertension are discussed in the next section of this chapter.

Airflow limitation is not usually routinely encountered in restrictive lung disease[44]. By contrast, increased lung elastic recoil can enhance expiratory flow. The exception to this rule is the development of traction bronchiectasis with advanced pulmonary fibrosis. Forces generated by the fibrotic process create a tethering effect on the adjacent bronchi, distorting their conformation. As with primary bronchiectasis, mucociliary clearance is affected, creating a secondary obstructive component. Sometimes the primary pathologic process is characterized by both lung restriction and lung obstruction. Diseases within this group include sarcoidosis, hypersensitivity pneumonitis, and eosinophilic granuloma. Because of the frequency of COPD with tobacco inhalation, individuals who smoke and develop a restrictive lung process often have COPD as a comorbid problem.

DISORDERS IN THE PULMONARY VASCULATURE

Under normal conditions, the pulmonary vascular system is a low-pressure circuit with a low vascular resistance[44]. Vascular resistance can be altered by disease. The mechanism depends on whether the vessel is a primary disease target. Box 32-3 shows the WHO Disease Classifications based on the cause of pulmonary hypertension. The distinction of etiology has both prognostic and therapeutic value.

Primary pulmonary hypertension (PPH) exemplifies the vessel wall as the primary disease target[44]. This disease is rare and mostly sporadic in occurrence, with only 10% of the cases demonstrating genetic linkage[44]. Risk factors predisposing to pulmonary artery hypertension include connective tissue diseases, chronic liver disease, HIV infection, cocaine or amphetamine use, and dietary agents such as fenfluramine and tryptophan. Diagnosis of PPH is complex, and readers are referred to McGoon et al.[54] for a detailed overview. The determination of disease severity of pulmonary hypertension follows the criteria used by the

BOX 32-3	**WHO Disease Classification of the Cause of Pulmonary Hypertension**

Pulmonary artery hypertension

Pulmonary venous hypertension

Extending from respiratory disease

Extending from thromboembolic disease

Extending from disease directly affecting pulmonary vascular

Adapted from Simonneau G, Galie N, Rubin LJ, et al: Clinical classification of pulmonary hypertension. J Am Coll Cardiol 43(suppl S):5S–12S, 2004.

American Heart Association outlined for congestive heart failure (Box 32-4)[55].

Secondary pulmonary hypertension demonstrates an indirect effect of disease on pulmonary vascular resistance. Diseases that can lead to the development of secondary pulmonary hypertension include pulmonary fibrosis, COPD, and left-sided heart disease[44]. Prognostic and therapeutic implications underscore the importance of making the distinction between primary and secondary pulmonary hypertension[44,55].

EXERCISE CONSIDERATIONS

Therapeutic considerations include both medical and surgical treatments for PPH[56,57] that may increase exercise performance. Exercise training in patients with PPH is controversial[58]. Pulmonary artery pressures are generally elevated during exercise, but pulmonary artery systolic pressure does not normally exceed 40 mm Hg[34]. In PPH, the increases in pulmonary artery pressures with exercise are likely to be exaggerated (see below). The vascular remodeling and endothelial dysfunction seen in

BOX 32-4	**WHO Classification of the Severity of Illness for Pulmonary Hypertension**
Class I	Asymptomatic, no physical limitations
Class II	Mild limitations with physical activity
Class III	Marked limitation with physical activity
	No discomfort at rest
Class IV	Unable to perform any physical activity
	Symptomatic at rest
	Right heart failure

Adapted from Simonneau G, Galie N, Rubin LJ, et al: Clinical classification of pulmonary hypertension. J Am Coll Cardiol 43(suppl S):5S–12S, 2004.

patients with PPH largely account for the increase in pulmonary vascular resistance, which affects right ventricular afterload[59]. In patients with PPH, pulmonary pressures can increase suddenly and dramatically during exercise, predisposing then to right ventricular decompensation and cardiovascular collapse[59]. Sudden death has been reported during exercise in individuals with PPH; the underlying mechanism is postulated as acute right ventricular pressure overload or cardiac arrhythmia. More recently, some investigators have suggested that exercise can be performed safely in patients with less severe PPH if the exercise is approached carefully[60].

Dyspnea is the major manifestation of these patients, with an incidence of at least 95%[59]. A reduced cardiac output relative to metabolic demands is one proposed mechanism[59-61]. This symptom is first evident with activity but progresses to the resting state as the disease advances. Fatigue and weakness also are important manifestations of PPH, also reflecting the inability to meet metabolic demands. Other symptoms include substernal chest pain, presyncope (dizziness), and syncope (loss of consciousness).

Hypoxemia is a major sign of pulmonary hypertension that can be detected during the physical examination[59]. Paralleling dyspnea, hypoxemia may be only seen during exercise with early disease but is eventually seen while resting as the disease progresses[59]. As the disease progresses, hypoxemia is seen under resting conditions and can be quite profound with exercise, often requiring supplemental oxygen[44].

V/Q mismatching is a major mechanism accounting for the hypoxia in pulmonary hypertension[44]. Remodeling of the vascular wall is a major contributor to V/Q mismatch and is present to variable degrees, depending on the cause and severity of pulmonary hypertension. Pulmonary arterial vasoconstriction also contributes to the V/Q mismatch[60]. Contributing factors include alveolar hypoxia and dysfunction of the vascular endothelium. Endothelial dysfunction is an important mechanism to consider in PPH because many of the more recent interventions are directed toward this abnormality. These mechanisms account for the reduced cross-sectional area for blood flow through the pulmonary circulation. As disease progresses, the cross-sectional area is progressively reduced[58,59,61]. Exercise augments the abnormality because pulmonary vascular recruitment is essential during exercise and limited in the setting of pulmonary hypertension[60].

Shunt is an important mechanism for the hypoxemia encountered in pulmonary hypertension because it is often the explanation for the refractory response to supplemental oxygen[60,61]. Many individuals have a patent foramen ovale, a congenital communication between the right and left atria. This communication remains closed after birth unless right-sided heart pressures become abnormally elevated. The pressure gradient favoring right-to-left intracardiac blood flow in pulmonary hypertension is often augmented by exercise. This venous admixture shunted into the left heart does not interface with ambient oxygen compared with blood flowing through the pulmonary capillary network. Thus, attempts at providing higher concentrations of supplemental oxygen are futile because that portion of blood does not travel through the intrapulmonary vascular network[59].

The increase in pulmonary vascular resistance with secondary pulmonary hypertension is largely induced by forces external or downstream to the pulmonary vascular network[44,60]. Examples include the tension created by lung fibrosis, air trapping induced by COPD, and vascular congestion extending from left heart dysfunction. Often the underlying lung disease causes a portion of the pulmonary capillary network to be destroyed. Blood vessel remodeling and endothelial dysfunction can occur with secondary pulmonary hypertension but do not seem to be as important as with PPH.

Different pathologic mechanisms accounting for the elevated pulmonary vascular resistance is likely to explain the differences in treatment and exercise response[59,60]. Exercise seems to be better tolerated with secondary pulmonary hypertension in comparison with PPH, particularly when the later is in the moderate to severe stage. A possible explanation is that acute right ventricular decompensation with exercise is more likely to occur with PPH, particularly in the moderate to severe stages. Even though exercise seems to be better tolerated with secondary pulmonary hypertension, the rate of improvement in the exercise response and endurance are still difficult. Many of these individuals have been shown to have significant cardiovascular limitations, suggested by the resting tachycardia observed in many of them[44,59]. The reduced endurance is further accentuated by the early development of anaerobic metabolism during exercise.

Disorders in Breathing Control

Ventilatory control is mediated either through metabolic or behavioral pathways[44]. Metabolic pathways are triggered by changes in carbon dioxide or oxygen tension or changes in acid–base balance (pH) detected by chemoreceptors. Chemoreceptors are located either centrally, such as in the brain, or peripherally, such as in the carotid bodies. Ventilatory control through behavioral pathway originates from the brain cortex and supramedullary region. Disorders in breathing control are classified as hyperventilation or hypoventilation syndromes.

HYPERVENTILATION SYNDROMES

The ventilatory drive for hyperventilation syndromes can originate either from metabolic or behavioral pathways[44]. Examples of hyperventilation that are metabolically induced include excessive acid ingestion (ethanol, methanol, aspirin) and poorly controlled diabetes mellitus (diabetic ketoacidosis). Anxiety disorder is the primary example of a behaviorally mediated pathway for hyperventilation. With regard to exercise, the importance of hyperventilation syndrome is that the individual has a lower breathing reserve[62]. Minute ventilation is already high at rest and sometimes near the ventilatory limit, leaving little margin to accommodate for exercise.

HYPOVENTILATION SYNDROMES

Hypoventilation mediated through a behavioral pathway is difficult to sustain with a conscious effort[44]. Arterial carbon dioxide tension increases with hypoventilation, creating a respiratory acidosis. To some extent, this category overlaps with the other lung categories, particularly when the disease is severe[44]. Severe OLD creates a physiologic restriction when a high degree of air trapping exists. The respiratory rate is the only means of compensating for the severely limited lung volumes seen with severe restriction but difficult to sustain because of limitations in ventilatory work.

Two syndromes within this category—obstructive sleep apnea and obesity hypoventilation syndrome—require consideration[44]. These two syndromes are frequently encountered within the morbidly obese population. Their importance largely relates to the contribution made by these two syndromes with regard to illness severity. Hypoxia is more likely to be problematic in obese individuals who have either one of these disorders. Additionally, these two syndromes predispose patients to cor pulmonale and right-sided heart failure.

Obstructive sleep apnea syndrome is characterized by increased airway resistance while sleeping and intermittent nocturnal airway collapse[63]. Nocturnal apneas sleep disruption, daytime hypersomnolence, and cognitive impairment are all classic manifestations of this disorder. Chronic hypoxia can be substantial and present while asleep and while awake for which supplemental oxygen is required. This disorder is frequently associated with systemic arterial hypertension. When systemic hypertension is present, additional hemodynamic exercise considerations include the reduced ventricular filling during diastole (i.e., diastolic dysfunction).

Obesity hypoventilation syndrome is exclusive seen in morbidly obese individuals[64]. Historically, this disorder was referred to as Pickwickian syndrome. Chronic hypoxemia and cor pulmonale are also seen with this disorder. This syndrome has an additional feature, chronic hypercapnia reflective of chronic respiratory failure. As predicted, many patients exhibit characteristics of both diagnoses by virtue of the population subset most likely affected and the similarity in signs and symptoms. In addition, patients with these syndromes are treated with assisted ventilation, particularly during sleep. Obstructive sleep apnea is appropriately treated with continuous positive airway pressure (CPAP) to prevent upper airway collapse, and obesity hypoventilation syndrome requires bilevel intermittent positive airway pressure (BiPAP) to augment alveolar ventilation. The consensus is that the diagnosis of "obesity hypoventilation syndrome" is reserved for individuals manifesting criteria but who do not have obstructive sleep apnea syndrome as diagnosed by a polysomnogram (overnight sleep study).

EXERCISE CONSIDERATIONS

The consequences of morbid obesity on exercise are multiple[34,65]. The restrictive effects that obesity has on lung function have already been described. The mechanical effects include limitation in ventilatory function because of the added weight on the chest wall and impaired diaphragmatic excursion[65]. Some additional features associated with obesity also have considerable impact on exercise. First, the energy expenditure in obese individuals is higher for them to do the same amount of work compared with lean individuals, predisposing obese individuals to respiratory muscle fatigue occurring at an earlier stage of exercise[64]. FRC is also reduced and approaches residual volume in extremely obese individuals[64]. This development coincides with collapse of peripheral lung units, a condition referred to as atelectasis. This effect is accentuated by body position. So, exercise in a recumbent position should be minimized in these individuals[65].

The Exercise Prescription

Determining the optimal exercise dose in lung disease is difficult (see GETP7 Chapter 9). Too little exercise means that reconditioning is hard to achieve. Too much exercise risks the potential for psychological anguish and respiratory failure. Signs and symptoms are the best parameters to use in determining the ideal exercise intensity, duration, and frequency. Coupling these parameters with many of the concepts used in pulmonary rehabilitation serve to guide this process.

Most of the symptoms and signs for lung disease (wheeze, cough, mucus production, presyncope, hypoxia) have been addressed in the sections on disease-specific considerations. One of the cardinal manifestations for lung disease that deserves more focus is dyspnea[66]. An accurate and detailed assessment of dyspnea cannot be overemphasized.

DYSPNEA

Dyspnea is defined as the "sensation of breathlessness"[66]. The underlying mechanism involves an imbalance between oxygen supply and demand. It is a nonspecific symptom, manifested when there is an uncoupling in pulmonary efficiency, cardiovascular function, or cellular metabolism. So, other diseases and illnesses outside of lung disease that directly impact oxygen supply must also be considered with the dyspnea evaluation[66].

Oxygen supply is determined by blood composition and blood delivery to the tissues[34]. Disease states are not a prerequisite because the fraction of inspired oxygen inhaled impacts blood composition, exemplified by high-altitudes conditions. Lung diseases affect oxygen supply, primarily through abnormal gas exchange[44]. Mechanisms linked to nonpulmonic processes include (a) reduced oxygen carrying capacity of the blood, such as with anemia and (b) reduced tissue perfusion, such as with congestive heart failure or vascular disease.

Oxygen demand is determined by end-organ function or the rate of cellular metabolism[34]. Exercise, fever, and thyroid and catecholamine hyperactivity can all increase in cellular metabolism. Cellular metabolism changes from aerobic to anaerobic conditions when the oxygen demand is not adequately met[34]. With chronic lung disease, exercise metabolism becomes reliant on anaerobic conditions at an earlier stage relative to what occurs in normal individuals[38,60]. Anaerobic conditions augment ventilatory requirement to compensate for the higher carbon dioxide output and eventual metabolic acidosis. In addition to increased ventilatory requirement, ventilatory capacity is low, thus limiting exercise performance. The significance of uncompensated metabolic acidosis is reduced muscle strength, reduced endurance, and a slower rate of recovery from exercise.

The cellular metabolism within muscles used for breathing requires additional consideration[34,38,61]. Under normal resting conditions, breathing accounts for less that 3% of the total body metabolism and does not require an active effort. In lung disease, the energy expenditure for breathing takes on a higher percentage. Obstacles such as air trapping and low lung compliance largely account for the relationship change. This relationship is further swayed by the higher acid production seen with anaerobic metabolism, which causes a secondary increase ventilatory work.

Assessment of Dyspnea

The consensus is to apply supplemental oxygen when exercise-induced hypoxia is detected[27]. Oxygen can facilitate reconditioning by enabling exercise to be performed at a higher intensity for a longer duration. A reduced lactic acid production has been linked to this response, lowering the ventilatory demand and level of dyspnea.

Consistency is a major objective to the dyspnea assessment[66]. The difficulty in achieving this objective is inherent to the nature this symptom largely attributable to different perceptions of dyspnea by each individual. Dyspnea scales can reduce the amount of variation encountered[67]. Several scales have been demonstrated to be valid and reproducible, but the Borg Dyspnea Index is one of the more commonly used scales. Visual analog scales can also be used to evaluate an individual's perception of dyspnea.

Dyspnea is a symptom reported by the individual, but there are multiple signs made by the observer that complement the dyspnea assessment. The degree of breathlessness can be estimated by the ease of speech during exercise[67,68], although some authors do not agree[69]. An inability to speak more than two or three words reflects a high degree of breathlessness. Additional signs include use of accessory muscles to assist with breathing[66,67]. Accessory muscles are primarily located in the neck and shoulder girdle. Flailing of the nares can also be seen with more severe levels of breathlessness. In the setting of airflow obstruction, a prolongation in the expiratory phase of the ventilatory cycle, greater than 1:3, usually reflects an increase in the amount of air trapping.

PERCEIVED LEVEL OF EXERTION

Fatigue and weakness are not mutually exclusive symptoms to the dyspnea assessment; rather, they are used to enhance the evaluation[66,67]. As opposed to the case in normal individuals, in those with chronic lung disease, HR is not the best indicator for maximum exercise intensity of energy expenditure[38]. Remember, resting HR is often elevated in individuals with chronic lung disease, particularly if their severity is advanced[60]. Ratings of perceived level of exertion have been found to be a better correlate for exercise intensity for this population, particularly because the direct measurement of $\dot{V}O_{2\,max}$ can be expensive and impractical[67]. Similar to the Dyspnea Index, several scales measuring the perceived level of exertion have been developed and demonstrated to be valid and reproducible. The Borg RPE scale was developed to rate perceived exertion (see GETP7 Table 4-7) Remember, making the distinction between perceived exertion and dyspnea is essential but difficult because they are not mutually exclusive[67]. The former represents the degree of peripheral muscle fatigue and weakness, and the latter represents the degree of breathlessness.

Often, there seems to be a reluctance to push exercise in individuals with moderate to severe lung disease. The key to estimating the maximum sustainable exercise intensity is: (a) recognize the difference between "perceived level of exertion" and "dyspnea;" (b) avoid sustained ventilatory loads close to ventilatory capacity, which would correlate to a "moderate" dyspnea index; and (c) aim for an exercise intensity level that is 60% to 80% of the maximum capability for that individual, which would approximate a 60% to 80% range on an "perceived level of exertion" scale. Sustained levels higher than these recommendations predispose to muscle fatigue and exhaustion. If the respiratory muscle fatigue is sustained, respiratory failure can ensue. Although skeletal muscle fatigue is better tolerated, it still influences the frequency at which exercise can be performed[38,67,68].

Pulmonary Rehabilitation

Pulmonary rehabilitation is a structured exercise program implemented in individuals with chronic respiratory illnesses that are associated with a progressive decline in

BOX 32-5	Goals of Pulmonary Rehabilitation

Reduce the work of breathing

Improve pulmonary function

Normalize arterial blood gases

Alleviate dyspnea

Increase efficiency of energy use

Correct poor nutrition

Improve exercise performance and activities of daily living

Restore a positive outlook

Improve emotional state

Decrease health-related costs

Lengthen survival

Adapted from Celli BR: Pulmonary rehabilitation for COPD: A practical approach for improving ventilatory conditioning. Postgrad Med 103:159–178, 1998.

performance status[70,71]. Both physical and psychological needs are addressed, and these programs facilitate a holistic approach to lung disease management (Box 32-5). The components of a comprehensive pulmonary rehabilitation are outlined in Box 32-6, and these components provide a general framework for approaching exercise in

BOX 32-6	Pulmonary Rehabilitation Exercise Prescription

1. Frequency
   a. Three to five sessions per week (program dependant)
2. Intensity
   a. Individualize targeted submaximal work capacity[a]
   b. Increase intensity every fifth session
   c. Increase work intensity as soon as submaximal targeted work is 20 to 30 minutes
3. Duration
   a. Starting pulmonary rehabilitation: Minimum of 30 min/session
   b. Near program completion: Minimum of 60 min/session

[a]Determined by maximal predicted heart rate coupled with 6-minute walk data when Cardiopulmonary Exercise Test (CPEX) not available. Most individuals can achieve 60% to 80% maximal work load. Severely debilitated individuals may need to start at 30% maximal work load. Individuals with resting tachycardia may need to start at 90% maximal work capacity unless contraindicated (e.g., angina, presyncope).

Adapted from Pulmonary rehabilitation: Joint ACCP/AACVPR evidence-based guidelines. ACCP/AACVPR Pulmonary Rehabilitation Guidelines Panel. American College of Chest Physicians. American Association of Cardiovascular and Pulmonary Rehabilitation. Chest 112:1363–1396, 1997.

patients with chronic lung disease (also see GETP7 Chapter 9). The algorithm found in Box 32-7 provides the foundation for exercise implementation. The building blocks for this foundation are the principles discussed throughout this chapter along with the observed responses to the exercise.

Substantial benefits resulting from pulmonary rehabilitation[72] have been identified (Box 32-8). The major premise underlying the metabolic improvements is that work performed is more efficient. Put another way, work performed before pulmonary rehabilitation results in lower energy expenditure during ADLs. Many studies have shown that pulmonary rehabilitation increases maximum workload, as measured by the $\dot{V}O_{2\ max}$. Therapeutic interven-

BOX 32-7	Components of Pulmonary Rehabilitation Program

PATIENT EDUCATION

Pulmonary anatomy, physiology, and disease pathophysiology

Diagnostic testing

Treatment, including oxygen, medications, surgery

Bronchial hygiene techniques

EXERCISE TRAINING

Breathing retraining

Endurance, strength, and flexibility training, including of the upper and lower extremities

Ventilatory muscle training

Energy conservation techniques

SELF-MANAGEMENT

Self-assessment and symptom management

Infection control (avoidance, early intervention, and immunization)

Environmental control

Indications for seeking medical advice and resources

Sleep disturbances

Sexuality and intimacy

Nutrition

Smoking cessation

PSYCHOSOCIAL INTERVENTION AND SUPPORT

Community services, including patient and family support groups

Advance care planning

Recreation and leisure activities and travel

Stress management

Adapted from Haynes JM: AARC clinical practice guideline: Pulmonary rehabilitation. Respir Care 47:617–625, 2002.

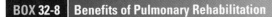

| BOX 32-8 | Benefits of Pulmonary Rehabilitation |

Large and significant increases in exercise endurance

Modest increase in exercise work capacity

Changes in biochemical muscle enzymes (the effects of which are controversial)

Significant reduction of dyspnea

Improved quality of life

Reduced health-related costs

Adapted from Celli BR: Pulmonary rehabilitation for COPD: A practical approach for improving ventilatory conditioning. Postgrad Med 103:159–178, 1998.

tions that reduce disease severity, improve airflow, or enhance lung compliance also impact this parameter because the maximum level of work directly relates to the disease process and disease severity[70,73]. The endproduct of improved work efficiency is a higher endurance, improved performance status, better quality of life, and a higher sense of well being. Studies that are more recent also demonstrate a reduction in health care utilization[73–76].

Multiple methods have been reported to be effective in pulmonary rehabilitation[70,74–76]. Aerobic exercise for endurance training is conventionally performed by stationary cycling and by walking on a track or treadmill. Some programs use water aerobics when a pool is available, which is advantageous when arthritis or morbid obesity is a comorbid condition. Strength training is an important complement to endurance training[76]. Resistance, light weights, and gravity are used to strength train in patients with lung disease. ADLs can be executed with greater ease, particularly with upper extremity strength training. Core muscle strength training should also be included in the program so that balance and posture are addressed, both of which are particularly problematic in these individuals. General principles of resistance training should be used (see Chapter 25 and GETP7 Chapter 7). For example, a practical resistance training program consists of two sets of exercises targeting the large agonist and antagonist muscles of the arms and legs. Each set should consist of eight to 10 repetitions. Most importantly, the resistance chosen should lead to fatigue within these eight to 10 repetitions.

The time frames used for pulmonary rehabilitation programs are variable. A program with 18 sessions is most frequently used. Shorter programs have been tried, but outcomes are not comparable to that seen after 18 sessions[70,76]. A significant training effect achieved during this time frame is not limited to individuals with mild to moderate disease; individuals with severe disease have demonstrated significant short- and long-term training effects through regimented exercise programs[77,78]. Aero-

bic training sessions should ideally be done three times weekly. It has been shown that twice-weekly sessions might not be effective. Resistance training, on the other hand, is best implemented twice weekly to allow for muscle recovery.

Summary

Exercise in chronic lung disease can be performed regardless of the illness severity level. Pulmonary rehabilitation principles should be used as the framework for the exercise prescription, but disease-specific principles should also be incorporated. Disease-specific principles can be easily identified with a basic understanding of lung pathophysiology as it relates to pattern recognition for each of the disease categories. These principles also facilitate identification of the proper therapeutic interventions. Incorporating modifications based on the individual's response to exercise can further augment individualization of the exercise program. The response to exercise is best judged by understanding basic pathophysiology and recognizing the meaning and measurement of certain signs and symptoms.

REFERENCES

1. American Thoracic Society: Standards for the diagnosis and care of patients with chronic obstructive pulmonary disease. Am J Respir Crit Care Med 152:S77–S121, 1995.
2. O'Donnell DE, Lam M, Webb A: Measurement of symptoms, lung hyperinflation, and endurance during exercise in chronic obstructive pulmonary disease. Am J Crit Care Med 158:1557–1565, 1998.
3. O'Donnell DE, D'Arsigny C, Fitzpatrick M, Webb KA: Exercise hypercapnia in advanced chronic obstructive pulmonary disease: The role of lung hyperinflation. Am J Respir Crit Care Med 166:663–668, 2002.
4. O'Donnell DE, Revill SM, Webb KA: Dynamic hyperinflation and exercise intolerance in chronic obstructive pulmonary disease. Am J Respir Crit Care Med 164:770–777, 2001.
5. Barnes PJ, Shapiro SD, Pauwels RA: Chronic obstructive pulmonary disease: Molecular and cellular mechanisms. Eur Respir J 22: 672–688, 2003.
6. Barnes PJ: Mechanisms in COPD: Differences from asthma. Chest 117(suppl):10S–4S, 2000.
7. Fraser RS, Colman N, Müller NL, Pare PD: Chronic obstructive pulmonary disease (pp. 2168–2243). In Fraser and Pare's Diagnosis of Disease of the Chest, 4th ed. Philadelphia: WB Saunders; 1999.
8. Desai TJ, Karlinsky JB: OPD: Clinical manifestations, diagnosis, and treatment (pp. 204–246) In Crapo JD, Glassroth J, Karlinsky J, King TE, eds. Baum's Textbook of Pulmonary Diseases, 7th ed. Philadelphia: Lippincott, Williams & Wilkins; 2004.
9. Bleecker ER: Similarities and differences in asthma and COPD. Chest 126:93S–995S, 2004.
10. Sciurba FC: Physiologic similarities and differences between COPD and asthma. Chest 126:117S–124S, 2004.
11. Soriano JB, Davis KJ, Coleman B, et al: The proportional Venn diagram of obstructive lung disease: Two approximations from the United States and the United Kingdom. Chest 124:474–481, 2003.
12. Sciurba FC: Physiologic similarities and differences between COPD and asthma. Chest 126:117S–124S, 2004.
13. Postma DS, Boezen HM: Rationale for the Dutch Hypothesis. Allergy and airway hyperresponsiveness as genetic factors and their interaction with environment in the development of asthma and COPD. Chest 126:96S–104S, 2004.

14. Barnes PJ: Asthma guidelines: Recommendations versus reality. Respir Med 98(suppl A):S1–S7, 2004.

15. Mannino DM, Homa DM, Akinbami LJ, et al: Chronic obstructive pulmonary disease surveillance—United States, 1971–2000. Morbid Mortal World Rep MMWR 51:1–16, 2002.

16. Hilleman DE, Dewan N, Malesker M, Friedman M: Pharmacoeconomic evaluation of COPD. Chest 118:1278–1285, 2000.

17. Nunn JF: Pulmonary ventilation: mechanisms and the work of breathing (pp. 117–128). In Nunn's Applied Respiratory Physiology 4th ed. Cambridge: Butterworth Heinmann; 1993

18. Pauwels RA, Buist AS, Ma P, et al: Global strategy for the diagnosis, management, and prevention of chronic obstructive pulmonary disease. NHLBI and WHO Global Initiative for Chronic Obstructive Lung Disease: Executive summary. Respir Care 46:798–825, 2001.

19. Global Initiative for Chronic Obstructive Lung Disease. Available at: http://www.goldcopd.com

20. Celli BR, Cote CG, Marin JM, et al: The body-mass index, airflow obstruction, dyspnea, and exercise capacity index in chronic obstructive pulmonary disease. N Engl J Med 350:1005–1012, 2004.

21. American Thoracic Society Statement: Lung function testing: Selection of reference values and interpretative strategies. Am Rev Respir Dis 144:1202–1218, 1991.

22. Nishimura K, Izumi T, Tsukino M, Oga T: Dyspnea is a better predictor of 5-year survival than airway obstruction in patients with COPD. Chest 121:1434–1440, 2002.

23. ATS Committee on Proficiency Standards for Clinical Pulmonary Function Laboratories: ATS statement: guidelines for the six-minute walk test. Am J Respir Crit Care Med 166:111–117, 2002.

24. Celli BR: Pathophysiology of chronic obstructive pulmonary disease (pp. 41–55). In Pulmonary Rehabilitation: Guidelines to Success, 3rd ed. Hodgkin JE, Celli BR, Connors GL, eds. Philadelphia: Lippincott, Williams & Wilkins; 2000.

25. Ferguson GT, Cherniack RM: Management of chronic obstructive pulmonary disease. N Engl J Med 328:1017–1022, 1993.

26. Tashkin DP, Cooper CB: The role of long-acting bronchodilators in the management of stable COPD. Chest 125:249–259, 2004.

27. Expert Panel Report 2: Guidelines for the diagnosis and management of asthma. Bethesda, MD: National Institutes of Health, National Heart, Lung, and Blood Institute. NIH Publication No. 97-4051; 1997.

28. National Institutes of Health Data Fact Sheet: Asthma, Statistics. Bethesda, MD: U.S. Department of Health and Human Services. NIH Publication No. 55-798; 1999.

29. Lange P, Parner J, Vestbo J, et al: A 15-year follow-up study of ventilatory function in adults with asthma. N Engl J Med 339:1194–2000, 1998.

30. Tiddens H, Silverman M, Bush A: The role of inflammation in airway disease: remodeling. Am J Respir Crit Care Med 162(2 Pt 2):S7–S10, 2000.

31. Busse W, Elias J, Sheppard D, et al: Effects of treatment on airway inflammation and thickening of basement membrane reticular collagen in asthma. A quantitative light and electron microscopic study. Am J Respir Crit Care Med 145(4 pt 1):890–899, 1992.

32. Sutherland ER, Kraft M, Crapo JD: Diagnosis and treatment of asthma (pp. 179–198). In Crapo JD, Glassroth J, Karlinsky J, King TE, eds. Baum's Textbook of Pulmonary Diseases, 7th ed. Philadelphia: Lippincott, Williams & Wilkins; 2004.

33. American Thoracic Society: Lung function testing: Selection of reference values and interpretative strategies Am Rev Respir Dis 146:1368–1369, 1992.

34. Wasserman K, Hansen JE, Sue DY, et al: Principles of Exercise Testing & Interpretation, 3rd ed. Philadelphia: Lippincott, Williams & Wilkins; 1999.

35. American Thoracic Society. ATS/ACCP statement on cardiopulmonary exercise testing. Am J Respir Crit Care Med 167:211–277, 2003.

36. Newman KB, Mason UG, Schmaling KB: Clinical features of vocal cord dysfunction. Am J Respir Crit Care Med 152:1382–1386, 1995.

37. Theodoropoulos DS, Pecoraro DL, Efstratiadis SE: The association of gastroesophageal reflux disease with asthma and chronic cough in the adult. Am J Respir Med 1:133–146, 2002.

38. Cooper CB: Exercise in chronic pulmonary disease: Limitations and rehabilitation. Med Sci Sports Exerc 33:S671–S679, 2001.

39. Donohue JF: Therapeutic responses in asthma and COPD: Bronchodilators. Chest 126 (2 suppl): 125S–137S, 2004.

40. Larj MJ, Bleeker ER: Therapeutic responses in asthma and COPD: Corticosteroids. Chest 126 (2 suppl): 138S–149S, 2004.

41. Barnes PJ: Asthma management: Can we further improve compliance and outcomes? Respir Med 98(suppl A):S8–S9, 2004.

42. Ryu JH, Myers JL, Swensen SJ: Bronchiolar disorders. Am J Respir Crit Care Med 168:1277–1292, 2003.

43. Silverman E, Ebright L, Kwiatkowski M, Cullina J: Current management of bronchiectasis: Review and 3 case studies. Heart Lung 32:59–64, 2003.

44. Murray JF, Nadel JA: Part 2: Manifestations and diagnosis of respiratory disease. In Textbook of Respiratory Medicine, 3rd ed. Philadelphia: WB Saunders; 2000.

45. Barnes PT, Drazen JM, Rennard S, Thompson NC: Asthma and COPD Basic Mechanisms and Clinical Management, 1st ed. Boston: Elsevier; 2000:467–468,.

46. Bradley J, Moran F, Greenstone M: Physical training for bronchiectasis. Cochrane Database Syst Rev(3):CD002166; 2002.

47. Nield M, Arora A, Dracup K, et al: Comparison of breathing patterns during exercise in patients with obstructive and restrictive ventilatory abnormalities. J Rehabil Res Dev 40:407–414, 2003.

48. Markovitz GH, Cooper CB: Exercise and interstitial lung disease. Curr Opin Pulm Med 4:272–280, 1998.

49. Harris-Eze AO, Sridhar G, Clemens RE, et al: Role of hypoxemia and pulmonary mechanics in exercise limitation in interstitial lung disease. Am J Respir Crit Care Med 154 (4 Pt 1):994–1001, 1996.

50. Marciniuk DD, Sridhar G, Clemens RE, et al: Lung volumes and expiratory flow limitation during exercise in interstitial lung disease. J Appl Physiol 77:963–973, 1994.

51. Marciniuk DD, Watts RE, Gallagher CG: Dead space loading and exercise limitation in patients with interstitial lung disease. Chest 105:183–189, 1994.

52. Mascolo MC, Truwit JD: Role of exercise evaluation in restrictive lung disease: New insights between March 2001 and February 2003. Curr Opin Pulm Med 9:408–410, 2003.

53. Neild M, Arora A, Dracup K, et al: Comparison of breathing patterns during exercise in patients with obstructive and restrictive ventilatory abnormalities. J Rehabil Res Dev 40:407–414, 2003.

54. McGoon M, Gutterman D, Steen V, et al: American College of Chest Physicians. Screening, early detection, and diagnosis of pulmonary arterial hypertension: ACCP evidence-based clinical practice guidelines. Chest 126(suppl):14S–34S, 2004.

55. Hunt SA, Baker DW, Chin MH, et al: American College of Cardiology/American Heart Association Task Force on Practice Guidelines (Committee to Revise the 1995 Guidelines for the Evaluation and Management of Heart Failure); International Society for Heart and Lung Transplantation; Heart Failure Society of America. ACC/AHA Guidelines for the Evaluation and Management of Chronic Heart Failure in the Adult: Executive Summary A Report of the American College of Cardiology/American Heart Association Task Force on Practice Guidelines Circulation 104:2996–3007, 2001.

56. Badesch DB, Abman SH, Ahearn GS, et al: American College of Chest Physicians. Medical therapy for pulmonary arterial hypertension: ACCP evidence-based clinical practice guidelines. Chest 126(suppl):35S–62S, 2004.

57. Doyle RL, McCrory D, Channick RN, et al: American College of Chest Physicians. Surgical treatments/interventions for pulmonary arterial hypertension: ACCP evidence-based clinical practice guidelines. Chest 126(suppl):63S–71S, 2004.

58. Barbera JA, Peinado VI, Santos S: Pulmonary hypertension in chronic obstructive pulmonary disease Eur Respir J 21:892–905, 2003.

59. Barst RJ, McGoon M, Torbicki A, et al: Diagnosis and differential assessment of pulmonary arterial hypertension. J Am Coll Cardiol 43(suppl):40S–47S, 2004.

60. Sietsema K: Cardiovascular limitations in chronic pulmonary disease. Med Sci Sports Exerc 33(suppl):S656–S661, 2001.

61. Gaine SP, Rubin LJ: Primary pulmonary hypertension. Lancet 352:719–725, 1998.

62. Shea SA, Andres LP, Shannon DC, Banzett RB: Ventilatory responses to exercise in humans lacking ventilatory chemosensitivity. J Physiol 468:623–640, 1993.

63. Guilleminault C, Abad VC: Obstructive sleep apnea syndromes. Med Clin North Am 88:611–630, viii, 2004.

64. Koenig SM: Pulmonary complications of obesity. Am J Med Sci 321:249–279, 2001.

65. Babb TG: Mechanical ventilatory constraints in aging, lung disease, and obesity: Perspectives and brief review. Med Sci Sports Exerc 31(suppl):S12–S22, 1999.

66. American Thoracic Society: Dyspnea: mechanisms, assessment, and management. A consensus statement. Am J Respir Crit Care Med 159:321–340, 1999.

67. Mahler DA, Horowitz MB: Perception of breathlessness during exercise in patients with respiratory disease. Med Sci Sports Exerc 26:1078–1081, 1994.

68. Sassi-Dambron DE, Eakin EG, Ries AL, Kaplan RM: Treatment of dyspnea in COPD. A controlled clinical trial of dyspnea management strategies. Chest 107:724–729, 1995.

69. Rotstein A, Meckel Y, Inbar O: Perceived speech difficulty during exercise and its relation to exercise intensity and physiological responses. Eur J Appl Physiol 92:431–436, 2004.

70. Lacasse Y, Brosseau L, Milne S, et al: Pulmonary rehabilitation for chronic obstructive pulmonary disease. Cochrane Database Syst Rev(3):CD003793; 2002.

71. Pulmonary rehabilitation: Joint ACCP/AACVPR evidence-based guidelines. ACCP/AACVPR Pulmonary Rehabilitation Guidelines Panel. American College of Chest Physicians. American Association of Cardiovascular and Pulmonary Rehabilitation. Chest 112: 1363–1396, 1997.

72. Celli BR: Pulmonary rehabilitation for COPD: A practical approach for improving ventilatory conditioning. Postgrad Med 103:159–178, 1998.

73. Berry MJ, Walschlager SA: Exercise training and chronic obstructive pulmonary disease: Past and future research directions. J Cardiopulm Rehabil 18:181–191, 1998.

74. Salman GF, Mosier MC, Beasley BW, Calkins DR: Rehabilitation for patients with chronic obstructive pulmonary disease: Meta-analysis of randomized controlled trials. J Gen Intern Med 18: 213–221, 2003.

75. Cambach W, Wagenaar RC, Koelman TW, et al: The long-term effects of pulmonary rehabilitation in patients with asthma and chronic obstructive pulmonary disease: a research synthesis. Arch Phys Med Rehabil 80:103–111, 1999.

76. Lacasse Y, Guyatt GH, Goldstein RS: The components of a respiratory rehabilitation program: A systematic overview. Chest 111: 1077–1088, 1997.

77. Casaburi R, Porszasz J, Burns MR, et al: Physiologic benefits of exercise training in rehabilitation of patients with severe chronic obstructive pulmonary disease. Am J Respir Crit Care Med 155: 1541–1551, 1997.

78. Puente-Maestu L, Luisa Sanz M, Sanz P, et al: Long-term effects of a maintenance program after supervised or self-monitored training programs in patients with COPD. Lung 181:67–78, 2003.

SELECTED REFERENCES FOR FURTHER READING

AACVPR Guidelines for Pulmonary Rehabilitation Programs, 2nd ed. Champaign, IL: Human Kinetics; 1998

Cooper CB, Storer TW. Exercise Testing and Interpretation: A Practical Approach. New York: Cambridge University Press; 2001.

Crapo JD, Glassroth J, Karlinsky J, King TE, eds. Baum's Textbook of Pulmonary Diseases, 7th ed. Philadelphia: Lippincott, Williams & Wilkins; 2004.

Durstine JL, Moore GE, ed: ACSM's Exercise Management for Persons with Chronic Diseases and Disabilities, 2nd ed. Champaign IL: Human Kinetics; 2002.

INTERNET RESOURCES

American Thoracic Society: Statements: http://www.thoracic.org/statements

GINA Workshop Reports: http://www.ginasthma.com/wr.html

Global Initiative for Chronic Lung Disease: http://www.goldcopd.com

National Asthma Education and Prevention Program Expert panel report 2: Guidelines for the diagnosis and management of asthma: http://www.nhlbi.nih.gov/guidelines/asthma/asthgdln.htm

National Clinical Guideline Clearinghouse: Pulmonary Rehabilitation: http://www.guideline.gov/summary/summary.aspx?doc_id=3211&nbr=2437&string=lung+and+exercise

LARRY S. VERITY

Diabetes mellitus is characterized by abnormal glucose metabolism resulting from defects in insulin release, action, or both[1]. This complex disease requires rigorous self-management, combined with an appropriate balance of nutritional intake, medications, and physical exercise for blood glucose control. Exercise is an important therapeutic intervention to assist in managing diabetes mellitus[2]. Regular exercise facilitates improved blood glucose control in type 2 diabetes and may offer similar benefit in gestational diabetes mellitus (GDM)[3,4]. Although regular exercise fails to favorably control glucose in type 1 diabetics[5], exercise can be a safe and effective adjunct therapy for diabetes management[6]. In those with diabetes, including type 1 diabetes, regular exercise has many benefits, including improvement of cardiovascular, metabolic, and psychological health; primary and secondary prevention of cardiovascular disease; and prevention of diabetes-specific complications[7].

This chapter focuses on the two most common forms of diabetes mellitus, types 1 and 2 diabetes, and also addresses GDM. Each type of diabetes is distinct in etiologic development and subsequent exercise programming. Safe and effective exercise recommendations are presented to assist in diabetes management and any accompanying complications. Chapter 16 reviewed assessments and exercise testing of patients with diabetes.

Epidemiology

In the United States, an estimated 18 million people have diabetes, and there are nearly 6 million undiagnosed cases[8]. Type 2 diabetes accounts for 90% to 95% of all cases of diabetes mellitus, and there is a greater prevalence in women[9]. The burden of diabetes disproportionately affects minorities: the prevalence rates are twofold greater in Hispanic Americans, African Americans, Native Americans, Asians, and Pacific Islanders compared with non-Hispanic whites. Type 1 diabetes accounts for 5% to 10% of all cases of diabetes, but it is the most common chronic diagnosed disease in children[9].

Pathophysiology and Etiology

Diabetes mellitus is a heterogeneous disease that can be divided into four major categories: type 1 diabetes, type 2 diabetes, gestational diabetes, and "other" specific types[1]. Diagnostic and classification criteria of diabetes focus on cause and pathogenesis[1]. The two major etiopathogenetic categories of diabetes are type 1 and type 2, and each has distinguishing characteristics (Table 33-1). These types of diabetes have as a common feature high blood glucose level, or **hyperglycemia**, caused by either an absolute or relative lack of insulin, along with abnormal protein and fat metabolism. Low blood glucose, or **hypoglycemia**, occurs most often in type 1 diabetes, but persons with type 2 diabetes and GDM can also experience episodes of hypoglycemia, although these are infrequent. Acute complications can occur when hypoglycemia or hyperglycemia are present for relatively short periods of time.

The presence of diabetes-related complications (DRCs) exacerbates morbidity and increases the likelihood of physical limitation or disability. Hyperglycemia for extended periods is linked with chronic DRCs that worsen macrovascular, microvascular, and neural disease processes. DRCs, shown in Box 33-1, can be quite serious. Because of the daily excursions in blood glucose that occur in diabetes mellitus, therapeutic interventions purposefully address effective blood glucose control and prevention of DRCs.

KEY TERMS

Autonomic neuropathy: Disease affecting the nerves innervating of the heart, it is also referred to as cardiovascular autonomic neuropathy

Glycosylated hemoglobin (HbA$_{1c}$): Test to assess glycemic control that reflects a time-averaged blood glucose concentration over the previous 2 to 3 months

Hyperglycemia: High blood glucose level

Hypoglycemia: Low blood glucose level

Insulin resistance: A condition in which there is a relative lack of insulin action in insulin-sensitive tissues to maintain normal glucose levels

Ketoacidosis: High level of ketones (β-hydroxybutyrate, acetoacetate)

Metabolic syndrome: A syndrome characterized by a constellation of disorders including insulin resistance, obesity, central adiposity, glucose intolerance, dyslipidemia, and hypertension

Nephropathy: A disease affecting the kidneys resulting in excessive urinary protein

Peripheral neuropathy: Disease affecting the nerves in the extremities, especially the lower legs and feet, resulting in loss of sensation

Retinopathy: A disease affecting the retina of the eye

Type 1 diabetes mellitus: Immune-mediated disease that selectively destroys the pancreatic β-cells, leading to a "central defect" in insulin release upon stimulation

Type 2 diabetes mellitus: Disease usually afflicting persons over the age of 30 years that is directly related to insulin resistance

TYPE 1 DIABETES MELLITUS

Type 1 diabetes mellitus usually afflicts persons younger than age 30 years and is an immune-mediated disease that selectively destroys the pancreatic β cells, leading to a "central defect" in insulin release upon stimulation, or hypoinsulinemia, and resultant hyperglycemia[10]. Serologic markers of pancreatic β-cell de-

struction (e.g., islet cell autoantibodies, insulin autoantibodies, glutamic acid decarboxylase, and human leukocyte antigens) are common at diagnosis and provide evidence for its autoimmune nature[1].

Onset of type 1 diabetes is usually abrupt and generally accompanied by "classic" signs of diabetes mellitus, including frequent urination (polyuria), constant hunger (polyphagia), excessive thirst (polydipsia), and unex-

TABLE 33-1. Major Characteristics of Type 1 and Type 2 Diabetes[26]

Factor	Type 1	Type 2
Age at onset	Usually early but may occur at any age	Usually over age 30 years but may occur at any age
Type of onset	Usually abrupt	Insidious
Genetic susceptibility	HLA-related DR3 and DR4, ICAs, IAAs	Frequent genetic background; not HLA related
Environmental factors	Virus, toxins, autoimmune stimulation	Obesity, nutrition, physical inactivity
Islet cell antibody	Present at onset	Not observed
Endogenous insulin	Minimal or absent	Stimulated response either adequate but delayed secretion or reduced but not absent; insulin resistance present
Nutritional status	Thin, catabolic state	Obese or normal
Symptoms	Thirst, polyuria, polyphagia, fatigue	Mild or frequently none
Ketosis	Common at onset, or during insulin deficiency	Resistant except during infection or stress
Control of diabetes	Often difficult, with wide glucose fluctuation	Variable; helped by dietary adherence, weight loss, exercise
Dietary management	Essential	Essential; may suffice for glycemic control
Insulin	Required for all	Required for ~40%
Oral hypoglycemics	Not effective	Effective
Vascular or neurological complications	Seen in most after 5 or more years of diabetes	Frequent

HLA = human leukocyte antigen; DR = D-related antigen; ICA = islet cell antibodies.

Adapted from Shulman CR: Diabetes mellitus: Definition, classification, and diagnosis. In Galloway JA, Potvin JH, Shulman CR, eds. Diabetes Mellitus, 9th ed. Indianapolis: Lilly Research Laboratories; 1988.

plained weight loss[1]. An absolute lack of insulin production in type 1 diabetes mellitus requires exogenous insulin administration (e.g., injections or pump) to maintain normal glucose level, minimize complications, and prevent **ketoacidosis**.

Ketoacidosis occurs when a high level of ketones (β-hydroxybutyrate, acetoacetate) are produced. Normally, ketones are a byproduct of fatty acid metabolism; however, the combination of deficient insulin and increased counterregulatory hormones (e.g., catecholamines, cortisol, glucagon) results in excessive ketone production and metabolic acidosis[3]. Diabetic ketoacidosis (DKA) can result from an infection but is more commonly linked with a lack of insulin, dehydration, and failure to manage glucose levels. Signs and symptoms of DKA include confusion, gastrointestinal (GI) upset, extreme thirst, lethargy, and a fruity breath odor[10,11]. If DKA is left untreated, it can result in coma or death.

TYPE 2 DIABETES MELLITUS

Type 2 diabetes mellitus usually afflicts persons older than age 30 years and is directly related to insulin resistance. The incidence of type 2 diabetes in children and adolescents has increased in recent years, presumably related to increased levels of obesity secondary to excess caloric intake and too little caloric expenditure. Although varying degrees of endogenous insulin production (e.g., normal or elevated) are present in type 2 diabetes, the disease is characterized by insulin resistance, which is a rela-

tive lack of insulin action in insulin-sensitive tissues to maintain normoglycemia (i.e., normal glucose levels).

Insulin resistance is considered a "peripheral defect" because of a decrease in insulin-mediated uptake and storage of glucose in the liver and skeletal muscle. Reduced insulin receptor binding at target tissues and impaired postreceptor activities related to insulin function manifest insulin resistance. Central to postreceptor deficiencies are abnormal translocation of muscle glucose transporters (GLUT-4) and insulin receptor substrates (IRS) that perform important intermediary phosphorylation processes[1]. Interestingly, these abnormalities are reversible with weight loss, diet, and physical activity[10]. The hyperglycemia present in type 2 diabetes suggests that insulin release is inadequate to compensate for the insulin resistance. Over time, the pancreas loses its ability to produce insulin, and the need for exogenous insulin to control blood glucose increases.

Control of glucose levels in type 2 diabetes is essential to prevent hyperosmolar hyperglycemic nonketotic syndrome (HHNS), which is an emergency condition in which blood glucose levels are very high accompanied by dehydration and ketones are not present in the blood or urine[11]. If not treated, HHNS can lead to coma or death.

Onset of type 2 diabetes is associated with genetic, environmental, and cultural factors. The risk of disease rises with family history, age, corpulence, and indolence. About 80% of persons with type 2 diabetes are obese and physically inactive, both of which are related to increased insulin resistance[9]. Lifestyle interventions focusing on weight loss and physical activity are essential strategies to manage diabetes, and lessen the onset of disease-related complications, and prevent onset of type 2 diabetes[12].

GESTATIONAL DIABETES MELLITUS

Gestational diabetes mellitus is an inability to maintain normal glucose or any degree of glucose intolerance during pregnancy despite being treated with either diet or insulin. GDM is occurs in about 7% of all pregnancies[1]. Several factors consistent with high risk for developing GDM include marked obesity, personal or family history of GDM, and glycosuria. GDM is usually diagnosed by an oral glucose tolerance test (OGTT) between 24 to 28 weeks of gestation. If GDM is diagnosed, then therapeutic strategies are used to monitor and manage maternal blood glucose to prevent fetal macrosomia and maternal complications[4]. GDM resolves postpartum, yet many women who experience GDM eventually develop type 2 diabetes. Although not identical in pathophysiology, GDM resembles etiologic features of type 2 diabetes, including obesity, insulin resistance, family history, and physical inactivity[4]. As in type 2 diabetes, GDM onset is related to genetic predisposition, insulin resistance, and subsequent deficient insulin release. Management of

GDM focuses on similar interventions that are commonly recommended in type 2 diabetes.

Clinical Features

The diagnosis of diabetes mellitus is based on any of the criteria shown in Box 33-2. After diagnosis, clinical emphasis is placed on frequent blood glucose monitoring (i.e., three to six glucose checks per day) in conjunction with diet and physical activity to control glucose levels and reduce risk of complications. Glycemic control is assessed using **glycosylated hemoglobin (HbA$_{1c}$)**, which reflects a time-averaged blood glucose concentration over the previous 2 to 3 months. The recommended HbA$_{1c}$ goal is set at less than 7.0%, which is approximately 1% above the nondiabetic range (HbA$_{1c}$ = 4.0% to 6.0%), and it is recommended that it is assessed every 3 to 4 months[10].

Assessment of overall health and identification of coexisting cardiovascular disease risk factors and DRCs are essential components of effective diabetes care[5,9]. Current recommendations focus on aggressive management of heart disease risk factors[10,13]. Glucose-lowering agents are the primary medications used in diabetes management, supplemented by indicated drugs to prevent coronary heart disease such as antihypertensive drugs, lipid-lowering agents, and antiplatelet medications.

Whereas body weight is usually normal in type 1 diabetes, obesity prevails in type 2 diabetes. Body mass index (BMI) often exceeds 30 kg·m^2 and abdominal girth is large (men $\geq$ 102 cm; women $\geq$ 88 cm) in type 2 diabetics, putting many patients at high risk for heart disease and cancer[14]. Therefore, weight loss is a primary treatment goal to improve insulin action in persons with type 2 diabetes[10].

THE METABOLIC SYNDROME

The **Metabolic syndrome**, also called *insulin resistance syndrome* or *syndrome X*, is commonly seen in type 2 diabetes[7] and is linked with physical inactivity, diet, and genetic factors[15]. The metabolic syndrome is characterized by a constellation of disorders, including insulin resistance, obesity, central adiposity, glucose intolerance, dyslipidemia, and hypertension[16]. The presence of the metabolic syndrome substantially increases the risk of

---

BOX 33-2 | Diagnostic Criteria of Diabetes Mellitus[1]

- Fasting blood glucose $\geq$ 126 mg·dL^{-1}
- Diabetes symptoms plus casual plasma glucose $\geq$ 200 mg·dL^{-1} (casual glucose is taken without regard for last meal);
- 2-hour glucose $\geq$ 200 mg·dL^{-1} during an oral glucose tolerance (OGTT) using a 75-g glucose load

---

BOX 33-3 | Criteria for the Diagnosis of the Metabolic Syndrome[16]

- Systolic BP $\geq$ 130 mm Hg or DBP $\geq$ 85 mm Hg
- Fasting glucose $\geq$ 110 mg·dL^{-1}
- Fasting HDL cholesterol < 40 for men < 50 mg·dL^{-1} for women
- Fasting triglycerides $\geq$ 150 mg·dL^{-1}
- Waist circumference $\geq$ 100 for men and $\geq$ 88 cm for women

BP = blood pressure; HDL = high-density lipoprotein.

---

developing both type 2 diabetes and cardiovascular disease. Three or more of the criteria in Box 33-3 are necessary for diagnosis of metabolic syndrome[16].

GLUCOSE REGULATION

Precise hormonal and metabolic events that normally regulate glucose homeostasis are disrupted in diabetes because of defects in insulin release, action, or both, and result in an excess release of counterregulatory hormones. Glucose control requires near-normal balance between hepatic glucose production and peripheral glucose uptake, combined with effective insulin responses. In diabetes, an inability to precisely match glucose production and use results in daily glucose excursions that require adjustments in the dosage of exogenous insulin dose or oral agent, combined with adjustments in dietary intake.

Insulin Injections

Type 1 diabetics and nearly 40% of all type 2 diabetics require multiple daily insulin injection therapy to control blood glucose[10]. An insulin pump (continuous subcutaneous insulin infusion [CSII]) can be used to manage some patients with type 1 diabetes and GDM. Insulin administered by syringe is injected into subcutaneous tissue, using a rotation of sites, including the abdomen (fastest absorption rate), upper arms, lateral thigh, and buttocks[17]. CSII is subcutaneously delivered only in the abdominal area. Insulin administered by syringe can be rapid acting (peak action: 0.5 to 1.0 hour), short acting (peak action: 2 to 3 hours), intermediate acting (peak action: 4 to 10 hours), or long acting (peak action: sustained for 20 to 24 hours). A mixed dose of different types of insulin produces a more normal glucose response, so it is most commonly used. Usually, rapid acting insulin is used with CSII.

Frequent adjustments in insulin administration are generally needed to effectively manage diabetes. These insulin adjustments involve a trial-and-error process that requires an understanding of insulin action and the impact of exercise, food intake, and medication on glucose excursions, combined with frequent routine self-blood glucose monitoring (SBGM)[17].

Before exercise sessions SBGM, is essential to make any adjustments in insulin or caloric intake for glucose management. When underinsulinized, insulin-stimulated glucose uptake in skeletal muscle is reduced, and exercise-induced hepatic glucose output is excessive, resulting in hyperglycemia, or elevated blood glucose (e.g., > 126 mg·dL^{-1}). After glucose levels exceed 250 to 300 mg·dL^{-1}, urinary ketones appear and represent excessive fat metabolism, and they contribute to DKA if glycemia remains uncontrolled. This scenario requires that insulin be given to lower the glucose level and reestablish normoglycemia. When overinsulinized, hepatic glucose production is blunted, and glucose uptake into exercising muscle is heightened by exercise when insulin is high. This scenario can result in hypoglycemia, or low blood glucose (e.g., blood glucose < 80 mg·dL^{-1}), and requires that insulin be reduced and rapidly absorbed and that carbohydrates (10 to 20 g) be ingested before exercise to increase the glucose level to an acceptable level[17].

Oral Hypoglycemic Agents

Oral agents are widely prescribed for type 2 diabetes when onset is recent and little (e.g., units < 20) or no insulin is taken[10]. As with insulin injections, oral agents are prescribed individually or in combination to optimize glucose control in type 2 diabetes. Three groups of oral agents are used to control glucose and are discussed below.

β-Cell Stimulants for Insulin Release

Sulfonylurea and meglitinide drugs are taken at mealtime to stimulate insulin release and manage postprandial glycemia. Because of insulin stimulation, these oral agents can lead to hypoglycemia. Sulfonylureas include chlorpropamide (Diabinese), glipizide (Glucotrol and Glucotrol XL), glyburide (Micronase, Glynase, and Diabeta), and glimepiride (Amaryl). Repaglinide (Prandin) is the only meglintinide currently on the market

Drugs to Improve Insulin Sensitivity

The hiazolidinediones (rosiglitazone [Avandia] and pioglitazone [Actose]) improve insulin sensitivity at muscle and adipose tissue, and the biguanides (metformin [Glucophage]) promote muscle glucose uptake and inhibit hepatic glucose output.

Drugs that Abate Intestinal Absorption of Carbohydrates

Alpha-glucosidase inhibitors (acarbose (Precose) and miglitol (Glyset)) decrease carbohydrate absorption rate and slow the increase in postprandial blood glucose level.

Treatment

The treatment of patients with diabetes mellitus involves a multidisciplinary team of specialists that includes the diabetes physician, diabetes nurse educator, registered dietician, and clinical exercise physiologist to facilitate patient education and necessary lifestyle changes to manage this disease. Intensive SBGM, combined with balancing diet, oral drugs or exogenous insulin (or both), and exercise are established cornerstones of therapy to facilitate near-normal to normal metabolic function[10]. In general, management of blood glucose level in diabetes involves a planned regimen of insulin or oral medication (or both), frequent SMBG, an individualized nutrition plan, and participation in a regular physical activity program. Self-management skills are essential to the successful management of diabetes.

The primary goal of therapy for all diabetics focuses on SBGM to achieve acceptable blood glucose control (HbA$_{1c}$ < 7.0%), thereby limiting the development and progression of DRCs. Both types 1[18] and 2 diabetics[19] show reduced risk for retinopathy, nephropathy, and neuropathy with intensive therapy and the potential for a reduction of cardiovascular disease with improved glycemic control. Glycemic control is best achieved through SBGM combined with nutrition, adjustment of medications, and physical activity.

Cardiovascular risk factors, along with symptomatic and asymptomatic coronary heart disease, are common in diabetics[7]. Identification of macrovascular disease and comorbidities of diabetes and aggressive intervention are crucial in minimizing their progression, particularly factors linked with the metabolic syndrome[13].

Effects of Disease or Condition on Exercise Responses and Physical Function

The favorable effects of regular exercise have been reported for types 1[5,6,20] and 2[3,5,6,21] diabetes mellitus (Table 33-2). Regular aerobic and resistance training combined with individualized diet therapy promotes improved cardiovascular function (e.g., $\dot{V}O_{2max}$), along with favorable changes in lipids and lipoproteins, blood pressure (BP), body mass, fat-free mass (maintain or increase), fat mass, body fat distribution, insulin sensitivity, glucose metabolic machinery, and postprandial thermogenesis[3,5,6,20]. These physiological changes usually result in lowering of daily medication dose (e.g., insulin or oral agent) for type 1 and type 2 diabetes.

Regular exercise training improves glucose control only in type 2 diabetics, primarily through increased insulin sensitivity[3,5,14,21]. Little or no improvement in glucose control has been demonstrated in type 1 diabetics after regular exercise training[5,14,20,22]. Although excessive carbohydrate ingestion on days of exercise may partially explain the lack of improvement in glucose control after training, the lack of vigilant management of blood glucose before *and* after exercise through SMBG is a more plausible explanation for the lack of glucose control in type 1 diabetics.

TABLE 33-2. Effects of Exercise in Diabetes Mellitus[3,6]

Parameter	Type 1	Type 2
Cardiovascular		
Aerobic capacity or fitness level	⇑	⇑/⇔
Resting pulse rate and rate–pressure product	⇓	⇓
Resting BP in mild-moderate hypertensives	⇓	⇓
HR at submaximal loads	⇓	⇓
Lipid and Lipoprotein Alterations		
HDL	⇑	⇑
LDL	⇓/⇔	⇓/⇔
VLDL	⇓	⇓
Total cholesterol	⇔	⇔
Risk ratio (total cholesterol/HDL)	⇓	⇓
Anthropometric Measures		
Body mass	⇓	⇓
Fat mass, especially in obese persons	⇓	⇓
Fat-free mass	⇑	⇑/⇔
Metabolic Parameters		
Insulin sensitivity and glucose metabolic machinery	⇑	⇑
HbA$_{1c}$	⇔	⇓
Postprandial thermogenesis or thermic effect of food	⇑	⇑
Presumed Psychological Aspects		
Self-concept and self-esteem	⇑	⇑
Depression and anxiety	⇓	⇓
Stress response to psychological stimuli	⇓	⇓

BP = blood pressure; HDL = high-density lipoprotein; HR = heart rate; LDL = low-density lipoprotein; VLDL = very-low-density lipoprotein. ↑ = increase; ↓ = decrease; ↔ = no change.

Regular exercise may also favorably alter stress-related psychological factors and cognitive function in diabetic[14,21]. Depression is common in diabetics, and regular exercise may assist in countering this debilitating psychoemotional state. Overall, regular exercise may offer quality of life improvements for diabetics that other therapies fail to achieve.

Disease-specific Exercise Prescription and Programming

Diabetes therapy must encourage participation in physical activity. Given the benefits of a physically active lifestyle, health care professionals must also recognize the associated risks. Identifiable limitations (e.g., presence of complications) and precautions (e.g., degree of metabolic control) must be addressed before an exercise program can be developed.

SCREENING

A thorough pre-activity screening of the patient's clinical status is recommended to ensure safe and effective participation[14]. Coexisting morbidities in the diabetes health profile are important to determine whether the clinical status is acceptable for safely engaging in exercise and to determine the need for monitoring of each session.

BOX 33-4	**Indications For Stress Testing with Diabetes[6,10]**

- Known or suspected cardiovascular disease (e.g., CAD, PAD)
- Age > 35 years
- Age > 25 years if duration of diabetes > 10 years for type 1 or > 15 years for type 2
- Presence of any additional risk factors for cardiovascular disease
- Microvascular disease
- Autonomic neuropathy

CAD = coronary artery disease; PAD = peripheral arterial disease.

Before commencing exercise, prudent screening for vascular and neurological complications, including silent ischemia, are warranted, along with identification of the presence of cardiovascular disease risk factors and metabolic syndrome. Persons with diabetes are stratified in the high-risk category, according to recommended guidelines (see GETP7 Chapter 2), and a stress test is strongly recommended before initiating moderate to vigorous exercise irrespective of the patient's cardiac risk profile. Specific indications for a stress test be administered include the presence of one or more of the criteria shown in Box 33-4[6,10].

EXERCISE PROGRAMMING

In type 1 diabetes without complications, exercise recommendations are closely aligned with guidelines for apparently healthy persons[5]. However, recommendations for type 2 diabetics are more closely aligned with obesity and hypertension guidelines[14] and focus on caloric expenditure. Resistance training should be recommended for diabetic without complications[3,5,22] and follow apparently healthy guidelines with age and experience as prime considerations in program development. Appropriate attention to modifying the intensity of the lifting session may lessen risk for elevations in BP, glucose, and onset of musculoskeletal injury[3,5]. Those who use insulin may prefer to engage in daily physical activity to improve the balance between insulin dose and caloric needs[3,5,17,21,22].

The exercise program development must consider personal interests as well as past and present activity habits. The goals and needs of a physical activity program are critical to determining whether the exercise habit will be sustained, especially in persons with type 2 diabetes[3,22]. Additionally, past exercise habits can provide important information regarding present exercise preferences and behaviors.

Finally, glucose control must be maintained in order for exercise to be safe and effective. SBGM is recommended so that further adjustments in medications, caloric intake, or both may occur to preserve normoglycemia. SBGM is recommended before and after each exercise session in persons with diabetes, and a blood glucose value ranging between 100 and 250 mg·dL^{-1} is recommended for safe exercise participation[3,5,6,17].

Risks and Precautions of Exercise in Diabetes

A safe and effective exercise program for diabetes minimizes the acute risks and long-term complications while maximizing the benefits for persons with diabetes. Two common risks associated with exercise in diabetics are hypoglycemia and hyperglycemia; however, precautions can be taken to lessen or avoid their onset. Essential to preventing risk onset is SBGM[6,9,17]. Exercise-induced hypoglycemia is most common for those who require exogenous insulin, has been observed in those taking oral sulfonylureas, and may exist for meglitinide[17]. To prevent its onset, glucose monitoring before and after exercise is required as well as reducing insulin dosage (e.g., 50% to 90% of daily dosage) based on duration and intensity, along with personal experience. Also, extra carbohydrates may need to be taken before, during, and after exercise. For those taking oral sulfonylureas, preventing exercise-induced hypoglycemia requires pre-exercise SBGM with adjustments that may require dose reduction of oral drug (and exogenous insulin) or increased carbohydrate ingestion.

Hyperglycemia is a common outcome in insulin-requiring and poorly managed diabetics and is a common outcome of an underinsulinized state[17]. If pre-exercise glucose is above 250 mg·dL^{-1}, the acute effect of exercise is to augment release of counterregulatory hormones (e.g., catecholamines, glucagon) causing excessive hepatic glucose production, which exceeds blood glucose uptake in skeletal muscle because of a lack of adequate insulin. Hence, those who require exogenous insulin need to postpone any exercise until their glucose level is better controlled because exercise worsens glucose levels and may contribute to excessive urinary ketones (e.g., metabolic byproducts of fatty acids) that can be dangerous and fatal in high levels (Table 33-3).

COMPLICATIONS OF DIABETES

Diabetes poses challenges for exercise professionals because of increased morbidity and mortality from vascular and neurological disease processes. Macrovascular (e.g., coronary, cerebrovascular, and peripheral), microvascular (e.g., retinal, kidney), and neural (e.g., peripheral and autonomic nerves) diseases are common and constitute the DRCs that develop and worsen with poor glucose control and diabetes management. The onset and progression of vascular and neural complications of diabetes often cause physical limitation and varying levels of disability and are linked with depression and cognitive deficits. Thus, the quality of life in those with diabetes can be adversely affected without aggressive management and intervention.

TABLE 33-3. Practical Recommendations for Exercises for Persons with Diabetes Mellitus

Do SBGM.	Check before and after each exercise session. Allows the patient to understand glucose response to physical activity. It is important to ensure that glucose is in relatively good control before beginning exercise. If blood glucose is: >250 mg·dL^{-1}: Exercise should be postponed <100 mg·dL^{-1}: Eat a snack consisting of easily absorbed carbohydrates (~10 to 20 g) 100–240 mg·dL^{-1}: Exercise is recommended
Keep a daily log	Record the time of day the SBGM values are obtained and the amount of any pharmacologic agent (e.g., oral drugs, insulin). Also, approximate the time (min), intensity (HR), and distance (miles or meters) of exercise session. Over time, this aids the patient in understanding the type of glucose response to anticipate from an exercise bout.
Plan for exercise sessions	How much (e.g., time and intensity) exercise is anticipated allows adjusting insulin or oral drugs. If needed, carry extra carbohydrate feedings (~10 to 15 g·30 min^{-1}) to limit hypoglycemia. Hydrate before and rehydrate after each exercise session to prevent dehydration.
Modify caloric intake accordingly	Through frequent SBGM, caloric intake can be regulated more carefully on days of and after exercise.
Adjust insulin accordingly	If using insulin, reduce rapid- or short-acting insulin dosage by 50% to limit hypoglycemia episodes.
Exercise with a partner	Affords a support system for the exercise habit. Initially, diabetics should exercise with a partner until their glucose response is known.
Wear a diabetes identification tag..	A diabetes necklace or shoe tag with relevant medical information should always be worn. Hypoglycemia and other problems can arise that require immediate attention.
Wear good shoes.	Always wear proper-fitting and comfortable footwear with socks to minimize foot irritations and limit orthopedic injury to the feet and lower legs.
Practice good hygiene.	Always take extra care to inspect feet for any irritation spots to prevent possible infection. Tend to all sores immediately, and limit any irritations.

HR = heart rate; SBGM = self-blood glucose monitoring.

Exercise Recommendations for Specific Diabetes-related Complications

Diabetes with complications requires careful screening. The presence of complications is not a contraindication for exercise, and the benefits of low- to moderate-intensity exercise generally outweigh the risks presented in diabetes. Although precautions and limitations must be recognized, with prudent modifications, a safe exercise plan can be achieved when the clinical status and existing complications are thoroughly assessed in the screening process. Discussion of exercise considerations for individuals with complicated diabetes follow, and a summary of considerations is shown in Table 33-4.

AUTONOMIC NEUROPATHY

This complication broadly affects the involuntary functions of the body, including the cardiac, vascular, GI, and genitourinary systems. When **autonomic neuropathy** affects the innervation of the heart, it is referred to as *cardiovascular autonomic neuropathy* (CAN), and its presence is linked with poor prognosis and premature mortality[23]. Clinical features of CAN include silent ischemia and infarction, tachycardia at rest and early in exercise, reduced maximal heart rate (HR) and exercise tolerance, exercise-induced hypotension after strenuous activity, thermoregulatory dysfunction, prone to dehydration, and hypoglycemia unawareness[5]. If postural hypotension is present, inadequate HR and BP responses are observed with incremental work. Consequently, physical activity for these persons should focus on lower intensity activities in which mild changes in HR and BP are more easily tolerated and lessen ventricular ectopy. Any exercise program for persons with CAN requires physician approval and should be viewed with caution and careful monitoring and may require a clinical setting for safe exercising.

PERIPHERAL NEUROPATHY

Peripheral neuropathy (PN) affects the extremities, especially the lower legs and feet, and results in loss of sensation, or desensate feet[3,5,10]. Poor wound healing and ulcerations leading to amputation are common. Proper daily hygiene is essential to limit sores from progressing from a poor-healing wound to ulceration. Exercise combined with loss of sensation can lead to musculoskeletal injury through overstretching, loss of balance, or falling, in addition to infection with minor irritations from footwear. Thus, persons with desensate feet require non–weight-bearing activities to lessen onset of foot ulcerations, bunions, and foot deformity.

Exercise for persons with PN should focus on low-intensity activities, as gauged by RPE, and range of motion (ROM) activities for major joints to prevent or minimize contractures and maintain function. Non–weight-bearing

TABLE 33-4. Special Precautions for Recommending Exercise for Patients with Complications of Diabetes

Complication	Precaution
Autonomic neuropathy[b]	Likelihood of hypoglycemia and abnormal BP ($\Uparrow$/$\Downarrow$). Abnormal resting HR ($\Uparrow$) and maximal HR ($\Downarrow$). Impaired SNS or PNS nerves yield abnormal exercise HR, BP, and SV. Use of RPE is suggested. Prone to dehydration and hypothermia.
Peripheral neuropathy	Avoid exercise that may cause trauma to the feet (e.g., prolonged hiking, jogging, or walking on uneven surfaces). Non–weight-bearing exercises (e.g., cycling, chair exercises, swimming) are most appropriate. Aquatics are not recommended if active ulcers are present. Regular assessment of the feet recommended. Keep the feet clean and dry. Choose shoes carefully for proper fit. Avoid activities requiring a great deal of balance.
Nephropathy	Avoid exercise that increases BP (e.g., weight lifting, high-intensity aerobic exercise) and refrain from breath holding. High BP is common. Lower intensity is recommended.
Retinopathy[a,b]	With proliferative and severe stages of retinopathy, avoid strenuous, high-intensity activities that involve breath holding (e.g., weight lifting and isometrics) or overhead lifting. Avoid activities that lower the head (e.g., yoga, gymnastics) or that risk jarring the head. Consult an ophthalmologist for specific restrictions and limitations. Use of RPE is recommended.
Hypertension	Avoid heavy weight lifting or breath holding.
	Perform primarily dynamic exercise using large muscle groups, such as walking and cycling at a low-to-moderate intensity.
	Follow BP guidelines. Use of RPE is recommended.
All patients	Carry identification with diabetes information.
	Rehydrate carefully (drink fluids before, during, and after exercise). Avoid exercise in the heat of the day and in direct sunlight (wear hat and sunscreen when in the sun).

[a]If patient has proliferative retinopathy and has recently undergone photocoagulation or surgical treatment or is not properly treated, exercise is contraindicated.

[b]Submaximal exercise testing is recommended for patients with proliferative retinopathy and autonomic neuropathy.

BP = blood pressure; HR = heart rate; RPE = rating of perceived exertion; PNS = parasympathetic nervous system; SNS = sympathetic nervous system; SV = stroke volume. $\uparrow$= increase; $\downarrow$= decrease.

Reprinted with permission from Campaigne BN, Lampman RL: Exercise in the Clinical Management of Diabetes Mellitus. Champaign, IL: Human Kinetics; 1994.

activities that improve balance and awareness of the lower extremities are encouraged for persons with PN[23]. Properly fitted and comfortable footwear and socks for walking are important to minimize the likelihood for undetectable sores in persons with PN, which can evolve into infections if unnoticed. Frequent visual inspection of the feet is also recommended.

NEPHROPATHY

This DRC affects the kidneys and is present when excessive urinary protein is present (microalbuminuria > 200 $\mu g \cdot min^{-1}$), accompanied by hypertension[1]. Hypertension is a precursor to progression of **nephropathy** and must be controlled. Controlled hypertension limits BP excursions with exercise as well as any resulting albuminuria. Glucose control is central to reducing presence of albuminuria and delaying the onset or progression of this complication to end-stage renal disease (ESRD). Exercise recommendations for persons with nephropathy focus on low- to moderate-intensity aerobic and resistance exercise, proper hydration strategies used for apparently healthy persons, and avoidance of activities that cause excessive elevation in BP (e.g., Valsalva maneuver, high-intensity aerobic or strength exercises). Specific exercise testing and training recommendations may be found in Chapter 34.

RETINOPATHY

Diabetic retinopathy occurs in varying degrees of severity in the form of either nonproliferative diabetic **retinopathy** (NPDR) or proliferative diabetic retinopathy (PDR)[24]. BP and glucose control are essential in limiting progression of retinopathy. Although physical activity increases systemic and retinal BP, few studies have shown a worsening of retinopathy related to exercise[24]. There are some recommended limitations to physical activity, as shown in Table 33-5. Research has shown that low-inten-

| BOX 33-5 | **Recommended Precautions for Exercise in Diabetes with Retinopathy[24]** |

- Limit systolic BP to < 170 mm Hg.
- Use of HR and RPE from BP increase during exercise to establish safe intensity;
- Avoid heavy or effortful exercise. which causes dramatic BP increases, as in strength training (use of Valsalva maneuver) or when using performing activities with the arms overhead.
- Annual eye examinations are needed to establish the level of retinopathy and its progression for exercise modification.

BP = blood pressure; HR = heart rate; RPE = rating of perceived exertion.

sity training in a mixed group of persons with types 1 and 2 diabetes with PDR improved cardiovascular function by 15% without adverse retinal outcomes[25]. Recommended precautions for exercise in patients with retinopathy are shown in Box 33-5[24].

Limitations and Contraindications

Because of the increased risk for vascular and neural diseases related to diabetes, it is imperative that safe limit of exercise are established and that onset and progression of DRCs are lessened. To this end, there are potential contraindications to exercise for those with diabetes that follow previously established guidelines[3]. Depending on the patient's clinical status, those with heart disease, in combination with advanced CAN, PN, nephropathy, or retinopathy, may be limited to lower intensity exercise, and more vigorous exercise is contraindicated. Also, poor glucose control above 250 mg·dL^{-1} with or without ketones is a contraindication for persons with diabetes to safely participate in exercise[3,14].

TABLE 33-5. Considerations for Activity Limitation in Patients with Diabetic Retinopathy[24]

Level of DR	Acceptable Activities	Discouraged Activities	Ocular and Activity Reevaluation
No DR	Dictated by medical status	Dictated by medical status	12 months
Mild NPDR	Dictated by medical status	Dictated by medical status	6–12 months
Moderate NPDR	Dictated by medical status	Activities that dramatically increase BP such as power lifting, heavy Valsalva maneuver	
Severe NPDR		Limit systolic BP, Valsalva maneuvers, active jarring, boxing, heavy competitive sports	2–4 months (may require laser surgery)
PDR	Low-impact cardiovascular conditioning: Swimming (not diving); walking; low-impact aerobics; stationary cycling; endurance exercises	Low-impact cardiovascular jarring: Weight lifting, jogging, high-impact aerobics, racquet sports, strenuous trumpet playing	1–2 months (may require laser surgery)

BP = blood pressure; DR = diabetic retinopathy; NPDR = nonproliferative diabetic retinopathy; PDR = proliferative diabetic retinopathy.

Reprinted with permission from Aeillo LP, Wong J, Cavallerano JD, et al: Retinopathy (pp. 401–413). In Ruderman N, Devlin J, Schneider S, Kriska A, eds. Handbook of Exercise in Diabetes, 2nd ed. Alexandria, VA: American Diabetes Association; 2002.

REFERENCES

1. Report of the Expert Committee on the Diagnosis and Classification of Diabetes Mellitus. Diabetes Care 27(suppl 1):S5–S35, 2004.
2. Riddell MC, Ruderman N, Berger M, Vranic M: Exercise physiology and diabetes: From antiquity to the age of the exercise sciences (pp. 3–15). In Ruderman N, Devlin J, Schneider S, Kriska A, eds. Handbook of Exercise in Diabetes, 2nd ed. Alexandria, VA: American Diabetes Association; 2002.
3. American College of Sports Medicine: Exercise and Type 2 Diabetes. Position Stand. Med Sci Sport Exerc 32:1345–1360, 2000.
4. American Diabetes Association: Gestational Diabetes Mellitus: Position Statement. Diabetes Care 27(suppl 1):S88–S93, 2004.
5. American College of Sports Medicine and American Diebetes Association. Diabetes Mellitus and Exercise: A joint position statement of the American College of Sports Medicine and The American Diabetes Association. Med Sci Sport Exerc 29:i–vi, 1997.
6. American Diabetes Association: Physical Activity/Exercise and Diabetes: Position Statement. Diabetes Care 27(suppl 1):S58–S64, 2004.
7. Grundy, S, Benjamin IJ, Burke GL, et al: Diabetes and cardiovascular disease: A Statement for Healthcare Professionals From the American Heart Association. Circulation 100:1134–1146, 1999.
8. Centers for Disease Control and Prevention. Diabetes is a growing public health problem. Available at: http//www.cdc.gov/nccdphp/aag/agg-ddt.htm
9. Centers for Disease Control and Prevention: National Diabetes Fact Sheet: National estimates and general information on diabetes in the United States. Atlanta, GA: U.S. Department of Health and Human Services, Centers for Disease Control and Prevention; 2003.
10. American Diabetes Association: Standards of Medical Care in Diabetes: Position Statement. Diabetes Care 27(suppl 1):S15–S35, 2004.
11. American Diabetes Association: Hyperglycemic crises in patients with diabetes mellitus. Diabetes Care 27(suppl 1):S94–S102, 2004.
12. Pan X, Li G, Hu Y, et al: Effects of diet and exercise in preventing NIDDM in people with impaired glucose tolerance: The Da Qing IGT and Diabetes Study. Diabetes Care 20:537–544, 1997.
13. Joint National Committee on Prevention, Detection, Evaluation, and Treatment of High Blood Pressure: The seventh report of the Joint National Committee on Prevention, Detection, Evaluation, and Treatment of High Blood Pressure (JNC-VII). JAMA 289:2560–2572, 2003.
14. Hornsby WG, Albright AL: Diabetes (pp. 133–41). In Durstine L, Moore G, eds. ACSM's Exercise Management for Persons with Chronic Disease and Disabilities, 2nd ed. Champaign, IL: Human Kinetics; 2003.
15. Ruderman N: A target population for diabetes prevention: The metabolically obese, normal-weight individual (pp. 235–49). In Ruderman N, Devlin J, Schneider S, Kriska A, eds. Handbook of Exercise in Diabetes, 2nd ed. Alexandria, VA: American Diabetes Association; 2002.
16. National Institutes of Health and National Heart, Lung, and Blood Institute: Clinical Guidelines on the Identification, Evaluation, and Treatment of Overweight and Obesity in Adults: Evidence Report. Bethesda, MD: NIH Publication No. 98-4083, 1998.
17. Berger M: Adjustment of insulin and oral agent therapy (pp. 365–381). In Ruderman N, Devlin J, Schneider S, Kriska A, eds. Handbook of Exercise in Diabetes, 2nd ed. Alexandria, VA: American Diabetes Association; 2002.
18. American Diabetes Association: Implications of the Diabetes Control and Complications Trial: Position Statement. Diabetes Care 26(suppl 1):S25–S27, 2003.
19. American Diabetes Association: Implications of the United Kingdom Prospective Diabetes Study: Position Statement. Diabetes Care 26(suppl 1):S28–S32, 2003.
20. Wasserman D, Zinman B: Exercise in Individuals with IDDM. Diabetes Care 17:924–937, 1994.
21. U.S. Department of Health and Human Services: Physical Activity and Health: A Report of the Surgeon General. Atlanta: U.S. Department of Health and Human Service Centers for Disease Control and Prevention, National Center for Chronic Disease Prevention and Health Promotion; 1996.
22. Gordon N: The exercise prescription (pp. 269–288). In Ruderman N, Devlin J, Schneider S, Kriska A, eds. Handbook of Exercise in Diabetes, 2nd ed. Alexandria, VA: American Diabetes Association; 2002.
23. Vinik AI, Erbas T: Neuropathy (pp. 463–496). In Ruderman N, Devlin J, Schneider S, Kriska A, eds. Handbook of Exercise in Diabetes, 2nd ed. Alexandria, VA: American Diabetes Association; 2002.
24. Aeillo LP, Wong J, Cavallerano JD, et al: Retinopathy (pp. 401–413). In Ruderman N, Devlin J, Schneider S, Kriska A, eds. Handbook of Exercise in Diabetes, 2nd ed. Alexandria, VA: American Diabetes Association; 2002.
25. Bernbaum M, Alber SG, Cohen JD, Drimmer A: Cardiovascular conditioning in individuals with diabetic retinopathy. Diabetes Care 12:740–742, 1989.
26. Shulman CR: Diabetes mellitus: Definition, classification, and diagnosis. In Galloway JA, Potvin JH, Shulman CR, eds. Diabetes Mellitus, 9th ed. Indianapolis: Lilly Research Laboratories; 1988.

SELECTED REFERENCES FOR FURTHER READING

American College of Sports Medicine: ACSM's Exercise Management for Persons with Chronic Disease and Disabilities, 2nd ed. Champaign, IL: Human Kinetics; 2003.

American Diabetes Association: Clinical practice recommendations: 2003. Diabetes Care 26(suppl 1):S1–156, 2003. Available at http://care.diabetesjournals.org/content/vol26/suppl_1/

American Diabetes Association: Clinical practice recommendations: 2004. Diabetes Care 27(suppl 1):S1–150, 2004. Available at http://care.diabetesjournals.org/content/vol27/suppl_1/

American Diabetes Association: Physical Activity/Exercise and Diabetes Mellitus: Position Statement. Diabetes Care 26(suppl 1):S73–S77, 2003.

Ruderman N, Devlin J, Schneider S, Kriska A, eds: Handbook of Exercise in Diabetes, 2nd ed. Alexandria, VA: American Diabetes Association; 2002.

INTERNET RESOURCES

American College of Sports Medicine Position Stands: http://www.acsm.org/publications/positionstands.htm

American Diabetes Association: Diabetes and Cardiovascular Disease: http://www.s2mw.com/heartofdiabetes/cardio.html

American Diabetes Association: http://www.diabetes.org/for-health-professionals-and-scientists/professionals.jsp

American Dietetic Association: http://www.eatright.org/Public/GovernmentAffairs/index_20150.cfm

American Society of Diabetes Educators: http://www.aadenet.org/ProfessionalEd/index.html

Centers for Disease Control and Prevention: National Center for Chronic Disease Prevention and Health Promotion: Diabetes Public Health Resource: http://www.cdc.gov/diabetes/index.htm

National Clinical Guideline Clearinghouse: http://www.guideline.gov

National Institutes of Health and National Heart, Lung, and Blood Institute: Clinical Guidelines on the Identification, Evaluation, and Treatment of Overweight and Obesity in Adults: http://www.nhlbi.nih.gov/guidelines/obesity/ob_home.htm

Exercise in Patients with End-stage Renal Disease

PATRICIA PAINTER

Chronic renal failure results from structural kidney damage and progressively diminished renal function. Once initiated, chronic renal failure (CRF) progresses to **end-stage renal disease (ESRD)**, requiring some form of **renal replacement therapy** such as **dialysis** or transplantation. There are approximately 308,000 patients with kidney failure in the United States[1]. Although it affects people of every age, race, and walk of life, 42% of the ESRD population is over the age of 60 years, and ESRD tends to be more prevalent in populations in the lower socioeconomic realms[2]. The incidence and prevalence of ESRD is anticipated to grow at a rapid pace that will be primarily driven by the aging population, increased rates of diabetes and changing racial distributions[1].

Before 1972, access to dialysis treatment was limited in the United States, and selection of patients for treatment was made by committees composed of medical professionals, clergy, and lay people. Essentially, they decided who would receive the lifesaving therapy of dialysis. In 1972, Congress passed landmark legislation that extended Medicare coverage to patients with ESRD. This legislation hinged on the expectation of successful vocational rehabilitation of these patients (an expectation that has not

been realized). The cost of renal replacement therapy is high, with the estimated cost of dialysis being about $60,000 per patient per year, and transplants costing less over time (~$12,000/year after the first year)[1]. Although the payment for renal replacement therapy has remained relatively constant since 1972, the population of patients with ESRD is increasing annually (100 individuals are diagnosed with ESRD each day); thus, the cost to the Medicare program is substantial for the number of patients involved. Additionally, ESRD patients are qualified for disability payments, another cost to government programs[2]. Access to treatment, payment for treatment, and preferences of treatment vary in other countries.

Although the overall outcomes and well being of patients with renal failure have been significantly improved by advances in technology and pharmacology, allowing for improved potential for rehabilitation, it is generally acknowledged that rehabilitation has not been addressed nationally in this patient group in a sustained, consistent, and integrated fashion[2]. Despite advances in technology and pharmacology, patients with renal failure still have low levels of physical functioning. And despite increased interest in rehabilitation, as evidenced by the designation by the United States Renal Data System (USRDS) of a special study section on rehabilitation and quality of life, physical rehabilitation has not been addressed nationally in a sustained, consistent, and integrated fashion that affords patients to rehabilitation services as a part of the routine medical therapy.

Pathophysiology of Chronic Renal Failure

Damage to the kidney can result from long-standing diabetes mellitus, hypertension, autoimmune diseases (i.e., lupus), **glomerulonephritis**, **pyelonephritis**, some inherited diseases (i.e., polycystic disease, Alport's syndrome), and congenital abnormalities. The damaged kidney initially responds with higher filtration and excretion rates per nephron. These compensatory mechanisms delay the onset of symptoms up to a point where only 10% to 15% of renal function remains. Progressive renal failure ultimately results in the loss of both excretory and regulatory functions, resulting in uremic syndrome. Uremia is characterized by fatigue, nausea, malaise,

KEY TERMS

Chronic renal failure: Gradual and progressive loss of the ability of the kidneys to function

Creatinine clearance: A standard test that estimates the glomerular filtration rate, or function of the kidney

Dialysis: A method of removing toxic substances from the blood when the kidneys are unable to do so

End-stage renal disease: A complete or near complete failure of the kidneys to function.

Glomerular filtration rate (GFR) study: A test that uses a radioactive tracer to measure how well the kidneys filter waste products

Glomerulonephritis: A type of kidney disease caused by inflammation of the glomeruli of the kidney, which may be a reversible or progressive condition. Progressive glomerulonephritis may result in destruction of the kidney glomeruli and chronic renal failure and end-stage renal

disease. The disease may be caused by specific problems with the body's immune system, but the precise cause of most cases is unknown.

Hemodialysis: A method of filtering toxins from the blood by circulating the blood through special filters

Peritoneal dialysis: A method of removing toxic substances from the blood by using the peritoneal membrane inside the abdomen as the semipermeable membrane

Pyelonephritis: An infection of the kidney and the ureters that usually occurs as a result of a urinary tract infection, particularly in the presence of vesicoureteric reflux, which is an occasional or persistent backflow of urine from the bladder into the ureters or kidney

Renal replacement therapy: Treatment to replace lost function of the kidneys; includes dialysis and transplantation

---

anorexia, and subtle neurologic symptoms. Patients present with these symptoms along with peripheral edema, pulmonary edema, congestive heart failure (CHF), or a combination of these symptoms. Diagnosis of CRF is made from elevated serum creatinine level, elevated blood urea nitrogen level, and reduced **glomerular filtration rate (GFR)**[3].

The loss of the excretory function of the kidney results in the buildup of toxins in the blood, any of which may negatively affect enzyme activities and inhibit systems such as the NA/K-ATPase system, resulting in altered active transport across cell membranes and altered membrane potentials. The loss of regulatory function of the kidneys results in the inability to regulate extracellular volume and electrolyte concentrations, which adversely affects cardiovascular and cellular functions. Most patients are volume overloaded, resulting in hypertension and often CHF. Other malfunctions in regulation include impaired generation of ammonia and hydrogen ion excretion (resulting in metabolic acidosis), and decreased production of erythropoietin, which is the primary cause of the anemia of ESRD[3,4].

Normal substances may be excessively produced or inappropriately regulated in response to renal failure. Parathyroid hormone (PTH) may be the most important of these. PTH is produced in excess secondary to hyperphosphatemia, reduced conversion of vitamin D to its most active forms, and malabsorption and impaired release of calcium ions from bone. The attempt to maintain adequate circulating calcium ion concentrations in the face of hypocalcemia results in hyperparathyroidism and renal osteodystrophy[3,4].

Other metabolic abnormalities are associated with uremia, including insulin resistance and hyperglycemia. In patients treated with dialysis, hyperlipidemia is characterized by hypertriglyceridemia with normal (or low) total cholesterol concentrations. Very low-density lipoprotein (VLDL) is elevated with low levels of High-density lipoprotein (HDL) concentrations and normal low-density lipoproteins (LDL) levels. After successful renal transplantation, the lipid profile becomes hypercholesterolemic, with elevation of LDL fractions. Several clinical interventions associated with the dialysis treatment or immunosuppression therapy (after transplantation) may contribute to these metabolic abnormalities[3,4].

Patients with ESRD are at higher risk for cardiovascular disease (CVD), and CVD is the leading cause of death in both dialysis and transplant recipients[5]. The incidence of CVD is fourfold higher in the transplant population than in the general population[6,7]. All known risk factors for CVD are prevalent in both dialysis and transplant patients. It is not known, however, whether the usual multiple CV risk interventions are effective in this population.

Clinical Features

Deterioration in renal function results in an overall decline in physical well being. Signs include anemia, fluid buildup in the tissues, loss of bone minerals, and hypertension. Patients experience symptoms of fatigue, shortness of breath, loss of appetite, restlessness, change in urination patterns, and overall malaise. Glomerular damage is progressive and results in the buildup of toxins in the blood. Renal function level is established with the clinical markers of serum creatinine and blood urea nitrogen. GFR may also be measured to determine the level of renal function. Renal biopsy may also be done to determine the cause of the disease. Renal scans or intravenous pyelograms may be performed to rule out obstruction or congenital abnormalities that may contribute to increased creatinine levels in the blood.

Treatment of Chronic Renal Failure

Management of patients with CRF is directed at minimizing the consequences of accumulated nitrogenous waste products normally excreted by the kidneys. Dietary measures play a primary role in the initial management, with very low-protein diets being prescribed to decrease the symptoms of uremia and possibly to delay the progression of the disease. In addition to protein restriction, dietary sodium and fluid restrictions are critical[4] because the fluid regulation mechanisms of the kidney are deteriorating in function. Any excess fluid taken remains in the system and, with progressing deterioration in renal function, ultimately results in peripheral edema, CHF, and pulmonary congestion. Very strict blood pressure (BP) control is also recognized as an important factor in slowing the progression.

End-stage Renal Disease

Progressive deterioration of renal function ultimately requires the initiation of some form of renal replacement therapy for maintenance of life. Treatment options include **hemodialysis** (performed in a center or at home), **peritoneal dialysis**, or transplantation. The decision to initiate dialysis is determined by many factors, including cardiovascular status, electrolyte levels (specifically, potassium), chronic fluid overload, severe and irreversible oliguria or anuria, significant uremic symptoms, and excessively abnormal laboratory values (usually creatinine > 8 to 12 mg·dL^{-1}; blood urea nitrogen [BUN] > 100 to 120 mg·dL^{-1}) and creatinine clearance (<5 mL·min^{-1}).

Creatinine clearance is a standard test that estimates the GFR, or function of the kidney. The test compares the level of creatinine in the urine with the creatinine level in the blood, usually based on measurements of a 24-hour urine sample and a blood sample drawn at the end of the 24-hour period. Clearance is often measured as milliliters per minute. The test works because creatinine is found in stable plasma concentrations and it is freely filtered and not reabsorbed by the kidneys. Therefore, creatinine clearance can be used to estimate the GFR.

The home setting (i.e., support for home dialysis or distance from a clinic) may also be a factor in determining the type of treatment initiated. Factors such as age and economic status are not considered in the United States since the passage of the End Stage Renal Disease Act of 1972[4]. Renal replacement therapy does not correct all signs and symptoms of uremia and often presents the patient with other concerns and troubling side effects.

Treatment Options in End-stage Renal Disease

HEMODIALYSIS

Hemodialysis is the most common form of renal replacement therapy in the United States, with approximately 63% of all patients treated in a center or at home. Other countries may prefer more home-based treatments such as peritoneal dialysis (see below). Hemodialysis is a process of ultrafiltration (i.e., fluid removal) and clearance of toxic solutes from the blood. It necessitates vascular access by way of a blood access placed in the subclavian vein or an arteriovenous connection, either using a prosthetic conduit or native vessels. Two needles are placed in the access: one directs blood out of the body to the artificial kidney (dialyzer), and the other directs blood back into the body. The action of a blood pump draws blood to the dialyzer at an average rate of 200 to 300 mL·min^{-1}. No more than 500 mL of blood is out of the body at any time. Sensors and filters are incorporated throughout the system to assure constant pressures, temperatures, and steady flow and to prevent air from entering the system. The dialyzer has a semipermeable membrane that separates the blood from a dialysis solution, which creates an osmotic and concentration gradient to clear substances from the blood. Factors such as the characteristics of the membrane, transmembrane pressures, blood flow, and dialysate flow rate all determine removal of substances from the blood. Manipulation of the blood flow rate, dialysate flow rate, dialysate concentrations, or time of the treatment can all be used to remove more or less substances and fluids[4].

The prescription of dialysis depends on the quantity of fluid to be removed and the required clearance of toxins. The duration of the hemodialysis treatment is determined by the degree of residual renal function, body size, dietary intake, and clinical status. A typical hemodialysis prescription is 3 to 4 hours three times per week. Special monitoring of blood parameters helps determine the adequacy of dialysis. Complications of the hemodialysis treatment include hypotension, cramping, problems with bleeding, and fatigue. Significant fluid shifts can occur between treatments if patients are not careful with dietary and fluid restrictions.

PERITONEAL DIALYSIS

Approximately 8% of patients in the United States are treated with peritoneal dialysis. Other countries tend to have a higher percentage of patients treated with this form of dialysis. This form of therapy is accomplished by introducing a dialysis fluid into the peritoneal cavity via a permanent catheter placed in the lower abdominal wall. The peritoneal membranes are effective for ultrafiltration of fluids and clearance of toxic substances in the blood of uremic individuals. The dialysis fluid is of a given osmotic and concentration to provide gradients to remove fluid and substances. The fluid is introduced either by a machine (cycler), which cycles fluid in and out over a 8- to 12-hour period at night or manually by 2- to 2.5-L bags that are attached to tubing and emptied by gravity into and out of the peritoneum. The latter process is known as continuous ambulatory peritoneal dialysis (CAPD) and allows the patient to dialyze continuously throughout the day. CAPD requires exchange of fluid every 4 hours using sterile techniques[4].

Patients may choose peritoneal dialysis so they can experience more freedom and less dependency on a center for use of a machine. It allows patients to travel and dialyze on their own schedule. Patients may also be placed on peritoneal dialysis because of cardiac instability because this kind of dialysis does not involve the major fluid shifts experienced with hemodialysis. Peritoneal dialysis may also be preferable for diabetic patients because they can inject insulin into their dialysate and achieve better glucose control.

Complications of peritoneal dialysis include problems with the catheter or catheter site, infection, hernias, low back pain, and obesity. Hypertriglyceridemia is a problem because of the exposure and absorption of glucose from the dialysate. Patients may absorb as many as 1200 calories from the dialysate per day, contributing to the development of obesity and hypertriglycemia[4].

RENAL TRANSPLANTATION

Transplantation of kidneys is the preferred treatment of ESRD. Approximately 12,000 kidney transplants are performed every year in the United States (28% of ESRD patients). The source of the kidneys available for transplant can be a living related or unrelated individual or a cadaver. Because of the shortage of organs available for transplantation and improvements in immunosuppression medications, living-nonrelated transplants are becoming more frequent. Patients considered for transplants are generally healthier and younger than the general dialysis population, although there are no age limits to transplantation. Patients with severe cardiac, cerebrovascular, or pulmonary disease and neoplasia are not considered candidates. Extensive immunologic studies are performed on recipients before transplant to minimize the immunologic response to the transplanted kidney. When an appropriately matched kidney is found, it is surgically placed in an extrailiac position.

After transplantation, patients are placed on immunosuppression medication, which includes combinations of glucocorticosteroids (prednisone), cyclosporine deriva-

tive, and monoclonal antibody therapy. New immunosuppression medications are constantly being developed, allowing for minimization of side effects by altering therapies and combinations of therapies. Patients may experience rejection early (acute) or later (chronic), which is detected by elevation of serum creatinine level. Rejection is treated immediately using increased dosing of immunosuppression (mostly prednisone), with a tapering back to maintenance dose. Patients must remain on immunosuppression for the lifetime of the transplanted organ. Nationwide 1-year survival of the transplanted kidney is 85%, and patient survival is 90%. Five-year rates are 67% graft survival and 85% patient survival. Causes of graft loss include chronic rejection (25%), cardiovascular deaths (20.3%), infectious deaths (8.7%), acute rejection (10.2%), technical complications (4.7%), and other deaths (10.2%). Patient deaths occur primarily because of cardiac vascular disease (51.1%). Short-term transplant survival has been improved with new immunosuppression medications, leaving the major challenges of long-term survival of grafts and patients to be investigated. Loss of kidney results in the need to return to dialysis[8]. Complications of kidney transplantation are primarily related to immunosuppression therapy and include infection, hyperlipidemia, hypertension, obesity, steroid-induced diabetes, and osteonecrosis.

Cardiovascular Disease

Cardiovascular disease is main cause of death in patients with renal failure, regardless of the treatment. The extremely high incidence of CVD has been characterized as epidemic, being from five to 30 times that of in the general population[5,9,10]. Traditional risk factors for CV disease, such as hypertension, dyslipidemia, and diabetes mellitus, are highly prevalent in the dialysis population[5,9,10]. In addition, patients with ESRD have other disease-related risk factors, such as anemia, hyperhomocysteinemia, hyperparathyroidism, oxidative stress, hypoalbuminemia, chronic inflammation, and prothrombotic factors, that are believed to contribute to increased CVD risk. Data suggest that a uremic factor or a factor related to renal replacement therapy or dialysis may be implicated in the pathogenesis of heart disease in patients treated by dialysis[11]. The incidence of atherosclerotic CVD is four times higher in kidney transplant recipients than in the general population, and cardiovascular risk factors are prevalent in the majority of patients. No studies have documented whether traditional cardiovascular risk intervention is effective in reducing cardiovascular risk in patients with ESRD. The National Kidney Foundation (NKF) has developed the Dialysis Quality Outcomes Initiative (DOQI), an evidenced-based report to be published in winter 2005 that includes several treatment guideline publications on various complications associated with renal failure, including guidelines for the treatment of CVD. These guideline documents are available from the NKF's website.

Exercise and Rehabilitation

EXERCISE CAPACITY AND EXERCISE TESTING

Most patients on dialysis are severely limited in their exercise capacity. Peak oxygen uptake is reported to be only 60% to 70% of normal age-expected levels and as low as 39%, whether treated with hemodialysis or peritoneal dialysis[12–23]. The limitation to exercise in these patients is difficult to determine because of the complex nature of uremia, which affects nearly every organ system of the body. It is almost certain that the reduced exercise capacity is multifactorial and is influenced by anemia, reduced muscle blood flow, reduced muscle oxidative capacity, and myocardial dysfunction as well as physical inactivity. Muscle function may be abnormal, affected by nutritional status, dialysis adequacy, hyperparathyroidism, and other clinical variables[24,25].

Most exercise studies that have measured oxygen uptake in patients with kidney disease have limited study groups to healthier patients with few comorbid conditions. In fact, the majority of patients are lower than this in their exercise capacity, and most may be unable to perform exercise testing. Information obtained from exercise testing in this patient group is usually not diagnostically useful because most patients do not achieve age-predicted maximal heart rates (HRs) and stop exercise because of leg fatigue. Many patients have abnormal left ventricular function, and most patients have conditions that make interpretation of stress electrocardiograms (ECGs) difficult, including left ventricular hypertrophy (LVH) with strain patterns, electrolyte abnormalities, and digoxin effects on the ECG. Thus, stress testing is not necessarily mandatory before initiation of exercise training, and requiring stress testing may present a barrier to getting these patients more physically active[26]. Because their exercise capacity is so low, most patients will not be training at levels that are much above the energy requirements of their daily activities; thus, risk associated with such training is minimal. Measurement of HR is not recommended for determining training intensity because of variability in taking antihypertensive medications and the effects of the fluid shifts on HRs. Thus, exercise testing is not needed for developing a training HR prescription.

PERFORMANCE-BASED AND SELF-REPORTED PHYSICAL FUNCTION MEASURES

Testing of physical performance may be more appropriate for dialysis patients using tests such as stair climbing, the 6-minute walk test, the sit-to-stand-to-sit test, or gait speed testing (also see Chapter 15). These tests have been standardized and used in many studies of elderly individuals and have been shown to be predictive of outcomes such as hospitalization, discharge to nursing home, and mortality[27]. A walking stair climbing test has been validated in hemodialysis patients by Mercer et al[28]. In hemodialysis patients, these test results are extremely low compared with age-expected normal values[29]. For instance, muscle strength levels, as indicated by the sit-to-stand test, average only 25% of normal age-expected values[29]. These tests have been are effective in demonstrating improvements from exercise counseling interventions[29]. Additionally, self-reported physical functioning scales such as those on the SF-36 Health Status Questionnaire[30,31] are highly predictive of outcomes (specifically, hospitalization and death) in dialysis patients[32]. The physical functioning scales on the SF-36 are also extremely low in dialysis patients, and they improve but do not normalize after transplantation.

After successful renal transplantation, exercise capacity increases significantly, to near normal sedentary predicted values[13,18,33]. Renal transplant recipients who were active and who participated in the 1996 U.S. Transplant Games had exercise capacity that averaged 115% of normal age-predicted values[34]. A randomized clinical trial on exercise after renal transplant indicates that those who participate in regular exercise have significantly higher $\dot{V}O_{2peak}$ and self-reported functioning at 1 year compared with those receiving usual care (which does not include any exercise counseling)[35]. Exercise testing using standard protocols is more appropriate for transplant recipients who are able to push themselves in their training programs above their daily levels of activity. Exercise HR responses are normalized after transplant. The major abnormality noted in transplant recipients is excessive BP response to exercise.

EXERCISE TRAINING RESPONSES IN DIALYSIS PATIENTS

Most studies showed an improvement in $\dot{V}O_{2max}$ after exercise training, with an average increase of 16.4% across all studies (range, 0% to 52%)[14,16,17,22,23,24]. Although the improvement is similar to that seen in healthy individuals, training does not normalize $\dot{V}O_{2max}$ and the posttraining values remain well below age-predicted values. In addition to the improvements in oxygen uptake, there are reports of improvements in hematocrit (before the availability of erythropoietin), BP control, and lipid profiles. Many of these improvements have not been duplicated in other studies, and most studies have included too few subjects to be conclusive[25]. None of these studies included measures of quality of life or self-reported functioning. Khouidi et al.[24] reported impressive improvements in muscle fiber size and improvement in atrophy after a program of cardiovascular exercise training plus sports activity and strengthening exercises. Deligianis et al.[36,37] have reported improved cardiac function after physical training.

Significant improvements have been reported in the performance-based tests (specifically, gait speed and sit to stand-to-sit test) after exercise counseling interventions for independent home exercise and in-center cycling have been provided. This study also reported significant improvements in the physical scales of the SF-36 Health Status Questionnaire[29].

One exercise training study has been reported in patients who are treated with peritoneal dialysis, which showed significant improvements in $\dot{V}O_{2peak}$ (16.2%) and physical functioning dimensions of quality of life [38].

EXERCISE TRAINING RESPONSES IN TRANSPLANT PATIENTS

Three studies have reported significant improvements in exercise capacity in renal transplant recipients[35,39,40]. In a randomized, controlled trial of independent home exercise over the first year of transplant, significant improvements were found in $\dot{V}O_{2peak}$ with home exercise (increase in $\dot{V}O_{2peak}$ to $30 \ mL \cdot kg^{-1} \cdot min^{-1}$ at 1 year) compared with those in the usual care group ($24 \ mL \cdot kg^{-1} \cdot min^{-1}$ at 1 year)[35]. The usual care group was not much different than values reported for high-functioning dialysis patients. It is not likely that exercise training alone improves patients' cardiovascular risk profiles. However, the multidisciplinary interventions typically implemented in cardiac rehabilitation programs are probably beneficial in modification of risk factors for CVD because most patients do not receive risk factor education or similar follow-ups after kidney transplantation.

EXERCISE PRESCRIPTION

An important resource for exercise prescription is *Exercise: A Comprehensive Program for Dialysis Patients*, which can be found on the Life Options website (see Internet Resources). This information provides information for exercise professionals as well as dialysis staff members and dialysis patients on exercise.

In the general dialysis population, the goal of *improvements* in exercise capacity may not always be realized. However, because the typical course over time is deterioration in physical functioning, *maintenance* of functioning is a positive outcome and a realistic expectation from exercise interventions in these patients. The primary goal for most patients is to maintain independence, so any intervention that accomplishes this should be considered positive[27].

The exercise prescription for patients on dialysis should include flexibility and range of motion (ROM), strengthening, and cardiovascular exercises. Weight management considerations may be needed for many transplant recipients. For dialysis patients, the key to prescription is understanding the multiple barriers to exercise that may exist. These include general feelings of malaise, time requirements of treatment, lack of encouragement or information provided by their nephrology health care workers, fear, and accustomization or adaptation of lifestyles of low levels of functioning. Thus, any prescription should start slowly and progress gradually in order to prevent discouragement and additional feelings of fatigue or muscle soreness[41].

Timing of Exercise

The timing of exercise in relation to the dialysis treatment should be considered. Hemodialysis patients can exercise any time, although they may feel best on their nondialysis days. Therefore, they may tolerate higher intensity or durations on the days when they do not undergo dialysis. Most of these patients feel extremely fatigued after their dialysis treatment, and there may be a problem with hypotension after the treatment when physical activity–induced vasodilatation occurs. Immediately before the dialysis treatment, some patients may have excessive fluid in their systems because they are unable to rid their bodies of fluid taken in between treatments. It is typically recommended that patients restrict their fluid intake to limit their weight gain to no more than 2 to 3 kg between treatments. Some patients are unable to restrict their fluid intake and present to dialysis with much higher pre-dialysis weights (i.e., 5 to 12 kg increase in weight, which is primarily excess fluid). Thus, they may not tolerate as much exercise before dialysis because of an increased volume overload on the left ventricle and increased BP at rest (and during exercise), which may increase ventricular preload and afterload and, in extreme cases, result in pulmonary congestion. Although most patients can tolerate exercise before dialysis, their tolerance may be reduced compared with exercise on nondialysis days. Exercise should be deferred if the patient is experiencing shortness of breath related to the excess fluid status. There are no specific guidelines as to the "upper limit" of fluid weight gain that would contraindicate exercise, although the guidelines established by the American College of Sports Medicine for BP are indicated (see GETP7 Boxes 3-5 and 5-2).

The ideal time to exercise, in terms of adherence and convenience, may be during the hemodialysis treatment. Stationary cycling, using the cycle from the lazy-boy chair used for dialysis, is safe and does not interfere with the dialysis treatment. Although many dialysis clinics are becoming interested in this activity, most are still unwilling to have cycles in the clinic for their patients. Thus, independent home exercise may be the best approach for exercise for these patients.

Cycling during dialysis is best tolerated during the first 1.0 to 1.5 hours of the treatment. Exercising later in the treatment may be preferable for some patients; however, many patients become hypotensive when sitting up in the chair, making it difficult for the set up of the cycle. This response is attributable to the continuous removal of fluid throughout the treatment, resulting in a decreasing cardiac output, stroke volume, and mean arterial pressure at rest[42]. Thus, the cardiovascular exercise response superimposed on the hemodynamic effects of dialysis is adequately stable during the first couple hours of treatment; however, after 2 hours of dialysis, cardiovascular decompensation may preclude exercise[42].

For patients treated with CAPD, the exercise may be best tolerated at a time when the abdomen is drained of fluid. Thus, the patient may choose to exercise in the middle of a dialysis exchange after draining fluid and before introducing the new dialysis fluid. This requires capping off the catheter for exercise, a technique that must be discussed with the dialysis nurse. Exercising empty allows for greater diaphragmatic excursion and less pressure against the catheter during exertion, reducing the risk of hernias or leaks around the catheter site[43].

Type of Activity

There is no restriction on the type of activity that can be prescribed for dialysis or transplant patients. ROM and strengthening exercises are critical for most patients because of their history of long periods of inactivity and resulting stiffness and weakness. Because many patients have weak muscles and joint discomfort, non–weight-bearing cardiovascular activity may be best tolerated. As in anyone, if jarring activity causes joint discomfort, then a change in mode of exercise is indicated. The access site for hemodialysis may be placed in the arm or upper leg. This should not inhibit activity at all, even though many patients are told not to use the arm with their fistula in it. This restriction is typically given by the vascular surgeon at the time of placement and pertains only to the time of healing (i.e., 6 to 8 weeks). The only precaution for the fistula is to avoid any activity that would close off the flow of blood (i.e., having weights lying directly over the top of the vessels). Although patients will (and should) be quite protective of their access sites, use of the extremity increases flow through it and actually helps develop muscles around the access site, which should make placement of needles easier.

Full sit-ups and activities that involve full flexion at the hip should be avoided for patients with peritoneal catheters. Abdominal strengthening can be accomplished using isometric contractions and crunches. Swimming may be a challenge for those with peritoneal catheters because the possibility of infection. Patients must be advised to cover the catheter with some protective tape and clean around the catheter exit site after swimming. Fresh-water lake swimming is not recommended; swimming in chlorinated pools and in the ocean involves less risk of infection.

Although transplant recipients are often told not to participate in vigorous activities, the main concern is any contact sport that may involve direct hit to the area of the transplanted kidney (i.e., football). Vigorous activities and non-contact sports are well tolerated by transplant recipients who have worked to build adequate muscle strength and cardiovascular endurance through a comprehensive general conditioning program.

Frequency of Exercise

Range of motion exercises should be encouraged daily. Hemodialysis patients will feel especially stiff after their dialysis session because of the 3 to 4 hours of sitting, the removal of fluid, and often cramping. Stretching during the dialysis treatment and afterwards may relieve this stiffness. Muscle strengthening should be done 3 days per week. Cardiovascular exercise should be prescribed for at least 3 days per week, although a prescription of 4 to 6 days per week may be most beneficial.

Intensity of Exercise

Cardiovascular exercise intensity should be prescribed using a rating of perceived exertion because HR is highly variable in dialysis patients because of fluid shifts and vascular adaptations to fluid loss during dialysis treatments. Many patients initially may only tolerate several minutes of very low-level exercise, making warm-up and cool-down intensities irrelevant. These individuals should just be encouraged to gradually increase duration at whatever level they can tolerate. After they achieve 20 minutes of continuous exercise, then warm-up, conditioning, and cool-down intensities can be incorporated, with an RPE of 9 to 10 for warm-up and cool-down phases and 12 to 15 for the conditioning time (on the 20-point scale [see GETP7 Table 4-7]).

Progression of Exercise

It is critical to start patients slowly and progress gradually. In practice, this means that the patient should determine the duration of activity that is comfortably tolerated during the initial sessions. This duration should be the starting duration of activity. If only 2 to 3 minutes is tolerated, the prescription may be for several intervals of 2 to 3 minutes, with a gradual decrease in the rest times to progress the patient to continuous activity. A progression in duration of 2 to 3 minutes per session or per week is recommended, depending on individual tolerance. Very weak patients may need to start with strengthening program of low weights and high repetitions and ROM exercise before initiating any cardiovascular activity. The progression should gradually work up to 20 to 30 (or more) minutes of continuous activity at an RPE of 12 to 15 (on the 20-point scale).

When starting a patient cycling during dialysis, the initial session is usually limited to 10 minutes, even if the patient is able to initially tolerate a longer duration. This precaution is to assure the dialysis staff and the patient that the cycling does not have any adverse effects on the dialysis treatment. The patient can then increase duration according to tolerance as described above in subsequent sessions. RPE is also used for intensity prescription during the dialysis treatment because removal of fluid from the beginning to the end of dialysis can result in resting and exercise HRs (standard submaximal level) varying by 15 to 20 beats[38].

Exercise prescription for patients with renal failure depends on their treatment and must be individualized according to the limitations presented by the patient. The prescription should include the type of exercise (cardiovascular, ROM, strengthening), frequency of exercise, timing of exercise in relation to treatment, duration, intensity (prescribed primarily based on RPE), and progression. The progression should be very gradual in those who are extremely debilitated. The starting levels and progression must be according to tolerance because fluctuations in well being, clinical status, and overall ability frequently change because changes in medical status. Often, hospitalization or a medical event (e.g. clotting of fistula or placement of a new fistula) will set back a patient in the progression of the program, requiring frequent evaluation of the prescription. The goal is for patients to become more active in general and, if possible, for them to work toward a regular program of 4 to 6 days per week of cardiovascular exercise, 30 minutes or more per session, at an intensity of 12 to 14 on the RPE scale. Strengthening exercise should be recommended three times per week.

SPECIAL CONSIDERATIONS

When patients are diagnosed with end-stage renal failure, most are never given information on exercise and physical activity. If they ask, they are typically told to "take it easy" or "just don't overdo it." These comments pose questions and doubt in the minds of patients and their families, who are very protective. They do not know how to gauge how much is "too much" activity and because they do not feel well and are fatigued, they opt for no activity. This inactive lifestyle is often reinforced by the dialysis staff who see the patients regularly for their treatments[44]. It is, therefore, not surprising that many patients are skeptical about becoming physically active, and the data clearly indicate that dialysis patients are physically inactive[45,46]. Patients have little interaction with others and thus receive little information about physical activity from others than their dialysis providers. Thus, it is very important for any exercise professional to take the time to learn about dialysis and transplant to understand what the patient must deal with daily or three times per week. This could entail watching a patient being put on the dialysis machine and visiting with a few patients during their treatments. Patient support groups are also a good source of information. Patients talk freely about their experiences, many of which help exercise professionals better motivate patients and understand more about patient responses to major changes in lifestyle such as initiating exercise. Exercise professionals

should reach out to dialysis staff members about how exercise might benefit their patients and assure them that the programs initiated will be safe and not interfere with the treatments[47]. This education should also include ideas of how the dialysis staff can encourage patients to be physically active. This additional encouragement and reinforcement can greatly facilitate patient efforts in rehabilitation. Likewise, lack of support and understanding on the part of the dialysis staff can sabotage efforts to increase activity in their patients.

Most exercise professionals practice in their own laboratories and depend on referrals of patients to their exercise facilities. It is important to understand that there are many patients who may be unable to participate in exercise at the designated facility but for whom counseling on home independent exercise can be extremely beneficial. Thus, exercise professionals are encouraged to reach out to other health care providers (other than cardiologists and pulmonologists), educate them on the services they can offer their patients, and discuss the benefits of exercise for their patient groups. Although there is growing interest in the nephrology community on improving physical functioning of their patients, most nephrologists and kidney transplant staff members are not well versed or familiar with how exercise may benefit their patients, how to evaluate physical functioning, or how to prescribe exercise. Thus, the services of a trained professional who knows about the problems associated with dialysis and transplant may be a welcome addition to the patient care team.

REFERENCES

1. USRDS, U.S. Renal Data System 2003 Annual Report: Atlas of End-Stage Renal Disease in the United States. Bethesda, MD: National Institute of Diabetes and Digestive and Kidney Diseases; 2003
2. Oberly E, ed: Renal Rehabilitation: Bridging the Barriers. Medical Education Institute: Madison, WI; 1994.
3. Brenner BM, Stein JH: Chronic Renal Failure. New York: Churchill Livingstone; 1981
4. Nissenson AR, Fine RN: Dialysis Therapy, 2nd ed. Philadelphia: Hanley & Belfus; 1993.
5. Levey AS, Beto JA, Coronado BE, et al: Controlling the epidemic of cardiovascular disease in chronic renal disease: What do we know? What do we need to learn? Where do we go from here? Am J Kidn Dis 32:853–906, 1998.
6. Kassiske BL: Risk factors for cardiovascular disease after renal transplantation. Mineral Electrolyte Metabolism 19:186–195, 1993.
7. Kassiske BL, Guijarro C, Massy ZA, et al: Cardiovascular disease after renal transplantation. J Am Soc Nephrol 7:158–165, 1996.
8. United Network for Organ Sharing: UNOS Update 1996. Richmond: Organ Procurement and Transplantation Network and Scientific Registry for Organ Transplantation; 1999.
9. Uhlig K, Levey AS, Sarnak MJ: Traditional cardiac risk factors in individuals with chronic kidney disease. Seminars in Dialysis, 16: 118–127, 2003.
10. Longnecker JC, Coresh J, Powe NR, et al: Traditional cardiovascular risk factors in dialysis patients compared with the general population. J Am Soc Nephrol 13:1918–1927, 2002.
11. Sarnak MJ: Cardiovascular complications in chronic kidney disease. Am J Kidn Dis 41(suppl 5): S11–S17, 2003.
12. Barnea N, Drory Y, Iaina A, et al: Exercise tolerance in patients on chronic hemodialysis. Isr J Med Sci 16:17–21, 1980.

13. Beasley RW, Smith A, Neale J: Exercise capacity in chronic renal failure patients managed by continuous ambulatory peritoneal dialysis. Aust NZ J Med 16:5–10, 1986.

14. Goldberg AP, Geltman EM, Hagberg JM, et al: Therapeutic benefits of exercise training for hemodialysis patients. Kidn Int 16(suppl): S303–S309, 1983.

15. Moore GE, Brinker KR, Stray-Gundersen J, Mitchell JH: Determinants of VO₂ peak in patients with end-stage renal disease: on and off dialysis. Med Sci Sports Exerc 25:18–23, 1993.

16. Moore GE, Parsons DB, Painter PL, et al: Uremic myopathy limits aerobic capacity in hemodialysis patients. Am J Kidn Dis 22:277–287, 993.

17. Painter PL, Nelson-Worel JN, Hill MM, et al: Effects of exercise training during hemodialysis. Nephron 43:87–92, 1986.

18. Painter PL, Messer-Rehak D, Hanson P, et al: Exercise capacity in hemodialysis, CAPD and renal transplant patients. Nephron 42:47–51, 1986.

19. Painter P: Exercise in end stage renal disease. Exercise and Sports Science Reviews; 16:305–339, 1988.

20. Painter P: The importance of exercise training in rehabilitation of patients with end stage renal disease. Am J Kidney Dis 24 (suppl 1):S2–S9, 1994.

21. Ross DL, Grabeau GM, Smith S, et al: Efficacy of exercise for end-stage renal disease patients immediately following high-efficiency hemodialysis: A pilot study. Am J Nephrol 9:376–383, 1989.

22. Shalom R, Blumenthal JA, Williams RS: Feasibility and benefits of exercise training in patients on maintenance dialysis. Kidn Int 25:958–963, 1984.

23. Zabetakis PM, Gleim GW, Pasternak FL, et al: Long-duration submaximal exercise conditioning in hemodialysis patients. Clin Nephrol 8:17–22, 1982.

24. Kouidi E, Albani M, Natsis K, et al: The effects of exercise training on muscle atrophy in haemodialysis patients. Nephrol Dial Transplant 13:685–699, 1998.

25. Johansen KL: Physical functioning and exercise capacity in patients on dialysis. Adv Ren Replace Ther 6:41–148, 1999.

26. Copley JB, Lindberg JS: The risks of exercise. Adv Ren Replace Ther 6:165–171, 1999.

27. Painter PL, Stewart AL, Carey S: Physical functioning: Definitions, measurement, and expectations. Adv Ren Replace Ther 6:110–123, 1999.

28. Mercer T, Naish PF, Gleeson NP, et al: Development of a walking test for the assessment of functional capacity in non-anemic maintenance dialysis patients. Nephrol Dial Transplant 13:2023–2026, 1998.

29. Painter PL, Carlson L, Carey S, et al: Physical functioning and health related quality of life changes with exercise training in hemodialysis patients. Am J Kidn Dis 35:482–492, 2000.

30. Ware J: SF-36 Health Survey: Manual and Interpretation Guide. Boston: The Health Institute; 1993.

31. Ware JE, Kosinski M, Keller SD: SF-36 Physical and Mental Health Summary Scales: a User's Manual, 2nd ed. Boston: Health Institute; 1994.

32. DeOreo PB: Hemodialysis patient-assessed functional health status predicts continued survival, hospitalization and dialysis-attendance compliance. Am J Kidn Dis 30:204–212, 1997.

33. Painter P, Hanson P, Messer-Rehak, D, et al: Exercise tolerance changes following renal transplantation. Am J Kidn Dis 10:452–456, 1987.

34. Painter PL, Luetkemeier MJ, Dibble S, et al: Health related fitness and quality of life in organ transplant recipients. Transplantation 64:1795–1800, 1997.

35. Painter PL, Tomlanovich SL, Hector LA, et al: A randomized trial of exercise training following renal transplantation. Transplantation 74:42–48, 2002.

36. Deligianis A, Kouidid E, Tassoulas E, et al: Cardiac response to physical training in hemodialysis patients: An echocardiographic study at rest and during exercise. In J Cardiol 70:253–266, 1999.

37. Deligiannis A, Kouidi E, Tourkantonis A: Effects of physical training on heart rate variability in patients on hemodialysis. Am J Cardiol 84:197–202, 1999.

38. Lo C, Li L, Lo WK: Benefits of exercise training on continuous ambulatory peritoneal dialysis [abstract]. Am J Kidn Dis 32:1011–1018, 1998.

39. Miller TD, Squires RW, Gau GT, et al: Graded exercise testing and training after renal transplantation: a preliminary study. Mayo Clin Proc 62:773–777, 1987.

40. Kempeneers G, Myburgh KH, Wiggins T, et al: Skeletal muscle factors limiting exercise tolerance of renal transplant patients: Effects of a graded exercise training program. Am J Kidn Dis 14:57–65, 1990.

41. Painter P, Blagg C, Moore GE: Exercise for the Dialysis Patient: A Comprehensive Program. Madison, WI: Medical Education Institute; 1995.

42. Moore GE, Painter PL, Brinker KR, et al: Cardiovascular response to submaximal stationary cycling during hemodialysis. Am J Kidn Dis 31:631–637, 1998.

43. Carey S, Painter P: An exercise program for CAPD patients. Nephrology News and Issues June:15–18, 1997.

44. Painter PL, Carlson L, Carey S, et al: Determinants of exercise encouragement practices in dialysis staff. J Am Nephrol Nurses Assoc in press.

45. O'Hare AM, Tawney K, Bacchetti P, Johansen KJ: Decreased survival among sedentary patients undergoing dialysis: results from the dialysis morbidity and mortality study wave 2. Am J Kidn Dis 41:447–454, 2003.

46. Johansen KL, Chertow GM, Ng AV, et al: Physical activity levels in patients on hemodialysis and healthy controls. Kidn Int 57:2564–2570, 2000.

47. Carlson L, Carey S: Staff responsibility to exercise. Adv Ren Replace Ther 6:172–180, 1999.

SELECTED REFERENCES FOR FURTHER READING

American College of Sports Medicine: ACSM's Resources for Clinical Exercise Physiology: Musculoskeletal, Neuromuscular, Neoplastic, Immunologic, and Hematologic Conditions. Baltimore: Lippincott, Williams & Wilkins; 2002.

Levey AS, Coresh J, Balk E, et al: National Kidney Foundation. National Kidney Foundation practice guidelines for chronic kidney disease: Evaluation, classification, and stratification. Ann Intern Med 139:137–147, 2003. Erratum in Ann Intern Med 139:605, 2003.

Levin A, Stevens L, McCullough PA: Cardiovascular disease and the kidney: Tracking a killer in chronic kidney disease. Postgrad Med 111:53–60, 2002.

Clinical algorithms on cardiovascular risk factors in renal patients. Nephrol Dial Transplant15(suppl 5):127–128, 2000.

INTERNET RESOURCES

American Heart Association: http://www.americanheart.org

Life Options Rehabilitation Program: http://www.lifeoptions.org

National Institutes of Digestive & Diabetes & Kidney Diseases: http://www.niddk.nih.gov

National Kidney Foundation: Clinical Practice Guidelines: http://www.kidney.org/professionals/kdoqi/guidelines.cfm

Osteoporosis and Exercise

DAVID L. NICHOLS AND EVE V. ESSERY

Epidemiology

Osteoporosis is a systemic disease characterized by low bone mass and deterioration of the bone tissue michroarchitecture, resulting in an increase in bone fragility and susceptibility to fracture[1]. Osteoporosis and low bone mass are a major public health threat, affecting about 44 million individuals age 50 and older in the United States[2]. Eighty percent of Americans with osteoporosis are women, and the disease more often affects white and Asian women than black or Hispanic women. It has been estimated that one of every two women and one in four men over 50 years of age will suffer from an osteoporosis-related fracture in their lifetime. To illustrate the risk, a woman's risk of hip fracture is equal to her combined risk of breast, uterine, and ovarian cancers[2].

Osteoporosis is a silent, preventable disease that can be diagnosed and treated before any fracture occurs. Preventive measures include diet and exercise components and, in some cases, pharmacological agents. The purpose of this chapter is to provide a brief overview of the etiology, clinical features, and treatment of osteoporosis. Special emphasis is placed on the effects of the disease on exercise responses and physical function as well as exercise prescription and programming. Throughout this chapter, *bone mineral density (BMD)* and *bone mineral content (BMC)* will be used to quantify mineral content per unit area of bone. BMD and BMC are often used as primary outcome measures in research studies and in clinical settings.

Etiology and Pathophysiology

Throughout the life span, bone is continuously subjected to a dynamic process of resorption and subsequent formation known as **remodeling**. The process of bone remodeling is depicted in Figure 35-1. Remodeling maintains the mechanical integrity of bone tissue by replacing fatigue-damaged older bone with new bone. Remodeling is also necessary to maintain mineral homeostasis within the body. Bone remodeling occurs through the actions of cells known as osteoclasts and osteoblasts. **Osteoclasts** are multinucleated cells responsible for the degradation or resorption of old bone, and **osteoblasts** build new bone to replace the bone that has been removed. Osteoclasts erode portions of the bone surface, creating cavities. Within the cavity, osteoblasts secrete a collagen matrix that is then mineralized to form new bone. Remodeling of old bone is different than modeling of growing bone. **Modeling** refers to new bone formation and is not preceded by resorption. Modeling is the predominant activity in growing bones in which bones gain mass and undergo structural modifications.

The changes in BMC of girls and women across the life span are displayed graphically in Figure 35-2. During childhood and adolescence, new bone is added more rapidly than old bone is removed. Bone formation continues at a faster pace than bone resorption until **peak bone mass** is attained at around 30 years of age. After peak bone mass is obtained, the process of remodeling becomes less efficient in the adult skeleton, resulting in small deficits in formation after each remodeling cycle. The accumulation of these deficits may be partially responsible for the losses in bone mass seen with aging. Bone loss at different bone sites is experienced at a rate of approximately 0.5% to 1.0% per year, depending on a variety of genetic and environmental factors[3].

During perimenopause, women lose bone mass at a rate of approximately 1.0% per year. At menopause, when ovarian function ceases and hormones are not replaced, estrogen deficiency results in rapid bone loss for 5 to 7 years after menopause[4]. Bone loss during the first 5 years postmenopause can reach 9% to 13%[5]. Other research has described a 20% to 30% decrease in lifetime bone density during the early postmenopausal period[6]. However, bone loss eventually returns to a slower rate similar to premenopausal losses after the woman has adapted to the hormone deficiency. Men also experience age-related bone loss. However, men experience bone loss at a lower rate than women[7], and men may have greater bone size and bone mass than women[8].

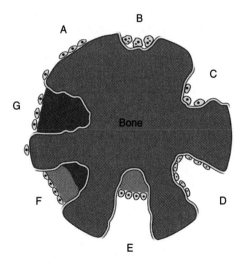

FIGURE 35-1. A. Resting trabecular surface. **B.** Multinucleated osteoclasts dig a cavity of approximately 20 μm. **C.** Completion of resorption to 60 μm by mononuclear phagocytes. **D.** Recruitment of osteoblast precursors to the base of the resorptive cavity. **E.** Secretion of new matrix by osteoblasts. **F.** Continued secretion of matrix with initiation of calcification. **G.** Completion of mineralization of new matrix. Bone has returned to a quiescent state, but a small deficit in bone mass persists.

Risk Factors

Risk factors associated with osteoporosis include female gender, white or Asian ethnicity, older age, small frame size, and family history of osteoporosis. Women are more likely to experience osteoporotic fractures than men primarily because of hormonal changes that they experience. When reproductive hormone status is compromised in women, such as with amenorrhea or menopause, reductions in BMD are observed[9,10]. Of particular concern are young women who experience amenorrhea coupled with reduced caloric intake and excessive energy expenditure. The female athlete triad is a syndrome that can occur in athletic girls and women that consists of amenorrhea, disordered eating, and osteoporosis[11]. Early intervention with amenorrheic athletes is necessary to prevent irreversible bone loss[12].

Osteoporosis risk increases as a result of low body weight, smoking, excessive alcohol consumption, and use of certain medications that affect bone metabolism. A low body mass index (BMI) is an important risk factor for osteoporosis and subsequent fractures[13]. Smoking has also been associated with low BMD and increased risk of fracture[14]. Use of medications such as glucocorticoids,

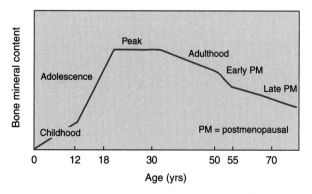

FIGURE 35-2. Model of bone mineral content changes with age in women. (Adapted with permission from Snow-Harter C: Exercise, calcium and estrogen: Primary regulators of bone mass. Contemporary Nutrition 17[4], 1992.)

anticonvulsants, glucocorticosteroids and adrenocorticotropin, gonadotropin-releasing hormone agonists, immunosuppressants, and long-term heparin has also been associated with the disease[15].

Poor nutrition is a risk factor for osteoporosis. Several dietary factors, including calcium, vitamin D, protein, phosphorus, and magnesium, are involved in the maintenance of the skeleton. Consumption of adequate amounts of calcium during childhood and adolescence has been associated with the development of greater peak bone mass[16]. It has also been suggested that bone mass may be enhanced by consuming adequate amounts of calcium during later stages of life[17]. Experimental studies have shown increases in bone acquisition as a result of the consumption of calcium supplements[18,19] and dairy products[20].

Bone is a mineral reservoir that is important in the maintenance of calcium homeostasis. Approximately 99% of the body's calcium is stored in bone, and the remaining calcium found in the body is involved in a variety of physiologic processes, including nerve transmission and muscle contraction. Maintaining adequate blood calcium levels is a high priority of the body. When dietary calcium is insufficient as a result of low consumption or poor absorption, calcium is removed from the bone for use in essential physiologic processes[21]. Thus, adequate calcium consumption is necessary. The recommendations for calcium intake from the Institutes of Medicine vary depending on the age of the individual. The recommended calcium intake of children 1 to 8 years of age is 500 to 800 mg·day^{-1}. Individuals from 9 to 18 years of age are recommended to consume 1300 mg·day^{-1} of calcium. Adults 19 to 50 years of age should consume 1000 mg·day^{-1} of calcium, and adults 51 years and older should consume at least 1200 mg·day^{-1} calcium[22].

Physical inactivity is another risk factor for osteoporosis. Cohort studies have generally found that physically active individuals and athletes have higher bone mass than sedentary control subjects. Athletes involved in sports with unilateral activity, such as tennis, demonstrate higher BMD in the dominant (playing) arm than in the nonplaying arm[23,24]. Athletes who perform activities that require high muscle forces and impact loads (e.g., gymnastics) appear to have higher bone mass than athletes in endurance training (e.g., distance running)[25]. Also, individuals who participate in activities without gravitational forces or impact (e.g., swimming) have lower BMD than those engaged in activities with a weight-bearing component[26]. Finally, athletes who regularly engage in resistance training typically have higher bone mass at the hip and spine than their non–weight training counterparts[27,28]. BMD has also been correlated with parameters of fitness. For example, lean body mass has been positively correlated with BMD[29]. Resistance, balance, and agility exercise training can also improve agility, strength, and balance among individuals at risk for osteoporosis and may reduce the risk of future falls[15,30–33].

Mechanical loading of bone can increase peak bone mass attained and attenuate age-related losses in bone mass. A 2-year high-impact jumping intervention within the school setting resulted in a substantial bone mineral accrual advantage in pubertal girls[34] with site-specific gains in bone strength of boys[35]. A 15-month resistance training program improved femoral neck BMD in female adolescents with no significant change observed in control subjects[36]. Physical activity transmits mechanical loads to the skeleton via gravitational forces and muscular pull at the sites of attachment. Bone responds to alterations in mechanical strain, and bone strength is a function of loads to which the skeleton is subjected. When strain is increased, as may occur during exercise, osteoblast activity increases and osteoclast activity remains constant, thus resulting in an increase in bone strength and density[37,38].

Diagnosis

Because there is no direct measure of bone strength, BMD is widely accepted as an indirect measure of bone strength[39]. BMD is used for the measurement of bone strength because it reflects the mineral content of the bone (responsible for an estimated 70% of bone strength), and it is directly associated with the load-bearing capacity of the hip and spine and the risk of fracture[40]. The World Health Organization (WHO)[40] and the National Institutes of Health (NIH)[39] have selected BMD measurements as the method of choice to establish the diagnosis of osteoporosis.

There are several different techniques available to assess BMD at single or multiple skeletal sites, including dual-energy x-ray absorptiometry (DXA), single-energy x-ray absorptiometry, quantitative ultrasound, peripheral computed tomography (CT), and radiographic absorptiometry[41]. DXA is currently considered to be the gold standard technique for BMD measurement and osteoporosis diagnosis[42], and the hip is the preferred site of assessment if a single site is selected[13]. However, a measurement of BMD at a specific joint is a better predictor of future fractures at that joint[39]. For example, a BMD measure at the spine is a better predictor of spine fracture than a measure on BMD at the hip[39]. For screening, calcaneal ultrasound and CT have been recommended to identify patients who may be at risk for fractures in the near future (i.e., 1 year)[43,44], but DXA is still recommended as the best method for following persons with osteoporosis[41]. Figure 35-3 shows an illustration of a DXA scan.

Some experts suggest that osteoporosis may be best diagnosed by combining risk factor assessment with a measure of BMD[40,43,45]. However, as the NIH Consensus statement[39] concedes, further study is needed before there can be consensus that the combined method of risk assessment and BMD measures is superior to BMD measurement alone. However, for exercise professionals, the use of an osteoporosis risk assessment questionnaire may be helpful in identifying persons at risk who may

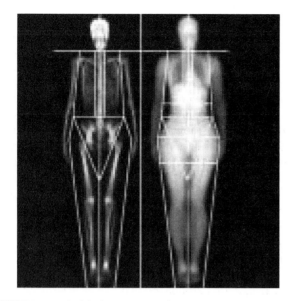

FIGURE 35-3. Typical dual-energy x-ray absorptiometry scan. (Courtesy GE Medical Systems.)

benefit from adaptations in the exercise prescription to minimize risk of fracture. Examples of two risk questionnaires that may be used to identify persons at high risk of osteoporosis include the Simple Calculated Osteoporosis Risk Estimation (SCORE)[46] and the Osteoporosis Risk Assessment Instrument[47].

The operational definition of osteoporosis proposed by the WHO is bone density that is 2.5 standard deviations below the mean[40]. The diagnostic criterion developed by the WHO compares the BMD value of an individual to the mean for young, normal, adult white women, and is expressed as a T score. The four general diagnostic categories of T scores used by the WHO for the assessment of BMD can be found in Table 35-1[40]. For example, if an elderly woman received a T score of -2.5, then her BMD value was 2.5 standard deviations below the mean for young normal adults, and she would be categorized as osteoporotic.

The diagnostic categories based on T score shown in Table 35-1 originated using data derived from DXA measurements of BMD at the hip, although the use of these categories has been extended to other skeletal sites and using technologies other than DXA[39]. Thus, the use

TABLE 35-1. Diagnostic Criteria for Osteoporosis

Classification	T score
Normal	1.0 and above
Osteopenia (low bone mass)	−1.0 to −2.5
Osteoporosis	below −2.5
Severe or established osteoporosis	below −2.5 in the presence of one or more fragility fractures

Note: Based on World Health Organization: Assessment of Fracture Risk and Its Application to Screening for Postmenopausal Osteoporosis. Geneva: World Health Organization; 1994, 1–129.

of the T score categories is not without controversy[39]. One obvious question is the appropriateness of the application of the WHO diagnostic criteria to sites other than the hip and to technologies other than DXA without supportive research data. Furthermore, few data have evaluated the application of a score developed on young white women to men, children, and persons of varying races and ethnicities, although the criteria are applied regularly to these groups. Combined with the problem of wide variability between different methods and instruments used to measure BMD, some experts believe that an improved, evidence-based diagnostic criteria should be developed[39].

Clinical Features

Fractures and their associated complications are the primary clinical features associated with osteoporosis. Individuals who suffer from a fracture may be able to fully recover, or the fracture may result in chronic pain, disability, deformity, or even death. More than 1.5 million fractures are associated with osteoporosis each year, primarily at the vertebrae (spine), proximal femur (hip), and distal forearm (wrist)[15]. Individuals with osteoporosis may experience fractures at other sites as well. However, a fracture is not required for an individual to be diagnosed with the disease. Some individuals are diagnosed with osteoporosis as a result of their BMD values, although they have not experienced a fracture.

An estimated 700,000 of vertebral fractures occurring each year are associated with osteoporosis[2]. Vertebral fractures can cause back pain, height loss, kyphosis, and even death[48]. Those who suffer from vertebral fractures may develop a "signature" Dowager's hump at the thoracic vertebrae fracture, resulting in a curve in the upper spine. Vertebral fractures may limit physical activity, range of motion, and balance. Vertebral fractures affecting posture can result in restrictive lung disease because of restriction of the thoracic cavity. Fractures in the lumbar vertebrae may also alter the abdominal anatomy, resulting in abdominal pain, distention, and constipation[15].

An estimated 300,000 hip fractures are associated with osteoporosis each year[2]. A hip fracture is actually a fracture at the neck of the femur, and it is often the most debilitating clinical feature associated with osteoporosis. Only 40% of individuals who suffer from an osteoporotic hip fracture fully regain their prefracture level of independence. One third of individuals who suffer a hip fracture also go on to fracture the opposite hip. Up to 25% of individuals who suffer from an osteoporotic hip fracture may require long-term nursing home care after the fracture, and 10% to 20% die within 1 year[15].

More than 250,000 osteoporotic wrist fractures occur annually, and approximately 300,000 fractures at other sites are associated with osteoporosis every year[2]. Although these fractures may not lead to the disability that accompanies fractures at the hip and spine, these fractures are associated with low bone mass and may indicate an increased risk for future fractures.

Treatment of Osteoporosis

Although treatment options for osteoporosis are available, there is no cure; thus, the primary focus should be prevention. If adequate bone mass is obtained during the first decades of life, the inevitable bone loss that seems to occur with aging need not be a problem. However, for individuals who fail to achieve an adequate bone mass or for those that have severe bone loss, medical treatment may become necessary. Several pharmacological treatments approved by the Food and Drug Administration (FDA) are available for osteoporosis (Table 35-2), and they can be broadly classified into two types: antiresorptive treatments and anabolic agents.

The majority of the currently available drugs with FDA approval for osteoporosis are considered antiresorptive drugs, which affect bone mass by inhibiting bone resorption. Thus, they slow the rate of bone loss and may result in a net increase in bone mass by altering the balance between bone resorption and bone formation. Increases in BMD are generally seen with the initiation of therapy and continue over the first 2 to 3 years of treatment. Thereafter, bone density is maintained as long as the therapy is continued. The increases seen in BMD with antiresorptive therapy are generally attributed to a filling in of the remodeling space that has occurred as a result of the excess bone resorption that occurred before the initiation of therapy. Decreases in fracture risk are of 10% to 40% are also seen with therapy. Antiresorptive drugs available include salmon calcitonin, bisphosphonates, selective estrogen receptor modulators (SERMs), and estrogen replacement therapy (ERT).

Salmon calcitonin is a drug derived from salmon that is the similar to the endogenous hormone that regulates calcium in the body. The drug comes in either in an injectable or nasal spray preparation and is effective in both increasing low bone mass and decreasing fracture risk in postmenopausal women[49–52]. Alendronate and risedronate are bisphosphonates that are used in the prevention and treatment of osteoporosis. Both alendronate and risedronate have been shown effective in reducing bone loss and decreasing fracture risk in postmenopausal women[50–54]. Alendronate has also been found effective in increasing BMD in men with osteoporosis[55,56], although large-scale studies in men are lacking. Bisphosphonates are among the newer osteoporosis drugs and are the most

TABLE 35-2. Medical Therapies Available for the Treatment or Prevention of Osteoporosis

Drug Class	Name of Drug	Brand Name
Estrogens[a]	Estrone sulfate	Ogen®
	Conjugated estrogen	Premarin®
	Transdermal estrogen	Estraderm®
	Estropipate	Ortho-Est®
	Esterified estrogen	Estratab®
	Conjugated estrogen +	Premphase®
	Medroxyprogestrone acetate[b]	PremPro®
		Activella®
Calcitonin[c]	Synthetic salmon calcitonin	MiaCalcin®
		Calcimar®
Bisphosphonates	Alendronate[d]	Fosamax®
	Risedronate[d]	Actonel®
	Etidronate[e]	Didronel®
SERMs	Raloxifene[f]	Evista®
	Tamoxifene	Nolvadex®
Others	Isoflavones (natural flavonoids)	
	Tibolone or ipriflavone (synthetic flavonoids)	
	Calcitriol or other vitamin d metabolites	
	Teriparatide[f] or other parathyroid hormones[g]	
	Sodium fluoride[g]	

SERM = selective estrogen receptor modulator.

[a]All estrogens have Food and Drug Administration (FDA) approval for prevention of osteoporosis, but only Premarin is approved for treatment.

[b]Premphase, PremPro and Activella are estrogen and progesterone taken in combination; Premphase and PremPro are FDA approved for the treatment of osteoporosis; Activella is approved for prevention of osteoporosis.

[c]Both calcitonins are approved for prevention, but only MiaCalcin is approved for treatment of osteoporosis.

[d]Alendronate and risedronate have FDA approval for both prevention and treatment of osteoporosis. Alendronate is also approved for treatment of osteoporosis in men.

[e]Etidronate has FDA approval but not with an osteoporosis indication in the United States.

[f]FDA-approved treatment of osteoporosis.

[g]Approval pending for an osteoporosis indication.

powerful of the antiresorptive drugs currently available. Etidronate is another biphosphate drug, but it is approved for use in Europe but not in the United States.

Selective estrogen receptor modulators are another antiresorptive agent for use in patients with osteoporosis. Raloxifene has FDA approval for use in prevention of osteoporosis, and other SERMs are under investigation. The increases in BMD that are shown when taking raloxifene or other SERMs are generally less than seen with other antiresorptive medication[57,58], but fracture risk reduction has been demonstrated. Results from the MORE (Multiple Outcomes of Raloxifene Evaluation) trial show a significant reduction in the risk of vertebral fracture with either a 60 or 120 mg·day^{-1} dose of raloxifine[59]. The major side effect of raloxifene use is an increased risk of venous blood clots, but favorable changes in serum lipids have been demonstrated[60]. Raloxifene has also been shown to reduce the risk of breast cancer[61]. Estrogen replacement therapy (estrogen alone) and hormone replacement therapy (HRT, estrogen in combination with progestin) have been used in the treatment and prevention of osteoporosis in postmenopausal women. Studies have shown that ERT or HRT can halt the loss of and often increase bone mass, but the effect on fracture risk is less well established[62–66]. Most of the studies demonstrating reductions in fracture risk with HRT were observational or retrospective studies. The Women's Health Initiative (WHI) is one of the few large-scale, randomized clinical trials done with ERT and HRT. Results from the WHI indicated a significant reduction in both vertebral and hip fracture risk with the use of both HRT and ERT[67,68]. However, the major finding of the WHI was that both HRT and ERT resulted in an increased risk of cardiovascular disease (CVD) morbidity and mortality, and HRT increased the risk for certain cancers[67,68]. As a result, the recommendation of HRT in the treatment of patients with osteoporosis must be reconsidered.

In summarizing the available antiresportive therapies, reductions in vertebral fractures have been consistently shown with each therapy. A few studies with bisphosphonates have found reductions in fracture risk at nonvertebral sites, but the results are not consistent. Therapies other than bisphosphonates have not demonstrated fracture risk reduction at sites other than the spine. The fracture risk reduction seen with antiresportive therapy is at least partially independent of the increase in BMD[69]. Finally, although HRT and ERT have long been used to treat patients with osteoporosis, based on the results from the WHI, which indicate that the risk of HRT or ERT use outweighs the benefits, they should probably no longer be recommended as a treatment for osteoporosis because other equally effective therapies are available[67,68,70].

Anabolic agents increase bone formation and usually result in increases in BMD that are much greater than those seen with antiresorptive therapy. However, the increase in bone formation also results in an increase in bone turnover, and it is thought that a reduction in overall bone turnover is important in reducing fracture risk[69]. Nevertheless, the one anabolic agent, teriparatide, that has received FDA approval for treatment of patients with osteoporosis has been found to increase BMD to twice the degree of aldendronate[71] and reduce fracture risk[72]. Other potential anabolic agents under investigation include sodium fluoride, growth hormone, insulinlike growth factor I, and statins; however, the results of these studies are not conclusive, and long-term trials evaluating fracture risk have not be conducted.

Calcium and vitamin D are nutrients necessary for bone health and are not considered antiresorptive or anabolic in effect. Both calcium and vitamin D alone and in combination have been used in patients with osteoporosis, although their effectiveness in increasing BMD is equivocal. Some studies have shown increases in BMD[73,74], but others have shown no effect[75,76]. Studies evaluating fracture risk reduction are scarce, particularly for calcium, but the available evidence suggests that calcium does not reduce fracture risk, although there have been promising results for vitamin D[77,78]. Another important finding regarding vitamin D is that it has been associated with a reduction in falls, presumably by increasing musculoskeletal function[79,80]. One thing to consider with regard to both calcium and vitamin D is that the vast majority of studies investigating other therapeutic modalities for osteoporosis (e.g., bisphosphonates, estrogen, exercise) have given calcium or vitamin D supplementation to the treatment and control groups. It is thought that the effectiveness of these therapies may be reduced without adequate intake of calcium and vitamin D.

Exercise Responses

The primary purposes of acute exercise testing are typically to aid in the detection and diagnosis of coronary artery disease (CAD) or to determine appropriate levels of exercise training. There are no studies evaluating the acute physiological responses to exercise in an osteoporotic population, but for patients who can tolerate exercise, there is no reason to believe their physiological responses would be different from the responses of individuals without osteoporosis. The only exception is in the presence of restrictive lung disease caused by thoracic deformity consequent to osteoporosis. The effects of restrictive lung disease on exercise responses are discussed in Chapter 32.

Osteoporosis can sometimes mask the presence of heart disease during exercise tests because the patient may be unable to exercise intensely enough to achieve the heart rate necessary for accurate diagnosis. The American College of Sports Medicine does not consider osteoporosis as an absolute contraindication to exercise testing (see GETP7 Box 3-5), although most would agree that a person with active fractures should not undergo an exercise test[81,82]. If an exercise stress test is to be performed in an individual with osteoporosis, a cycle ergometer protocol is recommended because it involves the least trauma and impact on the bones (see GETP7 Chapter 9). An upright posture should be maintained by the patient at all times because spinal flexion is contraindicated in people with osteoporosis because spinal flexion drastically increases the forces on the spine, increasing the likelihood of a fracture[83]. Treadmill protocols can be used, but a walking protocol is recommended, and care must be taken to ensure the patient does not trip or fall.

ACUTE EXERCISE RESPONSES: INTERACTIONS WITH MEDICATION

The majority of women and men diagnosed with osteoporosis, and postmenopausal women in general, take some form of calcium and vitamin D supplements. As discussed previously, drugs available for treatment or prevention of osteoporosis include ERT, HRT, bisphosphonates, calcitonin, SERMs, and teriparatide. Other less common agents include isoflavones (natural and synthetic) and sodium fluoride (see Table 35-1 for a more complete list). Isoflavones are plant-derived compounds that have a chemical structure similar to estrogen and thus have physiological effects that may be similar to estrogen. The effects of any of these drugs or nutrients on acute or chronic exercise responses have not been extensively studied. However, there is no clear reason why any of these agents would affect exercise responses, with the possible exception of estrogen. Estrogen (and the phytoestrogens, the isoflavones) has acute vasodilator action and thus may alter electrocardiographic responses to exercise during an exercise test. This effect has been seen in studies using large doses of estrogen[84], but it has not been demonstrated with doses normally used in ERT or HRT[85].

RESPONSE OF BONE MINERAL DENSITY TO CHRONIC EXERCISE

Long-term responses of BMD to exercise in patients with osteoporosis have been studied. The goals in prescribing exercise for persons with or at risk for osteoporosis are to increase or maintain BMD and to increase fitness, agility, and balance, which may aid in fall prevention[30–33]. A number of studies with postmenopausal women and a few with men have shown that exercise can increase bone density or prevent further bone loss compared with non-exercising control subjects[32,42,86–89]. Most studies of women have used exercise in combination with ERT or HRT, and the results typically indicate that exercise alone does not offset the bone loss that occurs without estrogen. One study has shown that exercise alone increases bone mass in postmenopausal women[87], but the magnitude of the increase was greater when estrogen and exercise were combined. Few data are available on the effects of exercise in combination with antiresorptive drugs or anabolic agents. One such study found that there was no effect of exercise, either alone or in combination with bisphosphonates[90].

Exercise Prescription and Programming

Although studies have shown that several forms of exercise training have the potential to increase BMD, the optimal training program for skeletal integrity has yet to be defined. Based on current experimental knowledge, it has been proposed that an osteogenic exercise regimen should include load-bearing activities at high magnitude (force) with few repetitions, create different types of strain distributions throughout the bone structure (i.e., stress the bone in directions to which it is unaccustomed), and be long term and progressive in nature[91,92]. Resistance training (weight lifting) probably offers the best opportunity to meet these criteria on an individual basis, requires little skill, and has the added advantage of being highly adaptable to changes in both magnitude and strain distribution (see Chapter 25 and GETP7 Chapters 7 and 9). In addition, increases in strength and muscle size have been demonstrated after resistance training, even in elderly individuals, which has the added benefit of reducing these patients' risk of falls[30,93].

No known studies have examined cardiovascular adaptations in patients with osteoporosis, but it is expected that these patients would have a normal response to training[94]. Older men and women with osteoporosis may also present with CVD and associated risk factors, so exercise endurance training to decrease CVD risk is recommended for these patients as well. Thus, resistance, balance, and agility training combined with cardiorespiratory training (e.g., bicycling or walking) is the optimal exercise program for patients with osteoporosis[30,32,42,86]. Not only will such a program increase overall fitness and perhaps BMD, but it will also aid greatly in reducing the risk of falling[30,32,42,95–98], which is one of the primary causes of fracture in osteoporosis.

The ACSM recommends that anyone older than age 50 years who wants to begin a vigorous exercise program should have a medically supervised stress test[99] (see GETP7 Table 2-1). For older women and men with osteoporosis who simply want to begin a moderate-intensity walking or resistance training program, this recommendation may be both impractical and unnecessary. However, the presence of other chronic diseases (e.g., CVD, diabetes mellitus) needs to be considered, and guidelines concerning those diseases should be followed[99,100]. Careful screening should be undertaken to identify which individuals need further evaluation by physicians[100,101].

Some recommendations specific to patients with osteoporosis should be considered when developing an exercise program (see GETP7 Chapter 9). In general, high-impact activities such as running, jumping, and high-impact aerobics should be avoided in patients with osteoporosis because of their risk of a fracture with little or no trauma. Another activity that absolutely must not be done by people with osteoporosis is spinal flexion, including sit-ups and toe touches[102,103]. Instead, spinal extension exercises along with exercises to improve scapular mobility are recommended[102,104]. Other activities to avoid are those that increase the chance of falling such as crossover stepping, trampolines, step aerobics, skating (ice or in-line), and exercising on slippery floors[97,103].

From the other perspective, there are certain exercises that are quite beneficial for osteoporotic patients. These include exercises designed to help with balance and agility in order to reduce falls[31,33,98,105]. For instance, exercises that strengthen the quadriceps muscles are helpful. Spine extension exercises can help strengthen the back muscles, which can help reduce the development of a dowager's hump and possibly reduce the risk of vertebral fracture[106]. However, these and all exercises done by patients with osteoporosis should be performed with slow and controlled movements, avoiding jerky, rapid movements. More complete information can be found on these and other exercises for osteoporotic patients (see Carter et al.[31], Liu-Ambrose et al.[33], Pearlmutter et al.[103], and Sinaki[107] or see the websites listed at the end of the chapter (e.g., National Osteoporosis Foundation, Mayo Foundation, Osteofit Program).

The goals of an exercise program for persons with osteoporosis should include an increase in cardiovascular fitness, increased muscular strength, improved balance and agility, and an increase in (or maintenance of) BMD. The 1996 Surgeon General's report on health and physical activity recommends approximately 30 minutes of moderate physical activity accumulated on most, if not all, days of the week[106]. This is a worthwhile goal for anyone, including those with osteoporosis. However, if the person with osteoporosis is just beginning an exercise program, the duration of exercise might need to be initially shortened to allow time for adjustment to the exercise. As the person's fitness level increases, the duration of exercise can be increased.

Weight training appears to offer the most benefits for increases in muscular strength and bone density. Current recommendations suggest a single set of 10–15 repetitions of eight to 10 exercises performed at least 2 days per week[99,100] (see GETP7 Chapter 7). This is a worthwhile goal for individuals with osteoporosis, but a less strenuous program may be needed initially with care taken to avoid the exercises mentioned above that are dangerous. In addition, some resistance training exercises have a tendency to cause spinal flexion, especially exercises for the upper and lower extremities, so it is important that during resistance training all exercise be done with an upright posture.

A program to increase flexibility can also benefit osteoporotic patients because decreased flexibility can cause problems with posture. Muscles such as the hamstrings that cross more than one joint are particularly important. However, many of the commonly prescribed exercises for increasing flexibility, especially of the hamstrings muscles, involve spinal flexion and must be avoided. There is little consensus on the optimal training program for increasing flexibility, but good suggestions are available from many sources including GETP7 Chapter 7, Pearlmutter et al.[104], and Internet Resources.

Exercise may be beneficial for both increasing bone density to help prevent osteoporosis and as a therapeutic modality for patients in whom osteoporosis is already present. However, caution must be observed in the type of exercise program to be used and the specific exercises performed. Exercise professionals should supervise patients with severe osteoporosis who are just beginning an exercise program until it is determined that they can perform the exercises safely.

REFERENCES

1. Peck WA: Consensus development conference: diagnosis, prophylaxis, and treatment of osteoporosis. Am J Med 94:646–650, 1993.
2. National Osteoporosis Foundation: America's Bone Health: The State of Osteoporosis and Low Bone Mass. Washington, DC: National Osteoporosis Foundation; 2002.
3. Marcus R, Kosek J, Pfefferbaum A, Horning S: Age–related loss of trabecular bone in premenopausal women: A biopsy study. Calcif Tissue Int 35:406–409, 1983.
4. Reeve J, Walton J, Russell LJ, et al: Determinants of the first decade of bone loss after menopause at spine, hip and radius. QJM 92:261–273, 1999.
5. Ravn P, Hetland ML, Overgaard K, Christiansen C: Premenopausal and postmenopausal changes in bone mineral density of the proximal femur measured by dual–energy X–ray absorptiometry. J Bone Miner Res 9:1975–1980, 1994.
6. Hedlund LR, Gallagher JC: The effect of age and menopause on bone mineral density of the proximal femur. J Bone Miner Res 4:639–646, 1989.
7. Burger H, de Laet CE, van Daele PL, et al: Risk factors for increased bone loss in an elderly population: The Rotterdam Study. Am J Epidemiol 147:871–879, 1998.
8. Seeman E: Osteoporosis in men. Osteoporos Int 9(suppl 2):S97–S110, 1999.
9. Richelson LS, Wahner HW, Melton LJ, Riggs BL: Relative contributions of aging and estrogen deficiency to postmenopausal bone loss. N Engl J Med 311:1273–1275, 1984.
10. Drinkwater BL, Nilson K, Chesnut CH III, et al: Bone mineral content of amenorrheic and eumenorrheic athletes. N Engl J Med 311:277–281, 1984.
11. Otis CL, Drinkwater B, Johnson M, et al: American College of Sports Medicine position stand. The Female Athlete Triad. Med Sci Sports Exerc 29:i–ix, 1997.
12. Keen AD, Drinkwater BL: Irreversible bone loss in former amenorrheic athletes. Osteoporos Int 7:311–315, 1997.
13. Kanis JA: Diagnosis of osteoporosis and assessment of fracture risk. Lancet 359:1929–1936, 2002.
14. Slemenda CW, Christian JC, Reed T, et al: Long-term bone loss in men: effects of genetic and environmental factors. Ann Intern Med 117:286–291, 1992.
15. National Osteoporosis Foundation. Physician's guide to prevention and treatment of osteoporosis. 2003. Washington, DC, National Osteoporosis Foundation.
16. Teegarden D, Lyle RM, Proulx WR, et al: Previous milk consumption is associated with greater bone density in young women. Am J Clin Nutr 69:1014–1017, 1999.
17. Ulrich CM, Georgiou CC, Snow-Harter CM, Gillis DE: Bone mineral density in mother-daughter pairs: Relations to lifetime exercise, lifetime milk consumption, and calcium supplements. Am J Clin Nutr 63:72–79, 1996.
18. Lee WT, Leung SS, Wang SH, et al: Double-blind, controlled calcium supplementation and bone mineral accretion in children accustomed to a low-calcium diet. Am J Clin Nutr 60:744–750, 1994.
19. Lloyd T, Andon MB, Rollings N, et al: Calcium supplementation and bone mineral density in adolescent girls. JAMA 270:841–844, 1993.

20. Cadogan J, Eastell R, Jones N, Barker ME. Milk intake and bone mineral acquisition in adolescent girls: Randomised, controlled intervention trial. BMJ 315:255–260, 1997.

21. Kanis JA: Calcium nutrition and implications for osteoporosis. Part I. Children and healthy adults. Eur J Clin Nutr 48:757–767, 1994.

22. National Academy of Sciences: New dietary reference intakes: Recommended levels for individual intakes 1997 and 1998, recommended dietary allowances, revised 1989. Nutr Today 33:257–259, 1998.

23. Haapasalo H, Kannus P, Sievanen H, et al: Effect of long-term unilateral activity on bone mineral density of female junior tennis players. J Bone Miner Res 13:310–319, 1998.

24. Kannus P, Haapasalo H, Sievanen H, Vuori I: The site-specific effects of long-term unilateral activity on bone mineral density and content. Bone 15:279–284, 1994.

25. Robinson TL, Snow-Harter C, Taaffe DR, et al: Gymnasts exhibit higher bone mass than runners despite similar prevalence of amenorrhea and oligomenorrhea. J Bone Miner Res 10:26–35, 1995.

26. Taaffe DR, Snow-Harter C, Connolly DA, et al: Differential effects of swimming versus weight-bearing activity on bone mineral status of eumenorrheic athletes. J Bone Miner Res 10:586–593, 1995.

27. Conroy BP, Kraemer WJ, Maresh CM, et al: Bone mineral density in elite junior Olympic weightlifters. Med Sci Sports Exerc 25:1103–1109, 1993.

28. Heinrich CH, Going SB, Pamenter RW, et al: Bone mineral content of cyclically menstruating female resistance and endurance trained athletes. Med Sci Sports Exerc 22:558–563, 1990.

29. Nichols DL, Sanborn CF, Bonnick SL, et al: Relationship of regional body composition to bone mineral density in college females. Med Sci Sports Exerc 27:178–182, 1995.

30. Robertson MC, Campbell AJ, Gardner MM, Devlin N: Preventing injuries in older people by preventing falls: a meta-analysis of individual-level data. J Am Geriatr Soc 50:905–11, 2002.

31. Carter ND, Khan KM, McKay HA, et al: Community-based exercise program reduces risk factors for falls in 65- to 75-year-old women with osteoporosis: Randomized controlled trial. CMAJ 167:997–1004, 2002

32. Pfeifer M, Sinaki M, Geusens P, et al: Musculoskeletal rehabilitation in osteoporosis: A review. J Bone Miner Res 19:1208–1214, 2004.

33. Liu-Ambrose T, Khan KM, Eng JJ, et al: Resistance and agility training reduce fall risk in women aged 75 to 85 with low bone mass: A 6–month randomized, controlled trial. J Am Geriatr Soc 52:657–65, 2004.

34. Mackelvie KJ, Khan KM, Petit MA, et al: A school-based exercise intervention elicits substantial bone health benefits: A 2–year randomized controlled trial in girls. Pediatrics 112:447, 2003.

35. Mackelvie KJ, Petit MA, Khan KM, et al: Bone mass and structure are enhanced following a 2-year randomized controlled trial of exercise in prepubertal boys. Bone 34:755–764, 2004.

36. Nichols DL, Sanborn CF, Love AM: Resistance training and bone mineral density in adolescent females. J Pediatr 139:494–500, 2001.

37. Buckwalter JA, Glimcher MJ, Cooper RR, Recker R: Bone biology. Part II: Formation, form, modeling, remodeling, and regulation of cell function. J Bone Joint Sur 77(suppl A):1276–1289, 1995.

38. Lanyon LE: Using functional loading to influence bone mass and architecture: Objectives, mechanisms, and relationship with estrogen of the mechanically adaptive process in bone. Bone 18:37S–43S, 1996.

39. National Institutes of Health: Osteoporosis Prevention, Diagnosis, and Therapy. NIH Consensus Statement 17:1–45, 2000. Available at http://consensus.nih.gov

40. World Health Organization: Assessment of Fracture Risk and Its Application to Screening for Postmenopausal Osteoporosis. Geneva: World Health Organization; 1994, 1–129.

41. U.S. Preventive Services Task Force: Clinical guidelines: Screening for osteoporosis in postmenopausal women: Recommendations and rationale. Ann Intern Med 137:526–528, 2002.

42. Kanis JA, Gluer CC: An update on the diagnosis and assessment of osteoporosis with densitometry. Committee of Scientific Advisors, International Osteoporosis Foundation. Osteoporos Int 11:192–202, 2000.

43. Moyad MA: Osteoporosis—Part I: Risk factors and screening. Urol Nurs 22:276–279, 2002.

44. Placide J, Martens MG: Comparing screening methods for osteoporosis. Curr Womens Health Rep 3:207–210, 2003.

45. Wei GS, Jackson JL, Hatzigeorgiou C, Tofferi JK: Osteoporosis management in the new millennium. Prim Care 30:711–741, vi–vii, 2003.

46. Lydick E, Cook K, Turpin J, et al: Development and validation of a simple questionnaire to facilitate identification of women likely to have low bone density. Am J Manag Care 4:37–48, 1998.

47. Cadarette SM, Jaglal SB, Kreiger N, et al: Development and validation of the Osteoporosis Risk Assessment Instrument to facilitate selection of women for bone densitometry. CMAJ 162:1289–1294, 2000.

48. Cummings SR, Melton LJ: Epidemiology and outcomes of osteoporotic fractures. Lancet 359:1761–1767, 2002.

49. Grigoriou O, Papoulias I, Vitoratos N, et al: Effects of nasal administration of calcitonin in oophorectomized women: 2-year controlled double-blind study. Maturitas 28:147–151, 1997.

50. Kapetanos G, Symeonides PP, Dimitriou C, et al: A double blind study of intranasal calcitonin for established postmenopausal osteoporosis. Acta Orthop Scand 275(suppl):108–111, 1997.

51. Chesnut CH, Silverman S, Andriano K, et al: A randomized trial of nasal spray salmon calcitonin in postmenopausal women with established osteoporosis: The prevent recurrence of osteoporotic fractures study. Am J Med 109:267–276, 2000.

52. Reginster JY, Deroisy R, Lecart MP, et al: A double-blind, placebo-controlled, dose-finding trial of intermittent nasal salmon calcitonin for prevention of postmenopausal lumbar spine bone loss. Am J Med 98:452–458, 1995.

53. Ensrud KE, Black DM, Palermo L, et al: Treatment with alendronate prevents fractures in women at highest risk: results from the Fracture Intervention Trial. Arch Intern Med 157:2617–2624, 1997.

54. McClung M, Clemmesen B, Daifotis A, et al: Alendronate prevents postmenopausal bone loss in women without osteoporosis. A double-blind, randomized, controlled trial. Ann Intern Med 128: 253–261, 1998.

55. Mortensen L, Charles P, Bekker PJ, et al: Risedronate increases bone mass in an early postmenopausal population: two years of treatment plus one year of follow-up. J Clin Endocrinol Metab 83:396–402, 1998.

56. Watts NB, Josse RG, Hamdy RC, et al: Risedronate prevents new vertebral fractures in postmenopausal women at high risk. J Clin Endocrinol Metab 88:542–549, 2003.

57. Wimalawansa, S. J. A four-year randomized controlled trial of hormone replacement and bisphosphonate, alone or in combination, in women with postmenopausal osteoporosis. Am J Med 104:219–226, 1998.

58. Gonnelli S, Cepollaro C, Montagnani A, et al: Alendronate treatment in men with primary osteoporosis: a three-year longitudinal study. Calcif Tissue Int 73:133–139, 2003.

59. Ringe JD, Faber H, Dorst A: Alendronate treatment of established primary osteoporosis in men: results of a 2–year prospective study. J Clin Endocrinol Metab 86:5252–5255, 2001.

60. Delmas PD, Bjarnason NH, Mitlak BH, et al:. Effects of raloxifene on bone mineral density, serum cholesterol concentrations, and uterine endometrium in postmenopausal women. N Engl J Med 337:1641–1647, 1997.

61. Lufkin EG, Whitaker MD, Nickelsen T, et al: Treatment of established postmenopausal osteoporosis with raloxifene: A randomized trial. J Bone Miner Res 13:1747–1754, 1998.

62. Ettinger B, Black DM, Mitlak BH, et al: Reduction of vertebral fracture risk in postmenopausal women with osteoporosis treated with raloxifene: Results from a 3–year randomized clinical trial. Multiple Outcomes of Raloxifene Evaluation (MORE) Investigators. JAMA 282:637–645, 1999.

63. Walsh BW, Kuller LH, Wild RA, et al: Effects of raloxifene on serum lipids and coagulation factors in healthy postmenopausal women. JAMA 279:1445–1451, 1998.

64. Cauley JA, Norton L, Lippman ME, S. et al: Continued breast cancer risk reduction in postmenopausal women treated with raloxifene: 4-year results from the MORE trial. Multiple outcomes of raloxifene evaluation. Breast Cancer Res Treat 65:125–134, 2001.

65. Ettinger BF, Genant HK, Cann CE: Long-term estrogen replacement therapy prevents bone loss and fractures. Ann Intern Med 102:319–324, 1985.

66. Hillard TC, Whitcroft SJ, Marsh MS, et al: Long-term effects of transdermal and oral hormone replacement therapy on postmenopausal bone loss. Osteoporos Int 4:341–348, 1994.

67. Kohrt WM, Birge SJJJ: Differential effects of estrogen treatment on bone mineral density of the spine, hip, wrist and total body in late postmenopausal women. Osteoporos Int 5:150–155, 1995.

68. Lees B, Pugh M, Siddle N, Stevenson JC: Changes in bone density in women starting hormone replacement therapy compared with those in women already established on hormone replacement therapy. Osteoporos Int 5:344–348, 1995.

69. Prestwood KM, Pilbeam CC, Burleson JA, et al: The short term effects of conjugated estrogen on bone turnover in older women. J Clin Endocrinol Metab 79:366–371, 1994.

70. Anderson GL, Limacher M, Assaf AR, et al: Effects of conjugated equine estrogen in postmenopausal women with hysterectomy: The Women's Health Initiative randomized controlled trial. JAMA 291:1701–1712, 2004.

71. Rossouw JE, Anderson GL, Prentice RL, et al: Risks and benefits of estrogen plus progestin in healthy postmenopausal women: Principal results from the Women's Health Initiative randomized controlled trial. JAMA 288:321–333, 2002.

72. Garnero P, Hauserr E, Chapuy MC, et al: Markers of bone resorption predict hip fracture in elderly women: The EPIDOS Prospective Study. J Bone Miner Res 11:1531–1538, 1996.

73. Solomon CG, Dluhy RG: Rethinking postmenopausal hormone therapy. N Engl J Med 348:579–580, 2003.

74. Body JJ, Gaich GA, Scheele WH, et al: A randomized double-blind trial to compare the efficacy of teriparatide [recombinant human parathyroid hormone (1–34)] with alendronate in postmenopausal women with osteoporosis. J Clin Endocrinol Metab 87:4528–4535, 2002.

75. Neer RM, Arnaud CD, Zanchetta JR, et al: Effect of parathyroid hormone (1–34) on fractures and bone mineral density in postmenopausal women with osteoporosis. N Engl J Med 344:1434–1441, 2001.

76. Baeksgaard L, Andersen KP, Hyldstrup L: Calcium and vitamin D supplementation increases spinal BMD in healthy, postmenopausal women. Osteoporos Int 8:255–260, 1998.

77. Dawson-Hughes B, Harris SS, Krall EA, Dallal GE: Effect of calcium and vitamin D supplementation on bone density in men and women 65 years of age or older. N Engl J Med 337:670–676, 1997.

78. Dawson-Hughes B, Dallai GE, Krall EA, et al: A controlled trial of the effect of calcium supplementation on bone density in postmenopausal women. N Engl J Med 323:878–883, 1990.

79. Riis B, Thomsen K, Christiansen C: Does calcium supplementation prevent postmenopausal bone loss: A double blind, controlled clinical trial. N Engl J Med 316:173–177, 1987.

80. Feskanich D, Willett WC, Colditz GA: Calcium, vitamin D, milk consumption, and hip fractures: A prospective study among postmenopausal women. Am J Clin Nutr 77:504–511, 2003.

81. Trivedi DP, Doll R, Khaw KT: Effect of four monthly oral vitamin D3 (cholecalciferol) supplementation on fractures and mortality in men and women living in the community: Randomised double blind controlled trial. BMJ 326:469, 2003.

82. Bischoff-Ferrari HA, Dawson-Hughes B, Willett WC, et al: Effect of Vitamin D on falls: A meta-analysis. JAMA 291:1999–2006, 2004.

83. Bischoff HA, Stahelin HB, Dick W, et al: Effects of vitamin D and calcium supplementation on falls: A randomized controlled trial. J Bone Miner Res 18:343–351, 2003.

84. American College of Sports Medicine: Position stand. Osteoporosis and exercise. Med Sci Sports Exerc 27:i–vii, 1995.

85. Kohrt WM, Ehsani AA, Birge SJ: HRT preserves increases in bone mineral density and reductions in body fat after a supervised exercise program. J Appl Physiol 84:1506–1512, 1998.

86. Bouxsein ML, Myers ER, Hayes WC: Biomechanics of age-related fractures (pp. 373–393). In Marcus R, Feldman D, Kelsey JL, eds. Osteoporosis. San Diego: Academic Press; 1996.

87. Rosano GM, Sarrel PM, Poole-Wilson PA, Collins P: Beneficial effect of oestrogen on exercise-induced myocardial ischaemia in women with coronary artery disease. Lancet 342:133–136, 1993.

88. Holdright DR, Sullivan AK, Wright CA, et al: Acute effect of oestrogen replacement therapy on treadmill performance in postmenopausal women with coronary artery disease. Eur Heart J 16:1566–1570, 1995.

89. Murphy NM, Carroll P: The effect of physical activity and its interaction with nutrition on bone health. Proc Nutr Soc. 62: 829–838, 2003.

90. Dalsky GP, Stocke KS, Ehsani AA, et al: Weight-bearing exercise training and lumbar bone mineral content in postmenopausal women. Ann Intern Med 108:824–828, 1988.

91. Kohrt WM, Snead DB, Slatopolsky E, Birge Jr SJ: Additive effects of weight-bearing exercise and estrogen on bone mineral density in older women. J Bone Miner Res 10:1303–1311, 1995.

92. Milliken LA, Going SB, Houtkooper LB, et al: Effects of exercise training on bone remodeling, insulin-like growth factors, and bone mineral density in postmenopausal women with and without hormone replacement therapy. Calcif Tissue Int 72:478–484, 2003.

93. Chilibeck PD, Davison KS, Whiting SJ, et al: The effect of strength training combined with bisphosphonate (etidronate) therapy on bone mineral, lean tissue, and fat mass in postmenopausal women. Can J Physiol Pharmacol 80:941–950, 2002.

94. Beck BR, Snow CM: Bone health across the lifespan—exercising our options. Exerc Sport Sci Rev 31:117–122, 2003.

95. Kannus P, Sievanen H, Vuori I: Physical loading, exercise, and bone. Bone 18:1S–3S, 1996.

96. Harridge SD, Kryger A, Stensgaard A: Knee extensor strength, activation, and size in very elderly people following strength training. Muscle Nerve 22:831–839, 1999.

97. Gregg EW, Cauley JA, Seeley DG, et al: Physical activity and osteoporotic fracture risk in older women. Study of Osteoporotic Fractures Research Group. Ann Intern Med 129:81–88, 1998.

98. Campbell AJ, Robertson MC, Gardner MM, et al: Randomised controlled trial of a general practice programme of home based exercise to prevent falls in elderly women. BMJ 315:1065–1069, 1997.

99. American College of Sports Medicine: The recommended quantity and quality for exercise for developing and maintaining cardiorespiratory and muscular fitness in healthy adults. Position Stand. Med Sci Sports Exerc 30: 975–991, 1998.

100. American College of Sports Medicine: Progression models in resistance training for healthy adults. Position Stand. Med Sci Sports Exerc 30:992–1008, 1998.

101. Evans WJ: Exercise training guidelines for the elderly. Med Sci Sports Exerc 31:12–17, 1999.

102 Sinaki M, Mikkelsen BA: Postmenopausal spinal osteoporosis: flexion versus extension exercises. Arch Phys Med Rehab 65: 593–596, 1984.

103. Bonnick SL: The Osteoporosis Handbook. Dallas: Taylor Publishing; 1997, 1–180.

104. Pearlmutter LL, Bode BY, Wilkinson WE, Maricic MJ: Shoulder range of motion in patients with osteoporosis. Arthritis Care Res 8:194–198, 1995.

105. Sinaki M, Lynn SG: Reducing the risk of falls through propriocep-

tive dynamic posture training in osteoporotic women with kyphotic posturing: A randomized pilot study. Am J Phys Med Rehabil 81:241–246, 2002.

106. Sinaki M, Wollan PC, Scott RW, Gelczer RK: Can strong back extensors prevent vertebral fractures in women with osteoporosis? Mayo Clin Proc 71:951–956, 1996.

107. Sinaki M: Postmenopausal spinal osteoporosis: physical therapy and rehabilitation principles. Mayo Clin Proc 57:699–703, 1982.

108. U.S. Department of Health and Human Services: Physical Activity and Health: A report of the Surgeon General. U.S. Department of Health and Human Services, Centers for Disease Control and Prevention, National Center for Chronic Disease Preventon and Health, Washington, D.C., 1996.

SELECTED REFERENCES FOR FURTHER READING

Bailey DA, Faulkner RA, McKay HA: Growth, physical activity, and bone mineral acquisition. Exerc Sport Sci Rev 24:233–266, 1996.

Khan K, McKay HA, Kannus P, et al: Physical Activity and Bone Health. Champaigne, IL: Human Kinetics; 2001.

INTERNET RESOURCES

American Academy of Physical Medicine and Rehabilitation: How PM&R Physicians Use Exercise to Prevent and Treat Osteoporosis: http://www.aapmr.org/condtreat/other/osteotreat.htm

American Medical Association CME Library Online: Managing Osteoporosis: http://www.ama–cmeonline.com/cstec_mgmt/

Mayo Clinic: Exercise and Osteoporosis: Staying Active Safely: http://www.mayoclinic.com/invoke.cfm?id=HQ00643

National Institute of Aging Exercise for Older Adults. http://www.niapublications.org/exercisebook/ExerciseGuideComplete.pdf

National Osteoporosis Foundation: http://www.nof.org

National Osteoporosis Foundation: Clinical Guidelines: http://www.nof.org/professionals/clinical.htm

National Osteoporosis Foundation: Exercise for Healthy Bones: http://www.nof.org/prevention/exercise.htm

NIH National Osteoporosis and Related Bone Diseases—National Resource Center: http://www.osteo.org

Osteofit: http://www.osteofit.org/osteofit.htm

Arthritic Diseases and Conditions

STEPHEN P. MESSIER

Epidemiology of Arthritis

Arthritis has reached epidemic proportions, creating widespread disability in American adults. It is the leading cause of disability in the United States, affecting about one third of adults[1]. This includes 22.4 million adults (10.6%) with physician-diagnosed arthritis, 20.9 million adults (10.0%) with chronic joint pain, and 26.5 million (12.4%) with both arthritis and chronic pain. Disability from arthritis results in 750,000 hospitalizations; 36 million outpatient visits; $51 billion in medical care costs; and $82 billion in total costs, including lost productivity per year[2]. Of the more than 100 known arthritic diseases and conditions, **osteoarthritis (OA)**, **fibromyalgia**, and **rheumatoid arthritis** are the most common[2]. This chapter reviews the epidemiology, clinical factors, etiology, and treatments for these common rheumatic diseases.

Osteoarthritis, or degenerative joint disease, is the most common form of arthritis, with a prevalence conservatively estimated at 21 million Americans or 12.1% of the adult population[3]. The knee is the most often affected weight-bearing joint and is second in prevalence only to the small joints of the hand[4,5]. Fibromyalgia has an overall preva-

lence of 2.0% in the United States, which represents approximately 6 million people. Similar to other rheumatologic conditions, fibromyalgia afflicts women more often than men: roughly 80% to 90% of individuals with fibromyalgia are women. Fibromyalgia affects about 3.4% of women and 0.5% of men. Rheumatoid arthritis affects approximately 2.1 million Americans[3]. The estimated yearly cost of rheumatoid arthritis is $2 billion in England and $8.7 billion in the United States[6,7]. Taking into consideration both direct and society costs, Lajas et al.[6] estimated the cost of rheumatoid arthritis at $10,419 per year per patient. This results in an estimated cost of $21.9 billion per year in the United States. There is two to three times greater mortality among rheumatoid arthritis patients than in the general population, and this trend has not changed in the past 40 years[8,9] The number of new cases of rheumatoid arthritis that occur in a population each year has decreased during the past few decades[10]. As shown in Figure 36-1, from 1955 to 1964 the incidence of rheumatoid arthritis was 61.2 per 100,000 persons and decreased to 32.7 per 100,000 persons from 1985 to 1994[11].

Osteoarthritis

CLINICAL FACTORS

Osteoarthritis is a degenerative disease that affects articular cartilage and the underlying subchondral bone. The cartilaginous surfaces become pitted, resulting in hypertrophic changes along the joint margins and reactive changes in the subchondral bone. Severe OA is characterized by joint space narrowing, absence of articular cartilage, increased density and stiffness of the subchondral bone (i.e., eburnation), and osteophyte (i.e., bone spur) formation along the joint margins[12] (Fig. 36-2).

The major symptoms of OA are pain and stiffness; however, only 25% to 50% of people with radiographic evidence of OA express these symptoms[4,5]. The clinical consequences of knee OA are decreased mobility leading to muscle atrophy; an accelerated decline in physical function; and eventually to inability to engage in activities of daily living (ADLs) requiring ambulation and transfer such as walking, climbing stairs, getting in and

KEY TERMS

COX-1: An enzyme that is necessary for normal physiologic function of the stomach, kidney, and platelets

COX-2: An enzyme involved in the production of prostaglandin, which produces inflammation and contributes to acute pain

Cytokines: Small proteins that can either step up or step down the immune response

Cyclo-oxygenase (COX): An enzyme found in two main forms, COX-1 and COX-2

Fibromyalgia: A rheumatologic syndrome characterized by chronic widespread pain in the muscles, ligaments, and joints

Osteoarthritis: A degenerative disease that affects the articular cartilage and the underlying subchondral bone

Rheumatoid arthritis: An inflammatory disease with the major symptoms of pain, swelling, stiffness, and reduced joint mobility

out of a chair, lifting, and carrying. OA often results in a loss of independence and a poor quality of life[4,5,13,14]. (Fig. 36-3).

ETIOLOGY

The etiology of primary (idiopathic) OA is unknown, although biomechanical and inflammatory mechanisms have been proposed as causative factors. Biomechanically, either structural abnormalities such as obesity or neuromuscular abnormalities may cause altered joint dynamics (i.e., changes in forces and moments), thereby increasing the load on the knee. Burr and Radin[15] suggest that failure to absorb these loads properly during ADLs causes microcracks in the subchondral tissue, reactivating the secondary center of ossification and causing thinning of the overlying articular cartilage, leading to increased stresses and eventual cartilage degradation. This, in turn, leads to increased subchondral bone density and a decrease in the shock-absorbing capability of the trabecular bone. As a result, the articular cartilage bears even greater

loads, which leads to further cartilage degradation, pain, decline in physical activity, and the sequelae of physical inactivity (loss of muscle strength, loss of physical function, and disability) [Figure 36-4].

No data support this hypothetical model of decline in physical function and increased physical disability in persons with OA. Messier et al.[16] found that persons with knee OA had poorer strength, flexibility, gait, and asymmetrical distribution of loads to the lower extremities. Others have found an association between abnormal external knee adduction moments and the severity of knee OA[17–19]. In addition, Al-Zahrani et al.[20] and Messier et al.[21] reported higher knee extension moments during gait in knee OA subjects, which, in the Messier study, were coupled with 8% greater knee compressive forces. The authors speculated that higher extension moments may increase knee joint forces and provide a pathway for the degeneration of articular cartilage. These increased loads, applied over the course of many years, are hypothesized to slowly degrade the articular cartilage and eventually result in knee OA[22].

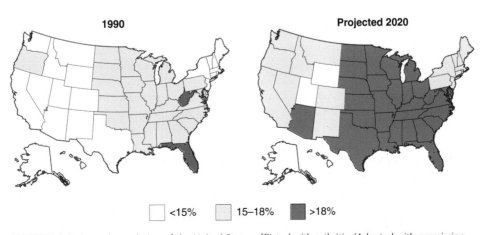

1990

Projected 2020

<15%   15–18%   >18%

FIGURE 36-1. Estimated population of the United States afflicted with arthritis. (Adapted with permission from Helmick CG, Lawrence RC, Pollard RA, Lloyd E, Heyse S: Arthritis and other rheumatic conditions: Who is affected now and who will be affected later? Arthritis Care and Research 8:203–211, 1995.)

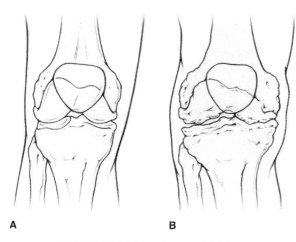

FIGURE 36-2. Healthy and osteoarthritic knees.

Recent studies have also demonstrated that low-grade inflammation plays a pathophysiological role in OA. Messier et al.[23] showed that the inflammatory cytokine interleukin-1 beta (IL-1beta) was present in the joint fluids of patients with OA. **Cytokines** are small proteins that can either step up or step down the immune response. IL-1beta is believed to play a role in mediating joint inflammation and cartilage degradation in OA. Likewise, an inflammatory component associated with OA can be detected in the circulation because serum concentrations of inflammatory markers such as cytokines (interleukin-6, IL-6; tumor necrosis factor alpha [TNF-alpha]) and the acute phase reactant C-reactive protein (CRP) are higher in persons with knee or hip OA compared with those without OA[24,25]. In addition, longitudinal studies demonstrate that high serum levels of CRP (note: this confounds the use of CRP as an emerging risk factor, as mentioned in Chapter 5) and TNF-alpha predict increased radiographic progression of knee OA as much as 5 years later[25–34]. Moreover, studies have shown that OA severity and physical function are associated with higher inflammatory markers in the blood[28,29]. Thus, mobility, pain, stiffness, and radi-

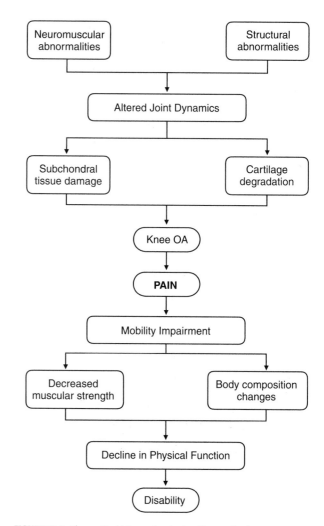

FIGURE 36-4. Theoretical biomechanical pathways for knee osteoarthritis (OA) and subsequent disability.

ographic progression are at least partly mediated by the level of chronic inflammation in OA patients[30]. Diffusion of cytokines from the synovial fluid into the cartilage nay contribute to the cartilage matrix loss observed in OA through stimulation of chondrocyte catabolic activity and inhibition of anabolic activity.

Because obese people have higher concentrations of inflammatory markers than lean persons and a large percentage of people with knee OA are overweight or obese, obese individuals with knee OA may have an even greater contribution of inflammation to functional limitation and disease progression[31]. Further work is needed to establish cause-and-effect relationships between these cytokines and knee OA. If these relationships exist, then clinical trials using pharmacologic and nonpharmacologic interventions should follow.

TREATMENTS

Treatment that affects the underlying disease process of OA is not currently available. The primary aim of therapies currently available is pain relief. Antiinflammatory

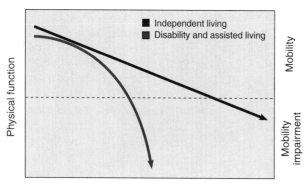

FIGURE 36-3. Osteoarthritis causes mobility impairment. Mobility impairment causes an accelerated decline in physical function (*yellow line*) that leads to an increase in disability and the need to rely on assisted living earlier in life.

medications and orthopedic procedures are the primary methods of treatment. More recently, exercise and weight loss have been used as therapeutic modalities for knee OA patients.

Nonpharmacologic Treatments

The difficulty patients with knee OA have with ADLs often results in activity avoidance[32]. Physical exercise, however, is an effective nonpharmacologic treatment. Several studies have shown that pain and disability improve with short-term (3 to 6 months) exercise. Short-term walking programs improve aerobic capacity, walking time, and self-reported function[33,34]. Similarly, lower extremity resistance training increases strength, decreases pain, and improves function in patients with OA[35,36]. More recently, long-term walking and resistance training programs have been effective in slowing the decline in physical function commonly seen in this disabled population (Fig. 36-5). A randomized clinical trial of 18-month walking and resistance training programs in 439 community-dwelling older adults with knee OA reduced disability and pain, improved balance, and improved physical performance relative to a health education control group[37]. A biomechanical gait analysis revealed that the improved mobility of the exercise treatment groups was associated with greater knee and ankle angular velocities and vertical and anteroposterior propulsive forces, characteristics that are related to faster walking speeds[38]. In a similar population, higher adherence to a physical activity program was associated with better mobility and self-reported physical function[39].

An important component of treatment for knee OA is the reduction of body weight in patients who are overweight or obese. Results of a randomized, controlled

TABLE 36-1. Dose Response to Weight Loss on WOMAC function for the ADAPT Trial[a]

% Weight Change	WOMAC Function	% Difference vs. gained	P (vs. gained)
Gained to −2.5%	21.5	—	—
−2.5% to −7.5 %	19.0	12%	0.04
−7.5% to −11.0%	17.0	21%	0.003

[a]Data represent means across the four intervention groups, diet, exercise, diet plus exercise, and healthy lifestyle control.

WOMAC = Western Ontario and McMaster University Arthrosis Index.

clinical trial have shown that a program of diet and exercise results in greater improvements in self-reported function, mobility, and pain than exercise only, diet only, or healthy lifestyle interventions[40]. A dose response to weight loss indicated that subjects who lost between 7.5% and 11.0% of their body weight exhibited significantly better self-reported function than subjects who exhibited more modest weight loss or no weight loss (Table 36-1).

Studies are beginning to show that weight loss decreases overall inflammation, reducing the cytokine activity that may be related to cartilage degradation. Nicklas et al.[31] showed that a 5% weight loss significantly reduced CRP, IL-6, and TNF-alpha receptor 1 concentrations compared with a weight-stable group. However, it is not yet known whether a specific amount of weight loss maximally reduces inflammatory markers or whether improvements in physical function, pain, and OA progression are related to declines in chronic inflammation with weight loss.

Exercise Prescription

Short- and long-term aerobic and resistance training programs are safe and effective treatments for knee OA[32]. Traditional 3 days/week, 1-hr/day programs have been the most common regimens studied. Unfortunately, little is known regarding the dose response to exercise in this older, mostly female, sedentary, and predominately overweight population. Continuous weight-bearing aerobic exercise such as walking can initially be difficult for patients with knee OA who experience significant pain. Starting with short bouts of exercise and inserting several rest periods when the patient has progressed to 30 or 40 minutes of walking improves adherence. Adding several resistance training exercises between periods of walking has proven effective and popular with patients[40]. The intensity of the exercise intervention may differ depending on the desired outcomes. If the goal is making exercise a part of a healthy lifestyle, then continued participation is more important than intensity. The exercise prescription should be flexible enough to accommodate periods of greater pain.

Pharmacologic Treatments

Initial therapy recommended by the American College of Rheumatology and the European League Against Rheumatism is acetaminophen for patients with mild to

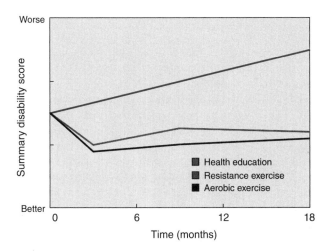

FIGURE 36-5. Summary disability scores for older adults with knee osteoarthritis randomly assigned to health education, resistance training, or aerobic exercise groups. (Adapted from Ettinger WH Jr, Burns R, Messier SP, et al: A randomized trial comparing aerobic exercise and resistance exercise with a health education program in older adults with knee osteoarthritis. The Fitness Arthritis and Seniors Trial (FAST). JAMA 277:25–31, 1997.)

moderate pain[41]. However, high doses of greater than 2 g per day increase the risk of upper GI bleeding. Antiinflammatory medications have also become increasing popular as an initial therapy for OA. The most common of these medications are the nonsteroidal antiinflammatory drugs (NSAIDs). NSAIDs include aspirin, ibuprofen, and naproxen. They exert antiinflammatory and usually analgesic actions. The mechanism of NSAIDs is to inhibit the enzyme **cyclo-oxygenase (COX)**, which is found in two main forms, **COX-1** and **COX-2**. COX-1 is necessary for normal physiologic function of the stomach, kidney, and platelets, and COX-2 is involved in the production of prostaglandin, which produces inflammation and contributes to acute pain. Lack of the COX-1 enzyme increases GI bleeding. Most NSAIDs are nonselective; that is, they inhibit to a certain degree the production of both COX-1 and COX-2. COX-2 inhibitors (Vioxx, Celebrex) avoid the COX-1 inhibitory effect, thereby reducing GI side effects. The COX-2 inhibitors are associated with increased risk of cardiovascular disease events (e.g., myocardial infarction) and should be prescribed with caution[42]. Renal toxicity, hypertension, and limb edema, however, must be continually monitored[43,44]. Interestingly, although acetaminophen and selective and nonselective NSAIDs are commonly considered the first-line of defense for mild to moderate OA, Fraenkel et al.[45] reported that many patients with symptomatic knee OA preferred a topical pain medication (Capsaicin) because of its negligible side effects. Hence, patients were willing to accept a less effective treatment in exchange for a much lower risk of side effects.

The dietary supplements glucosamine and chondroitin, separately and in combination, have gained widespread use for the treatment of OA. Glucosamine is derived from chitin in crustacean shells and is thought to promote proteoglycan and glycosaminoglycan synthesis, important components of cartilage, by inhibiting the proinflammatory cytokine IL-1beta. IL-1beta reduces proteoglycan and glycosaminoglycan synthesis, thereby inhibiting cartilage repair. Chondroitin, manufactured from shark and bovine cartilage, is responsible, with collagen and noncollagenous glycoproteins, for giving cartilage its resiliency and inhibiting synovial degradative enzymes[46].

Previous clinical trials that compared glucosamine (which come in the form of glucosamine sulfate and glucosamine hydrochloride) with a placebo suggest that it is moderately effective in reducing pain from knee OA[47,48]. Hauselmann[47] found the effect sizes (ES) for pain in five randomized, controlled trials ranged from 0.28 to 1.0 with a median effect size of 0.58, suggesting that glucosamine has a moderate effect on pain. One long-term study showed significant improvements in self-reported physical function scores and joint space narrowing after 3 years of taking glucosamine; however, the effect was small (ES = 0.28).

Mazieres et al.[49] enrolled 120 patients with knee or hip OA into a 5-month randomized, controlled trial and found that patients using chondroitin used fewer NSAIDs, had less pain, and showed improved function compared with a placebo control group. Although the results were significant, the ES (0.32) of the intent-to-treat analysis was small. Smaller studies that did not use an intent-to-treat analysis showed greater effects, with a mean effect size of 1.37. McAlindon et al. noted in their meta-analysis that many of these studies suffer from methodological problems, but overall it seems probable that glucosamine and chondroitin have some efficacy in treating the symptoms of OA with few reported side effects[47,48].

Several studies have combined glucosamine with chondroitin, attempting to create a synergistic effect of improved production (i.e., the glucosamine effect) and inhibited degradation (i.e., the chondroitin effect) of proteoglycan and glycosaminoglycan[50,51]. Using a rabbit model, the combination of glucosamine and chondroitin stimulated glycosaminoglycan synthesis compared with either preparation alone[52]. Human studies of combination therapy of glucosamine and chondroitin have shown reductions in pain in adults with OA, although each study has used supplements in addition to glucosamine and chondroitin. Two studies of patients with knee OA found combination therapy along with manganese ascorbate was effective in reducing pain after 4 and 6 months[45,52], respectively. Another study added vitamin C to show reduced temporomandibular joint pain in 40 of 50 participants[54]. Das and Hammad[46] reported that 52% of their intervention group (i.e., a combination of glucosamine, chondroitin, and manganese ascorbate) reported greater than 25% improvement in function and pain compared with 28% of the placebo group ($P = 0.04$). As with many nonsurgical treatments of OA, the best results occur in patients with mild to moderate disease[48].

Surgical Treatment

When non-invasive treatments of knee OA fail to relieve pain and improve function, several surgical treatment options may be considered. Several of the surgical methods involve arthroscopic surgery that usually involves a method to "clean out" the joint. Débridement is a method to trim torn and damaged cartilage and may be combined with joint lavage, or "washing" of the joint. Joint lavage may also be performed alone. Lavage and débridement are the most common surgical procedures for mild to moderate knee OA, accounting for approximately 650,000 procedures at an estimated total cost of $3.25 billion annually[55]. The success of these procedures varies, but approximately 50% of the patients report pain relief from either procedure[56]. A randomized, controlled trial comparing arthroscopic débridement with lavage found no difference in clinical (range of motion [ROM], tenderness, swelling), functional (self-reported pain, function, physical activity, social activity, depression, anxiety, 50-foot walk test), patient overall well being, and blinded physician (disease activity assessment) global outcomes between the groups. After 1 year, 44% of the patients who

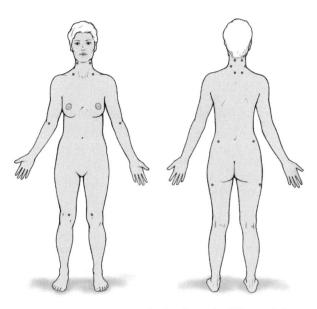

FIGURE 36-6. Tender points for the diagnosis of fibromyalgia.

underwent surgery reported improvements in their global assessment versus 58% for the lavage group[57]. A randomized, placebo-controlled trial to determine the efficacy of arthroscopic lavage and débridement using a simulated arthroscopic débridement procedure as a placebo surgery found no difference in pain or function between the lavage, débridement, and placebo surgery groups[56].

The second category of surgical procedures commonly used in patients with OA is total joint replacement (TKR) or arthroplasty. TKR is most commonly performed in knees with severe OA. The most common age range for TKR is 60 to 75 years. Patients younger than 55 years will increase the stress placed on a TKR, increasing the likelihood of a second procedure. Hence, younger patients are usually considered for alternative procedures such as unicompartmental knee replacement (partial knee

replacement) or osteotomy to improve alignment. TKR is a safe and effective treatment for end-stage knee OA. The mortality rate is 0.5%, and improvements in pain, function, and health-related quality of life appear rapid and substantial in 90% of the patients[58].

Fibromyalgia

CLINICAL FEATURES

Fibromyalgia is a rheumatologic syndrome characterized by chronic widespread pain in muscles, ligaments, and joints as well as a heightened tenderness at discrete anatomical locations called "tender points" (Fig. 36-6)[1]. Individuals with fibromyalgia have a decreased pain threshold (allodynia) during digital palpation or dolorimetry at these tender points. Besides chronic pain and tender points, individuals with fibromyalgia frequently have additional symptoms, including sleep disturbance, chronic fatigue, psychological distress, morning stiffness, and irritable bowel syndrome[59].

The American College of Rheumatology (ACR) 1990 Criteria for the Classification of Fibromyalgia continues to serve as the primary guidelines for the diagnosis of fibromyalgia[59]. The main criteria are widespread pain for at least 3 months, bilateral pain, and pain on palpation with a force of 4 kg at 11 or more of 18 tender point sites (Table 36-2).

Although the ACR criteria serve as the main diagnostic guidelines, they have received numerous criticisms. First, the ACR criteria fail to address the fact that the population of fibromyalgia patients is heterogeneous in type, degree, and location of their pain. Second, critics have noted problems with consistency in diagnosis; that is, can physicians be expected to be both accurate and consistent in the administration of a force of 4 kg[60]? Finally, Clauw and

TABLE 36-2. American College of Rheumatology 1990 Criteria for Fibromyalgia

Criterion	Definition
1. History of widespread pain	Pain is considered widespread when all of the following are present: pain in the left side of the body, pain in the right side of the body, pain above the waist, and pain below the waist. In addition, axial skeletal pain (cervical spine or anterior chest or thoracic spine or low back) must be present. In this definition, shoulder and buttock pain is considered as pain for each involved side. "Low back" pain is considered lower segment pain.
2. Pain in 11 of 18 tender point sites on digital palpation (see Fig. 36-5)	Pain, on digital palpation must be present in at least 11 of the following 18 tender point sites: • **Occiput:** Bilateral, at the suboccipital muscle insertions • **Low cervical:** Bilateral, at the anterior aspects of the intertransverse spaces at C5–C7 • **Trapezius:** Bilateral, at the midpoint of the upper border • **Supraspinatus:** Bilateral, at origins above the scapula spine near the medial border • **Second rib:** Bilateral, at the second costochondral junctions, just lateral to the junctions on upper surfaces • **Lateral epicondyle:** Bilteral, 2 cm distal to the epicondyles • **Gluteal:** Bilateral, in upper outer quadrants of the buttocks in the anterior folds of muscle • **Greater trochanter:** Bilateral, posterior to the trochanteric prominence • **Knee:** Bilateral, at the medial fat pad proximal to the joint line Digital palpation should be performed with an approximate force of 4 kg. For a tender point to be considered "positive," the subject must state that palpation was painful. "Tender" is not to be considered "painful."

Crofford[1] contend that tender points do not accurately assess the tenderness of fibromyalgia patients because patients become anxious and tend to recoil as pressure is applied. The current definition of fibromyalgia is thought to capture only 20% of individuals with chronic widespread pain. One solution may be to apply the stimuli in a random fashion. This would eliminate psychological status, most notably in people with a high level of distress.

ETIOLOGY

Historically, fibromyalgia has been diagnosed by the process of elimination. Specifically, fibromyalgia is diagnosed when the subject experiences widespread chronic pain in the absence of other identifiable pathology. No definite causal mechanism has been identified, but many have been hypothesized. Most of these hypotheses focus on the abnormal levels of nociceptive hormones and neurotransmitters in subjects with fibromyalgia. Particular attention has been paid to the function of the hypothalamic-pituitary-adrenal (HPA) axis and its associated chemical pain mediators, which include (among others) cortisol, growth hormone, insulin-like growth factor-1, substance P, and serotonin[61]. Additionally, genetics and environmental factors (e.g., muscle trauma, certain infections such as hepatitis C, Lyme disease, Epstein-Barr virus) are possible mechanisms in the development of fibromyalgia[1].

Glucocorticoid deficiency may result in pain, and individuals with fibromyalgia exhibit moderate basal hypocortisolism[61,62]. It remains unclear, however, whether low cortisol levels represent a cause or effect of chronic pain. Moreover, low levels of growth hormone in fibromyalgia subjects could be related to sleep disturbances. Growth hormone is secreted primarily during stages 3 and 4 of non-REM sleep[63], and fibromyalgia patients exhibit an abnormal sleep pattern, particularly for stages 3 and 4[64].

Substance P is a peptide that may be important in the neurotransmission of pain. Numerous human studies have shown two- to threefold average increases in substance P in the cerebrospinal fluid of subjects with fibromyalgia[65–69]. Moreover, a prospective study showed that increases in medication-free substance P concentration were directly related to increased levels of pain and tenderness in fibromyalgia patients[67]. Finally, recent studies have shown a probable reason for the efficacy of antidepressants in the treatment of fibromyalgia. A study of the effects of tricyclic antidepressants (TCAs) on rats showed a downregulation of substance P in the limbic system[70], and a human study of the antidepressant St. John's wort showed a dose-dependent decrease in substance P[71].

Patients with fibromyalgia have abnormalities in collagen metabolism that are related to increased inflammation. More specifically, Salemi et al.[72] found that abnormalities in collagen metabolism were correlated with increased levels of IL-1beta, IL-6, and TNF-alpha in roughly one third of fibromyalgia subjects. These data suggest that there is a connection between collagen abnormalities and pain-inducing inflammation in a subset of the fibromyalgia population, which may help explain why some fibromyalgia sufferers experience pain relief from NSAIDs.

TREATMENTS

There is currently no cure for fibromyalgia. Treatment is focused on the management of pain and associated symptoms using nonpharmacologic and pharmacologic therapies separately or in combination[73].

Nonpharmacologic Treatments

Common nonpharmacologic treatments for fibromyalgia include education programs, cognitive behavior therapy with a focus on psychosocial issues, acupuncture, and exercise therapy. Exercise therapy is the most common treatment, although much debate still exists regarding the optimal frequency, duration, and intensity of exercise therapy in individuals with fibromyalgia. The most effective treatment is a combination of these therapies carried out by an interdisciplinary team that includes physicians, nurses, physical therapists, occupational therapists, psychologists, and others. This section focuses on clinical trials that have examined the effects of exercise on fibromyalgia.

Short-term aerobic exercise interventions are generally successful in improving function and pain in patients with fibromyalgia. Richards and Scott[74] examined the effects of a 3-month, 2 d·wk^{-1} aerobic exercise intervention in 136 patients and found significant improvements in self-reported global assessment of well being compared with a flexibility and relaxation attention control group. Tender point count was not significantly different at the end of the intervention period; however, a 1-year follow-up revealed improved pain levels in the aerobic group. Compliance for both groups was low, with only 53% of the participants attending at least one third of the sessions. Fatigue, pain, and Medical Outcomes Study Questionnaire Short Form (SF-36) scores did not differ between the groups. Gowans et al.[75] randomized 51 fibromyalgia patients into either a 23-week aerobic exercise program or a control group and found the exercise group significantly improved mood, 6-minute walk distance, and self-efficacy relative to the control group. A meta-analysis of 16 randomized, clinical trials that compared various forms of aerobic exercise with control groups found a significant treatment effect with improvements in aerobic performance, tender point pain threshold, and pain[76]. However, the exercise interventions were of short duration, lasting 24 weeks or less.

Speculation that fibromyalgia was related to muscle trauma limited the number of clinical trials that used strength training as a primary intervention[77]. Recent studies, however, suggest that strength training may attenuate the accelerated decline in physical function common in patients with fibromyalgia. Jones et al.[78] enrolled 68 women with fibromyalgia into either a 12-week strength training or a flexibility program. There were no significant differences between the groups in isokinetic strength, number of tender points, pain, fatigue, sleep, depression, anxiety, or quality of life. In contrast, Hakkinen et al.[79] found significant differences in leg strength between FM patients randomized to a progressive strength training intervention and a control group. The authors concluded that strength training is a safe and effective intervention for patients with fibromyalgia. Finally, Geel and Robergs[80] found between 43 and 51% improvements in fibromyalgia patients after an 8-week strength training intervention; however, the lack of control group severely limits the interpretation of the results.

Taken together, it appears that aerobic—and to a lesser extent, resistance training—result in short-term improvements in function, mood, self-efficacy, and pain in fibromyalgia patients. Future investigations need to examine the long-term benefits of aerobic and resistance training in fibromyalgia patients.

Exercise Prescription

The most fundamental rule for recommending exercise for patients with fibromyalgia is to individualize the prescription. Individuals with fibromyalgia are a diverse group, but a common feature is deconditioning. Exercise prescription should ideally begin with a detailed assessment that includes both the individual's fitness level and pain and then follows a progression so that severe pain from overexertion is avoided at all times. Many of the exercise clinical trials that reported low adherence indicated that the intervention exacerbated patients' pain. Gowans et al.[75] began a 23-week, graduated aerobic exercise program with 6 weeks of warm water exercises followed by walking and eventually jogging. Only 22% of the participants failed to attend at least 45% of the exercise classes. Clearly, more study is needed regarding adherence and the type, intensity, and duration of exercise that is most appropriate for this population[78].

Pharmacologic Treatment

Antidepressants are a common pharmacologic treatment for FM. The most popular include TCAs, selective serotonin reuptake inhibitors (SSRIs), and dual reuptake inhibitors. This class of drugs increases neurotransmission and has a positive analgesic effect. TCAs improve sleep, pain, and fatigue, but their effect on mood is less definitive[73]. SSRIs have proven effective for major depressive disorders, but their effectiveness for fibromyalgia patients has been inconsistent and appears less effective than TCAs[81,82]. Dual reuptake inhibitors are similar pharmacologically to TCAs but have a better analgesic effect and diminished side effects. One open-label and one randomized, placebo-controlled trial produced conflicting results, with differences in dosage likely a major factor[83,84]. Further testing of high dosage dual reuptake inhibitors is needed before their efficacy is known.

NSAIDs have also been used to treat fibromyalgia. Goldenberg et al.[85] used a 2×2 factorial design to compare naproxen, amitriptyline (a TCA), and the combination of naproxen and amitriptyline with a placebo in patients with fibromyalgia. The authors found no significant effect of naproxen; however, amitriptyline was significantly better than the placebo on all outcomes, including pain, sleep difficulties, fatigue, and tender point scores. There was no significant interaction effect. Several other trials have also failed to find significant improvements in pain using NSAIDs in the treatment of fibromyalgia[86,87]. Hence, it appears that NSAIDs are of limited use in the treatment of fibromyalgia.

Rheumatoid arthritis

CLINICAL FEATURES

Rheumatoid arthritis (RA) is an inflammatory disease whose major symptoms are pain, swelling, stiffness, and reduced joint mobility. Table 36-3 describes each clinical symptom associated with RA. RA is an autoimmune disorder in which there is an attack on a person's own cells inside the joint capsule. Inflammatory periods are characterized by an abnormal increase in the cells of the synovial membrane, a thickening of this membrane, and a further

TABLE 36-3. Revised 1987 American College of Radiology Criteria for Rheumatoid Arthritis

Criterion[a]	Definition
1. Morning stiffness	Morning stiffness in and around the joints, lasting at least 1 hour before maximal improvement
2. Arthritis of three or more joint areas	Swelling of at least three joint areas for at least 6 weeks. The 14 possible areas are right or left PIP, MCP, wrist, elbow, knee, ankle, and MTP joints.
3. Arthritis of hand joints	Swelling of the wrist, MCP or PIP joint for at least 6 weeks
4. Symmetrical arthritis	Simultaneous involvement of the same joint areas (as defined in #2) on both sides of the body (bilateral involvement of PIPs, MCPs or MTPs is acceptable without absolute symmetry)
5. Rheumatoid nodules	Subcutaneous nodules over bony prominences or extensor surfaces or in juxta-articular regions
6. Serum rheumatoid factor	Detected by a method positive in not more than 5% of normal control subjects
7. Radiographical changes	Radiographical changes typical of rheumatoid arthritis on posteroanterior hand and radiographs, which must include erosions or unequivocal bony decalcification localized in or most marked adjacent to the involved joints

[a]At least four criteria must be fulfilled for classification as rheumatoid arthritis.

MCP = metacarpophalangeal; MTP = metatarsophalangeal; PIP = proximal interphalangeal.

increase in joint swelling. As the disease progresses, cartilage and bone that participate in joint articulations are degraded. In severe cases, the bones fuse together, resulting in a further loss of function and increased pain and deformity (Fig. 36-7).

Chronic inflammatory diseases such as RA cause premature aging[88]. Diseases that take decades to advance during normal aging, such as atherosclerosis, osteoporosis, muscle wasting, and sleep disorders, change dramatically within a few months in those with RA. Women are affected two to three times more often than men, with the peak incidence occurring between the sixth and seventh decades of life[11] (Fig. 36-8).

The rheumatoid factor (RF) is a blood test used to diagnosis RA, although a positive RF test result can also indicate the presence of other diseases such as Sjögren's syndrome, systemic lupus, and systemic sclerosis[89]. Approximately 80% of patients with RA have a positive RF test result. RF is an antibody that attaches to immunoglobulin G (IgG), forming an immune complex that can activate inflammatory processes in the body.

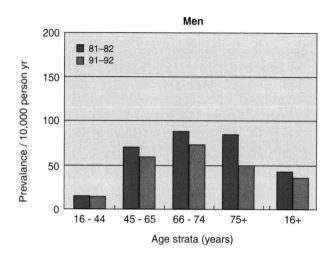

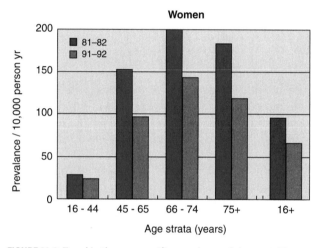

FIGURE 36-8. Trend in the age-specific prevalence of rheumatoid arthritis (annual consulting rate per 10,000) for men and women from the last two morbidity surveys by the Royal College of General Practitioners (1981 to 1982 and 1991 to 1992)[128]

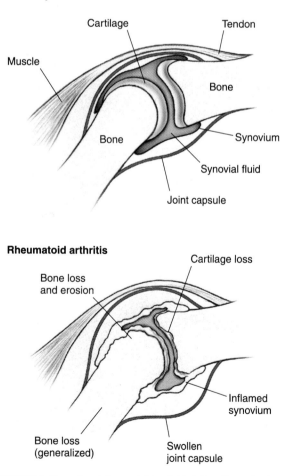

FIGURE 36-7. Normal and rheumatoid arthritic joints. (From the National Institutes of Health: Handout on Health: Rheumatoid arthritis: http://www.niams.nih.gov/hi/topics/arthritis/rahandout.htm.)

ETIOLOGY

The development of RA has both genetic and environmental (i.e., nongenetic) determinants. The genetic contribution is estimated at 60%[90]. Studies that have advanced our understanding of RA genetics include a 1978 study by Stastny[91], who found a link between the human leukocyte antigen system (specifically HLA-DR4) and RA and Gregersen et al.[92] in 1987 who advanced the case for a genetic link by finding a one in six chance of developing a higher risk in individuals who are homozygous for a polymorphism of the HLA gene (*HLA-DRB*0408*).

Environmental, or nongenetic, factors linked to the occurrence of RA include age, hormonal factors, infection, smoking, and obesity[93]. More specifically, the incidence of RA increases with age, is rare in women before menarche, has declined in women with the increased use of oral contraception, is widely believed to be linked to some type of infection, and is higher in smokers and in individuals with a body mass index of 30 kg/m^2 or above. After the onset of RA has occurred, the severity of the disease is related to the DR4 alleles, which are alternative forms of the HLA gene; onset after the age of 60 years; being female; and smoking, which initially decreases pain but ultimately increases the risk for lung and blood vessel involvement[94].

Treatments

NONPHARMACOLOGIC TREATMENT

Patients with RA have reduced muscle strength and compromised joint ROM that decreases mobility and increases pain[95,96]. Before the 1960s, the recommended nonpharmacologic treatment for RA was bed rest. Patients with acute disease reported better mobility and reduced disease activity. The negative effects of bed rest, which include muscle atrophy, decreased bone density, and cardiovascular deconditioning, were eliminated with the introduction of therapeutic exercise programs for RA patients.

Long-term dynamic strength training has a positive effect on muscle strength, self-reported physical function, and physical performance in women with RA[96]. As little as 1.4 exercise sessions per week for 24 months provided these positive effects without exacerbating disease activity. Aerobic exercise also appears to have a positive effect on similar outcomes. A 12-month aerobic weight-bearing exercise program significantly improved self-reported function and activity level, and bone mineral density and disease activity remained unchanged[39].

Of concern with RA patients is the potential inappropriate activation of the immune system that would exacerbate the chronic inflammation associated with the disease[97]. In a study of RA patients, young exercises, healthy elderly exercises, and healthy elderly control subjects, Rall et al.[97] found no significant increase in the inflammatory biomarkers TNF-alpha and IL-1beta in the RA patients after 12 weeks of resistance exercise relative to the healthy exercise and control groups. Hence, the benefits of both aerobic and resistance exercises in RA patients appears to have few negative side effects and important physiologic benefits.

Exercise Prescription.

An analysis of 15 randomized, clinical trials suggests that aerobic exercises (e.g., walking, aquatics, bicycling) performed three times per week for 30 to 60 minutes per session at an intensity of 60% to 85% of maximum heart rate successfully improves aerobic capacity and muscle strength. Furthermore, resistance training (e.g., use of weight machines, dumbbells, elastic bands) performed two to three times weekly at 50% to 80% of a maximal voluntary contraction improves strength and does not have a detrimental effect on pain[98] (also see GETP7 Chapter 9).

Pharmacologic Treatment

A mainstay of the treatment of RA is pharmacologic therapy[98]. Pharmacologic therapy for the treatment of RA includes NSAIDS, disease-modifying antirheumatic drugs (DMARDs), glucocorticoids (steroids), and biologic therapies. NSAIDs reduce swelling, pain, and inflammation but have some serious side effects, including stomach bleeding and ulcers. DMARDs include injectible or oral gold, hydroxychloroquine, penicillamine, sulfasalazine, methotrexate, azathioprine, cyclosporine, and lefluomide. This classification of drugs also works to suppress the immune system and is thought to slow the progression of the disease and reduce cartilage degradation. Possible side effects include liver and kidney damage. Glucocorticoids (steroids) such as prednisone, methylpredinsone, cortisone, and hydrocortisone reduce inflammation and suppress the immune response. The most serious side effect is the increased risk of infection. Biologic therapies work to suppress joint inflammation that is thought to play a role in cartilage degradation by blocking the action of certain cytokines, specifically, TNF[99].

Randomized clinical trials, primarily of short duration, have shown nine pharmacologic agents to be effective in slowing the radiographic progression of RA compared with a control group[100]. Infliximab (a biologic therapy) and high-dose corticosteroids showed the greatest efficacy followed closely by cyclosporine, sulphasalazine, leflunomide, methotrexate, parenteral gold, corticosteroids, auranofin, and IL-1 receptor antagonist. Other pharmaceuticals that have shown trends toward improvement but have not produced significant results include D-penicillamine, hydroxychloroquine, pamidronic acid, minocycline, chloroquine, and cyclophosphamide. Of the trials that have shown significant radiographic improvements versus a placebo, all have confidence limits that overlapped, suggesting that pharmaceutical agents that produce better results than a placebo (see list above) all produce similar radiographic results[101]. Therefore, patient acceptance, cost, and toxicity may govern the choice for each patient. Large randomized clinical trials are necessary to determine if a combination of the effective drugs produces better results than a single drug alone.

Several clinical trials have reported a number of side effects, including cytopenias or nephritic syndrome (parental gold), GI symptoms (sulphasalazine), skin rash and abnormal taste (penicillamine), and liver disease (methotrexate)[102]. Table 36-4 lists the general categories of drugs used in the treatment of RA.

Surgical Treatment

Age, disease severity, degree of disability, and the combination of involved joints are important considerations in the timing of orthopedic interventions. Less definitive orthopedic procedures include synovectomy (excision of inflamed synovial tissue), tendon realignment, and arthro-

TABLE 36-4. Medications Used in the Treatment of Rheumatoid Aarthritis

Category	Examples (Trade Names)
NSAIDs	Aspirin
	Ibuprofen (Advil, Motrin IB)
	Ketoprofen (Orudis)
	Naproxen (Naprosyn)
	Celecoxib (Celebrex)
	Rofecoxib (Vioxx)
DMARDs	Gold, injectable or oral
	Antimalarials (Plaquenil)
	Penicillamine (Cuprimine, Depen)
	Sulfasalazine (Azulfidine)
	Methotrexate (Rheumatrex)
	Azathioprine (Imuran)
	Cyclosporine (Sandimmune, Neoral)
	Lefluomide (Arava)
Gulcocorticoids (steroids)	Prednisone (Deltasone, Orasone)
	Methylprednisone (Medrol)
Biologic therapy	Etanercept (Enbrel)

DMARDs = disease-modifying antirheumatic drugs; NSAIDs = nonsteroidal antiinflammatory drugs.

scopic débridement. These procedures can improve alignment, reduce synovial tissue, control pain, provide stability, and improve function in some RA patients. These techniques can also prolong periods of good function and delay the need for replacement procedures[95]. After all other options have been exhausted, joint replacement results in vastly improved function and reduced pain[103].

Summary

Arthritis and chronic joint symptoms affect more than 70 million Americans, and its 100 various forms are the leading cause of disability[2] Arthritis increases pain and obesity, reduces strength, restricts mobility, and lowers health-related quality of life. There are no known cures for arthritis; however, exercise appears to improve the clinical symptoms of a variety of rheumatic diseases, including OA, fibromyalgia, and RA. Pharmacologic therapies are effective, but many have potentially serious side effects. The most effective surgical procedure is joint replacement. Less definitive surgical procedures provide temporary relief and delay joint replacement surgery.

Projections by the Centers for Disease Control and Prevention suggest that arthritis will continue to afflict a greater portion of our population over the next 20 years. Funding of research on the prevention and rehabilitation of patients with arthritis should be a priority for both private and governmental agencies concerned with the health of our adult population[2].

REFERENCES

1. Clauw DJ, Crofford LJ: Chronic widespread pain and fibromyalgia: What we know, and what we need to know. Best Pract Res Clin Rheumatol 17:685–701, 2003.
2. Center for Disease Control and Prevention: Targeting Arthritis: The Nation's Leading Cause Of Disability, Atlanta: Department of Health and Human Services; http://www.cdc.gov/nccdphp/adg_arthritis.htm 2004.
3. Lawrence RC, Helmick CG, Arnett FC, et al: Estimates of the prevalence of arthritis and selected musculoskeletal disorders in the United States. Arthritis Rheum 41:778–799, 1998.
4. Davis MA, Ettinger WH, Neuhaus JM. The role of metabolic factors and blood pressure in the association of obesity with osteoarthritis of the knee. J Rheumatol 15:1827–1832, 1988.
5. Felson DT, Naimark A, Anderson J, et al: The prevalence of knee osteoarthritis in the elderly. The Framingham Osteoarthritis Study. Arthritis Rheum 30:914–918, 1987.
6. Lajas C, Abasolo L, Bellajdel B, et al: Costs and predictors of costs in rheumatoid arthritis: A prevalence-based study. Arthritis Rheum 49:64–70, 2003.
7. Yelin E: The costs of rheumatoid arthritis: Absolute, incremental, and marginal estimates. J Rheumatol 44(suppl):47–51, 1996.
8. Gabriel SE, Amadio PC, Ilstrup DM, et al: Change in diagnosis among orthopedists compared to non-orthopedists in the management of acute knee injuries. J Rheumatol 27:2412–2417, 2000.
9. Harney S, Wordsworth BP: Genetic epidemiology of rheumatoid arthritis. Tissue Antigens 60:465–473, 2002.
10. Symmons DP: Epidemiology of rheumatoid arthritis: Determinants of onset, persistence and outcome. Best Pract Res Clin Rheumatol 16:707–722, 2002.
11. Doran MF, Pond GR, Crowson CS, et al: Trends in incidence and mortality in rheumatoid arthritis in Rochester, Minnesota, over a forty-year period. Arthritis Rheum 46:625–631, 2002.
12. Martin DF: Pathomechanics of knee osteoarthritis. Med Sci Sports Exerc 26:1429–1434, 1994.
13. Bunning RD, Materson RS: A rational program of exercise for patients with osteoarthritis. Semin Arthritis Rheum 21:33–43, 1991.
14. Jokl P: Prevention of disuse muscle atrophy in chronic arthritides. Rheum Dis Clin North Am 16:837–844, 1990.
15. Burr DB, Radin EL: Microfractures and microcracks in subchondral bone: Are they relevant to osteoarthrosis? Rheum Dis Clin North Am 29:675–685, 2003.
16. Messier SP, Loeser RF, Hoover JL, et al: Osteoarthritis of the knee: Effects on gait, strength, and flexibility. Arch Phys Med Rehabil 73:29–36, 1992.
17. Baliunas AJ, Hurwitz DE, Ryals AB, et al: Increased knee joint loads during walking are present in subjects with knee osteoarthritis. Osteoarthritis Cartilage 10:573–579, 2002.
18. Hurwitz DE, Sumner DR, Andriacchi TP, Sugar DA: Dynamic knee loads during gait predict proximal tibial bone distribution. J Biomech 31:423–430, 1998.
19. Sharma L, Hurwitz DE, Thonar EJ, et al: Knee adduction moment, serum hyaluronan level, and disease severity in medial tibiofemoral osteoarthritis. Arthritis Rheum 41:1233–1240, 1998.
20. Al Zahrani KS, Bakheit AM: A study of the gait characteristics of patients with chronic osteoarthritis of the knee. Disabil Rehabil 24:275–280, 2002.
21. Messier SP, Devita P, Cowan RE, et al: Do older adults with knee osteoarthritis place greater loads on the knee during gait? A preliminary study. Arch Phys Med Rehabil 2004.
22. Radin EL, Yang KH, Riegger C, et al: Relationship between lower limb dynamics and knee joint pain. J Orthop Res 9:398–405, 1991.
23. Messier SP, Loeser RF, Mitchell MN, et al: Exercise and weight loss in obese older adults with knee osteoarthritis: A preliminary study. J Am Geriatr Soc 48:1062–1072, 2000.
24. Otterness IG, Swindell AC, Zimmerer RO, et al: An analysis of 14 molecular markers for monitoring osteoarthritis: Segregation of the markers into clusters and distinguishing osteoarthritis at baseline. Osteoarthritis Cartilage 8:180–185, 2000.
25. Spector TD, Hart DJ, Nandra D, et al: Low-level increases in serum C-reactive protein are present in early osteoarthritis of the knee and predict progressive disease. Arthritis Rheum 40:723–727, 1997.
26. Goldring MB: Osteoarthritis and cartilage: The role of cytokines. Curr Rheumatol Rep 2:459–465, 2000.

27. Sharif M, Shepstone L, Elson CJ, et al: Increased serum C reactive protein may reflect events that precede radiographic progression in osteoarthritis of the knee. Ann Rheum Dis 59:71–74, 2000.

28. Otterness IG, Weiner E, Swindell AC, et al: An analysis of 14 molecular markers for monitoring osteoarthritis. Relationship of the markers to clinical end-points. Osteoarthritis Cartilage 9:224–231, 2001.

29. Wolfe F: The C-reactive protein but not erythrocyte sedimentation rate is associated with clinical severity in patients with osteoarthritis of the knee or hip. J Rheumatol 24:1486–1488, 1997.

30. Pelletier JP, Martel-Pelletier J, Abramson SB: Osteoarthritis, an inflammatory disease: Potential implication for the selection of new therapeutic targets. Arthritis Rheum 44:1237–1247, 2001.

31. Nicklas BJ, Ambrosius W, Messier SP, et al: Diet-induced weight loss, exercise, and chronic inflammation in older, obese adults: A randomized controlled clinical trial. Am J Clin Nutr 79:544–551, 2004.

32. Ettinger WH Jr, Afable RF: Physical disability from knee osteoarthritis: The role of exercise as an intervention. Med Sci Sports Exerc 26:1435–1440, 1994.

33. Kovar PA, Allegrante JP, MacKenzie CR, et al: Supervised fitness walking in patients with osteoarthritis of the knee. A randomized, controlled trial. Ann Intern Med 116:529–534, 1992.

34. Minor MA, Hewett JE, Webel RR, et al: Efficacy of physical conditioning exercise in patients with rheumatoid arthritis and osteoarthritis. Arthritis Rheum 32:1396–1405, 1989.

35. Fisher NM, Gresham G, Pendergast DR: Effects of a quantitative progressive rehabilitation program applied unilaterally to the osteoarthritic knee. Arch Phys Med Rehabil 74:1319–1326, 1993.

36. Fisher NM, Pendergast DR: Effects of a muscle exercise program on exercise capacity in subjects with osteoarthritis. Arch Phys Med Rehabil 75:792–797, 1994.

37. Ettinger WH Jr, Burns R, Messier SP, et al: A randomized trial comparing aerobic exercise and resistance exercise with a health education program in older adults with knee osteoarthritis. The Fitness Arthritis and Seniors Trial (FAST). JAMA 277:25–31, 1997.

38. Messier SP, Thompson CD, Ettinger WH: Effects of long-term aerobic or weight training regimens on gait in an older, osteoarthritic population. J Appl Biomech 13:205–225, 1997.

39. Westby MD, Wade JP, Rangno KK, Berkowitz J: A randomized controlled trial to evaluate the effectiveness of an exercise program in women with rheumatoid arthritis taking low dose prednisone. J Rheumatol 27:1674–1680, 2000.

40. Messier SP, Loeser RF, Miller GD, et al: Exercise and dietary weight loss in overweight and obese older adults with knee osteoarthritis: The Arthritis, Diet, and Activity Promotion Trial. Arthritis Rheum 50:1501–1510, 2004.

41. Hochberg MC, Dougados M: Pharmacological therapy of osteoarthritis. Best Pract Res Clin Rheumatol 15:583–593, 2001.

42. Psaty BM, Furberg CD: COX-2 inhibitors-lessons in drug safety. N Eng J Med Feb 15 [Epubahead of print], 2005.

43. Burris JE: Pharmacologic approaches to geriatric pain management. Arch Phys Med Rehabil 85:S45–S49, 2004.

44. Schnitzer TJ: Osteoarthritis management: The role of cyclooxygenase-2-selective inhibitors. Clin Ther 23:313–326, 2001.

45. Fraenkel L, Bogardus ST Jr, Concato J, Wittink DR: Treatment options in knee osteoarthritis: The patient's perspective. Arch Intern Med 164:1299–1304, 2004.

46. Das A Jr, Hammad TA: Efficacy of a combination of FCHG49 glucosamine hydrochloride, TRH122 low molecular weight sodium chondroitin sulfate and manganese ascorbate in the management of knee osteoarthritis. Osteoarthritis Cartilage 8:343–350, 2000.

47. Hauselmann HJ: Nutripharmaceuticals for osteoarthritis. Best Pract Res Clin Rheumatol 15:595–607, 2001.

48. McAlindon TE, LaValley MP, Gulin JP, Felson DT: Glucosamine and chondroitin for treatment of osteoarthritis: A systematic quality assessment and meta-analysis. JAMA 283:1469–1475, 2000.

49. Mazieres B, Loyau G, Menkes CJ, et al: Chondroitin sulfate in the treatment of gonarthrosis and coxarthrosis. 5-months result of a multicenter double-blind controlled prospective study using placebo. Rev Rhum Mal Osteoartic 59:466–472, 1992.

50. Pujalte JM, Llavore EP, Ylescupidez FR: Double-blind clinical evaluation of oral glucosamine sulphate in the basic treatment of osteoarthrosis. Curr Med Res Opin 7:110–114, 1980.

51. Reginster JY, Deroisy R, Rovati LC, et al: Long-term effects of glucosamine sulphate on osteoarthritis progression: A randomised, placebo-controlled clinical trial. Lancet 357:251–256, 2001.

52. Lippiello L, Woodward J, Karpman R, Hammad TA: In vivo chondroprotection and metabolic synergy of glucosamine and chondroitin sulfate. Clin Orthop 229–240, 2000.

53. Leffler CT, Philippi AF, Leffler SG, et al: Glucosamine, chondroitin, and manganese ascorbate for degenerative joint disease of the knee or low back: A randomized, double-blind, placebo-controlled pilot study. Mil Med 53.

54. Shankland WE: The effects of glucosamine and chondroitin sulfate on osteoarthritis of the TMJ: A preliminary report of 50 patients. Cranio 16:230–235, 1998.

55. Owings MF, Kozak LJ: Ambulatory and inpatient procedures in the United States, 1996. Vital Health Stat 13:1–119, 1998.

56. Moseley JB, O'Malley K, Petersen NJ, et al: A controlled trial of arthroscopic surgery for osteoarthritis of the knee. N Engl J Med 347:81–88, 2002.

57. Chang RW, Falconer J, Stulberg SD, et al: A randomized, controlled trial of arthroscopic surgery versus closed-needle joint lavage for patients with osteoarthritis of the knee. Arthritis Rheum 36:289–296, 1993.

58. Rankin EA, Alarcon GS, Chang RW, et al: The orthopaedic forum: NIH consensus statement on total knee replacement December 8–10, 2003. J Bone Joint Surgery 86-A:1328–1335, 2004.

59. Wolfe F, Ross K, Anderson J, et al: The prevalence and characteristics of fibromyalgia in the general population. Arthritis Rheum 38: 19–28, 1995.

60. Quintner JL, Cohen ML: Fibromyalgia falls foul of a fallacy. Lancet 353:1092–1094, 1999.

61. Demitrack MA, Crofford LJ: Evidence for and pathophysiologic implications of hypothalamic-pituitary-adrenal axis dysregulation in fibromyalgia and chronic fatigue syndrome. Ann N Y Acad Sci 840: 684–697, 1998.

62. Buchwald D: Fibromyalgia and chronic fatigue syndrome: Similarities and differences. Rheum Dis Clin North Am 22:219–243, 1996.

63. Bennett RM: Beyond fibromyalgia: Ideas on etiology and treatment. J Rheumatol 19(suppl):185–191, 1989.

64. Moldofsky H, Scarisbrick P, England R, Smythe H: Musculosketal symptoms and non-REM sleep disturbance in patients with "fibrositis syndrome" and healthy subjects. Psychosom Med 37:341–351, 1975.

65. Bradley LA, Alarcon GS: Is Chiari malformation associated with increased levels of substance P and clinical symptoms in persons with fibromyalgia? Arthritis Rheum 42:2731–2732, 1999.

66. Liu Z, Welin M, Bragee B, Nyberg F: A high-recovery extraction procedure for quantitative analysis of substance P and opioid peptides in human cerebrospinal fluid. Peptides 21:853–860, 2000.

67. Russell IJ, Fletcher EM, Vipraio GA et al: Cerebrospinal fluid (CSF) substance P (SP) in fibromyalgia; changes in CSF SP over time parallel changes in clinical activity. J Musculoskeletal Pain 1998.

68. Vaeroy H, Helle R, Forre O, et al: Elevated CSF levels of substance P and high incidence of Raynaud phenomenon in patients with fibromyalgia: New features for diagnosis. Pain 32:21–26, 1988.

69. Welin M, Bragee B, Nyberg F, Kristiansson M: Elevated substance levels are contrasted by a decrease in met-enkephalin-arg-phelevels in CSF from fibromyalgia patients. J Musculoskeletal Pain 1995.

70. Shirayama Y, Mitsushio H, Takashima M, et al: Reduction of substance P after chronic antidepressants treatment in the striatum, substantia nigra and amygdala of the rat. Brain Res 739:70–78, 1996.

71. Fiebich BL, Hollig A, Lieb K: Inhibition of substance P-induced cytokine synthesis by St. John's wort extracts. Pharmacopsychiatry 34 Suppl 1:S26–S28, 2001.

72. Salemi S, Rethage J, Wollina U, et al: Detection of interleukin 1beta (IL-1beta), IL-6, and tumor necrosis factor-alpha in skin of patients with fibromyalgia. J Rheumatol 30:146–150, 2003.

73. Rao SG, Bennett RM: Pharmacological therapies in fibromyalgia. Best Pract Res Clin Rheumatol 17:611–627, 2003.

74. Richards SC, Scott DL: Prescribed exercise in people with fibromyalgia: Parallel group randomised controlled trial. BMJ 325: 185, 2002.

75. Gowans SE, DeHueck A, Voss S, et al: Effect of a randomized, controlled trial of exercise on mood and physical function in individuals with fibromyalgia. Arthritis Rheum 45:519–529, 2001.

76. Busch A, Schachter CL, Peloso PM, Bombardier C: Exercise for treating fibromyalgia syndrome. Cochrane Database Syst Rev CD003786, 2002.

77. Clarke SR, Jones KD, Burckhardt CS, Bennett RM: Exercise for patients with fibromyalgia :Risk versus benefits. Curr Rheumatol Rep 3:135–146, 2001.

78. Jones KD, Burckhardt CS, Clark SR, et al: A randomized controlled trial of muscle strengthening versus flexibility training in fibromyalgia. J Rheumatol 29:1041–1048, 2002.

79. Hakkinen A, Hakkinen K, Hannonen P, Alen M: Strength training induced adaptations in neuromuscular function of premenopausal women with fibromyalgia: Comparison with healthy women. Ann Rheum Dis 60:21–26, 2001.

80. Geel SE, Robergs RA: The effect of graded resistance exercise on fibromyalgia symptoms and muscle bioenergetics: A pilot study. Arthritis Rheum 47:82–86, 2002.

81. Arnold LM, Hess EV, Hudson JI, et al: A randomized, placebo-controlled, double-blind, flexible-dose study of fluoxetine in the treatment of women with fibromyalgia. Am J Med 112:191–197, 2002.

82. Miller LJ, Kubes KL: Serotonergic agents in the treatment of fibromyalgia syndrome. Ann Pharmacother 36:707–712, 2002.

83. Dwight MM, Arnold LM, O'Brien H, et al: An open clinical trial of venlafaxine treatment of fibromyalgia. Psychosomatics 39:14–17, 1998.

84. Zijlstra TR, van de Laar MA:. The lack of a placebo effect in a trial of fluoxetine in the treatment of fibromyalgia. Am J Med 113:614–615, 2002.

85. Goldenberg DL, Felson DT, Dinerman H: A randomized, controlled trial of amitriptyline and naproxen in the treatment of patients with fibromyalgia. Arthritis Rheum 29:1371–1377, 1986.

86. Lautenschlager J: Present state of medication therapy in fibromyalgia syndrome. Scand J Rheumatol 113(suppl):32–36, 2000.

87. Miller LJ, Kubes KL: Serotonergic agents in the treatment of fibromyalgia syndrome. Ann Pharmacother 36:707–712, 2002.

88. Straub RH, Scholmerich J, Cutolo M: The multiple facets of premature aging in rheumatoid arthritis. Arthritis Rheum 48:2713–2721, 2003.

89. Hess EV: Rheumatoid Arthritis. Schumacher HR, ed. Atlanta: Arthritis Foundation, 1988; pp. 83–96.

90. MacGregor AJ, Snieder H, Rigby AS, et al: Characterizing the quantitative genetic contribution to rheumatoid arthritis using data from twins. Arthritis Rheum 43:30–37, 2000.

91. Stastny P: Association of the B-cell alloantigen DRw4 with rheumatoid arthritis. N Engl J Med 298:869–871, 1978.

92. Gregersen PK, Silver J, Winchester RJ: The shared epitope hypothesis. An approach to understanding the molecular genetics of susceptibility to rheumatoid arthritis. Arthritis Rheum 30:1205–1213, 1987.

93. Kaipiainen-Seppanen O, Aho K, Isomaki H, Laakso M: Shift in the incidence of rheumatoid arthritis toward elderly patients in Finland during 1975–1990. Clin Exp Rheumatol 14:537–542, 1996.

94. Symmons DP: Epidemiology of rheumatoid arthritis: Determinants of onset, persistence and outcome. Best Pract Res Clin Rheumatol 16:707–722, 2002.

95. Gerber LH: Exercise and arthritis. Bull Rheum Dis 39:1–9, 1990.

96. Hakkinen A, Haanonan P, Nyman K, Hakkinen K. Aerobic and neuromuscular performance capacity of physically active females with early or long-term rheumatoid arthritis compared to matched healthy women. Scand J Rheumatol 31:345–350, 2002.

97. Rall LC, Roubenoff R, Cannon JG, et al: Effects of progressive resistance training on immune response in aging and chronic inflammation. Med Sci Sports Exerc 28:1356–1365, 1996.

98. Stenstrom CH, Minor MA. Evidence for the benefit of aerobic and strengthening exercise in rheumatoid arthritis. Arthritis Rheum 49:428–434, 2003.

99. Moreland LW, Baumgartner SW, Schiff MH, et al: Treatment of rheumatoid arthritis with a recombinant human tumor necrosis factor receptor (p75)-Fc fusion protein. N Engl J Med 337:141–147, 1997.

100. American College of Rheumatology: Guidelines for the management of rheumatoid arthritis: 2002 update. Arthritis Rheum 46:328–346, 2002.

101. Jones G, Halberti J, Crotty M, et al: The effect of treatment on radiological progression in rheumatoid arthritis: A systematic review of randomized placebo-controlled trials. Rheumatology 42:6–13, 2003.

102. van Schaardenburg D: Rheumatoid arthritis in the elderly. Prevalence and optimal management. Drugs Aging 7:30–37, 1995.

103. McCoy TH, Salvati EA, Ranawat CS, Wilson PD, Jr: A fifteen-year follow-up study of one hundred Charnley low-friction arthroplasties. Orthop Clin North Am 19:467–476, 1988.

SELECTED REFERENCES FOR FURTHER READING

Brandt KD: Osteoarthritis (Rheumatic Disease Clinics of North America). Philadelphia: Elsevier Science Health Science; 2003

Brent S, Wilk KE: Clinical Orthopaedic Rehabilitation, 2nd ed. Philadelphia: Mosby; 2003

Center for Disease Control and Prevention: Prevalence of doctor-diagnosed arthritis and possible arthritis-30 states, 2002. MMWR 53:383–388, 2004.

Fransen M, McConnell S, Bell M. Exercise for osteoarthritis of the hip or knee. Cochrane Database Syst Rev. 2003;(3):CD004286.

Green WB, Snider RK: Essentials of Musculoskeletal Care, 2nd ed. Rosemont, IL: American Academy of Orthopaedic Surgeons; 2001

Hakkinen A: Effectiveness and safety of strength training in rheumatoid arthritis. Curr Opin Rheumatol 16:132–137, 2004.

Jordan KM, Arden NK, Doherty M, et al: Standing Committee for International Clinical Studies Including Therapeutic Trials ESCISIT. EULAR Recommendations 2003: An evidence based approach to the management of knee osteoarthritis: Report of a Task Force of the Standing Committee for International Clinical Studies Including Therapeutic Trials (ESCISIT). Ann Rheum Dis 62:1145–1155, 2003.

Haq I, Murphy E: Dacre osteoarthritis J Postgrad Med J 79:377–383, 2003.

Jette AM, Keysor JJ: Disability models: Implications for arthritis exercise and physical activity interventions. Arthritis Rheum 49:114–120, 2003.

Krebs D, Herzog W, McGibbon CA, Sharma L: Work group recommendations: 2002 Exercise and Physical Activity Conference. St. Louis. Arthritis Rheum 49:261–262. 2003.

O'Dell JR: Therapeutic strategies for rheumatoid arthritis. N Engl J Med 350:2591–2602, 2004.

Roubenoff R: Exercise and inflammatory disease. Arthritis Rheum 49:263–266, 2003.

Sahrmann S: Diagnosis and Treatment of Movement Impairment Syndromes. Philadelphia: Mosby; 2001

Symmons D, Turner G, Webb R, et al: The prevalence of rheumatoid arthritis in the United Kingdom: New estimates for a new century. Rheumatology (Oxford) 41:793–800, 2002.

van Gool CH, Penninx BWJH, Kempen GIJM, et al: Effects of exercise adherence on osteoarthritis-related performance and disability. Arthritis Care Res 53:24–32, 2005.

INTERNET RESOURCES

American College of Rheumatology Treatment Guidelines: http://www.rheumatology.org/publications/guidelines/index.asp?aud=prs

Arthritis Foundation: Bulletin on the Rheumatic Diseases: http://www.arthritis.org/research/bulletin/archives.asp

Arthritis Foundation: Research Update: http://www.arthritis.org/research/ResearchUpdate/archives.asp

HealthTalk Rhematoid Arthritis: http://www.healthtalk.com/rheumatoidarthritis/index.cfm

National Guidline Clearinghouse: Exercise Prescription for Older Adults with Osteoarthritis Pain: Consensus Practice Recommendations: http://www.guideline.gov/summary/summary.aspx?doc_id=3188&nbr=2414&string=arthritis

National Guideline Clearinghouse: Osteoarthritis: AAOS Clinical Guideline on Osteoarthritis of the Knee: http://www.guideline.gov/summary/summary.aspx?doc_id=3856&nbr=3069&string=arthritis

National Guideline Clearinghouse: Osteoarthritis: AAOS Clinical Guideline on Osteoarthritis of the Knee (Phase II). http://www.guideline.gov/summary/summary.aspx?doc_id=4584&nbr=3374&string=arthritis

Neuromuscular Diseases and Exercise

JANET A. MULCARE AND KURT JACKSON

Multiple Sclerosis

EPIDEMIOLOGY

Multiple sclerosis (MS) is a chronic, often disabling, disease characterized by a destruction of the myelin sheath (i.e., demyelination) that surrounds the nerve fibers of the central nervous system (CNS). Lesions representing areas of inflammatory demyelination can be present in any part of the brain and spinal cord. Much of the permanent disability results from axonal destruction of the long pathways of the pyramidal tracts that supply motor and sensory input to the lower extremities[1]. Worldwide, the incidence of MS varies. Estimates from the National Multiple Sclerosis Society indicate between 250,000 and 350,000 individuals in the United States have MS[2]. The worldwide distribution of MS varies, and the prevalence of MS is associated with specific degrees of latitude north: high (37° to 52°), medium (30° to 33°), and low (12° to 19°)[3]. A similar latitude-specific prevalence rate can be seen in the southern hemisphere in Australia and New Zealand. In Asia and Africa, with the exception of the white South African population, prevalence rates are in the low range[4]. Epidemiological studies have shown that people who are born in a geographic area with a high risk for MS and move to an area with lower risk acquire the risk associate with that of their new home, if the move occurs before the age of 15 years[4].

The incidence of MS in women surpasses men by a ratio of three to one. Eighty-five percent of patients are diagnosed in the third through sixth decade of life, with 5% diagnoses occurring before age 21 and less than 10% after age 50 years[5]. MS is most prevalent in whites; however, where good data are available, the less susceptible racial groups (e.g., Asians and Africans) appear to share the geographic gradient of whites, with higher frequencies of the disease in high-risk areas[6].

ETIOLOGY

The etiology of MS is currently not known; however, much of the scientific research indicates that a combination of factors may be involved. The major scientific theories regarding the etiology of MS are based on immunologic, environmental, viral, and genetic factors. It is generally accepted that MS involves an autoimmune process. Furthermore, it has long been hypothesized that a viral infection may be the "triggering" factor for MS. More than a dozen viruses have been studied, but it has yet to be proven that any one virus triggers MS[7].

Although MS is not hereditary, the risk of the disease in a child or sibling of an affected individual is much higher than in the general population. For instance, a child of a parent with MS has a one in 40 chance of acquiring MS, and the risk for identical twins is one in three. It should be noted that 80% of people with MS have no first-degree relative with the disease; therefore, a definitive conclusion regarding a genetic link is limited. Some neurologists have theorized that MS develops because a person is born with a genetic predisposition to react to some environmental agent, which, upon exposure, triggers an autoimmune response[7].

TYPES OF MULTIPLE SCLEROSIS

Each case of MS displays one of several different patterns and is characterized by great variability. Experts now con-

KEY TERMS

Basal ganglia: A group of related nuclear masses located deep within the cerebrum that play a major roll in motor output as well as numerous other functions

Bradykinesia: Significant slowness of movement

Dyskinesia: Abnormal involuntary movement, often a side effect of long-term use of dopaminergics

Freezing: A sudden loss of the ability to move, often associated with gait

Festination: A gait pattern characterized by an increasing step cadence and decreasing step length which can ultimately lead to loss of balance

Idiopathic: A disease that develops without an apparent or known cause

On–off phenomenon: Sudden changes in the motor response of an individual to L-dopa, generally associated with long-term use

cede that there are four major clinical subtypes based on disease pattern[8]. The four types, incidence, and pattern of progression are presented in Table 37-1.

DIAGNOSIS

For a definite diagnosis of MS, two or more distinct areas of demyelination at two different time points must be detected. This is usually accomplished through a careful clinical history in conjunction with laboratory tests such as magnetic resonance imaging (MRI) and analysis of cerebrospinal fluid. To evaluate neurologic function, evoked potential tests are often administered. Evoked potential tests measure electrical activity in certain areas of the brain in response to stimulation of specific sensory nerve pathways. These tests are often used to help make a diagnosis of MS because they can indicate dysfunction along these pathways that is too subtle to be noticed by the person or

TABLE 37-1. Types, Incidence, and Description of the Four Types of Multiple Sclerosis

Type	Incidence, %	Description
Relapsing–remitting	51	Series of attacks, each followed by complete or partial remission. A minority (10% to 20%) of this group has "benign" form with little or no disability for 25 years after diagnosis.
Primary–progressive	9	Characterized by a gradual clinical decline with no distinct remissions.
Secondary–progressive	31	Begins with a relapsing–remitting course followed by a later primary–progressive course 5 to 15 years after diagnosis.
Progressive–relapsing	5	The disease takes a progressive path, punctuated by acute attacks.

to show up on neurologic examination. The main types of evoked potential tests are (a) visual evoked potentials (VEPs,), in which the patient sits before a screen on which an alternating checkerboard pattern is displayed; (b) brainstem auditory evoked potentials (BAEPs,), in which the patient hears a series of clicks in each ear; and (c) sensory evoked potentials (SEPs), in which short electrical impulses are administered to an arm or leg. These types of clinical tests are extremely important in the diagnosis of MS because they can confirm the presence of a "suspected" lesion or identify "unsuspected" lesion that has produced no symptoms[9,10].

CLINICAL FEATURES

The most frequent initial symptom of MS is an acute or subacute onset of numbness or tingling in one or more limbs. The symptoms usually begin distally in the limbs and expand proximally. Occasionally, the symptoms migrate from one side to the other, which is believed to represent the transverse expansion of lesions in the spinal cord[9]. In some patients, a paroxysmal sensory symptom in the back or lower limbs brought on by flexing the head forward (Lhermitte's symptom) may precede the persistent sensory symptoms or may occur in isolation[9]. Optic neuritis (inflammation of the optic nerve) is also common, and patients report blurred vision, diplopia, or reduction in visual fields. Symptoms that are less likely to appear initially but are common as the disease progresses are muscle weakness, bowel and bladder dysfunction, heat intolerance, pain, ataxia, movement disorders, depression, and higher cortical function disorders. The latter often presents as a decrease in short-term memory, as well as difficulty with "executive function" processing (e.g., planning, prioritizing, sequencing, self-monitoring, self-correcting; inhibiting, initiating, controlling or altering behavior).

Complications resulting from several of these symptoms are often referred to as "secondary symptoms," and they include joint contractures, urinary tract infection, osteoporosis, muscle atrophy, and skin breakdown[10]. Spasticity, the involuntary increased tone in muscles, is also common and can lead to joint stiffness and muscle spasms.

Fatigue is the most common symptom of MS, affecting 75% to 90% of persons with MS, with 50% to 60% reporting it as their worst symptom[11-13]. The cause of fatigue is unknown, but multiple factors have been proposed, including "twitch decline"[14]; reduced central motor drive[15] abnormalities in peripheral motor function[16,17]; and factors related to neuroendocrine function, abnormal cerebral glucose metabolism, and glucose availability[18]. Excessive energy use during walking associated with muscle weakness; spasticity and ataxia[19] may also contribute to the overall feeling of fatigue. Deconditioning, medication side effects[20,21], depression[22], and nocturia[23] are other secondary problems that may increase fatigue level in these individuals. Krupp et al.[24] have published a comprehensive review of this topic.

Approximately 80% of persons with MS report heat intolerance, whether generated by ambient conditions or internally (e.g., fever, thermogenesis, exercise)[25]. In most clinical research, patients are rated on the Kurtzke Expanded Disability Scale (EDSS)[26] as a basis of characterizing the level of impairment at a particular point in time. The scale provides an ordinal rating of impairment between 0 and 10, derived through a standard neurologic examination and subsequent scoring of symptoms in eight specific categories relating to CNS function. In studies in which subjects with MS have been placed in high ambient temperatures, 60% report symptoms not previously experienced. Elimination of the heat source usually reverses the symptoms. The mechanisms for sensitivity to heat have been investigated for more than 100 years using a wide range of approaches and summarized by several authors[25,27]. The presently accepted neuroblockage hypothesis, spearheaded by Davis and colleagues[28-30] over several years of research, proposes that temperature elevations and other noxious stimuli can reduce the "safety factor" of neural transmission. When several nodes of Ranvier are demyelinated, even the smallest elevation in tissue temperature can temporarily block conduction[30]. There is no evidence that the brain or spinal cord are actually heated during the occurrence of heat sensitivity; therefore, the validity of this hypothesis remains questionable. The focus of more recent studies has been to examine the relationship between heat sensitivity, fatigue, and physical activity (i.e., from exercise). Experimental perturbations have included total body surface cooling using an external cooling garment[31-33], full-body water immersion prior to exercise[34], cooling garment during chronic exercise[35], as well has heating with a heating garment during exercise[36]. In each instance, the cooling or heating perturbations have been used to evaluate the effects of cooling and heat on physical performance and symptoms, more specifically, "fatigue." In most clinical research, MS patients are characterized using the EDSS[26]. This scale provides a numerical rating of the level of impairment at that particular point in time. The ordinal rating of impairment (range, 0 to 10) is derived through a standard neurologic examination and subsequent scoring of symptoms in eight categories relating to CNS function. In addition to using the EDSS as a means of tracking changes in impairment over time, it also offers a common variable for comparison of samples across studies.

AUTONOMIC NERVOUS SYSTEM DYSFUNCTION IN MULTIPLE SCLEROSIS

The myelinated pathways of the autonomic nervous system (ANS) within the brain and spinal cord may be involved in MS; however, the symptoms associated with the somatic nervous system often divert attention away from these disturbances. The ANS plays an important role in increasing heart rate (HR), maintaining blood pressure (BP), and regulating cutaneous blood flow and sweating[37]. Research of ANS function using clinical tests indicates that abnormalities in HR and BP are common in approximate 30% of the MS population[38,39]. BP abnormalities have been demonstrated in response to isometric exercise[40], as well as incremental dynamic exercise[41,42].

Cartlidge[43] reported abnormal sweat response in persons with MS when they are immersed in hot water. A more recent study, found abnormal sweating in 50% of the MS patients examined during submaximal steady-state exercise[35]. Another feature of ANS disturbance in persons with MS is postural dizziness[44]. Bladder dysfunction may be characterized by urgency of micturation or difficulty voiding. Bowel dysfunction presents most frequently as severe constipation, but frequent diarrhea may also occur[45]. Medications used in the management of MS may have possible side effects on ANS function. A summary of common drugs used to treat MS symptoms is presented in Table 37-2. For example, amantadine HCl, which is often prescribed for fatigue, can cause peripheral vasodilation and orthostatic hypotension. Tricyclic antidepressants and selective serotonin reuptake inhibitors, prescribed for depression and neuropsychological symptoms, respectively, may also cause hypotension. It is important that a complete history of medications be included before patient evaluation and exercise prescription with this population.

CLINICAL TREATMENT

Most treatments for MS are directed toward treating symptoms. Various studies of complimentary alternative medicine (CAM) show that between 30% and 67% of persons with MS use some form of alternative medicine in conjunction with conventional medicine[46]. The National Center for Complimentary and Alternative Therapy[47] places the types of CAM used by persons with MS in six categories: specific practices, enhancement therapies, ingested or injected substances, toxic removal therapy, special diets, and other therapies. An extensive list is available

TABLE 37-2. A Summary of Medications Commonly Used to Treat Multiple Sclerosis–Related Symptoms that May Affect Exercise Tolerance or Response

Medication	Symptom	Special Considerations
Amantadine HCl	Temporarily reduces fatigue	May cause dizziness, peripheral vasodilation, and orthostatic hypotension.
Baclofen	Reduces spasticity	High dosage may cause tachycardia, constipation, bladder dysfunction, muscle weakness and fatigue.
Tricyclic antidepressenats	Depression	May cause tremor, dizziness, lightheadedness, hypotension, tachycardia, constipation, bladder dysfunction, and abnormal gait
Prednisone	Acute exacerbation	May cause muscle weakness, loss of muscle mass, hypertension, and osteoporosis (in chronic use); increased appetite, weight gain, aggressiveness, and irritability.
Modafinil	Fatigue (off label)	May interact with other drugs commonly used by patients with multiple sclerosis. Side effects include anxiety, headache, nausea, nervousness, and insomnia.
Selective serotonin reuptake inhibitors	Neuropsychological symptoms	Hypotension and tachycardia

from Mulcare and Jackson[48]. Unfortunately, no scientific evidence supports most of the claims associated with these therapies. Furthermore, there are fundamental risks in using many of these products without medical supervision, risks that are not recognized by patients.

In recent years, clinical trials have demonstrated that interferons, as well as immune-modulating drugs reduce the number of new lesions and exacerbations in patients with relapsing–remitting MS. The Food and Drug Administration has approved several drugs: interferon beta-1a (Avonex), interferon beta-1b (Betaseron), interferon beta 1a (Rebif), and copaxone (Glatiramer acetate). The side effects of the interferon drugs vary slightly, but all result in a flulike syndrome consisting of fever, chills, muscle aches, and malaise[49]. Although there has been no research as to whether these drugs affect exercise capacity, tolerance, or the safety of exercise, there appears to be no reason why patients cannot engage in regular physical activity.

EXERCISE RESPONSE IN PERSONS WITH MULTIPLE SCLEROSIS: MAXIMAL AEROBIC POWER

Establishing a baseline aerobic fitness level for patients with MS can help provide a foundation for developing a program of regular exercise and increasing physical activity. Depending on the level and nature of the physical impairment, modifications in modality, equipment, and protocol may be necessary to ensure an effective and safe method of exercise testing and training. Experts generally recommend the use of a bicycle ergometer for evaluating aerobic fitness in this population because of problems with balance[50–53]. Most research using the bicycle method with patients with MS has reported corresponding HR maximums that vary between 90% and 96% of the expected age-related maximum. Thus, in the absence of expensive metabolic equipment, an inexpensive HR monitor is helpful in estimating a maximal effort based on the

attainment of at least 90% of age-predicted maximal HR. It is also important to note that in more than 100 tests of maximal aerobic power, there has never been the occurrence of an existing MS symptom or provocation of a new symptom, with the exception of post-exercise fatigue.

Nevertheless, some clinicians may feel uncomfortable stressing MS patients to a maximal level and wonder whether submaximal HR can be used with existing prediction equations. Limited research has shown that the use of existing regression models (e.g., the Astrand-Rhyming Nomagram) for predicting $\dot{V}O_{2peak}$ from submaximal values can result in an error greater than 15%[50]. Part of the reason for the error of prediction may be related to a "blunting" of the HR response during submaximal exercise related to ANS dysfunction in some patients with MS[42].

There is no standard protocol that "best" suits the MS population because of the diversity of abilities, but subjective reports from some MS patients show a preference for an abbreviated, submaximal, ramping protocol. A discontinuous protocol can provide brief rest periods between progressively more difficult workloads, which may provide psychological benefit to patients.

Beginning the exercise test with an initial stage of "no-resistance" pedaling is helpful as a warm-up period; however, individuals with lower extremity spasticity may have difficulty pedaling without resistance because this type of movement often elicits ankle clonus. Toe clips and heel straps prevent the feet from slipping off the pedals in this situation, and the addition of resistance in subsequent stages generally results in resolution of the clonus response.

When designing a protocol, one should consider the gender, anatomical size, and level of neurologic impairment based on the patient's disability level. The stages should last between 3 and 5 minutes, with increments often depending on the level of impairment. Most research has used increments of 12 to 15 Watts for more severely impaired subjects; however, for larger individuals with minimal disability, the workloads will probably need to be adjusted upward (e.g., 25 Watt). Also, persons who exhibit more neurologic impairment are capable of lower maximal workload and have been shown to experience less of a benefit from training over a specific length of time[33].

EXERCISE PROGRAMMING OPTIONS

Endurance Training

The primary goal of endurance training in MS patients is similar to the goal in nondisabled adults: to increase physical function and improve health. Activities such as stationary cycling; walking; and low-impact, chair, and water aerobics are good choices depending on personal interest and the level and nature of physical impairment. Patients with impaired balance or proprioceptive deficits may find that either the buoyancy offered in water aerobics or the stability of an increased base of support in chair aerobics is a better choice than trying to maintain balance while performing standard low-impact aerobics. Walking in a climate-controlled area such as an indoor track or mall provides stable temperatures, a level surface, and the opportunity to rest when needed. Stationary cycling is a more appropriate option for non-ambulatory MS patients, and it offers a controlled environment and standardized workloads. Table 37-3 summarizes MS symptoms and corresponding considerations when selecting a form of exercise as they relate to each symptom, which should be discussed with patients when selecting a mode of exercise. Exercise HR should be generally maintained at 60% to 75% of age-predicted maximal HR (HR_{max}), according to guidelines from the American College of Sports Medicine (ACSM); however, more severely impaired, elderly individuals may need to exercise between 50% and 65% of age-predicted HR_{max} until they have reached a higher level of fitness. Because MS symptoms can vary day to day, a perceptual scale is recommended to monitor intensity. Work rates should be adjusted to daily symptoms and energy levels.

Ideally, people with MS should try to incorporate some form of moderate physical activity into each day[54]; however, a more realistic and achievable goal for structured exercise is three times per week for a minimum of 30 minutes. The 30 minutes can be distributed over three 10-minute or two 15-minute sessions, which is a valuable option to those with very low initial fitness levels or low resistance to fatigue. The balance of the days on which exercise is not performed may be reserved for completion of household or leisure activities, which places a fairly high demand on most individuals with physical impairment[55].

A supervised program of aerobic exercise for as little as 15 weeks can improve aerobic fitness level (i.e., $\dot{V}O_{2max}$) in some persons with MS. For example, Petajan et al.[56] reported a 22% increase in $\dot{V}O_{2max}$ and a 48% improvement in physical work capacity. Ponichtera-Mulcare et al.[31] found similar improvements in persons with equivalent impairment level (+19%) but less dramatic for those more severely impaired (+7%) after a 24-week supervised program. This raises an important issue regarding the development of realistic expectations based on the baseline impairment level of the individual. Subtle neurologic changes may not be observable to the clinician. However, small, unnoticeable changes may affect exercise training outcomes. It is important to carefully monitor neurologic changes by periodically interviewing clients regarding subjective impressions of their disease status. Training outcomes observed under strict supervision may not be similar to an unsupervised or a home exercise program. When developing an exercise training program for persons with MS, two other important issues to address are heat sensitivity and hydration.

Heat Sensitivity

There is ample research documenting the presence of heat sensitivity in most persons with MS. The use of fans, wet neck wraps, and spray bottles may help reduce the perception of overheating, but they do not actually lower core temperature. Surface cooling via water immersion (16° to 17°C) before exercise (i.e., pre-cooling) has been shown to

TABLE 37-3. Summary of Symptoms and Considerations for Choosing a Mode of Ergometry and Designing Protocols for Exercise Testing and Training

Symptom	Special Consideration
Spasticity	• May cause ankle clonus, which makes foot stability during cycling difficult. • Agonist/antagonist co-contraction may impair treadmill walking or appear as muscle weakness of the agonist group. • Hip adductor and abductor spasticity may interfere with bicycle ergometry
Lack of coordination	• Combined arm/leg ergometers that are not mechanically synchronized may be difficult to coordinate.
Ataxia	• May make treadmill walking difficult without handrail support.
Sensory	• Lower extremity sensory or proprioceptive deficits could make treadmill walking difficult.
Muscle weakness	• Lower extremity muscle weakness may limit workload increments using a bicycle ergometer.
Foot drop	• Weakness in the tibialis anterior muscle group is common and results in "foot drop" as fatigue ensues after continuous walking. If not corrected with an ankle and foot orthotics, treadmill walking could be dangerous.
Visual disturbances	• Central scotoma and loss of peripheral vision may necessitate modifications during treadmill walking and use of handrails.

significantly reduce core temperature, as well as improve aerobic endurance, reduce submaximal exercise HR, and reduce the perceived level of exertion[34]. In addition, the reduction in core temperature that occurs immediately after cooling has been shown to persist for several hours and is associated with significantly less perceived fatigue. Furthermore, this strategy, coupled with exercising early in the day to take advantage of the lower circadian body temperature, might pose less physiologically and psychologically stress. Subjective reports from many individuals with MS indicate there is a general decline in energy level during the afternoon hours, with the occurrence of fatigue and other MS-related symptoms. Most individuals, not just MS patients, are at their highest circadian temperature (i.e., core temperature) in the later afternoon hours.

Hydration

Many people with MS experience symptoms that affect bladder function. Because of problems with bladder urgency and exertional incontinence, MS clients may severely limit their daily intake of fluids. This can result in chronic dehydration and may contribute to the general fatigue experienced by some individuals. Current recommendations for proper hydration before exercise and rehydration published by the ACSM[57] may be difficult to apply, since both the intensity and duration of activity completed by most individuals with MS is well-below the level to which the recommendations apply.

STRENGTH TRAINING

Muscle weakness is one of the most common manifestations of MS and is frequently reported as an initial symptom. It has been estimated that at least half of persons with MS experience some form of muscle weakness, as well as the phenomenon of motor fatigue[58]. Weakness can have a profound impact on an individual's functional independence. Basic activities such as walking, rising from a chair, and climbing stairs can become difficult over time because residual weakness often increases after repeated exacerbations. Although strengthening does not alter the disease process itself, compensatory strengthening of uninvolved muscle groups and prevention of weakness secondary to disuse may improve function.

Little research has been done regarding the effects of training on muscle performance in persons with MS. The available research shows that there is a carryover effect of aerobic training to improved muscle strength after a supervised program of aerobic exercise training, as well as an unsupervised program of free weights[53]. Petajan et al.[52] reported a mean improvement of 17% in upper extremity isometric strength and an 11% improvement in lower extremity isometric strength in a sample of 21 MS subjects. Mulcare et al.[33] observed a 29% improvement in power output during leg cycling after 24 weeks of supervised aerobic exercise training.

Before patients start training, it is important to evaluate their baseline strength levels for proper exercise prescription. Traditional methods of strength testing such as manual muscle testing, an estimated one-repetition maximum (1RM), isokinetic dynamometry, or a functional strength assessment are all appropriate methods. Special modifications may need to be made when an individual has significant spasticity or joint contracture. These adaptations should be documented so that follow-up testing can be performed in the same manner. When testing, it is often useful to perform several repetitions to assess muscular endurance because strength can often appear normal but quickly deteriorate after just a few repetitions. Functional testing such as the sit-to-stand test, get-up-and-go test, or physical performance test often provides the most useful information about a person's ability to accomplish various activities of daily living (ADLs). For example, sit-to-stand performance has been shown to correlate well with isokinetic measures of lower extremity strength, walking speed, and balance[56,59].

Unfortunately, very little research has been done that guide us in this process as it relates to individuals with MS. Kraft et al.[60] investigated the effects of a 3-month, 3-day-per-week strength training program in persons with mild and severe MS. During the study, subjects performed three sets of 10 repetitions of each exercise with 60 seconds of rest between exercises. After training, subjects demonstrated significant improvements in strength, walking velocity, and stair climbing ability, with the mildly affected group showing the greatest improvement. In addition, no MS-related exacerbations were reported during

---

BOX 37-1 | Other Recommendations Specific to the Multiple Sclerosis Population

- Optimize strength in the unaffected muscle groups to allow for effective compensation and stabilization.
- When possible, make exercises functional (e.g., partial squats for working quadriceps simulates everyday bending as opposed to seated knee extensions).
- Allow adequate rest time between exercises, especially when working weaker muscle groups.
- Educate patients regarding temporary fatigue and discomfort associated with exercise versus profound fatigue or pain.
- Emphasize larger proximal (i.e., core) muscle groups.
- During exacerbations of symptoms, focus on stretching and gentle active range of motion rather than strengthening.
- Weight machines are often helpful for patients with poor balance and coordination because they allow for more controlled movement and postural stability.
- When instructing a patient in a home exercise program, give clear written instructions because short-term memory impairment is common.

TABLE 37-4. Common Muscle Groups Prone to Developing Tightness and Contracture in Persons with Multiple Sclerosis

Muscle Group	Motion Restricted	Functional Limitations
Iliopsoas	Hip extension	Inability to achieve trailing limb posture during walking, which shortens stride length and increases energy expenditure. Can cause forward trunk lean, affecting posture and balance.
Hamstrings	Knee extension when hip flexed	Limits step length during walking, difficulty bending over to dress, pick objects off floor or perform household activities such as loading laundry.
Gastrocnemius	Ankle dorsiflexion, especially with knee extended	Limits gait if less than 10 degrees of dorsiflexion. Difficulties with sit to stand transfers. Decreased ability to use ankle strategy for balance.
Anterior trunk: pecs, intercostals, rectus abdominus	Trunk extension, rib elevation, shoulder flexion and external rotation	Inability to achieve erect posture. Reduced pulmonary function. Difficulty with dressing and grooming.

the training. In general, it appears that strength training of major muscle groups performed 2 or 3 nonconsecutive days per week using one to three sets of 10 to 15 repetitions appears relatively safe and effective. See Box 37-1 for other recommendations.

FLEXIBILITY

There has been little research on the effects of stretching in persons with MS. A study by Brar et al.[61] demonstrated that regular stretching may enhance the effects of medication in the management of spasticity. The most common muscle groups prone to developing tightness and contracture are the iliopsoas, hamstrings, gastrocnemius and pectoralis major and minor The muscle groups are most commonly affected when a person spends prolonged periods of time in a seated position or lying in bed with his or her head elevated and pillows propped under the knees. A summary of the most common muscle groups affected and the resultant functional limitations are presented in Table 37-4.

Although the literature provides limited guidelines regarding stretching parameters, it is generally accepted that flexibility exercises should be performed one to two times per day depending on the patient's level of activity and degree of spasticity. Most stretches are held for a period of 30 to 60 seconds and repeated three to five times. Persons with severe spasticity or contracture may require stretching of much longer duration. In these cases, low-load, prolonged stretches of 20 minutes to several hours using dynamic splints or weights may be needed to induce plastic deformation of connective tissue.

Parkinson's Disease

EPIDEMIOLOGY

Parkinson's disease (PD) is a progressive neurodegenerative disorder involving the **basal ganglia (BG)** and its associated pathways and is one of the most common neurologic conditions affecting older adults. It is estimated that at least 500,000 individuals in the United States have PD and that about 1.5% to 2.5% of the population older

than age 70 years are affected[62,63]. Disease frequency varies dramatically across age groups. It is rarely seen before the age of 30 years and has a peak age of onset in the sixth decade of life[63,64]. Mortality rates for persons with PD are higher than the general population, but average life expectancy has risen since the introduction of effective drug therapies, increasing from 67 to 69 years to 72 to 74 years[65–72]. With an increasing life expectancy for individuals with PD and a rapidly growing elderly population, one can expect to see dramatic increases in its incidence and prevalence.

ETIOLOGY

Parkinson's disease and its constellation of symptoms were first described in 1817 by James Parkinson. Despite intensive research and advances in science and medicine, the cause or causes of PD remain unknown. It is widely believed that most cases of the disease are caused by an interaction of environmental and genetic factors[73].

There has long been speculation that an environmental toxin (or toxins) may cause PD, but no specific agent has been discovered. Evidence for an environmental source includes examples of specific drug (1 methyl-4-phenyl-1,2,3,6-tetrahydropyridine [MPTP]) and pesticide and viral exposures that cause destruction of dopamine-producing neurons[74]. In most cases of PD, there is no family history of the disease; however, a number of rare genetic forms of the disease have recently been discovered[75,76]. It is hoped that by understanding the pathophysiology of these toxic and rare hereditary forms of the disease that the degenerative process involved in the more common **idiopathic** PD might be elucidated.

PATHOPHYSIOLOGY

Parkinson's disease is an age-related progressive neurologic disorder that involves the loss of the neurotransmitter dopamine within the BG. The BG are a group of interrelated nuclear masses deep within the brain and brainstem that play an important role in the output of voluntary movement and associated postural adjustments. The five fundamental components of the BG are the caudate nucleus, putamen, globus pallidus, substantia nigra, and subthalamic nucleus. The primary role of these nuclei is to modulate the flow of information through the BG, including motor commands from the cortex.

The primary pathologic process associated with PD is the loss of dopaminergic neurons in the substantia nigra, a vital component of the BG circuitry. Symptoms typically do not occur until there is a 70% to 80% loss of these cells. In addition to the loss of dopaminergic neurons, intracytoplasmic inclusions known as Lewy bodies form as the disease progresses. Neurodegeneration can also be found in other regions, including the locus ceruleus, nucleus basalis, hypothalamus, cerebral cortex, and autonomic ganglia[77].

CLINICAL MANIFESTATIONS

Rest tremor, bradykinesia, rigidity and postural instability are often referred to as the four cardinal signs of PD. Although these are the most common direct motor impairments associated with the disease, there is great variability among individuals in their clinical manifestations and disease progression.

Tremor is frequently the initial symptom of PD. It is often confined to one upper extremity early in the disease but can spread to all four limbs. A parkinsonian tremor is more obvious when the limb is at rest and is often ameliorated with voluntary movement. Although tremor may be disconcerting for the patient, it generally does not affect exercise testing and training in a significant way.

The slow and hesitant movement associated with PD is called **bradykinesia**. In addition to speed, amplitude and scaling of movement become impaired. Problems with fine motor skills, including small writing (micrographia) and garbled low-volume speech, are related to these movement deficits. Akinesia refers to a lack of initiation of movement and is manifested by a decrease in natural automatic movements associated with body and facial gestures.

Rigidity is an increased resistance to passive stretch of both the agonist and antagonist muscle groups surrounding a joint. Similar to tremor, it often begins in one limb and eventually spreads to other limbs as well as the trunk. When assessing rigidity, if there is jerky quality to the resistance, it is often referred to as *cogwheel rigidity*. A constant, slow, sustained resistance to passive movement is called *lead-pipe rigidity*. When rigidity significantly affects the trunk, rotation and extension of the spine become limited, postural reflexes are impaired, and there is a decreased ability to perform functional activities that require coordinated movements of the trunk and extremities. Although the exact cause of rigidity remains unclear, it appears to be related to abnormal responses of central mechanisms to stretch[78].

Postural instability and abnormal postural reflexes can dramatically affect the gait and balance of individuals with PD. The posture in individuals with PD can generally be referred to as "stooped" with increased thoracic kyphosis, a forward head, and hip and knee flexion. This posture can shift the center of gravity forward and decrease the person's ability to deal with various postural challenges effectively. When balance is challenged, especially in an unexpected manner, there is a delayed response, and patients have difficulty using normal postural synergies to recover[79].

In addition to the common movement impairments mentioned above, there are numerous non-motor problems associated with PD. These non-motor problems are attributable to the diverse and complex connections of the BG. Box 37-2 lists some of the more common motor and non-motor impairments that may affect exercise testing and training.

CLASSIFICATION

Parkinsonism refers to a group of disorders associated with abnormalities in BG function that can lead to symptoms that are parkinsonian in nature. PD also known as idiopathic or primary parkinsonism is by far the most common disorder and is the focus of this chapter. Secondary parkinsonism includes a number of disorders with identifiable causes that can produce parkinsonian symptoms along with other neurologic signs. The term *parkinsonism-plus syndrome* refers to another group of neurodegenerative disorders that can produce parkinsonian symptoms along with other neurologic signs.

BOX 37-2	**Common Manifestations of Parkinson's Disease Affecting Exercise Testing and Prescription**

PRIMARY OR DIRECT IMPAIRMENTS
Tremor
Bradykinesia, akinesia
Rigidity
Postural instability
Autonomic dysfunction
Cognitive impairment

SECONDARY AND COMPOSITE IMPAIRMENTS
Poor balance
Abnormal gait (freezing, festination)
Incoordination
Fatigue
Sleep disorders
Decreased Strength
Decreased joint range of motion
Swallowing and communication dysfunction
Impaired vision
Pain
Depression
Orthostatic hypotension
Respiratory dysfunction

Movement disorder is the hallmark of PD and is frequently used for classification and diagnosis. Koller and Hubble[80] categorized persons with PD into three distinct subgroups based on clinical symptoms: tremor predominant; postural instability and gait difficulty, and akinetic rigidity predominant. Patients falling into the last two categories often require special considerations for exercise testing and training.

The Hoehn and Yahr[70] classification is a five-stage scale used by neurologists and researchers to describe the level of disability associated with PD. Although the validity and reliability of this scale is not strong, it is the most commonly used clinical scale for describing physical symptoms and progression of the disease. The Unified Parkinson's Disease Rating Scale (UPDRS) is a comprehensive assessment tool that examines cognition, ADLs, motor function, and complications of drug therapy. This scale has established reliability and validity and can be useful for measuring disability and disease progression[80]. This scale can be cumbersome to administer in the clinical setting because of its length. However, subcomponents of the scale can be scored individually to meet the needs of the clinician.

MEDICAL MANAGEMENT

There is no cure for PD, and treatment is focused on managing the symptoms of the disease. Pharmacologic therapy is the primary intervention for alleviating the disabling symptoms, but the side effects of long-term drug therapy can present their own unique problems. The primary goal of pharmacologic treatment is to correct the neurochemical imbalances associated with PD. Drug management can generally be divided into two phases: (1) a protective phase aimed at slowing the progression of neuronal degeneration and (2) a symptom-alleviating phase directed at the disabling movement impairments associated with the middle and later stages of the disease.

The most common drug classifications used for treatment include the dopaminergics, anticholinergics, monoamine oxidase type B (MAO-B) inhibitors, and catechol-O-methyl transferase (COMT) inhibitors. Table 37-5 lists these classifications, common medications in each category, and side effects that can impact exercise testing and training.

Levodopa (L-dopa) remains the single most effective drug in the treatment of most patients. Patients, especially those with bradykinesia and rigidity, generally have dramatic improvements in symptoms when taking the drug. Unfortunately, with prolonged use, the effectiveness of L-dopa decreases and the potential for severe side effects increases. Approximately 80% of individuals taking L-dopa experience significant **dyskinesias**. Some also begin to experience distinct fluctuations in their response to L-dopa (**on–off phenomenon**). For patients receiving L-dopa, physical activity should be scheduled to coincide with peak effects of drug therapy, approximately 1 hour after a dose has been taken, although there is wide variability in absorption and degradation times.

Although pharmacologic treatment is the primary means of medical management, recent advances in stereotactic surgical techniques have made this a viable option for some patients who are not helped by medical management.

TABLE 37-5. Pharmacology of Parkinson's Disease

Drug Classification	Common Medications	Side Effects of Drug Group
Dopaminergics		
Dopamine replacement	Levodopa/carbidopa (Sinemet®)	Nausea and vomiting
		Orthostatic hypotension
		Cardiac arrhythmias
		Dyskinesias
		Behavioral changes
		On–off phenomena
Dopamine agonists	Pergoglide (Permax®)	Nausea and vomiting
	Bromocriptine(Parlodel®)	Orthostatic hypotension
	Ropinirole (Requip®)	Confusion or hallucinations
	Pramipexole (Mirapex®)	
Anticholinergics	Trihexyphenidyl (Artane®)	Cardiac irregularities, mood changes,
	Ethopropazine (Parsidol®)	confusion, hallucinations, blurred vision
		dry mouth, nausea and vomiting
Monoamine Oxidase Type B Inhibitor	Selegiline (Eldepryl®)	Insomnia, headaches, sweating
Other		
Antiviral	Amantadine (Symmetrel®)	Nausea, confusion, dyskinesia
Catecholo-methyltransferase (COMT) inhibitors	Entecapone (Comtan®)	Nausea, dizziness, orthostatic hypotension, dyskinesia, confusion
	Tolcapone (Tasmar®)	Dizziness, orthostasis, diarrhea

EXERCISE TESTING AND PRESCRIPTION FOR PERSONS WITH PARKINSON'S DISEASE

Cardiorespiratory endurance is often decreased in individuals with PD because of their long-term inactivity and deconditioning. Obstructive and restrictive pulmonary dysfunction may also occur in individuals with PD and is probably related to the bradykinetic functioning of the respiratory muscles, loss of musculoskeletal flexibility of the trunk, and postural changes[82].

Autonomic nervous system dysfunction can be present in persons with PD. These problems can be directly related to the disease or side effects of medications. Common problems include excessive or reduced perspiration, greasy skin, increased salivation, postural hypotension, thermoregulatory abnormalities, and bowel and bladder dysfunction. Cardiac arrhythmias can also result form L-dopa toxicity. Therefore, patients' vital signs should be monitored closely until a consistent exercise response is established.

Cardiorespiratory Exercise Testing

Limited research has been done on cardiorespiratory exercise testing for individuals with PD. In two separate studies, Stanley et al.[83,84] compared the aerobic exercise performance of individuals with mild to moderate PD with healthy normal subjects using an incremental exercise protocol of either lower or upper extremity ergometry. Results from this research indicate that although maximal oxygen consumption (VO_{2max}) did not differ significantly from healthy normal subjects, persons with PD demonstrated higher submaximal oxygen consumption and HR as well as a lower peak power. A small investigation of the reliability of exercise testing for persons with mild to moderate PD showed that VO_{2max}, peak and submaximal HRs, and rate of perceived exertion (RPE) were all highly reproducible using a semi-recumbent leg cycle[85].

When choosing a mode of cardiorespiratory exercise testing, it is important take into consideration each patient's specific impairments and limitations. For persons with balance problems, use of a safety harness may be required for treadmill testing or the use of a stationary or semi-recumbent bike may be more appropriate. Toe clips or ace wraps may be needed for persons with severe dyskinesias or tremors to maintain foot and hand contact on an upper or lower extremity ergometer. When using open circuit spirometry, subjects with PD may have difficulty using a traditional mouthpiece secondary to increased salivation and swallowing difficulties. In these cases, a mask or a mouthpiece with a saliva collector would be preferable.

In general, guidelines for cardiorespiratory exercise testing should be followed as outlined by the ACSM (see Chapter 14 and GETP7 Chapter 5. A submaximal evaluation such as the 6-minute walk test may be a preferable measure of endurance for patients who are greatly deconditioned[86,87] (see Chapter 15).

Cardiorespiratory Endurance Training

Several studies have evaluated the effects of cardiorespiratory exercise training in persons with PD[88–90]. Results from these studies indicate that patients with mild to moderate PD experience similar training effects as age-matched normal individuals. Improvements in motor function and quality of life have also been reported in these studies.

Safety should be the first priority when deciding on an exercise modality. If the patient is ambulatory, walking is the preferred mode of exercise. Use of a stationary, recumbent, or upper extremity ergometer may be more appropriate for persons with postural instability. The Air-Dyne™ (Schwinn®, Madison, WI) can be a good choice because it encourages trunk rotation and distributes work to all four extremities. If a treadmill is used, a safety harness may be needed for fall protection or to provide consistent body weight support. Miyai et al.[91] demonstrated a 17% improvement in over-ground walking speed after 4 weeks of harness-supported treadmill training. Another novel approach for a walking program involves the use of "trekking" poles. These lightweight poles that are usually used for hiking on uneven terrain can help in the maintenance of good balance and posture while allowing for an increase in gait speed and trunk rotation[92]. For individuals who have frequent episodes of **freezing** or **festination** during ambulation, visual cues such as strips of tape to step over and auditory prompts using music or a metronome can be helpful. Swimming and other forms of water exercise can also be effective forms of aerobic activity.

With respect to frequency, duration, intensity, and exercise progression, the GETP7 Chapters 7, 8, and 9 provides appropriate parameters when age and comorbidities such as heart disease are taken into account (also see Chapters 24 and 31).

Muscular Performance Testing

Although muscle weakness is often considered an insignificant clinical problem in individuals with PD, this is not generally the case, and it should be an area of concern for exercise professionals. Muscle weakness can be overlooked because rigidity often masks the loss of voluntary force production. It also appears that some clinical measures of muscle strength (e.g., manual muscle testing) are generally too insensitive to detect the weakness associated with mild to moderate PD.

When compared with healthy age-matched subjects, electromyographic (EMG) firing patterns of persons with PD show inconsistent discharge rates, activation of excessive motor units at lower forces, and increased coactivation of agonist and antagonist muscles. Additionally, there is a delay in the rate of muscle force production[93,94]. There is also some evidence that trunk and proximal limb muscles may initially be more affected than distal ones[95].

As mentioned previously, assessing muscle strength using manual muscle testing can be difficult in persons with PD. Measures of muscle performance that may identify more subtle changes include isokinetic testing, handheld dynamometry, and 1RM. Muscular endurance can be evaluated using resistance training equipment with a predetermined submaximal workload and counting the number of repetitions to fatigue (see Chapter 13). Functional measures of motor performance such as the repetitive sit-to-stand test or timed up-and-go test (TUG) can often be more useful for identifying muscular impairments that are likely to impact ADLs[59,96,97].

Muscular Strength and Endurance Training

Research on the independent effects of strength training for persons with PD is lacking. Scandalis et al.[98] demonstrated significant increases in lower extremity strength, gait speed, and stride length in 14 individuals with PD (Hoehn and Yahr stages 2–3) after a progressive resistive exercise program. This program was performed two times per week for 8 weeks with an initial resistance of 60% of 1RM.

Based on our current knowledge, strength training guidelines established by the ACSM appear suitable for most persons with PD when their individual impairments are taken into consideration (see Chapter 25 and GETP7 Chapter 7). Some disease-specific strength training considerations are listed in Box 37-3.

BOX 37-3 | **Strength Training Considerations for Patients with Parkinson's Disease**

- Ensure that the client performs adequate warm-up and flexibility activities just before strength training.
- Emphasize muscle groups that extend the trunk or lower extremities (e.g., erector spinae, rhomboids, middle and lower trapezius, gluteus maximus, gastrocnemius, quadriceps).
- Perform exercises in functional positions when possible (e.g., standing partial squats and heel raises).
- After the initial training period (4 to 6 weeks), it may be appropriate to add some exercises that emphasize rate of force development by increasing the speed of contraction and decreasing weight (if necessary) or incorporating some simple plyometric activities.
- Use auditory cues such as clapping, counting, or a metronome to help with timing of repetitions.
- Ensure good posture during all strength training activities.

Flexibility and Posture

Loss of flexibility and changes in posture can have serious consequences for individuals with PD, including respiratory complications, an increased risk of falling, and a loss of functional mobility[99]. Rigidity and lack of movement can lead to the characteristic stooped posture of PD. Eventually, this flexed posture can cause contracture formation in various muscle groups. Patients are likely to present with losses in range of motion (ROM) of hip and knee extension, ankle dorsiflexion, shoulder flexion, shoulder external rotation, trunk extension, and axial rotation[95,100].

An assessment of musculoskeletal ROM and flexibility is an important part of an initial examination and can be used to guide exercise prescription (see Chapter 13 and GETP7 Chapter 4). Goniometric and tape measurements are most common ways to assess ROM. Inclinometer systems can be quite useful for measuring segmental spinal motion. The sit-and-reach, functional reach, and functional axial rotation (FAR) tests can be used to measure the flexibility of multiple body segments[99].

Limited research has been done on the effectiveness of flexibility training for individuals with PD. Schenkman et al.[97] conducted a randomized, controlled trial of spinal flexibility training involving 51 subjects with early to midstage PD. After the program, which took place for 10 weeks, three times per week, the intervention group demonstrated improvements in spinal flexibility and functional reach but no changes in the time required to move from a supine to sitting position[101]. Another small study involving group flexibility and coordination training for the trunk and extremities did find improvements in transitional movements such as standing from a chair and moving in bed[102].

When designing a flexibility program for clients with PD, the two most important factors to consider are: the extent of ROM loss and how long the restriction has been present. Patients with mild tightness of relatively short duration may respond to a general stretching program following parameters as outlined in the GETP7 Chapter 7 (also see Chapter 25). Patients with more severe long-standing contractures require a more aggressive proactive approach involving longer (several minutes to several hours) positional stretches or the use of dynamic splints. Using modalities such as moist heat or ultrasound before or during the stretch may also be helpful. When prescribing a program for improving flexibility, emphasis should be place on exercises that promote extension of the trunk, hips, and knees. Axial rotation and thoracic cage mobility are also critical to maintain. Equipment such as large exercise balls and foam rolls can be especially useful for trunk flexibility activities.

FUNCTIONAL TRAINING

A detailed description of functional training and assessment is beyond the scope of this chapter. However, it is important to understand that the primary goal of any exercise program for persons with PD is an improvement in physical function. Whenever possible, exercises should be functional in nature and mimic normal activities to enhance motor learning and carry-over effect. For additional information on functional training, refer to O'Sullivan[100].

Summary

Exercise training is an essential component of treatment for individuals with PD and should be considered a first line of defense in symptom management. Although limited, research has consistently demonstrated improvements in various measures of fitness, function, and quality of life[88–92,98,101,103].

For most persons with mild to moderate disease, a general fitness program following ASCM guidelines is probably appropriate. As the disease progresses, a more individualized program that emphasizes functional activities such as transfers, gait, and balance is necessary. This requires the expertise of a team of health professionals that includes (but is not limited to) a physician, physical therapist, occupational therapist, and exercise physiologist.

Although exercise has not been shown to directly affect the progressive neurodegeneration associated with PD, it may slow or prevent many of the secondary impairments and complications[100]. Long-term compliance is vital to the success of any exercise program and is of even greater importance for persons with PD. Education of both the client and family is essential for maintaining an active lifestyle. Most communities have PD organizations that can provide information regarding local exercise groups. These groups can provide much needed motivation and socialization for patients and their families.

REFERENCES

1. Herndon RM: Pathology and pathophysiology (p. 43). In Burks JS, Johnson KP, eds. Multiple Sclerosis: Diagnosis, Medical Management and Rehabilitation. Demos Publications; 2000.
2. National Multiple Sclerosis Society: Sourcebook—Epidemiology; 2003. Available at http://www.//nationalmssociety.org/sourcebook-epidemiology.asp
3. Kurtzke JF: The geographic distribution of multiple sclerosis: An update with special reference to Europe and the Mediterranean region. Acta Neurol Scand 62:65–80, 1980.
4. Kurtzke JF: The epidemiology of multiple sclerosis (pp. 91–139). In: Raine CS, McFarland H, Tourtellotte WW, eds. Multiple Sclerosis: Clinical and Pathogenetic Basis. London: Chapman & Hall; 1997.
5. National Multiple Sclerosis Society: Who Gets MS; 2003. Available at http://www.nationalmssociety.org/who%20gets%20ms.asp
6. Kurtzke JF, Wallen MT: Epidemiology (pp. 49–71). In Burks JS, Johnson KP, eds. Multiple Sclerosis: Diagnosis, Medical Management and Rehabilitation. Demos Publications; 2000.
7. National Multiple Sclerosis Society: Sourcebook—Etiology; 2003. Available at http://www.nationalmssociety.org/sourcebook-etiology.asp
8. Coyle PK: Diagnosis and classification of inflammatory demyelinating disorders (p. 84). In Burks JS, Johnson KP, eds. Multiple Sclerosis: Diagnosis, Medical Management and Rehabilitation. Demos Publications; 2000.

9. Paty DW, Noseworthy JH, Ebers GC: Diagnosis of multiple sclerosis. In Paty DW, Ebers GC, eds. Multiple Sclerosis. Contemporary Neurology Series. Philadelphia: FA Davis; 1997.
10. Britell CW, Burks JS, Schapiro RT: Introduction to symptom and rehabilitation management: Disease management model (p. 215). In Burks JS, Johnson KP, eds. Multiple Sclerosis: Diagnosis, Medical Management and Rehabilitation. Demos Publications; 2000.
11. Fisk JD, Pontefract A, Ritvo PG, et al: The impact of fatigue on patients with multiple sclerosis. Can J Neurol Sci 21:9–14, 1994.
12. Freal JE, Kraft GH, Coyell JK: Symptomatic fatigue in multiple sclerosis. Arch Phys Med Rehabil 65:135–148, 1984.
13. Bergamaschi R, Romani V, Versino M, et al: Clinical aspects of fatigue in multiple sclerosis. Functional Neurol 12:247–251, 1997.
14. Sheehan GL, Murray NMF, Rothwell JC, et al: An electrophysiological study of the mechanism of fatigue in multiple sclerosis. Brain 120:299–315, 1997.
15. Latash M, Kalugina E, Orpet NJ, et al: Myogenic and central neurogenic factors in fatigue in multiple sclerosis. Mult Scler 1:236–241, 1996.
16. Sharma KR, Kent-Brown J, Mynhier MA, et al: Evidence of an abnormal intramuscular component of fatigue in multiple sclerosis. Muscle Nerve 18:1403–1411, 1995.
17. Kent-Braun J, Sharma KR, Miller RG Weiner MW: Postexercise phosphocreatine resynthesis is slowed in multiple sclerosis. Muscle Nerve 17:835–841, 1994.
18. Roelcke U, Kappos L, Lechner-Scott J, et al: Reduced glucose metabolism in the frontal cortex and basal ganglia of multiple sclerosis patients with fatigue: A 18F-fluorodeoxyglucose positron emission tomography study. Neurology 48:1566–1571, 1997.
19. Olgiati R, Jacquet J, DiPrampero PE: Energy cost of walking and exertional dyspnea in multiple sclerosis. Am Rev Respir Dis 134:1005–1010, 1986.
20. Quesada JR, Talpaz M, Rios A, et al: Clinical toxicity of interferons in cancer patients, a review. J Clin Oncol 4:234–243, 1986.
21. Neilly LK, Goodin DS, Goodkin DE, Hause SL: Side effect profile of interferon beta-1b in MS: Results of an open label trial. Neurol, 46:552–554, 1996.
22. Archibald CJ, McGrath P, Ritvo PG, et al: Pain in multiple sclerosis: Prevalence, severity, and impact on mental health. Pain 58:89–93, 1994.
23. Taphoorn MJ, van Someren E, Snoeck FJ, et al: Fatigue, sleep disturbances, and circadian rhythm in multiple sclerosis. J Neurology 240:446–448:1993.
24. Krupp LB, et al: Fatigue in multiple sclerosis. Curr Neurol Neurosci Rep 1:294–298, 2001.
25. Guthrie TC, Nelson DA: Influence of temperature changes on multiple sclerosis: Critical review of mechanisms and research potential. J Neurol Sci 129:1–8, 1995.
26. Kurtzke JF: Rating neurological impairment in multiple sclerosis: an expanded disability status scale (EDSS). Neurology 33:1444–1452, 1983.
27. Ponichtera-Mulcare JA: Exercise and multiple sclerosis. Med Sci Sport Exerc 25:451–465, 1992.
28. Davis FA: Axonal conduction studies based on some considerations of temperature effects in multiple sclerosis. Electroenceph Clin Neurophysiol 28:281–286, 1970.
29. Davis FA, Jacobson S: Altered thermal sensitivity in injured and demyelinated nerve: A possible model of temperature effects in multiple sclerosis. J Neurol Neurosurg Psychiatry 34:551–561, 1971.
30. Schauf CL, Davis FA: Impulse conduction in multiple sclerosis: A theoretical basis for modification by temperature and pharmacological agents. J Neurol Neurosurg Psychiatry 37:152–161, 1974.
31. Ponichtera-Mulcare JA, Glaser RM, Mathews T, Camaione DN: Maximal aerobic exercise in persons with multiple sclerosis. Clin Kinesiol 46:12–21, 1992.
32. Ponichtera JA, Glaser RM, Camaione DN, Mathews T: Physiologic responses to prolonged recumbent cycling of individuals with mul-

tiple sclerosis and able-bodied individuals. Med Sci Sport Exerc 20:S123, 1990.

33. Mulcare JA, Mathews T, Barrett PJ, Gupta SC: Changes in aerobic fitness of patients with multiple sclerosis during a 6-month training program. Sport Med Train Rehabil Internat J 7:265–272, 1997.

34. White AT, Wilson TE, Davis SL, Petajan JH: Effect of precooling on physical performance in multiple sclerosis. Multiple Sclerosis 6:176–180, 2000.

35. Mulcare JA, Webb P, Mathews T, et al: The effect of body cooling on the aerobic endurance of persons with multiple sclerosis following a 3-month aerobic training program. Med Sci Sport Exerc 29:S83, 1997.

36. Mulcare JA, Webb P, Mathews T, Gupta SC: Sweat response in persons with multiple sclerosis during submaximal aerobic exercise. Int J MS Care 3:33–38, 2001.

37. Guyton AC: The autonomic nervous system: Cerebral blood flow and cerebralspinal fluid (pp. 459–463). In Guyton AC, ed. Human Physiology and Mechanisms of Disease. Philadelphia: WB Saunders, 2000.

38. Drory VE, Nisipeanu PF, Kroczyn AD: Tests of autonomic dysfunction in patients with multiple sclerosis. Acta Neurol Scand 92:356–360, 1995.

39. Nordenbo AM, Boesen F, Anderson EB: Cardiovascular autonomic function in multiple sclerosis. J Auton Nerv Syst 26:77–84, 1989.

40. Pepin EB, Hicks RW, Spencer MK, et al: Pressor response to isometric exercise in patients with multiple sclerosis. Med Sci Sport Exerc 28:656–660, 1996.

41. Senaratne MP, Carroll D, Warren KG, Kappagoda T: Evidence for cardiovascular autonomic nerve dysfunction in multiple sclerosis. J Neurol Neurosurg Psychiat 47:947–952, 1984.

42. Ponichtera JA, Mathews T, Glaser RM, Ezenwa BN: A test to determine dynamic exercise capacity and autonomic cardiovascular function in individuals with multiple sclerosis. Proc IEEE 12–14, 1992.

43. Cartlidge NE: Autonomic function in multiple sclerosis. Brain 95:661–664, 1972.

44. Andersen EB, Nordenbo AM. Sympathetic vasoconstritor responses in multiple sclerosis with thermo-regulatory dysfunction. Clin Auton Res 7:13–16, 1997.

45. Eidelman BH: Autonomic disorders (p. 473). In Burks JS, Johnson KP, eds. Multiple Sclerosis: Diagnosis, Medical Management and Rehabilitation. Demos Publications; 2000.

46. Eisenberg DM, Davis RV, Ettner SL, et al: Trends in alternative medicine use in the United States 1990–1997: Results of a follow-up national survey. JAMA, 280:1569–1575, 1998.

47. National Institutes of Health: National Center for Complementary and Alternative Medicine. Available at: http://nccam.nih.gov/health/whatiscam

48. Mulcare JA: Multiple sclerosis (pp. 267–268). In ACSM's Exercise Management for Persons with Chronic Diseases and Disabilities, 2nd ed. Champaign, IL: Human Kinetics; 2003.

49. National Multiple Sclerosis Society: Library & Literature—Brochures: Comparing the Disease-Modifying Drugs. Available at: http://nmss.org

50. Ponichtera-Mulcare JA, Mathews T, Glaser RM, Gupta SC: Maximal aerobic exercise of individuals with multiple sclerosis using three modes of ergometry. Clin Kinesiol 49:4–12, 1995.

51. Shapiro RT, Petajan JH, Kosich D, et al: Role of cardiovascular fitness in multiple sclerosis. J Neurol Rehabil 2:43–49, 1988.

52. Petajan JH, Gappmeir E, White AT, et al: Impact of aerobic training on fitness and quality of life in multiple sclerosis. Ann Neurol 39:432–441, 1996.

53. Mostert S, Kesselring J: Effects of a short-term exercise training program of aerobic fitness, fatigue, health perception and activity level of subjects with multiple sclerosis. Mult Scler 8:161–168, 2002.

54. U.S. Dept. Health and Human Services: Healthy People 2010, vol II. Objectives for Improving Health Part B: Focus Areas 15–28. International Medical Publishing, Inc; 2000: 22–29.

55. Mulcare JA, Mathews T: Physical activity in persons with multiple sclerosis. Final Report—B1939R. United Stated Department of Veterans Affairs, Rehabilitation Research and Development. http://vard.org/va/02/mulcare.htm

56. Petajan JH: Weakness (pp. 307–321). In Burks JS, Johnson KP, eds. Multiple Sclerosis: Diagnosis, Medical Management and Rehabilitation. Demos Publications; 2000.

57. American College of Sports Medicine: Exercise and Fluid Replacement Position Stand. Med Sci Sports Exerc 28:i–vii, 1996.

58. Convertino VA, Armstrong LE, Coyle EF, et al: Exercise and fluid replacement. Med Sci Sport Exerc 28:i–vii, 1998.

59. Bohanan RW: Sit to stand test for measuring performance of lower extremity muscles. Percep Motor Skill 80:163–166, 1995.

60. Kraft GH, Alquist AD, de Lateur BJ: Effect of resistive exercises on strength in patients with multiple sclerosis. Rehabilitation R&D Progress Reports 33:328–330, 1995.

61. Brar SP, Smith MB, Nelson LM, Franklin GM, Cobble ND. Evaluation of treatment protocols on minimal to moderate spasticity in multiple sclerosis. Arch Phys Med Rehabil 72:186–189, 1991.

62. Tanner CM, Ben-Schlomo Y: Epidemiology of Parkinson's disease (pp. 153–157). In Stern GM, ed. Parkinson's Disease: Advances in Neurology, vol. 80. Philadelphia: Lippincott and Williams; 1999.

63. Martilla RJ: Epidemiology (pp. 35–57). In Koller WC, ed. Handbook of Parkinson's Disease, 2nd ed. New York: Marcel Dekker; 1992.

64. Adams RD, Victor M: Principles of Neurology, 5th ed. New York: McGraw Hill; 1993:975.

65. Sweet RD, McDowell FH: Five years' treatment of Parkinson's disease with levodopa. Ann Intern Med 83:456–463, 1975.

66. Yahr MD: Evaluation of long-term therapy in Parkinson's disease (pp. 435–443). Mortality and therapeutic efficacy. In Birkmayer W, Hornykiewicz O, eds. Advances in Parkinsonism. Basel: Editiones Roche; 1976.

67. Martilla RJ, Rinne UK, Siirtola T, Sonninen V: Mortality of patients with Parkinson's disease treated with levodopa. J Neurol 216:147–153, 1977.

68. Shaw KM, Lees AJ, Stern GM: The impact of treatment with levodopa on Parkinson's disease. Q J Med 49:283–293, 1980

69. Pritchard PB, Netsky MG: Prevalence of neoplasms and cause of death in aralysis agitans. Neurology 23:215–222, 1973

70. Hoehn MM, Yahr MD: Parkinsonism: Onset, progression, and mortality. Neurology 17:427–442, 1967.

71. Daimond SG, Markham CH, Hoehn MM, et al: An examination of male-female differences in progression and mortality of Parkinson's disease. Neurology 40:763–766, 1990.

72. Martilla RJ, Rinne UK: Epidemiology of Parkinson's disease—An overview. J Neural Transm 51:135–148, 1981.

73. Guttman M, Kish SJ, Furukawa Y: Current concepts in the diagnosis and management of Parkinson's disease. CMAJ 168:293–301, 2003.

74. Langston JW, Tanner CM: Etiology (pp. 369–381). In Koller WC, ed. Handbook of Parkinson's disease, 2nd ed. New York: Marcel Dekker; 1992.

75. Valente EM, Brancati F, Ferraris A, et al: PARK6-linked parkinsonism occurs in several European families. Ann Neurol 51:14–18, 2002.

76. Van Duijin CM, Dekker MCJ, Bonifati V, et al: Park 7, a novel locus for autosomal recessive early-onset parkinsonism, on chromosome 1p36. Am J Hum Genet 69:629–634, 2001.

77. Forno L: Pathology of Parkinson's disease: The importance of the substantia nigra and Lewy bodies (pp. 185–238). In Stern GM, Parkinson's Disease. Baltimore: Johns Hopkins University Press; 1990.

78. Stelmach GE, Phillips JG: Parkinson's disease and other involuntary movement disorders of the basal ganglia (p. 433). In Fredricks CM, Saladin LK, ed. Pathophysiology of the Motor Systems: Principles and Clinical Applications. Philadelphia FA Davis; 1996.

79. Horak FB, Nutt JG, Nashner LM: Postural inflexibility in parkinsonian subjects. J Neurol Sci 111:46–58, 1992.

80. Koller WC, Hubble JP: Classification of parkinsonism (pp. 59–103). In Koller WC, ed. Handbook of Parkinson's Disease, 2nd ed. New York: Marcel Dekker; 1992.

81. Fahn S, et al: The Unified Parkinson's Disease Rating Scale (pp. 153–163, 293–304). In Fahn S, Marsden CD, Calne DB, Goldstein M, eds. Recent Developments in Parkinson's Disease, vol 2. Floorham Park, NJ: Macmillan Healthcare Information; 1987.

82. Sabate M: Obstructive and restrictive pulmonary dysfunction increases disability in Parkinson's disease. Arch Phys Med Rehabil 77:29–34, 1996.

83. Stanley RK, Protas EJ, Jankovich J: Exercise performance in those having Parkinson's disease and healthy normals. Med Sci Sports Exerc 31:761–766, 1999.

84. Protas EJ, Stanley RK, Jankovich J, MacNeill B: Cardiovascular and metabolic responses to upper- and lower-extremity exercise in men with idiopathic Parkinson's disease. Phys Ther 76:34–40, 1996.

85. Hooker SP, Foudray CK, Mckay LA, et al: Heart rate and perceived exertion measures during exercise in people with Parkinson's disease. J Neurol Rehabil 10:101–105, 1996.

86. American College of Sports Medicine: ACSM's Exercise Management for Persons with Chronic Diseases and Disabilities, 2nd ed. Champaign, IL: Human Kinetics; 2003.

87. Light KE, Behrman AL, Thigpen M, Triggs WJ: The 2-minute walk test: A tool for evaluating walking endurance in clients with Parkinson's disease. Neurology Report 21:136–139, 1997.

88. Bridgewater KJ, Sharpe MH: Aerobic exercise and early Parkinson's disease. J Neuro Rehab 10:233–241, 1996.

89. Bergen JL, Toole T, Elliot RG, et al: Aerobic exercise intervention improves aerobic capacity and movement initiation in Parkinson's disease patients. NeuroRehabilitation 17:161–168, 2002.

90. Reuter I, Englehardt M, Stecker K, Baas H: Therapeutic value of exercise training in Parkinson's disease. Med Sci Sports Exerc 31:1544–1549, 1999.

91. Miyai I, Fujimoto Y, Ueda Y, et al: Treadmill training with body weight support: its effect on Parkinson's disease. Arch Phys Med Rehabil. 81:849–852, 2000.

92. Baatile J, Langbein WE, Weaver F, et al: Effects of exercise on perceived quality f life of individuals with Parkinson's disease. J Rehabil Res Dev 37:529–534, 2000.

93. Glendinning DS, Enoka RM: Motor unit behavior in Parkinson's disease. Phys Ther 74:61–70, 1994.

94. Stelmach GE, Teasdale N, Phillips J, Worringham CJ: Force production characteristics in Parkinson's disease. Exp Brain Res 76:165–172, 1989.

95. Bridgewater KJ, Sharpe MH: Trunk muscle performance in early Parkinson's disease. Phys Ther 78:566–576, 1998.

96. Podsialdo D, Richardson S: The timed "Up & Go": A test of basic functional mobility for frail elderly persons. J Am Geriatr Soc 39:142–148, 1991.

97. Csuka M, McCarty DJ: Simple method for measurement of lower extremity muscle strength. Am J Med 78:77–81, 1985.

98. Scandalis TA, Bosak A, Berliner JC, et al: Resistance training and gait function in patients with Parkinson's disease. Am J Phys Med Rehabil 80:38–43, 2001.

99. Schenkman M, Morey M, Kuchibhatla M: Spinal flexibility and balance control among community-dwelling adults with and without Parkinson's disease. J Gerontol Biol Sci Med Sci 55:441, 2000.

100. O'Sullivan SB: Parkinson's disease (p. 760). In O'Sullivan SB, Schmitz TJ, eds. Physical Rehabilitation: Assessment and Treatment, 4th ed. Philadelphia: FA Davis; 2001.

101. Schenkman M, Cutson TM, Kuchibhatla M et al: Exercise to improve spinal flexibility and function for people with Parkinson's disease: a randomized, controlled trial. J Am Geriatr Soc 46:1207, 1998.

102. Viliani T, Pasquetti P, Magnolfi S, et al: Effects of physical training on the straightening-up process in patients with Parkinson's disease. Disabil Rehabil 21:68–73, 1999.

103. Curtis CL, Bassile CC, Cote LJ, Gentile AM: Effects of exercise on the motor control of individuals with Parkinson's disease: Case studies. Neurology Report 25:2–12, 2001.

SELECTED REFERENCES FOR FURTHER READING

American College of Sports Medicine. ACSM's Resources for Clinical Exercise Physiology: Musculoskeletal, Neuromuscular, Neoplastic, Immunologic, and Hematologic Conditions. Baltimore: Lippincott, Williams & Wilkins; 2002.

Burks JB, Johnson KJ, eds: Multiple Sclerosis: Diagnosis, Medical Management and Rehabilitation. Demos Publications; 2000.

Melnick ME: Basal ganglia disorders: Metabolic, hereditary, and genetic disorders in adults (p. 606). In Umphred DA, ed. Neurological Rehabilitation, 3rd ed. St. Louis: Mosby; 1995.

O'Sullivan SB, Schmitz TJ, eds. Physical Rehabilitation: Assessment and Treatment, 4th ed. Philadelphia: FA Davis; 2001.

Siderowf A, Stern M: Update on Parkinson's disease. Ann Intern Med 8:651–658, 2003.

Stelmach GE, Phillips JG: Basal ganglia and their connections (p. 212). In Fredricks CM, Saladin LK, ed. Pathophysiology of the Motor Systems: Principles and Clinical Applications. Philadelphia: FA Davis; 1996.

Umphred DA, ed: Neurological Rehabilitation, 3rd ed. St. Louis: Mosby; 1995.

INTERNET RESOURCES

National Institute of Neurological Disorders and Stroke: NINDS Parkinson's Disease Information Page: http://www.ninds.nih.gov/disorders/parkinsons_disease/parkinsons_disease.htm

National Multiple Sclerosis Society: Professional Resource Center: http://www.nationalmssociety.org/prc.asp

National Parkinson's Disease Foundation: Allied Team Training for Parkinson's Disease: http://www.parkinson.org/site/pp.asp?c=9dJFJLPwB&b=71403

NCPAD: Disabilities and Conditions: http://www.ncpad.org/disability/?PHPSESSID=3782bbb6fc49265506dea2b77751c5a4

NOAH—New York Online Access to Health—Multiple Sclerosis: http://www.noah-health.org/eng/bjm/ms/

NOAH—New York Online Access to Health—Parkinson's Disease: http://www.noah-health.org/eng/bns/disorders/parkinson

Immunological Conditions

DAVID C. NIEMAN AND KERRY S. COURNEYA

Overview of the Immune System

From birth, humans are exposed to a continuous onslaught of bacteria, viruses, and other disease-causing organisms. Without an effective shield, every person would soon succumb to infectious disease and cancer. In the battle with microbial invaders, protection is provided through a complex array of defensive measures collectively identified as the immune system.

The immune system is a remarkably adaptive and complex defense entity. It is able to generate an enormous variety of cells and molecules capable of recognizing and eliminating a limitless variety of foreign invaders. White blood cells (WBCs or leukocytes) are a type of cell in the immune system that helps the body fight infection and disease. A basic outline of the major types of WBCs is depicted in Figure 38-1. Cells of the immune system operate in two functional divisions: **innate immunity**, which refers to the basic resistance to disease that we are born with, acting as a first line of defense, and **acquired immunity**, which when activated, produces a specific reaction and immunological memory to each infectious

agent[1]. This section emphasizes immune parameters that are most influenced by exercise.

INNATE IMMUNITY

The innate immune system includes anatomic and physiologic barriers (skin, mucous membranes, body temperature, low pH, and special chemical mediators such as complement and interferon), specialized cells (natural killer cells and phagocytes, including neutrophils, monocytes, and macrophages, which can engulf, kill, and digest whole microorganisms), and inflammatory barriers[1]. When the innate immune system fails to effectively combat an invading pathogen, the body mounts an acquired (specific) immune response.

Neutrophils are important components of the innate immune system, aiding in the phagocytosis of many bacterial and viral pathogens and the release of cytokines[1]. Neutrophils are the body's most effective phagocyte and are critical in the early control of invading infectious agents. Neutrophil function can be expressed as a measure of the ability to engulf pathogens (phagocytosis) and the facility to kill the pathogens once engulfed (the oxidative burst). *Cytokines* are low molecular weight proteins and peptides, including interleukins (ILs), which help control and mediate interactions among cells involved in immune responses. Cytokines can be categorized as anti-inflammatory (e.g., IL-6, IL-10, and IL-1ra), proinflammatory (tumor necrosis factor alpha [TNF-α] and IL-1β), and immunomodulatory (IL-2, IL-12, interferon (IFN)-γ, and IFN-α).

Natural killer (NK) cells are large granular lymphocytes that can mediate cytolytic reactions against a variety of cancer and virally-infected cells[1]. NK cells also exhibit key noncytolytic functions and can inhibit microbial colonization and the growth of certain viruses, bacteria, fungi, and parasites. Natural killer cell activity (NKCA) is measured with a 4-hour ^{51}Cr-release assay, in which certain types of cancer or virally infected cells are mixed with blood lymphocytes and monocytes. NK cells, which represent about 10% to 15% of blood lymphocytes, respond quickly and within 4 hours, they can lyse a significant proportion of the ^{51}Cr-labeled target cells. The released ^{51}Cr is collected into filters and then measured with a gamma counter.

KEY TERMS

Acquired immune deficiency syndrome (AIDS): A syndrome of the immune system characterized by opportunistic diseases caused by the human immunodeficiency virus, which is transmitted by exchange of body fluids (notably blood and semen). Hallmark of the immunodeficiency is depletion of $CD4^+$ helper/inducer lymphocytes.

Acquired immunity: Resistance resulting from previous exposure of an individual to an infectious agent or antigen. This may be active and specific as a result of naturally acquired infection or intentional vaccination or it may be passive, being acquired from transfer of antibodies from another person or from an animal.

Bone marrow transplant: A procedure in which high doses of anticancer drugs or radiation are used to kill cancer cells. The bone marrow is also destroyed by treatment and needs to be replaced by marrow taken from the patient before treatment (autologous) or donated by another person (allogeneic).

Cancer: Diseases in which abnormal cells divide without control. Cancer cells can invade nearby tissues and can spread through the bloodstream and lymphatic system to other parts of the body (i.e., metastasize).

Cancer control: The conduct of basic and applied research in the behavioral, social, and population sciences that, independently or in combination with biomedical approaches, reduces cancer risk, incidence, morbidity, and mortality and improves quality of life. Any activity that reduces the burden of cancer.

Cancer recurrence: Return of the same cancer after treatment. Cancer recurrence can be local (i.e., the cancer has recurred at the original site), regional (i.e., the cancer has recurred in the lymph nodes near the original site), or distant (i.e., the cancer has recurred in organs or tissues further from the original site).

5-year relative survival rate: The percentage of persons who are alive 5 years after a cancer diagnosis after adjustment for normal life expectancy (i.e., other causes of death). The statistic includes persons cured of cancer, in remission, under treatment, and with advanced disease.

Human immunodeficiency virus (HIV): A cytopathic retrovirus that is the etiologic agent of acquired immunodeficiency syndrome (AIDS)

Innate immunity: Resistance manifested by an individual who has not been immunized by previous infection or vaccination. Innate immunity is nonspecific and is not stimulated by specific antigens.

Upper respiratory tract infection: Infection that involves inflammation of the respiratory mucosa from the nose to the lower respiratory tree, not including the alveoli. In addition to malaise, it causes localized symptoms that constitute several overlapping syndromes: sore throat (pharyngitis), rhinorrhea (common cold), facial fullness and pain (sinusitis), and cough (bronchitis).

The secretory immune system of the mucosal tissues of the upper respiratory tract is considered the first barrier to colonization by pathogens[1]. Secretory IgA antibodies provide protection against pathogens at mucosal surfaces via several mechanisms that limit viral replication, attachment, and entry into the body.

ADAPTIVE IMMUNITY

The acquired immune system includes special cells called B and T lymphocytes, which are capable of secreting a large variety of specialized chemicals (i.e., antibodies and cytokines) to regulate the immune response[1]. T lymphocytes can also engage in direct cell-on-cell warfare. Antibodies are specialized proteins produced by the immune system in response to the presence of antigens. Antibodies help enable the immune system to defend the body against substances identified by the immune system as potentially harmful. Antigens are large molecules (usually proteins) on the surface of cells, viruses, fungi, bacteria,

and some non-living substances such as toxins, chemicals, drugs, and foreign particles. The immune system recognizes antigens and produces antibodies that destroy substances containing antigens.

Determination of the proliferative response of human lymphocytes upon stimulation with various activators (mitogens) in vitro is a well-established test to evaluate the functional capacity of T and B lymphocytes. Mitogen stimulation of lymphocytes in vitro using optimal and suboptimal doses is believed to mimic events that occur after antigen stimulation of lymphocytes in vivo. When lymphocytes are exposed to a foreign pathogen, their ability to "divide and conquer" is an important component of the adaptive immune system. In the laboratory, researchers expose lymphocytes to various types of mitogens for 3 days and then add thymidine (methyl)-^{3}H during the last 4 hours before harvesting. The thymidine (methyl)-^{3}H is incorporated into the DNA of the dividing lymphocytes and then counted using a liquid scintillation beta counter.

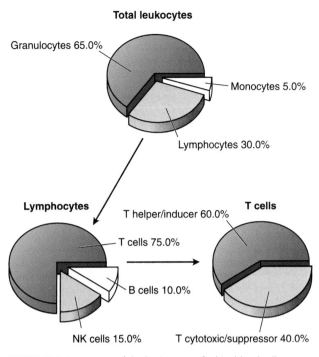

FIGURE 38-1. A summary of the basic types of white blood cells (WBCs) in circulation. Percentages in the first pie chart refer to average proportions of WBCs in humans, in the second pie chart to the average proportions of blood lymphocytes, and in the third chart to blood T lymphocytes. NK = natural killer.

Influence of Exercise on Immune Function

Does physical activity influence immune function and as a consequence risk of certain types of cancer and infection from the common cold and other **upper respiratory tract infections (URTIs)**? Does the immune system respond differently to moderate compared with intense physical exertion? These important questions are explored in this chapter section, with physical activity and lifestyle guidelines provided to support augmentation of one's immunity (also see GETP7 Chapter 9).

CHRONIC EXERCISE AND RESTING IMMUNE FUNCTION

Is immune function augmented through a regular physical activity regimen? One strategy used by exercise immunologists to answer this question is the comparison of immune function in athletes and nonathletes when resting in the laboratory. Surprisingly, in the rested state, immune function in athletes and nonathletes is more similar than disparate[2–5]. Of all immune measures, only NK cell activity has emerged as a somewhat consistent indicator differentiating between the immune systems of athletes and nonathletes. Several studies of elite female rowers, male cyclists, and marathon runners have shown elevated NKCA comparison with nonathletic control subjects[3,4].

ACUTE EXERCISE AND ASSOCIATED CHANGES IN IMMUNITY

Although chronic exercise has little effect on immune function, acute exercise bouts cause numerous changes. During moderate exercise (i.e., an exercise intensity of 40% to 60% $\dot{V}O_{2max}$), several positive changes occur in the immune system[5,6], and stress hormones and cytokines (indicative of intense metabolic activity and physiologic stress) are not elevated. Although the immune system returns to pre-exercise levels very quickly after the exercise session is over, each session represents a boost in immune surveillance that appears to reduce the risk of infection over the long term.

In contrast, prolonged and intensive exercise that lasts 90 minutes or more causes multiple negative changes in immunity in lymphoid compartments throughout the body. During this "open window" of altered immunity (which may last between 3 and 72 hours, depending on the immune measure), viruses and bacteria may gain a foothold, increasing the risk of subclinical and clinical infection (Fig. 38-2). Changes in immune function after heavy exertion that is sustained for 90 minutes and more are listed in Box 38-1[4,5,7].

The data in Box 38-1 suggest that immune function in several body compartments exhibits transient signs of stress or suppression after prolonged endurance exercise. Thus, it makes sense that infection risk may be increased when endurance athletes go through repeated cycles of unusually heavy exertion; have been exposed to novel pathogens; and have experienced other stressors to the immune system, including lack of sleep, severe mental stress, malnutrition, or weight loss[8].

Investigations are currently underway to test the hypothesis that athletes showing the most extreme immune suppression after heavy exertion are who contract infec-

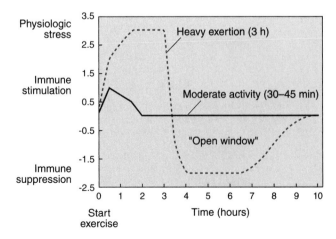

FIGURE 38-2. The "open window" theory indicates that sustained, heavy exertion results in physiologic stress and immune suppression. In contrast, moderate activity causes a mild immune stimulation during each exercise bout.

BOX 38-1	Changes in Immune Function After Heavy Exertion Sustained for 90 Minutes or More

- Neutrophilia (high blood neutrophil counts) and lymphopenia (low blood lymphocyte counts), induced by high plasma catecholamines, growth hormone, and cortisol
- Increase in blood granulocyte and monocyte phagocytosis and activation markers (reflecting an inflammatory response caused by substances released from injured muscle cells) but a decrease in nasal neutrophil phagocytosis and blood granulocyte oxidative burst activity
- Decrease in natural killer cell cytotoxic activity (an important antiviral measure), and mitogen-induced lymphocyte proliferation (a measure of T-cell function)
- Decrease in the delayed-type hypersensitivity response (DTH), a complex immunological process that involves several different cell types (including T lymphocytes) and chemical mediators and is manifested by firm, red skin indurations
- Increase in plasma levels of three antiinflammatory cytokines: IL-6, IL-10, and IL-1ra. Plasma levels of IL-8, a neutrophil chemotactic, and activation protein, also increase after prolonged, intense exercise. Post-exercise plasma levels are slightly increased for the proinflammatory cytokines, tumor necrosis factor alpha (TNF-α), and IL-1β, with negligible changes reported for the immunomodulatory cytokines, IL-2, IL-12, interferon (IFN)-γ, and IFN-α. Muscle tissue is an important source of IL-6 during heavy exertion.
- Decrease in nasal and salivary IgA concentration and nasal mucociliary clearance, indicating an impaired ability of the upper respiratory tract to clear external pathogens
- Blunted major histocompatibility complex (MHC) II expression and antigen presentation in macrophages. The MHC antigens are essential for reactions of immune recognition. After phagocytosis and antigen processing, small antigenic peptides are bound to MHC II and presented to T lymphocytes, an important step in adaptive immunity. Thus, heavy exertion blunts macrophage expression of MHC II, negatively affecting the process of antigen presentation to T lymphocytes and thus their ability to respond to a challenge by viruses.

Adapted from Nieman DC. Endurance exercise and the immune response. In Shephard RJ, Astrand P-O. Endurance in Sport, 2nd ed. Oxford, UK: Blackwell Science; 2000; Mackinnon LT: Advances in Exercise Immunology. Champaign, IL: Human Kinetics; 1999; and Nieman DC. Immune response to heavy exertion. J Appl Physiol 82:1385–1394, 1997.

tions during the following 1 to 2 weeks. This link must be established before the "open window" theory can be wholly accepted in humans[9,10].

Exercise and Infection

The relationship between exercise workload and infection can be modeled in the form of a "J" curve (Fig. 38-3). This model indicates that although the risk of URTI may de-

crease below that of a sedentary individual when one engages in moderate exercise training, risk may increase above average during periods of excessive amounts of high-intensity exercise.

MODERATE EXERCISE AND INFECTION

People who exercise regularly report fewer colds than their sedentary peers. Numerous surveys of fitness enthusiasts, runners, and master athletes indicate that between 60% and 90% believe that they experience fewer colds than their sedentary peers[11].

Data from three randomized studies support the viewpoint that near-daily physical activity reduces the number of days with sickness[12–14]. In these studies, women in the exercise groups walked briskly fro 35 to 45 minutes, five days a week, for 12 to 15 weeks during the winter and spring or fall; the control groups remained physically inactive. The results were similar to those reported by fitness enthusiasts: walkers experienced about half the days with cold symptoms of the sedentary control subjects. Several epidemiological studies involving large numbers of adults have also shown that the odds for URTI are reduced by 25% to 50% when comparing physically active and inactive participants[15–17].

The data on the relationship between moderate exercise, enhanced immunity, and lowered risk of sickness are consistent with guidelines urging the general public to

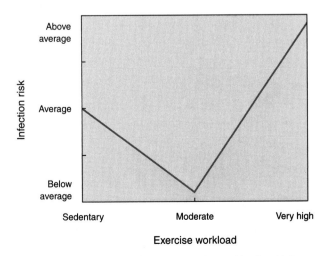

FIGURE 38-3. The relationship between exercise workload and infection can be modeled in the form of a "J" curve.

engage in near-daily brisk walking and other forms of aerobic activity.

OVERTRAINING AND INFECTION

In contrast, growing evidence suggests excessive exercise workloads increase URTI incidence rates. A common perception among elite endurance athletes and coaches is that overtraining lowers resistance to URTI such as the common cold and sore throats[11] (also see Box 28-7).

The results of epidemiological studies generally support the belief that URTI risk is elevated during periods of heavy training and in the 1- to 2-week period after participation in competitive endurance races[11,18]. A high percentage of self-reported illnesses occurs when elite athletes exceed their individually identifiable training thresholds, mostly related to the strain of training[19]. The majority of endurance athletes, however, do not report URTIs after competitive race events. When athletes train hard but avoid overreaching and overtraining, URTI risk is typically unaltered[3].

Together, these data indicate that a relationship exists between exercise workload and infection. Most endurance athletes should experience low to normal URTI risk during periods of regular training, with URTI increasing rising during periods of overreaching or overtraining and competition.

SPORTS AND INFECTIOUS DISEASE OUTBREAKS

Participation in competitive sports has been linked with infectious disease outbreaks, and these have been related to person-to-person, common-source, and airborne routes[20]. The risk of infection can be high among athletes when several factors converge, as listed in Box 38-2.

Practical Guidelines to Reduce the Risk of Immunosuppression and Infection

Whether one gets sick with a cold after a sufficient amount of the virus has entered the body depends on many factors that affect the immune system other than just physical activity. Poor nutrition, older age, cigarette smoking, mental stress, and lack of sleep have all been associated with impaired immune function and an increased risk of infection[5,11,20]. Cold viruses are spread by both personal contact and breathing the air near sick people. Therefore, if at all possible, athletes should avoid being around sick people before and after important events. If an athlete is competing during the winter months, an influenza vaccination is recommended.

For most fitness enthusiasts, good immune function can be maintained by regular physical activity, eating a well-balanced diet, keeping life stresses to a minimum, avoiding overtraining and fatigue, and obtaining adequate

---

BOX 38-2 | **Factors That Increase the Risk of Infectious Disease Outbreaks Among Athletes**

- Athletes often perform in environments where certain pathogenic microorganisms are particularly widespread.
- Depending on the type of sport, abrasions or other tissue injuries may be more likely, allowing the transfer of microbial agents.
- Athletes may experience cross-infection from others with whom they are in close contact (e.g., sharing of contaminated drinking utensils).
- Exposure to alien environmental pathogens may occur during foreign travel when there is a lack of specific immunity.
- The potential for immunosuppression from both psychosocial and physiological stress is high during periods of heavy training and competition.

Adapted from Nieman DC: Exercise, the immune system, and infectious disease (pp. 177–190). In Garrett WE, Kirdendall DT, eds. Exercise and Sport Science. Philadelphia: Lippincott, Williams & Wilkins 2000.

---

sleep. Immune function is suppressed during periods of very low caloric intake and quick weight reduction, so weight loss should be gradual to maintain good immunity.

NUTRITION CONCERNS

Nutrition impacts the development of the immune system in growing fetuses and in the early months of life[21]. Nutrients are also necessary for the immune response to pathogens so that cells can divide and produce antibodies and cytokines.

Should nutrient and herbal supplements be used to enhance immune function above and beyond the effects of physical activity? Despite all of the hype about supplements such as phytochemicals, antioxidants, flavonoids, carotenoids, glutamine (an amino acid), ginseng, and echinacea, there is insufficient evidence to warrant taking high doses in the belief they will prevent or cure ailments ranging from the common cold to cancer. In fact, extremely large doses of these supplements may lead to health problems rather than confer benefits[21]. The best practice is to eat a varied and balanced diet in accordance with energy needs and the U.S. Food Guide Pyramid and be assured that vitamin, mineral, and phytochemical intake is adequate for both health and immune function[21].

For athletes, the influence of a growing list of nutritional supplements on the immune and infection response to intense and prolonged exercise has been assessed[21]. Of these, only carbohydrate has emerged as a useful nutritional countermeasure to exercise-induced immunosuppression.

Several studies with runners and cyclists have shown that carbohydrate beverage ingestion plays a role in attenuating changes in immunity when an athlete experiences physiologic stress and depletion of carbohydrate stores in response to high intensity ($\approx 75\%$ to 80% $\dot{V}O_{2max}$) exercise bouts lasting longer than 2 hours[22,23]. In particular, carbohydrate ingestion (about 1 L·hr^{-1} of a typical sports drink) compared with a placebo has been linked to significantly lower blood cortisol and epinephrine levels, a reduced change in blood immune cell counts, and lower pro- and antiinflammatory cytokines. These data suggest that endurance athletes ingesting carbohydrates during race events should experience much lower perturbations in hormonal and immune measures compared with athletes avoiding carbohydrates.

REST OR EXERCISE DURING SICKNESS?

Fitness enthusiasts are often uncertain of whether they should exercise or rest during sickness. Human studies are lacking to provide definitive answers. Animal studies, however, generally support the finding that one or two periods of exhaustive exercise after injection of an animal with certain types of viruses or bacteria leads to a more frequent appearance of infection and more severe symptoms[9,24].

With athletes, it is well established that the ability to compete is reduced during sickness[25]. Also, several case histories have shown that sudden and unexplained downturns in athletic performance can sometimes be traced to a recent bout of sickness. In some athletes, exercising when sick can lead to a severely debilitating state known as "postviral fatigue syndrome"[26,27]. The symptoms can persist for several months, and they include weakness, an inability to train hard, easy fatigability, frequent infections, and depression.

Concerning exercising when sick, recommendations of most clinical authorities in the area of exercise immunology are shown in Box 38-3[5,25]. In two studies using nasal sprays of a rhinovirus leading to common cold symptoms, subjects were able to engage in exercise during the course of the illness without any negative effects on severity of symptoms or performance capability[28,29].

Conclusions and Recommendations

Exercise immunology is a relatively new area of scientific endeavor, with 80% of articles published during the past decade. Even though exercise immunology is a new science, convincing evidence indicates that physical activity does influence immune function and risk of infection. By far, the most important finding that has emerged from exercise immunology studies is that positive immune changes take place during each bout of moderate physical activity. Over time, this translates to fewer days of sickness with the common cold and other respiratory infections.

Many components of the immune system exhibit adverse change after prolonged, heavy exertion lasting longer than 90 minutes. During this "open window" of impaired immunity (which may last between 3 and 72 hours, depending on the immune measure), viruses and bacteria may gain a foothold, increasing the risk of subclinical and clinical infection. URTI risk can increase when athletes push beyond normal limits and is amplified when other factors related to immune function are present, including exposure to novel pathogens during travel, lack of sleep, severe mental stress, malnutrition, and rapid weight loss.

Exercise and HIV Infection

Acquired immune deficiency syndrome (AIDS) is a major public health problem of this generation, first recognized in the United States as a distinct syndrome in 1981, and has since become a major worldwide epidemic[30,31].

HIV/AIDS EPIDEMIOLOGY

More than 790,000 cases of AIDS have been reported in the United States since 1981, and as many as 900,000 Americans may be infected with the human immunodeficiency virus (HIV)[30,31]. The epidemic is growing most rapidly among minority populations and is a leading killer of African American men ages 25 to 44 years. According to the U.S. Centers for Disease Control and Prevention (CDC), AIDS affects nearly seven times more African Americans and three times more Hispanics than whites.

According to the Joint United Nations Program on HIV/AIDS, 42 million people are estimated to be living with HIV/AIDS throughout the world today. An estimated 5 million people acquired HIV in 2002, and AIDS caused the deaths of an estimated 3.1 million people. Women are becoming increasingly affected by HIV and now represent approximately 50% of all adults living with HIV or AIDS worldwide[30].

BOX 38-3	Recommendations for Exercise During Illness[5,25]

- If one has common cold symptoms (e.g., runny nose and sore throat without fever or general body aches and pains), intensive exercise training may be safely resumed a few days after the resolution of symptoms.
- Mild- to moderate-intensity exercise (e.g., walking) when sick with a common cold does not appear to be harmful.
- With symptoms of fever, extreme tiredness, muscle aches, and swollen lymph glands, 2 to 4 weeks should probably be allowed before resumption of intensive training.

TRANSMISSION OF HIV

AIDS is caused by the **human immunodeficiency virus (HIV)**[30,31]. By killing or damaging cells of the body's immune system, HIV progressively destroys the body's ability to fight infections and certain cancers. People diagnosed with AIDS may get life-threatening diseases called opportunistic infections, which are caused by microbes such as viruses or bacteria that usually do not make healthy people sick.

According to the CDC, transmission of HIV occurs through several avenues (Box 38-4)[30,31]. Having unprotected sex with an infected partner spreads HIV most commonly. The virus can enter the body through the lining of the vagina, vulva, penis, rectum, or mouth during sex. HIV frequently is spread among injection drug users by the sharing of needles or syringes contaminated with very small quantities of blood from someone infected with the virus. HIV also is spread through contact with infected blood. Before donated blood was screened for evidence of HIV infection and before heat-treating techniques to destroy HIV in blood products were introduced, HIV was transmitted through transfusions of contaminated blood or blood components. Today, because of blood screening and heat treatment, the risk of getting HIV from such transfusions is extremely small. Women can transmit HIV to their babies during pregnancy and birth. HIV also can be spread to babies through the breast milk of mothers infected with the virus.

Although researchers have found HIV in the saliva of infected people, there is no evidence that the virus is spread by contact with saliva. Scientists also have found no evidence that HIV is spread through sweat, tears, urine, or feces. Studies of families of HIV-infected people have shown clearly that HIV is not spread through casual contact such as the sharing of food utensils, towels and bedding, swimming pools, telephones, or toilet seats. Biting insects such as mosquitoes or bedbugs do not spread HIV.

STAGES OF HIV INFECTION

Many people do not have any symptoms when they first become infected with HIV. Some people, however, have a flulike illness within 1 or 2 month after exposure to the virus. These symptoms usually disappear within 1 week to

1 month and are often mistaken for those of another viral infection. During this period, people are very infectious, and HIV is present in large quantities in genital fluids[30,31].

More persistent or severe symptoms may not appear for 10 years or more after HIV first enters the body in adults, or within 2 years in children born with HIV infection. This period of "asymptomatic" infection is highly individual. Some people may begin to have symptoms within a few months, but others may be symptom free for more than 10 years.

Even during the asymptomatic period, the virus is actively multiplying, infecting, and killing cells of the immune system. HIV's effect is seen most obviously in a decline in the blood levels of CD4$^+$ T helper cells, the immune system's key infection fighters. At the beginning of its life in the human body, the virus disables or destroys these cells without causing symptoms.

As the immune system worsens, a variety of complications start to take over. Often, the first sign of infection is swollen lymph nodes that may be enlarged for more than 3 months. Other symptoms often experienced months to years before the onset of AIDS include lack of energy, weight loss, frequent fevers and sweats, persistent or frequent yeast infections (oral or vaginal), persistent skin rashes or flaky skin, pelvic inflammatory disease in women that does not respond to treatment, and short-term memory loss.

The term *AIDS* applies to the most advanced stages of HIV infection. The CDC's definition of AIDS includes all HIV-infected people who have fewer than 200 CD4$^+$ T helper cells per cubic millimeter of blood[30,31]. (Healthy adults usually have CD4$^+$ T-cell counts of 1000 or more.) In addition, the definition includes 26 clinical conditions that affect people with advanced HIV disease. Most of these conditions are opportunistic infections that generally do not affect healthy people. In people with AIDS, these infections are often severe and sometimes fatal because the immune system is so ravaged by HIV that the body cannot fight off certain bacteria, viruses, fungi, parasites, and other microbes.

Symptoms of opportunistic infections common in people with AIDS include coughing and shortness of breath, seizures and lack of coordination, difficult or painful swallowing, mental symptoms such as confusion and forgetfulness, severe and persistent diarrhea, fever, vision loss, nausea, abdominal cramps, vomiting, weight loss and extreme fatigue, severe headaches, and coma. People with AIDS are particularly prone to developing various cancers, especially those caused by viruses such as Kaposi's sarcoma and cervical cancer as well as cancers of the immune system known as lymphomas. These cancers are usually more aggressive and difficult to treat in people with AIDS. Signs of Kaposi's sarcoma in light-skinned people are round brown, reddish, or purple spots that develop in the skin or in the mouth. In dark-skinned people, the spots are more pigmented.

BOX 38-4	Methods Of Transmission of HIV[30,31]

- Unprotected sex
- Sharing of needles by drug users
- Contact with infected blood
- Transmission from mother to baby

DIAGNOSIS OF HIV INFECTION

Because early HIV infection often causes no symptoms, a doctor or other health care provider can usually diagnose it by testing a person's blood for the presence of antibodies to HIV. HIV antibodies generally do not reach detectable levels in the blood for 1 to 3 months after infection[30,31]. It may take the antibodies as long as 6 months to be produced in quantities large enough to show up in standard blood tests. People exposed to the virus should get an HIV test as soon as they are likely to develop antibodies to the virus, within 6 weeks to 12 months after possible exposure to the virus.

TREATMENT OF HIV INFECTION

The U.S. Food and Drug Administration (FDA) has approved a number of drugs for treating HIV infection. The first group of drugs used to treat HIV infection, called nucleoside reverse transcriptase (RT) inhibitors, interrupts an early stage of the virus' making copies of itself. Included in this class of drugs (called nucleoside analogs) are AZT (azidothymidine), ddC (zalcitabine), ddI (dideoxyinosine), d4T (stavudine), 3TC (lamivudine), abacavir (ziagen), and tenofovir (viread). These drugs may slow the spread of HIV in the body and delay the start of opportunistic infections[30,31].

Health care providers can prescribe non-nucleoside reverse transcriptase inhibitors (NNRTIs), such as delvaridine (Rescriptor), nevirapine (Viramune), and efravirenz (Sustiva), in combination with other antiretroviral drugs.

More recently, the FDA has approved a second class of drugs for treating HIV infection. These drugs, called protease inhibitors, interrupt virus replication at a later step in its life cycle. They include ritonavir (Norvir), saquinivir (Invirase), indinavir (Crixivan), amprenivir (Agenerase), nelfinavir (Viracept), and lopinavir (Kaletra).

Because HIV can become resistant to any of these drugs, health care providers must use a combination treatment to effectively suppress the virus. When RT inhibitors and protease inhibitors are used in combination, it is referred to as *highly active antiretroviral therapy* (HAART), and it can be used by people who are newly infected with HIV as well as people with AIDS.

Highly active antiretroviral therapy has been a major factor in significantly reducing the number of deaths from AIDS in this country. Although HAART is not a cure for AIDS, it has greatly improved the health of many people with AIDS, and it reduces the amount of virus circulating in the blood to nearly undetectable levels. HIV, however, remains present in hiding places, such as the lymph nodes, brain, testes, and retina of the eye, even in patients who have been treated.

HIV EXERCISE PRESCRIPTION

Most HIV/AIDS exercise investigators have used American College of Sports Medicine (ACSM) exercise pre-scription guidelines in their studies and have concluded that aerobic and progressive resistive exercise programs are safe and beneficial for adults living with HIV/AIDS. Exercise prescriptions for all HIV-infected individuals should be made on an individual basis, with appropriate initial screening[20,32–42]. The exercise prescription should emphasize both cardiorespiratory and musculoskeletal training components and be adapted to the stage of disease. Box 38-5 summarizes exercise testing and prescription recommendations for individuals with HIV/AIDS.

Pertinent questions have been raised regarding HIV transmission during sports that require close physical contact[32–42]. Most patients diagnosed with active AIDS are acutely and chronically ill and are not likely to participate in athletic endeavors. For each patient with clinically apparent AIDS, however, there are many more who are HIV infected and free of clinical manifestations who may be capable of normal participation in sports[20,32].

There are several situations in which the transmission of HIV is of concern in athletic settings. In sports in which athletes can be cut, such as in boxing or wrestling, or in other contact sports such as football, basketball, and baseball, risk of HIV transmission exists when the mucous membranes of a healthy athlete are exposed to the blood of an infected athlete. At present, the feeling is that testing all athletes before sports participation is impractical, unethical, and unrealistic[20,32]. Therefore, team physicians and athletic trainers are urged to provide information about the transmission of HIV, recommended behavior to reduce risks, and referral for care or diagnosis[20,40–42]. It should be the responsibility of any athlete participating in a combative sport who has a wound or other skin lesion to report it immediately to a responsible official and seek medical attention. Athletes who know they are HIV infected should seek medical counseling about further participation in sports, especially in sports such as wrestling or boxing that involve a high theoretical risk of contagion to other athletes. Each coach and athletic trainer should receive training in how to clean skin and athletic equipment surfaces exposed to blood or other body fluids.

EFFECT OF EXERCISE ON HIV/AIDS DISEASE PROGRESSION AND IMMUNITY

Can exercise training be used as a method to delay the progression from HIV infection to AIDS? Few investigators have published results in this area, but a growing consensus is that exercise training does not counter HIV-induced immunosuppression or decreases in T helper cell counts[38,39]. Moderate exercise training, on the other hand, does not have a detrimental effect on plasma HIV levels or immune function[32–39]. Exercise training is recommended, however, because it has been linked to multiple benefits for HIV-infected individuals, including improvement in psychological coping, increases in both cardiorespiratory and musculoskeletal fitness, enhanced

| BOX 38-5 | Exercise Testing and Prescription Guidelines for Individuals with HIV/AIDS |

- Individuals with HIV infection range from asymptomatic to critically ill. Thus, individuals with HIV/AIDS must be evaluated on an individual basis. Evaluations should include a medical history, physical examination, and tests for all components of fitness (body composition, muscular fitness, and aerobic fitness). As HIV progresses to AIDS, several physiological changes occur, including loss of strength and muscle mass; increased fatigue and weakness; gain in fat tissue in the abdominal area; loss of fat in the arms, legs, and face (lipodystrophy); and decrease in physical activity and aerobic capacity.
- Submaximal and maximal exercise testing provide useful information for exercise prescription. Asymptomatic individuals in the early phases of the disease using appropriate medications can undergo maximal exercise testing using commonly accepted test termination criteria. Exercise testing is contraindicated if an individual with HIV/AIDS is experiencing severe medication side effects (e.g., diarrhea, electrolyte imbalance) or fatigue and neuromuscular complications during advanced stages of the disease.
- Moderate exercise training is safe and efficacious in individuals with HIV/AIDS. Guidelines from the American College of Sports Medicine for moderate cardiorespiratory and resistance training should be followed. The goal is to enhance aerobic and muscular fitness and improve overall health and quality of life. Until more is known, prolonged and intense exercise is not recommended in order to avoid immunosuppression. Specific cardiorespiratory and resistance training protocols are described in the reference listed below.
- As HIV/AIDS progresses to the symptomatic stage, the goal is to remain physically active to the extent the illness allows. The individual with HIV/AIDS, the physician, and other health care professionals should carefully select and monitor the mode, intensity, and volume of exercise to optimize health and functional status. Exercise programs and testing should not be performed when an individual with HIV/AIDS has a fever higher than 100°F or any acute symptoms such as nausea, vomiting, uncontrolled diarrhea, or dehydration.

Source: American College of Sports Medicine. ACSM's Resources for Clinical Exercise Physiology: Musculoskeletal, Neuromuscular, Neoplastic, Immunologic, and Hematologic Conditions. Baltimore: Lippincott Williams & Wilkins; 2002.

quality of life and functional status, attenuation of lipodystrophy (abdominal fat gain with peripheral subcutaneous fat atrophy), and reduction of fatigue[32–39].

Exercise and Cancer

Cancer is a group of more than 100 diseases characterized by uncontrolled growth and spread of abnormal cells. Most cancers fall into four major classifications based on the type of cell from which they arise. Carcinomas are cancers that develop from epithelial cells that line the surfaces of the body, glands, and internal organs. They comprise 80% to 90% of all cancers and include prostate, colon, lung, cervical and breast. Cancers can also arise from the cells of the blood (i.e., leukemias); the immune system (i.e., lymphomas); and connective tissues such as bones, tendons, cartilage, fat, and muscle (i.e., sarcomas).

CANCER EPIDEMIOLOGY

Over their lifetime, Americans have about a 41% probability of developing some form of invasive cancer[43]. In 2003 alone, approximately 1.3 million Americans will be diagnosed with an invasive cancer[43]. Moreover, cancer accounts for 25% of all deaths in the United States, with an expected 550,000 deaths in 2003[43]. Prostate, breast, colorectal, and lung cancer account for more than 50% of all cancer cases and deaths (Table 38-1).

TABLE 38-1. Estimated New Cancer Cases and Deaths Overall and for the Most Common Cancer Sites by Gender, United States, 2003[a]

Site	Estimated New Cases			Estimated New Deaths		
	Total	Male	Female	Total	Male	Female
All Sites	1,334,100	675,300	658,800	556,500	285,900	270,600
Prostate	220,900	220,900	—	28,900	28,900	—
Breast	212,600	1300	211,300	40,200	400	39,800
Lung	171,900	91,800	80,100	157,200	88,400	68,800
Colorectal	147,500	72,800	74,700	57,100	28,300	28,800

[a] Excludes basal and squamous cell skin cancers and in situ carcinomas except urinary bladder.

Adapted from the American Cancer Society: Cancer Facts & Figures. Atlanta: American Cancer Society, 2003.

TABLE 38-2. Five-Year Relative Survival Rates for the Most Common Cancers by Stage at Diagnosis, United States, 1992–1998[a]

Site	All Stages (%)	Local (%)	Regional (%)	Distant (%)
Prostate	97	100	100	34
Breast	86	97	78	23
Colorectal	62	90	65	9
Lung	15	49	22	3

[a] Rates are adjusted for normal life expectancy and are based on persons diagnosed from 1992 to 1998 followed through 1999.

Adapted from the American Cancer Society: Cancer Facts & Figures 2003. Atlanta: American Cancer Society; 2003.

BOX 38-6 | **Physical Activity Guidelines for Cancer Prevention**

- **Adults:** Engage in at least moderate activity for 30 minutes or more on 5 or more days of the week; 45 minutes or more of moderate to vigorous activity on 5 or more days per week may further enhance reductions in the risk of breast and colon cancer.
- **Children and adolescents:** Engage in at least 60 minutes per day of moderate to vigorous physical activity at least 5 days per week.

Adapted from American Cancer Society: Cancer Prevention and Early Detection. Atlanta: American Cancer Society; 2003.

Early detection and improved treatments for cancer have resulted in increased survival rates over the past few decades[43]. The **5-year relative survival rate** across all cancers and disease stages is 62%[43]. This figure soars to more than 90% for some of the most common cancers (e.g., prostate, breast, and colon) if they are detected early (Table 38-2). Currently, there are almost nine million cancer survivors living in the United States[43]. Physical exercise may play an important role in **cancer control** across the entire cancer experience[44].

CANCER PREVENTION

The causes and risk factors for human cancer are diverse, but lifestyle is very important[45–48]. The American Cancer Society[48] has provided the key guidelines for cancer prevention. Research on physical inactivity as a risk factor for cancer has increased dramatically over the past decade based on a number of plausible biological mechanisms[47]. Generally, the evidence indicates that physical activity may significantly reduce the risk of developing some cancers. The most convincing evidence comes from research on colon and breast cancer, in which the risk reduction may be as much as 30% to 50%[47]. Moreover, evidence is also available to suggest that physical activity may have a protective effect against prostate cancer, lung cancer, and endometrial cancer, although definitive conclusions cannot be made at this time[47]. Evidence for other cancers (e.g., ovarian, pancreas, stomach) is currently too sparse to make even tentative conclusions[47]. The American Cancer Society[48] has provided physical activity guidelines for cancer prevention (Box 38-6).

CANCER DETECTION AND DIAGNOSIS

A key to improving survival rates from cancer is identifying the disease in its early stages. Screening techniques can identify abnormalities that may be cancer before physical signs and symptoms develop, and screening tests are available for many of the most common cancer sites, including the prostate, breast, colorectal system, uterus, skin, oral cavity, and testes[48]. The effects of exercise on the accuracy of screening and diagnostic tests for cancer are largely unknown. Interestingly, one study[49] found a threefold increase in prostate-specific antigen (PSA) concentration in serum after a 15-minute session of cycle ergometer exercise. Consequently, the authors suggested that extensive exercise should be avoided before PSA blood sampling for prostate cancer screening is done.

CANCER TREATMENTS

Many different cancer treatments can be used to cure cancer, to prolong life when a cure is not possible, or to improve quality of life (i.e., symptom relief). The most common treatment modalities for cancer are surgery, radiation therapy, and systemic therapy (i.e., drugs). Details of these medical interventions and their implications for exercise are presented elsewhere[50]. Surgery is the oldest form of cancer treatment and, depending on the location and extent of the operation, significant morbidity can occur (e.g., wound complications, infections, loss of function, decreased range of motion, diarrhea, dyspnea, pain, numbness, lymphedema). Radiation therapy is typically delivered in repeated small doses (i.e., fractions) over a 5- to 8-week period in order to maximize the killing of cancer cells and minimize the damage to normal cells. Nevertheless, toxicity to normal tissue does occur but is dependent on the site that is irradiated (e.g., pain, blistering, reduced elasticity, decreased range of motion, nausea, fatigue, dry mouth, diarrhea, lung fibrosis, cardiomyopathy).

The three major types of systemic therapy are chemotherapy, endocrine or hormone therapy, and biologic or immunotherapy[50]. Chemotherapy is usually administered intravenously or orally and is given in repeated courses or cycles 2 to 4 weeks apart over a 3- to 6-month period. Chemotherapy may cause various adverse events, including fatigue, anorexia, nausea, anemia, neutropenia, thrombocytopenia, peripheral neuropathies, ataxia, and cardiotoxicity. Hormone therapy is usually administered orally (continuously or intermittently) for many years and can have significant side effects such as weight gain, muscle loss, proximal muscle weakness, fat accumulation in the trunk and face, osteoporosis, fatigue, hot flashes, and increased susceptibility to infection. Lastly, biologic therapies are the newest treatments, and they influence the body's own defense mechanisms to act against cancer cells or potentiate the effects of other drugs. These treatments tend to be better tolerated but can still produce significant side effects.

No studies have examined the possible interaction of exercise with cancer treatment efficacy. Consequently, it is unknown whether exercise during cancer treatments potentiates, impedes, or is unrelated to treatment efficacy. Research into this question is needed, but there does not appear to be any compelling reason to believe that exercise may undermine cancer treatment efficacy.

EXERCISE IN CANCER SURVIVORS

Research into the effects of exercise on cancer survivors is of relatively recent vintage compared with research examining exercise and cancer prevention. The earliest studies were published in the mid- to late 1980s, and progress was sporadic throughout the late 1980s and early 1990s. In the mid- to late 1990s, several groups in North America and Europe initiated research programs in the area. This upsurge in research led to several early[51–53] and more recent[54–60] reviews on the topic. Readers are directed to these reviews for a more detailed analysis. In this chapter, a brief overview of the effects of exercise in cancer survivors is provided and is divided into disease outcomes and quality of life.

Effects of Exercise on Recurrence, Second Cancers, Other Diseases, and Overall Survival

Very little human research has been done to examine the effects of exercise on **cancer recurrence**, second cancers, other diseases, and overall survival in cancer survivors. Nevertheless, a relationship between exercise and disease outcomes in cancer survivors seems plausible. For cancers in which exercise has been implicated in their primary prevention (e.g., colon, breast), it seems reasonable to suggest that exercise may also play a role in the recurrence of the disease or second cancers. With respect to other major diseases and conditions (e.g., heart disease, diabetes), it is well documented that exercise plays a strong role in risk reduction in other populations. Consequently, it seems reasonable to suggest that such relationships should also hold for cancer survivors. Moreover, compelling data suggest that body mass index is an independent predictor of cancer recurrence and survival in breast and colon cancer survivors[61]. To the extent that exercise can reduce obesity in cancer survivors, it may also be expected to reduce the risk of recurrence and extend survival. Lastly, effects on recurrence, second cancers, and other diseases would be expected to confer an overall survival advantage. Nevertheless, the issue of whether postdiagnosis exercise may influence tumor growth, disease progression, recurrence, other chronic diseases, or survival is a controversial and unanswered question.

Effects of Exercise on Symptom Management and Overall Quality of Life

More than 50 studies have examined the relationship between physical exercise and quality of life in cancer survivors[54]. About half of these studies have examined exercise during cancer treatment, and the other half has examined exercise posttreatment. Just over half of the studies focused on breast cancer survivors, with the next largest study population being **bone marrow transplant** survivors. The vast majority of studies tested interventions, and most of these studies used supervised exercise programs.

Moreover, almost all studies tested aerobic exercise programs, although several combined aerobic and resistance training programs. Most of the early studies were pilot or feasibility studies with significant methodological limitations. Nevertheless, despite these limitations, the studies have consistently demonstrated that exercise has beneficial effects on a wide variety of physical fitness and quality of life outcomes, including exercise capacity, muscular strength, body weight and composition, flexibility, fatigue, nausea, diarrhea, pain, physical well being, functional well being, depression, anxiety, vigor, anger, mood, self-esteem, satisfaction with life, and overall quality of life. These studies have resulted in exercise being recommended as a therapy for fatigue in cancer survivors[62].

Exercise Motivation and Adherence

The effectiveness of exercise for cancer survivors depends to a large extent on the motivation and adherence of participants. Exercise adherence is a major challenge for health professionals, and the significant morbidity caused by cancer and its treatments makes it likely that exercise adherence is even more difficult in cancer survivors. Not surprisingly, the amount of exercise performed by cancer survivors decreases significantly during treatments and does not appear to return to prediagnosis levels even years after treatment[63–65]. Nevertheless, many cancer survivors are quite receptive to health promotion programs, including exercise, and desire information soon after diagnosis. The key point for fitness professionals is that cancer survivors present with unique incentives and barriers to exercise that need to be understood and addressed[66–69]. Creative exercise programming and adherence strategies for this population are required.

EXERCISE PRESCRIPTION GUIDELINES FOR CANCER SURVIVORS

Before initiating an exercise program, it is important to have cancer survivors complete a cancer history questionnaire in addition to other usual exercise and medical history questionnaires (e.g., Revised Physical Activity Readiness Questionnaire [PAR-Q], see GETP7 Figure 2-2). The cancer history questionnaire should assess important diagnostic and treatment variables such as time since diagnosis, type and stage of disease, type of surgery and adjuvant therapy, and known or suspected side effects of treatment (e.g., ataxia, cardiomyopathy, pulmonary complications, orthopedic conditions). The survivor's cancer care team may need to be consulted to provide complete and accurate information.

Challenges and Precautions

Specific exercise prescription guidelines for cancer survivors are challenging because cancer is not a uniform disease with singular treatment options that elicit predictable responses. Rather, cancer consists of more than 100 different diseases with myriad treatment protocols that produce a unique constellation of side effects for each individual. Moreover, the lack of information on the underlying mechanisms of exercise benefit in cancer survivors precludes the prescription of a precise mode, frequency, intensity, and duration of exercise. Consequently, the appropriate exercise prescription varies depending on the cancer site (e.g., breast, prostate, colon), the treatment protocol (e.g., surgical procedure, specific drugs), individual responses to treatment (e.g., level of fatigue, nausea, pain, cachexia, ataxia), and baseline fitness. To date, information is available on two cancer/treatment combinations: early-stage breast cancer survivors treated with surgery and chemotherapy and mixed-cancer survivors treated with dose-dense chemotherapy and bone marrow transplant. Even for these cancer/treatment combinations, however, the optimal type, frequency, duration,

intensity, and progression of exercise are unknown because all intervention studies have compared single exercise prescriptions with nothing at all. Clearly, determining the optimal exercise prescription for each cancer/treatment combination is a large challenge awaiting future research.

There are several important exercise precautions for cancer survivors in addition to those based on age (Table 38-3). One of the most important exercise precautions in cancer survivors is the presence of metastatic bone disease, which occurs at some point in about 50% of all survivors. The bone metastases most commonly occur in the vertebra, pelvis, femur, and skull, although the most common site of major fracture is the hip. Cancer survivors with hip pain that is worse on activity should be referred back to their cancer care team.

Type, Volume, and Context

The key point when prescribing exercise to cancer survivors is to take into account any acute or chronic physical impairments that may have resulted from medical treatment. Presently, no evidence suggests that one type of exercise is superior to another for the general rehabilitation of cancer survivors. From a clinical perspective, it is probably safest to prescribe walking or cycle ergometry. Walking is the preferred exercise of cancer survivors[70], and it has direct implications for activities of daily living. The advantages of cycle ergometry include a sitting position with leg exercises that minimize the effects of ataxia (i.e., coordination and balance problems) and limitations in upper extremity movement. Although evidence for the efficacy of weight training is only beginning to emerge[71], the optimal rehabilitation program

TABLE 38-3. Special Precautions When Prescribing Exercise for Cancer Survivors

Complication	Precaution
Complete Blood Counts	
Hemoglobin level <8.0 g·dL^{-1}	Avoid activities that require significant oxygen transport (e.g., high intensity).
Absolute neutrophil count <0.5 × 10^9/l	Avoid activities that may increase the risk of bacterial infection (e.g., swimming).
Platelet count <50 × 10^9/l	Avoid activities that increase the risk of bleeding (e.g., contact sports or high impact exercises).
Other	
Fever >38°C and >40°C	May indicate systemic infection and should be investigated. If neutropenic, avoid exercise altogether. If not neutropenic, avoid high intensity exercise if fever >38°C and all exercise if fever >40°C.
Ataxia, dizziness, peripheral	Avoid activities that require significant balance and sensory neuropathy coordination (e.g., treadmill).
Severe cachexia (loss of >35% of premorbid weight)	Loss of muscle mass usually limits exercise to mild intensity, depending on the degree of cachexia.
Dyspnea	Investigate etiology. Exercise to tolerance.
Bone metastases or pain	Avoid activities that increase risk of fracture at the location of the bone pain or metastases (e.g., contact sports or high impact exercises).
Severe nausea	Investigate etiology. Exercise to tolerance.
Extreme fatigue or muscle weakness	Investigate etiology. Exercise to tolerance.
Severe lymphedema	Avoid upper extremity exercises with the affected arm.
Dehydration	Ensure adequate hydration.

Modified from Courneya KS, Mackey JR, Jones LW: Coping with cancer: Can exercise help? Phys Sportsmed 28:49–73, 2000.

for cancer survivors likely combines aerobic and weight training. Table 38-4 provides general aerobic exercise guidelines for cancer survivors that need to be modified based on morbidity.

The volume of exercise (i.e., frequency, intensity, and duration) prescribed for cancer survivors has closely followed the ACSM's[72] recommendations. Most studies have prescribed moderate-intensity exercise performed 3 to 5 days per week for 20 to 30 minutes per session. This prescription appears appropriate for most cancer survivors but may need to be modified based on current medical treatments, comorbid conditions, and fitness level. Many cancer survivors do not feel like exercising at certain times during their treatments because of significant sickness and fatigue. The key point is to build flexibility into the exercise prescription so that cancer survivors are able to modify the frequency, intensity, or duration of their exercise depending on how well they tolerate treatment.

It is also important to recognize that cancer survivors exercise as much for psychological outcomes as for disease outcomes. Consequently, it is important to take psycho-logical benefits into account when prescribing exercise for cancer survivors. As a general guideline, fitness professionals should prescribe exercise that is enjoyable, builds confidence, facilitates perceptions of control, develops new skills, incorporates social interaction, and takes place in an environment that engages the mind and spirit[57].

Summary

Almost 9 million Americans are cancer survivors, and this number will increase in the coming decades. Guidelines for exercise prescription in this population need to take into account the significant and diverse morbidity that results from cancer treatments. Facilitating exercise adherence among cancer survivors requires a good understanding of the unique incentives and barriers in this population and the application of creative behavior change strategies.

TABLE 38-4. General Aerobic Exercise Recommendations for Otherwise Healthy Cancer Survivors

Parameter	Guidelines and Comments
Mode	Most exercises involving large muscle groups are appropriate, but walking and cycling are especially recommended. The key is to modify exercise mode based on acute or chronic treatment effects from surgery, chemotherapy, or radiation therapy.
Frequency	At least three to five times per week, but daily exercise may be optimal for deconditioned survivors performing lighter intensity or shorter duration exercises.
Intensity	Moderate intensity depending on current fitness level and severity of side effects from treatments. Guidelines include 50% to 75% $\dot{V}O_{2max}$ or $HR_{reserve}$, 60% to 80% HR_{max}, or 11 to 14 RPE. $HR_{reserve}$ is best guideline if HR_{max} is estimated rather than measured.[a]
Duration	From 20 to 60 continuous minutes, but this goal may have to be achieved through multiple intermittent shorter bouts (e.g., 5 to 10 minutes) with rest intervals in deconditioned survivors or those experiencing severe side effects of treatment.
Progression	Initial progression should be in frequency and duration, and intensity be increased only when these goals are met should. Progression should be slower and more gradual for deconditioned survivors and those experiencing severe side effects of treatment.

HR = heart rate; RPE = rating of perceived exertion.

[a] $HR_{reserve}$ = maximal heart rate (HR_{max}) minus standing resting heart rate (HR_{rest}). Multiply $HR_{reserve}$ by 0.60 and 0.80. Add each of these values to HR_{rest} to obtain the target heart rate range.

HR_{max} can be estimated as 220 - age (years).

Reprinted with permission from: Courneya KS, Mackey JR, Jones LW: Coping with cancer: Can exercise help? Phys Sportsmed 28:49–73, 2000.

REFERENCES

1. Roitt I, Delves PJ: Roitt's Essential Immunology, 10th ed. Oxford, UK: Blackwell Publishing; 2001.
2. Nieman DC: Exercise effects on systemic immunity. Immunol Cell Biol 78:496–501, 2000.
3. Nieman DC, Nehlsen-Cannarella SL, Fagoaga OR, et al: Immune function in female elite rowers and nonathletes. Br J Sports Med 34:181–187, 2000.
4. Nieman DC. Endurance exercise and the immune response. In Shephard RJ, Astrand P-O. Endurance in Sport, 2nd ed. Oxford, UK: Blackwell Science; 2000.
5. Mackinnon LT: Advances in Exercise Immunology. Champaign, IL: Human Kinetics; 1999.
6. Nehlsen-Cannarella SL, Nieman DC, Balk-Lamberton AJ, et al: The effects of moderate exercise training on immune response. Med Sci Sports Exerc 23:64–70, 1991.
7. Nieman DC. Immune response to heavy exertion. J Appl Physiol 82:1385–1394, 1997.
8. Konig D, Grathwohl D, Weinstock C, et al: Upper respiratory tract infection in athletes: influence of lifestyle, type of sport, training effort, and immunostimulant intake. Exerc Immunol Rev 6:102–120, 2000.
9. Davis JM, Kohut ML, Colbert LH, et al: Exercise, alveolar macrophage function, and susceptibility to respiratory infection. J Appl Physiol 83:1461–1466, 1997.
10. Nieman DC, Henson DA, Fagoaga OR, et al: Change in salivary IgA following a competitive marathon race. Int J Sports Med 23:69–75, 2002.
11. Nieman DC: Is infection risk linked to exercise workload? Med Sci Sports Exerc 32 (suppl 7):S406–S411, 2000.
12. Nieman DC, Nehlsen-Cannarella SL, Markoff PA, et al: The effects of moderate exercise training on natural killer cells and acute upper respiratory tract infections. Int J Sports Med 11:467–473, 1990.
13. Nieman DC, Henson DA, Gusewitch G, et al: Physical activity and immune function in elderly women. Med Sci Sports Exerc 25:823–831, 1993.
14. Nieman DC, Nehlsen-Cannarella SL, Henson DA, et al: Immune response to exercise training and/or energy restriction in obese females. Med Sci Sports Exerc 30:679–686, 1998.
15. Matthews CE, Ockene IS, Freedson PS, et al: Moderate to vigorous physical activity and risk of upper-respiratory tract infection. Med Sci Sports Exerc 34:1242–1248, 2002.
16. Kostka T, Berthouze SE, Lacour J, et al: The symptomatology of upper respiratory tract infections and exercise in elderly people. Med Sci Sports Exerc 32:46–51, 2000.

17. Strasner A, Barlow CE, Kampert JB, Dunn AL: Impact of physical activity on URTI symptoms in Project PRIME participants. Med Sci Sports Exerc 33(suppl):S304, 2001.

18. Nieman DC, Johansen LM, Lee JW, et al: Infectious episodes in runners before and after the Los Angeles Marathon. J Sports Med Phys Fit 30:316–328, 1990.

19. Foster C: Monitoring training in athletes with reference to overtraining syndrome. Med Sci Sports Exerc 30:1164–1168, 1998.

20. Nieman DC: Exercise, the immune system, and infectious disease (pp. 177–190). In Garrett WE, Kirdendall DT, eds. Exercise and Sport Science. Philadelphia: Lippincott, Williams & Wilkins 2000.

21. Nieman DC, Pedersen BK: Nutrition and Exercise Immunology. Boca Raton, FL: CRC Press; 2000.

22. Nieman DC: Exercise immunology: Nutritional countermeasures. Can J Appl Physiol 26(suppl):S45–S55, 2001.

23. Gleeson M, Lancaster GI, Bishop NC. Nutritional strategies to minimise exercise-induced immunosuppression in athletes. Can J Appl Physiol 26(suppl):S23–S35, 2001.

24. Gross DK, Hinchcliff KW, French PS, et al: Effect of moderate exercise on the severity of clinical signs associated with influenza virus infection in horses. Equine Vet J 30:489–497, 1998.

25. Friman G, Wesslen L: Special feature for the Olympics: effects of exercise on the immune system: infections and exercise in high-performance athletes. Immunol Cell Biol 78:510–522, 2000.

26. Maffulli N, Testa V, Capasso G: Post-viral fatigue syndrome. A longitudinal assessment in varsity athletes. J Sports Med Phys Fit 33:392–399, 1993.

27. Parker S, Brukner P, Rosier M: Chronic fatigue syndrome and the athlete. Sports Med Train Rehab 6:269–278, 1996.

28. Weidner TG, Anderson BN, Kaminsky LA, et al: Effect of a rhinovirus-caused upper respiratory illness on pulmonary function test and exercise responses. Med Sci Sports Exerc 29:604–609, 1997.

29. Weidner T, Cranston T, Schurr T, Kaminsky L: The effect of exercise training on the severity and duration of a viral upper respiratory illness. Med Sci Sports Exerc 30:1578–1583, 1998.

30. Centers for Disease Control and Prevention: HIV/AIDS. Available at: http://www.cdc.gov/hiv/stats/2003surveillancereport.pdf

31. Chin J.:Control of Communicable Diseases Manual, 17th ed. Washington DC: American Public Health Association; 2001.

32. Nixon S, O'Brien K, Glazier RH, Tynan AM: Aerobic exercise interventions for adults living with HIV/AIDS. Cochrane Database Syst Rev 2:CD001796; 2001.

33. Roubenoff R, Schmitz H, Bairos L, et al: Reduction of abdominal obesity in lipodystrophy associated with human immunodeficiency virus infection by means of diet and exercise: case report and proof of principle. Clin Infect Dis 34:390–393, 2002.

34. Roubenoff R, Wilson IB: Effect of resistance training on self-reported physical functioning in HIV infection. Med Sci Sports Exerc 33:1811–1817, 2001.

35. Yarasheski KE, Roubenoff R: Exercise treatment for HIV-associated metabolic and anthropometric complications. Exerc Sport Sci Rev 29:170–174, 2001.

36. Smith BA, Neidig JL, Nickel JT, et al: Aerobic exercise: effects on parameters related to fatigue, dyspnea, weight and body composition in HIV-infected adults. AIDS 15:693–701, 2001.

37. Roubenoff R, Skolnik PR, Shevitz A, et al: Effect of a single bout of acute exercise on plasma human immunodeficiency virus RNA levels. J Appl Physiol 86:1197–1201, 1999.

38. Terry L, Sprinz E, Ribeiro JP: Moderate and high intensity exercise training in HIV-1 seropositive individuals: A randomized trial. Int J Sports Med 20:142–146, 1999.

39. Rigsby LW, Dishman RK, Jackson AW, et al: Effects of exercise training on men seropositive for the human immunodeficiency virus-1. Med Sci Sports Exerc 24:6–12, 1992.

40. Goldsmith MF: World Health Organization consensus statement. Consultation on AIDS and sports. JAMA 267:1312–1314, 1992.

41. American Academy of Pediatrics, Committee on Sports Medicine and Fitness: Human immunodeficiency virus [acquired immunodeficiency syndrome (AIDS) virus] in the athletic setting. Pediatrics 88:640–641, 1991.

42. Brown LS, Phillips RY, Brown CL, et al: HIV/AIDS policies and sports: the National Football League. Med Sci Sports Exerc 26:403–407, 1994.

43. American Cancer Society: Cancer Facts and Figures 2003. Atlanta: American Cancer Society; 2003.

44. Courneya KS, Friedenreich CM: Framework PEACE: An organizational model for examining physical exercise across the cancer experience. Ann Behav Med 23:263–272, 2001.

45. Harvard Center for Cancer Prevention: Harvard report on cancer prevention volume 1: Causes of human cancer. Cancer Causes Control 7:S3–S59, 1996.

46. Calle EE, Rodriguez C, Walker-Thurmond K, Thun MJ: Overweight, obesity, and mortality from cancer in a prospectively studied cohort of U.S. adults. N Engl J Med 348:1625–1638, 2003.

47. Friedenreich CM: Physical activity and cancer prevention: From observational to intervention research. Cancer Epidemiol Biomarkers Prev 10:287–301, 2001.

48. American Cancer Society: Cancer Prevention and Early Detection. Atlanta: American Cancer Society; 2003.

49. Oremek GM, Seiffert UB: Physical activity releases prostate-specific antigen (PSA) from the prostate gland into blood and increases serum PSA concentrations. Clin Chem 42:691–695, 1996.

50. Courneya KS, Mackey JR, Quinney HA: Neoplasms (pp.179–191). In Myers JN, Herbert WG, Humphrey R, eds. ACSM's Resources for Clinical Exercise Physiology: Musculoskeletal, Neuromuscular, Neoplastic, Immunologic, and Hematologic Conditions. Baltimore: Lippincott, Williams & Wilkins;, 2002.

51. Friedenreich CM, Courneya KS: Exercise as rehabilitation for cancer patients. Clin J Sports Med 6:237–244, 1996.

52. Mock V: The benefits of exercise in women with breast cancer. In Dow KH, ed. Contemporary Issues in Breast Cancer. Sudbury, MA: Jones & Bartlett; 1996.

53. Smith SL: Physical exercise as an oncology nursing intervention to enhance quality of life. Oncol Nurs Forum 23:771–778, 1996.

54. Courneya KS: Exercise in cancer survivors: An overview of research. Med Sci Sports Exerc, 35:1846–1852, 2003.

55. Courneya KS, Friedenreich CM: Physical exercise and quality of life following cancer diagnosis: A literature review. Ann Behav Med 21:171–179, 1999.

56. Courneya KS, Mackey JR, Jones LW: Coping with cancer: Can exercise help? Phys Sportsmed 28:49–73, 2000.

57. Courneya KS, Mackey JR, McKenzie DC: Exercise for breast cancer survivors: Research evidence and clinical guidelines. Phys Sportsmed 30:33–42, 2002.

58. Courneya KS, Mackey JR, Rhodes RE: Exercise and cancers other than breast. In LeMura LM, von Duvillard SP, eds. Clinical Exercise Physiology: Application and Physiological Principles. Baltimore: Lippincott, Williams & Wilkins, 2003.

59. Fairey AS, Courneya KS, Field CJ, Mackey JR: Physical exercise and immune system function in cancer survivors: a comprehensive review and future directions. Cancer 94:539–551, 2002.

60. Pinto BM, Maruyama NC: Exercise in the rehabilitation of breast cancer survivors. Psychooncology 8:191–206, 1999.

61. Chlebowski RT, Aiello E, McTiernan A: Weight loss in breast cancer patient management. J Clin Oncol 20:1128–1143, 2002.

62. Jacobsen PB, Thors CL: Fatigue in the radiation therapy patient: Current management and investigations. Semin Radiat Oncol 13:372–380, 2003.

63. Courneya KS, Friedenreich CM: Relationship between exercise during cancer treatment and current quality of life in survivors of breast cancer. J Psychosoc Oncol 5:120–127, 1997.

64. Courneya KS, Friedenreich CM: Relationship between exercise pattern across the cancer experience and current quality of life in

colorectal cancer survivors. J Altern Complement Med 3:215–226, 1997.

65. Keats MR, Courneya KS, Danielsen S, Whitsett SF: Leisure-time physical activity and psychosocial well-being in adolescents after cancer diagnosis. J Pediatr Oncol Nurs 16:180–188, 1999.

66. Ajzen I: Nature and operation of attitudes. Annu Rev Psychol 52:27–58, 2001.

67. Courneya KS, Friedenreich CM, Sela RA, et al: Correlates of adherence and contamination in a randomized controlled trial of exercise in cancer survivors: An application of the theory of planned behavior and the five factor model of personality. Ann Behav Med 24:257–268, 2002.

68. Courneya KS, Keats MR, Turner AR: Social cognitive determinants of hospital-based exercise in cancer patients following high dose chemotherapy and bone marrow transplantation. Int J Behav Med 7:189–203, 2000.

69. Courneya KS, Friedenreich CM: Utility of the theory of planned behavior for understanding exercise during breast cancer treatment. Psychooncology 8:112–122, 1999.

70. Jones LW, Courneya KS: Exercise counseling and programming preferences of cancer survivors. Cancer Pract 10:208–215, 2002.

71. Segal R, Reid RD, Courneya KS, et al: Resistance exercise in men receiving androgen deprivation therapy for prostate cancer. J Clin Oncol 21:1653–1659, 2003.

72. American College of Sports Medicine: The recommended quantity and quality of exercise for developing and maintaining cardiorespiratory and muscular fitness and flexibility in healthy adults. Position Stand. Med Sci Sports Exerc 30:975–991, 1998.

SELECTED REFERENCES FOR FURTHER READING

American College of Sports Medicine. ACSM's Resources for Clinical Exercise Physiology: Musculoskeletal, Neuromuscular, Neoplastic, Immunologic, and Hematologic Conditions. Baltimore: Lippincott, Williams & Wilkins; 2002.

Courneya KS, Friedenreich CM, Sela RA, et al: The group psychotherapy and home-based physical exercise (group-hope) trial in cancer survivors: Physical fitness and quality of life outcomes. Psychooncology 12:357–374, 2003.

Courneya KS, Mackey JR, Bell GJ, et al: Randomized controlled trial of exercise training in postmenopausal breast cancer survivors: Cardiopulmonary and quality of life outcomes. J Clin Oncol 21:1660–1668. 2003.

Cunningham AJ, Edmonds CV, Jenkins GP, et al: A randomized controlled trial of the effects of group psychological therapy on survival in women with metastatic breast cancer. Psychooncology 7:508–517, 1998.

Fairey AS, Courneya KS, Field CJ, et al: Effects of exercise training on fasting insulin, insulin resistance, insulin-like growth factors, and IGF binding proteins in postmenopausal breast cancer survivors: A randomized controlled trial. Cancer Epidemiol Biomarkers Prev 12:721–727, 2003.

Friedenreich CM, Orenstein MR: Physical activity and cancer prevention: Etiologic evidence and biological mechanisms. J Nutr 132(11 suppl):3456S–3464S, 2002.

Nieman DC: Exercise Testing and Prescription: A Health-Related Approach. New York: McGraw-Hill; 2003.

Rohan TE, Fu W, Hiller JE: Physical activity and survival from breast cancer. Eur J Cancer Prev 4:419–424, 1995.

INTERNET RESOURCES

American Cancer Society:
http://www.cancer.org

Centers for Disease Control: Divisions of HIV/AIDS Prevention:
http://www.cdc.gov/hiv

International Society of Exercise and Immunology:
http://www.isei.de

National Cancer Institute:
http://www.nci.nih.gov

Human Behavioral Principles Applied to Physical Activity

SECTION EDITOR: LEONARD A. KAMINSKY, PhD, FACSM

Acknowledgments
Thank you to John M. Jakicic, Ph.D., FACSM who developed the organization of this section and selected the authors for the chapter in this section.

Principles of Health Behavior Change

MELISSA A. NAPOLITANO, BETH LEWIS, JESSICA A. WHITELEY, AND BESS H. MARCUS

This chapter addresses KSAs from the following content areas:

1 Exercise Physiology and Related Exercise Science
2 Pathophysiology and Risk Factors
3 Health Appraisal, Fitness, and Clinical Exercise Testing
4 Electrocardiography and Diagnostic Techniques
5 Patient Management and Medications
6 Medical and Surgical Management
7 Exercise Prescription and Programming
8 Nutrition and Weight Management
9 Human Behavior and Counseling
10 Safety, Injury Prevention, and Emergency Procedures
11 Program Administration, Quality Assurance, and Outcome Assessment

This chapter provides information to help guide your work with clients. To do so, the chapter introduces behavior change theories, gives examples of research applications of each theory, and provides amples of how to apply the theoretical principles to your work with your clients. (Readers should also consult Chapter 44 because the theories that are mentioned in this chapter are also covered there, and Chapter 44 provides even more practical applications for working with clients.)

THE IMPORTANCE OF THEORIES

Physical activity is a complex behavior that involves many steps and a series of skills to adopt and maintain. It is impossible to consider all possible influences on physical activity; therefore, psychological theories and models of behavior change can be important to help guide both research and clinical practice[1]. Theories provide a framework for understanding the process through which a complex behavior, such as physical activity, changes and is sustained over time. Theories can also provide guidance to practitioners in helping people make behavior changes by understanding the connection between theo-

ries and results[1]. Theories can help provide techniques and shed light on potential pitfalls in becoming more physically active.

This chapter provides an overview of the theories that have been applied to help understand and guide changes in physical activity behavior in healthy and clinical populations[1,2]. The theories covered in this chapter include the stages of change for motivational readiness (or the transtheoretical model), decision-making theory, social-cognitive theory, health belief model (HBM), social ecology theory, theories of reasoned action and planned behavior, and relapse prevention model. The theories were selected for this chapter based on their clinical and research applications. Each of these theories has been applied to studies of physical activity determinants, as well as in studying other health behavior changes[1]. Some of the theories (e.g., social cognitive theory [SCT]) have more predictive utility than other theories (e.g., theory of reasoned action [TRA])[3]. Although we acknowledge that there may be some theories that are not included in this review (e.g., health action process approach)[4], the theories addressed in this chapter are ones that have been applied most often in relation to physical activity[1,2]. For an additional overview of these models, please see the books by Marcus and Forsyth, *Motivating People to Be Physically Active*[5], and Sallis and Owen, *Physical Activity and Behavioral Medicine*[1]. The first part of each subsection provides a general overview of each theory followed by research applications of the theory.

INCORPORATING THEORY-BASED TECHNIQUES AND PRINCIPLES INTO WORK WITH CLIENTS

A large body of research addresses the importance of using theory to help guide individuals through behavior changes. Although not all theories or aspects of theories can be applied to all individuals at a given time, theories can be helpful in designing an intervention and in selecting evaluation measures at the time you are assessing the patient's progress. The approach can incorporate such considerations as a clients' readiness for change, the environment in which they live, and their social context.

THE IMPORTANCE OF UNDERSTANDING THE PRINCIPLES OF BEHAVIOR CHANGE

It may be a challenge to directly apply research findings while working in community settings, cardiac rehabilitation facilities, school settings, as a personal trainer, or as an exercise physiologist. Therefore, the last part of each subsection provides a clinical application, which essentially transfers the research findings and applies them to real-world examples that a practitioner might encounter in working with clients.

Theories of Behavior Change

THE STAGE OF MOTIVATIONAL READINESS FOR CHANGE MODEL

The stages of motivational readiness for change model (SOC), or the transtheoretical model (TTM), consists of numerous components, including the **stages of change** and **processes of change**. In addition, components of other theories are used in conjunction with the SOC model. These examples include decisional balance from decision making theory[6], and self-efficacy, which is a key concept of SCT[7], both of which are described in detail in other sections of the chapter.

Stages

The SOC model postulates that individuals move through a series of stages and face common barriers when making behavior changes and that intervention approaches may vary by the client's identified stage of change[8]. Several researchers have applied this model to individuals adopting and maintaining physical activity (e.g., Dunn et al.[9]; Marcus et al.[10]). The stages include precontemplation, contemplation, preparation, action, and maintenance (see GETP7 Box 7-2 and Figure 7-7). The precontemplation

stage includes individuals who are inactive and not thinking about becoming active. Individuals in the contemplation stage are inactive but are thinking about becoming active. The preparation stage includes individuals who are physically active but not at the recommended levels (30 minutes or more of moderate intensity physical activity on most, preferably all, days of the week[2,11]). The action stage includes individuals who are physically active at the recommended levels but have been active at this level for less than 6 months. Individuals in the maintenance stage are physically active at the recommended levels and have been for more than 6 months.

The movement across stages may be conceptualized as cyclical rather than linear given that it takes many individuals numerous attempts before successfully adopting and maintaining physical activity. A self-report four-item questionnaire is available to identify an individual's stage of change, including such statements as, "I intend to become more physically active in the next 6 months," and "I currently engage in regular physical activity"[5,12] (see Chapter 44 for the measure and scoring information).

Processes of Change

The SOC model also posits that individuals use a variety of processes of change as they progress through the stages. Five behavioral and five cognitive processes have been identified[10]. The behavioral processes include rewarding yourself (e.g., doing something nice for yourself when achieving a physical activity goal), substituting alternatives (e.g., participating in physical activity to decrease fatigue and increase energy), committing yourself (e.g., making promises to be physically active), reminding yourself (e.g., posting reminders to be physically active at work), and enlisting social support (e.g., having someone to depend on when having problems sticking with a physical activity program). Cognitive processes include being aware of risks (e.g., thinking that physical inactivity can be harmful), increasing knowledge (e.g., thinking about physical activity information obtained from articles), comprehending benefits (e.g., believing that physical activity would make one healthy), increasing healthy opportunities (e.g., awareness of physical activity programs), and caring about consequences to others (e.g., wondering how inactivity affects family and friends). The use of cognitive processes typically peaks in the preparation stage, and the use of the behavioral processes typically peaks in the action stage. A self-report 40-item measure has been developed to assess the 10 processes of change (see Marcus and Forsyth[5] and Marcus et al.[10]).

A recent meta-analysis of the processes of change for physical activity[13] highlighted some interesting results. In general, the results indicated that all 10 processes of change are used across the stages when individuals are actively making behavior changes. They found that the cognitive processes of change peaked in action, and the behavioral processes peaked during maintenance. Additionally, the transition from precontemplation to contemplation and from preparation to action was marked by the sharpest increases in the use of behavioral processes.

INTEGRATING THE COMPONENTS OF THE STAGES OF MOTIVATIONAL READINESS FOR CHANGE MODEL

Although some of the components of the SOC model can be examined separately, research and practice applications are most effective when combining the different components. Therefore, a summary of the research findings that integrate the different aspects of the model and practice applications for integrating the model are presented below.

Research Findings

An excellent example of research that is guided by the theoretical framework of the SOC is a study by Marcus et al[14]. This study used information that was targeted and information that was tailored to the individual. Targeting refers to defining and intervening with a subgroup of the population based on one common characteristic (e.g., gender)[15]. Targeting assumes that individuals have similar enough characteristics to be influenced by the same message[15]. Alternatively, tailoring incorporates a higher level of specificity, and interventions that are tailored use information on characteristics unique to an individual person[15].

Marcus et al[14]. randomly assigned sedentary individuals ($n = 194$) to an intervention targeted to stage of change and tailored to other theory-based constructs believed to be important for behavior change or to a standard treatment group not targeted to stage of change. The tailored group reported a significantly greater number of physical activity minutes per week than individuals in the nontailored self-help group at 6 months. This increase in

physical activity minutes was also maintained at the 12-month follow-up[16].

Practice Applications

To follow is a summary of strategies to help individuals increase or maintain physical activity, based on the SOC model. One way to integrate the different components is to provide different types of intervention strategies depending on an individual's stage of change, although there may be some overlap across the stages. (For further information, see Chapter 44.)

Precontemplation

The precontemplation stage includes individuals who are not active and are not thinking about becoming active. Therefore, the goal for this stage is for the individual to begin thinking about physical activity. The pros and cons of becoming physically active should be discussed with the individual. Specifically, the individual should write down what the benefits of physical activity would be in addition to the disadvantages of physical activity. Specific barriers to physical activity should also be assessed such as lack of time, lack of energy, environmental constraints (e.g., lack of access to physical activity facilities), and fear of injury.

Another important behavioral strategy for this stage is goal setting. For example, a stage-appropriate goal for this stage would be set aside time for reading a pamphlet about physical activity to learn more about the benefits of regular physical activity. You might want to have your client think about how personally relevant these benefits are for her. Another strategy for working with a client who is in this stage is to have your client write down her reasons for not being physically active and what gets in her way. The goal for an individual in the precontemplation stage is to start thinking about becoming physically active. Evidence suggests that an individual in precontemplation can progress in the stage of change. For instance, studies have shown that 65% of individuals who were provided stage-targeted information progressed one or more stages[17].

Contemplation

The contemplation stage includes individuals who are not physically active but are thinking about becoming active. The aim for this stage is for the individual to begin taking steps to become physically active and to think about setting goals. Individuals in this stage should also weigh the pros and cons of physical activity as well as read materials describing how to start a physical activity program. The individual can then make specific physical activity goals after he decides on which physical activity he would most prefer. Personal preference for specific activities as well as positive experience with certain activities should be considered when developing a program. For example, if a person has found walking to be an enjoyable activity because she is able to spent time with her husband, then a walking program that incorporates planned time with her husband would be an effective incentive for this person. The individual should also implement a reinforcement program in that he rewards himself for meeting his specific physical activity goals. Because research indicates that social support is important for becoming physically active (e.g., Tessaro et al.[18]), individuals might identify one or two people who could be supportive and enlist their support for starting and maintaining a physical activity program.

Preparation

The preparation stage includes individuals who are currently engaging in some physical activity but not at the recommended level[5,10]. The goal for this stage is to increase physical activity behavior to the recommended level. Specifically, the goal is to engage in physical activity of at least moderate intensity on most, preferably all, days of the week for 30 minutes or more each day. Several of the strategies used in the previous stages can also be used in this stage, including weighing the pros and cons of physical activity, choosing an appropriate physical activity program, and implementing a reinforcement schedule. Identifying and overcoming the barriers that prevent the individual from increasing their physical activity to the recommended level is the key for this stage. Goal setting can play an instrumental role in gradually increasing physical activity to the intended level. At this stage, self-monitoring of physical activity also becomes very important. Specifically, the individual could be encouraged to join an exercise group and keep a physical activity log in which the type of activity, intensity, and duration are documented.

Action

The action stage includes individuals who are physically active at the recommended level but have been for less than 6 months. The goal of this stage is to continue to make physical activity a regular part of the client's life. Important strategies for this stage include setting up a plan for self-monitoring physical activity and making short-term goals (e.g., "I will walk on Monday, Wednesday and Friday after work with my coworkers and then walk on Saturday and Sunday with my husband"). In addition, it might be helpful to suggest that your client try a new activity or find a walking or running race that is going to take place in the future for which your client can train. Talking with your client about relapse prevention (discussed later in this chapter) is also very useful at this stage.

Maintenance

The maintenance stage includes individuals who have been physically active at the recommended level and have been for 6 or more months. The goal for this stage is to

prepare for future setbacks and to continue to increase enjoyment for physical activity. Therefore, some of the same suggestions that apply to individuals in the action stage will also apply to individuals in the maintenance phase. It is important to continue to help your clients find ways to avoid boredom, either by trying out new activities or by enlisting social support (e.g., walking with a neighbor). Also, it might be helpful to have your clients reflect on the benefits they have already achieved from physical activity because as these might be powerful rewards.

DECISION-MAKING THEORY

Decision-making theory postulates that individuals decide whether to engage in a particular behavior based on their comparison of the perceived benefits versus the perceived costs of the behavior[6]. Specifically, individuals are more likely to be physically active if they perceive that the benefits (e.g., sleeping better) outweigh the costs (e.g., time lost to other activities[1,6]). **Decisional balance** is another important component that is used in conjunction with the SOC model[19]. Research has shown that in later stages of motivational readiness for behavior change (e.g., action, maintenance), individuals perceive more benefits for being physically active. In contrast, individuals who are in earlier stages (e.g., precontemplation) perceive that there are more disadvantages than advantages[19]. An example of an advantage of physical activity is, "I would have more energy for my family and friends if I were regularly physically active," and an example of a disadvantage is, "I think I would be too tired to do my daily work after being physically active." A 16-item self-report measure has been developed to assess decisional balance. Examples of these include: "I would feel more confident if I were regularly physically active" and "Regular physical activity would take up too much of my time"[5,19].

Research Findings

An intervention study of 355 patients participating in a physician-based counseling intervention (intervention $n = 181$; control $n = 174$; mean age, 65.6 years) was conducted[20]. The intervention was based on the SOC and incorporated components of SCT and health education theory. After 6 weeks of intervention, the intervention group had significant changes in decisional balance, self-efficacy, and processes of change. Specifically, individuals increased their view of the benefits of physical activity, were more confident about their ability to perform the behavior, and were using more strategies to assist them in their behavior change. Therefore, intervention studies that are grounded in SOC theory show intermediate changes in variables such as decisional balance.

Practice Implications

The use of decisional balance can be a helpful way to begin to engage participants, particularly those who are in the precontemplation and contemplation stages. The goal of decisional balance is to have a client identify the pros (or the benefits) of being physically active (e.g., sleep better, more energy) and the cons (or the negative aspects) of being physically active (e.g., time constraints, lack of interest). By helping your clients identify the pros and cons, you can assist them by working on increased attention to the pros and minimizing the cons. (Chapter 44 provides a more detailed description on how to assess decisional balance and ways to intervene using this theoretical approach.)

SOCIAL COGNITIVE THEORY

Social cognitive theory has had the most success in its application to changing physical activity behavior[3,7,21]. This model states that behavior change is influenced by the interactions between the environment, personal factors, and the behavior itself[7,21]. This is called the model of reciprocal determinism[21]. Components of this model are shown in Figure 39-1.

Self-efficacy

An important construct of SCT is **self-efficacy**. Self-efficacy is one's beliefs about his or her capabilities to exercise control over particular or specified life events.[7] For example, someone with high self-efficacy for physical activity would endorse having the confidence to continue to exercise despite barriers (e.g., bad weather). Efficacy beliefs influence health behavior choices in that people tend to pursue tasks that they feel competent to perform and avoid those about which they feel incompetent[21,22]. The most commonly measured and cited type of self-efficacy, barriers self-efficacy, is related to the level of effort and

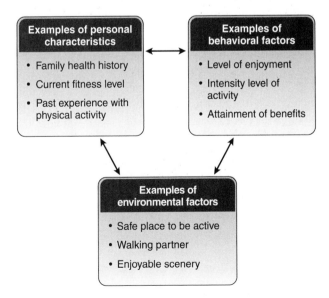

FIGURE 39-1. Reciprocal determinism. (Adapted with permission from Marcus BH, Forsyth LH: Motivating People to be Physically Active. Champaign, IL: Human Kinetics; 2003.)

persistence expended when faced with adverse situations or barriers to attaining the desired outcome. Self-efficacy to perform the behavior itself (e.g., how confident are you that you can walk 30 minutes five times per week) has also been measured. Research indicates that self-efficacy level predicts participation in physical activity promotion programs[23,24].

Differences in self-efficacy have been found for individuals in different stages of change[25,26]. Cross-sectional studies indicate that as the stages of change progress from precontemplation to maintenance, a corresponding increase in self-efficacy for physical activity takes place. A five-item self-report measure has been developed to examine self-efficacy for physical activity in different situations (e.g., feeling fatigued, inclement weather; see Marcus and Forsyth[5] and Marcus et al.[25]).

Bandura[21] has listed the four influences on self-efficacy as performance of mastery experiences, vicarious experiences, verbal persuasion regarding one's capabilities, and inferences from physiological and affective responses. The two that are discussed in this chapter are performance accomplishments and vicarious experience. The sense of efficacy that arises from performance accomplishments is based on personal mastery experiences. That is, success increases feelings of mastery, which, in turn, promotes the behavior and increases the likelihood of setting new and more challenging goals. Also, setting smaller, accomplishable goals helps a person feel more confident (or self-efficacious) and helps build more challenging goals. Personal experience is the strongest influence on feelings of self-efficacy. For example, if a person is able to be physically active again after an illness, he or she should have a resulting increase in self-efficacy.

The second influence on self-efficacy, vicarious experience or modeling, involves improvements in self-efficacy caused by observing others perform the activity (e.g., watching a demonstration or video). Individuals increase their self-efficacy by observing others succeed at being physically active. This type of efficacy expectation is of particular interest in group sessions: if one participant is doing extraordinarily well, this can improve the self-efficacy of the others and further motivate them. For example, in a cardiac rehabilitation setting, if one patient is doing well with her physical activity program, then this might serve to increase the self-efficacy of others in that setting.

Outcome Expectations

Another important SCT construct is **outcome expectations**, which refers to the potential results that one anticipates after performing a particular behavior[7]. This distinction is exemplified in that an individual can anticipate or understand that exercise will have positive health consequences (e.g., more energy) yet not have the self-efficacy to execute the behavior (e.g., exercise regularly to accrue benefits). As would be expected, the extent to which individuals perceive they will be able to perform a behavior is related to the outcomes they anticipate. Three major forms of outcome expectations have been identified: positive and negative physical effects, positive and negative social effects, and positive and negative self-evaluative reactions to the change in behavior[21]. Within each major form, positive expectations function as incentives and the negative expectations function as disincentives toward making behavior change.

Self-regulatory Strategies

Self-regulation is the ability to mobilize oneself to perform a behavior regularly in the face of a variety of personal, situational, or social barriers. Bandura[7] states that the major process of self-regulation includes self-monitoring, proximal goal setting, strategy development, and self-motivating incentives. A person's self-regulatory efficacy is crucial for adherence to a behavior such as exercise in that those with low self-regulatory efficacy tend to drop out of programs more quickly and are less able to exercise at the intensity, duration, and frequency needed to accrue health benefits.

According to Bandura, goals do not directly regulate motivation and action. Instead, self-efficacy beliefs influence people's choices of goals and persistence of behavior when they face challenges and obstacles[21]. Goals provide direction and reference points against which people can monitor their progress[22]. Through self-monitoring, people can develop efficacy beliefs about their current level of competence and expectancies regarding their rate of improvement[27]. Bandura[7] states that goal specificity, challenge, and proximity are the most important qualities of goals to enhance motivation and persistence.

Research Findings

Several studies have examined the efficacy of SCT-based interventions (e.g., Trost et al.[3]). The majority of research has examined only the SCT construct of self-efficacy; therefore, research on self-efficacy is the primary focus of this section.

As already mentioned, SCT incorporates personal influences, cognitions, and environmental factors as variables that influence each other as well as influence behavior[4]. Hofstetter et al.[28] investigated correlates of exercise self-efficacy to study the extent to which childhood experience with exercise would affect exercise self-efficacy later in life. They found that environmental variables (e.g., barriers to exercise, the availability of home equipment, facilities), cognitive variables (e.g., benefits and barriers, normative beliefs), and social variables (e.g., social support) all influenced self-efficacy. Therefore, this research supports the notion that self-efficacy is malleable and can be influenced by additional factors such as the context in which the individual is located.

A more recent study[29] was conducted to examine the effect of walking and stretching or toning on changes in self-efficacy in 174 previously sedentary older adults (mean age, 65.5 years). Results indicated that there was a nonsignificant increase in barriers self-efficacy from baseline to month 2, which declined at montsh 4 and 6. For exercise self-efficacy, there was a reported decline in efficacy over the four time points (week 2, month 2, month 4, and month 6). It is interesting that efficacy cognitions declined in the context of an exercise intervention rather than increased. These results highlight the temporal relationship of self-efficacy and show that it can vary during the course of an exercise program. The authors conclude that it is important to target different sources of efficacy information (e.g., one's beliefs about exercise such as "I might become injured if I exercise" or the barriers related to exercise such as not having enough time or the weather, which might have implications for the long-term maintenance of physical activity). One area that may be important to target is assessing feelings of confidence and working to build self-efficacy at the end of a program to help individuals maintain their behavior changes.

Practice Implications

The research findings cited above underscore the importance of helping clients make intermediate steps towards behavior change. Some of these intermediate steps include increasing self-efficacy, learning how to set goals, planning for physical activity, and having realistic expectations for behavior change. Chapter 44 gives more examples of incorporating SCT principles when working with your clients.

Self-efficacy is a powerful component of SCT, and it can be influenced in two primary ways: performance accomplishments and vicarious experience or modeling[30]. Thus, one way for SCT to be applied to clinical practice is to assist clients in improving their self-efficacy. Someone who has had a cardiac event might learn to make exercise a part of his life by watching others like himself participate in cardiac rehabilitation. Another way to help a person increase her self-efficacy is to set small goals and "try out" activities. Therefore, for someone who does not exercise, the strategy might be to have her begin to walk for 2 minutes at a time. As soon as this client begins to feel confident with the short duration of a walking bout, her self-efficacy is likely to increase, and then she might have the confidence to walk for an even longer distance.

An outcome expectation is a person's belief that certain behaviors will lead to specific outcomes. Therefore, another way to assist your clients in becoming more physically active is to work on developing realistic expectations of physical activity behavior change. For example, it might be helpful to educate your client about the short-term benefits of being physically active (e.g., having more energy, sleeping better), as well as some of the long-term benefits (e.g., prevention of cardiovascular disease). In addition, many people have an outcome expectation that significant weight loss will result from being physically active. In order to establish realistic outcome expectations, it might be important to talk with your client about the synergy between physical activity and diet, in that dietary changes in conjunction with physical activity are usually necessary for weight changes.

HEALTH BELIEF MODEL

The HBM was designed to explain and predict why people engage in preventive health practices[31,32]. Generally, the HBM hypothesizes that the extent to which individuals engage in a health action is determined by their readiness to take action coupled with their belief of the threat of not taking action. There are four main components of the HBM that serve to explain a system of beliefs individuals hold while attempting to avoid disease. The components are (a) the person perceives being susceptible to a particular disease; (b) the consequences of the disease appear serious enough to warrant action; (c) there are benefits to taking action; and (d) there would not be insurmountable barriers such as cost, inconvenience, pain, or embarrassment associated with taking action[31,33]. In 1984, Janz and Becker[34] modified the HBM to incorporate self-efficacy into the barriers component of the HBM, which some researchers have suggested as a positive move because it places limits on the barriers dimension, which tended to be a "catch-all" category, and it suggests more areas for future research[32].

Research Findings

The HBM has not received as much consistent research support as have the SCT and SOC models[1]. However, some evidence has been found for the use of the HBM in predicting health actions. For example, the HBM has been used to predict compliance with a cardiac rehabilitation program. Oldridge and Streiner[35] found that after a 6-month exercise rehabilitation program for cardiac patients, the only difference in HBM factors between individuals who complied and those who dropped out (52% dropout rate) was that the compilers had greater scores on perceived severity. Other components of the HBM also have provided predictive usefulness. For example, two studies of postsurgery coronary artery disease patients found that a significant portion of the variance in exercise compliance was accounted for by the concept of perceived barriers (financial costs, side effects)[36,37]. Another study investigated which components of the HBM were associated with attendance at a supervised exercise program for the prevention, detection, and treatment of coronary heart disease. General health motivation and perceived severity of cardiovascular disease were associated with attendance at the program. However, perceived benefits were negatively associated, with higher benefits reported being associated with lower attendance rates[38]. Therefore, overall, the HBM has not received consistent support as a useful model for intervention studies of physical activity, although subcomponents of the model have shown potential utility.

Practice Implications

It may be useful for practitioners to assess the components of the HBM in working with their clients[32]. One way to do this is to first assess the educational needs of your clients. Is your client interested in health matters? Does your client feel susceptible to serious health problems? Does your client believe threat could be reduced by engaging in preventive health practices? Does your client believe that there are major barriers to making behavior changes? These needs assessments are important for understanding clients' perceptions of risk and their likelihood of engaging in and maintaining preventive health behaviors. It is important for the practitioner to ask these types of questions in order to better understand the perceptions and beliefs that are held by their clients. For instance, the practitioner may think that, given a client's family history of cardiovascular disease and the client's own individual risk factors, the client is susceptible to developing some form of cardiovascular disease. However, without assessing the client's own perceptions, the practitioner would not know if the client held these same beliefs, which might influence the strength and conviction with which a person would opt to make behavior changes. There has been little intervention research on the HBM in healthy populations. It appears that the HBM has most of its utility for understanding the beliefs that clients hold and for helping them set goals based on their health beliefs.

SOCIAL ECOLOGY THEORY

Social ecology theory underscores the importance of the constant interaction between an individual's behavior and his or her environment. This model emphasizes social, institutional, and cultural contexts as they relate to an individual's health. It is this interaction between the environment (e.g., geographic, architectural, technological features) as well as sociocultural factors that influence one's health and health choices. The assumption of this model is that human health and behavior change are a dynamic process such that both the physical and the social environment influence the healthfulness of a situation and the individual embedded in that situation. For example, many workplaces are designed in a way that limits physical activity. In some workplaces, the elevators are centrally located and the stairs are difficult to find and tend to be less well maintained. Thus, for an individual to try to accumulate lifestyle activity, he or she must make an extra effort to seek out the stairs. These environmental factors, such as workplace design, are also mediated by personal factors such as genetics, temperament, and behavioral patterns of the individual[39]. For example, someone who has a history of cardiovascular disease in her family may be more likely to seek out the stairs in this example because she knows the health importance of accumulating bouts of physical activity throughout the day.

TABLE 39-1. Examples of the Ecological Model

| | | Physical Environmental Factors | |
| | | Natural Environment | Built Environment |
Intrapersonal Factors	Interpersonal Factors		
Demographics (e.g., age, race or ethnicity)	Supportive behaviors (e.g., friends or family encouraging activity)	Weather (e.g., temperature, precipitation)	Urban or suburban environment (e.g., crime, safety)
Personal barriers (e.g., lack of time, lack of energy)	Perceptions of community leaders (e.g., incentives and policies, crime, traffic, access to trails, parks)	Geography (e.g., hills)	Architectural environment (e.g., sidewalks, lighting)
Participant perceptions about the environment (e.g., hills, safety, traffic, access to trails, parks)	Participant ratings of policies governing incentives (e.g., time during workday to exercise)		Transportation environment (e.g., traffic)
	Participants ratings of policies governing resources and infrastructure (e.g., requiring physical education in schools)		Recreation infrastructure (e.g., trails, parks)

Adapted with permission from Sallis JF, Owen N: Physical Activity and Behavioral Medicine. Thousand Oaks, CA: Sage Publications; 1999.

Social ecology emphasizes multiple influences on behavior and suggests that the most successful programs are the ones that combine and target these multiple influences on behavior. Therefore, it is important to develop individual skills for changing behavior as well as having physical environments and policies that are supportive of physical activity. Examples of the components of social ecology are represented in Table 39-1.

Research Findings

Researchers postulate that to maximize the efficacy of interventions, programs need to combine environmental components with individual and community-based physical activity promotion efforts[40]. There are numerous advantages of multilevel interventions with behavioral and environmental components, including the potential to be more efficacious for improving public health[39,40].

Intrapersonal

Intrapersonal factors related to physical activity have been researched extensively. Some examples of these factors are demographic factors (e.g., age, gender, race, health status), personal barriers (e.g., motivation level, childcare), cognitive perceptions (e.g., perceived lack of time, self-efficacy), and behavioral factors[39].

Some recent population-based, cross-sectional studies have examines correlations among perceived environmental and policy variables and physical activity behavior[40,41]. These studies have found that the intrapersonal barriers that were inversely related to physical activity included having too little time, being too tired, lacking energy, lacking motivation, having less education, and not liking physical activity (also see Chapter 42).

Interpersonal

To a lesser degree, interpersonal factors have begun to be researched. Interpersonal factors such as one's living area (where many people exercise), friends who encouraged exercise, and having at least one friend with whom to exercise have been shown to be related to physical activity[41]. Similarly, another study[42] found the infrequent observation of others exercising in one's neighborhood was associated with inactivity. Additionally, policy factors were examined in relation to physical activity, and most of the respondents were supportive of these policy approaches[41]. For example, 71% of respondents believed the employers should provide time during the workday for employees to exercise, and 95% believed physical education should be required in schools. The policy variables that were positively associated with physical activity were believing one's employer should provide time for exercise and supporting the use of local government funds for walking and jogging trials.

Physical Environment

The relationships between environmental settings and support for physical activity are not as well understood as personal, cognitive, social, and physiological barriers[43]. Older adults in Australia ($n = 449$) were interviewed and asked a series of questions related to physical activity behavior, social cognitive, and perceived environmental factors[43]. This study found that the presence of paths that are safe for walking and access to facilities such as recreation centers, gym, or parks were associated with being more physically active[41] Respondents who reported engaging in some physical activity reported that they were active in the following locations: 66% on neighborhood streets, 37% at shopping malls, 30% at parks, 25% on walking and jogging trials, 25% on treadmills, and 21% at indoor gyms. When the environmental variables were examined in relation to physical activity behavior, access to parks, indoor gyms, and treadmills was associated with physical activity behavior. Neighborhood characteristics such as the presence of sidewalks, enjoyable scenery, heavy traffic (which may relate to higher levels of activity in urban than suburban areas), and hills were positively associated with physical activity. In the King et al.[42] study, lack of hills in one's neighborhood and absence of enjoyable scenery were associated with inactivity.

Research in the areas of environmental factors and physical activity has largely been cross-sectional in nature and has assessed perceived environmental barriers. This information can be useful for understanding the social and environmental contexts in which individuals live and are physically active.

Practice Implications

Social ecology has been shown to be most effective on a larger scale than what might be possible when working with individuals. However, understanding clients' social and physical environments can help you to work with them toward maximizing their activity. To help clients make behavior changes, it is important to assist them in understanding that numerous factors can be related to physical activity behavior. For instance, many people might not recognize that their environment can function as a facilitator or a barrier to making behavior changes. Therefore, it may be helpful to point out ways that individuals can work within the parameters of their neighborhoods or social structures. For example, someone may need to seek out a park or other recreational facility in his neighborhood if an adequate place to walk is not in close proximity to his home or work. It may also be important for someone to find social support to walk in a neighborhood or to start a walking group that meets at the local school track on an appointed day and time each week. Finally, building awareness of policies related to creating physical activity friendly environments can be an important factor from an advocacy perspective. For instance, there may be local advocacy and campaigns regarding the construction of bike lanes and sidewalks. These proposals, although also improving the aesthetics of one's environment, also serve to create physical activity friendly environments. Finally, individuals should be empowered to begin working with local transportation departments in their communities, as well as schools, community organizations, and public works groups to increase the availability and accessibility of programs and physical activity opportunities.

THE THEORY OF REASONED ACTION

The TRA was developed as a way of understanding and predicting an individual's behavior[44,45]. For the purposes of this theory, the behavior must be clearly specified, volitional in nature, and performed in a specific situation. This theory postulates that a person who believes that a given behavior will result in a positive outcome will most likely hold a favorable attitude toward performing that behavior. According to the TRA, intention is the sole and immediate predictor of behavior[44], and intention mediates the effect of attitude toward the behavior and the subjective normative beliefs (NBs) toward the behavior[46–48].

There has been limited support of the TRA when applied to physical activity[1,3,49]. To date, it has been found that the basic variables in this model only account for a fraction of the variance in exercise behavior[49]. Also, the TRA has been found to be most useful[50,51] when behaviors are completely under volitional control, meaning no practical constraints or barriers to executing the behavior are present. It has been shown that for exercise, perceived barriers are variables that influence exercise intention and behavior[24,25], which may help to explain the lack of support of the TRA within the physical activity literature. To account for perceived limitations or barriers[50,51], developed the theory of planned behavior (TPB), which includes a measure of perceived behavioral control.

THE THEORY OF PLANNED BEHAVIOR

The TPB[52] is an extension of the TRA that includes perceived behavioral control as a third exogenous variable. Perceived behavioral control is similar to the concept of self-efficacy[30,53] because it reflects one's belief as to the likelihood of difficulty to be encountered when adopting a particular behavior and the perceived availability of resources and opportunities that may be beneficial in adopting a particular behavior. It has been stated that the TPB is most useful for describing behaviors that are entirely under volitional control, or ones with no perceived barriers present[50,51]. Alternatively, a lack of control exists when adoption of the behavior requires opportunities, resources, or skills that are not readily available to the individual. Intuitively, most behaviors (including exercise) fall somewhere on the continuum between total control to complete lack of control[44,54]. A representation of this model is:

Attitude
Subjective norm ⟶ Behavioral intention ⟶ Behavior
Perceived behavioral control

Thus, perceived behavioral control has a direct and indirect (through behavioral intention) effect on behavior. The theory postulates that perceived behavioral control can affect behavioral intention through motivation. The TPB also proposes that individuals intend to perform a behavior if they evaluate it positively, believe that others think it is important, and perceive the behavior to be under their control[51].

Research Findings

Although research has indicated that the inclusion of perceived behavioral control as an exogenous variable enhances the prediction of intentions and target behaviors[52], the research applying the TRA and the TPB to physical activity has been limited. Most of the studies to date have tended to combine or compare the efficacy of the two theories rather than directly test their predictive utility[1,3].

In a literature review of studies on the predictive utility of the TRA and TPB for exercise between the years 1980 and 1995, Blue[55] cited 16 studies that used the TRA and seven studies that used the TRB. Cross-sectional designs were used most frequently, and the majority of studies conducted used young, healthy middle-aged adults. Findings from this review indicate that the TRB was better than the TRA for predicting exercise behavior. According to Blue[55], this was because the TPB has more predictive qualities for exercise intention and the TPB does not assume that the exercise behavior is entirely under the volitional control of the individual. Blue does state, however, that this finding should be interpreted with caution because of the limited number of studies in this area. These findings are consistent with more recent meta-analyses, which have found perceived behavioral control to be associated with exercise behavior[47,48].

Godin et al.[56] conducted two similar studies in different populations to evaluate the utility of the construct of perceived behavioral control for predicting exercising behavior in a group of healthy adults (130 men and 217 women) and in 136 pregnant women. The pertinent TPB variables (i.e., exercise behavior, intention, attitude, subjective social norm, and perceived behavioral control) were measured in both samples. The healthy adults were followed for 6 months after initial assessments, and the pregnant women were followed 8 to 9 months after baseline, at which time they completed behavioral measures to assess how many times within that time-frame they had engaged in one or more physical activities for at least 20 minutes per session. Structural equation modeling was used to analyze the data. For the healthy adults, results indicate that intention to exercise directly influenced exercise behavior. Perceived behavioral control influenced exercise behavior only through the effects it had on intention. For the pregnant women, none of the TPB constructs were associated with exercising behavior. These two studies provide mixed support for utility of using the TPB for predicting exercise behavior.

A more recent study[57] examined the utility of the TPB for understanding exercise adherence during phase II cardiac rehabilitation. In this study, 215 patients completed questionnaires that included TBP constructs before beginning phase II cardiac rehabilitation. The results of this study indicated that the TBP constructs of attitude, subjective norm, and perceived behavioral control accounted for 30% of the variance in exercise intention. Exercise intention accounted for 12% of the variance in explaining exercise adherence (i.e., number of sessions prescribed divided by the number of sessions attended). Although this study provided some support for the predictive utility of the TBP for use in understanding adherence to cardiac rehabilitation, overall, the model only accounted for a small portion (12%) of the variance in explaining exercise behavior.

The results of the present studies have indicated mixed findings with respect to the usefulness of the TRA or TPB in the area of intervening on exercise behaviors, with estimates of intentions contributing at most 30% of the variance in exercise behaviors. The TRA and TPB have provided some theoretical information for understanding health behaviors, such as exercise, and the postulated relationships between the variables have been supported[47,48]. The theories, however, are limited in their applicability to interventions related to changing physical activity behavior. Intentions may be an important prerequisite for exercise adoption, but they are not solely sufficient for predicting regular physical activity. In sum, the TRA and TPB intuitively have some merit but have limitations in their application for the field of exercise adoption and maintenance.

PRACTICE APPLICATIONS

Although the research findings relating to the TRA and TPB have been mixed, components of these theories may be useful for assisting clients in making changes in their physical activity. For instance, in helping a client make behavior change, many times the first step is to understand the framework under which the individual is operating. For example, it is helpful to understand clients' attitudes toward physical activity, the value that they and other people in their lives place on physical activity, and their sense or belief that they have control over the behavior. It is possible that a client may hold certain beliefs towards exercise (e.g., "I have never been athletic, so I can't exercise") or their family members may not understand the importance of being physically active and, therefore, not value it, which may negatively impact your client. By assessing these factors initially, the practitioner can help anticipate potential barriers and help the client problem solve to address those barriers.

Additionally, an important component of the TPB is perceived behavioral control, which is similar to the concept of self-efficacy. The methods for helping clients improve their self-efficacy are similar to those that could be used for helping them increase their sense of perceived behavioral control. For instance, clients could be encouraged to think about the realistic barriers they might encounter when making behavior changes and about the resources available to them for helping overcome those barriers. An example is a client who thinks she does not have a safe place to exercise. The practitioner could help the client think about other options for overcoming this barrier, including finding a walking "buddy," finding a mall in which to walk indoors, or finding other locations (e.g., a YMCA).

RELAPSE PREVENTION

The **relapse prevention (RP)** model was developed to help understand relapse behavior in individuals who were seeking to remain abstinent from a negative health behavior (e.g., smoking, drinking). However, the components of the relapse prevention model can be applied to other health behaviors, such as at the beginning of a physical activity program. The overall goal of RP is to assist individuals in maintaining long term behavior change by anticipating potentially high-risk situations and devising strategies to cope with these high-risk situations[5,58]. The RP model is a combination of behavioral skills training, cognitive intervention, and lifestyle change. therefore, it is an important model for use with physical activity behavior maintenance. The RP model makes two very important distinctions in defining the terms lapse and relapse. Whereas *lapse* is defined as a slight error or slip (e.g., missing one exercise session) *relapse* is a return to former behavior patterns (e.g., not being physically active for an extended period of time).

The RP model cautions against viewing behavior change as either a complete success or a failure. This dichotomous approach ignores the potential influence of situational and psychological factors as determinants in relapse and reinforces the idea that someone who experiences a relapse lacks personal control[58]. Furthermore, establishing the dichotomy of success (e.g., exercising 5 days per week for 30 minutes each time) or failure (e.g., not exercising at all) can also set up an individual for a "abstinence violation effect," which is one's tendency to give up if even a small slip has occurred. For instance, if someone has missed her exercise sessions for the week due to work demands, she may think, "Why should I bother now? I am already out of my routine." Instead, the RP model encourages people to view a lapse as a "fork in the road"[58] that could either lead back to successful behavior maintenance or a return to earlier behavior patterns. For example, someone would be using relapse prevention strategies if he or she thought in advance about a high-risk situation such as a vacation and devised a plan for exercising during the vacation (i.e., locating a walking path near the hotel).

Research Findings

Although many experts cite the importance of relapse prevention strategies for helping individuals maintain behavior changes, little research has focused specifically on relapse prevention for *physical activity*. A large body of literature focuses on relapse prevention for weight loss[59]; however, for physical activity, the focuses on relapse pre-

vention tends to be incorporated with a variety of other strategies. One study investigated the use of relapse prevention to promote exercise adherence among 120 women who were previously sedentary[60]. In this study, subjects were randomly assigned to either a control group or one of two experimental groups (relapse prevention or reinforcement/lottery); all groups participated in an 18-week exercise program. The relapse prevention group consisted of focusing on potential high-risk situations, developing coping responses, and using a planned relapse. The reinforcement group consisted of rewarding participants for consistent attendance. Results indicated that compared with the control group, the relapse prevention group attended significantly more sessions during the first 9 weeks of the program; the reinforcement group was not significantly different from the control group ($P < 0.01$). However, by 18 weeks and at the 2-month post-treatment assessment, there were no differences between the groups. Marcus and Stanton[60] cite some potential considerations when examining the relapse prevention approach for physical activity. They state that factors such as the convenience of class schedule, group cohesion, and the strength of the intervention may have been mitigating factors to help explain the lack of longer term efficacy of the relapse prevention approach.

Practice Implications

Relapse prevention is an important aspect of any behavior change program. Marlatt and Gordon[58] stress the importance of establishing a collaborative relationship with the client and focusing on using a few techniques at a time rather than trying to incorporate all techniques at once. The research of Marcus and Stanton[60] provides an excellent framework for practitioners who are working with clients trying to maintain physical activity behavior change. The RP model has a series of strategies that can be used by clients to learn how to anticipate and cope with the possibility of relapse. For instance, the first stage helps clients reflect on the importance of regular exercise and the importance of being flexible in their thinking regarding the need to miss a session, if necessary. In addition, the next phase is to work with clients to help them identify situations in which they were able to successfully overcome a potential barrier and the challenges faced when they were not successful. Reflecting a situation in which client were successful can help them understand that they have a skill set, or a "tool-box" of skills that they have successfully engaged in the past.

Next, it is important to teach clients how to identify high-risk situations that may trigger a relapse. It may be helpful in this step to identify some examples of potential relapse situations, which can be combined into two main categories: intrapersonal and interpersonal[40]. Examples of intrapersonal determinants include negative emotional states, negative physical states, and positive emotional states. Interpersonal determinants include social pressure and interpersonal conflict. One intrapersonal state that tends to be common is stress. Clients who have difficulty managing stress should be encouraged to take a walk or do some other physical activity. Even if the client only has 10 minutes in between scheduled meetings during a busy day, a brisk walk can help clear the mind, provide some relaxation, and reduce stress. An interpersonal state that clients might identify is having many demands on their time and feeling unable to devote the time to being physically active. One suggestion that might assist clients with these types of high-risk situations is to see if the client might be able to fit in shorter bouts of activity (e.g., 10 minutes in length three times a day) rather than trying to block out a full 30 minutes each day. By dividing the time into smaller bouts, this can help clients feel like they have more control over ways to "fit in" the activity.

After identifying high-risk situations, the next step is to anticipate those situations, and problem solve around effective coping strategies. Using the example above, you might suggest to a client who has multiple demands that if she is feeling unsure about how to fit in physical activity that she can try to do 10 minutes first thing in the morning, 10 minutes at lunch, and 10 minutes right after dinner. By dividing a longer bout into smaller pieces, this can be an effective coping strategy to address a potential high-risk situation and avoid a relapse. More examples of how to incorporate this model into working with your clients are presented in Chapter 44.

Summary

This chapter has provided an overview of the theories of behavior change that have been applied most successfully to physical activity. This information should be useful for helping to understand the factors that influence the complicated process through which individuals decide to begin and maintain a physical activity program. This chapter has provided you with several theoretical frameworks for understanding the strategies and skills associated with adopting a new behavior and with some ways to help your clients prevent relapse. This chapter also has provided you with the research applications of these theories, as well as practical implications for everyday interactions with individuals wanting to become more physically active. The information provided in this chapter should serve as a reference point for helping individuals become and stay physically active in order to live a healthier lifestyle and prevent disease.

REFERENCES

1. Sallis JF, Owen N: Physical Activity and Behavioral Medicine. Thousand Oaks, CA: Sage Publications; 1999.
2. U.S. Department of Health and Human Services: Physical Activity and Health: A Report of the Surgeon General. Atlanta: U.S. Department of Health and Human Services, Centers for Disease Control and Prevention, National Center for Chronic Disease Prevention and Health Promotion; 1996.
3. Trost SG, Owen N, Bauman AE, et al: Correlates of adults' participation in physical activity: Review and update. Med Sci Sports Exerc 34:1996–2001, 2002.
4. Schwarzer R: Self-efficacy in the adoption and maintenance of health behaviors: Theoretical approaches and a new model (pp. 217–242). In Schwarzer R, ed. Self-efficacy: Thought Control of Action. Washington, DC: Hemisphere; 1992.
5. Marcus BH, Forsyth LH: Motivating People to be Physically Active. Champaign, IL: Human Kinetics; 2003.
6. Janis IL, Mann L: Decision Making: A Psychological Analysis of Conflict, Choice and Commitment. New York: Free Press; 1977.
7. Bandura A: Self-efficacy: The Exercise of Control. New York, NY: W.H. Freeman; 1997.
8. Prochaska JO, DiClemente CC: The stages and processes of self-change in smoking: Towards an integrative model of change. J Consul Clin Psychol 51:390–395, 1983.
9. Dunn AL, Marcus BH, Kampert JB, et al: Reduction in cardiovascular disease risk factors: 6-month results from Project ACTIVE. Prev Med 26, 883–892, 1997.
10. Marcus BH, Rossi JS, Selby VC, et al: The stages and processes of exercise adoption and maintenance in a worksite sample. Health Psychol 11:386–395, 1992.
11. Pate RR, Pratt M, Blair SN, et al: Physical activity and public health: A recommendation from the Centers for Disease Control and Prevention and the American College of Sports Medicine. JAMA 273:402–407, 1995.
12. Marcus BH, Simkin LR: The stages of exercise behavior. J Sports Med Phys Fitness 33:83–88, 1993.
13. Marshall SJ, Biddle SJH: The transtheoretical model of behavior change: a meta-analysis of applications to physical activity and exercise. Ann Behav Med 23:229–246, 2001.
14. Marcus BH, Bock BC, Pinto BM, et al: Efficacy of an individualized, motivationally-tailored physical activity intervention. Ann Behav Med 20:174–180, 1998.
15. Marcus BH, Nigg CR, Riebe D, Forsyth LH: Interactive communication strategies: Implications for population-based physical activity promotion. Am J Prev Med 19:121–126, 2000.
16. Bock BC, Marcus BH, Pinto B, Forsyth L: Maintenance of physical activity following an individualized motivationally-tailored intervention. Ann Behav Med 23:79–87, 2001.
17. Marcus BH, Emmons KM, Simkin-Silverman LR, et al: Evaluation of motivationally tailored vs. standard self-help physical activity interventions at the workplace. Am J Health Promot 12:246–253, 1998.
18. Tessaro I, Campbell M, Benedict S et al: Developing a worksite health promotion intervention: Health works for women. Am J Health Behav 22, 434–442, 1998.
19. Marcus BH, Rakowski W, Rossi RS: Assessing motivational readiness and decision-making for exercise. Health Psychol 11:257–261, 1992.
20. Goldstein MG, Pinto BM, Marcus BH, et al: Physician-based physical activity counseling for middle-aged and older adults: A randomized trial. Ann Behav Med 21:40–47, 1999.
21. Bandura A: Social Foundations of Thought and Action: A Social Cognitive Theory. Englewood Cliffs, NJ: Prentice-Hall; 1986.
22. Maibach EW, Cotton D: Moving people to behavior change. A staged social cognitive approach to message design. In Maibach E, Parrot RL, eds. Designing Health Messages. Approaches from Communication Theory and Public Health Practice. Thousand Oaks, CA: Sage Publications, 1995.
23. Bandura A: Exercise of personal agency through the self-efficacy mechanism (pp. 3–38). In Schwarzer R, ed. Self-efficacy: Thought Control of Action. Washington, DC: Hemisphere; 1992.
24. Sallis JF, Hovell MF, Hofstetter CR et al: A multivariate study of determinants of vigorous exercise in a community sample. Prev Med 18:20–34, 1989.
25. Marcus BH, Selby VC, Niaura RS, Rossi JS: Self-efficacy and the stages of exercise behavior change. Res Q Exerc Sport 63:60–66, 1992.

26. Marcus BH, Owen N: Motivational readiness, self-efficacy, and decision-making for exercise. J Appl Soc Psychol 22:3–16, 1992.

27. Maddux JE: Self-efficacy, Adaptation, and Adjustment: Theory, Research, and Application. New York: Plenum Press; 1995.

28. Hofstetter CR, Hovell MF, Sallis JF: Social learning correlates of exercise self-efficacy: Early experiences with physical activity. Soc Sci Med 31:1169–1176, 1990.

29. McAuley E, Jerome GJ, Marquez DX, et al: Exercise self-efficacy in older adults: Social affective and behavioral influences. Ann Behav Med 25:1–7, 2003.

30. Bandura A: Self-efficacy: toward a unifying theory of behavior change. Psychol Rev 84:192–215, 1977.

31. Becker MH, ed: The health belief model and personal health behavior. Health Educ Monogr 2:324–508, 1974.

33. Rosenstock IM: Historical origins of the health belief model. Health Educ Monogr 2:328–335, 1974.

32. Rosenstock IM, Strecher VJ, Becker MH: Social learning theory and the health belief model. Health Educ Q 15:175–183, 1988.

34. Janz NK, Becker MH: The Health Belief Model: A decade later. Health Educ Quarterly 11:1–47, 1984.

35. Oldridge NB, Streiner DL: The health belief model: Predicting compliance and dropout in cardiac rehabilitation. Med Sci Sports Exerc 22:678–683, 1990.

36. Tirrell BE, Hart LK: The relationship of health beliefs and knowledge to exercise compliance in patients after coronary bypass. Heart Lung 9:487–493, 1980.

37. Roberston D, Keller C: Relationships among health beliefs, self-efficacy and exercise adherence in patients with coronary artery disease. Heart Lung 21:56–63, 1992.

38. Mirotznik J, Feldman L, Stein R: The Health Belief Model and adherence with a community center-based supervised coronary heart disease exercise program. J Community Health 20:233–247, 1995.

39. Stokols D: Establishing and maintaining healthy environments: Toward a social ecology of health promotion. Am Psychol 47:6–22, 1992.

40. Sallis JF, Owen N: Ecological models of health behavior. In Glanz K, Rimer BK, Lewis FM, eds. Health Behavior and Health Education: Theory, Research and Practice, 3rd ed. San Francisco: Jossey-Bass; 2002.

41. Brownson RC, Baker EA, Houseman RA, et al: Environmental and policy determinants of physical activity in the United States. Am J Public Health 91:1995–2003, 2001.

42. King AC, Castro C, Wilcox S, et al: Personal and environmental factors associated with physical inactivity among different racial-ethnic groups of U.S. middle-aged and older-aged women. Health Psychol 19:354–364, 2000.

43. Booth ML, Owen N, Bauman A, et al: Social-cognitive and perceived environment influences associated with physical activity in older Australians. Prev Med 31:15–22, 2000.

44. Fishbein M: A theory of reasoned action: Some applications and implications. Nebraska Symposium on Motivation 27:65–116, 1979.

45. Fishbein M: Belief, Attitude, Intension, and Behavior. Boston: Addison-Wesley; 1975.

46. Ajzen I, Fishbein M: Understanding Attitudes and Predicting Social Behavior. Englewood Cliffs, NJ: Prentice-Hall; 1980.

47. Hausenblas HA, Carron AV, Mack DE: Application of the theories of reasoned action and planned behavior to exercise behavior: A meta-analysis. J Sport Exerc Psychol 19:36–51, 1997.

48. Hagger MS, Chatzisarantis NLD, Biddle SJH: A Meta analytic review of the theories of reasoned action and planned behavior in physical activity: Predictive validity and the contribution of additional variables. J Sport Exerc Psychol 24:3–32, 2002.

49. Godin G: Theories of reasoned action and planned behavior: Usefulness for exercise promotion. Med Sci Sports Exerc 26:1391–1394, 1994.

50. Ajzen I: From intentions to actions: A theory of planned behavior (pp. 11–39). In Kuhl J, Beckman J, eds. Action-Control: From Cognition to Behavior. New York Springer-Verlag, 1985.

51. Ajzen I: Attitudes, Personality and Behavior. Chicago: Dorsey Press; 1988.

52. Madden TJ, Ellen PS, Ajzen I: A comparison of the theory of planned behavior and the theory of reasoned action. Pers Soc Psychol Bull 18:3–9, 1992.

53. Bandura A: Social Learning Theory. New Jersey: Prentice Hall; 1977.

54. Godin G: Social-cognitive models (pp. 113–136). In Dishman RK, ed. Advances in Exercise Adherence. Champaign, IL: Human Kinetics; 1994.

55. Blue CL: The predictive capacity of the theory of reasoned action and the theory of planned behavior in exercise research: An integrated literature review. Res Nurs Health 18:105–121, 1995.

56. Godin G, Valois P, Lepage L: The Miriam Hospital pattern of influence of perceived behavioral control upon exercising behavior: An application of Ajzen's theory of planned behavior. J Behav Med 16:81–101, 1993.

57. Blanchard CM, Courneya KS, Rodgers WM, et al: Is the Theory of Planned Behavior a useful framework for understanding exercise adherence during Phase II cardiac rehabilitation? J Cardiopulm Rehabil 23:29–39, 2003.

58. Marlatt GA, Gordon JR: Relapse Prevention: Maintenance Strategies in the Treatment of Addictive Behaviors. New York: Guilford Press; 1985.

59. Brownell KD, O'Neil PM: Obesity (pp. 318–361). In Barlow D, ed. Clinical Handbook of Psychological Disorders; 1993.

60. Marcus BH, Stanton AL: Evaluation of relapse prevention and reinforcement interventions to promote exercise adherence in sedentary females. Res Q Exerc Sport 64:447–452, 1993.

SELECTED REFERENCES FOR FURTHER READING

Maddux JE. Self-efficacy, Adaptation, and Adjustment: Theory, Research, and Application. New York: Plenum Press; 1995.

Marcus BH, Forsyth LH: Motivating People to be Physically Active. Champaign, IL: Human Kinetics; 2003.

Marlatt GA, Gordon JR: Relapse Prevention: Maintenance Strategies in the Treatment of Addictive Behaviors. New York: Guilford Press; 1985.

Rosenstock IM, Strecher VJ, Becker MH: Social learning theory and the health belief model. Health Educ Q 15:175–183, 1988.

Sallis JF, Owen N: Ecological models of health behavior. In Glanz K, Rimer BK, Lewis FM, eds. Health Behavior and Health Education: Theory, Research and Practice, 3rd ed. San Francisco: Jossey-Bass; 2002.

INTERNET RESOURCES

Behavior Change Theories and Models: http://www.csupomona.edu/;jv-grizzell/best_practices/bctheory.html

Centers for Disease Control and Prevention: Theories and Models Used in Physical Activity Promotion: http://www.cdc.gov/nccdphp/dnpa/physical/handbook/appendix3.htm

Centers for Disease Control and Prevention: Understanding and Promoting Physical Activity: http://www.cdc.gov/nccdphp/sgr/chap6.htm

Environmental Approaches to Promote Physical Activity: http://www.cdc.gov/nccdphp/dnpa/dnpalink.htm#Environmental

Stage of Change: http://fitness.gov/Reading_Room/Digests/march2003digest.pdf

Channels for Delivering Behavioral Programs

JUDITH J. PROCHASKA AND JAMES F. SALLIS

This chapter addresses KSAs from the following content areas:

1 Exercise Physiology and Related Exercise Science
2 Pathophysiology and Risk Factors
3 Health Appraisal, Fitness, and Clinical Exercise Testing
4 Electrocardiography and Diagnostic Techniques
5 Patient Management and Medications
6 Medical and Surgical Management
7 Exercise Prescription and Programming
8 Nutrition and Weight Management
9 Human Behavior and Counseling
10 Safety, Injury Prevention, and Emergency Procedures
11 Program Administration, Quality Assurance, and Outcome Assessment

An important consideration when developing a behavioral program for physical activity promotion relates to how it will **reach** the target population. Reach refers to the extent to which the **message** or program is delivered to the target population. The greater the reach, the greater the potential for impacting health. This chapter focuses on the modes or **channels** for delivering behavioral programs.

Only very motivated or strongly encouraged individuals seek out information and training from exercise professionals. More commonly, exercise professionals use one or more communication strategies to attract and engage the target population. Program objectives may include increasing the demand for, availability of, and access to physical activity programs as well as enhancing social norms that promote a physically active lifestyle.

With advances in technology and interactive communications, a multitude of channels are available. A communication framework can help with channel selection (Table 40-1). Factors that influence the choice of channel delivery include the message and program objectives, the source, the target **audience**, and the **context** or setting. The message may focus on a health supporting (e.g., walking, aerobic activity, strength training, stretching) or

health compromising (e.g., television watching) behavior. The source of the message may be an authoritative voice (e.g., exercise professional, teacher, physician) or organization (e.g., American College of Sports Medicine [ACSM], Centers for Disease Control and Prevention [CDC]), a famous figure (e.g., athlete, actor), or layperson (e.g., peers). The target audience is the receiver of the message and may be defined by demographic (e.g., age, gender), geographic, social, cultural, or psychological factors. The message or program may occur in a variety of contexts or settings, such as a school, home, or work.

Characteristics of each factor influence the strategies chosen in delivering behavioral programs. Ideally, the selected channel should reflect the target audience's preferred format and context. It should also provide a feasible medium for delivering the message or program. For example, a program to increase vigorous physical activity (message) among adolescents (target audience) at school (context) might be delivered via the Internet or an after-school program (channels). But a program developed for disabled older adults (target audience) to promote strength training (message) in assisted living programs (context) may select a very different delivery channel (e.g., individualized personal training, video).

This chapter focuses on channels for delivering behavioral programs and health promotion messaging. Individual delivery channels are presented by modality followed by a discussion of approaches for integrating them across multiple channels. Repeated presentation of information and behavior change strategies is often key to the adoption and maintenance of physical activity, and a multilevel approach is recommended. As much as possible, the strategies presented are evidence based—that is, they are drawn from the research literature. Chapter 46 covers settings and marketing aspects related to the delivery of exercise programs.

Channels for Health Behavior Change

PERSONAL COMMUNICATION

The oldest, most traditional channel is personal communication delivered individually in small groups, to organizations, or to entire communities. Program objectives often include teaching participants specific behavioral

KEY TERMS

Advocacy: Communication directed at policymakers to promote policies and programs to support (health behavior) change

Audience: The intended receiver of a communication or health program

Channel: A mode of communication or access for delivering a health program

Context: The setting where people may be reached with communications or programs

Message: Information that is intended to be communicated

Policy: An organizational statement or rule meant to influence behavior

Reach: The extent to which a message or program is delivered to the target population

skills to incorporate regular physical activity participation into their daily routines. Personal communications may be delivered in a variety of contexts, including an individual's home, school, worksite, church, community or commercial agency, primary care setting, or health fair.

In developing the U.S. *Guide to Community Preventive Services*, an extensive review was conducted of physical activity programs organized by channel delivery[1]. The document reported strong evidence in support of individually based health behavior change programs, school-based physical education, and social support interventions in community settings. School-based physical education programs have been effective at increasing the amount of class time students spend engaged in physical activity with the benefit of reaching large groups of youths. Programs encouraging a decrease in sedentary activity (e.g., television watching, video games) also show promise. Strong evidence supports the use of interventions in community settings that focus on building, strengthening, and maintaining social networks for supporting physical activity involvement. Examples include setting up "buddy" systems with peers, community walking groups, and social contracts. Insufficient evidence was found for classroom-based health education focused on information provision, college-based health education and physical education, or family-based social support programs.

Personal communications are often the most personalized—but time intensive—of delivery channels. The result is often limited reach and costly dissemination. To reach a greater number of individuals, print and electronic media can be used alone or as an adjunct to personal communications.

PRINT MEDIA

Print media can take the form of informational pamphlets and brochures, newsletters, articles and newspaper inserts, advertisements, self-help materials and books, exercise diaries, direct mailings, and poster and billboard displays (Figure 40-1). Messages can be informative, persuasive, or promote the use of specific behavioral strategies (e.g., self-monitoring, personal fitness contracts). A variety of print materials are available free or at low cost from professional organizations such as the ACSM, the CDC, and other fitness, sport, or physical activity agencies.

A simple form of print media with demonstrated efficacy is the use of point-of-decision prompts that encourage people to use the stairs instead of elevators and escalators. In five studies reviewed, increases in stair climbing exceeded 50%[1]. Collaborations with local news agencies and commercial entities are another method of disseminating health messaging and program promotion. An innovative example is the ACSM's partnership with General Mills to include physical activity messaging on the back of Wheaties cereal boxes. Importantly, print media can be used as a "pull" strategy, creating interest and

TABLE 40-1. Options for Applying a Communications Model

Source	Delivery Channel	Target Audience	Context/Setting
• Celebrity • Health professional • Peer • Organization	• Personal (individual, group, curricula) • Print (brochures, books, tip sheets) • Electronic (telephone, radio, video, television, computer, cell phone, personal digital assistant)	• Age based • Race or ethnicity based • Geography based (e.g., city, neighborhood) • Culturally based • Psychological profile-based (e.g., readiness to change)	• Home • School • Worksite • Community organization • Religious institution

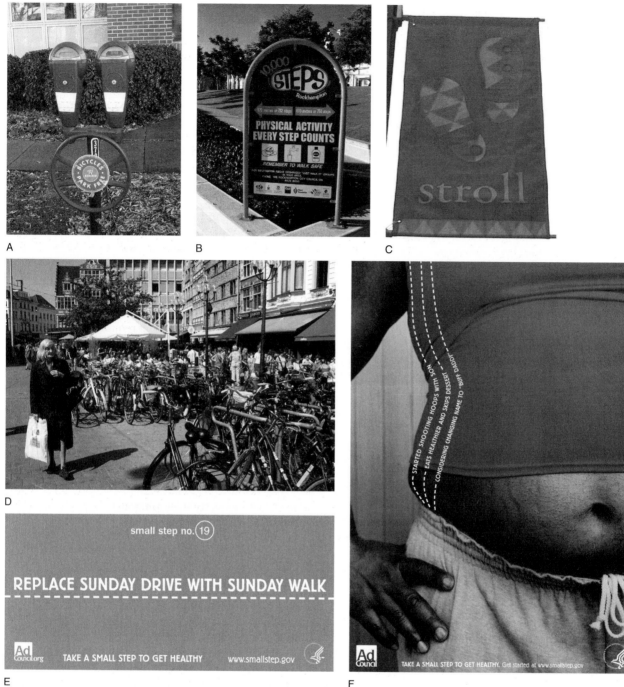

FIGURE 40-1. A. A sign supporting a policy of free parking for bicycles shows one of the multiple roles of communication. **B.** A multi-faceted community intervention in Rockhampton, Australia, included this informational sign. **C.** A banner on a light pole in the Dupont Circle section of Washington, DC. **D.** A communications programs may work better in a culture that supports physical activity and in an environment that makes it easy to bike and walk. **E** and **F.** The Small Steps campaign included television and print advertisements. (Photo credit for A-D, James Sallis; image credit for E, F, public campaign of the Ad Council and the U.S. Department of Health and Human Services).

consumer demand, in concert with a "push" strategy delivered by exercise professionals or interactive media channels.

Whereas traditional mass print media campaigns once took a one-size fits all approach, more recent efforts have focused on the development of targeted or tailored print communications. Targeted messages and materials are directed at a specific segment of the population, usually defined by one or more demographic or other shared characteristics, such as age, gender, race or ethnicity, or disease group. Tailored communications, on the other hand, are designed to reach specific individuals based on an assessment of their unique characteristics. As one moves from mass print media to targeted and tailored print communications, the message salience and relevance increases along with the program complexity and associated costs. Although tailored communications can be delivered as print media—a personalized handwritten prescription is a simple example—the advance of interactive technologies has made tailoring of health messages more feasible and cost effective.

ELECTRONIC MEDIA

Electronic media include radio, video, telephone, and computers. Recent years have seen a dramatic growth in the variety of electronic media channels available, including email, the Internet, chat rooms, text paging, mobile phones, personal digital assistants, Web-enabled television, and other emerging technologies. The immediate advantage of electronic media is the potential for mass distribution to maximize reach. Interactive media also allow for dynamic tailoring of messages based on assessment of the target audience's characteristics and individual needs.

A number of clinical trials have been conducted with demonstrated success to evaluate use of telephone-assisted counseling for physical activity promotion[2]. Diverse population groups have been studied, including healthy adults, men with uncomplicated postmyocardial infarction, older female caregivers of relatives with dementia, and adults with knee osteoarthritis. Telephone-based programs have the advantage of convenience, time efficiency, ready availability, and reduced burden associated with travel. In actuality, most programs have included telephone counseling as an adjunct or follow-up to an initial face-to-face contact. Whether used alone or in conjunction with other channels, the evidence supports telephone delivery of physical activity programming. The California Department of Health Services is translating research into public health practice, funding more than 15 communities to develop and deliver local telephone-based physical activity programs throughout the state. The next generation of telephone-mediated physical activity programs is examining the use of automated systems using keypad data entry for assessment of participants' exercise goals and progress over time.

An example of interactive computer-mediated technologies is the Patient-centered Assessment and Counseling for Exercise plus Nutrition (PACE+) programs developed for adolescents and adults[3]. The programs, delivered over the Internet, include a brief assessment of current physical activity involvement, as well as perceived benefits and barriers. Participants are then guided to develop an individually tailored plan for increasing their physical activity participation; relapse prevention plans are created by participants already meeting recommended levels of physical activity. The plan is printed for review with participants' health care providers. Computer-based delivery channels can be a useful mode of efficiently as-

sessing individual needs and providing personally relevant recommendations. With the capacity to add email messaging and hosted chat rooms, delivery channels such as the Internet expand the possibilities for communication between exercise professionals and their clients.

In 2002, 73 million Americans used the Internet for health-related reasons, which reflected 59% growth in health-related Internet seeking activity since the year 2000[4]. Nevertheless, limited access to new technologies can reduce reach and contribute to health disparities. Commonly referred to as the "digital divide," persons with less education, certain racial and ethnic groups, low income, and residing in rural households are less likely to have Internet access. An identified goal for the nation is to increase the proportion of households with Internet access at home from 26% in 1998 to 80% by 2010[5]. Lastly, the explosion of growth and the popularity of the Internet increase the risk of poor quality health information[6] as well as risks to privacy and confidentiality of personal health information. As with other channels of delivery, use of electronic media requires careful consideration of message development and characteristics of the target population.

Integrating Across Multiple Channels

Because inactive lifestyles are so common and specific programs reach only a minority of people, it is widely believed that coordinated, long-term, community-wide intervention approaches are needed to increase physical activity levels in the population[7]. There is no standard approach to community-wide programs, but they provide opportunities for integrating interventions using a variety of communication channels in several settings to reach numerous subgroups of people. The most extensive community-wide physical activity interventions were the heart disease prevention programs conducted during the 1980s in the United States. Although physical activity tended to be a low priority of these multiple risk factor studies that emphasized smoking and dietary change, the studies serve as examples of ways to integrate physical activity messages across multiple channels. Each of the three studies used a different mix of channels and settings with messages from a variety of sources. The target audience encompassed entire communities, so widespread reach was critical. The interventions spanned several years, with program sustainability an important factor.

All the programs used extensive print media that included booklets; books; self-help kits; tip sheets to post on refrigerators; newspaper columns and stories; billboards; and advertising to promote products, programs, and events. Some of the studies extensively used television commercials, programs, and news stories. Radio was used to target specific subgroups, such as Spanish speakers, with advertisements, news stories, and even health-related drama series. Personal communication was delivered in health counseling sessions, lectures to community groups, health fairs, and courses in schools and colleges. The projects engaged media experts to coordinate the development and delivery of messages, and investigators assured the accuracy and usefulness of the materials by pretesting draft materials and evaluating the impact of the materials and programs on users. Other staff members worked with representatives of worksites, schools, and community organizations to deliver information and programs in various settings. Limited efforts were made to improve resources or change policies that might promote physical activity. The three U.S. programs that pioneered many of these approaches are briefly profiled here.

The Stanford Five-City Project (FCP) relied heavily on the delivery of information using electronic and print mass media, along with face-to-face activities such as classes and contests. Coalitions were formed to provide structures in the community to continue the interventions. Examples of interventions included a self-help "Walking Kit" and physical activity contests between companies. Young et al.[8] reported modest but statistically significant changes. Men in the intervention communities were more likely to take part in at least one vigorous physical activity. Small but significant increases in moderate-intensity activities were noted among women.

The Minnesota Heart Health Program (MHHP) concentrated more on promoting physical activity through local health professionals and community organizations. Personal, intensive, and multiple-contact programs were used to directly influence physical activity behaviors though teaching behavior change skills. Large proportions of the communities participated in risk factor screenings, followed by feedback, personal counseling, and printed materials. The MHHP found small but significant physical activity intervention effects over the first 3 years of the program, which disappeared as the control communities became more active in subsequent years[9].

The Pawtucket Heart Health Project (PHHP) was built around partnerships with community organizations, churches, schools, and worksites. Physical activity information was included in a variety of printed materials, counseling sessions, and school curricula. Three distinct programs targeted physical activity change. The ExerCity program was run by the Department of Recreation and provided training of activity leaders, promoted use of community resources (e.g., trails) for activity, and created new programs throughout the community. GetFit! used mainly printed media and personal communications in a 6-week campaign at worksites. Because GetFit! participants were mainly already active, the Imagine ACTION approach featured printed materials designed for all stages of change. The PHHP did not have any significant effects on physical activity in the population[10].

All three major community-wide intervention trials reported weak and inconsistent changes in physical activity. Because substudies indicated that many of the component materials and programs were effective in helping people change, the disappointing results may be partly explained by insufficient numbers of people who were exposed to the materials or participated in programs (i.e., insufficient reach). The complexity of intervening on multiple risk factors in multiple communities was found to present many challenges to the investigators. Thus, most subsequent community interventions have had more modest goals and have identified carefully defined target communities.

Six rural counties in Missouri were targeted for a multiple risk factor heart health project that was built around community coalitions. Coalitions included voluntary health organizations, government agencies, and interested citizens. The investigators provided data, materials, and modest resources to support the coalitions. The coalitions mainly organized events, with the most common being walking clubs and exercise classes. It can be assumed the events were promoted through unpaid print and electronic media. Some coalitions built walking trails. Adults in counties with active coalitions increased their physical activity levels[11]. This project is interesting because the intervention used the organizational work of coalitions instead of traditional communication media to achieve change throughout the community.

A project in Wheeling, West Virginia, was built around paid media advertising but used several other media in a coordinated fashion. The target population was older adults in a small town, and the target behavior was simply walking, making the intervention more focused than the earlier community interventions. Two paid television ads were shown 683 times on network television over an 8-week period, and radio advertisements were broadcast 1988 times on 12 stations. Newspaper advertising space was bought repeatedly. Weekly press conferences and coverage of campaign-related events created an even greater media presence. Printed information on walking was distributed at worksites, a website allowed people to log their walking, prescription pads for walking were distributed to physicians, and lectures were given to community organizations. Because the media market was small, the project was able to buy enough television commercials so the average household was exposed more than 50 times to the walking message. Among adults aged 50 to 64 years who were sedentary at baseline, 32% in the intervention community met physical activity guidelines at the end of the campaign compared with 18% in a control community[12]. This study may have had stronger effects than previous community interventions because of the high intensity of the media campaign and the limited focus of the targeted behavior (walking) and population (older adults).

Policy and Environmental Approaches

Most of the community-wide programs described in this chapter may be criticized because they rarely went beyond efforts to motivate and educate the individual to make behavior changes. Strengths of all the studies were the variety of communication channels and community change strategies used to maximize reach and sustainability. However, relatively few attempts were made to change policies or environments that could help people be active over the long term. Ecological models of health behavior state that because there are multiple levels of influence on behavior, the most effective interventions should change all levels of influences, including psychological, social, **policy**, and environmental factors[13]. Adopting an ecological model suggests several strategies for planning physical activity interventions. The application of ecological models to physical activity is recent, and there are few examples of successful approaches. However, it may be useful to consider the possibilities.

Physical activity must be done in a specific place. Whether it is on a home treadmill, at a health club, or on a trail, the availability of convenient and attractive facilities is expected to enhance the effectiveness of communication approaches. For example, when a walking trail was developed in a rural community and promoted through various media, a substantial number of sedentary adults became physically active[11]. Educational campaigns can motivate people to be active, but accessible and attractive facilities make it easier for them to follow through. Various media channels can be used to inform the community about the availability of physical facilities.

Policies reflect decisions made by governments and private groups that can have major implications for physical activity[14]. Policies control incentives for behavior. Examples of incentives for physical activity include insurance discounts for active individuals and a similar reimbursement for workers who walk or ride bikes on company business. Policies also control the physical environment. Relevant policies may include requiring parks and playgrounds in new developments, mandating that a percentage of transportation funds be spent on pedestrian and cycling facilities, and requiring schools to be opened for community use in the evenings and on weekends.

Consideration of policy changes and environmental approaches suggests that target audiences and messages need to be expanded. The same communication channels, however, of print, electronic media, and personal communication still apply. Communication to the lay public can provide information on the benefits of changing policies as well as motivate **advocacy** of these changes to policymakers. Policymakers themselves become critical audiences for communication. Because policies that affect physical activity can be made by those with responsibility for transportation, real estate, public safety, recreation, education, and health care[14,15], there are many relevant audiences.

There are few documented examples of communication strategies applied to policy change related to physical activity, but this is likely to be an area of focus for the future. Those who design physical activity interventions are challenged to expand the messages to include motivation and skills instruction for behavior change as well as advocacy for policy and environment change (see Chapter 42).

For substantial population improvements in physical activity, it may be necessary for those designing interventions to communicate not only with subgroups of the general public but also with policymakers in government and the private sector.

Summary

Delivery channels are the media through which physical activity messages and programs are transmitted. Formats include print and electronic media and personal communications. Channel selection is guided by consideration of the target audience's preferred format and context as well as characteristics of the program to be delivered. With the dramatic increases in communication technology, a wide variety of delivery channels is available. To increase physical activity in large populations, it is necessary to use a variety of communication channels to deliver an array of messages to multiple target audiences. Supplementing communications with other intervention strategies and advocating for policy and environmental changes are important adjuncts to consider.

The community-wide heart health studies provide an example of how different communication channels can be integrated in a coordinated approach. The Wheeling Walks campaign had particularly promising short-term effects, perhaps because the "walking" message was simple and the communications were targeted to a single target audience of older adults. Communications can be used for multiple purposes, including motivating and educating individuals, promoting other physical activity interventions, and encouraging individuals to advocate for policy and environmental changes. The rural Missouri study showed that creating the environmental change of a walking trail, in combination with media-based promotion, had important effects on the community's walking behavior[16]. This study suggests that there is value in expanding our targets for communication to include both individuals and policymakers.

To maximize the reach of behavioral programs, the use of multiple channels is encouraged. With greater expansion of delivery channels, however, there comes the greater potential for inaccurate or poor quality messaging. When multiple channels are used, monitoring the consistency, reliability, and credibility of delivered program content is crucial.

REFERENCES

1. Kahn EB, Ramsey LT, Brownson RC et al: The effectiveness of interventions to increase physical activity. Am J Prev Med 22(suppl): 73–107, 2002.
2. Castro CM, King AC: Telephone-assisted counseling for physical activity. Exerc Sport Sci Rev 30:64–68, 2002.
3. Prochaska JJ, Zabinski MF, Calfas KJ, et al: PACE+: Interactive communication technology for behavior change in clinical settings. Am J Prev Med 19:127–131, 2000.

4. Pew Internet & American Life: America's Online Pursuits: The Changing Picture of Who's Online and What They Do. Available at: http://www.pewinternet.org/reports/toc.asp?Report=106

5. U.S. Department of Health and Human Services: Healthy People 2010: Understanding and Improving Health, 2nd ed. Washington, DC: U.S. Government Printing Office; 2000. Available at: http://www.healthypeople.gov/Document/HTML/volume1/11Healt hCom.htm

6. Doshi A, Patrick K, Sallis JF, Calfas K: Evaluation of physical activity web sites for use of behavior change theories. Ann Behav Med 25:105–111, 2003.

7. King AC: Community and public health approaches to the promotion of physical activity. Med Sci Sports Exerc 26:1405–1412, 1994.

8. Young DR, Haskell WL, Taylor CB, Fortmann SP: Effect of community health education on physical activity knowledge, attitudes, and behavior: The Stanford five-city project. Am J Epidemiol 144:264–274, 1996.

9. Luepker RV, Murray DM, Jacobs DR, et al: Community education for cardiovascular disease prevention: Risk factor changes in the Minnesota Heart Health Program. Am J Public Health 84:1383–1393, 1994.

10. Eaton CB, Lapane KL, Garber CE, et al: Effects of a community-based intervention on physical activity: The Pawtucket Heart Health Program. Am J Public Health 89:1741–1744, 1999.

11. Brownson RC, Housemann RA, Brown DR, et al: Promoting physical activity in rural communities: Walking trail access, use, and effects. Am J Prev Med 18:235–241, 2000.

12. Reger B, Cooper L, Booth-Butterfield S, Smith H, et al: Wheeling Walks: A community campaign using paid media to encourage walking among sedentary older adults. Prev Med 35:285–292, 2002.

13. Sallis JF, Owen N: Ecological models of health behavior (pp. 462–484). In Glanz K, Rimer BK, Lewis FM, eds. Health Behavior and Health Education: Theory, Research, and Practice, 3rd edition. San Francisco: Jossey-Bass; 2002.

14. Sallis JF, Bauman A, Pratt M: Environmental and policy interventions to promote physical activity. Am J Prev Med 15:379–397, 1998.

15. King AC, Stokols D, Talen E, et al: Theoretical approaches to the promotion of physical activity: Forging a transdisciplinary paradigm. Am J Prev Med 23(suppl 2):15–25, 2002.

16. Brownson RC, Smith CA, Pratt M, et al: Preventing cardiovascular disease through community-based risk reduction: The Bootheel Hearth Health Project. Am J Public Health 86:206–213, 1996.

SELECTED REFERENCES FOR FURTHER READING

Centers for Disease Control and Prevention: Promoting Physical Activity: A Guide for Community Action. Champaign, IL: Human Kinetics 2; 1999

Donovan RJ, Owen N: Social marketing and population interventions. In Dishman RK, ed. Advances in Exercise Adherence (pp. 249–290). Champaign, IL: Human Kinetics; 1994.

Marcus BH, Owen N, Forsyth LH, et al: Physical activity interventions using mass media, print media, and information technology. Am J Prev Med 15:362–378, 1998.

Sallis JF, Owen N: Interventions to promote physical activity in communities and populations (pp. 153–174). In Physical Activity & Behavioral Medicine. Thousand Oaks, CA: Sage Publications; 1999.

Weinreich NK: Hands-on Social Marketing: A Step-by-Step Guide. Thousand Oaks, CA: Sage Publications; 1999.

INTERNET RESOURCES

Active Living Network: Communications Toolkit: http://www.activeliving.org/index.php/Communications_Toolkit/80

American Heart Association: JustMove.org: http://www.justmove.org

Centers for Disease Control and Prevention: Increasing Physical Activity: A Report on Recommendations of the Task Force on Community Preventive Services: http://www.cdc.gov/mmwr/preview/mmwrhtml/ rr5018a1.htm#top

Getting Australia Active: http://www.ausport.gov.au/fulltext/2002/npha/gaa.pdf

National Coalition for Promoting Physical Activity: Resource Guide: http://www.ncppa.org/resources.asp

Factors Associated with Regular Physical Activity Participation

ABBY C. KING AND CYNTHIA CASTRO

This chapter addresses KSAs from the following content areas:

1   Exercise Physiology and Related Exercise Science
2   Pathophysiology and Risk Factors
3   Health Appraisal, Fitness, and Clinical Exercise Testing
4   Electrocardiography and Diagnostic Techniques
5   Patient Management and Medications
6   Medical and Surgical Management
7   Exercise Prescription and Programming
8   Nutrition and Weight Management
9   Human Behavior and Counseling
10 Safety, Injury Prevention, and Emergency Procedures
11 Program Administration, Quality Assurance, and Outcome Assessment

An explosion of interest, by both the public and health professionals, has emerged with respect to **physical activity** as a means for achieving positive benefits related to health, functioning, and quality of life. Despite this increased interest, available evidence indicates that close to half of Americans do not exercise regularly (i.e., on 4 or more days per week) and one fourth or more do not exercise at all[1,2]. In the United States as well as in a number of other industrialized nations, a number of subgroups remain underactive[1], most notably individuals who are older (particularly women), from ethnic minority groups, less educated, smokers, and overweight. Of the 10% (or less) of initially sedentary adults who begin regular physical activity in a year, as much as 50% may drop out within 3 to 6 months, and the recidivism rates are similar among those who were already active. For "high-risk" individuals enrolled in secondary prevention programs, 50% have been reported to drop out within 12 months.

Such statistics indicate that assisting individuals to stay regularly physically active is a challenge that requires creativity and patience. In addition, finding ways to encourage extremely sedentary individuals to adopt a more active lifestyle represents an increasingly important public health goal. Exercise professionals can take advantage of the current public enthusiasm for becoming more active, as well as the growing literature suggesting strategies that can be effective for enhancing participation in physical activity.

The Adherence Problem

In some ways, physical activity is a unique health behavior, governed by factors that may differ, to at least some extent, from other health behaviors. Certainly, the demand for regularity in performing physical activity to obtain benefits throughout life calls for innovative methods of studying the process that makes regular physical activity habitual. Additionally, factors or **determinants** that influence initial adoption and early participation in physical activity may differ from those that affect subsequent long-term maintenance. Stage of change models that take into account motivational readiness for change (e.g., the transtheoretical model[3]) may better identify strategies that work for individuals in different stages and at different levels of physical activity participation (e.g., sedentary persons contemplating joining a physical activity program, those in the early stage of physical activity adoption, those committed to maintaining a program across the long term) [see Box 44-4 and GETP7 Figure 7-7 and Box 7-2][3]. Such models draw extensively from social cognitive theory and other theories of behavior change[4,5]. Although the understanding of the behavior change and maintenance process continues to develop, a number of potentially important cognitive, behavioral, social, and environmental variables influencing both initial adoption and longer term maintenance of physical activity patterns have been identified[6,7]. These variables are noted in the next section.

Social Cognitive Theory

Although no single theory allows full explanation of why individuals become or stay active, efforts to understand such health behaviors have been helped by placing them in the context of a social learning/social cognitive model of health behavior change (see Chapter 39). The social cognitive approach, broadly defined, views such behavior as being initiated and maintained through a complex interaction of

KEY TERMS

Adherence: The percent of physical activity participation, derived by comparing the amount of physical activity engaged in (numerator) with the amount of physical activity recommended or prescribed (denominator)

Determinant: A variables or factor that is significantly associated with the outcome of interest (e.g., physical activity) and that may be targeted in intervention efforts. Such variables may or may not be part of the causal chain with respect to physical activity participation and may require

examination to specifically determine their causal impact.

Physical activity: Any form of repetitive movement, typically involving large muscle groups, that results in energy expenditure

Predictor: A variable or factor that is associated prospectively with physical activity levels or changes in physical activity over time

personal, behavioral, and environmental factors and conditions[4]. Factors that may play a role in influencing how active an individual is include their experiences with physical activity; attitudes and perceptions of physical activity in general and different forms of activity in particular; the extent of current activity-related knowledge, skills, and beliefs; and the influence of surrounding physical and social environments or perceptions of those environments that either help or hinder efforts to increase physical activity.

The social learning/social cognitive theoretical approach emphasizes the individual's ability to self-regulate behavior through setting goals, monitoring progress toward these goals, and modifying resources in the physical and social environment (as well as one's own thoughts or beliefs, as appropriate) to support the goals. Observational learning and modeling by others are important influences. Self-efficacy (i.e., the level of confidence in one's ability to successfully perform a specific behavior or activity) and outcome expectancies (i.e., one's belief that the behavior leads to a desired outcome) are identified to be the critical factors that influence which behaviors are attempted and with how much effort before a person gives up.

In addition to social cognitive theory, other conceptual models or approaches that have been applied include the health belief model; the locus of control model; relapse prevention models; the theory of reasoned action or planned behavior; expectancy value decision theories; and, recently, self-determination theory[6,8]. To date, few have been as heuristic as the social cognitive perspective in helping to shape effective intervention, although more efforts are being made to test the utility of these models.

Social cognitive theory and related approaches to understanding physical activity behavior have been supplemented in recent years with an increased appreciation for the role of motivational readiness in changing physical activity patterns. An individual's motivational readiness to become more active interacts with and can be influenced by the types of personal, behavioral, program-related, and environmental factors described below.

PERSONAL FACTORS

Among the *demographic* factors found to be associated with physical activity participation are the following[7]:

Gender

Women generally participate less in vigorous activity, especially at younger and older ages, relative to men. Women often find moderate-intensity regimens and activities (e.g., brisk walking) more appealing and may be more successful, as a group, in adopting and maintaining moderate-intensity activities relative to more vigorous activity[9].

Age

Increasing age is generally associated with lower levels of physical activity, particularly vigorous forms of physical activity. The decline in activity with age may be partly caused by physical or mobility impairments often associated with older age, although many studies demonstrate that older adults can preserve or improve physical functioning through regular physical activity. As a group, older adults, in particular, prefer more moderate-intensity activities[10].

Educational Attainment

Educational level is positively associated with leisure time physical activity. That is, more years of education are linked to greater amounts of reported physical activity, in a continuous fashion.

Household Income

Household income is also positively associated with increased leisure time physical activity. The reasons for this (and the other relationships already discussed) have not been well studied.

Meanwhile, demographic factors such as occupation and race or ethnicity have less consistent relationships with leisure time physical activity. Although relatively few studies have specifically examined differences by ethnicity, some have demonstrated that African American and Hispanic women are consistently less active than white women[11]. There is some evidence that physical activity levels may, to some extent, "run in families;" however, the reasons for this (i.e., genetic, behavioral, environmental, or some combination of these factors) are currently unclear.

Health factors have been shown to have consistent relationships with physical activity level. People with medical problems or disabilities are more likely to be inactive. Health-related barriers and concerns have been found to be particularly important in older age groups, in whom fears of physical activity-related injury often increase[10]. Smoking status is related to lower levels of physical activity in some, although not all populations, as well as associated with higher dropout rates from vigorous leisure time exercise programs.

Overweight and obese individuals have been consistently found to be less active across a range of activities, including both leisure time and routine activities such as walking and taking stairs. Why overweight and obese individuals are less active, however, is not generally well understood. The epidemiological evidence generally indicates an inverse association between physical activity levels and body weight in most populations, beginning in youth, suggesting that inactivity is a factor in weight gain[12,13]. It is also possible that engaging in physical activity is more aerobically challenging and physically difficult for already overweight individuals and may lead to increased stress and strain on the musculoskeletal and cardiovascular systems. Additionally, some evidence suggests that attending exercise classes or engaging in physical activity is stressful for some subgroups of overweight individuals who are dissatisfied with their physical appearance[14]. People may be more dissatisfied (about their appearance) when they are in situations that elicit thoughts about appearance, so they may actively avoid situations that exacerbate these feelings of dissatisfaction[15]. Exercise, especially in groups with a focus on appearance and social comparison, may be one such situation. Cognitive strategies such as correcting size and weight estimates of self relative to peers, norms, and objective standards, as well as behavioral strategies such as incremental exposure to a target situation, have been demonstrated to improve body image for normal weight individuals[16].

In addition to demographic and health factors, *cognitive and experiential* variables negatively influencing initial participation in regular physical activity include the following[7,9] negative experiences with physical activity; negative perceptions of one's own health status as well as physical activity ability and skills; lower self-efficacy beliefs, defined as the level of confidence in the ability to successfully perform a specific physical activity regimen or program; limited outcome efficacy beliefs (i.e., belief that physical activity has value for health, fitness, or re-

lated desired outcomes); low levels of perceived physical activity enjoyment and satisfaction; negative perceptions related to access to exercise facilities, convenience of the physical activity behavior being attempted, lack of time, and physical activity intensity; limited understanding of how increased physical activity relates to personal benefits, both in the short term and the long term; and limited perceived value of the benefits of physical activity relative to the "costs" or burden required to undertake a physical activity program.

In addition, level of self or intrinsic motivation (i.e., internal desires for achievement), as described in self-determination theory and similar perspectives[17,18], may be positively related to continued participation in physical activity. Importantly, intrinsic motivation may be learned when one finds personal, self-identified rewards for behavior (e.g., personal achievement, the satisfaction obtained in reaching one's physical activity goals) independent of external or extrinsic rewards (e.g., social support) available for that behavior[8]. Such approaches typically involve the acknowledgment of the client's perspective and feelings about the proposed change; providing a rationale for the change; providing a choice of alternative behaviors, which is intended to reduce conflicts regarding making the change; and affirming the importance of the client's own preferences and experiences[19]. This concept of motivation is preferable to definitions of motivation that place responsibility for nonadherence on internal processes related to "personality" or similar constructs that are assumed to be immutable and relatively unaffected by learning. These latter definitions, aside from typically being unfair to the individual by ignoring externally controlled or extrapersonal influences on behavior (e.g., the environment), do not provide exercise professionals with a firm direction for intervention.

Although many of the above-mentioned factors are associated with initial participation in physical activity, relatively few appear to substantially influence length of maintenance of a physical activity regimen. Factors that may influence longer term physical activity maintenance are smoking status, body weight, perceived lack of time, and perceptions of success in achieving one's expected benefits from being physically active[20]. Other factors likely to have an effect on continued participation are ongoing enjoyment of or satisfaction with the physical activity program or regimen; support from others; and the ability to overcome barriers such as scheduling, illness, travel, and other factors that can impede ongoing participation in physical activity (also see Chapter 42).

BEHAVIORAL FACTORS

Behavioral factors include the skills to carry out physical activity to facilitate health and quality of life benefits while minimizing injury and boredom. Such skills include knowledge and use of behavioral and psychological strategies that assist in the negotiation of barriers and pitfalls that inevitably interfere with regular activity.

A useful behavioral skill may be as simple as knowing how to plan ahead by identifying and preparing for periods when disruption of physical activity is likely (e.g., during holidays). This type of strategy is known as relapse prevention. Studies applying relapse prevention strategies, either alone or in combination with other behavioral strategies, suggest their utility in the promotion, adoption, and maintenance of physical activity[21,22]. Another potentially effective strategy is implementation of a decision balance sheet, whereby careful evaluation of expected or experienced benefits and costs of participating are compared. Other self-regulatory skills that appear to promote physical activity participation if used regularly are self-monitoring of progress, realistic short- and longer term goal setting coupled with ongoing feedback related to success, and the giving oneself rewards[6,7]. Also, stimulus control or structuring the immediate environment to remind or encourage one to be active (e.g., through the use of visual or auditory reminders or prompts) can be helpful (also see Chapter 42).

ENVIRONMENTAL AND PROGRAM FACTORS

A number of environmental and program-based factors can influence initial participation as well as longer term **adherence**[23,24] (see GETP7 Box 7-3). These include family influences and support (e.g., individuals reporting spouses to be neutral or unsupportive of physical activity are more likely to drop out); proximity, access to, and affordability of facilities (for those who prefer facility-based activities); weather; regimen flexibility (type of activity, intensity, location, timing, frequency); convenience and ease of scheduling of the activity (real or perceived); immediate visual or auditory cues and prompts in the environment promoting physical activity (e.g., reminders to exercise); and immediate consequences of physical activity for the individual (e.g., discomfort).

The *social environment* can have also a major impact on both physical activity adoption and maintenance. Family participation and support as well as parental or family level of physical activity are associated with increased physical activity in some population groups[25–27]. Social support from friends or coworkers may also have a positive effect. In addition, physicians and other health professionals can positively influence physical activity behavior. Although surveys suggest that physician advice is considered to be potentially important with respect to health behaviors, relatively few physicians routinely discuss physical activity practices with patients[28,29]. Barriers to physician counseling on physical activity include lack of confidence in ability to effectively advise patients (often stemming from lack of knowledge or training), lack of time, lack of knowledge related to the most appropriate referral sources in the community, and limited

reimbursement for these services. As part of Project PACE (Patient-centered Assessment and Counseling for Exercise), funded by the Centers for Disease Control and Prevention, a physician-based brief physical activity assessment and counseling protocol is available for use in the clinical setting for a variety of patient populations[30].

In addition to the social environment, there has been an increasing appreciation of how tangible aspects of the *physical environment* can impact people's physical activity levels throughout the day. For example, research has begun to shed light on the potential association of physical activity patterns and preferences with such environmental characteristics as the layout and design of neighborhood streets and thoroughfares, as well as the presence or absence of such things as sidewalks, streetlights, stray dogs, and neighborhood crime[23,31]. As physical activity researchers increasingly collaborate with experts in urban planning, transportation, and environmental development to better understand the influence of these physical environmental factors, our ability to harness such factors in facilitating increases in physical activity participation will increase.

With respect to *program-related* factors, the type of physical activity (e.g., swimming, brisk walking, aerobic dance), as well as intensity, duration, and frequency can influence subsequent participation levels. The format in which the activity is offered (e.g., class, home-based, with or without partners) may also have an important effect on both initial participation and longer term adherence. Although the majority of community-based physical activity programs are offered in a class or group format, evidence indicates that the public generally prefers programs offered outside of a formal group or facility[31]. There are important benefits to long-term adherence with adequately structured home-based regimens[32]. The mode, intensity, frequency, duration, and location of physical activity must meet the needs of differing groups of individuals. For example, women generally report a stronger preference for videotaped exercise and aerobic dance than men. Similarly, the workplace has been shown to be a preferred location for undertaking physical activity in some groups, though not in others[33,34].

Immediate consequences, including observance of physical activity–related benefits and enjoyment of activity, are other program-related factors likely to have a strong impact on participation levels[20]. Conversely, sedentary people persist in inactive patterns principally because sedentary activities are immediately reinforcing and attempts to become physically active are likely to result in immediate aversive sensory or physiological consequences. Thus, the task of health professionals is to ensure that initial attempts to become more physically active are perceived as generally pain free, enjoyable, and reinforcing through encouraging gradual, progressive increases in physical activity duration, frequency, and intensity, while keeping in mind the individual's physical and psychological readiness to progress. Although time constraints are typically noted as major reasons for inactivity, regular exercisers complain as much as persons who are not regularly active about such constraints. Thus, perceived available time may reflect, in large part, one's current priorities related to being active or time management skills rather than actual time limitations (also see Chapter 42).

FACTORS INFLUENCING FORMS OF PHYSICAL ACTIVITY IN ADDITION TO LEISURE ACTIVITY

The current focus on increasing the public's participation in moderate-intensity activities, as well as more vigorous forms of physical activity, has opened the door to investigations focusing on **predictors** that influence a variety of physically active pursuits in addition to the leisure forms of activity that have typically been the target of study. Forms of physical activity that are increasingly being studied include physical activities used for transportation purposes, for household and yard maintenance, as well as the routine forms of physical activity occurring naturally throughout the day (e.g., taking the stairs, walking to accomplish routine errands). Our understanding of factors influencing the performance of such activities is currently in its infancy. Although several recent intervention studies have provided evidence related to the potential utility of teaching groups of individuals ways for becoming more physically active throughout the day[35], evidence that the individuals participating in such programs increased their physical activity levels primarily through their participation in such routine forms of activity (e.g., taking stairs, walking to do errands) remains lacking. The field will continue to benefit from advances in physical activity measurement that allow us to better capture the more routine, intermittent forms of light- and moderate-intensity physical activity being targeted in such approaches. Similarly, most of the behavioral research in the field has focused on endurance forms of physical activity, as opposed to other types of physical activity, such as strengthening and flexibility exercises, that have been increasingly recognized as important to overall health and functioning, particularly as people age[36].

IDENTIFYING FACTORS OF IMPORTANCE TO SPECIFIC POPULATION SUBGROUPS

A growing area of interest in the field pertains to identifying personal, program-related, and environmental factors that may be particularly influential for specific population subgroups. By identifying the most useful combination of factors predicting future physical activity participation in different population segments, individuals can be better matched with a program that may particularly suit their preferences and needs. For example, one 2-year study examined 269 healthy, initially sedentary middle-aged men and women who had been randomly assigned to one of three different physical activity programs. There were six different clinically meaningful subgroups of people, based on a combination of baseline characteristics and variables, who were at either low, moderate, or high risk of poor adherence by the second year of their physical activity program[14]. In this investigation, persons who had been initially assigned to a community-based exercise class offered three times per week throughout the study period and who had a body mass index (i.e., body weight in kg/height in m^2) of 27 or greater were at particularly high risk for poor adherence throughout the 2-ear study period (i.e., only 7.7% of this subgroup achieved exercise adherence rates of at least 66% or greater by the second year). In contrast, individuals who had been initially assigned to a supervised home-based physical activity program and who reported low initial stress levels were at relatively lower risk for poor exercise adherence throughout the 2-year study period (i.e., more than half of this subgroup achieved exercise adherence rates of at least 66% or greater across the 2-year period).

Continued research in this area using applications of such clinical decision-making approaches will help to further refine our understanding of those subgroups of people, defined through a combination of biologic, psychosocial, behavioral, and exercise program–specific factors, for whom tailored interventions are particularly indicated. One such methodological approach, applied in the above study, involves applications of signal detection techniques to the physical activity field[37]. A strength of signal detection in behavioral research is that it allows for full use of all data available for each variable being evaluated, thereby eliminating problems related to missing data that accompany the use of multiple regression approaches. Applications of such approaches will continue to shed light on the most important combinations of physical activity–relevant factors that may be targeted in future interventions.

Summary

The factors that most strongly influence initial adoption are likely different, to at least a certain degree, from those that affect maintenance[7,38]. The variables described in this chapter clearly represent only some of the constellation of relevant factors that influence physical activity levels, many of which have yet to be identified. Because of the complex interrelationships among these variables, many individuals may have difficulty explaining problems with starting or maintaining physical activity without some self-monitoring of their activity. Some factors identified as predictive of inactivity (e.g., being a smoker or overweight) are present in those who may reap the most benefits from regular physical activity. Finally, the variety of factors implicated indicates the importance of developing programs and strategies that fit the needs and preferences of different population groups. The types of "tailoring" or "matching" approaches can be contrasted with more typical methods of fitting individuals into existing generic programs. By tailoring physical activity to the population group or individual, physical activity professionals may positively influence initial dropout rate (during the critical period, which is the first 3 to 6 months) as well as during later periods. Systematic research evaluating specific methods of tailoring programs is increasingly indicated. In addition, knowledge in this area obtained from studies of endurance exercise should be systematically applied to other dimensions of physical activity, including strength and flexibility training, which to date have received much less systematic behavioral attention.

The use of linear regression methodologies to define factors associated with physical activity participation has limited our understanding of the manner in which various personal, behavioral, program-specific, and environmental factors combine to identify subgroups at particular risk for poor physical activity participation. Recent applications of clinical decision-making approaches, such as signal detection analysis, show promise in helping to meaningfully define subgroups of people at risk for poor physical activity participation, for whom tailored programs may be especially effective.

Acknowledgments

This work was supported in part by PHS grants #AG-16587, #MH58853, and #HL72489 from the National Institutes of Health awarded to Dr. King.

REFERENCES

1. U.S. Department of Health and Human Services: Physical Activity and Health: A Report of the Surgeon General. Atlanta: U.S. Department of Health and Human Services, Centers for Disease Control and Prevention, National Center for Chronic Disease Prevention and Health Promotion; 1996.
2. U.S. Department of Health and Human Services: Healthy People 2010: Understanding and Improving Health. Washington, DC: U.S Department of Health and Human Services; 2000.
3. Marcus BH, Simkin LR: The transtheoretical model: Applications to exercise behavior. Med Sci Sports Exerc 26:1400–1404, 1994.
4. Bandura A: Social cognitive theory: An agentic perspective. Ann Rev Psychol 52:1–26. 2001.
5. Bandura A: The anatomy of stages of change. Am J Health Promot 12:8–10, 1997.
6. Young DR, King AC: Exercise adherence: Determinants of physical activity and applications of health behavior change theories. Med Exerc Nutr Health 4:335–348, 1995.
7. Marcus BH, Dubbert PM, Forsyth LH, et al: Physical activity behavior change: Issues in adoption and maintenance. Health Psychol 19:32–41, 2000.
8. King AC, Friedman R, Marcus B, et al: Harnessing motivational forces in the promotion of physical activity: The Community Health Advice by Telephone (CHAT) Project. Health Education Research 17:627–636, 2002.
9. King AC, Blair SN, Bild DE, et al: Determinants of physical activity and interventions in adults. Med Sci Sports Exerc 24(suppl 6): S221–S236, 1992.
10. King AC, Rejeski WJ, Buchner DM: Physical activity interventions targeting older adults: a critical review and recommendations. Am J Prev Med 15:316–333, 1998.
11. Taylor WC, Baranowski T, Young DR. Physical activity interventions in low-income, ethnic minority, and populations with disability. Am J Prev Med 15:334–343, 1998.
12. NHLBI Obesity Education Initiative Expert Panel: Clinical guidelines on the identification, evaluation, and treatment of overweight and obesity in adults: The evidence report. Obesity Research 6(suppl 2):515–2105, 1998.
13. Takahaski E, Yoshida K, Sugimori H, et al: Influence factors on the development of obesity in 3-year-old children based on the Toyama study. Prev Med 28:293–296, 1999.
14. King AC, Kiernan M, Oman RF, et al: Can we identify who will adhere to long-term physical activity? Application of signal detection methodology as a potential aid to clinical decision-making. Health Psychology 16:380–389, 1997.
15. Haimovitz D, Lansky LM, O'Reilly P: Fluctuations in body satisfaction across situations. Int J Eat Disord 13:77–84, 1993.
16. Rosen JC, Saltzberg E, Srebnik D: Cognitive behavior therapy for negative body image. Behav Ther 20:393–404, 1989.
17. Deci EL, Ryan RM: Intrinsic Motivation and Self-determination in Human Behavior. New York: Plenum; 1985.
18. Mullan E, Markland D, Ingledew D: A graded conceptualisation of self-determination in the regulation of exercise behavior: Development of a measure using confirmatory factor analytic procedures. Pers Individ Dif 23:745–752, 997.
19. Deci EL, Ryan RM: the support of autonomy and the control of behavior. J Pers Soc Psychol 53:1024–1037, 1987.
20. Neff KL, King AC: Exercise program adherence in older adults: The importance of achieving one's expected benefits. Med Exerc Nutr Health 4:355–362, 1995.
21. King AC, Frederiksen L: Low-cost strategies for increasing exercise behavior: Relapse preparation training and social support. Behavior Modification 8:3–21, 1984.
22. King AC, Haskell WL, Taylor CB, et al: Group- versus home-based exercise training in healthy older men and women: A community-based clinical trial. JAMA 266:1535–1542, 1991.
23. Sallis JF, Bauman A, Pratt M: Environmental and policy interventions to promote physical activity. Am J Prev Med 15:379–397, 1998.
24. Sallis JF, Owen N: Physical activity and behavioral medicine. Thousand Oaks, CA: Sage Publications; 1999.
25. Treiber FA, Baranowski T, Braden DS, et al: Social support for exercise: Relationship to physical activity in young adults. Prev Med 20: 737–750, 1991.
26. Oka RK, King AC, Young DR: Sources of social support as predictors of exercise adherence in women and men ages 50 to 65 years. Women's Health: Research on Gender, Behavior, and Policy 1:161–175, 1995.
27. McAuley E, Blissmer B, Marquez DX, et al: Social relations, physical activity, and well-being in older adults. Prev Med 31:608–617, 2000.
28. Eaton CB, Menard LM: A systematic review of physical activity promotion in primary care office settings. Br J Sports Med 32:11–16, 1998.
29. Damush TM, Stewart AL, Mills KM, et al: Prevalence and correlates of physician recommendations to exercise among older adults. J Gerontol A Biol Sci Med Sci 54:M423–M427, 1999.
30. Calfas KJ, Long BJ, Sallis JF, et al: A controlled trial of physician counseling to promote the adoption of physical activity. Prev Med 25: 225–233, 1996.
31. King AC, Castro C, Wilcox S, et al: Personal and environmental factors associated with physical inactivity among different racial/ethnic groups of U.S. middle- and older-aged women. Health Psychol 19: 354–364, 2000.
32. Castro CM, King AC: Telephone-assisted counseling for physical activity. Exerc Sport Sci Rev 30:64–68, 2002.
33. King AC, Carl F, Birkel L, Haskell WL: Increasing exercise among blue-collar employees: The tailoring of worksite programs to meet specific needs. Prev Med 17:357–365, 1988.

34. King AC, Taylor CB, Haskell WL, DeBusk RF: Identifying strategies for increasing employee physical activity levels: findings from the Stanford/Lockheed exercise survey. Health Educ Q 17:269–285, 1990.

35. Dunn AL, Marcus BH, Kampert JB, et al: Comparison of lifestyle and structured Interventions to increase physical activity and cardiorespiratory fitness: A randomized trial. JAMA 281:327–334, 1999.

36. American College of Sports Medicine: ACSM position stand on exercise and physical activity for older adults. Med Sci Sports Exerc 30:992–1008, 1998.

37. Kraemer HC: Assessment of 2×2 association: Generalization of signal detection methods. Am Stat 42:37–49, 1988.

38. Rothman AJ: Toward a theory-based analysis of behavioral maintenance. Health Psychol 19:64–69, 2000.

SELECTED REFERENCES FOR FURTHER READING

Giles-Corti B, Donovan RJ: The relative influence of individual, social and physical environment determinants of physical activity. Soc Sci Med 54:1793–1812, 2002.

King AC, Bauman A, Calfas K, eds: Innovative approaches to understanding and influencing physical activity. Am J Prev Med 23(suppl): 1–108, 2002.

King AC, Kiernan M, Oman RF, et al: Can we identify who will adhere to long-term physical activity? Application of signal detection methodology as a potential aid to clinical decision-making. Health Psychol 16:380–389, 1997.

Kraemer HC, Stice E, Kazdin A, et al: How do risk factors work together? Mediators, moderators, and independent, overlapping and proxy risk factors. Am J Psychiatr 158:848–856, 2001.

Sallis JF, Owen N: Physical Activity and Behavioral Medicine. Thousand Oaks, CA: Sage Publications; 1999.

INTERNET RESOURCES

Active Living By Design: http://www.activelivingbydesign.org

Health Canada: Physical Activity Unit: http://www.phac-aspc.gc.ca/pau-uap/paguide/

National Center for Bicycling & Walking: http://www.bikewalk.org

National Coalition for Promoting Physical Activity: http://www.ncppa.org

University of South Carolina: Physical Activity Links: http://prevention.sph.sc.edu/palinks

42 Behavioral Strategies to Enhance Physical Activity Participation

ABBY C. KING, JOHN E. MARTIN, AND CYNTHIA CASTRO

This chapter addresses KSAs from the following content areas:

1 Exercise Physiology and Related Exercise Science
2 Pathophysiology and Risk Factors
3 Health Appraisal, Fitness, and Clinical Exercise Testing
4 Electrocardiography and Diagnostic Techniques
5 Patient Management and Medications
6 Medical and Surgical Management
7 Exercise Prescription and Programming
8 Nutrition and Weight Management
9 Human Behavior and Counseling
10 Safety, Injury Prevention, and Emergency Procedures
11 Program Administration, Quality Assurance, and Outcome Assessment

---

A growing number of health behavior change theories and models has been applied in systematic attempts to change physical activity behavior, with varying results[1]. Among the most heuristic of these approaches is the application of social learning/social cognitive theories[2]. These theories, described previously (see Chapter 41), focus on the dynamic relationship between personal attributes and resources, the behavior targeted for change, and influences of the physical and social environment in shaping the **physical activity adoption** and **physical activity maintenance** of the targeted behavior. Along with similar conceptual approaches, these theories provide a framework for development of physical activity **intervention strategies**.

It is important to note, however, that social cognitive theory and similar approaches, as well as stage-based approaches to intervention, have not often been applied in a comprehensive fashion in physical activity intervention research. In addition, the majority of physical activity intervention studies focus on endurance exercise, often ignoring other forms of activity, such as strength and flexibility training, that are important components of fitness. Although more systematic work is needed in this area, some promising strategies—drawn primarily from social

cognitive, stage of change, and similar approaches—for facilitating **physical activity participation** in different stages of physical activity acquisition have been identified.

Increasing Adoption and Early Adherence

Adoption of increased physical activity patterns can be enhanced through paying particular attention to factors in the personal, behavioral, environmental, and program-related spheres described in Chapter 41.

PERSONAL AND BEHAVIORAL FACTORS

With respect to personal factors, previous experience with physical activity should be explored, along with unreasonable beliefs and misconceptions about physical activity (e.g., the "no pain, no gain" fallacy or myths that older individuals should not be active because they need to "conserve their energy"). For example, many inactive individuals believe that exercise is inherently or unavoidably painful and, therefore, aversive; these individuals must be convinced and shown that this statement is untrue. Sedentary individuals are often unaware of the utility of moderate activities (e.g., brisk walking) that may be more appealing and comfortable than more structured, vigorous activity regimens (e.g., high-impact aerobics). Behaviorally, many sedentary individuals benefit from specific instruction (accompanied by actual rehearsal and feedback) on appropriate ways of performing specific activities at a safe, beneficial pace or intensity (e.g., jogging, striding, brisk walking, cycling, and warm-up exercises) to obtain health-related benefits while avoiding injury.

In addition to physical activity–related attitudes, knowledge, and skills, a physical activity program should be personally relevant, both in terms of type of activity (or activities) and goals. For example, if stress reduction is a motivating factor, activities that can be helpful in reducing stress (i.e., not overly competitive, noisy, or demanding) should be targeted. Examples of such activities include brisk walking, jogging, or bicycling conducted outdoors in pleasant surroundings that allow time to "get away from it all."

Additional useful strategies include structuring appropriate expectations concerning physical activity (what can

KEY TERMS

Adherence: The percent of physical activity participation, derived by comparing the amount of physical activity engaged in (numerator) with the amount of physical activity recommended or prescribed (denominator)

Intervention strategies: Any technique or approach that aims at enhancing physical activity participation; these strategies can span a range of domains, from individual to policy level

Physical activity adoption: The initiation of or initial increases in physical activity that often accompany an

intervention or that can occur naturally by an individual. Often, the adoption period is considered to be the initial 3 to 6 months of an intervention or program.

Physical activity maintenance: Sustained physical activity participation that occurs over extended periods of time (i.e., 1 year or longer).

Physical activity participation: The amount of physical activity engaged in more generally, including structured and unstructured (e.g., routine) forms of physical activity

and cannot be accomplished and when results should be expected) as early as possible, stressing the many benefits of making physical activity changes, as well as exploring perceived barriers to increasing physical activity (e.g., unreasonable expectations concerning time or program intensity, fear of embarrassment, failure, boredom). A simple questionnaire or checklist regarding expectations can provide exercise professionals with early clues to such expectations and areas for important problem solving and planning[3].

An underlying goal of many of these strategies is to enhance an individual's early feelings of *self-efficacy* (i.e., confidence in one's abilities to successfully undertake physical activity on a regular basis). Self-efficacy expectations appear to be particularly potent predictors of physical activity participation early on[4]. Thus, it behooves physical activity professionals to focus on clients' initial feelings of self-efficacy and to help to increase their efficacy expectations through shaping early successes. This can be accomplished by helping individuals set realistic, readily accomplishable physical activity goals, providing regular positive feedback and support related to the client's physical activity efforts, and teaching clients to monitor their own physical activity levels as a way of gauging accomplishments and helping them take charge of their programs. Helping clients to think ahead in planning for inevitable lapses in physical activity participation (i.e., relapse prevention) is another means of encouraging clients to take charge of their own programs and enhance their self-efficacy levels in the face of barriers to their physical activity programs[5,6].

PROGRAM-RELATED AND ENVIRONMENTAL FACTORS

Numerous environmental and program-related variables enhance initial adoption and early **adherence** to physical activity (also see GETP7 Box 7-3). These include the factors discussed below.

Convenience

Three factors related to convenience are important to successful initiation and maintenance of an exercise program. First, it is clear that the greater the effort required to prepare for physical activity (i.e., a long drive to and from an exercise facility and other location-related issues; having to change clothes before and after activity), the greater the potential for dropping out[6]. Facilities should be easily accessed. Alternatively, encouraging methods of being physically active in or around the home (the place where many people prefer to exercise) can make convenience less of a deterrent to adherence. Participation in a physical activity program (i.e., joining a spa or health club) close to home or work or conveniently located between these settings should be encouraged. Second, time is often the primary factor leading to perceptions of inconvenience. If a physical activity program is offered within a class structure, several time options may be helpful. For some people with extreme time constraints (e.g., working mothers), alternatives to a class format are often necessary if childcare is not available or affordable at home or at the community facility offering the program. A practical alternative is to emphasize ways that individuals can build regular physical activity into their daily routines, such as through using transportation alternatives that facilitate more walking or bicycling, taking stairs, and walking to do errands. It is becoming increasingly recognized that to optimize the benefits one can obtain from an active lifestyle, participating in both structured as well as routine, functional forms of physical activity is important for many people. Third, modes of physical activity that require special, costly, or time-consuming preparation (e.g., skiing, swimming) may adversely affect adoption and adherence.

Location (or facility), time, and mode can be critical factors during early stages of acquisition. Choices should be carefully evaluated by both the participant and the physical activity professional before initiating a physical activity program. This helps to mitigate the negative impact of such factors.

Behavioral Shaping

For sedentary persons, the major objective is to establish a successful physical activity habit that will lead to the accomplishment of the individual's goals while decreasing opportunities for failure. The initial activity prescription should fall well within the capabilities of the individual and should be easily accomplished, given preferences, motivation, skills, and life circumstances. For some individuals, shaping may translate into a simple initial increase in activities of daily living (ADLs), for example, walking more at work and at home or taking stairs. For others, the initial prescription may involve some less frequent, structured endurance activity with a concomitant increase in routine activity until more vigorous activity is indicated.

A key consideration in all physical activity program planning should be *gradual* shaping of the physical activity behavior toward the ultimate goal set forth by the client and physical activity professional. When behavior shaping is violated, adherence is almost always negatively affected. The rate of injury and dropout increases significantly when beginning exercisers are exposed to physical activities of higher intensity relative to their capacity, frequency (e.g., five or more days per week), or duration (e.g., 45 or more minutes per session) [see Chapter 28]. In contrast, after an individual is beyond the initial stages of his or her program, higher intensity, frequency, and duration are often appropriate.

The physical activity regimen should thus be initially easy to undertake and gradually incremented, ensuring success at each stage (see GETP7 Table 7-1). As noted earlier, exercise professionals (and beginning exercisers) should focus primarily on shaping and maintaining the physical activity habit for approximately 6 to 12 weeks rather than rapidly establishing what may eventually be the optimal regimen for desired benefits. This approach of first establishing behavioral control of the habit implies that physical activity professionals should encourage beginners to simply show up (e.g., "No matter how little you may feel like doing or are able to do, remember that we are working on reinforcing the habit of regular physical activity; the benefits will come, if you can form the habit").

Several methods might be considered in properly shaping the behavior to avoid excessive physical activity (of either undue intensity or duration) during the early stages of a program. Maintaining an intensity during which talking is possible is one method. This level can be easily monitored and assessed by the participant and the physical activity professional. In contrast, simply telling participants to "take it easy" in class- or group-based physical activity programs, when the instructor and most of the class are working at a higher level of intensity, is often ineffective. A more effec-

tive strategy is to provide an additional rolemodel who demonstrates a lower intensity alternative. Individuals can also be taught distraction techniques (e.g., music, reading, or TV watching when using indoor equipment), when relevant, to help refocus their attention from aversive aspects of activity (e.g., increased exertion and sweating).

Heart rate (HR) is a good index of physiological intensity. Pulse rates can be monitored manually or with portable HR monitors. Rating of perceived exertion (RPE) tracks perception of intensity, which may be as important as physical work[7] (GETP7 Table 4-7). In practice, these measures can be used together. For example, an initial RPE of 12 or less and a HR of 70% or less of maximum is recommended in underactive participants for optimal enjoyment and establishment of a habit. In fact, it has been shown that even relatively low levels of exercise intensity (e.g., <60% of maximum HR) can be associated with significant health improvements and disease risk reduction (see Chapter 7). This is particularly true in special populations such as older individuals and those with hypertension[8].

Goal Setting

The success of behavioral shaping is based on the determination of realistic goals that provide the individual with some motivational challenge but that are likely to be successfully achieved, thus leading to increases in self-efficacy. Some physical activity professionals use the acronym SMART to delineate appropriate goal-setting principles (i.e., specific, measurable, attainable, realistic or recorded, timeframe specific).

Enjoyability

For most individuals, it is critically important for adherence that the activity be enjoyable. The physical discomfort that often accompanies early stages of increased activity should be minimized or at least moderated by positive factors and normalized with respect to the individual's expectations if a physical activity habit is to be established. Methods for enhancing enjoyability include tailoring of the types of activities, the actual physical activity regimen or program, and the format of the regimen (group vs. individual, facility or home based). One method of assessing enjoyability is to ask participants to note their level of enjoyment on a range of values from "very unenjoyable" to "very enjoyable" (e.g., scale of 1 to 5). If two or more sessions are "unenjoyable," the exercise regimen should be modified or varied and accompanied, if appropriate for the individual, by additional rewards or incentives.

External Rewards and Incentives

As noted previously, the initial steps involved in becoming more physically active are found by many persons to be anything but rewarding. Often it is not until several months into a regular physical activity program that participants begin to report experiencing positive benefits from physical activity on a regular basis. In fact, the longer the period of inactivity and the more unfit the individual, the longer the period may be before any physical activity becomes intrinsically reinforcing (i.e., feels good). Therefore, beginners may need external rewards early in the program for encouragement and motivation.

Use of such rewards is consistent with the process of behavioral shaping in which early approximations of goal or target behaviors require ample reinforcement or rewards for optimal acquisition (i.e., adoption). For highly unfit, overweight individuals or smokers, for example, beginner status might extend to 6 months or 1 year, and special external incentives may need to be programmed throughout that time. For other, more fit persons, the beginner phase may occur for only a short time, perhaps as little as 2 to 3 weeks. Generally, the choice of which rewards or incentives to use should reside with the participant (because which incentives people find motivating varies from person to person). However, it is important to help participants identify rewards that will not be counterproductive to desired health goals (i.e., high-fat snacks or days off from exercise should be discouraged as rewards).

One valuable and reinforcing form of reward is *social support*. Social support is a powerful motivator for many people. It can be delivered in a variety of forms, including through an instructor, exercise partners, family members, coworkers, or neighbors who encourage increased activity, as well as through telephone contacts or letter or email prompts from a health professional. Praise is a critical component of social support, especially for inexperienced, beginning exercisers and completely relapsed former exercisers. To be most effective, encouragement should be both immediate (during or very shortly after the physical activity episode, if possible) and specific. For example: "Your effort level is great! You'll be able to keep that pace for some time!" or "Great going! Your attendance has been perfect over the past month!" Praise from physical activity professionals, family members, and fellow participants should occur consistently and frequently during the early stages of acquisition. Families of beginning exercisers should also be encouraged to exercise with them if appropriate or to accompany them whenever possible to enhance support. (However, others' physical activity pace must be appropriate for the beginner. If not, both frustration and the chance of injury are often increased.) When support from significant others is active and ongoing, exercisers are more likely than those with little or no social support to persist in a physical activity program[9]. Counselors, family members, and helpers should all be cautioned, however, against even well-intentioned nagging or use of other aversive procedures (e.g., using guilt) designed to induce a reluctant person to become more physically active. Minimal data exist to support the notion that instilling guilt or fear has a beneficial, motivating effect on physical activity. These counterproductive actions almost inevitably increase the punishing

characteristics of physical activity as well as potentially impairing the partnership between the individual and the supportive agent, thus further upsetting the often delicate balance between the motivation to become physically active and remaining inactive.

The use of social support can also be extended and formalized using *written contracts* between the individual and a significant person. Contracts are written, signed agreements that specify the physical activity-related goals in a public format and for which there is value exchange, much like a legal contract (Fig. 42-1 for a sample behavioral contract). They typically specify short-term, concrete goals and the types of positive consequences that occur upon reaching the goals. The contract should be flexible so that rigid daily goals that may be difficult or impossible to meet are avoided (see the next section). In the earlier stages of a program, an appropriate goal might be related to attendance or participation rather than performance. These contracts often work best if they are developed in tandem with an interested person or helper. Such contracts can help to increase personal responsibility and commitment. Those managing physical activity programs should also consider using contingency management, in which more highly rewarding or preferred activities are made contingent on achieving a particular goal (e.g. watching a favorite television program only after a physical activity session is completed).

An alternative to the value–exchange contract is a written agreement through which the participant agrees in writing to perform or complete certain behaviors or activities. An agreement can be useful for persons who refuse or are reluctant to sign a behavioral contract.

The use of appropriate and consistent physical activity models in the environment (i.e., other individuals who may be observed engaging in relevant forms of physical activity) can also motivate people to begin and continue exercise. These models should be as similar as possible to the targeted individuals (some programs use successful graduates as future participant assistants for maximal effectiveness)[6,10]. Furthermore, when possible, the physical activity professional or therapist should set an appropriate example by exercising with participants and displaying other behaviors that are consistent with an active lifestyle (e.g. taking stairs, walking to accomplish errands, adhering to appropriate exercise safeguards such as stretching and hydration).

Another important form of social support is *feedback* regarding progress in relevant or important dimensions of activity. Feedback stimulates a positive, reactive effect on a wide variety of behaviors. For example, short-term reduction of caloric intake usually results when it is monitored. Similarly, the physical activity habit is frequently enhanced when attendance, general physical activity adherence or performance, or the results of the physical activity program are systematically monitored. One simple way to bring this reactive effect of feedback to bear,

Date: _____

Client Responsibilities:

1. Over the next 4 weeks, I will walk at least 4 days per week, for a total of at least 30 minutes per day. (I understand that I can break the 30 minutes up into two 15-minute episodes or walk continuously for 30 minutes).

2. For each week that I attain the above set of goals, I will reward myself by putting aside $5 to be used to treat myself to an article of clothing, a movie, or a similar reward.

3. For each week that I don't meet the above set of goals, I will forego watching a favorite TV show (and I will use that time to walk, if possible).

4. I will record my data on my physical activity calendar at the end of each day, and I will evaluate the success of this set of goals (and revise if necessary) on _____ (date)_____ .

My helper in supporting and reminding me about my goals is:

_____

My signature: _____   Date: _____

Helper signature: _____   Date: _____

FIGURE 42-1. Sample behavioral contract.

especially in those having difficulty engaging in a systematic physical activity program, is to provide an inexpensive pedometer, step-counter, or movement sensor to track walking and related physical activities. Current pedometers have been found to be a cost efficient, valid, and reliable means for providing motivational feedback across a variety of populations[11].

Feedback can also be delivered by another person or generated through use of self-recorded monitoring sheets, an activity diary, or a graph showing progress in one or more variables, plotted HRs, and attendance and adherence across time. Computer-generated feedback letters that summarize progress made in the program over time show promise as an efficient, systematic method for providing personalized feedback on a regular basis. When used in conjunction with goals that are reasonable, personally relevant, and short term, feedback can be a powerfully motivating factor.

Behavioral Success

Continued adherence usually results from behavioral success rather than education or changes in knowledge; that is, engaging in an activity on a regular basis subsequently shapes beliefs and attitudes about continuing the activity, rather than vice versa. This may help explain why many

individuals, despite being knowledgeable about exercise, are not active. Physical activity professionals can help by pointing out the changes and gains being made, no matter how modest. Participants should be shaped such that they engage in some form of regular physical activity regardless of the presence of negative subjective feelings (barring illness or injury) or attitudes. Such regular, successful participation often produces appropriate feelings of mastery and perhaps enjoyment, as well as positive attitudes toward physical activity, a process that enhances the probability of maintaining physical activity.

Self-management

Successful behavior change often correlates with early training in self-management strategies and an understanding of the importance of taking personal responsibility and accountability for physical activity. Individuals must recognize the importance of taking charge of physical activity as a lifelong goal rather than as something that ends when a 12-week class or program is over. Such programs should be thought of as a vehicle for establishing a lifelong habit rather than the means by which physical activity should be defined. Early in all programs, methods to prompt and successfully engage participants in alternate forms of physical activity in a variety of settings and under

BOX 42-1	Methods for Engaging Participants in Physical Activity

Suggestions for Planning Physical Activity

- Carry your exercise clothes or walking shoes in the car; place a pair of walking shoes at work; pack a bag with a set of exercise clothes and shoes so it will be ready when you need it.
- Leave your exercise clothes or shoes by the bed or the front door.
- Formally schedule physical activity into your weekly planner or calendar.
- Spend time with other physically active people.
- Park your car and walk; take stairs whenever possible.
- Only make decisions concerning whether or not to be physically active or how much to exercise *after* arriving at the designated physical activity site or locale.
- Develop a plan or program for high-risk situations (e.g., travel, holidays) to assist with maintaining physical activity.

Suggestions for a Missed Session (Relapse Prevention)

- Admit responsibility for the slip.
- Develop a restart plan, including appropriate goals.
- Call physical activity "buddy" for support and motivation.
- Arrange reinforcements or rewards to help restart the activity.
- Simplify or change regimen to accommodate temporary changes in availability or time.
- Begin by simply visiting the usual physical activity place or locale.

a variety of circumstances should be outlined, along with relevant relapse prevention tips (Box 42-1). In addition, forming a partnership with each individual that fosters the individual's feelings of autonomy and control with respect to the physical activity program has been increasingly recognized as a potentially important means for facilitating long-term participation[12].

Enhancing Maintenance

In addition to sedentary individuals who may have difficulty initiating physical activity, some individuals spend significant time *restarting* physical activity programs that have been terminated for various reasons. Often individuals stop exercising completely after an inevitable break because of illness or injury, travel, holidays, inclement weather, or increased work demands. One useful step is to prepare in advance (both psychologically and behaviorally) for breaks or slips in activity that may lead to a full-blown relapse (and a return to the previous sedentary lifestyle)[5,6,13]. It should be emphasized that such breaks are inevitable and do not indicate laziness or failure. Early identification of high-risk situations that might lead to

inactivity as well as devising strategies to prepare for slips and for restarting the physical activity program can be effective. Useful relapse preparation plans include identification of alternate activities (e.g., brisk walking) that can be undertaken in place of the usual activity, planning to exercise as soon as possible after a break, arranging to exercise with someone else, and resetting goals to an easier level to avoid discouragement. Other methods that may be used for enhancing maintenance include those below.

REMINDERS OF BENEFITS

It is generally worthwhile to provide continued evidence of relevant personal benefits (physical, social, and psychological) from being regularly active. Physical activity professionals should regularly inquire about benefits and positive outcomes experienced from the current physical activity program. For persons at particular risk for dropping out, these questions should be posed frequently (e.g., one or more times per month). If an individual cannot define the positive aspects of physical activity or, alternatively, provides a number of negatives, there is serious risk of dropout. Such participants should be targeted for increased attention and support. Having participants regularly engage in defining their cost–benefit or decisional balance sheet can be a useful means for reinforcing their personal commitments to be active, as well as a prelude for revising the physical activity plan to increase the benefits portion of the equation. In addition, training individuals in simple field methods for evaluating changes in their own fitness or physical functioning levels can serve as a powerful motivator for continued physical activity participation[14].

GENERALIZATION TRAINING

From an instructional standpoint, it is generally wise to avoid discontinuing physical activity programs suddenly, especially if no generalization training has been provided. Generalization training involves expanding the behavior initiated in a setting or a set of circumstances to a different setting to link the behavior with cues or stimuli in the second setting that may help to facilitate ongoing participation. To ensure adherence, the physical activity habit must be generalized or reestablished in new (e.g., home) environments before discontinuing programmed, facility-based sessions[15]. Generalization may be accomplished in several ways, including requiring offsite, home exercise sessions from the beginning or at an early stage of the program (stimulus generalization); involving family or significant others in physical activity sessions; and adding additional exercises before graduation (response generalization) that are easily maintained in the home environment.

Ideally, the responsibility for session supervision, reinforcement, and feedback should be gradually transferred from the instructor to the participants, as well as to helpers in the home environment as the change date approaches. This more closely approximates the conditions likely to be experienced in the new (maintenance) setting.

REASSESSMENT OF GOALS

Regular reassessment of physical activity goals provides an opportunity to verify that they are relevant, realistic, and motivating. Goals that are too long term (e.g., months) or vague (e.g., "I will exercise more") do not provide sufficient motivation to maintain behavior through difficult periods. During the early stages of a physical activity program (i.e., 1 to 6 months), goals should be adjusted as frequently as necessary (i.e., once every 2 weeks) to maintain physical activity behavior.

SOCIAL SUPPORT

Continued use of a variety of social support mechanisms is valuable for continued physical activity maintenance. For instance, if the format is a class or group situation, the leader can call participants who miss two classes in a row (one class in high-risk participants). The purpose of such calls is to let individuals know that they are missed and that others notice and care. Other individuals in the class can assume this type of responsibility as well (a "buddy system"). If physical activity is conducted outside of a formal class or group, the physical activity professional may continue support in the form of periodic telephone calls, letters, emails, or newsletters. Family members, coworkers, neighbors, and friends should continue to encourage and support the physical activity program. (Written materials or newsletters that target these natural support persons can be useful, as can training and encouraging participants to continue to enlist positive support from these persons.) In addition, it may be helpful to schedule special sessions to train helpers in supporting (prompting, modeling, and reinforcing) physical activity. Most importantly, individuals should be encouraged to be proactive about seeking out and identifying their own meaningful sources of support; this increases their feeling of ownership and their role in sustaining their physical activity regimen and resources.

RELEVANT REWARDS

Rewards should change periodically to maintain motivating impact if they are used in conjunction with physical activity goals. Reward systems may include such things as points accumulated as exercise continues to be maintained. Material rewards (e.g., a new exercise outfit, dinner out, a small trip) or small rewards such as free time (to read or engage in other enjoyable activities) may ensue from the accumulation of points. Other examples are requiring a monetary deposit that is returned contingent upon achievement of goals (especially behavioral goals such as attendance and participation) or reducing program fees based on program adherence.

FEEDBACK

Self-monitoring and other forms of feedback are useful for noting progress and enhancing motivation. Research in the field continues to support the utility of regular self-monitoring of physical activity for long-term maintenance. This point notwithstanding, few behavioral strategies evoke more resistance from participants than the prospect of long-term self-monitoring. Individuals should fully participate in designing the self-monitoring strategies that will be the easiest and most convenient for them to maintain. Such strategies can be as simple as noting the number of minutes of moderate-intensity or more vigorous physical activity undertaken throughout the week on a calendar or personal scheduler. As noted earlier, for some, feedback may take the additional form of self-administered fitness tests (e.g., field tests) or professional fitness assessments. Such assessments can be used as a yardstick to measure current compared with past levels of fitness or function.

CONTRACTS

Personal contracts should be updated and changed frequently, if necessary, and should include specific goals, rewards, and helpers. Contracts that are too easy do not provide the challenge needed to motivate many individuals. In contrast, contracts that are too difficult lead to frustration; discouragement; and, potentially, injury.

AVOIDING BOREDOM

Individuals should be encouraged to monitor enjoyment and to be responsible for making activity more enjoyable, especially if it is not meeting their needs or expectations. Physical activity professionals can collaborate to help individuals achieve this goal (e.g., through assisting in suggestions related to new activities, environments, goals, or partners). With a wide variety of physical activities and a diversity of settings in which to conduct activities, the "I'm bored" response should not be allowed to persist and extinguish behavior. Individuals who have achieved improvements in their aerobic conditioning may renew their motivation by trying activities or intensities with a higher level of physical challenge. For some individuals, boredom may be resolved through a regimen involving a variety of activities. For others, one activity conducted in varied settings and formats may be more appropriate. Often, enjoyable competition (e.g., walkathons) can help to stimulate maintenance and reinvigorate a stale program or regimen.

IMPORTANCE OF ROUTINE ACTIVITIES

An increase in ADLs can provide a useful backdrop to help maintain individual activity levels or fitness, especially during times when more structured or vigorous activity is not performed. It is important for many individuals to understand that health benefits obtained from physical activity can be more effectively realized by becoming more active in a variety of ways, both within and outside of formal exercise programs. One method of doing this is to help individuals become aware of times in their daily routines when lower valued, sedentary activities are being engaged in with little thought or planning (e.g., indiscriminant television viewing). After such time periods are identified, more suitable, physically active alternatives can be devised (e.g., going for a walk with family members or dog).

MOTIVATIONAL COUNSELING TO ENHANCE PHYSICAL ACTIVITY PARTICIPATION

Attention has recently been paid to the application of brief motivational interviewing approaches[16] for health behaviors such as physical activity. Motivational interviewing was initially developed as a brief and effective method of helping those with addictive behaviors (primarily alcohol abuse and subsequently smoking) increase their motivational readiness to make positive behavior changes. Some promising work with such techniques has recently begun to occur in the physical activity area as well. Key components of this approach include acknowledging, normalizing, and gently working through the person's ambivalence concerning physical activity participation; stressing the individual's freedom to choose not to be physically active while at the same time encouraging acceptance of responsibility for change and the consequences of not changing; developing an internal discrepancy for remaining inactive through strategic reflections, feedback, and questions from the counselor; and encouraging the client to evaluate the pros and cons (i.e., decisional balance) of remaining inactive versus becoming more active[16]. Such motivational strategies can be applied via telephone as well as through face-to-face encounters (also see Chapter 44).

Summary

Assisting individuals to initiate and maintain increased levels of physical activity can be a challenge to even the most enterprising or creative physical activity professional. Such a task requires continued creativity and flexibility in developing and modifying programs to meet the changing needs of participants. Physical activity professionals may be more effective in these efforts by applying the following guidelines for changing and maintaining behavior:

1. Behavior (including physical activity) is strongly influenced by its immediate consequences rather than distal, long-term consequences. Increasing the immediately rewarding aspects of behavior and decreasing the negative or punishing aspects increases the likelihood that a behavior will occur.
2. Individual choice concerning rewards and incentives is personally motivating.
3. It is important to set mutually agreed-upon and realistic physical activity–related goals and regularly update and modify those goals as necessary.
4. It is useful to encourage individual tailoring of and flexibility in physical activity goal setting, with the emphasis placed on behavioral adherence or attendance initially rather than performance or change in physical outcomes (e.g., body weight). Although participation in physical activity behavior is under the direct control of the individual, factors leading to successful weight loss as well as other physiological changes are often complex and often not well understood.
5. Given the above point, it is critical that the structuring of appropriate and realistic expectations concerning physical activity–related benefits and outcomes be addressed up front during the initial stage of a program to prevent subsequent disappointment and disillusionment.
6. Providing relevant feedback whenever possible is strongly indicated. It is typically helpful to encourage and teach participants to plot and display their progress visually to enhance and maintain their motivation.
7. In order to gradually "shape" an initially difficult behavior, it is useful to have individuals start with less demanding activity goals in order to ease into the habit of being physically active.
8. Preparing participants for inevitable lapses or breaks in their regimens or programs should be encouraged via planning and forethought. In doing so, unexpected breaks in programs can more easily be put into perspective.
9. Whenever possible, it is advisable to offer choices as a means of tailoring physical activity programs to fit the changing needs and preferences of participants and to provide participants with a sense of personal control and autonomy related to their program.
10. Research has shown that encouraging public expression of commitment to being physically active through the use of written contracts, decision balance sheets, and other strategies can promote participation.
11. Teaching individuals how to use environmental or social prompts, cues, and reminders can set the stage for regular participation.
12. To facilitate sustained participation over time, it is useful to foster, from an early point in the program, the use of self-management strategies, including ongoing use of behavioral self-monitoring, decision balance, public declarations, self-assessment, reward systems, and other strategies.
13. It is recommended that individuals enlist and use as many types and sources of social support as possible for their physical activity program. When relevant, it is strongly recommended that individuals be prepared for changes in exercise instructors to minimize disruptions to the class, group, or program.

14. The physical activity program should be used as an opportunity to model and promote a healthy lifestyle that includes and extends beyond physical activity.

15. When appropriate, one can consider the application of motivational interviewing strategies and other client-centered approaches when counseling and interacting with more resistant, inactive individuals and those struggling with ambivalence concerning becoming more active.

16. Helping the individual to explore beliefs, misconceptions, expectations, and barriers early on in the program sets the stage for realistic goal setting and minimizes disappointment and frustration with the program.

Finally, applying a *public health perspective* within which to consider physical activity adoption and maintenance activities can provide a valuable reminder concerning thinking about and targeting *all* members of a community rather than just those who are already reasonably active or motivated to be active. Such a broad perspective emphasizes the importance of inspiring a large number of individuals in a community to engage in at least some physical activity on a regular basis. Striving to motivate sedentary individuals to increase their general activity through more moderate, convenient ADLs is a worthwhile endeavor from both a public health and clinical perspective[17]. Health professionals must remain open to the increasing options for enhancing physical activity, particularly on a community-wide, cost-efficient basis.

Acknowledgments
This work was supported in part by PHS grants #AG-16587, #MH58853, and #HL72489 from the National Institutes of Health awarded to Dr. King.

REFERENCES

1. Young DR, King AC: Exercise adherence: Determinants of physical activity and applications of health behavior change theories. Med Exerc Nutr Health 4:335–348, 1995.
2. Bandura A: Social cognitive theory: an agentic perspective. Ann Rev Psychol 52:1–26, 2001.
3. Neff KL, King AC: Exercise program adherence in older adults: The importance of achieving one's expected benefits. Med Exerc Nutr Health 4:355–362, 1995.
4. Oman RF, King AC. Predicting the adoption and maintenance of exercise participation using self-efficacy and previous exercise participation rates. American Journal of Health Promotion 12:154–161, 1998.
5. Marcus BH, Stanton AL. Evaluation of relapse prevention and reinforcement interventions to promote exercise adherence in sedentary females. Research Quarterly for Exercise and Sport 64:447–452, 1993.
6. Marcus BH, Dubbert PM, Forsyth LH, et al. Physical activity behavior change: Issues in adoption and maintenance. Health Psychology 19:32–41, 2000.
7. Borg GAV. Borg's perceived exertion and pain scales. Champaign, IL: Human Kinetics; 1998.
8. Patten CA, Martin JE: Exercise interventions for older adults with high blood pressure: From efficacy to adherence. J Prevent Intervent Commun 13:111–142, 1996.
9. Oka RK, King AC, Young DR: Sources of social support as predictors of exercise adherence in women and men ages 50 to 65 years. Women's Health: Research on Gender, Behavior, and Policy 1:161–175, 1995.
10. Martin JE, Dubbert PM, Katell AD, et al: Behavioral control of exercise in sedentary adults: Studies 1 through 6. J Consult Clin Psychol 52:795–811, 1984.
11. Bassett DR Jr, Ainsworth BE, Leggett SR, et al: Accuracy of five electronic pedometers for measuring distance walked. Med Sci Sports Exerc 28:1071–1077, 1996.
12. King AC, Friedman R, Marcus B, et al: Harnessing motivational forces in the promotion of physical activity: The Community Health Advice by Telephone (CHAT) Project. Health Educ Res 17:627–636, 2002.
13. King AC, Frederiksen L: Low-cost strategies for increasing exercise behavior: Relapse preparation training and social support. Behav Mod 8:3–21, 1984.
14. Rikli RE, Jones CJ: Development and validation of a functional fitness test for community-residing older adults. J Aging Phys Act 7:129–161, 1999.
15. Rejeski WJ, Brawley LR: Shaping active lifestyles in older adults: A group-facilitated behavior change intervention. Ann Behav Med 19(suppl):S106, 1997.
16. Rollnick S, Mason P, Butler C: Health Behavior Change: A Guide for Practitioners. London/New York: Churchill Livingstone; 1999.
17. Pate RR, Pratt M, Blair SN, et al: Physical activity and public health: A recommendation from the Centers for Disease Control and Prevention and the American College of Sports Medicine. JAMA 273:402–407, 1995.

SELECTED REFERENCES FOR FURTHER READING

Blair SN, Morrow JR Jr, eds: Physical activity interventions [theme issue]. Am J Prev Med 15:255–440, 1998.
Carron AV, Hausenblas HA, Estabrooks PA: The Psychology of Physical Activity. St. Louis: McGraw-Hill; 2002.
King AC: Interventions to promote physical activity in older adults. J Gerontol A Biol Sci Med Sci 56A(special issue II):36–46. 2001.
Marcus BH, Dubbert PM, Forsyth LH, et al: Physical activity behavior change: Issues in adoption and maintenance. Health Psychol 19:32–41, 2000.
Taylor WC, Baranowski T, Young DR: Physical activity interventions in low-income, ethnic minority, and populations with disability. Am J Prev Med 15:334–343, 1998.

INTERNET RESOURCES

Active Living By Design:
http://www.activelivingbydesign.org

Health Canada: Physical Activity Unit:
http://www.phac-aspc.gc.ca/pau-uap/paguide/

National Center for Bicycling & Walking:
http://www.bikewalk.org

National Coalition for Promoting Physical Activity:
http://www.ncppa.org

University of South Carolina: Physical Activity Links:
http://prevention.sph.sc.edu/palinks

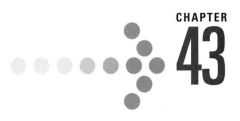

Psychopathology

ANDREA L. DUNN AND HEATHER O. CHAMBLISS

This chapter addresses KSAs from the following content areas:

1   Exercise Physiology and Related Exercise Science
2   Pathophysiology and Risk Factors
3   Health Appraisal, Fitness, and Clinical Exercise Testing
4   Electrocardiography and Diagnostic Techniques
5   Patient Management and Medications
6   Medical and Surgical Management
7   Exercise Prescription and Programming
8   Nutrition and Weight Management
9   **Human Behavior and Counseling**
10 Safety, Injury Prevention, and Emergency Procedures
11 Program Administration, Quality Assurance, and Outcome Assessment

---

Defining Mental Illness

Disturbances in psychological functioning, ranging from mild or moderate to severe, are commonly encountered by exercise professionals working with clients. Some disorders are more common in certain client populations. Understanding and identifying mental disorders is important because of their effects on exercise participation and overall health and well being. For example, population studies consistently show that persons who have more depressive symptoms are less like to be physically active. Furthermore, numerous studies demonstrate that individuals with more depressive symptoms are more likely to develop chronic diseases (e.g., cardiovascular disease) compared with those who have fewer symptoms. Also, when individuals have chronic disease and depressive symptoms, they are more likely to have worse outcomes than are those with chronic disease and few depressive symptoms[1].

Mental health and mental illness are considered part of a continuum of mental functioning. Mental health involves being able to engage in useful work, join in productive relationships with others, and be able to cope with change and adversity. Disruptions in mental health are likely to occur in most people at least once in their lifetime. These disruptions can be transient or chronic and can range from mild to severe. Some may require referral to treatment by a specialist or support group, or the disruptions may resolve over time[1]. In this chapter, the most common mental health problems that are likely to be encountered by exercise professionals are discussed. Terminology established by the most recent *Surgeon General's Report on Mental Health* that differentiates between "mental health problems" and "mental illness" is used in this chapter. Also, criteria for diagnosis for mental disorders established by the fourth edition of the American Psychiatric Association in the *Diagnostic and Statistical Manual of Mental Disorders* (DSM-IV) are the basis for describing symptoms[2]. Discussions are limited to disorders described in DSM-IV.

Mental illness refers to mental disorders that are diagnosable and involve alterations in thinking, mood, or behavior or some combination of these and are associated with impaired functioning. *Mental health problems* are signs and symptoms that are not of sufficient intensity and duration that they can be diagnosed[1]. Each type of mental health problem or mental disorder, including signs and symptoms, according to the DSM-IV; methods of assessment; effective treatments and when to refer to other health specialists are described here. It is important that exercise professionals understand that there are a number of effective treatments for most mental illnesses and mental health problems and to be able to recognize symptoms of mental health problems, so they can refer individuals to appropriate treatment resources.

RECOGNIZING STRESS: SYMPTOMS, ASSESSMENT, TREATMENT, AND REFERRAL

Psychological stress is something everyone experiences to varying degrees. The causes of stress may be specific life events, such as the death of a loved one or the loss of a job, or stress may be caused by less identifiable triggers such as daily hassles or difficult work. Symptoms of stress often overlap those of more severe depression and anxiety disorders (Box 43-1).

KEY TERMS

Anorexia nervosa: An eating disorder that involves intake of calories that is insufficient to maintain normal age and height body weight

Binge-eating disorder: An eating disorder that involves recurrent binge eating episodes at least 2 days per week over 6 months without compensatory behaviors to prevent weight gain

Bipolar disorder: A disorder of mood that involves periods of depressive symptoms and mania

Bulimia nervosa: An eating disorder that involves recurrent binge eating episodes and purging or compensatory behaviors to prevent weight gain

Generalized anxiety disorder (GAD): A type of anxiety disorder characterized by chronic, exaggerated worry that is more extreme than expected by the actual situation

Major depressive disorder (MDD): A mood disorder characterized by depressed mood or loss of interest or

pleasure most of the day, nearly every day for at least 2 weeks; weight loss or weight gain; insomnia or hypersomnia; psychomotor retardation or agitation; fatigue; feelings of worthless or guilt; inability to think; and recurrent thoughts of death

Panic attacks: A type of anxiety disorder characterized by sudden feeling of loss of control or fear, including heart palpitations, sweating, difficulty breathing, chest pain, dizziness, or gastrointestinal distress

Substance abuse: A type of substance use disorder characterized by repeated substance use that results in impairment in functioning or distress

Substance dependence: A type of substance use disorder characterized by cognitive, behavioral, and physiological symptoms that are the result of continued substance use despite problems

Physical symptoms of acute stress include autonomic nervous system activation such as elevated heart rate (HR) and blood pressure (BP), and prolonged stress may impair the immune system, resulting in susceptibility to illness. In addition, persons experiencing high levels of stress often report higher pain ratings and may be at increased risk for injury. High levels of stress may negatively influence health behaviors, including smoking, exercise, diet, and medication use[3].

Formal assessment of stress typically involves the administration of questionnaires to measure an individual's experience and appraisal of stressful life events. A reliable and valid questionnaire that is commonly used to measure an individual's perception of stress is the perceived stress scale (http://www.mindgarden.com)[4]. This instrument quantifies the degree to which individuals appraise their lives as unpredictable, uncontrollable, and overloaded.

Interventions for stress often include using social support networks, including family and friends, religious services, and self-help groups as well as participating in physical activity or relaxation exercises. In addition, assisting individuals in developing problem-focused coping skills can enable them to identify solutions to their problems and enhance feelings of controllability. High levels of stress place individuals at risk for developing more serious mental or physical disorders[2]. Therefore, more formal interventions, including psychotherapy or biofeedback training, may be needed to help individuals develop appropriate coping strategies.

Exercise professionals should be able to recognize when stress is negatively impacting a client's daily functioning or is causing health problems. Many people find relief from stress by participating in exercise, and exercise professionals can work with their clients to determine the most appropriate types of activities for stress relief.

BOX 43-1 | Symptoms of Stress

Symptoms of stress are often similar to symptoms of depression and anxiety and include:

- Difficulty sleeping and fatigue
- Muscle tension and soreness
- Changes in appetite
- Headaches or gastrointestinal problems

RECOGNIZING DEPRESSION: SYMPTOMS, ASSESSMENT, TREATMENT, AND REFERRAL

The burden of depressive disorders is significant. According to the Global Burden of Disease Study conducted by the World Health Organization, major depression ranks second behind ischemic heart disease in the significance of disease burden worldwide[2]. The lifetime prevalence of **major depressive disorder** is approximately 16% in the United States with an estimated 13 million adults suffering from depression each year[5].

| BOX 43-2 | Symptoms of Major Depressive Disorder |

Symptoms of depression include the following:

- Persistent feelings of sadness or irritability
- Loss of interest in previously enjoyed activities
- Feelings of guilt, worthless, or helplessness
- Fatigue or decreased energy
- Difficulty thinking or concentrating
- Sleep disturbances including insomnia or oversleeping
- Changes in appetite; weight gain or loss
- Psychomotor agitation or retardation
- Thoughts of death or suicide

Depression occurs twice as often in women as men, and the gender differences are seen as early as adolescence. However, depression affects both men and women of all age groups, ethnicities, and socioeconomic categories. Certain populations may be at increased risk for depression, including women in the perinatal or menopausal periods; individuals who have experienced a stressful life event; and people with certain medical conditions, including heart disease and diabetes[1]. Depressive disorders are diagnosed according to clinical criteria such as the DSM-IV[2] (Box 43-2).

Mood disorders also include **bipolar disorders**, which are characterized by periods of both depression and mania. Symptoms of mania include extreme elation or irritability, increased energy and decreased need for sleep, grandiose ideas, inflated self-esteem, distractibility, physical agitation, and poor judgment or inappropriate behavior.

Questionnaires such as the Beck Depression Inventory (BDI)[6,7] and Center for Epidemiological Studies Depression Scale (CES-D)[8] are commonly used to assess symptoms of depression. Self-report instruments assess the frequency or severity of symptomatology and commonly include items relating to emotional, cognitive, or physical symptoms of depression. Although questionnaires can give a good indication of presence of depressive symptoms, depressive disorders can only ascertained using standard diagnostic criteria such as the DSM-IV[2]. Consultation with a psychiatrist, psychologist, or physician is important to rule out any other potential causes of symptoms, such as medication or illness, and to develop an appropriate treatment plan.

Effective treatments for depression are available, but many individuals do not seek treatment or receive inadequate treatment. Treatment of depression depends on the type and severity of symptoms and patient preference. Effective treatments include classes of antidepressant medications such as selective serotonin reuptake inhibitors (SSRIs), tricyclic antidepressants (TCAs), and monoamine oxidase inhibitors (MAOIs). Newer antidepressant medications that act on the neurotransmitter sys-

tems serotonin, norepinephrine, or dopamine generally have fewer side effects than TCAs or MAOIs[9,10]. Antidepressant pharmacotherapy takes several weeks before symptoms begin to decrease, and often the dosage must be adjusted for optimal therapeutic effect. Psychotherapy may be used alone or in combination with antidepressant medication to treat depression. Some types of psychotherapy have also been found to be effective and include cognitive-behavioral therapy (CBT) and interpersonal psychotherapy[11,12]. In cases of severe depression or when depression persists despite treatment, electroconvulsive therapy (ECT) may be used and has been found to be effective[11]. Regardless of the treatment modality, it is important that patients are regularly assessed throughout the course of treatment to ensure full remission of depressive symptoms[12]. For individuals who do not respond to the initial course of treatment, it may be necessary to use a combination of treatments, change medication dose, or switch treatment modalities. This process often requires long-term follow-up and continued treatment.

Exercise professionals working with individuals who are receiving antidepressant treatment should be aware the type of medication and any potential somatic or cardiac effects[9,10]. Although most antidepressant medications should not affect response to exercise, some medication side effects such as weight change or sleep disturbances may be relevant to exercise participation. In addition, research suggests that exercise may be useful in reducing depressive symptoms and can be recommended as an adjunctive therapy; thus, patients should inform their mental health providers of their exercise participation.

If untreated depression is suspected, individuals can be referred to a number of community resources that are able to provide diagnostic and treatment services[13] (Box 43-3).

Rarely, an exercise professional may encounter someone who expresses such hopelessness or depression that suicidal risk is suspected[14]. It may be necessary to directly inquire if a person is thinking about suicide. Simply

| BOX 43-3 | First-line Resources for Local Mental Health Services |

- Mental health practitioners, including psychiatrists, psychologists, social workers, or mental health counselors
- Family practice physicians
- Community mental health centers
- Hospital psychiatry departments and outpatient clinics
- Family service, social agencies, religious organizations, and clergy

More information on depression and local treatment resources is available from the Depression and Bipolar Support Alliance (1-800-826-3632 or http://www.dbsalliance.org).

asking: "You seem pretty depressed. Have you had any recent thoughts of harming yourself?" can be a good gauge of suicidal threat. People usually respond honestly, and asking this allows the opportunity to gauge the seriousness of such thoughts. Immediate action is needed if a person communicates planned suicidal intentions. If the person is not under the care of mental health provider, he or she can be referred to a local suicide or crisis center or be taken directly to a hospital emergency room. It is important to make sure that the person is accompanied to the treatment center and that the person is not left alone until professional help is available. The National Hopeline Network (1-800-SUICIDE) is a 24-hour hotline that connects individuals to trained counselors at local crisis centers.

RECOGNIZING ANXIETY: SYMPTOMS, ASSESSMENT, TREATMENT, AND REFERRAL

The most prevalent type of mental disorders is anxiety disorders, with an estimated prevalence of approximately 16% among adults[15]. As with depression, women are twice as likely as men to suffer from anxiety disorders. In contrast to the feelings of anxiety that people experience during stressful events, anxiety disorders are characterized by chronic symptoms that may worsen if left untreated (Box 43-4). Types of anxiety disorders include panic disorder, specific phobias, generalized anxiety disorder (GAD), obsessive-compulsive disorder (OCD), posttraumatic stress disorder (PTSD), and social anxiety disorder; the disorders are diagnosed according to DSM-IV symptom profile and etiology[2].

Panic attacks are characterized by the sudden experience of intense feelings of fear or loss of control. Symptoms include palpitations, sweating, difficulty breathing, chest pain, dizziness, and gastrointestinal (GI) distress. The attacks have an abrupt onset and peak within 10 to 15 minutes, but during that time, individuals often feel as if they are having a heart attack, dying, or "going crazy."

Specific phobias are anxiety disorders in which individuals experience intense fear and avoidance around objects or situations that present no actual danger. In some individuals, exposure to the object may induce a panic attack.

BOX 43-4 | **Common Symptoms of Anxiety Disorders**

- Intense anxiety, worry, fear, or dread
- Difficulty sleeping
- Sympathetic nervous system activation with physical symptoms such as dry mouth, increased heart rate, sweating, trembling, agitation, or gastrointestinal distress

---

Depending on the phobia, the disorder may or may not interfere with daily functioning.

Generalized anxiety disorder (GAD) is characterized by chronic, exaggerated worry and anxiety. An individual with GAD may worry over everyday situations, but the concerns are constant and more extreme than the situation actually presents. Symptoms often include difficulty concentrating and irritability as well as physical complaints such as fatigue, headaches, muscle aches and tension, GI distress, trembling, and sweating.

Obsessive-compulsive disorder involves the experience of disturbing and irrational thoughts (obsessions) and the need to engage in repeated behaviors or rituals (compulsions) to prevent or relieve the anxiety. Individuals with OCD usually recognize that their thoughts and behaviors are senseless, but they are controlled by the troubling thoughts and the urgent need to engage in rituals. Rituals often involve counting, checking, or washing and may significantly interfere with daily functioning.

Posttraumatic stress disorder develops after experiencing or witnessing an intense, terrifying event such as a violent attack, serious accident, natural disaster, or abuse. Symptoms include repeated disturbing thoughts of the trauma, nightmares, sleep disturbances, emotional detachment, irritability, and exaggerated startle response. Persons with PTSD may also experience sudden flashbacks of the event and avoid triggers, or situations that cause memories of the incident. The disorder usually begins within 3 months of the event but may not develop until years later.

Social anxiety disorder is also known as social phobia. This disorder is characterized by intense anxiety and self-consciousness during normal social situations. Individuals with this disorder have a persistent, excessive fear of being watched and evaluated by others and worry of being embarrassed or humiliated. Social anxiety disorder can be specific to certain situations such as speaking or eating in public or be generalized to any social setting.

As with depressive disorders, questionnaires are commonly used to assess symptoms of anxiety. Self-report instruments such as the State/Trait Anxiety Inventory (STAI) typically assess the frequency or intensity of symptoms, including emotional, cognitive, or physical domains[16]. Although questionnaires can give a good indication of presence of symptoms of anxiety, they typically do not categorize symptoms to indicate type of anxiety disorder (e.g., social phobia, GAD) Thus, the presence of an anxiety disorders can only determined by trained professionals using standard diagnostic criteria[2]. Referral to a psychiatrist, psychologist, or physician is important to develop an appropriate treatment plan, which may include psychotherapy, medication, or both.

Common medications for anxiety include antidepressants, benzodiazepines, and beta-blockers. SSRI antidepressant medications are often prescribed for panic disorder, OCD, PTSD, and social phobia; however, this class of medications takes several weeks to achieve full therapeutic effect and is not useful for acute anxiety symptom relief. Benzodiazepines quickly reduce anxiety symptoms and are commonly used in the treatment of patients with panic disorder, social phobia, and GAD. However, people develop tolerance to benzodiazepines and may become dependent on them; symptom rebound may also occur when medication is discontinued. Beta-blockers, which are typically used to treat heart conditions, may be indicated when an anxiety-provoking event is anticipated to minimize physical symptoms[15].

Targeted psychotherapy is often indicated for anxiety disorders[15]. CBT has been found to be particularly useful for treatment of patients with panic disorder and social phobia. Exposure therapy, a type of behavioral therapy, is often used to treat specific phobias, OCD, and PTSD. This technique involves exposing individuals to the feared object or situation in a safe environment so that they can practice controlling their anxiety and responding in more appropriate and productive ways. Relaxation training, including breathing exercises and biofeedback, may also be used as a component of anxiety treatment. Treatment plans for an anxiety disorder should also include evaluation and treatment of comorbid mental disorders because depression, substance abuse, and other anxiety disorders often occur concomitantly.

If a person exhibits symptoms of anxiety, he or she can be referred to the same community mental health resources that treat depression. However, mental health professionals with specialized training in CBT and anxiety treatment may provide the most comprehensive treatment options. Additionally, self-help groups are often particularly helpful for people with anxiety disorders because people find it comforting to share their experiences with people who can understand their concerns and problems.

As with antidepressant medications, exercise professionals working with individuals who are receiving anti-anxiety medication should be aware the type of medication and any potential side effects. Some types of medication may affect the sympathetic nervous system's response to exercise so that HR or BP may not increase as expected. As with depressive symptoms, research suggests that exercise may be useful in reducing symptoms of stress and anxiety[17,18]. Although individuals with panic disorder may avoid participating in exercise for fear of inducing a panic attack, the attacks are not more likely to occur during physical activity than during other daily activities[17,18]. By understanding a person's individual concerns, exercise professionals can work to create a safe and comfortable environment by minimizing potential exposure to anxiety-inducing situations. The Anxiety Disorders Association of America (240-485-1001 or http://www.adaa.org) can provide additional information on anxiety disorders and local treatment services[15].

RECOGNIZING EATING DISORDERS: SYMPTOMS, ASSESSMENT, TREATMENT, AND REFERRAL

Disordered eating comprises a spectrum of behavioral, cognitive, and emotional symptoms involving disturbances in eating and body image. Eating disorders are diagnosed according to standard criteria and include the disorders of anorexia nervosa, bulimia nervosa, and binge-eating disorders[2]. Eating disorders are more common in women than in men, and disorders often develop in adolescence or young adulthood. Because eating disorders can cause significant health problems and even death, early recognition and treatment are critical (Box 43-5).

Anorexia nervosa is characterized by insufficient caloric intake to sustain body weight, below-normal weight for age and height, intense fear of becoming fat, distorted body image, and disturbances in menstrual cycles. Health complications of this disorder include osteoporosis, muscle atrophy, electrolyte imbalances, and cardiac arrhythmias, sometimes resulting in death[19,20].

Bulimia nervosa involves episodes of binge eating, or consuming large amounts of food within a discrete period of time and purging, or compensatory behaviors to prevent weight gain such as self-induced vomiting, use of diuretics or laxatives, fasting, and excessive exercise. Individuals with this disorder are often of normal body weight but may express intense body dissatisfaction and a desire to lose weight. Health consequences of bulimia nervosa include GI disturbances, electrolyte imbalances, esophageal ruptures, pancreatitis, and erosion of tooth enamel[19,20].

Binge-eating disorder involves recurrent binge eating episodes, at least 2 days per week over 6 months, without compensatory behaviors to prevent weight gain. The episodes often involve eating more rapidly than usual, feeling uncomfortably full, eating when not hungry, eating alone, and feelings of guilt or disgust[19,20].

Symptoms of disordered eating are often readily recognizable to outside observers. However, determining the

---

BOX 43-5 | **Symptoms of Eating Disorders**

- Extreme eating patterns including restriction and overeating
- Body weight loss or gain
- Purging behaviors, including vomiting, laxative use, or excessive exercise
- Unusual eating behaviors, including preferences or phobias of certain foods and obsessive rituals
- Excessive weighing or avoidance of weighing
- Distorted body image, low self-esteem, feelings of guilt and self-disgust

extent of the problem is often difficult because individuals with eating disorders are often very good at hiding their behaviors and resist intervention. Professional assessment of eating disorders involves multiple components, including medical evaluation to assess body weight and health problems, psychological evaluation to assess the severity of the eating disorder and the presence of comorbid mental disorders, and nutritional consultation to evaluate current eating habits.

Treatment is a multifaceted process that often involves a team of health care professionals, including physicians, psychologists or counselors, and nutritionists. Severe eating disorders are often treated in an inpatient setting so that weight can stabilized and medical conditions treated. Psychotherapy is an important component of treatment to reduce inappropriate eating behaviors and explore psychological issues such as body image, self-esteem, and interpersonal relationships. Nutritionists and exercise professionals can play an important role on the intervention team to regulate energy balance through appropriate caloric intake and energy expenditure. Finally, SSRI medications may be helpful in the treatment of eating disorders.

Exercise professionals can play an important role in recognizing symptoms of eating disorders and referring individuals to treatment. When working with clients who have symptoms of disordered eating, care should be taken to monitor energy balance, modify exercise prescriptions to accommodate any medical problems, use sensitivity when weighing or conducting body composition measurements, and communicate appropriate messages to protect body image and self-esteem. More information on eating disorders can be found from the National Association of Anorexia Nervosa and Associated Disorders (847-831-3438 or http://www.anad.org).

RECOGNIZING ALCOHOL AND DRUG ABUSE: SYMPTOMS, ASSESSMENT, TREATMENT, AND REFERRAL

Substance use disorders include any disorders related to problems associated with the use of alcohol, drugs of abuse, prescribed or over-the-counter medications, and toxins. Substance use disorders include substance abuse and substance dependence[1].

Substance abuse refers to a condition in which repeated substance use results in significant adverse effects that produce impairment in functioning or distress. Use of the substance may interfere with role obligations, occur in hazardous situations, result in legal problems, or occur despite interpersonal or social problems[2].

Substance dependence is characterized by cognitive, behavioral, and physiological symptoms that result when an individual continues substance use despite problems. Specific symptoms of substance dependence include tolerance to the substance so that more is needed to achieve an effect and withdrawal symptoms in the absence of the substance. Additional symptoms that characterize dependence include the inability to control use of the substance, using more than intended, neglect of activities, significant time spent using or recovering from effects of the substance, and continued use despite psychological or health problems.

Professional assessment of patients with substance use disorders is critical to ensure the safety of the individual and to implement appropriate treatment. Substance abuse commonly occurs with other mental disorders such as depression, and treatment may involve a combination of individual therapy, group therapy, medication, or a combination. Local hospitals and substance abuse centers can provide medical and psychological evaluation and treatment in inpatient or outpatient settings.

Exercise professionals are most likely to recognize symptoms of substance use during acute intoxication or when the client reports questionable behaviors such as recurrent binging or blackouts. Written food diaries used in nutrition counseling may also provide evidence of substance abuse. Often individuals with drug or alcohol problems may deny a problem and resist treatment; however, they may be open to receiving referrals if the information is presented in a professional and caring manner. The Substance Abuse Treatment Facility Locator service (1-800-662-HELP or http://findtreatment.samhsa.gov) provides information on local substance abuse treatment services, and community chapters of Alcoholics Anonymous and Narcotics Anonymous can also provide information and resources.

Summary

Mental disorders are common problems affecting people of all ages and backgrounds. If recognized, mental health problems can be readily treated, with significant improvement in psychological functioning, physical health, and quality of life. In most cases, exercise is a useful adjunctive therapy to the treatment of mental disorders and may be effective in preventing symptoms of disorders such as anxiety and depression. Exercise professionals should be able to recognize symptoms of mental disorders and refer clients to appropriate community services for treatment.

REFERENCES

1. U.S. Department of Health and Human Services: Mental Health: A Report of the Surgeon General. Rockville, MD: U.S. Department of Health and Human Services, Substance Abuse and Mental Health Services Administration, Center for Mental Health Services, National Institutes of Health, National Institute of Mental Health; 1999.
2. American Psychiatric Association: Diagnostic and Statistical Manual of Mental Disorders, 4th ed. Washington, DC: American Psychiatric Association; 1994.
3. Cohen S, Schwartz JE, Bromet EJ, Parkinson DK: Mental health, stress, and poor health behaviors in two community samples. Prev Med 20:306–315, 1991.
4. Cohen S, Kamarck T, Mermelstein R: A global measure of perceived stress. J Health Soc Behav 24:385–396, 1983.

5. Kessler RC, Berglund P, Demler O, et al: The epidemiology of major depressive disorder: Results From the National Comorbidity Survey Replication (NCS-R). JAMA 289:3095–3105, 2003.

6. Beck AT, Ward CH, Mendelson M, et al: An inventory for measuring depression. Arch Gen Psychiatr 4:561–571, 1961.

7. Beck AT, Steer RA, Garbin MG: Psychometric properties of the Beck Depression Inventory: Twenty-five years of evaluation. Clin Psychol Rev 8:77–100, 1988.

8. Radloff LS: The CES-D Scale: a Self-report depression scale for research in the general population. App Psychol Meas 1:385–401, 1977.

9. Glassman AH, Roose SP, Bigger JT Jr: The Safety of tricyclic antidepressants in cardiac patients. Risk-benefit reconsidered. JAMA 269:2673–2675, 1993.

10. Roose SP, Laghrissi-Thode F, Kennedy JS, et al: Comparison of paroxetine and nortriptyline in depressed patients with ischemic heart disease. JAMA 279:287–291, 1998.

11. Rush AJ, Golden WE, Hall GW, et al: Depression in Primary Care: Volume 1. Detection and Diagnosis. Clinical Practice Guideline., Number 5. 93-0550 ed. Rockville, MD: U.S. Department of Health and Human Services, Public Health Service, Agency for Health Care Policy and Research; 1993.

12. Rush AJ, Golden WE, Hall GW, et al: Depression in primary care: Volume 2. Treatment of Major Depression. Clinical Practice Guideline, no. 5, 2nd ed. Rockville, MD: U.S. Department of Health and Human Services, Public Health Service, Agency for Health Care Policy and Research; 1993.

13. National Institutes of Mental Health: Depression. Available at: http://www.nimh.nih.gov/healthinformation/depressionmenu.cfm

14. Brown GK: A review of suicide assessment measures for intervention research with adults and older adults. National Institute of Mental Health. Available at http://www.nimh.nih.gov/suicideresearch/adultsuicide.pdf.

15. National Institute of Mental Health: Anxiety disorders. Available at: http://www.nimh.nih.gov/healthinformation/anxietymenu.cfm

16. Spielberger CD, Gorsuch RL, Lushene R, et al: Manual for the State-Trait Anxiety Inventory (STAI) Form Y. Palo Alto, CA: Consulting Psychologsits Press; 1983.

17. Byrne A, Byrne DG: The effect of exercise on depression, anxiety and other mood states: A review. Health Psychol 12:292–300, 1993.

18. Cameron OG, Hudson CJ: Influence of exercise on anxiety level in patients with anxiety disorders. Psychosomatics 27:720–723, 1986.

19. Foster DW: Anorexia nervosa and bulimia. In Wilson JD, Braunwald E, Isselbacher KJ, et al. (eds) 12th ed. Harrison's Principles of Internal Medicine New York: McGraw-Hill, 1981.

20. National Institutes of Mental Health: Eating Disorders. Available at: www.nimh.gov/publicat/eatingdisorders.cfm

SELECTED REFERENCES FOR FURTHER READING

Brownell KD, Fairburn CG: Eating Disorders and Obesity: A Comprehensive Handbook. New York: Guilford Press; 1995.

Johnson VE: Intervention: How to Help Someone Who Doesn't Want Help. Center City, MN Hazelden Publishing; 1986.

Leahy RL, Holland SJ: Treatment Plans and Interventions for Depression and Anxiety Disorders. New York: Guilford Press; 2000.

Morgan WP: Physical Activity and Mental Health. Washington, DC: Taylor & Francis; 1997.

Sapolsky RM: Why Zebras Don't Get Ulcers: An Updated Guide to Stress, Stress-Related Diseases, and Coping. New York: W.H. Freeman & Company; 1998.

INTERNET RESOURCES

Anxiety Disorders Association of America:
http://www.adaa.org

Depression Screening:
http://www.depression-screening.org

National Eating Disorders Association:
http://nationaleatingdisorders.org

National Institutes of Mental Health:
http://www.nimh.nih.gov

Substance Abuse and Mental Health Services Administration
http://www.samhsa.gov

JESSICA A. WHITELEY, BETH LEWIS, MELISSA A. NAPOLITANO, AND BESS H. MARCUS

This chapter discusses some fundamental counseling skills and some steps for applying them with clients. In doing so, the chapter borrows from several of the theoretical principles mentioned in Chapter 39. Specifically, the transtheoretical model[1], social cognitive theory[2,3], and the relapse prevention model[4] are discussed. In addition, the chapter introduces some strategies from motivational interviewing[5]. The intention is to teach some strategies that blend a client-centered approach[6,7], in which the counselor listens and follows what clients say, and a directive approach, which include constructive discussions regarding behavior change[7]. The strategies do not include giving advice. Advice giving, although effective in some instances, can be detrimental to behavior change in others[7]. Some clients perceive advice giving as condescending or presumptuous, in that the client might perceive that you are telling them what to do, thereby undermining their autonomy and possibly generating resistance[7]. Instead, this chapter focuses on a client-centered approach that incorporates the counseling skills of rapport building, active listening, reflective listening, and empathy. These counseling skills can then be the tools that are used with a directive approach in which discussions regarding self-

monitoring, benefits and barriers, confidence, feedback, and relapse prevention can take place.

Health Counseling Techniques

The "**client-centered approach**"[6–9] takes the client's perspective into account when making decisions about behavior change. Box 44-1 lists what Stewart et al.[9] have described as several of the key elements of the client-centered approach. This approach, when used by physicians, has been shown to be related to higher client satisfaction, increased medication compliance, a reduction in clients' concerns, and a reduction in actual symptoms such as raised blood pressure[9]. Rollnick et al.[7] summarize the goals of the client-centered approach as encouraging clients to express concerns, helping them to be more active in the consultation, allowing them to state what information they need, giving them more control of the decision making, and reaching joint decisions. One caveat to this approach is that if you have a very limited amount of time with a client (e.g., one 15-minute consultation), the client-centered approach is more difficult. In this case, you may need to be more directive. However, whenever possible we recommend trying to incorporate the techniques discussed below.

In order to achieve these goals, the practitioner needs to adopt a set of counseling skills that are nonjudgmental. Practitioners need to establish rapport, be encouraging, be interested in the client's perspective, ask open-ended questions, and be good active listeners.

ESTABLISHING RAPPORT

The first important aspect in using the client-centered approach in working with clients is establishing **rapport**. Rapport is the relationship you establish with your client. It is built on trust and mutual respect. If a strong therapeutic relationship is established from the beginning, the behavior change process is more likely to succeed. One strategy for establishing rapport is to ask the client open-ended questions. For example, Rollnick et al.[7] suggest asking clients to describe a typical day. This is meant to allow clients to tell you about activities that occur throughout the day while providing you with a number of facts regarding how they spend their time. This may be

KEY TERMS

Active listening: A process whereby a practitioner tries to understand the underlying meaning of what a client is saying

Client-centered approach: A counseling style that takes the client's perspective into account, features collaboration between the client and counselor, and includes genuine respect for the client's opinions

Decisional balance: The comparison of the benefits of making a behavior change versus the costs

Empathy: The understanding that is conveyed by a counselor to a client

Processes of change: The strategies that individuals use as they are adopting and maintaining behavior changes; five behavioral (e.g., obtaining social support) and five cognitive processes (e.g., increasing knowledge) have been identified

Rapport: The positive relationship counselors establish with their clients

Reflective statements: Statements that repeat back to client what the counselor has heard and understood the client to say. If done in conjunction with active listening, these statements reflect the underlying meaning of what they client is saying.

Relapse prevention: The process by which one maintains long-term behavior change by anticipating potentially high-risk situations and devising strategies to cope with these situations

Self-efficacy: An individual's belief and confidence about his or her ability to make specific behavior changes

Stages of change: A model that postulates that individuals move through a series of stages and face common barriers when making a behavior change

helpful in identifying opportunities for decreasing sedentary behavior and increasing active behavior.

INTEREST AND EMPATHY

Conveying interest and **empathy** also helps to establish rapport. The process of listening and conveying understanding, or empathy, is not a passive process. If you are listening carefully to your client, you can convey that you are hearing what she is saying by either repeating what you heard her say, summarizing her statements, or asking questions for clarification. For example, a client might be telling you about how she was active in sports as a child, but as she had children of her own and continued her full-

| BOX 44-1 | Key elements of the Client-centered Approach[9] |

- Approach the client with unconditional positive regard.
- Behavior change is based on a genuine, respectful relationship.
- Assessment of the client occurs when the practitioner seeks to enter the world of the client to understand his or her unique perspective.
- The client and the practitioner work together to define the problem and to establish the goals and the roles of the client and practitioner.
- Each contact between the practitioner and the client is an opportunity to build the therapeutic relationship for health promotion.

time job, she had less time to be physically active and wonders if she will enjoy it now that her life circumstances have changed. You might summarize this by saying, "Let me just make sure I am following you, Jane. You played sports as a child, but as you have gotten older, you have had fewer opportunities to be active and aren't sure if you will enjoy it anymore. Is that right?" This demonstrates that you were listening and gives both you and the client a chance to make sure you understand one another. This helps to build rapport with your client.

ACTIVE LISTENING

Another client-centered technique is called **active listening**. Active listening is a process wherein the practitioner tries to understand the *underlying meaning* of what the client is saying. The practitioner then makes **reflective statements** to convey that she has heard and understood this underlying meaning. This is a more advanced counseling skill and typically takes some practice. Reflecting back the underlying meaning can help to establish rapport and empathy in that it demonstrates your understanding of the client's perspective. In the example above, a response that combines a reflective statement, an empathetic statement, and an open-ended question would be: "It sounds like you are a little apprehensive about exercising right now [reflective statement]. This is common when you haven't been active in a long time [empathetic statement]. What are some of your concerns [open-ended question]?" This reflective statement reflects the understanding of the underlying emotional meaning that the client is worried or perhaps afraid but does so in a way that is intended to be nonthreatening. By asking the client to state her concerns through an open-ended question, you have begun a conversation about her barriers to being physically active. We will discuss this in more detail later.

SUMMARY OF HEALTH COUNSELING TECHNIQUES

Through the use of a few counseling techniques that are client-centered, you may be able to increase satisfaction and compliance among your clients. Rollnick et al.[7] summarize these techniques found in Box 44-2. To know if you are practicing these techniques correctly, there will be a few clues from the client. These are summarized by Rollnick et al.[7] in Box 44-3.

Behavior Change Strategies

The health counseling skills described above can be used within the framework of behavior change strategies. These strategies are more directive but can be accomplished through conversations in which you use the client-centered techniques of summarizing, clarifying, active listening, reflective statements, and empathy. To maximize success for your clients, it is important to use techniques and strategies that have been shown to be effective. Thus, the behavior change strategies that are presented here offer ways of working with clients to assess their readiness for behavior change, determine the strategies that are appropriate for them given their stage of change, track their progress, and set goals to achieve progress.

STAGES OF CHANGE

As is described in Chapter 39, the transtheoretical model offers both a means of assessing readiness to change as well as a number of cognitive and behavioral processes to promote with your clients. In brief, the transtheoretical model postulates that individuals move through a series of stages as they become physically active[1,10]. These stages include

---

BOX 44-2	Summary of Client-centered Techniques[7]

- Ask simple, open-ended questions (i.e., questions that elicit details, not simple yes-or-no responses).
- Listen and encourage with verbal and nonverbal prompts.
- Clarify and summarize. Check your understanding of what the client said and check to see that the client understood what you said.
- Use reflective listening. This involves making statements that aim to bridge the gap between what that client is saying and the meaning behind the statements.

BOX 44-3	How You Know When You Are Using the Client-centered Approach[7]

- You are speaking slowly.
- The client is talking more than you.
- The client is talking about behavior change.
- You are listening intently and directing the conversation when appropriate.
- The client appears to be making realizations and connections that he or she had not previously considered.
- The client is asking you for information or advice.

---

precontemplation (not intending to make changes), contemplation (considering a change), preparation (making small changes), action (actively engaging in the behavior), and maintenance (sustaining the change over time) [see GETP7 Box 7-2 and Figure 7-7]. As participants move through the **stages of change**, they engage in cognitive and behavioral processes. The **processes of change** were translated from the terms first created by Prochaska and DiClemente[1] for physical activity and to make them more readily accessible for participants. The cognitive processes include increasing knowledge, warning of risks, caring about consequences to others, comprehending benefits, and increasing healthy opportunities[11]. Behavioral strategies include substituting alternatives, enlisting social support, rewarding yourself, committing yourself, and reminding yourself[11].

Although there are a few different versions of how to assess the stages of change, we recommend using the version in Box 44-4[12]. Moderate-intensity physical activity is defined for the individuals. Then clients indicate a "yes" or "no" to four statements: "I am currently physically active," "I intend to become more physically active in the next 6 months," "I currently engage in regular physical activity," and "I have been regularly physically active for the past 6 months." The algorithm shown in Box 44-4 is used to identify the stage for a specific individual. In working with your client, you could ask these questions conversationally to assess the client's motivational readiness, or you might have the client fill out the questionnaire.

Knowing a person's stage of change suggests different strategies for working with that particular person. It is possible to target an intervention to an individual's stage of change[10]. It has been shown that individuals who are in the earlier stages of change—precontemplation and contemplation—are more likely to use the cognitive processes of change such as increasing knowledge and comprehending the benefits. As people move into the later stages, they start to use more behavioral processes of change such as enlisting social support and substituting alternatives. Matching the change processes to the participant's stage is another important component of a client-centered approach. This conveys that you understand how ready a client is to change. Chapter 39 provides a number

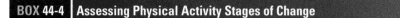

| BOX 44-4 | Assessing Physical Activity Stages of Change |

PHYSICAL ACTIVITY STAGES OF CHANGE

INSTRUCTIONS: For each question below, please fill in the circle Yes or No. Please be sure to follow the instructions carefully.

	Yes	**No**
1. I am currently physically active.	Y	N
2. I intend to become more physically active in the next 6 months.	Y	N

For activity to be regular, it must add up to a total of 30 or more minutes per day and be done at least 5 days per week. For example, you could take one 30-minute walk or three 10-minute walks each day.

	Yes	**No**
3. I currently engage in regular physical activity.	Y	N
4. I have been regularly physically active for the past 6 months.	Y	N

	ITEM			
Stage	1	2	3	4
Precontemplation	No	No	—	—
Contemplation	No	Yes	—	—
Preparation	Yes	—	No	—
Action	Yes	—	Yes	No
Maintenance	Yes	—	Yes	Yes

Modified with permission from Marcus BH, Forsyth LH: Motivating People to be Physically Active. Champaign, IL: Human Kinetics; 2003.

of examples of how the change processes vary by stage. This chapter focuses on some examples of how you might counsel your clients with a stage-based approach.

In addition to knowing your client's stage of change, it will also be important to understand how the client tends to spend his time and what factors will influence his decision to be physically active. It is important to identify both the benefits and barriers to physical activity. For many people, time will be their number one barrier. When clients talk about their barriers, it is important to use the counseling skills of empathy and reflective listening to allow them to discuss these barriers with you. If the client feels understood and if you engage in problem solving to effectively deal with barriers (to be described in more detail below), the client is more likely to remain engaged in the behavior change process.

TRACKING ACTIVITY

Another strategy to assess daily activities is to have your clients track their daily behaviors on self-monitoring forms. There are many ways to do this, and you can tailor the tracking form to an individual's needs. For example, if a client is in contemplation, she may need to track how she spends her time on a daily basis. This means writing down her activities, including sedentary activities (e.g., time spent watching television, driving, sitting while eating, sitting at the computer) and the time spent at each activity. Box 44-5 provides an example of a self-monitoring log. If the client keeps track of this for several days over the course of the week, you can review the monitoring form together the following week. This allows somewhat of a directive framework for your discussion while still using your client-centered counseling strategies. It is important to identify opportunities for decreasing sedentary behavior, increasing physical activity, and what the benefits and barriers might be for both. For instance, if the client finds she is sitting at her computer for many hours at a time, it may be possible for her to start incorporating short walks to break up this computer time. From a client-centered perspective, you would initiate a conversation about the inactivity of her computer time in which she comes to the

BOX 44-5	Tracking Form

EXAMPLE

Date: _____

TIME	ACTIVITY	MINUTES SPENT DOING	NOTES
7:00am	Got ready for work	60	
8:00am	Drove to work	45	
8:45am	Walked in to work	3	Walked slowly
8:50am	At my desk for computer work	180	Wow!

YOUR TURN

Date: _____

TIME	ACTIVITY	MINUTES SPENT DOING	NOTES

conclusion that this might be an opportunity for change (rather than your pointing this out to her). Finding small instances for the client to become less sedentary can provide the first building block of activity for an individual who has been inactive.

In contrast, if a person is in the preparation stage, the tracking might be quite different. The person in preparation may not need to record his activity throughout the day but may focus instead on his bouts of moderate or vigorous activity while identifying opportunities for increasing the behaviors in which he is already engaged. This self-monitoring form would include the day of the week the activity is done, the time spent doing the activity, and perhaps the time of day. Again, the self-moni-

toring form can then provide the framework for a discussion regarding physical activity. You can review with your client any patterns of behavior that may arise and work with him to think of ways to increase his activity level. For instance, in tracking his activity, a client may have 2 days when he was physically active. In an attempt to clarify and understand this, you may ask, "What is different about the days when you weren't physically active versus the days you were?" The client may then describe that on the days when he was inactive, he had planned to go to the fitness facility *after work*. However, he often was too tired after work and went home instead. Thus, he may recognize that he was more successful going to the fitness center before work. The natural tendency is to advise the client based on this information. However, using the client-centered approach, it would be important for the client to come to his own realizations about changing his behavior. By listening carefully, reflecting, and emphasizing the positive, the client might make the connections that you hope he will make (i.e., "I should be physically active in the mornings or make a plan to go the gym even if I am tired"). In some cases, the client may understand what is not working but is unsure of what to do to change the situation. In these situations, the technique of problem solving, as described later, may be used.

DECISIONAL BALANCE

Another strategy for motivating behavior change is to have your client identify the benefits and barriers of being physically active, or her **decisional balance**. To do this, you might have an open-ended conversation about this or you can have your client make a list where the pros, or benefits, are listed on one side and the cons, or barriers, are listed on the other (Box 44-6). It is important that the client list the factors that are important to her rather than what she knows should be important. For example, a client may know that one of the benefits of physical activity is decreasing the risk of osteoporosis, but this might not be important to her. However, feeling less fatigued may be more motivating factor for this particular client. Information obtained from this list can to provide the framework for another conversation about behavior change while continuing to use your counseling techniques. Another resource for a similar measure is the decisional balance questionnaire, which is found in Marcus and Forsyth[12].

Benefits

This list of benefits, or pros, can be important to discuss as a means of affirming the reasons why the client is interested in behavior change. This list can also be important to keep in mind when working with your client if his motivation or behavior is low in the future. You can ask your client to recount why he would like to be physically active. For a client who feels tired after work, remembering that one of the pros he listed was increased energy and that he will feel more energetic after exercising may give him the motivation he needs to make that decision in the moment. In addition, if you are working with a client over time, you can emphasize progress with positive statements that will help to reinforce or increase the behavior. For example, if you see the client looking less fatigued, you might comment, "It looks like you have more energy these days." This helps to reaffirm the benefits of his activity.

Barriers

The list of barriers, or cons, is important to address to determine the obstacles that may stand in the way of your client's making progress. If your client is having difficulty identifying her barriers or it seems the list is incomplete, you may find that self-monitoring may provide insight into the client's barriers. For example, if the client takes a walk on the day her neighbor is available to walk with her but not on the days when she would need to walk alone, you might have a discussion about this. As discussed earlier, you should find a way to allow the client to come to her own conclusion. Examples of what you might say include: "It seems as though you really enjoy walking with your neighbor" or "What do you enjoy about your walks with your neighbor?" In this way, you may be able to gently

---

BOX 44-6	Pros and Cons Worksheet

Pros	Cons
_____	_____
_____	_____
_____	_____
_____	_____
_____	_____
_____	_____
_____	_____
_____	_____
_____	_____
_____	_____

direct the client to realize that walking alone is a barrier and having someone to walk with is a facilitator to being active. The goal is to work with your client to determine her unique barriers to increase physical activity. In doing so, you may need to refer to the self-monitoring form, and you may need to help the client determine which barriers are more or less difficult to overcome. It is particularly important to be nonjudgmental in this process so that the client feels comfortable and confident to problem solve solutions to the barriers.

PROBLEM SOLVING

After the barriers have been determined, an important skill to help your client develop is problem solving. Problem solving can be done to determine solutions for the barriers that your client has identified. The *process* of problem solving is more important to learn than a set of solutions for any one barrier, so that the client will know how to tackle barriers in the future. Problem solving, therefore, fosters independent thinking and self-confidence in one's abilities to remain physically active. Problem solving involves several different steps[12]. The acronym IDEA has been developed to identify the four steps of Identifying the problem, Developing a list of solutions, Evaluating the solutions, and Analyzing how well the plan worked. See Box 44-7 for an example of this.

The first step involves identifying the problem. From the list of barriers that your client has been able to identify, have your client pick one that is most pressing. In identifying the problem, it will be important to think through the problem fully to determine the key element or elements. In our example above of the woman who only walked when her neighbor was available, you should ask her to identify why this occurred. As the client starts to talk about this, she may realize that she needs social support to be active. There are often many layers to any one problem, and it may be necessary to probe further to determine what about obtaining social support is important. In doing so, you may learn that walking with her neighbor is enjoyable, the time passes quickly, she feels safer, and she feels more motivated because she knows her friend is going to be meeting her.

The second step is to develop a list of solutions. This is a brainstorming session in which the client thinks of any and all solutions while withholding any evaluation of them until later. This is a time to be creative. You may help your client with a few if he or she is having trouble getting started. It is likely that you will need to remind your client that you do not evaluate the ideas at this stage. Have the client write down all of the solutions that are generated. Possible solutions for the female walker include seeing if her neighbor can walk more often, joining a class at a gym, walking with her spouse, starting a walking club, or finding other friends who are available on other days.

The third step is to evaluate the solutions. Some solutions will be more realistic and address more of the details of the problems than others. You can work with your client to determine which of the solutions seem most appropriate. It may be that starting a walking club is too daunting but asking her neighbor to walk more often seems feasible. Whatever the solutions, work with your client to set goals and make a concrete plan about how the solution will be implemented.

The final step is to analyze how well the plan worked. If a plan worked well, then praise the client for a job well done. Many times, however, the plan will not have worked as was intended. It is important to emphasize that problem solving is a process that allows for learning and it is not uncommon to need to fine-tune the solution. In some cases, attempts to implement a solution elicit new details regarding the problem or new barriers. This information is critical to correctly identifying all of the important aspects of a problem and searching for a solution that addresses these aspects. Clients may be discouraged with their progress. It is important to emphasize the positive of what the client did accomplish, emphasize the importance of learning from what does not work, and work together to generate new solutions and plans.

GOAL SETTING

Another important skill for clients to develop is the ability to set goals. It is important to identify several characteristics of goal setting, including setting goals that are specific, short term, and challenging yet realistic[3]. It also is also important to make goals measurable, develop a way to track goals through self-monitoring, and provide feedback regarding success or failure to achieve goals. In the context of the stages of change, the goals that are appropriate for clients vary by stage. For example, a person in precontemplation may read about the benefits of physical activity over the coming week, and a person in preparation may set a physical activity goal. Chapter 39 provides more details about stage-appropriate strategies.

Setting goals that are specific is the first important characteristic of a goal. This might initially require some coaching. Clients may set a goal of "I will try to be more physically active." Although this is a good start and should be reinforced, actually getting the client to fill in the details increases the likelihood of success. Therefore, work with your client to establish the frequency, duration, intensity, and type of activity. As the specifics are delineated, help your client make the goal both short term and realistic. Consider individual circumstances and possible physical limitations. For example, keep the goal limited to the following week. Also help your client to evaluate how realistic the goal is for her situation. If a client knows she needs to take care of her sister's children in the following week, it may not be realistic to think she can go from 2 days of 20 minutes of activity each day to 5 days of 20 min-

BOX 44-7 | **Problem-solving Worksheet**

IDEA
1. Identify the problem
2. Develop solutions
3. Evaluate the solutions
4. Analyze the plan

EXAMPLE
1. Identify the problem: Don't want to exercise by myself
   Details of the problem: Prefer the company, need the accountability, feel safer
2. Develop solutions

SOLUTIONS	EVALUATION	SELECT
Walk with my neighbor		
Walk with other friends		
Join an aerobics class		

3. Evaluate the solutions

SOLUTIONS	EVALUATION	SELECT
Walk with my neighbor	She is too busy	
Walk with other friends	Offers company, safety, accountability	X
Join an aerobics class	Offers company, safety, and accountability but is too expensive	

4. Analyze the solution: Two friends agreed and I went on one walk with one friend and two walks with another friend. Seem to be working. _____

YOUR TURN:
1. Identify the problem: _____
   Details of the problem: _____
   _____

2. Develop solutions
3. Evaluate solutions

SOLUTIONS	EVALUATION	SELECT

4. Analyze plan: _____

Modified with permission from Marcus BH, Forsyth LH: Motivating People to be Physically Active. Champaign, IL: Human Kinetics; 2003.

utes of activity in the coming week. It is better to set a goal that can be accomplished. Accomplishing goals increases self-confidence and the likelihood that a client will set more challenging goals in the future. On the other hand, it is also important to make sure the goal is challenging and not too easy to accomplish because more difficult goals can provide increased motivation. Therefore, for the woman who walked 2 days for 20 minutes, perhaps she can increase this to 3 days of 20 minutes, 2 days of 30 minutes, or simply maintain her activity in the face of a hectic week. It is important to use the counseling techniques and be directive when necessary to ensure that goals meet these important characteristics.

Writing down the goal and then recording activity is an important way for the client to see his or her progress and to continue to identify barriers. The monitoring sheets provide feedback to the client (see Box 44-5). You can also provide positive feedback if this is not something that comes naturally to a client. Ideally, clients learn how to give themselves feedback and feel proud of their accomplishments. In addition, the monitoring forms can provide opportunities for identifying barriers and problem-solving opportunities. Another technique is to have your client post his or her goals around the home.

CONFIDENCE

Self-efficacy, or confidence in one's abilities to be physically active, is very important for behavior change[3]. Confidence can be increased through reinforcement, watching others be successful at the behavior, and correctly interpreting the body's physiological reaction to a situation as well as through guided mastery experiences[3]. You can help clients with all of these components by encouraging their successes and by having them think of others who were successful. Additionally, encourage them to think of other areas in which they have been successful and how information from these experiences can help them with this new behavior change by guiding them to self-monitor, problem solve, set goals, and receive feedback. In this way, clients increase their confidence and become better equipped to problem solve new obstacles. The use of a client-centered approach and matching the activity to clients' particular stages of change also help in increasing clients' confidence in being physically active. See Marcus and Forsyth[12] for a self-efficacy assessment.

RELAPSE PREVENTION

Another area that can be helpful in working with your clients is that of **relapse prevention**[4]. Chapter 39 details this principle. Preventing relapse (i.e., reverting to inactivity) is a proactive approach to problem solving future obstacles or for managing temporary lapses (i.e., temporary periods of inactivity). If you have a client who has a life event coming up during which it will be difficult to remain active, you can identify the problem and engage in problem solving just as you would any other barrier. These times are often referred to as "high-risk situations." Examples include times of bad weather, vacations, visitors, or other situations that might make it difficult to engage in physical activity.

There may also be times when you notice that your client's activity level has dropped. Helping your client see this as a temporary lapse and not a relapse can be helpful in getting the client back into a routine of activity. To do this, you can problem solve and set goals but also let the client know that although it is not unusual to have times of decreased activity, it is important to get back on track as soon as possible.

There may be times, however, when you find that your clients are experiencing difficulties that are making physical activity hard to accomplish. In some cases, a person may be experiencing depression, anxiety, or other mental health issues. Some of the symptoms of depression and anxiety are lack of energy and difficulty concentrating, both of which make attending to physical activity difficult. In these cases, it may be important to determine if there is a need to refer the person for additional help. For suspected depression, you can ask the person, "Are you feeling so sad or down that it is making it difficult to perform your daily activities?" For anxiety, you can ask, "Are you feeling so nervous or anxious that it is making it difficult to perform your daily activities?" If the client answers yes, then it is appropriate to recommend seeking help from a physician or a mental health professional. In some cases, you may suspect that a person is very depressed or anxious. In the event that you suspect a person may need medical or psychological assistance, you should refer the client to other health care providers as necessary.

Summary

Health counselors have the opportunity to develop rapport and facilitate behavior change with their clients. This chapter discussed the client-centered approach, which emphasizes techniques such as empathy, listening, active listening, and reflective statements. These skills can be used by counselors to understand the perspective of their clients. These counseling techniques can also be used when using behavior change techniques such as tracking progress, problem solving, increasing confidence, goal setting, and providing feedback. Long-term success for clients will be enhanced as they become increasingly self-sufficient with these behavior change strategies.

REFERENCES

1. Prochaska JO, DiClemente CC: Stages and processes of self-change of smoking: Towards an integrative model of change. J Consult Clin Psychol 51:390–395, 1983.
2. Bandura A: Social Foundations of Thought and Action: A Social Cognitive Theory. Englewood Cliffs, NJ: Prentice Hall; 1986.
3. Bandura A: Self-Efficacy: The Exercise of Control. New York: W.H. Freeman and Company; 1997.

4. Marlatt GA, Gordon JR: Relapse Prevention: Maintenance Strategies in the Treatment of Addictive Behaviors. New York: Guilford Press; 1985.

5. Miller WR, Rollnick S: Motivational Interviewing: Preparing People to Change Addictive Behavior. New York: Guilford Press; 1991.

6. Rogers CT: A theory of therapy, personality, and interpersonal relationships as developed in the client-centered framework. In Kock S, ed. Psychology: The Study of a Science, vol 3. Formulations of the Person and the Social Context. New York: McGraw Hill; 1959.

7. Rollnick S, Mason P, Butler C: Health Behavior Change. A Guide for Practitioners. New York: Churchill Livingstone; 1999.

8. Grueninger UL, Duffy FD, Goldstein MG: Patient education in the medical encounter: How to facilitate learning, behavior change, and coping, In Lipkin M, Putnam S, Lazare A, ed., The Medical Interview. New York: Springer-Verlag; 1995.

9. Stewart M, Stewart M, Belle Brown J, et al: Patient-centered medicine: Transforming the clinical method. Thousand Oaks, CA: Sage Publications; 1995.

10. Marcus BH, Lewis BA: Stages of motivational readiness to change physical activity behavior. President's Council on Physical Fitness and Sports Research Digest 4:1–8, 2003.

11. Dunn AL, Marcus BH, Kampert JB, et al: Reduction in cardiovascular disease risk factors: 6-month results from Project Active. Prev Med 26:883–892, 1997.

12. Marcus BH, Forsyth LH: Motivating People to be Physically Active. Champaign, IL: Human Kinetics; 2003.

SELECTED REFERENCES FOR FURTHER READING

American College of Sports Medicine: ACSM Fitness Book, 3rd ed; Champaign, IL: Human Kinetics; 2003.

Marcus BH, Forsyth LH: Motivating People to be Physically Active. Champaign, IL: Human Kinetics; 2003.

Marcus BH, Lewis BA: Stages of motivational readiness to change physical activity behavior. President's Council on Physical Fitness and Sports Research Digest 4:1–8, 2003.

Proper KI, Hildebrandt VH, Vander Book AJ, et al: Effect of individual counseling on physical activity fitness and health: a randomized controlled trial in a workplace setting. Am J Prev Med 24:218–226, 2003.

Rollnick S, Mason P, Butler C: Health Behavior Change. A Guide for Practitioners. New York: Churchill Livingstone; 1999.

Stewart M, Stewart M, Belle Brown J, et al: Patient-centered medicine: Transforming the clinical method. Thousand Oaks, CA: Sage Publications; 1995.

INTERNET RESOURCES

American Heart Association: Exercise (physical activity) counseling. http://www.americanheart.org/presenter.jhtml?identifier=4534

Cancer Control Planet. Physical Activity: 5 Steps to Effective Cancer Control Planning. http://cancercontrolplanet.cancer.gov/physical_activity.html

Centers for Disease Control and Prevention: National Center for Chronic Disease Prevention and Health Promotion. Nutrition & Physical Activity. http://www.cdc.gov/nccdphp/dnpa/physical/index.htm

Exercise Program Administration

SECTION EDITOR: KIMBERLY A. BONZHEIM, MS

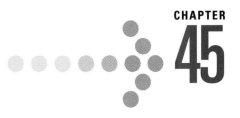

Exercise Program Professionals and Related Staff

BARRY A. FRANKLIN

This chapter addresses KSAs from the following content areas:

1   Exercise Physiology and Related Exercise Science
2   Pathophysiology and Risk Factors
3   Health Appraisal, Fitness, and Clinical Exercise Testing
4   Electrocardiography and Diagnostic Techniques
5   Patient Management and Medications
6   Medical and Surgical Management
7   Exercise Prescription and Programming
8   Nutrition and Weight Management
9   Human Behavior and Counseling
10   Safety, Injury Prevention, and Emergency Procedures
11   Program Administration, Quality Assurance, and Outcome Assessment

. . . all parts of the body which have a function, if used in moderation and exercised in labours in which each is accustomed, become thereby healthy, well-developed and age more slowly, but if unused and left idle they become liable to disease, defective in growth, and age quickly.

—Hippocrates

We doctors can now state from our experience with people, both sick and well, and from a growing series of scientific researches that "keeping fit" does pay richly in dividends of health and longevity.

—Paul Dudley White, MD

From a public health perspective, the emphasis on getting sedentary adults to become moderately active is highly appropriate; the evidence shows that on a populationwide basis, this is where the majority of the health benefits are to be obtained.

—Steven N. Blair, PED

Smoking, body-mass index, and exercise patterns in midlife and late adulthood are predictors of subsequent disability. Not only do persons with better health habits survive longer, but in such persons, disability is postponed and compressed into fewer years at the end of life.

—James F. Fries, MD

Epidemiologic data have established that physical inactivity increases the incidence of at least 17 unhealthy conditions, almost all of which are chronic diseases, resulting in approximately 250,000 premature deaths in the U.S. each year[1]. One meta-analysis of 43 studies that examined the relationship between physical activity and the incidence of **coronary heart disease (CHD)** reported that the relative risk of CHD in relation to physical inactivity ranged from 1.5 to 2.4, with a median value of 1.9[2]. Two important findings emerged: first, an inverse association between physical activity and the incidence of CHD was consistently observed, especially in better designed studies, and second, the relative risk of a sedentary lifestyle appeared to be similar in magnitude to that of other major coronary risk factors (e.g., hypertension, hypercholesterolemia, cigarette smoking). Although regular physical activity and improved cardiorespiratory fitness are widely believed to be cardioprotective, a recent meta-analysis concluded that these variables had significantly different relationships to cardiovascular disease[3]. The risk decreased linearly with increasing levels of physical activity; in contrast, there was a precipitous decrease in risk as one moved from the lowest to the second lowest fitness category. Beyond this demarcation, the reductions in relative risk paralleled those observed with increasing physical activity but were approximately twice as great for cardiorespiratory fitness (i.e., only a 30% decline from the least to most physically active vs. a 64% decline in cardiovascular disease risk from the least to most fit). Thus, it appears that extremely low aerobic fitness warrants consideration as a risk factor[4] (also see Chapter 7).

Numerous studies in persons with and without coronary artery disease have identified a low level of **aerobic fitness**, expressed as **metabolic equivalents** (METs;

KEY TERMS

Aerobic fitness: A measure of cardiorespiratory fitness, expressed as mL O_2/kg/min or METs; generally synonymous with the maximal oxygen consumption or aerobic capacity

Coronary heart disease: Blockage of the coronary arteries from a buildup of low-density lipoprotein cholesterol and fibrous calcified tissue on the inner portion of the artery wall

Exercise compliance: Steady devotion to a structured exercise program, as prescribed (frequency, intensity, duration, type), for at least 6 months

Exercise physiologist: Professional who uses exercise testing or training in the evaluation and management of a broad spectrum of healthy and diseased patients

Metabolic equivalent (MET): The rate of energy expended at rest (1 MET ~ 3.5 mL $O_2 \cdot kg^{-1} \cdot min^{-1}$); used to categorize activities in multiples above rest

1 MET = 3.5 mL $O_2 \cdot kg^{-1} \cdot min^{-1}$), as an independent risk factor for all-cause and cardiovascular mortality[5–7]. Fortunately, a low aerobic fitness level can be improved by regular endurance exercise at an intensity corresponding to only 30% to 45% of oxygen uptake reserve[8,9], depending on the initial aerobic capacity, with each 1-MET increase in exercise capacity conferring an 8% to 12% reduction in mortality[6,10,11]. There are multiple mechanisms by which moderate to vigorous physical activity and improved cardiorespiratory fitness may decrease morbidity and mortality rates associated with cardiovascular disease (Fig. 45-1), including antiatherosclerotic, anti-ischemic, antiarrhythmic, antithrombotic, and psychosocial effects[12]. The challenge for physicians and other health care providers, including exercise professionals, is to engage increasing numbers of patients with and without chronic disease, in home-, club-, or medically based exercise programs so that many more individuals may realize the cardioprotective and general health benefits that regular physical activity can provide.

Meeting Manpower and Training Needs

The expansion of modern medicine has contributed immensely to the early detection and treatment of chronic diseases, especially CHD. Mortality and recurrent events have declined, and patients' quality of life has improved. Technologic, medical, preventive, and rehabilitative developments are largely responsible.

One of the most impressive gains in the management of patients with chronic disease has been the establishment of the benefits of structured exercise and physical activity interventions and their progressive incorporation into the mainstream of contemporary medical care. Recently, increased attention has been directed toward the role of exercise for improving the health, physical fitness, and rehabilitation potential of patients who are coping with CHD[13], including congestive heart failure[14]. Patients afflicted with cardiovascular or pulmonary disease commonly experience a constellation of challenges, including a reduced functional capacity, associated symptomatol-

Potential cardioprotective effects of regular physical activity

Anti-atherosclerotic	Psychologic	Anti-thrombotic	Anti-ischemic	Anti-arrhythmic
Improved lipids	↓ Depression	↓ Platelet adhesiveness	↓ Myocardial O_2 demand	↑ Vagal tone
Lower BPs	↓ Stress	↑ Fibrinolysis	↑ Coronary flow	↓ Adrenergic activity
Reduced adiposity	↑ Social support	↓ Fibrinogen	↓ Endothelial dysfunction	↑ HR variability
↑ Insulin sensitivity		↓ Blood viscosity		
↓ Inflammation				

FIGURE 45-1. A structured endurance exercise program sufficient to maintain and enhance cardiorespiratory fitness may provide multiple mechanisms to reduce nonfatal and fatal cardiovascular events. BP = blood pressure; ↑ = increased; ↓ = decreased; O_2 = oxygen. Also see GETP7 Boxes 1-1 and 1-2.

ogy, depression, anxiety, job and economic stress, and (for some) an overwhelming sense of uncertainty. Common medical conditions such as stroke, multiple sclerosis, muscular dystrophy, and traumatic injury to the central nervous system can elicit muscle paralysis, paresis, or spasticity. Special deficits or defects resulting from congenital deformities, musculoskeletal, neoplastic, immunological, or hematological anomalies and the needs and contraindications imposed by these conditions must also be taken into account. A superimposed sedentary lifestyle can exacerbate the associated disease-specific sequelae, causing these patient subsets to experience secondary complications such as reduced cardiorespiratory fitness, muscle atrophy, osteoporosis, and impaired circulation to the lower extremities, leading to potential thrombus formation and decubitus ulcers. Consequently, physicians have increasingly embraced the use of exercise in the prevention, diagnosis, and treatment of these clinical conditions and other chronic health problems.

The emergence of this new specialty—that is, the essential medical role of exercise testing and training in the evaluation and management of a broad spectrum of healthy and diseased patients—has created the need for educating and training physicians and allied health personnel to provide these services. Numerous professional organizations, including the American Heart Association, American College of Cardiology, American Medical Association, American College of Physicians, and American College of Chest Physicians, have responded through the sponsorship of conferences, establishment of committees, writing of position stands and scientific statements, and the development of educational materials. Over the past 2 decades, however, cost containment initiatives and time constraints on physicians have encouraged more extensive use of specially-trained health-care professionals (e.g., nurses, exercise physiologists, physician assistants, and physical therapists) to directly provide many of the diagnostic and treatment services under the overall direction of physicians. Indeed, in the current era of managed health care, the judicious use of specialized health care professionals has been shown to be a safe and cost-effective alternative for many hospitals and medical centers[15]. Although several professional organizations have responded by providing clinically oriented exercise physiology continuing education workshops or certifications, including the American Council on Exercise (ACE) and the American Society of Exercise Physiologists (ASEP), perhaps the greatest recent emphasis placed on this area has been within the American College of Sports Medicine (ACSM).

The seventh edition of *ACSM's Guidelines for Exercise Testing and Prescription* represents another step in the evolution of this text first published by the ACSM in 1975[16]. Paralleling the evolution of the guidelines has been the development of a "certification process," incorporating written and practical examinations, for certain individuals involved in the administration of graded exercise testing,

| BOX 45-1 | **Content Matter for American College of Sports Medicine Certifications** |

- Exercise Physiology and Related Exercise Science
- Pathophysiology and Risk Factors
- Health Appraisal, Fitness, and Clinical Exercise Testing
- Electrocardiography and Diagnostic Techniques
- Patient Management and Medications
- Medical and Surgical Management
- Exercise Prescription and Programming
- Nutrition and Weight Management
- Human Behavior and Counseling
- Safety, Injury Prevention, and Emergency Procedures
- Program Administration, Quality Assurance, and Outcome Assessment

with or without concomitant myocardial perfusion imaging, pharmacologic stress testing, and physical conditioning programs, categorized by "tracks." The health/fitness instructor title is designed primarily for individuals involved in fitness assessment and exercise programming of a preventive nature for apparently healthy individuals and persons with controlled disease. The exercise specialist and registered clinical **exercise physiologist** (RCEP) titles are designed for exercise professionals who may work with high-risk or diseased individuals as well as apparently healthy persons. The ACSM has published a complete listing of the current knowledge, skills, and abilities that comprise the foundations of these certification examinations, as well as the minimum requirements for experience, level of education, and recommended competencies (see Appendix B). The content matter for the varied certifications is shown in Box 45-1; a potential staffing plan for health/fitness and clinical services is depicted in Figure 45-2.

Personnel for Exercise Services

Qualified allied health care personnel, including health and fitness and clinical exercise professionals, provide the treatment plans and services for structured exercise training and physical activity interventions. The collective knowledge, skills, and abilities of the staff must reflect the multidisciplinary competencies necessary to effect the desired treatment outcomes. Depending on individual client or patient needs, personnel must guide interventions for restoring and enhancing functional capacity, reducing body weight and fat stores, improving the coronary risk factor profile, and promoting attitudes and behaviors that lead to long-term **exercise compliance**. Accordingly, exercise professionals must also address the myriad of factors that may present the major impediment to regular exercise participation, including psychosocial variables (e.g., perception of the program), personal convenience factors, and the family environment, such as

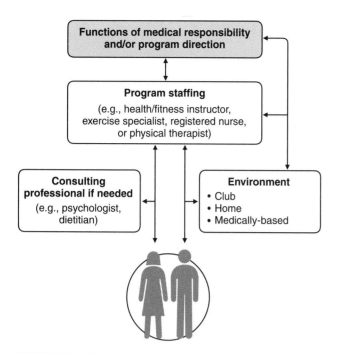

FIGURE 45-2. Staffing plan for an adult fitness or exercise-based cardiac rehabilitation program.

spousal support. Staff must also assure safe and appropriate monitoring using the necessary clinical skills and medicolegal provisions, provide educational programming that reinforces health behaviors and safe and effective exercise practices, and review the progress of each individualized treatment plan.

Working as a team, exercise professionals should:

- Conduct an individualized functional capacity assessment that considers the patient's medical history and current health status (e.g., associated comorbidities) as well as psychosocial characteristics, personal goals, and potential barriers to the maintenance of a structured exercise commitment, including lifestyle physical activity[17,18].
- Establish treatment goals through collaboration with the referring or primary care physician and other responsible staff (e.g., psychologist, registered dietitian, health and fitness instructor, exercise specialist) to meet the client's/patient's needs.
- Implement individualized exercise-based interventions via the "readiness to change" model[19] using strategies to promote safety and effectiveness, improve functional status and prognosis, promote independent self-management of exercise and health behaviors, and deal with hypokinetic lapses or relapses (i.e., the temporary cessation of structured physical activity) [see Chapter 39 and GETP7 Figure 7-7 and Box 7-2].
- Monitor progress, conduct outcome evaluation in consultation with other responsible staff, provide "updates" to the referring physician (when appropri-

ate), and encourage pleasurable activities in a supportive social environment to help individuals maintain their exercise commitments.

The number, disciplinary background, and professional specialization of the staff may include licensed and unlicensed health care professionals, depending on the nature of the exercise program. Nevertheless, the collective knowledge base of those assigned to provide diagnostic testing or exercise treatment services must include a comprehensive and up-to-date understanding of varied topic areas (see Box 45-1). The professions most frequently represented in preventative and rehabilitative exercise programs include physicians (e.g., family practitioners, internists, physiatrists, cardiologists), specially trained nurses, exercise specialists, clinical exercise physiologists, health/fitness instructors, nutritionists, health educators, health psychologists, vocational rehabilitation counselors, physical therapists, corrective therapists, occupational therapists, and pharmacists. The minimum and preferred experience and educational qualifications for these disciplines are available in previously published sources, as are staff-to-patient ratios[20] (see GETP7 Table 7-3). In smaller programs with only a few individuals assigned to services on a full- or part-time basis, it is important for staff members to assume multidisciplinary roles and participate in continuing education activities. Ongoing recertification of personnel also assures the maintenance of competence.

One of the most important challenges in establishing a state-of-the-art exercise-based preventative or rehabilitative program is hiring personnel with the competencies and knowledge to provide a safe, effective, viable, financially sound, and successful program (see Chapter 46). The staff is generally the first interface with clients and patients, family, and physicians in the application of these services. An "internship program" provides an ideal way to recruit and hire future staff members who are knowledgeable about program services, policies, and procedures and who have already developed a good rapport with existing staff members and clients and patients. Staff interviews for potential part-time or permanent positions should be thorough and comprehensive and attempt to evaluate a number of personal and professional characteristics, including adaptability, competence, experience, interpersonal skills, manageability, initiative, attitude, stability, maturity, emotional control, integrity, and values. References should be carefully checked, ideally over the phone. Managers and supervisors should also engage existing staff members in the final selection process and provide their recommendations for hire (e.g., having staff nurses interview the top two or three nurse candidates, as identified by management). Preferred candidates are those who are either positive or neutral when referring to their relationships with previous employers and supervisors and those whose answers indicate that they are more likely to work well with others.

Emergence of the Clinical Exercise Physiology

Since 1975, ACSM workshops and certifications have served as the "gold standard" in professional development and continuing education, helping physicians and allied health professionals counsel their patients and clients with and without cardiopulmonary disease and other medical conditions regarding the benefits of a physically active lifestyle. Although the ACSM provides certification for exercise professionals interested in preventive exercise programming (i.e., the health fitness instructor designation), the ACSM has also, for many years, highlighted the utility of the ACSM exercise specialist certification, which is primarily designed for professionals who plan to administer and supervise exercise programs for patients with cardiovascular or pulmonary disease, as well as other common clinical conditions (e.g., hypertension, peripheral vascular disease, diabetes mellitus, obesity).

To more clearly define the benefits and limitations of exercise testing and training in the clinical evaluation and management of an even broader spectrum of patients, including those with stroke, cerebral palsy, multiple sclerosis, Parkinson's disease, spinal cord injury, post-polio and Guillain-Barré syndrome, muscular dystrophy and other myopathies, peripheral neuropathy and chronic neurogenic pain, head injury, osteo- and rheumatoid arthritis and fibromyalgia, chronic back pain, osteoporosis, vertebral disorders, amputation, neoplasms, immune system and hematological disorders, HIV infection, and chronic fatigue syndrome[21], in 1998 the ACSM developed a registry of clinical exercise physiologists. The prerequisites for an ACSM RCEP include a minimum of a master's degree in exercise physiology, exercise science, or physiology along with more than 600 hours of clinical experience, preferably across varied disease states and clinical conditions[22]. Goals of the RECP are to improve visibility and acceptance of clinical exercise physiologists among the public and other health professionals and to support the need for future licensure (i.e., using nursing or physical therapy as models).

Strategies to Increase Exercise Compliance

Although many persons can be encouraged to initiate an exercise program, motivating them to continue can have a favorable impact on public health. Unfortunately, exercise testing and exercise prescription are often emphasized more than education and motivation[23]. Consequently, negative variables often outweigh the positive variables contributing to sustained participant interest and enthusiasm (Fig. 45-3). Such an imbalance leads to a decline in adherence as program effectiveness diminishes.

Adult fitness and exercise-based cardiac rehabilitation programs have typically reported dropout rates ranging from 9% to 87% (mean, 45%)[24,25]. Thus, it appears that ex-

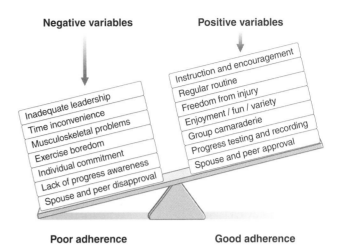

FIGURE 45-3. Programmatic and related variables affecting long-term exercise compliance. Negative variables often outweigh the positive variables, resulting in poor adherence.

ercise is similar to other health-related behaviors (e.g., medication compliance) in that typically half or less of those who initiate the behavior will continue (Fig. 45-4), irrespective of initial health status or type of program. Others (i.e., compliers) who do not technically meet the definition of an "exercise dropout" may continue the program, but at a subthreshold intensity, frequency, or duration.

To understand why people sometimes lack the motivation for regular physical activity, one must first acknowledge a simple yet important fact: exercise is voluntary and time consuming. Therefore, it may extend the day or compete with other valued interests and responsi-

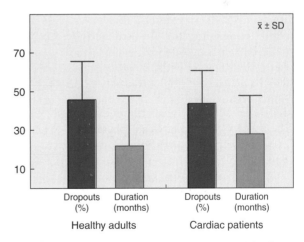

FIGURE 45-4. Relationship between the dropout rate and the duration of exercise training in studies of healthy adults and cardiac patients. (Adapted from Franklin BA: Program factors that influence exercise adherence: practical adherence skills for clinical staff (pp. 237–258). In Dishman R, ed. Exercise Adherence: Its Impact on Public Health. Champaign, IL: Human Kinetics; 1988 and Oldridge NB: Compliance with exercise rehabilitation (pp. 283–304). In Dishman R, ed. Exercise Adherence: Its Impact on Public Health. Champaign, IL: Human Kinetics; 1988.)

bilities of daily life. In one study, patients undergoing gymnasium-based exercise training spent more time in their cars going to and from the programs than patients in a home-training comparison group spent on their cycle ergometers[26].

Research and empiric experience suggest that certain program modifications and educational and motivational strategies may enhance participant interest and compliance[27] (also see Chapters 41 and 42 and GETP7 Box 7-3). These components are responsibilities of exercise professionals, and they include:

- **Emphasize the educational component.** Education of participants should serve as an integral part of the exercise program and include substantive information on body mechanics, energy expenditure, exercise prescription, importance of the warm-up and cool-down periods, exercise myths and misconceptions, guidelines on appropriate exercise clothing and shoes, nutrition, and the effects of ambient temperature and humidity on performance. Several programmatic features can be used to promote the educational component, including films, lectures, group discussions, bulletin boards, a regular newsletter, and websites.

  Client education may be provided by the use of written materials, audio compact discs, group education, and one-on-one counseling. One innovative approach provides a computer-generated report detailing the patient's coronary risk factor profile[28], the goal level for each risk factor based on national guidelines, and an individualized lifestyle management action plan for achieving these goals based on several behavior change models (i.e., social learning theory, stages of change, and single-concept learning theory).

- **Recruit physician referrals and encourage physicians' counseling on physical activity.** According to recent clinical studies, the single most important factor determining patients' participation in exercise was receiving a strong recommendation from their primary care physician[29]. Unfortunately, surveys of primary care physicians indicate that only 30% of them routinely provide counseling on physical activity to their sedentary patients[30]. To assist in this regard, a five-step counseling plan has been suggested to help patients initiate and maintain a regular exercise program: (a) Ask all patients about their current physical activity habits to determine whether they are sufficient to confer fitness or health benefits; (b) assist patients in formulating an exercise program, considering their occupational demands and recreational habits, current medications, response to graded exercise testing (if appropriate), and degree of direct medical supervision (if necessary); (c) encourage increased physical activity in daily living; (d) emphasize the short- and long-term benefits of regular exercise participation; and (e) plan follow-up contact to reinforce

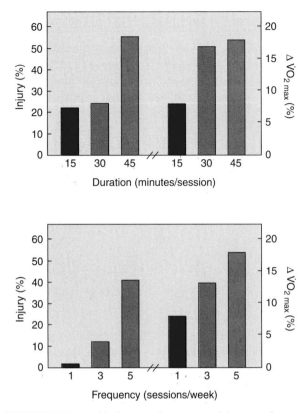

FIGURE 45-5. Relationship between frequency and duration of exercise training, improvement in aerobic capacity ($\dot{V}O_{2max}$) and the incidence of orthopedic injury. Above an exercise duration of 30 min/session or a frequency of three sessions/wk, additional improvement in $\dot{V}O_{2max}$ is small, yet the injury rate among novice exercisers increases disproportionately. (Adapted from Pollock ML, Gettman L, Milesis C, et al: Effects of frequency and duration of training on attrition and incidence of injury. Med Sci Sports 9:31–36, 1977.)

efforts and devise ways to overcome barriers to regular activity (also see Chapter 44).

- **Minimize injury with a written, moderate-intensity exercise prescription.** Inordinate physical demands, particularly during the initial weeks of an exercise program, often result in muscle soreness, orthopedic injury, and attrition (see Box 28-6). Exercise professionals should recognize that excessive frequency ($\geq$5 days/ week), duration ($\geq$45 minutes/session), or intensity ($\geq$90% aerobic capacity) offer participants little additional gain in aerobic fitness but disproportionately increase the incidence of musculoskeletal injury (Fig. 45-5)[31,32]. Using an exercise prescription form (Fig. 45-6) provides a standardized method of ensuring your recommendations.

- **Provide alternatives to supervised group programs.** Although traditional supervised group programs are associated with increased cost and extended travel time, considerable data are available regarding the safety, efficacy, and cost effectiveness of this model, especially in persons at increased risk for exercise-

MD _____

Name _____ Age _____ Starting Date _____

Clinical Status: Normal
Arrhythmia   Angina   CABG   CAD   HTN   MI   PTCA   VR

Note: This prescription is valid only if you remain on the same medications (type and
      dose), and you are in the same clinical status as on the day your exercise test
      was conducted.

Contraindications: Angina at rest, fever, illness
                   Temperature and weather extremes (below 30°F or more than 80°
                   with high humidity)

Activities to avoid: Sudden strenuous lifting or carrying
                     Exertion that leads to holding your breath

Exercise Type: Aerobic types of exercise that are continuous, dynamic and repetitive
               in nature

Frequency: _____ times/day _____ days/week

Duration: Total duration of exercise session: _____ min

To be divided as follows:

   Warm-up: (light flexibility/stretching routine) _____ min

   Aerobic training activity: _____ to _____ min

   Cool-down: (slow walking and stretching): _____ min

Intensity:

   Target heart rate _____ to _____ beats/min

                     _____ to _____ beats/10 sec

                  Perceived exertion should not exceed "somewhat hard"
                                    Re-evaluation

Your next graded exercise test is due: _____
Call our office to schedule an appointment. Phone: _____

Exercise Physiologist _____ _____

FIGURE 45-6. Exercise prescription form. CABG = coronary artery bypass graft; CAD = coronary artery disease; HTN = hypertension; MI = myocardial infarction; PTCA = percutaneous transluminal coronary angioplasty; VR = valve replacement.

related complications. Such programs also facilitate patient education; provide variety and recreational opportunities; and offer staff reassurance and the potential for enhanced adherence, safety, and surveillance[33].

Home exercise should be promulgated as an alternative, however, because of its lesser cost, increased practicability, convenience, and potential to promote independence and self-responsibility, especially for apparently healthy and low-risk individuals[26]. A variety of techniques may be used to facilitate monitoring and communication between clients managed at home and exercise staff, including regular telephone contact, mail (e.g., completion of activity logs), fax, video recording, email, and transtelephonic electrocardiographic monitoring (if appropriate)[33].

- **Emphasize variety and enjoyment.** Calisthenics, when relied on too heavily in an physical conditioning regimen, readily become monotonous and boring, leading to poor exercise adherence. Programs that are most successful are those that are pleasurable and offer the greatest diversification. In structured group programs, game modifications that serve to minimize skill and competition and maximize participant success are particularly important[24]. For example, volleyball played allowing one bounce of the ball per side serves to facilitate this objective.

- **Consider gender differences and incorporate specific activities for women.** Some women may be uncomfortable participating in a male-dominated physical conditioning program, and others may harbor fears because of lack of prior exercise experience[34]. Most programs offer classes and equipment geared to the majority of their clientele—that is, middle-aged and older men—and few provide specific exercises or educational offerings for women[35]. Exercise professionals should incorporate specific activities (e.g., aerobic dance, water aerobics, yoga, t'ai chi) that may be especially appealing to women.

- **Provide positive reinforcement through periodic testing.** Exercise testing, body fatness assessment, and serum lipid profiling should be performed before the start of the conditioning program and at regular intervals thereafter to assess the individual's response to the exercise stimulus. Favorable changes in these evaluations can serve as powerful motivators that produce renewed interest and dedication.

- **Recruit spouse support of the exercise program.** The importance of this influence became evident in one study that showed that the husband's adherence to the exercise program was directly related to the wife's attitude toward it[36]. Of men whose spouses had a positive attitude toward the program, 80% demonstrated a good to excellent adherence pattern. However, when the spouses' attitudes were neutral or negative, only 40% of the men showed good to excellent adherence patterns (Fig. 45-7). Similar observations have been reported in exercise-based cardiac rehabilitation programs[37].

- **Use progress charts to record exercise achievements.** Research substantiates the importance of immediate positive feedback on reinforcement of health-related behaviors. A progress chart that permits participants to record their daily exercise achievements can facilitate this objective.

- **Recognize individual accomplishments through a system of extrinsic rewards.** Peer recognition is a powerful motivator. To this end, an annual awards ceremony or banquet is recommended. Recognition of

TABLE 45-1. Traits and Skills of Successful Exercise Leaders

Traits	Skills
Regard for fellow leaders	Ability to establish rapport
Alert to social environment	Articulate orally and in writing
Cooperative	Creative and innovative
Decisive	Knowledgeable and intelligent
Dependable	Organized
Empathetic	Physically talented
Flexible	Tactful
Energetic and enthusiastic	Adapts programs when appropriate
Self-confident	
Willing to assume responsibility	

participant accomplishments can be made in the form of inexpensive trophies, plaques, or certificates.

- **Provide quality, enthusiastic exercise leaders.** Although numerous variables affect participant exercise compliance, perhaps the most important is the exercise leader[24]. Exercise leaders should be well-trained, highly motivated, innovative, and enthusiastic. Certain leadership traits and skills that appear to be especially important are listed in Table 45-1. The participants and their individual needs, including mastery, attention, recognition, social acceptance, security of health, and social interaction, should receive the highest priority.

Exercise leaders should program activities to correspond to stages of the life cycle. For individuals who are in their 20s or early 30s, physical challenges strengthen the ego and serve as a buffer against stress. Such participants often view exercise as a means of controlling their weight and improving their appearance. From the mid-30s through the 50s, health and the avoidance of chronic disease become potentially powerful motivators. Finally, individuals who are in their 60s and older often view exercise as a means of counteracting the inevitable decline in function that accompanies biological aging.

Summary

Exercise professionals are presented the opportunity to provide safe, beneficial, and enjoyable physical activity for the clients they serve. This can be accomplished by increasing the physical skills of the participants and by instilling in them a positive attitude toward exercise and recreation. To this end, exercise professionals must possess knowledge of a variety of physical activities, recognize individual differences and adapt programs accordingly, motivate participants to make long-term exercise commitments, and cultivate personal associations. The relationship between the exercise leader and the program participant appears to be particularly important. Box 45-2 lists

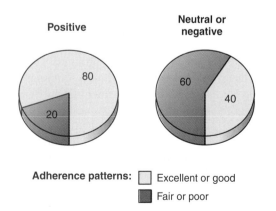

FIGURE 45-7. Relation of wives' attitudes to husbands' adherence to an exercise training program (values are %). (Adapted from Heinzelman F, Bagley RW: Response to physical activity programs and their effects on health behavior. Public Health Rep 85:905–911, 1970.)

BOX 45-2	**Behavioral Strategies of Good Exercise Leaders**

1. Show a sincere interest in the participants. Learn why they have gotten involved in your program and what their health and fitness goals are.
2. Be enthusiastic in your instruction and guidance.
3. Develop a personal association and relationship with each participant; exchange names and take a genuine interest in each participant.
4. Consider the various reasons why adults exercise (i.e., health, recreation, weight loss, social, personal appearance) and allow for individual differences.
5. Initiate participant follow-up (e.g., postcards or telephone calls) when several unexplained absences occur in succession. Novice exercisers should be advised that an inevitable slip in attendance does not imply failure.
6. Practice what you preach. Participate in the exercise sessions yourself. Good posture and grooming are essential to projecting the desired self-image. Cigarette smoking should be prohibited, and drinking or eating on the gymnasium floor should be prohibited.
7. Honor special days (e.g., birthdays) or exercise accomplishments with extrinsic rewards such as t-shirts, ribbons, or certificates.
8. Attend personally to orthopedic and musculoskeletal problems. Provide alternatives to floor exercise.
9. Counsel participants on proper foot apparel and exercise clothing.
10. Avoid constant references to complicated medical or physiological terminology and attempt to convey information in practical, user-friendly terms. Concentrate on a few selected terms to provide a little education at a time.
11. Arrange for occasional visits by personal physicians.
12. Provide a constant flow of newspaper or magazine articles to the participants on topics related to physical activity and other pertinent information.
13. Encourage an occasional visitor or participant to lead an activity.
14. Have a designated area for participant counseling and pay some attention to decor. Also, avoid trying to converse with clients while performing another task simultaneously.
15. Display your continuing education certifications and educational degrees. You are more likely to be successful at modifying behavior if you are perceived to be an expert.
16. Introduce first-time exercisers on the gymnasium floor or in the locker room. This orientation will encourage a sense of belonging to the group.
17. Reinforce participants by complimenting them on their appearance as they are exercising. Your conversation during exercise can also serve as a distracter from any unpleasant sensations they may be experiencing.
18. Consider entering city- or business-sponsored road races to pace your participants. Also show your interest and enthusiasm by participating with clients at community fitness events.

Adapted from Franklin BA: Program factors that influence exercise adherence: Practical adherence skills for clinical staff (pp. 237–258). In Dishman R, ed. Exercise Adherence: Its Impact on Public Health. Champaign, IL: Human Kinetics, 1988.

recommended behavioral strategies of good exercise leaders. Exercise professionals can play a critical role in favorably modifying the physical activity habits of the persons they counsel. The challenge is a formidable one.

REFERENCES

1. Booth FW, Gordon SE, Carlson CJ, et al: Waging war on modern chronic diseases: Primary prevention through exercise biology. J Appl Physiol 88:774–787, 2000.
2. Powell KE, Thompson PD, Caspersen CJ, et al: Physical activity and the incidence of coronary heart disease. Annu Rev Public Health 8: 253–287, 1987.
3. Williams PT: Physical fitness and activity as separate heart disease risk factors: A meta-analysis. Med Sci Sports Exerc 33:754–761, 2001.
4. Franklin BA: Survival of the fittest: Evidence for high risk and cardioprotective fitness levels. Curr Sports Med Rep 1:257–259, 2002.
5. Blair SN, Kampert JB, Kohl HW III, et al: Influences of cardiorespiratory fitness and other precursors on cardiovascular disease and all-cause mortality in men and women. JAMA 276:205–210, 1996.
6. Myers J, Prakash M, Froelicher V, et al: Exercise capacity and mortality among men referred for exercise testing. N Engl J Med 346: 793–801, 2002.
7. Gulati M, Pandey DK, Arnsdorf MF, et al: Exercise capacity and the risk of death in women. The St. James Women Take Heart Project. Circulation 108:1554–1559, 2003.
8. Swain DP, Franklin BA: VO$_2$ reserve and the minimal intensity for improving cardiorespiratory fitness. Med Sci Sports Exerc 34:152–157, 2002.
9. Swain DP, Franklin BA: Is there a threshold intensity for aerobic training in cardiac patients? Med Sci Sports Exerc 34:1071–1075, 2002.
10. Blair SN, Kohl HW III, Barlow CE, et al: Changes in physical fitness and all-cause mortality: A prospective study of healthy and unhealthy men. JAMA 273:1093–1098, 1995.
11. Dorn J, Naughton J, Imamura D, et al: Results of a multicenter randomized clinical trial of exercise and long-term survival in myocardial infarction patients. The National Exercise and Heart Disease Project (NEHDP). Circulation 100:1764–1769, 1999.
12. Franklin BA, de Jong A, Kahn JK, et al: Fitness and mortality in the primary and secondary prevention of coronary artery disease: Does the effort justify the outcome? Am J Med Sports 6:23–27, 2004.

13. Taylor RS, Brown A, Ebrahim S, et al: Exercise-based rehabilitation for patients with coronary heart disease: Systematic review and meta-analysis of randomized controlled trials. Am J Med 16:682–692, 2004.

14. Smart N, Marwick TH: Exercise training for heart failure patients: A systematic review of factors that improve patient mortality and morbidity. Am J Med 116:693–706, 2004.

15. Franklin BA, Gordon S, Timmis GC, et al: Is direct physician supervision of exercise stress testing routinely necessary? Chest 111:262–265, 1997.

16. American College of Sports Medicine: ACSM's Guidelines for Exercise Testing and Prescription, 7th ed. Baltimore: Lippincott, Williams & Wilkins; 2005.

17. Gordon NF, Kohl HW III, Blair SN: Life style exercise: A new strategy to promote physical activity for adults. J Cardiopulm Rehabil 13:161–163, 1993.

18. Franklin BA: Lifestyle activity: A new paradigm in exercise prescription. ACSM's Health & Fitness Journal 5:33–35, 2001.

19. Prochaska J, Di Clemente C: Transtheoretical therapy, toward a more integrative model of change. Psych Theory Res Prac 19:276–288, 1982.

20. American Association of Cardiovascular and Pulmonary Rehabilitation: Guidelines for Cardiac Rehabilitation and Secondary Prevention Programs, 4th ed. Champaign, IL: Human Kinetics; 2004.

21. American College of Sports Medicine: ACSM's Resources for Clinical Exercise Physiology: Musculoskeletal, Neuromuscular, Neoplastic, Immunologic, and Hematologic Conditions. Philadelphia: Lippincott, Williams & Wilkins; 2002.

22. Ehrman J, Gordon P, Visich PS, Keteyian S, eds: Clinical Exercise Physiology. Champaign, IL: Human Kinetics; 2003.

23. Wilmore JH: Individual exercise prescription. Am J Cardiol 33: 757–759, 1974.

24. Franklin BA: Program factors that influence exercise adherence: Practical adherence skills for clinical staff (pp. 237–258). In Dishman R, ed. Exercise Adherence: Its Impact on Public Health. Champaign, IL: Human Kinetics; 1988.

25. Oldridge NB: Compliance with exercise rehabilitation (pp. 283–304). In Dishman R, ed. Exercise Adherence: Its Impact on Public Health. Champaign, IL: Human Kinetics; 1988.

26. De Busk RF, Haskell WL, Miller NH, et al: Medically directed at-home rehabilitation soon after clinically uncomplicated acute myocardial infarction: A new model for patient care. Am J Cardiol 55: 251–257, 1985.

27. Franklin BA: Motivating patients to exercise: Strategies to increase compliance. Sports Medicine Digest 16:1–3, 1994.

28. Gordon NF, Salmon RD, Mitchell BS, et al: Innovative approaches to comprehensive cardiovascular disease risk reduction in clinical and community-based settings. Curr Atheroscler Rep 3:498–506, 2001.

29. Ades PA, Waldmann ML, Mc Cann WJ, et al: Predictors of cardiac rehabilitation participation in older coronary patients. Arch Intern Med 152:1033–1035, 1992.

30. Franklin BA, Sanders W:. Reducing the risk of heart disease and stroke. Phys Sportsmed 28:19,20,26, 2000.

31. Pollock ML, Gettman L, Milesis C, et al: Effects of frequency and duration of training on attrition and incidence of injury. Med Sci Sports 9:31–36, 1977.

32. Mann G, Garrett H, Farhi A, et al: Exercise to prevent coronary heart disease: An experimental study of the effects of training on risk factors for coronary disease in man. Am J Med 46:12–27, 1969.

33. Franklin BA, Hall L, Timmis GC: Contemporary cardiac rehabilitation services. Am J Cardiol 79:1075–1077, 1997.

34. Caras DS, Wenger NK: Exercise rehabilitation of women with coronary heart disease. J Myocard Ischemia 5:42–52, 1993.

35. Durstine JL, Thomas RJ, Miller NH, et al: Women and cardiac rehabilitation programming. Read before the Vth World Congress of Cardiac Rehabilitation, Bordeaux, France, July 5–8, 1992.

36. Heinzelman F, Bagley RW: Response to physical activity programs and their effects on health behavior. Public Health Rep 85:905–911, 1970.

37. Oldridge NB: Compliance and exercise in primary and secondary prevention of coronary heart disease: A review. Prev Med 11:56–70, 1982.

SELECTED REFERENCES FOR FURTHER READING

Andler EC: Winning the Hiring Game. Springfield, IL: The Smith Collins Company; 1992.

Johnson S, Blanchard K: Who moved my cheese? An amazing way to deal with change in your work and in your life. New York: Putnam; 1998.

McGinnis AL: Bringing Out the Best in People. Minneapolis: Augsbury Publishing House;, 1985.

INTERNET RESOURCES

American Association of Cardiovascular and Pulmonary Rehabilitation (AACVPR): http://www.aacvpr.org

American College of Sports Medicine (ACSM): http://www.acsm.org

American Council on Exercise (ACE): http://www.acefitness.org

National Academy of Sports Medicine (NASM): http://www.nasm.org

National Strength and Conditioning Association (NSCA): http://www.nsca.org

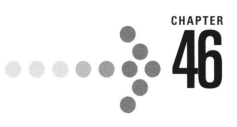

Health and Fitness Program Development and Operation

JAMES A. PETERSON, STEPHEN J. THARRETT, AND CEDRIC X. BRYANT

This chapter addresses KSAs from the following content areas:

1   Exercise Physiology and Related Exercise Science
2   Pathophysiology and Risk Factors
3   Health Appraisal, Fitness, and Clinical Exercise Testing
4   Electrocardiography and Diagnostic Techniques
5   Patient Management and Medications
6   Medical and Surgical Management
7   Exercise Prescription and Programming
8   Nutrition and Weight Management
9   Human Behavior and Counseling
10 Safety, Injury Prevention, and Emergency Procedures
11 Program Administration, Quality Assurance, and Outcome Assessment

---

The benefits of a physically active lifestyle are both extensive and well documented. As such, most individuals are aware of the fact that fitness is important and engaging in an exercise program on a regular basis can have multiple positive consequences in their lives. On the other hand, research reveals that less than 20% of adults exercise regularly. Obviously, it is not sufficient to merely be aware of the importance of a physically active lifestyle. Individuals must match their actions with their beliefs and attitudes. One of the key determinants in that regard is having access to a well-designed, well-run health and fitness program. This chapter presents an overview of the critical factors that health and fitness professionals should consider when developing and operating health and fitness programs that are appropriate for the individuals they are intended to serve. The chapter also reviews individual attitudes and behaviors toward health and fitness as they relate to health and fitness programming.

Understanding Health and Fitness Consumers

Individuals engage in health and fitness programs in a variety of organizational settings. Why people exercise and the settings they choose are affected by a number of factors, including cost, convenience, values, interests, and needs. By the same token, individuals stop exercising for any number of reasons, both personal and facility driven. The key point to keep in mind is that the better health and fitness professionals understand consumers (i.e., their potential clients), the more prepared they will be to develop and operate well-conceived health and fitness programs for the individuals with whom they are working. Furthermore, they will also be better prepared to design and execute retention strategies that will enhance their ability to retain the members that they have.

ORGANIZATIONAL SETTINGS

The health and fitness marketplace is composed of a diverse array of organizational settings. Each setting tends to be differentiated by a relatively unique combination of key factors, including business model, location, staffing, facilities, and equipment. In each instance, these factors impact on the menu of programs offered within that particular organizational setting.

Cumulatively, the number of individuals who engage in organized health and fitness programs tends to vary from country to country. For example, as Figure 46-1 illustrates, the United States has the largest percentage of its population as members of a health and fitness facility of the seven industrialized nations. In that regard, more than 34 million individuals are members of health and fitness facilities in the United States[1].

By far the largest segment in the health and fitness facility industry in the United States involves commercial clubs (48% of all facilities). In the past 2 decades, for example, the number of commercial health and fitness clubs in the United States has grown threefold from just over 6000 to almost 18,000. In descending order (as a percentage of all health and fitness facilities), the next 10 largest U.S. organizational settings are YMCAs/JCCs (17%), university based (6%), hospital based (5%), residential (5%), corporate based (4%), municipal (4%), military (2%), country clubs (2%), hotels and resorts (1%), and private studio (1%). Despite their comparatively low numbers, membership in residential, municipal, university-based, and hotel and resort fitness facilities has increased

Financial plan: A written statement that addresses the financial issues attendant to a particular organization or program, including financial objectives and priorities (both short and long term), budget benchmarks, and the identification of actual and projected sources of revenue

Retention strategy: A systematic plan that involves actions and steps that should be undertaken to enhance the likelihood that individuals who currently belong to a facility will retain their membership

Risk management: A concerted effort to undertake specific steps to minimize undue risk of injury to a facility's participants, identify and address any potentially

unsafe conditions, and maximize the ability of facility personnel to respond appropriately to emergency situations

Strategic plan: A planning tool that is designed to address strategic decisions concerning key issues such as short- and long-term goals for the organization; what steps need to be undertaken to achieve each particular goal; a time line for reaching each goal; and an allocation and prioritization of time, energy, and resources to each goal

Target audience: A well-defined, specific segment of the population to whom an organization attempts to market and promote a particular service, product, or program offering

substantially in the past few years. During the same period, the number of individuals who use corporate fitness facilities has dropped by more than 10%[2].

Demographically, the composition of the individuals who join health and fitness facilities has also changed in recent years. Being aware of and reacting to these changes can aid health and fitness professionals in their efforts to develop and operate successful health and fitness programs. Among the more pertinent demographic trends that have occurred recently are the following[2]:

- Fifty-three percent of the individuals who are members of health and fitness facilities are women.
- Men and women, as a percentage of the total U.S. population, are equally likely to join health and fitness clubs.
- The number of individuals who are 55 or older who become members of health and fitness facilities has increased from 9% to nearly 25% since 1987.
- The population age 55 years and older is the most active users of health and fitness facilities, with an average of 97 visits per person per year.

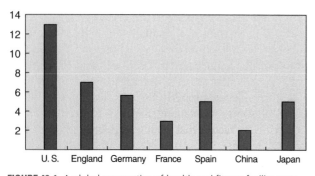

FIGURE 46-1. A global perspective of health and fitness facility numbers as a percentage of a country's population. (Adapted from the International Health, Racquet, and Sportsclub Association, Boston, MA [IHRSA] Global Report: State of the Health Club Industry; 2002).

- Individuals who are 35 to 54 years old represents the largest membership segment at 37%, having grown 143% since 1987.
- The number of individuals younger than age 18 years who use health and fitness facilities has increased by more than 180% since 1987.
- Individuals age 18 to 34 years have shown the least growth in membership over the past 25 years but still represent 34% of the total industry membership.
- For men, the highest membership penetration rates are for those age 25 to 34 years; for women, it is age 35 to 44 years.
- The average health and fitness facility member has an income of $76,000.
- Forty-six percent of all facility members earn over $75,000.
- Fifty-five percent of all facility members have at least a 4-year degree, with 25% of those individuals having an advanced degree.
- More than 15% of the individuals with advanced degrees in the United States hold facility memberships compared with 12% of those with 4-year degrees and less than 4% of those individuals who do not have a high school degree. Overall, 13.2% of the U.S. population is health club members.
- The Western section of the United States represents the largest segment of memberships, with more than 33% of all health and fitness facility memberships.
- In the past few years, memberships in the West and South have grown the fastest.

LEARNING WHAT INDIVIDUALS WANT

At least four primary tools exist for health and fitness professionals to develop meaningful insight into what their clients (actual and prospective) want from their involvement with a health and fitness facility. These tools are focus groups, surveys, interviews, and feedback systems. The ways health and fitness professionals use the information gained from these tools can impact their ability to attract, serve, and retain members.

Focus Groups

This particular learning tool offers a qualitative approach to learning about the attitudes, behaviors, and need of a particular market. As a rule, focus groups can serve several purposes, including gaining an understanding of individual attitudes and where they originate;, generating ideas, testing ideas, educating, uncovering problems, and helping to build a survey tool.

To maximize the information obtained by conducting focus groups, health and fitness professionals should take several steps, including:

- Take notes of what is said.
- Look for patterns and note them.
- Identify the most common answers and input because this information can serve as the foundation for a subsequent survey.
- Realize that the comments made by the individuals within the focus group do not necessarily represent universal opinion. Rather, these comments provide a foundation by which a greater understanding of universal thought can be gained.

Health and fitness professionals can enhance the effectiveness of the focus groups they are conducting by:

- Assigning a moderator who is impartial (i.e., someone who is not impacted by the information).
- Inviting between 10 and 15 individuals to participate in the focus group in order to get at least eight to 10 people who are willing (and able) to be part of the group.
- Making sure that the individuals invited to be part of the focus group appropriately reflect diversity in order to obtain a cross-pollination of ideas and input.
- Conducting a minimum of three sessions on any one particular topic.
- Conducting the sessions at times that are convenient to the group's participants.
- Keeping each focus group session to 1 hour or less.
- Holding the sessions in a private area.
- Focusing on open-ended questions that cannot be answered with a "yes" or "no."
- Ensuring that the moderator of the focus group stays neutral and keeps the session moving.
- Sending a thank you note to each member of the group after the group's sessions have concluded.

Surveys

Surveys provide a quantitative approach that health and fitness professionals can use to learn about their market and to help them develop their business models. In that regard,

surveys can serve several purposes, including assessing the participants' level of interest in a quantitative fashion; obtaining specific information on the clients' interests; determining information concerning such key topics as pricing, hours of operation, program choices, and so on; gaining information to use in developing business assumptions; and getting a sense of what the membership feels.

Health and fitness professionals should adhere to the following steps in order to enhance the effectiveness of the survey process:

- Ideally, survey the entire membership or target audience. If the number of individuals is too large, then randomly identify a sample audience to be surveyed (e.g., at least 20% of the entire group).
- If a written survey or an e-mail survey is used, use an introductory letter.
- If the process involves a written survey, provide a convenient, easy way for participants to return the completed survey at no cost.
- Use incentives to help gain greater rates of return.
- Make sure that the survey format matches the identified objectives for conducting the survey.
- Focus on closed-end questions such as multiple choice and true and false questions.
- Keep the questions to those areas that are of greatest importance and interest.
- Target a return rate that provides statistically valid information.

The following guidelines should be used when tabulating the results of a survey:

- Use a statistics package to analyze the results, if possible.
- Tabulate the results in easily understandable constructs, such as averages, percentages, and frequencies.
- Review the survey's results with other individuals and compare the results with information gained from other surveys (if available) in order to identify reliable assumptions for business models.

Interviews

Interviews offer an in-depth approach to learning specific attitudes, behaviors, and needs of clients (actual and prospective). Interviews are a type of a survey in which the information is typically obtained either in person or over the telephone. Each method has its own advantages and disadvantages with regard to the ease of administering, cost, the amount of information that can be obtained, and so on. If conducted properly, both approaches provide an effective means for obtaining useful information.

Among the factors that health and fitness professionals should consider when conducting interviews are the following:

- Ask relevant, pertinent questions.
- Conduct the interviews at an appropriate time that is convenient for the people being interviewed.

- Be clear, direct, and articulate when conducting interviews.
- Have a specific agenda of questions that will collectively elicit the desired information.
- Hear silence as it is intended.
- Speak with an appropriate level of formality or informality.
- To relax the respondents, start with the easier questions.
- Ask individuals for opinions rather than facts if the goal of the interview is to draw out the respondents.
- Do not ask a question simply to ask a question.
- Take copious notes or record the respondents' answers. If permission is granted, tape the sessions.
- Keep the time to conduct the interviews to an appropriate level (i.e., not excessive).
- Follow up with a thank you note to the individuals who participated in the interview process.
- Have a predetermined strategic plan on how the information obtained from the interviews is to be analyzed and used.

Feedback Systems

This particular learning tool involves multiple approaches to gaining input from consumers in a non-intimidating, personal fashion. One possible approach is to establish a Web-based "comment box" to which individuals could provide feedback in an anonymous manner. The health and fitness professionals who are responsible for administering this tool could then post the individuals' feedback and their responses to each point raised in the feedback.

Why Consumers Join Health and Fitness Facilities

Understanding why individuals join health and fitness facilities can affect the decisions that health and fitness professionals make concerning such key factors as what business model to use, what activities should be included in a facility's program offering, and what operational guidelines should govern a particular facility.

Box 46-1 presents an overview of the top overall and specific reasons that individuals join health and fitness facilities. In reality, consumers can have several reasons for becoming members of a particular facility. The priority given to each reason can vary from person to person and circumstance to circumstance[3].

Gender can also play a role in why individuals join health and fitness facilities. Table 46-1 and Box 46-2, respectively, present an overview of the gender gap that exists between men and women concerning why they join health and fitness facilities and what critical variables affect men and women when they are deciding whether to become members of a particular facility.

BOX 46-1	Top Reasons Consumers Join Health and Fitness Facilities

TOP OVERALL REASONS	TOP SPECIFIC REASONS
To get in shape (84%)	To get in shape (64%)
To stay in shape (79%)	Need a place to exercise (54%)
Need a place to exercise (73%)	To stay in shape (49%)
Equipment availability (72%)	Equipment availability (40%)
Liked facility (71%)	Need motivation (33%)
Friendly staff (63%)	Liked facility (30%)
Good price (61%)	Good price (29%)
Need motivation (60%)	Friendly staff (22%)

Why An Individual Quits a Health and Fitness Facility

For a variety of reasons, every year, more than 31% of the individuals who belong to a health and fitness facility drop their membership[2–4]. Although no one (except the person involved) can say for absolute certainty why a particular individual quits a health and fitness facility, the most frequently reported reasons for such behavior include could not afford the expense (30%), overcrowded facility (27%), time (26%), inconvenient location (18%), lost interest (17%), moved (16%), and switched to exercising outdoors (15%). As Box 46-3 illustrates, the primary reasons for quitting a health and fitness facility can either be personal or facility driven.

Why Members Stay

The previous two sections addressed why individuals join and then some subsequently drop their memberships in health and fitness facilities. Although useful, such information is not enough for health and fitness professionals who want to maximize participation in their wellness programs in an effective and efficient manner. They also need

TABLE 46-1. The Gender Gap Concerning the Top Reasons for Joining Health and Fitness Facilities[3]

Reasons	Men (%)	Women (%)
Place to exercise	60	50
Need motivation	28	38
Friendly staff	17	26
Friends joined	17	25
Participate in classes	4	20

BOX 46-2 | **Gender Differences Concerning the Critical Decision-making Variables for Why People Join Health and Fitness Facilities**[2,3]

MEN

Location, location, location (fitness facility needs to be within 12 to 15 minutes of home or work)

Convenience

Quality and quantity of facilities and equipment.

Price–value equations

Availability of equipment

Staff quality and service delivery

Competitive environment

WOMEN

Location, location, location (within 2 to 15 minutes of home or work)

Convenience

Cleanliness of the facility

Group exercise programs

Friends are members

Non-intimidating environment

Staff quality and service delivery

Program for kids

Price–value equation

to know why individuals remain members of health and fitness facilities. Research suggests that a number of variables influence the membership retention levels in health and fitness facilities. Being aware of these factors can have a meaningful impact on the decision-making processes that directly or indirectly help affect whether individuals retain their facility memberships. In that regard, the variables that impact a person's decision concerning membership include the following[5-7]:

- The staff-to-member relationship. The better the relationship, the more likely members are to remain.
- Positive first impressions with the facility and the staff.
- Attendance. The more frequent the number of visits by the individual to the facility during the first 30 days and then the next 90 days, the more likely he or she is to remain.
- Initial connection and integration over the first 90 days.
- Achieving expressed fitness and health goals.
- Social connection with other members.
- Age and education (older and more educated members are more likely to remain).

- The enrollment or joining fee (the more an individual pays, the more likely that person is to stay).
- Method of payment (the retention rate is typically higher for an annual payment than a monthly one).

It is essential that health and fitness professionals are aware of the fact a serious disparity often exists between the perception that individuals have of a health and fitness facility and the reality of the situation. As Box 46-4 illustrates, how disconnect can have important decision-making implications for individuals who manage health and fitness facilities.

Given the aforementioned information concerning why individuals join, quit, and remain as members of health and fitness facilities, it is important for health and fitness professionals to realize that they can undertake certain **retention strategies** to increase the likelihood that members will retain their facility memberships. In that regard, the following steps have been shown to be effective:

- Provide each member with an immediate connection and orientation to the facility's programs, services, staff, and other members.
- Personalize the orientation around the member's own needs and interests (keeping in mind the differences between genders).

BOX 46-3 | **Facility-driven and Personal Reasons for Quitting Health and Fitness Facilities**

FACILITY-DRIVEN REASONS

Overcrowding

Dissatisfied with staff

Lack of attention by staff

Unresponsive management

Favorite staff member left

Facility was not clean

Culture of the facility

Equipment was not well kept

Dishonest business practices

PERSONAL REASONS

Did not make enough use of the facility

Lost interest or motivation

Did not have a partner

Switched to home exercise

Switched to exercising outdoors

Did not achieve desired results

BOX 46-4	The Disconnect Between Perception and Reality Concerning Why Individuals Join and Quit Health and Fitness Facilities

PERCEPTION OF FACILITY	JOIN FOR	LEAVE FOR
Worth the money	Good price	Overcrowded
Fun	Availability of equipment	Lost interest
Knowledgeable staff	Get in shape or stay in shape	Could not afford
For fit people	Staff quality or service	No partner
For young people	Cleanliness (women)	Results not achieved
Overcrowded	Friends are members (women)	Lack of attention by staff
	Non-intimidating environment	Culture of club
	Group exercise program (women)	Poor programs
		Dissatisfied with staff
		No connection

- Help establish realistic goals for members and then provide a program that allows individuals to achieve these goals.
- During an individual's initial 90 days of membership, provide extra staff interaction and follow-up.
- Track membership usage of the facility. Contact non-users and low users. Focus particularly on an individual's first 90 days as a member, but continue the process going forward.
- Survey the members of the facility in order to make sure that the facility is offering the right services and programs.
- Create member-driven activities so that members can connect with other members.
- Recognize the success and accomplishments of the members through newsletters, bulletin board postings, awards, and so on.
- Provide a very clean facility (a factor that is particularly important if the facility is attempting to attract and retain female members).
- Make sure to have enough equipment that is in good condition.
- Do not oversell memberships.
- Keep in mind that appropriately high dues and fees can have a positive impact on not only profit margins but also membership retention levels.
- At a minimum, make sure that at least a portion (more if feasible) of the facility has a non-intimidating environment.
- Make sure that everything in the facility is as convenient as possible for the members. If it is not, find out what that involves and then take steps to implement it.
- Create both a system that allows members to communicate their feelings about the positive and negative aspects involving the facility and a system for promptly responding to those concerns.

Developing a Health and Fitness Program

A number of factors should be taken into consideration when developing a health and fitness program. None is more important than designing a program that is consistent with the **strategic plan** of the facility or organization. Although providing people with the opportunity to achieve the innumerable benefits of exercising is undeniably a very worthy undertaking, expecting key matters (e.g., being able to pay the bills and meet the long-term objectives of the facility) to simply work themselves out over time would be naïve at best and disastrous at worst. Rather, detailed planning is required, not the least of which involves giving appropriate attention to the facility's health and fitness program.

ENHANCING THE FACILITY'S OPPORTUNITY FOR SUCCESS

Success is not a matter of desire; rather, it is the byproduct of preparation and hard work. In almost every human endeavor, the more preparation undertaken and the greater the effort expended, the more likely that the venture will be successful. Developing and operating a health and wellness program is no different.

A sound plan for developing a health and wellness program should address several factors, including finances, staffing, necessary facilities, equipment, risk management, and target markets. After the plan is developed, the decisions relating to the health and wellness program become an integral part of the health and fitness facility's business plan.

From a practical standpoint, a business plan for a health and fitness facility typically involves a "vision" of the future for that facility and how that "vision" will be achieved. In order to be viable, the "vision" must meet several criteria. First and foremost, it must be achievable. It must also be tangible. Finally, it must meet the expectations of those responsible for the future of the facility.

The business plan should also detail the parameters of the path that the facility will take in achieving its articulated vision. In this regard, the two most commonly used guideposts are goals and objectives. As a rule, goals are positive statements that delineate what needs to be accomplished over the long run to achieve the "vision" of the facility, and objectives are clear, relatively specific statements, the completion of which will lead to the achievement of the facility's goals. Unlike objectives, goals are purposely stated in generalities (e.g., to be the largest health and fitness facility in town within 5 years). Objectives, on the other hand, are generally short-range, challenging (but realistic) statements of a facility's intentions that focus on immediate accomplishments that are consistent with an organization's long-range goals (e.g., achieve a 4% net growth in the facility's membership in the current fiscal year).

A responsible business plan specifies a **financial plan** for how the facility will be viable going forward. This projection includes detailing what resources will be available (currently and in the future) and to what items those resources will be allocated. An appropriate business plan also outlines the strategic steps for implementing the plan, including cataloging what the facility will do if things do not go as planned (a process typically referred to as contingency planning).

IDENTIFYING TARGET AUDIENCES

The health and fitness program offering in some organizational settings (e.g., YMCAs, JCCs, hospital-based groups) is influenced by the expressed mission of the organization involved. For those organizations, the mission essentially defines the facility's menu of services and activities. The family orientation of YMCAs, for example, mandates that YMCAs offer a significant number of activities that are geared toward families, particularly children. By the same token, hospital-based programs tend to focus primarily on rehabilitation-directed offerings

Although all health and fitness facilities have a degree of freedom in deciding what services and activities to include in their program offerings, none has more latitude than commercial health and fitness clubs (collectively a group that represents almost half of the health and fitness facilities in the United States). Strategically, the key issue for health and fitness clubs is to identify **target audiences** that will be interested in using (i.e., pay for) the services and activities offered by the clubs. How well they determine that has a major impact on their ability to succeed.

In reality, health and fitness clubs vary the way that they evaluate the appropriateness of a particular market for them. As a rule, the typical approach is to analyze the market by specific variables. This analysis allows the clubs to segment the market according to a variable-driven structure. As a rule, three major ways exist to segment a market: geographic (location, density, urban vs. rural), demographic (age, gender, family size, family cycle, income, occupation, education, religion, race, nationality, social class), and psychographic (lifestyle, personality, benefits sought, user status, user rate, loyalty status, readiness stage).

Because psychographic segmentation tends to focus more on individuals and their attitudes and behaviors, health and fitness clubs tend to favor this approach over the other two options. Psychographics factors have been found to be effective as tools for recognizing market opportunity and addressing individual needs. Research on attitudes toward health and fitness has enabled investigators to categorize individuals according to their psychographic portraits. These portraits potentially have substantial implications for health and fitness professionals who are responsible for attracting and retaining members. According to this research, individuals fall into one of six categories[3]:

1. Balanced holistics (13%)
   - Take a balanced approach to exercise; exercise regularly; and exercise for both emotional and physical reasons, including "to get centered"
   - Feel badly if they do not exercise
   - Twice as likely to be health club members (approximately 26% of the population)
   - Describe themselves as socially confidant, goal oriented, intelligent, energetic, and health conscious
   - Are considered "hard-core" exercisers
2. Conscientious preventers (8%)
   - Take a balanced approach to exercise; are more focused on exercise as a way to prevent health problems and treat existing medical conditions
   - Place a high level of importance on fitness
   - Twice as likely to be health club members (approximately 26% of the population)
   - Describe themselves as health conscious, family-oriented, energetic, religious, and perfectionistic
   - Are considered "hard-core" exercisers
3. Social competitors (20%)
   - Prefer social, competitive, and relationship-engaging activity
   - Equally likely to be a health club member as the general public (13%)
   - Describe themselves as professionally ambitious, competitive, outgoing, risk taking, and a sports fan
4. Abracadabras (14%)
   - Are out of shape; do not exercise and have no desire to do so
   - Hate to exercise; if they do exercise, it is to lose weight
   - Half as likely to be health club members (6.5%)
   - Describe themselves as energetic, socially skillful, health conscious, and less outgoing
   - Considered to be part of the "indifferent"
5. Woulda–shoulda's (12%)
   - Do exercise, but less than general public
   - Are self-conscious; tend to be out of shape
   - Do not hate exercise; rather, lack self-discipline

- As likely as the general public to be health club members
- Describe themselves as emotional, bookish, shy, and professionally ambitious
- Considered to be part of the "uninitiated believers"

6. Sitcom skeptics (12%)
   - Believe that individuals who exercise are self-absorbed
   - Believe that a good diet and clean living negate the need to exercise
   - Some do exercise occasionally and are equally likely to be health club members as the general public
   - Describe themselves as not falling for the fitness craze
   - Considered to be part of the "indifferent"

DETERMINING THE PROGRAM OFFERING

Perhaps no decision has more important ramifications for the ability of a health and fitness facility to fulfill its vision than the determination of the services and activities that it will offer to its members. Such a decision can impact not only the facility's short-term financial health but also its ability to survive in the long term.

The business plan is the basic foundation underlying the decisions of what to include in the program offerings. Collectively, the offerings must be appropriate for the short- and long-term goals and objectives of the organization. How the offerings address this lofty aspiration may require a strategic balancing act because one decision may be more appropriate than another for the organization in the short term or in a particular set of ever-changing circumstances.

Within the context of adhering to the business plan, the next preeminent factor that must be considered when developing a health and fitness program is meeting the needs and interests of the consumers (actual and potential) that the facility is intended to serve. As previously discussed, a number of tools for helping to determine those needs and interests exist, including surveys, focus groups, and questionnaires.

Two additional tools that can be used to help identify the services and activities that should be offered in a facility's health and wellness program are fitness assessments and pre-activity health screening instruments (see Chapter 5 and GETP7 Chapter 2). Properly used, both devices can provide information that can help "personalize" the program offering specifically to an individual's needs. Not only can the information gained from the two tools offer insight concerning what activities an individual should undertake, but they also can be used to help health and fitness professionals prioritize those activities for that person. The primary aim in this regard is to ensure that the activity programming takes into account the unique characteristics of the participants who are engaged in the activity.

Another factor that should be weighed when determining the services and activities that a facility should include in its health and wellness program offering is the degree to which changing individual attitudes toward fitness affect individuals' behavior as it concerns health and fitness programming. Obviously, these changes can influence what a facility does or does not decide to include in its health and wellness program. For example, in the past decade, the following macro trends have occurred involving fitness activities[2,8]:

- Aerobic dancing participation has declined by 40%.
- High-impact aerobic activity participation has declined by 50%.
- Low-impact aerobic activity participation has declined by 40%.
- Step aerobic participation has declined by 30%.
- Treadmill participation has increased by more than 100%.
- Stair climbing participation has declined by 40%.
- Cross-country skiing participation has declined by 50%.
- Stationary cycling participation has declined by 30%.

In the past 3 to 5 years, the following changes in activity participation have transpired, each of which could affect how a health and fitness facility decides to allocate its resources[2,8]:

- Spinning participation has declined by just over 10%.
- Elliptical participation has increased by over 100%
- Free weight participation has increased by over 10% (while increasing by 50% over the past decade).
- Resistance equipment participation has remained flat (while declining 30% in the past decade).
- Yoga participation has increased 100%.
- Pilates participation has increased by more than 150%.

EVALUATING THE PROGRAM OFFERINGS

A process should be established to evaluate whether the various parts of the health and wellness program (i.e., services and activities) are making their expected contribution to the business plan of the facility. Among the factors that health and fitness professionals should consider to ensure that such an evaluation is conducted in an appropriate way are the following:

- Specific criteria that are consistent with the parameters detailed in the business plan (e.g., financial, growth, total participation, community service) should be identified.
- The evaluation should be undertaken with both short- and a long-term goals and objectives in mind.
- Industry participation trends should be considered when analyzing the evaluation results.
- The process of evaluation should be conducted on an ongoing basis.

Operating a Health and Wellness Program

Similar to every effort directed at achieving the goals and objectives of the organization, operating a health and wellness program requires strategic planning, the ability to adapt to circumstances, competent management, accountability, and keen attention to detail. Among the administrative matters that health and fitness administrators must be concerned with are staffing, facilities and equipment, finances, marketing and sales, customer service, and **risk management**.

STAFFING

Competent staff must be hired to supervise all of the various elements of the health and wellness program (see GETP7 Table 7-3). Ideally, overall responsibility for the program is assigned to an individual with a college degree in health and fitness or a related exercise science degree. Preferably, that person will also hold a current certification from a reputable professional organization (see Appendix B). All applicable local, state, and federal regulations and laws concerning staffing should be strictly followed. In addition, professionally trained instructors who have demonstrable expertise in the activity being taught should conduct all exercise classes. By the same token, trained personnel should periodically monitor all activity areas on a regular basis. Furthermore, people who are fully qualified to conduct the training should administer all fitness testing. Finally, every employee who is involved with the health and fitness program should have a current CPR/AED certification.

FACILITIES AND EQUIPMENT

All activities conducted in facilities should be appropriate for the activity being offered and that meet all local, state, and federal codes, regulations, and laws. All facilities should be well lighted, with an appropriate level of temperature, humidity, and ventilation. Every activity area should be clean, well kept, and regularly inspected to ensure that no condition involving an undue risk of injury to participants exists.

Similar to the facility areas, all equipment used in a particular activity should be appropriate for that activity. To the extent feasible and appropriate to the business plan of the organization, a variety of equipment should be provided that addresses each of the major components of fitness. Among the criteria that should be considered when purchasing equipment are durability, serviceability, value, appropriate for the intended users, and safety. Whenever possible, equipment should be purchased from reputable companies with demonstrable records of responsible, ethical behavior with regard to making user-friendly equipment and honoring their service commitments.

All equipment should be well maintained (i.e., at a minimum, strictly adhere to the maintenance guidelines prescribed in the owner's manual provided by the equipment's manufacturer) and regularly inspected to ensure that the equipment does not present a potential risk to individuals who use it. Furthermore, when appropriate, all equipment should have instructional signage posted in an appropriate place (e.g., attached to or adjacent to the particular piece of equipment) that details how to safely use each piece of equipment.

FINANCES

A detailed plan is needed for addressing all of the financial issues involving the health and wellness program (both required expenditures and anticipated revenues generated by the program). This step involves not only formulating a financial plan of the program but also evaluating the various elements of the plan after it has been put into action and making changes when appropriate, as discussed in Chapter 48. The financial planning process should include establishing financial objectives and priorities (both short- and long term), budgeting, and identifying actual and projected sources of funds.

Individuals responsible for the financial health of the organization must be knowledgeable about key financial issues. The information that they have concerning the finances of the organization must be accurate and up to date. They should also be aware of industry benchmarks for revenues and expenses because such information will help them validate their budget assumptions.

MARKETING AND SALES

Relatively speaking, very little (if any) truth exists concerning the old axiom "build a better mousetrap, and the world will beat a path to your door." Rather, steps have to be undertaken to make the world aware of the fact that such a device exists and how such a mousetrap can meet the needs and expectations of individuals who might otherwise be interested in an apparatus for dealing with mice. The same argument holds true for promoting the services and activities offered by health and wellness programs.

Promoting a health and wellness program requires systematic planning; an understanding of the potential markets for the menu of services and programs offered by the program; and a concerted, well-conceived effort to reach the targeted markets. Responsibility for each step in the particular effort to promote the program should be specifically defined, including overall accountability for each specific marketing effort undertaken.

Depending on the circumstances, a variety of tools can be used to promote a health and wellness program, either as a whole or in part, including direct mail, signage, member incentives, telephone, e-mails, radio, television, word of mouth, sponsorships, and endorsements. Which means are used in a given situation depends on such factors as the organization's strategic plan, the available resources, the accessibility and sophistication of the **targeted audiences**, and the competition for the attention and resources of the targeted audiences by other factors (e.g., organization, people, activities). The key point to keep in mind is that marketing and promotion of a health and wellness program are an ongoing process that tends to directly or indirectly involve everyone in the organization.

Within some health and fitness organizational settings, particularly health clubs, a key focal point of the marketing process is the sales of memberships. As a rule, membership sales tend to follow a three-step pathway. The first stage involves identifying individuals who are referred to as *leads*. Leads are individuals who have demographics or characteristics that match the targeted audience of the health club. Leads have not expressed any interest or been shown to have an interest in becoming a club member.

The second level of the membership pathway involves individuals who are typically known as prospects. Prospects either have shown an interest in the club or have been identified as being more suitable candidates for membership.

The third and final stage of the pathway to membership involves individuals who have decided to actually become members of the club. The obvious goal of the process is to capture leads, turn them into prospects, and ultimately convince them to become members of the club.

Health and fitness clubs use a variety of strategies to build their memberships. Among the more popular steps that are used in this regard are the following:

1. Membership referral
   - The focus is on generating prospects and members.
   - The process involves existing members providing the names of potential new members.
   - Members are provided with referral cards to hand in the names of prospects. Incentives are typically given to members for providing referrals.
   - As a program, it is usually conducted once a year.
   - High-end clubs often make this strategy one of their major sales focuses by using committees and getting referrals from all new members.
   - This approach is the most focused strategy.
2. Lead boxes
   - This strategy primarily serves as a source for leads (names).
   - As a rule, because this strategy does not generate quality leads, low-price and high-volume clubs often use it.
   - The boxes are placed in business locations that tend to serve customer bases that are demographically similar to the targeted audiences (e.g., sporting good stores, restaurants)
   - Businesses are given awards for allowing the lead boxes to be placed in their locales.
   - This strategy produces a very low rate of return.
3. Advertising
   - In general, this strategy is designed to enhance the image of the organization, create leads, or occasionally generate prospects.
   - This technique is a scatter-gun approach to reaching a facility's market (versus a sharpshooter method).
   - Cable television, radio, newspapers, billboards, and external or internal signage are examples of this method.
   - The most effective type of advertising for generating leads or prospects focuses on engaging the audience to act via such devices as coupons, raffles, and so on.
   - It is important to know the audience before the advertising medium is selected.

4. Alliances with homeowner associations (HOAs) and realtors
   - This strategy is a good source for qualified leads (and even prospects). HOAs and realtors whose customers match the organization's target market should be engaged in the process.
   - HOAs and realtors can provide the names of new people in the area.
   - As a rule, the strategy involves providing some complementary club memberships or guest passes for the HOAs or realtors to use.
   - Another option is to pre-sell club memberships to the HOA or builder so that when a home is purchased, the new owner is already a member of the club.
5. Direct mail
   - This strategy is primarily a technique for creating leads or turning leads into prospects.
   - This method is a more focused technique than advertising.
   - Mailing lists from agencies should be used. Very targeted lists can be obtained to best match the desired market area and demographics of the coveted audience.
   - The piece that is mailed is typically simple, with an attention-grabbing call for action.
   - The recipient of the piece normally incorporates some incentive into the mailed piece to generate an action response.
   - The return rate for this technique is usually 1% to 3% for mailed pieces and 7% to 15% for e-mails.
6. Community involvement
   - This strategy focuses on creating relationships to uncover prospects.
   - The technique involves creating a specific image in the community and becoming recognized as an integral part of the community.
   - An example of this approach is to become active in community organizations, such as the local chambers of commerce, the Rotary, church groups, and so on.
   - Another option is to host community events in the club or sponsor community events at other locations.
   - Service and relationship-driven clubs use this strategy most often.
7. Cold calling
   - This strategy is used to turn leads into prospects.
   - The technique can use general or targeted lists of names, including referral names.
   - Telemarketing, phone call solicitation, and cold calling on homes and businesses are examples of this approach.
   - This approach normally includes some incentives to get action-oriented responses.
   - This strategy typically gets a low rate of return.
   - Individuals who are contacted often consider this technique intrusive.
8. Reputation management
   - This strategy is used to enhance the public image of the organization.
   - Over time, this approach can be a great source for prospects.
   - The technique involves developing a press kit on the club (e.g., a background, fact sheet).
   - This strategy requires establishing positive relationships with the local media.

- The approach requires regularly issuing press releases of human interest involving the club and following up with the media.
9. Promotional materials
   - This strategy is normally used to assist converting leads to prospects or prospects to members.
   - The materials are designed to create a positive image of the club and to help educate consumers on the club.
   - Websites, print brochures, and video brochures are examples of this technique.
   - These materials are normally given to leads and more often to prospects.
10. Strategic alliances
    - This strategy is designed to create partnerships between businesses and organizations with similar target audiences.
    - This technique is good at bringing in leads and prospects.
    - The approach involves cross-marketing between the businesses.
    - The customers of each business become potential customers for the other partner (alliance group).
    - This method is frequently used in an effective, strategic manner by relatively large, multiple-club organizations.

CUSTOMER SERVICE

Without question, one of the most important factors in the effort by health and fitness clubs to get an adequate number of members is to keep the customers that they already have. Accordingly, every club should make an absolute commitment to customer service. Integral to this commitment is a clean, well-run facility that is responsive to the needs and interests of the members. Furthermore, all staff members should be pleasant, relatively well groomed and appropriately attired, and exhibit an attitude that providing good service to the members is an integral part of their job. In addition, every health and fitness facility should implement a specific system for soliciting and responding to feedback provided by the members.

RISK MANAGEMENT

Every health and fitness facility should take specific steps to minimize the risk of unsafe conditions and to maximize the ability of facility personnel to respond to emergency events (see Chapter 28). Among the actions that can enhance the safety level of the health and fitness program participants are qualified staff; pre-activity screening; adequate levels of activity supervision; regular maintenance of all equipment and facilities; attention accorded to physical plant safety issues; appropriate signage; and requiring all activities to be conducted in an appropriate, safety-conscious manner.

Health and fitness facilities must also have emergency plans that ensure that events involving the health or safety of participants are handled in an appropriate manner[9]. An emergency plan should be developed and implemented to provide specific guidelines concerning how the staff members should react when emergency incidents occur. Staff members should conduct themselves in a manner that minimizes the consequences of the incidents. In practical terms, emergency plans help to ensure that minor incidents do not become major incidents and that major incidents do not lead to fatalities[10].

An emergency plan should include several elements, including provisions for physical access to all areas of the facility, as well as a basic plan for dealing with any bystanders who might need treatment. In addition, the emergency plan should include detailed instructions for securing and using specific protocols and emergency supplies. Steps must also be undertaken to ensure that the emergency supplies (including automated external defibrillators) are positioned in easily accessible locations that are well known to all staff personnel. Furthermore, the emergency plan should include specific information on how to contact outside assistance from predetermined sources.

Health and fitness facilities should put their emergency plans in writing and ensure that all staff members are fully aware of the emergency procedures to be followed in the case of untoward incidents, particularly concerning how to use the existing emergency supplies and how to quickly contact outside medical resources. Finally, the emergency plan should include provisions for documenting all emergency incidents to provide a basis for the orderly evaluation of the situation after it occurs and for identifying the follow-up actions that subsequently should be undertaken (see Chapter 49 for more detailed information).

Summary

Developing and operating health and wellness programs is a multifaceted process that involves giving appropriate consideration to a number of factors, including the business plan of the health and fitness facility and the needs and interests of the participants. The process should be undertaken in a systematic, thoughtful manner to ensure that the effort is both prudent and effective.

REFERENCES

1. International Health, Racquet & Sportsclub Association: IHRSA Global Report 2002: State of the Health Club Industry. Boston, MA; 2002.
2. International Health, Racquet & Sportsclub Association/ASD. Health Club Trend Report: 1987–2002. Boston, MA; 2002.
3. International Health, Racquet & Sportsclub Association: (prepared by Roper Starch): Fitness American-Style: A Look at How and Why Americans Exercise. Boston, MA; 2001.
4. International Health, Racquet & Sportsclub Association: 2002 Profiles of Success. Boston, MA; 2002.
5. International Health, Racquet & Sportsclub Association: Why People Quit. Boston, MA; 1998.
6. International Health, Racquet & Sportsclub Association: Why People Stay. Boston, MA; 2000.
7. Fitness Industry Association: Winning the Retention Battle (Parts 1–3). Boston, MA; 2001.
8. American Sports Data: Sports Participation Report. Boston, MA; 2003.

9. American College of Sports Medicine: Recommendations for cardio-vascular screening, staffing, and emergency policies at health/fitness facilities. A joint position statement with the American Heart Association. Med Sci Sports Exer 30:1009–1018, 1988.
10. Peterson J, Tharrett S, eds: ACSM's Health/Fitness Facility Standards and Guidelines, 2nd ed. Champaign, IL: Human Kinetics; 1997.

SELECTED REFERENCES FOR FURTHER READING

Grantham B, Patton R, York T, Winick M: Health Fitness Management: Champaign, IL: Human Kinetics; 1998.
McCarthy, J, ed:. IHRSA's Guide to Lenders and Investors, 2nd ed. Boston: IHRSA; 2003.
Plummer T: The Business of Fitness: Understanding the Financial Side of Owning a Fitness Business. Monterey, CA: Healthy Learning; 2003.
Plummer T: Making Money in the Fitness Business. Monterey, CA: Healthy Learning; 1999.

INTERNET RESOURCES

ACE: American Council on Exercise: http://www.acefitness.org

American College of Sports Medicine: http://www.acsm.org

FitnessManagement: http://www.fitnessmanagement.com

IDEA Health & Fitness Association: http://www.ideafit.com

International Health, Racquet & Sportsclub Association: http://www.ihrsa.org

Clinical Exercise Program Development and Operations

JEANNE E. RUFF

Clinical exercise services are expanding beyond traditional cardiac and pulmonary rehabilitation programs to include other patient populations such as those with peripheral vascular disease, cancer, multiple sclerosis, and diabetes. As the field of clinical services diversifies and expands, so do the roles of exercise specialists and registered clinical exercise physiologists. Their scopes of practice, skills, and competencies must span a broader range of knowledge to accommodate varying patient populations. Cardiac and pulmonary rehabilitation program models also need to be adapted to encompass the expanding patient needs. The challenge of clinical exercise program management is to incorporate the standards of care delivered by appropriately credentialed staff while also fulfilling medical necessity and insurance guidelines for delivering safe and effective treatment.

Reimbursement

Typically, clinical rehabilitation programs are hospital based and generate revenue via third-party reimbursement. Therefore, the underlying program format needs to comply with the rules and regulations of the insurers to be a viable clinical service. A physician initiates a patient's clinical exercise program by providing the following:

- A signed prescription or referral to the program
- A diagnosis or sign or symptom (ICD-9 code) that establishes medical necessity appropriately paired with a Current Procedure Terminology (CPT) code for the services provided
- Ideally, the individual's insurance coverage description includes the service as a benefit or, if not a covered benefit, the patient agrees to pay out of pocket

Clinical exercise professionals need to be well versed in the steps necessary to secure insurance coverage for the services offered. Typically, reimbursement concerns are discussed with the patient and agreed upon before service is initiated.

The largest payer of both cardiac and pulmonary rehabilitation services is the Centers for Medicare and Medicaid Services (CMS)[1]. Currently, these services are billed "incident to the physician," which means that the services of nonphysician personnel (i.e., nurses, exercise physiologists) must be furnished under the direct supervision of a physician. Direct supervision means that a physician must be in the exercise program area and immediately available and accessible for an emergency at all times the exercise program is conducted. These guidelines from CMS are further interpreted and implemented by the local Medicare Intermediaries, which may have some variability in different states or regions. Some of the local Medicare Intermediaries state that a physician does not need to be physically present in the exercise room, but others insist that a physician must be in the room or within a certain radius of the room. The "incident to physician" service is a complex issue and is currently under scrutiny by CMS by means of audits for compliance with the established guidelines.

Centers for Medicare and Medicaid Services also determines the medical necessity for the services for which they provide reimbursement. So far, CMS has only approved three diagnoses for cardiac rehabilitation: myocardial infarction, bypass surgery within the past 12 months, and stable angina. The diagnosis of stable angina is being closely evaluated through audits. CMS has clarified that to use stable angina, it must be further supported by clinical symptoms and records from the referring physician or documentation supporting the diagnosis. Stable angina cannot be the principle diagnosis after patients undergo coronary artery stent placement or other percutaneous coronary intervention. If the patient's symptoms return after the intervention and are deemed stable, the patient would then be considered as a candidate for cardiac rehabilitation.

In addition, a national policy decision from CMS for Pulmonary Rehabilitation Services has been pending since the late 1990s, even though pulmonary rehabilitation was an integral part of their lung volume reduction surgery evaluation. The American Association of Cardiovascular and Pulmonary Rehabilitation (AACVPR) provides the most up-to-date information on the various national and regional reimbursement guidelines. This information is available on their website (http://www.aacvpr.org). Other insurance carriers tend to follow the lead of CMS; therefore, a clinical program based on the published CMS rules will tend to be compliant with others insurance carriers' requirements.

Program Certification

Although not yet a requirement for reimbursement, the AACVPR has established a program certification process for cardiac rehabilitation and pulmonary rehabilitation programs. The impetus for the establishment of this certification process was to have a standard of minimal requirements or operations that all cardiac and pulmonary rehabilitation programs would follow. Certification by the AACVPR is designed to provide patients with the highest **standards of care.** The application process includes submitting information regarding the following criteria:

- Individual staff credentials (e.g., current certifications and licenses, competencies, annual appraisals)
- Facilities, equipment, and supplies
- Methods of documentation (e.g., policies and procedures; medical records; medical emergencies; and outcome assessments in three domains, clinical, behavioral, and health)

- Methods of patient care (e.g., assessments, therapeutic plan or individual plan of care, interventions and treatment components, evaluations, discharge, follow-up)

Since 1998, more than 1000 programs from across the United States have been awarded certification. The program certification process is an excellent guide for new programs or as a periodic program review or update. Program certification is granted for 3 years, after which a recertification application process and review must be completed.

Accreditation

Hospital-based clinical exercise programs are under additional scrutiny by the Joint Commission on Accreditation of the Healthcare Organizations (JCAHO). The JCAHO is an organization to which health care entities may apply for accreditation in order to provide services and meet reimbursement criteria from federal agencies (i.e., CMS)[2].

Many of the JCHAO standards required for accreditation are strategically included in the AACVPR program certification application process. Of similarity and importance to JCAHO and AACVPR program certification is the tracking of clinical outcomes or quality indicators. JCAHO requires that dimensions of performance (DOP) relating to procedures, treatments, tests, or services include the following:

1. **Efficacy:** The degree to which the care of the patient has been shown to accomplish the desired or projected outcome
2. **Appropriateness:** The degree to which the care provided is relevant to the patient's clinical needs, given the current state of knowledge
3. **Availability:** The degree to which appropriate care is available to meet the patient's needs
4. **Timeliness:** The degree to which care is provided to the patient at the most beneficial or necessary time

5. **Effectiveness:** The degree to which care is provided in the correct manner, given the current state of knowledge, to achieve the desired or projected outcome for the patient

6. **Continuity:** The degree to which care for the patient is coordinated among the practitioners, among organizations, and over time

7. **Safety:** The degree to which the risk of an intervention and risk in the care environment are reduced for the patient and others, including the health care provider

8. **Efficiency:** The relationship between the outcomes (results of care) and the resources used to deliver patient care

9. **Respect and caring:** The degree to which the patient or a designee is involved in his or her own care decisions and to which those providing services do so with sensitivity and respect for the patient's needs, expectations, and individual differences

These dimensions of performance are then identified in a specific clinical or service improvement initiatives that are department specific or cross-functional (i.e., involving other departments). Figure 47-1 is an example of a quality improvement summary whereby the topic at hand is identified, followed by the dimension of performance, baseline findings, an action plan to improve the process, and data-driven improvement results. The rationale for tracking clinical outcomes is to evaluate the effectiveness of the delivery of the clinical services. The evaluation is based on objective data and national **benchmarks** from which current processes or practices will continue or new processes or practices will be implemented.

Outcomes

The traditional outcome measures within clinical programs have focused on physiological responses to the exercise therapy. For example, changes in metabolic equivalents at a given submaximal heart rate, hemodynamic responses at rest and with exercise, lipid levels benchmarked to national standards, or body weight are used to track improvement. More recently, psychosocial and quality of life indices have been added to outcome lists and have been tracked with demonstrated improvements. Examples of these are perception of health and anxiety and depressions scales[3].

QUALTIY IMPROVEMENT ANNUAL SUMMARY

Department / Service _____

Preparer: _____

Page _____ of _____

Time Frame _____

FOCUS		ANALYZE	DEVELOP	EXECUTE
Q.I. TOPIC	D.O.P	BASELINES, FINDINGS TRENDS	ACTIONS OR PLAN	IMPROVEMENT RESULTS

Annual Reappraisal: _____

_____

_____

FIGURE 47-1. Example of a quality improvement annual summary.

Program professionals should select outcome variables to measure in a variety of domains within the core components of program services. Often, program professionals measure outcome variables at the start of the program, the end of the initial exercise program (i.e., phase II), and 6 and 12 months thereafter. These findings provide valuable information for quality improvement, accreditation, and reimbursement and are critical for providing feedback to patients regarding their progress. The AACVPR program certification requires documentation of outcome assessments in three domains: health (morbidity, mortality, quality of life, **risk stratification,** status of cardiovascular disease [CVD] symptoms), clinical (physical, psychological, medical utilization, social), and behavioral (compliance with medical regimen, recognition and reporting). A fourth domain is service, which includes the reporting of patient satisfaction as well as financial and economic data. Finally, a fifth domain reflects education or the level of knowledge a patient has about his or her disease. The data from outcome tracking provide valuable information for quality improvement, accreditation, reimbursement, and program effectiveness.

Core Components

Core components to cardiac rehabilitation and secondary prevention programs have been thoroughly outlined in the American Heart Association (AHA)/AACVPR Scientific Statement[4]. The objectives of the statement are to optimize cardiovascular risk reduction, foster health behaviors and compliance to these behaviors, reduce disability, and promote an active lifestyle for patients with CVD. The purpose of the statement is to present specific information regarding evaluation, intervention, and expected outcomes in each of the core components of cardiac rehabilitation and secondary prevention programs:

- Baseline patient assessment
- Nutritional counseling
- Risk factor management (lipids, hypertension, weight, diabetes, and smoking)
- Psychosocial management
- Physical activity counseling
- Exercise training

These recommendations are intended to assist clinical staff in the design and development of their programs and to assist health care providers, insurers, policymakers, and consumers in the recognition of the comprehensive nature of such programs[4].

STAFF COMPETENCY

The key to a successful clinical exercise program is having competent and motivated staff. The collective knowledge, skills, and clinical experience of the staff are essential to building a multidisciplinary team. This blend of knowledge and technical skills brings about optimal care for the patients being serviced. Licensed and unlicensed health care professionals are included in the multidisciplinary team. The knowledge base of the staff should include a comprehensive understanding of CVD and pulmonary disease, cardiovascular emergency procedures, nutrition, exercise physiology, pharmacology, behavior modification strategies, health psychology, and medical and educational strategies for risk factor management. The professionals typically represented in the clinical team included specially trained nurses, exercise physiologists, dietitians, psychologists, physical therapists, pharmacists, occupational therapists, respiratory therapists, and physicians. Core standards, functions, and adequate emergency response capabilities are the basis of clinical competencies. The AACVPR **Core Competencies** document provides a thorough summary of standards and competencies for clinical staff members.

Staff competency assessments, training, and continuing education are ongoing and require validation yearly, along with documentation in each staff member's personnel files. A competency assessment plan should include the following documentation:

- Copies of current licenses, registrations, and certifications that are required by the job description
- Documentation of hospital and department orientation using a comprehensive competency-based orientation program to ensure the proper training of new employees
- Hospital-wide competence assessment, including fire safety, electrical safety, confidentiality, corporate compliance, disaster training, and universal precautions
- Department competence assessment, including emergency procedures, skill validation, in-service attendance, and participation in staff meetings
- Annual performance appraisals that are completed based on a competency-driven job description

Parameters used in the selection of core competencies to measure include:

- New procedures and practice guidelines
- New equipment (department specific)
- High-risk and low-volume issues
- Quality improvement, outcome findings, and sentinel events
- Customer satisfaction
- Age-related development issues
- Patient safety concerns

Figure 47-2 is a development checklist that may be used to organize and plan educational competencies. Employees should be aware of their annual competence requirements and be provided with opportunities to comply with these requirements. Job descriptions should describe the competencies for each position, and the annual performance appraisal should include an evaluation of the staff person's competency.

Competency Development Checklist

I. Prior to developing a competency:

☐ Identify the competency facilitator: _____

☐ How was the need for competency identified?

   ____ New procedure/practice, ____ New equipment, ____ High risk/low volume,

   ____ Customer service

   ____ QA & I findings/sentinel event, ____ other: _____

☐ Target skill level (i.e. RN, rad tech, secretary, etc.): _____

☐ Goal of competency: _____

II. All competencies must include the following:

☐ The name/title of the competency: _____

☐ A space for the learner to write his/her name, unit, badge number, and date

   Directions for completion of the competency:

☐   a. How to complete the competency—Example: circle the correct answer, fill in the blank, correctly demonstrate,

☐   b. Provide the date for completion of competency

☐   c. List whom to return the completed competency

☐   d. Standard statement to appear on all competencies: "Documentation of successful completion of this competency will be entered on your personal transcript."

III. Competency Content

☐   a. Objectives for competency

☐   b. Include age-appropriate information in the content as applicable.

☐   a. Standard statement to include on skills review competencies: *"All of the following items must be reviewed and/or demonstrated by the employee and signed off by the department head/supervisor/designee. All information reviewed and skills assessed are based on the department policy and procedure manuals."*

☐   b. When formatting an observational skills checklist type competency, all items that have a sign-off space must be initialed and dated by the department head/supervisor/designee when completed. (NOTE: If an employee is unable to demonstrate skill or competence, further documentation is needed as to how competence was evaluated.)

☐   c. All observational skills checklist type competencies must include this final statement and a signature line at the completion of the competency. *"My signature below indicates that the above information/skills have been covered and that I have fully demonstrated understanding/competence."*

_____   _____

Signature of Employee   Date

(over)

FIGURE 47-2. Example of a competency development checklist.

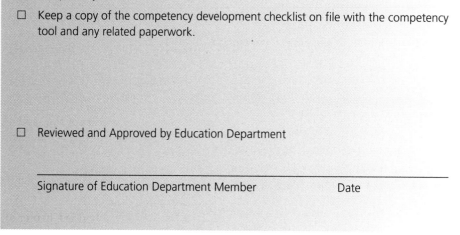

d. Initials Validation—Observational skills checklist type competencies often require more than one person to validate a learner's skills. When this occurs, a space for initials validation needs to be included with enough lines so that all persons who have initialed the competency have room to identify their initials and name.

_____ _____   _____ _____
Initials   Signature   Initials   Signature

_____ _____   _____ _____
Initials   Signature   Initials   Signature

IV. Competency Evaluation

☐ Select a method of evaluation for this competency that is compatible with the tool you are using (e.g., observational skills checklist for skills demonstration, written test for knowledge verification)

☐ Scoring guidelines:

   a. The minimum passing score for <u>any</u> competency posttest is 80%, however, based on the critical nature of the content, the facilitator may select a higher passing score.

   b. The score written on the actual posttest must be in the form of a percentage.

   <u>For Observational Skills Checklist type Competencies:</u>

   All competence statements must be successfully completed to pass the competency.

The competency facilitator is to:

☐ Keep a copy of the competency development checklist on file with the competency tool and any related paperwork.

☐ Reviewed and Approved by Education Department

_____
Signature of Education Department Member   Date

FIGURE 47-2. Continued.

Proper documentation is required by JCAHO. Additional information regarding clinical competencies can be found in Chapter 49.

PHYSICAL ENVIRONMENT

The physical environment and equipment needs for primary and **secondary prevention** programming must be well planned for the patient population served. The environment should allow for safe and easy patient movement and flow. General guidelines suggest floor space of approximately 40 to 45 square feet per patient, temperature controls between 65 and 72°F, humidity level at approximately 65%, ceiling height at a minimum of 10 feet, water source available, no food or drink allowed near exercise or monitoring equipment, confidentiality of the patient records, patient privacy maintained, and regularly tested telephone and emergency call system available[3]. The Fourth Edition of *The AACVPR Guidelines for Cardiac Rehabilitation and Secondary Prevention Programs*[3] is an excellent resource for additional facility considerations and suggested equipment needs for clinical programming.

Because of the diversified patient populations with several **comorbidities** (i.e., chronic obstructive pulmonary disease, diabetes, peripheral vascular disease, arthritis) attending clinical exercise programs, facilities need to have the following equipment available in order to assess and monitor the safe implementation of exercise therapies and risk factor changes:

- Chair and examination table or cart suitable for recumbent positions
- Portable oxygen or supplemental oxygen source
- A blood glucose meter and glucose supplies
- Emergency equipment, including a portable defibrillator with cardioversion and external pacing capabilities, portable suction, intubation supplies, blood pressure measurement equipment, first-line medications in accordance with the AHA's advanced cardiac life support (ACLS) standards, and intravenous fluid administration access equipment
- Body weight scale and protocol for determining body composition
- Quality stethoscope, portable sphygmomanometer, electrocardiographic (ECG) surveillance capabilities, pulse oximeter, rating of perceived exertion, and pain and discomfort scales
- Telephone, and emergency signal system

Specific exercise equipment selection is individualized to each program based primarily on available space, budget guidelines, and patients' needs and preferences. General exercise equipment should include weight-bearing (e.g., treadmills) and non–weight-bearing (e.g., recumbent cycle ergometers, arm and leg ergometers, stationary cycles ergometers, upper body ergometers, rowing machines) modalities. Other potential exercise equipment includes resistance training equipment with adjustable benches, seats, and arm settings; dumbbells in pairs; and elastic bands.

STAFFING PATTERNS

With the facility and equipment needs in place, staffing patterns must be planned for and implemented. The AACVPR guidelines[3] suggest the following:

- Early post-hospital discharge outpatient programs should have a maximum patient-to-staff ratio of five to one; a second staff person should be available for emergencies.
- Intermediate and maintenance programs that do not involve continuous ECG monitoring should have a maximum patient-to-staff ratio of 15 to one.
- For intermediate- and high-risk patients, an even lower patient-to-staff ratio may be warranted.

- For high-risk patients and in accordance with insurance guidelines, a supervising physician must be immediately available.

The staffing guidelines outlined reference largely cardiac and pulmonary rehabilitation settings. However, staffing patterns for other patient populations need to be individualized to the clinical setting, the knowledge and experience of the staff, the functional level of the patients, and the guidelines outlined for the specific billing parameters and reimbursement guidelines.

DOCUMENTATION

The next parameter for effective clinical programming management is documentation. The requirements for documentation should reflect the evaluation, intervention, and measured outcomes of the clinical services. This is essential for describing the therapy provided, education reviewed, and the patient's response to these interventions. The content for documentation should emphasize the following.

Initial Assessment

The initial assessment compiles patient demographics, insurance information, written and signed physician referral, informed consent, signed release of medical information, initial evaluation (i.e., medical history; symptoms; risk factors; comorbidities; medications; work history; psychosocial history; exercise history; recent illnesses, surgical procedures, and hospitalizations), and physical examination and exercise test results.

Care Plan

The care plan should include an identification of desired outcomes, a description of the methodology to achieving the objectives, the manner in which each objective will be measured, an exercise prescription, a specific risk factor intervention, and the timeline for modifications to the plan. The care plan should be customized for the specific disease population for which it is intended. An example of a care plan can be found in Chapter 49.

Provision of Service

The provision of service documentation encompasses daily progress notes; education flow sheets; the discharge summary; progress notes for the patient, referring physician, and (if warranted) third-party payers; documentation of changes in the clinical profile of the patient; and tracking or documentation of emergent interventions, untoward events, and hospital admissions.

Exercise Training

As outlined in an exercise prescription, exercise training includes intensity, frequency, duration, and modality; a quantification of the exercise therapy; support measures used during exercise; and any adverse responses, including the action taken and the results.

Discharge Evaluation

The discharge evaluation is the description of the outcomes achieved and the specific plan for maintaining the desired goals, including a follow-up schedule. In all circumstances, patient information is confidential. The program's policies and procedures manual should define the content, usage, and storage of the patient's records. Chapters 49 and 50 address confidentiality and privacy rights.

Expanding Patient Populations

As programs and professionals look to diversify from the traditional cardiac rehabilitation programs, the clinical core will remain the same. However, staff competence, equipment availability, patient assessment, core components, and outcome measurements will need to be modified to better reflect the specific needs of the patients to be treated.

For example, a 6-minute walk test would be conducted in pulmonary rehabilitation not only as a measure of fitness for outcome documentation but to also ascertain whether the patient's oxygen saturation level would decrease with activity, establishing the need for supplemental oxygen during exercise (i.e., oxygen saturation level < 90%). An exercise tolerance test with the measurement of expired gases is extremely helpful in determining the pulmonary patient's cause for exercise limitation as well as for determining an exercise prescription for the training program. Purse-lipped breathing and diaphragmatic breathing would be taught and monitored for compliance and efficiency during the actual exercise session. The educational topics presented during the pulmonary rehabilitation session would focus on topics unique to the disease, including pulmonary disease, use of inhalers, breathing techniques, and performance of activities of daily living. The second edition of the *AACVPR Guidelines for Pulmonary Rehabilitation Programs*[5] provides a detail account for the delivery of a comprehensive pulmonary rehabilitation program. Chapter 32 provides a more detailed account of the pathophysiology of pulmonary disease and the application of exercise therapy for this patient population.

Diabetes is a common comorbidity in both cardiac and pulmonary rehabilitation patients that many programs choose to aggressively address. Chapter 33 outlines the etiology, pathology, and clinical application of exercise for diabetic patients. Operational aspects of a traditional rehabilitation programs need to be enhanced to best serve this patient population. Suggestions for the successful management of patients with diabetes in clinical exercise programs[6] includes staff members' knowing the signs, symptoms, and management of hypoglycemia, including the medications that tend to mask or exacerbate the effects. Sources of glucose need to be immediately available. A glucometer should be accessible. Documentation of staff training and competency in performing blood glucose tests is expected. A certified diabetes educator or dietician is an important person to have as part of the care team. The patient education that this individual could provide regarding diet and insulin management is critical to patients' success. The exercise equipment available to diabetic patients should take into consideration the neuropathies associated with this disease. Moreover, it is important that the clinical exercise program management of these patients with various comorbidities takes into account all aspects of the disease and looks for ways to optimize patient outcomes within the clinical exercise program.

A current limitation for nontraditional patient populations is the lack of insurance coverage except for a very select group of cardiac and pulmonary diagnoses. Clinical research supports exercise therapy for the nontraditional patient groups; however, third-party payers tend to move very slowly when adding additional coverage or diagnoses eligible for service to their policies. For example, many believe that patients with congestive heart failure, peripheral artery disease, and arrhythmias would benefit from a structured program with medical surveillance to ensure the safe and effective delivery of the exercise therapy for a limited duration. However, the current CMS guidelines do not cover these patient diagnoses in the traditional cardiac rehabilitation programs. Therefore, fee-for-service or self-pay models can be established for these patients to meet their needs as well as provide alternative revenue sources for the program. Often, working with the medical director and the referring physicians, patients may be safely stratified into programs with less intensive monitoring and staffing to help minimize the patient's out-of-pocket costs. Chapters 34 to 38 provide a comprehensive review of the pathophysiology of these chronic diseases and disabilities. The application of exercise therapy for these patient populations is also presented, which is invaluable for the multidisciplinary team members in their implementation and management of effective exercise programs.

Clinical exercise programs must broaden their services to meet the needs of the growing patient populations who benefit from therapeutic exercise and to incorporate alternative revenue sources to help cover operating costs. As noted in this text, the ACSM exercise specialist certification and the registry examination for clinical exercise physiologists are two examinations professionals can take to reflect their clinical competencies for the design and implementation of safe and effective exercise programs for patients with various medical conditions (see Appendix B).

As patients transition from acute care settings to subacute care and then to outpatient rehabilitation settings, their continuum of care for a lifetime of exercise therapy can often be accomplished by participating in medically-based fitness and wellness centers. These centers incorporate the mission statements of many hospitals by promoting the prevention of disease and the promotion of health. A strategy for the development of a medical fitness center would be to have a facility for existing clinical services to expand to. Examples of clinical services include cardiology, pulmonary, orthopedics, physical medicine, neuromuscular, women's services, senior services, oncology services, pain management, and employee health. These clinical specialties could all benefit by having continuing services housed within an affiliated medical fitness center. Physician practices could also be based or located adjacent to the medical fitness center. This concept of clinical programs in close alignment with a fitness center can enhance referrals to all service lines. But more impressively, this concept of a medically-based fitness center can provide the model of continuity and continuum of care throughout the medical model and to the community. This expansion of clinical services and the "retail" component of a medical fitness center would also be a new outpatient revenue sources for the institution. Planning a medically based fitness center requires a thorough market analysis and comprehensive business plan to ensure the feasibility that such a venture would be cost effective and be well received by the community. The Medical Fitness Association is a nonprofit organization that serves as a resource to hospitals and medical centers engaging in the dual concept of fitness and clinical services under one roof, and it is very accessible at its website (http://www.medicalfitness.org).

Daily Operations of Clinical Exercise Services

General day-to-day operations of the clinical exercise services would be similar to any outpatient service line or medical practice. Key operational strategies that need to be determined and addressed include the daily hours of operation, services to be offered, staffing mix and assignments, a central office staff to receive and process referrals, charting and documentation standards, operational budgets, productivity standards, and, patient satisfaction measures. The financial aspects of the service must be well thought out to ensure financial stability. Billing, procedure codes, insurance verification, and fee-for-service collections are the foundation from which the financial basis of the clinical service line is based. The determination of a clinical exercise service must ensure a financial base to offset expenses and to generate a means of revenue. Meeting patients' and customers' needs is of key importance because without a patient base or customers, there is no service. Quality service ensures repeat and satisfied customers who will continue to come to your health care facility for all of their needs.

Summary

The management of clinical exercise programs requires a diversified manager who has an understanding of the clinical parameters for special populations, knows how to implement management principles, understands insurance criteria for reimbursement, and obtains financial viability. Quality care is imperative to programming success. The pinnacle for quality care is having a competent staff to deliver the program services. Ongoing education, certification, and incorporating nationally endorsed core programming components ensure a competent staff. Clinical exercise professionals who understand all aspects of clinical programs, including the management rationale discussed and the financial aspects highlighted in Chapter 48 will be the most prepared to function in the dynamic and challenging health care environment.

REFERENCES

1. Centers for Medicare and Medicaid Services: Medicare Preventive Services. Available at: http//www.hcfa.gov/quality/3q2.htm
2. Joint Commission on Accreditation of Healthcare Organization. Hospitals. Available at: http://www.jcaho.org/
3. American Association of Cardiovascular and Pulmonary Rehabilitation: Guidelines for Cardiac Rehabilitation and Secondary Prevention Programs, 4th ed. Champaign, IL: Human Kinetics; 2004.
4. Balady GJ, Ades PA, Comoss PM, et al: Core components of cardiac rehabilitation/secondary prevention program. Circulation 102: 1069–1073, 2000.
5. American Association of Cardiovascular and Pulmonary Rehabilitation: Guidelines for Pulmonary Rehabilitation Programs, 3rd ed. Champaign, IL. Human Kinetics; 2004.
6. Gordon NF: The exercise prescription (pp. 70–82). In The Health Professional's Guide to Diabetes and Exercise. Alexandria, VA: American Diabetes Association; 1995.

SELECTED REFERENCES FOR FURTHER READING

American College of Cardiology/American Heart Association: Clinical competence statement on stress testing. Circulation 102:1726–1738, 2000.

American College of Cardiology/American Heart Association: Guidelines for the evaluation and management of chronic heart failure in the adult: Executive summary. J Am Coll Cardiol 38:2102–2112, 2001.

American College of Cardiology/American Heart Association: Guidelines for the management of patients with acute myocardial infarction. J Am Coll Cardiol 28:1328–428, 1996.

American College of Cardiology/American Heart Association: 2002 guidelines for the management of patients with chronic stable angina: Summary article. Circulation 107:149–158, 2003.

American College of Sports Medicine ACSM's health/fitness facility standards and guidelines. Champaign, IL: Human Kinetics; 1997.

American Diabetes Association: Clinical practice recommendations: Summary of revisions for the 2005 clinical practice recommendations. Diabetes Care 2005:28–53(suppl 1).

American Heart Association: Cardiac rehabilitation and secondary prevention of coronary heart disease. AHA scientific statement. Circulation 111:369–376, 2005.

Expert Panel on the Identification, Evaluation, and Treatment of Overweight and Obesity in Adults: Executive summary of the Clinical Guidelines on the Identification, Evaluation, and Treatment of Overweight and Obesity in Adults. Arch Internal Med 1998; 158:1855–1867.

Joint National Committee on Prevention, Detection, Evaluation, and Treatment of High Blood Pressure: Seventh report of Joint National Committee on Prevention, Detection, Evaluation, and Treatment of High Blood Pressure. JAMA 289:2560–2572, 2003.

National Cholesterol Education Program (NCEP): Executive summary of the third report of the Expert Panel on Detection, Evaluation and Treatment of High Blood Cholesterol in Adults (Adult Treatment Panel III). JAMA 285:2486–2497, 2001.

Smith SC Jr, Blair SN, Bonow RO, et al: Guidelines for preventing heart attack and death in patients with atherosclerotic cardiovascular disease: 2001 update: A statement for healthcare professionals from the AHA/ACC. Circulation 104:1577–1579, 2001.

United States Department of Health and Human Services, Centers for Disease Control and Prevention: Physical Activity and Health: A Report of the Surgeon General. Washington, DC: National Center for Chronic Disease Prevention and Health Promotion; 1996.

United States Department of Health and Human Services, Public Health Services, Agency for Health Care Policy and Research, and the National Heart, Lung and Blood Institute: Guide for smoking cessation specialists. AHCPR Publication No. 96-0693. Rockville, MD; April 1996.

Wenger NK, Froelicher ES, Smith LK, et al: Cardiac Rehabilitation. Clinical Practice Guidelines No. 17. Rockville, MD: US Department of Health and Human Services, Public Health Service, Agency for Health Care Policy and Research, and the National Heart, Lung, and Blood Institute. AHCPR Publication No. 96-0672. October 1995.

INTERNET RESOURCES

The American Association of Cardiovascular and Pulmonary Rehabilitation:
http://www.aacvpr.org

American Heart Association:
http://www.americanheart.org

American Lung Association:
http://www.lungusa.org

Joint Commission on Accreditation of the Healthcare Organizations:
http://www.jcaho.org

Medicare:
http://www.medicare.gov

National Institutes of Health:
http://ww.nih.gov

Preventive Cardiovascular Nurses Association:
http://www.pcna.net

Financial Considerations

SARA J. MCGLYNN

The financial considerations of any organization, including health care entities in hospital and clinical, university, and private settings, are often the driving force behind major decisions. Exercise professionals too often view the bottom line as a necessary evil for which someone else is responsible. Although exercise professionals are primarily concerned with clinical protocols and procedures and the health and welfare of the patients, this would not be possible over the long term without maintaining a positive bottom line. Therefore, successful exercise professionals must understand and incorporate certain financial concepts into their everyday activities and decisions. This chapter discusses these financial concepts.

Terms and Principles

FINANCIAL STATEMENTS AND BUDGETS

Financial management in the health and fitness field is essentially no different from that of any other industry. However, one of the notable differences is the responsibility a publicly held corporation may have to stockholders.

Few companies in the health and fitness industry are publicly held; therefore, they do not have such an obligation. Recently, however, firms such as Bally's Total Fitness and Sports Club Company of Los Angeles have made initial public offerings (IPOs) with limited success[1]. The employees of the organizations that are not publicly held have a responsibility to keep the organizations financially solvent for the well being of the community or the interests of the private owners.

GROSS REVENUE AND NET REVENUE

Although health and fitness organizations and hospital departments generate revenue like other business organizations, the specifics behind the generation of this revenue vary significantly depending on whether the revenue comes from private sources or is received from third-party payers (e.g., insurance companies, Medicare, Medicaid). Health clubs generally rely on payment directly from club members and, thus, operate like other corporate entities in that revenue equals fees charged to members. However, health care facilities, whether independent or affiliated with a hospital organization, are usually dependent on third-party insurance companies for reimbursement for services rendered. It is important to note that insurance companies rarely pay health care organizations the amount charged for services rendered. This lesser amount is usually determined by individual contracts.

Clinical health care organizations have two very distinct revenue numbers. The first is **gross revenue**, which consists of the total of charges for services rendered. The second is **net revenue**, which consists of the total of payments received or expected to be received for services rendered. Net revenue is typically less and often significantly less than gross revenue depending on the payment rates of third-party payers. The difference between gross and net revenue is called the **contractual allowance**. For example, a health care facility may charge $1000 for an exercise stress test, and the insurance company may pay the health care facility $400 for the test. The $1000 is gross revenue, the $400 is net revenue, and the contractual allowance is $600. Health care organizations usually accept payment from insurance companies at contracted amounts as payment in full for services rendered and

---

KEY TERMS

Assets: Resources owned by an organization

Contractual allowance: The difference between gross revenue and net revenue

Fixed costs: Costs that remain the same regardless of volume

Gross revenue: Total charges for services rendered

Liabilities: Obligations of an organization

Net loss: The sum of variable costs and fixed costs exceed net revenue

Net profit: Operating profit minus fixed costs when net revenues exceed variable costs and fixed costs

Net revenue: Total payments received or expected to be received for services rendered

Operating profit: Net revenue minus variable costs

Variable costs: Costs that may change with volume

Working capital: Current assets minus current liabilities

---

cannot bill the patient for additional amounts. Net revenue must be greater than the total expenses for the clinical organization to remain profitable.

NET REVENUE (REIMBURSEMENT) AND CODING

In clinical settings, receiving payment from third-party payers for services rendered is a complex process both for inpatient and outpatient cases. The method of determining payment for services is one of the more significant differences between finances for the clinical health care industry and other industries.

If services such as cardiac rehabilitation, stress testing, or other procedures commonly performed by exercise professionals in a hospital setting are provided to inpatients, the hospital will most often not be paid directly for these services. Medicare and many other insurance companies pay health care organizations for inpatient visits based on the diagnosis of each admission commonly referred to as payment by diagnosis-related groups (DRGs). DRGs were established as part of the Medicare Prospective Payment System established in 1983. Since then, many other insurance companies have adopted this payment methodology. As of 2004, there were 540 DRGs, each of which is assigned a set payment amount. Each inpatient case is assigned to one of these DRGs determined by the diagnosis code (e.g., coronary artery disease) and the primary procedure code (e.g., bypass surgery) assigned to the case (see discussion on ICD-9 codes below). The hospital receives one DRG payment for the entire hospital stay. The number of days spent in the hospital or the number of different services provided during the inpatient stay does not change this payment. The DRG payment methodology transfers financial risk (i.e., the risk that the cost of the patient's hospital stay will be greater than the reimbursement received) to the hospital. The hospital must try to provide the patient with the necessary care while keeping total expenses relating to resource consumption at or below the expected payment from the insurance company.

Other forms of inpatient payment include per diem and capitated plans. Under a per diem payment plan, the hospital is paid a set amount per day of the patient's hospital stay regardless of the resources expended each day. Under capitated insurance plans, the health care organization is paid a set amount per member per month regardless of the number of patients admitted during the month. Both of these types of insurance arrangements also transfer financial risk related to the patient's hospital stay to the hospital.

Although third-party insurance payment methodology is different in an outpatient setting, the majority of the financial risk still lies with the health care provider. In 2000, Medicare established the ambulatory payment classification (APC) system as part of the outpatient prospective payment system. Under this methodology, a case is assigned one or more APCs depending on the CPT-4/HCPCS codes associated with the procedures done. (*HCPCS* is the acronym for the Health Care Financing Administration Common Procedure Coding System. *CPT-4* is the acronym for the *Physician's Current Procedural Terminology*, fourth edition, published by the American Medical Association.)[2] Although a case may be assigned more than one APC, Medicare designated many HCPCS codes as zero payment amounts under the assumption that these procedures are always done in conjunction with other procedures assigned a payment amount. Medicare has also categorized some APCs so that the payment is reduced if they occur in conjunction with other procedures. Crucial to proper payment under the APC system is assignment of the correct HCPCS code to each procedure done. Without an HCPCS code, a procedure cannot be assigned to an APC, and it will not be paid for by Medicare. Also, a case can be assigned more than one APC; however, not all HCPCS codes result in additional APC assignment and payment.

Often, third-party payers pay the health care organization a set fee determined by the third-party payer for the service rendered. Similar to APCs, a fee-for-service methodology is also based on HCPCS. However, unlike the APC methodology, each HCPCS is assigned a payment amount or assigned a "no payment" status. Under a fee-for-service arrangement, HCPCS are not categorized into APCs, and fees are not reduced when performed in conjunction with other HCPCS. Under this type of arrangement, the health care provider is paid a set amount for each service provided regardless of the other services performed at the same time.

Essential to both inpatient and outpatient payment is the assignment of ICD-9-CM diagnosis codes. ICD-9-CM (commonly referred to as ICD-9) is the acronym for *The International Classification of Diseases*, 9th revision, Clinical Modification[3]. The ICD-9 system also includes procedure codes. The ICD-9 diagnosis codes and procedures codes assigned to an inpatient stay determine the DRG under which that the case will be paid. ICD-9 diagnosis codes are also essential for outpatient payment because insurance companies use these codes to determine if the HCPCS codes assigned (as described above) are appropriate for the diagnoses indicated. ICD-9 diagnosis codes are assigned to each procedure on an outpatient visit, unlike an inpatient visit, in which they are assigned to the visit. Preferably, ICD-9 codes for outpatient diagnostic testing originate when the physician orders the test. If the diagnosis is not available at the time the order is placed, a diagnosis determined as a result of the test may be used. If the insurance company determines that the ICD-9 diagnosis code is not an appropriate reason for the test, the claim may be denied for payment. Most insurance companies, including Medicare, do not cover orders that are written to rule out a diagnosis. Instead, the order must state the sign or symptom indicating the reason for the test.

Some insurance companies pay the health care organization for outpatient services on a percentage of charge arrangement often in the range of 50% to 80% of charges. Outpatient services may also be part of a capitated arrangement between the health care organization and the third-party payer. Although these types of arrangements may still require ICD-9 diagnosis codes, the payments are not dependent on the assignment of HCPCS.

Medicare may determine that certain procedures are not "medically necessary" (e.g., preventive care, unapproved diagnoses such as obesity) and, thus, will not reimburse for services. If Medicare subscribers elect to receive services that are not covered by Medicare, the health care provider has the responsibility to properly inform the subscriber of his or her responsibility to pay. Payment for noncovered services provided to Medicare subscribers requires the processing of an advanced beneficiary notice (ABN). In such cases, the patient must be notified in writing using the ABN form that Medicare will not cover the procedure or service and told how much he or she will have to pay out of pocket. This notification must occur before the patient receives the service. If the patient is not notified and the service is rendered, the hospital is not entitled to payment for the procedure and may be at risk of fraudulence.

Although Medicare is a federal program, Medicare contracts with certain insurance companies or other organizations by region of the United States (determined by state or geography) to administer the Medicare program. These contracted organizations are fiscal intermediaries of the Medicare program. Although they must follow Medicare policy, many specifics are left to the discretion of the regional carrier or intermediary. The fiscal intermediaries establish local medical review policies (LMRPs) to manage insurance claims in their respective areas. Thus, something that may be covered in one region or state may not be covered in another region or state. LMRPs are made available by regional carriers or intermediaries to health care professionals and beneficiaries via the Internet or various publications and software products.

A thorough understanding of this complex reimbursement process is necessary to ensure proper payment for services rendered. Most clinical health care facilities have professional medical coders, billers, and revenue teams to facilitate proper billing. However, the clinical staff provides the documentation of procedure performed and often the diagnosis code supporting the procedure. Proper payment is dependent on documentation of information before and during the visit. Without proper documentation and resultant coding, the facility will not receive payment for services rendered.

EXPENSES

The concept of expense in the health care or fitness club setting is the same as it is in other business or personal settings. An expense is incurred when resources are used in the activities of the organization or individual. In the health fitness setting, the most significant expenses usually consist of the salary cost of the staff and the depreciation resulting from the cost of the facility and equipment. Other costs may consist of employee benefits, including FICA (Federal Insurance Contributions), office supplies, rent, telephone, and marketing costs.

Expenses or costs can be designated as **variable costs**, which may change with volume, and **fixed costs**, which remain the same regardless of volume. Some examples of variable costs are staff salaries when staffing levels can be altered based on patient volume, medications, and medical supplies. Some examples of fixed costs are administrative staff salaries (e.g., costs for managers and supervisors), depreciation on the facility and equipment, rent, and insurance. Depreciation is an allocated expense reported to estimate the devaluation of large items such as facility, furniture, and equipment using generally accepted accounting principles, a formal set of rules established by the accounting profession.

Expenses can also be designated as direct or indirect expenses. Direct expenses are those that are incurred and controlled within the department such as staff and department management salaries, towels, drugs and medications, forms, and office supplies. Indirect expenses are those that are incurred on an organization-wide basis or in a department that benefits more than one other department. Some examples of indirect expenses are electricity, water, building repairs, billing costs when performed by a hospital billing department, housekeeping costs when performed by a centralized housekeeping department, and maintenance costs when performed by a centralized maintenance department. Indirect expenses are allocated to the respective departments benefiting from the incurrence of the expense.

NET PROFIT OR LOSS

Net profit or loss is calculated using information from costs (variable and fixed) and revenue as illustrated:

- **Operating profit**: Net revenue minus variable cost
- **Net profit**: Operating profit minus fixed costs when revenue exceeds variable costs and fixed costs
- **Net loss**: Occurs when the sum of variable costs and fixed costs exceed net revenue

BREAK-EVEN POINT

When evaluating a prospective, planned, or existing facility financially, the break-even point occurs when revenue is equal to expenses. In Figure 48-1, the break-even point occurs in year 2. This is also when a net profit results.

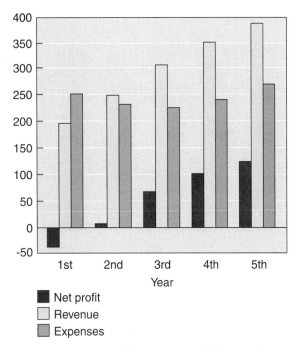

FIGURE 48-1. Sample break-even profitability graph.

TABLE 48-1. Sample Balance Sheet

Assets	Liabilities
Short-term	Short-term
Cash	Accounts payable
Marketable securities	Short-term debt (notes payable)
Accounts receivable	Accruals (taxes due, salaries, wages)
Inventory	
Long-term	Long-term
FF&E, plant	Debt
Less: Depreciation	Preferred stock
Net: FF&E, plant	Equity (owner's equity)
	Stock
	Retained earnings
Total Assets	**Total Liabilities**

FF&E furniture, fixtures, and equipment.

ASSETS, LIABILITIES, AND EQUITY

Assets are the resources owned by the organization. **Liabilities** are financial obligations of the organization. Both assets and liabilities can be short term (expected to be converted to cash within 1 year) or long term. Short-term assets consist of cash, marketable securities (cash equivalent investments or stocks), accounts receivable (billed services awaiting payment), inventory, and prepaid expenses. Long-term assets include furniture, fixtures and equipment, and marketable securities that mature beyond 1 year. Short-term liabilities consist of accounts payable (expenses owed for services/product received), short-term debt (payable within 1 year), and accrued expenses. Long-term liabilities consist of debt payable after 1 year. Assets, liabilities, and equity are presented on the organization's balance sheet (Table 48-1).

REAL ASSETS

Real assets consist of tangible and intangible assets. Tangible assets are such things as furniture, fixtures, equipment, and buildings. Intangibles include technical expertise, trademarks, and patents.

FINANCIAL ASSETS

Financial assets include cash, accounts receivable, and investments in stocks and bonds.

WORKING CAPITAL

Working capital is current assets minus current liabilities. Current assets are assets that are or will be converted to cash within 1 year. Current assets, including cash in checking or savings accounts and accounts receivable, make up a portion of total assets (see Table 48-1). Current liabilities are liabilities that are due within 1 year. Examples of current liabilities are accounts payable, accrued taxes, and accrued salaries.

Working capital is necessary to maintain the day-to-day operations of an organization. In a start-up organization, working capital must be obtained through investors, donations, personal savings, or bank loans to finance a net loss until revenues exceed variable and fixed expenses.

EQUITY

Equity is the difference between assets and liabilities on the balance sheet. In the case of a for profit entity, equity consists of stockholder equity, contributed capital, and retained earnings. In its simplest form, retained earnings are the cumulative results of operations over the existence of the organization. In a not-for-profit entity, equity is called fund balance. Fund balance is not owned by stockholders but is retained by the organization. Equity is measured at historical cost and not market value.

FINANCIAL STATEMENTS

The two financial statements that are the most important to fitness professionals are the balance sheet and the statement of operations (also known as the income statement). The balance sheet is a snapshot at a point in time of the resources (assets), obligations (liabilities), and equity or net worth of an organization. Assets must equal total liabilities plus equity on the balance sheet (see Table 48-1). The income statement or statement of operations is a summary of sales and costs for a specific period of time. Both statements are essential in determining the financial well being of an organization and are prepared retrospectively after revenue has been earned and expenses have been incurred.

BUDGET

A budget is a forecast of revenue and expenditures for a period of time in the future. Budgets are necessary to forecast financial expectations and goals, provide accountability, track progress of actual versus projected results, and allow for justification and scrutiny. Budgets should be prepared well in advance of the fiscal period for which they are being prepared.

Operating Budget

An operating budget is a plan detailing expected revenues and expenses to operate a business. The format of the operating budget should mirror the format of the statement of operations (income statement). Ideally, projected revenue should exceed projected expenses. Start-up facilities may be the exception. Expenses are usually broken down into two categories, operating and fixed. See Table 48-2 for a sample budget. A reliable litmus test against industry norms would be to compare the budget against key financial ratios as determined by industry financial experts (Table 48-3).

Capital Budget

The difference between a capital budget and an operating budget is in its purpose. The capital budget does not mirror any of the financial statements. A capital budget is developed to plan for large-scale purchases such as furniture, fixtures, and equipment and building improvements for 1 year or more. Exercise equipment, renovations, and expansion plans are addressed in this type of budget. Expenses for major facility changes (commonly referred to as project expenses) are detailed in the capital budget as well and should be carefully monitored and implemented. Managers or owners should regularly plan for a portion the organization's profits to be invested in capital expenditures to ensure that facility and equipment are competitive and consistent with industry standards.

Assumptions for the Budget

A critical component of the budget process is the development of assumptions. In this attachment to the budget, an item-by-item (e.g., enrollment fees, payroll increases, cost of uniforms) explanation with supporting calculations is included. Table 48-4 shows an example of assumptions that correspond to line items on the budget.

Although perhaps initially tedious, the process is worth the effort. During budgetary approval, all parties privileged to the justification of the proposed budget are able to make informed decisions. This process is useful for preparing the budget, explaining variances throughout the year, and planning for the next year.

Development, evaluation, revision, and approval of a budget are usually lengthy processes, and adequate time should be allotted (typically 3–4 months before the start of the fiscal year). Before each budget meeting, the director should gather general ledgers, current financial statements, and assumption pages for the current and projected years[4]. Additionally, it is a good strategy to include department supervisors, administrators, and key staff in the budget development process. Incorporating the feedback from others not only provides opportunities for improved budget planning but also increases employee participation and buy-in to the department's overall success.

REVENUE AND EXPENSE MANAGEMENT

Analysis of financial statements should be conducted monthly and should include all staff members involved with budget preparation (see above). Variance reports should be developed to explain deviations from budget and action plans written to outline strategies for avoiding unfavorable variances in upcoming months. The statement of operations typically includes a comparison between actual versus budgeted revenues and expenses, as well as comparisons between current versus prior year activity. Assumptions pages and general ledgers can be used to

TABLE 48-2. Sample Budget

ACSM Fitness Center						
Existing Clients	Monthly	New	Avg Fee	Cancels	Total Clients	Total Revenue
ENROLLMENT PROJECTIONS						
Jan	700	$ 45	50	$ 150	0	750	$ 39,000
Feb	750	$ 45	75	$ 150	22	803	$ 44,010
Mar	803	$ 45	75	$ 150	25	853	$ 46,260
Apr	853	$ 45	65	$ 150	25	893	$ 47,010
May	893	$ 45	55	$ 150	27	921	$ 47,220
June	921	$ 45	50	$ 150	28	943	$ 47,685
July	943	$ 45	50	$ 150	28	965	$ 48,675
Aug	965	$ 45	50	$ 150	29	986	$ 49,620
Sept	986	$ 45	60	$ 150	29	1017	$ 52,065
Oct	1017	$ 45	65	$ 150	31	1051	$ 54,120
Nov	1051	$ 45	70	$ 150	31	1090	$ 56,400
Dec	1090	$ 45	50	$ 150	33	1107	$ 55,065

TOTAL MEMBERSHIP REVENUE: **$ 587,130**

OTHER REVENUE

Smoking cessation	$ 1,200
Massage	$ 16,200
Guest Fees	$ 35,000
1–1 Training	$ 32,400
Weight management	$ 12,000
Pro-shop	$ 1,200
Rest	$ 3,000
Welness programs	$ 1,200
Misc.	$ 10,000
TOTAL OTHER REVENUE	**$ 112,200**
MEMBERSHIP REVENUE	$ 587,130
TOTAL REVENUE	**$ 699,330**

PAYROLL PROJECTIONS

General Manager	$ 35,000
Sales 1	$ 35,000
Administrator	$ 20,000
Fitness Director	$ 26,000
FT Fitness 1	$ 22,000
FT Fitness 2	$ 20,000
PT Fitness	$ 21,840
Receptionist	$ 25,000
Aerobics	$ 18,000
Nutrition	$ 9,500
Cleaning	$ 24,000
Bonus	$ 8,000
TOTAL PAYROLL	**$ 264,340**
TAXES	$ 34,364
BENEFITS	$ 18,240
TOTAL SALARIES	**$ 316,944**

TOTAL OPERATING EXPENSES

Salary, Tax & Benefits	$ 316,944
Marketing	$ 48,000
Maintenance/Repair	
HVAC	$ 1,500
Equipment	$ 2,400
Exterminate	$ 1,200
Other	$ 500
TOTAL MAINTENANCE	$ 5,600
Operating Supplies	
Cleaning	$ 1,200
Locker Rm	$ 3,000
Other	$ 1,500
Towels	$ 2,000
TOTAL SUPPLIES	$ 7,700
Utilities	
Electric	$ 36,000
Gas	$ 4,800
Water	$ 2,000
TOTAL UTILITIES	$ 42,800
Rent	$ 70,705
Other Expenses	
Printing	$ 3,600
Postage	$ 3,000
Travel	$ 2,000
Uniforms	$ 6,000
Programs	$ 500
Office Supp.	$ 600
Telephone	$ 7,200
Misc	$ 1,000
TOTAL OTHER EXPENSES	$ 23,900
Corporate Expenses	
Amort/Dep	$ 24,000
Debt	
Insurance	
Leasing	
Mgmt Fees	
TOTAL CORPORATE	$ 108,400
TOTAL EXPENSES	**$ 624,049**
NET PROFIT/(LOSS)	**$ 75,281**

TABLE 48-3. Key Ratios, 1997–1998

Revenue growth (annual)	9.6%
Payroll (% of gross revenue)	42.0%
Retention (annual)	69.0%
Net membership growth (annual)	8.4%
Revenue/member ($)	$871.00
Sq. ft./member	23
Revenue/sq. ft. ($)	$45.00
Revenue not from dues	27.0%

Adapted with permission from Profiles of Success: Industry Data Survey. Boston, 2000.

explain variances and to generate action points. Clinical personnel should consider working with finance personnel to better understand variances and to develop action plans for avoiding unfavorable variances in the future.

Comparisons of actual financial results with the budget should be used as a guide for evaluating fiscal performance. It is important to note that although budgets are reviewed monthly, understanding activity trends throughout the fiscal year (e.g., seasonal occurrences) may provide a better understanding of the bigger financial picture. Anticipating and planning for monthly shortfalls and surpluses are essential practices for sound budget management. Although not generally popular, making difficult choices (e.g., reducing staffing levels, changing staff mix, restricting educational or travel benefits) to better control expenses may be necessary at times.

Financial statements reflect both revenue- and expense-related problems. Over time, reducing expenses to offset revenue shortfalls may become a serious problem of diminishing returns. Continual expense cutting affects service, customer satisfaction, retention, and ultimately, revenue.

When faced with such a challenge, the sense of urgency to generate revenue cannot be overstated. This is an area with which much time and effort should be concentrated. Referral recruitment and marketing efforts should be planned properly and the results diligently tracked in order to measure effectiveness. New revenue sources

such as Pilates or t'ai chi classes, ballroom or line dancing, spa services, scuba lessons, or group trips (e.g., sporting or theater events) can be developed to fill revenue gaps.

There are many ways to manage expenses, but it is essential to have a thorough understanding of general ledgers, assumptions pages, and operational cost issues. The following are some techniques used by health fitness and clinical professionals to manage financial challenges.

Expense Control

- Review facility and equipment contracts semiannually.
- Review program attendance and consider reducing or eliminating poorly attended programs.
- Conduct cost–benefit evaluations on all programs and complementary services (e.g., laundry, daycare, parking)
- Evaluate equipment repair costs and consider the benefits of new purchases.
- Consider less costly new-hire staff recruitment strategies such as implementing referral incentives for existing staff members, hosting job fairs, or networking with colleges and universities.
- Review job responsibilities and consider changes to job descriptions or job classifications that do not impact the quality of care to maximize use of lesser-compensated employees (e.g., employing undergraduate versus graduate level professionals).
- Restrict use of supplies and equipment (e.g., office and medical supplies, uniforms, postage, long-distance telephone use) and consider limiting staff access to storage areas and systems by implementing code or key access.
- Consider regular review of supply and inventory costs and obtain competitive bids from several vendors, including Internet options.
- Implement a well-organized purchase order system with management authorization.
- Check unit costs regularly. Watch for abrupt increases with regular vendors. Ask for price lists semiannually.

TABLE 48-4. Assumptions for Budget Preparation

Line Item	Assumptions
Revenue	
New enrollment fees	Each new member pays 50% of current months dues plus one full month and an average enrollment fee of $75 each.
Guest fees	Project 10 members/day paying $10/visit 7 days/week for 52 weeks.
Expenses	
Payroll: reception	4 part-time employees, each working 20 hours for $6.00/hr for 52 wk. Each will receive a 5% raise in June.
Uniforms	10 new full uniforms at $50/uniform (jacket, pants, shorts, shirt) three times/year. Staff pays via payroll deduction for seconds.
Insurance	Increased $100/month compared to last year at $1,500/month.

Revenue Control

- Develop meaningful and ongoing relationships with referral sources (e.g., physicians and other health care providers, schools, corporations, present customers).
- Evaluate the cost–benefit of outsourcing services versus providing in house (e.g., publications, Web page management, food and beverages, laundry).
- Consider collaboration on marketing initiatives with local vendors and community agencies.
- When planning for new facility locations, use independent market feasibility analysis. Superior services, equipment, facilities, and staff cannot overcome a poor location[5].

BUSINESS ORGANIZATION

There are various types of business organizations, each with specific defining criteria (e.g., tax status, liability). The major business classifications are defined below.

Sole Proprietorship

Sole proprietorship is a business owned by one individual. This is the simplest, least expensive form of business to start. Often, only a license or registration is required to begin operation. Few government regulations apply, and earnings are subject to personal income tax. The major disadvantages to this type of organization are the difficulty in obtaining significant capital to start or expand such a business and the extensive personal liability for debt.

Partnership

A partnership is a business organization owned by two or more entities. A partnership can be either an informal agreement or a formal written document filed with the state government. Partnerships have limited governmental constraints, and the partners are personally taxed in proportion to their share of ownership. This form of business can consolidate the skills and resources of each partner, but transfer of ownership or the death of a partner may become a complicated process to resolve. Partnership does carry financial liability, including exposure to risk of loss of personal assets if other partners cannot meet obligations.

Corporation

A corporation is a formal establishment and is heavily influenced by laws and regulations. The charter and bylaws govern the operations of a corporation. A corporation is a legal entity that is completely separate from managers and owners. Changes in management and ownership do not affect the charter or bylaws. Corporations can be organized as for-profit or not-for-profit entities. For profit corporations are owned by shareholders. The risk to owners is limited, and a wide variety of investors may be attracted to the business. Transfer of ownership of corporations is less complicated than transfers with partnerships or sole proprietorships. Corporations may also be not-for-profit entities. Not-for-profit corporations do not issue stock or have external ownership. Most not-for-profit corporations are not subject to income taxes. Some fitness facilities and most hospitals are not-for-profit corporations.

Subchapter S Corporation

The subchapter S corporation (S corporation) is a hybrid of a partnership and a corporation. This entity combines the advantages of a sole proprietorship, a partnership, and a corporation without the accompanying disadvantages. There is limited risk and exposure of personal assets, and partners cannot be taxed twice on salary and business income. Partners are free to distribute dividends, avoiding the complexities of a partnership.

Limited Liability Company

A limited liability company (LLC) is another form of business organization that is a hybrid between a partnership and a corporation. One of the main differences between an LLC and an S corporation is the increased flexibility in ownership structure in an LLC.

CAPITAL INVESTMENTS

Capital is money available for new equipment and facility improvements. Funding of capital may come from the facility's financial assets or from external sources. The investor may use a return on investment (ROI) valuation to determine whether the return is worth the investment before making the investment. ROI is determined by dividing the average annual cash flow (e.g., new program income adjusted for non-cash expenses such as depreciation) generated over the life of the project by the initial investment outlay (e.g., purchase of new equipment). ROI is sometimes referred to as a return on assets (ROA). For example, if the average annual cash flow is \$80,000 over 5 years (each respectively at \$50,000, \$60,000, \$70,000, \$100,000, \$120,000) and the initial investment is \$400,000, the ROI is 20% (\$80,000 ÷ \$400,000). Unless the ROI is very near or exceeds what an investor can get in the market, obtaining private or bank financing will be difficult. An investor generally decides on a balance between risk and reward. A high ROI with limited risk or investment is generally preferred. An average ROI of 15% to 20% is considered excellent.

TAXES

A noteworthy trend is the attention the Internal Revenue Service is now paying to tax-exempt organizations. Fitness facilities, similar to other health care organizations, may be organized as either taxable or tax-exempt entities[5]. The primary advantage a tax-exempt entity enjoys is simply in tax savings, which is often significant and carries a competitive advantage over commercial facilities. However, certain restrictions are placed on tax-exempt organizations, including continuing proof of benefit to the community. In addition, these entities should provide services that cannot be found in for-profit settings within the community. Furthermore, organizations labeled as tax exempt must restrict revenue-generating activities unrelated to the organization's primary purpose[6].

PEOPLE

The principles of finance include people because real assets and financial assets alone do not constitute a successful facility. Assets, although tangible, are not brought to life without the cooperation, teamwork, and support of people who must carry out the business. Although there is a fiduciary responsibility to understand and manage the financial aspects of a business, one must not lose sight of the people-driven dynamics of business.

Financial Industry Trends

The fitness industry has many organizations that monitor and support financial performance. The International Health Racquet Sports Association (IHRSA) is well recognized by commercial for-profit facilities. The IHRSA performs and provides analysis of industry trends to clubs. Some of the more significant trends noted by the IHRSA in 2001 include[7]:

- About 53,800,000 people in the United States use health clubs.
- There were 18,203 clubs.
- California, Texas, New York, Florida, and Pennsylvania had the most participants.
- The most commonly offered programs were personal training, fitness evaluation, step or bench aerobics, strength training, child care, yoga, nutritional counseling or classes, weight management, exercise prescription, and massage.
- The largest age group exercising in facilities in 2001 was 35 to 54 years old at 37%; 34% of those exercising in facilities were in the 18- to 34-age group, and 12% were in the 55+ age group.
- Some 24% of revenue came from programming not covered by dues.
- The most profitable clubs had low attrition rates and high revenue–generating participants.
- The average attrition rate was 31%.
- Payroll was 40% of gross revenue.
- Net growth in membership from 2000 to 2001 was 4.3%.
- Revenue per member per year was $598.
- Revenue per square foot was $49, a 9% 4-year growth trend.

Factors That Affect Decisions

Not every decision can or should be made in a purely financial fashion using only budgetary or financial data. Haste in decision making may lead to some of the biggest mistakes. The day-to-day process of dealing with multiple situations, being consumed by multiple priorities, and having days filled with endless interruptions lends credence to the axiom that haste makes waste.

Lack of planning contributes to poor decisions. Little time dedicated to thinking about planning precipitates disregard for planning. With the fiscal tasks required in a health fitness program, including budgeting, financial statement review, program evaluation, staff allocation, market analysis, and community development, planning

cannot be successfully performed without quiet and dedicated time.

Following are three examples of how this quiet time might be used to make important decisions concerning operations that contain financial and non-financial considerations.

- **Decision 1:** Consider transferring patients from a clinical setting to a health club setting for long-term health maintenance. A health club setting is generally lower cost than a clinical setting and will result in better use of clinical staffing. This arrangement can be a win–win situation in that referrals may also be made from the health club to the clinical program for individuals who require clinical care.
- **Decision 2:** Staff positions can be examined for level of contribution and whether hiring or layoff is necessary. Examine staff mix, performance reviews, and scheduling grids to ensure maximum staffing levels. Hire fewer people and expect more from them. Higher pay may be possible to help retain key personnel. Brainstorming can generate ideas that may lead to solutions.
- **Decision 3:** The marketing department may project from competitive market analysis that bicycle spinning classes would create a competitive advantage and attract new members. If the number of new enrollments caused by providing spinning classes exceeds the cost of the bikes, instructors, and other equipment within a short time, the decision is clear. The major variable is the confidence in enrollment projections. However, the capital budget may be reduced by 10%, forcing close scrutiny of spinning over, for example, replacing a chlorinating system for the pool. Space may be at a premium, so a program, although financially beneficial, may not be possible. Formal planned evaluations of programs are necessary to justify the time and money being used. Attendance, cost of materials, and revenue generated should be considered during evaluation of a program.

    Another kink in this spin scenario is that current members may prefer another use for the space. If staff members are not in tune with existing and prospective members' needs, the addition of such classes may be a mistake. (See Chapter 46 for methods of determining program needs.) Also, if retention improves because existing members' needs are met or exceeded by adding space for stretching weight bars, resistance balls, or spinning classes, this additional revenue may be made available for other capital items.

The constant barrage of decisions for a facility is commonplace. It is wise to seek feedback of superiors, subordinates, and members. After all such input is digested, a director sometimes uses his or her instincts to make the right decision.

One must also consider obligations to the community. Hospitals, universities, and health clubs are giving back to the community and educating the public. If the fitness industry is to be a torchbearer for exercise and health, proactive involvement with local charities or business chambers must occur.

Summary

The competition among the various types of rehabilitation and fitness organizations is increasing. Each entity is under scrutiny from constituents. Not-for-profit entities are under continual pressure from declining reimbursement rates, increasing costs, and the demand for high quality service. Shareholders, taxpayers (in some cases), and investors in commercial facilities all demand justification for dollars spent. The pressure to justify costs and enhance financial performance is shared by all types of entities. Business success requires nothing less than an organizational commitment to ensure quality care in a fiscally responsibly manner.

It is no longer sufficient to be the best exercise professional on the floor, to influence morale and productivity of an organization, or to decrease absenteeism and health care costs of participants. The bottom line knows no bias when it comes to facilities and organizations. Success may depend on open-minded, basic financial knowledge and

fear that a poor bottom line may result. Financial considerations have become as important as influencing behavior to increase the exercise habit. The more this is accepted, the better all facets of the organization can be coordinated and directed toward success.

Acknowledgments

The author acknowledges Frank Ancharski, author of Chapter 24 in the 4th edition for his previous contributions.

REFERENCES

1. Caro R, King D, Davis N: Developing an Exit Strategy. San Diego: International Health Racquet Sports Association National Convention; 1996.
2. American Medical Association: CPT 2004. Chicago: AMA Press; 2003.
3. Hart A (Ed.): International classification of diseases, 9th revision, clinical modification. Hopkins, CA: Ingenix St. Anthony, 2004.
4. Weston JF, Copeland TE: Managerial Finance. New York: CBS College; 1986. Profiles of Success: Industry Data Survey. Boston: International Health, Racquet & Sportsclub Association; 2000.
5. Sattler TP, Doniek CA: Trim the extra fat from your facility. Fitness Manage April 1996.
6. McCarthy J: Fund allocation has become critical. Club Bus Int 1990.
7. Coopers, Lybrand: Tax Implications of Hospital Owned Fitness Facilities. Boston: International Health, Racquet & Sportsclub Association; 1996.

SELECTED REFERENCES FOR FURTHER READING

Rosenbloom J: Cardiovascular Coding Reference Guide. Reseda, CA: JR Associates; 2003.
Gapenski LC: Financial Analysis & Decision Making for Healthcare Organizations. New York: McGraw-Hill; 1996.

INTERNET RESOURCES

American Institute of Certified Public Accountants:
http://www. aicpa.org

American Medical Association:
http://www.ama-assn.org

Centers for Medicare & Medicaid Services:
http://www.cms.gov

Healthcare Financial Management Association:
http://www.hfma.org

International Health, Racquet & Sportsclub Association:
http://www.ihrsa.or

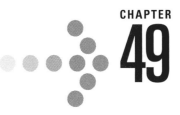

Policies and Procedures for Program Safety and Compliance

SUE BECKHAM AND VALERIE BISHOP

Although there is always risk associated with exercise, research suggests that the benefits outweigh the risks[1]. These risks can, however, be reduced through adherence to guidelines promulgated by organizations such as the Joint Commission on Accreditation of Healthcare Organizations (JCAHO), American Public Health Association, American College of Sports Medicine (ACSM), Commission on Accreditation of Rehabilitation Facilities (CARF), and American Association of Cardiovascular and Pulmonary Rehabilitation (AACVPR). These organizations have or are developing certification procedures or guidelines for facilities and programs that address quality control, staff licensure and certification, appropriateness of care, policies and procedures, and outcome measurement—in essence, everything in the conduct of business. In addition, organizations such as hospitals and hospital-based ambulatory care programs must meet JCAHO accreditation standards to receive reimbursement from federal agencies[2].

The information in this chapter is intended as a template for developing **policies and procedures** specific to safety, clients' rights, staff, information management, client assessment, and program evaluation for clinical and health and fitness programs. Clinical and health and fitness facilities must continually review and redesign their scope of services and policies and procedures in order to comply with updated guidelines and to remain a viable part of the health care service community.

Also, appropriate medical and legal personnel should regularly review the policies and procedures so they may serve as the immediate line of defense for a program in the event of legal claims or lawsuits[3]. In addition, this chapter reviews other aspects often included in policies and procedures, including emergency protocols, prevention of injuries, and contraindicated or high-risk exercises (also see Chapter 28).

Steps for Developing a Policies and Procedures Manual

Before writing policies and procedures for clinical or health and fitness programs, several important steps should be taken. These include development of a vision and mission statement, identification of other similar programs with excellent industry reputations, review of published standards and guidelines, and examination of existing policies and procedures within the organization.

VISION AND MISSION STATEMENTS

All preventive and rehabilitative programs should develop vision and mission statements that define the philosophy and purpose of the program or center. A vision statement is a broad, powerful, forward-looking description of the ideal state that a center may achieve; the mission statement describes how the vision will be accomplished. The major thrust of these statements should be to provide the best possible programs, producing positive outcomes that can be benchmarked against local, regional, and national programs. As with all aspects of a program, the vision and mission statements should be regularly reviewed and rewritten in response to changing circumstances. A copy of the vision and mission statements should be placed in the policies and procedures manual as it defines program direction and goals.

PUBLISHED STANDARD AND GUIDELINES

Collect and review the most recent publications of standards and guidelines promulgated by national

KEY TERMS

Health Insurance Portability and Accountability Act of 1996 (HIPAA): An act that protects the privacy and security of patient records

Policies and procedures: An atlas that includes guidelines for employee conduct and ethics, facility compliance, protection of client privacy, safety and

emergency procedures, operations, patient care, and performance evaluations

Sudden cardiac arrest: A cardiac emergency in which an individual develops an abnormal heart rhythm, preventing the effective pumping of blood

organizations. It is important to understand the distinction between guidelines and standards. A standard is a practice that gives rise to duties for all health and fitness or clinical programs[4]. Standards represent the baseline performance criteria necessary to satisfy facility obligations to provide a relatively safe environment. Guidelines, however, do not give rise to duties of care; rather, they are recommendations designed to enhance facility design and operating procedures that improve the quality of service to clientele. Publications such as ACSM's *Health/Fitness Facility Standards and Guidelines*[4]; *ACSM's Guidelines for Exercise Testing and Prescription*; *Guidelines for Cardiovascular Rehabilitation and Secondary Prevention Programs*[5]; and *Guidelines for Pulmonary Rehabilitation Programs*[6] provide guidelines and standards for health and fitness, cardiopulmonary rehabilitation, and exercise testing facilities. Position statements published by these and other organizations such as the American Heart Association (AHA) also provide recommendations for client screening, staffing, and emergency procedures[7]. There are also federal, state, and local agency documents and standards to which a program or facility may be held accountable.

Policies and procedures for programs and facilities should not fall below local, state, regional, or national standards. When legal liability may be in question, these gold standards have been, and continue to be, used as the baseline for determining the standard of care against which the issue in question will be compared.

ORGANIZATIONAL POLICIES AND PROCEDURES MANUALS

Collect policies and procedures manuals within the parent organization. For example, the policies and procedures manuals generally available in most hospitals are listed in Box 49-1.

Comprehensively review these manuals before attempting to write policies and procedures for programs, facilities, or staff. If a standard or guideline in these manuals or in the state, regional, or national guideline is exactly what will be followed, there is no need for duplication; rather, cite the standard or guideline in the departmental

policy manual. Policies and procedures manuals from other similar programs or facilities that are respected and well managed can also serve as a template for new programs that do not have policies and procedures manuals from a parent organization.

Policies and Procedures for Preventive, Exercise Testing, and Rehabilitative Exercise Programs

When identifying and writing policies and procedures for delivery of preventive, exercise testing, and rehabilitative services, basic standards of care and program implementation guidelines for all staff in operating the facility, dealing with clients, and applying therapy should become standard operating procedure. Hence, policies and procedures should be placed in a central location where all staff members have access to program and facility policies and procedures manuals, as well as state, regional, and national guidelines and standards. This area contains the directional atlas for the facility, programs, and staff. During orientation, new staff members should read the policies and procedures manuals and be trained to apply it. This manual must identify the right thing to do and define how to do it. Leadership must be sure that the staff members follow these procedures. After training has been completed, a competency checklist should be filled out and placed in the personnel file. Many facilities require employees to sign a statement acknowledging that they have read the corporate policies and procedures manuals.

BOX 49-1 | **Common Policy and Procedure Manuals Found in Hospitals**

- Infection control and hazardous waste
- Human resource management
- Emergency preparedness
- Hospital policies and procedures manual
- Standards of nursing practice

LEADERSHIP

Providing excellent services to clients requires effective leadership. Effective leadership is based on planning, designing, and evaluating programs, facility use, staff growth, marketing, and program development. Leadership is responsible for directing, integrating, and coordinating services. Possible types of leadership include a board of directors, a president or vice president, or a medical director. An organizational chart designating lines of authority should be placed at the beginning of the policies and procedures manual.

ENVIRONMENTAL MANAGEMENT AND INJURY PREVENTION

Policies and procedures regarding management of the environment are aimed at providing safe, functional, and effective surroundings for program delivery. The components should include those listed in Box 49-2.

These policies should reflect national, state, and local regulations, and all staff members should be aware of them. Facilities with cardiovascular and resistance equipment need environmental management policies that address equipment maintenance and injury prevention. Many injuries that occur in the fitness setting can be prevented with regular maintenance of equipment, training of personnel, and formal member orientations regarding equipment use, weight room etiquette, and safety policies.

Outlined hereafter are precautions to ensure members' and employees' safety. The *ACSM's Health/Fitness Facility Standards and Guidelines*[4] contains a detailed list of guidelines. The following recommendations for maintenance and safety apply to both preventive and rehabilitative programs:

- Free-weight exercises, such as squats and bench presses, should be performed with a properly trained spotter. Two spotters are recommended for heavily loaded free weight exercises. Racks and Smith machines used for free weight exercises should have appropriate safety features such as adjustable bench and bar heights, safety pins, and levers; members should be required to use these safety features.
- The buddy system is ideal for resistance training. One individual monitors form and biomechanics and provides feedback to the partner. In the event of an emergency, a rapid response is ensured.
- Routine inspection and maintenance of resistance and cardiovascular equipment are necessary to reduce the risk of injury resulting from equipment malfunction. Maintenance should be documented and frequently replaced parts kept in inventory.
- A copy of the manufacturer's recommendations for equipment maintenance should be placed in the policies and procedures manual.
- Facilities should follow the design standards outlined in the Americans with Disabilities Act (http://www.usdoj.gov/crt/ada/adahom1.htm).
- A facility should provide at least 20 to 40 square feet for each piece of exercise equipment[4]. In addition, any electrical cords should be secured to prevent falls.
- Weights and other accessories (pads, attachments, locks, pins, mats, and exercise balls) must be racked or properly stored after use.
- Participants should be oriented to the equipment, including proper lifting technique, controlled speed of movement, adjustments required for proper alignment, appropriate amount of weight, and number of sets and repetitions. Any policies that limit use of cardiovascular equipment should be clearly posted with any required sign-up procedures.
- Weight room etiquette should be shared with clients to facilitate courteous flow through the weight room. Allowing others to rotate in during the rest period, racking weights, and wiping equipment with towels to decrease the risk of transmitting viral or bacterial infections are examples of such courtesy.
- Staff members should clean all pads daily with antifungal and antibacterial agents.
- Equipment should be arranged in a manner consistent with the appropriate order of training.

STAFFING PLAN

The program should have a master staffing plan based on a thorough evaluation of the complexity of client care, delivery of services, information management, fiscal

---

BOX 49-2 | Important Components for Policy and Procedures Related to Environmental Management

- Planning the use of space
- Acquisition and maintenance of equipment and dispersal of resources
- Reduction and control of environmental hazards and risks
- Prevention of accidents and injuries
- Maintenance of safe conditions, including signage in exercise, pool, and spa area
- Provision for emergency response, training, and practice programs
- Training staff for emergencies such as disasters, bomb threats, fires, earthquake, hazardous waste, and power failures
- Climate control
- Smoking policy
- Storage, control, and emergency management of hazardous waste and materials
- Ongoing records and documentation of safety and security management

| BOX 49-3 | **Policy and Procedure Components Related to Staffing** |

- Job descriptions for each position with baseline educational requirements and knowledge. The job description outlines primary responsibilities and required competencies, certifications, and degrees and includes a description of the physical demands and working conditions (e.g., Occupational Safety and Health Administration rules, bloodborne pathogens, lifting, carrying, job classification).
- An orientation process and formal 90-day evaluation period to ensure proper training of new employees
- The annual performance appraisal of employees and a mechanism of remuneration in each employee's file
- Completed competency and skills checklist for each specific job description. Competence must be assessed, maintained, demonstrated, and continually improved. Core skills are defined by each facility and must be assessed annually. The program manager must have a signed competency report for employee files, as required by JCAHO.
- Policies for telephone manners, confidentiality, leave of absence, breaks, and sick days should be clearly defined
- Required staff certifications and licenses; current staff should have copies of credentials on file
- A written grievance policy outlining proper process and specific lines of communication. In addition, documentation of any counseling or termination should be placed in each employee's file.
- Guidelines for employee dress code and appearance
- Policies that address outside work by employees
- Policies regarding part-time and contract employees
- Statement of required continuing education and inservice training. A number of national guidelines require monthly inservice training for emergency education and skill training. Surveying agencies may review documentation of departmental meetings, agendas, inservice training, educational programs, and certifications. The policies and procedures manual should describe what, when, how, and where these should be delivered, evaluated, and recorded.
- Regularly scheduled and documented staff meetings and inservice training with attendance records
- Equal Opportunity Employment statement
- Non-harassment policy
- Clearly delineated staff rights

management (including purchasing, billing, membership sales, insurance precertification, marketing, and financial resource management), and facility maintenance. As with all aspects of a program, the staffing plan should address continual analysis and evaluation of performance within the context of scientific knowledge. The mechanism for continual performance improvement should mirror the plan within the parent organization. In addition, policies and procedures should include a plan for informing staff members of new policies and procedures through e-mail, mail, and signage. Verification should be documented vie e-mail responses or the employee signatures. Policies and procedures manuals should be reviewed regularly to ensure comprehensiveness and accuracy (required every 2 years by the JCAHO) and include the items listed in Box 49-3.

SAFETY AND EMERGENCY PROTOCOLS

All facilities should have written emergency plans for medical complications. These plans should list specific responsibilities of each staff member, emergency equipment, and a predetermined contact for emergency response. Emergency plans, including numbers for emergency medical services, police, building security (if applicable), and the fire department should be posted next to all telephones. First aid kits, first-responder bloodborne pathogen kits, latex gloves, a blood pressure kit with stetho-

scope, an automated external defibrillator (AED)[8] or defibrillator, oxygen, crash cart with medications and supplies, cardiopulmonary resuscitation (CPR) masks, and resuscitation bags as recommended based on the level of the facility as outlined in the ACSM/AHA Joint Position Statement[7] must be readily available and transportable. Defibrillators, AEDs, crash carts (supplies and medication), and first aid kits should be checked daily, and their storage areas should be clearly labeled with appropriate signage.

Regular periodic review of the emergency plan by a medical professional is recommended to ensure that all appropriate steps are outlined. The plan should be practiced with both announced and unannounced drills on a quarterly basis or more often depending on staff turnover. Strategies for coping with potential and common injuries in the exercise, rehabilitation, and exercise testing settings should be rehearsed. During the rehearsal or practice sessions, the supervisor presents a mock emergency, giving the staff information about the victim as the emergency unfolds; drills are practiced until the staff can effectively manage the emergency in a timely manner. Completion of a written report, including an evaluation of the drill and recommendations for any necessary changes, should be done each emergency drill. In addition, daily records documenting the function of emergency equipment such as defibrillators, AEDs, and suction should be maintained. Other daily documentation should include volume checks on oxygen tanks, expiration dates for pharmacologic agents, and inventory of other disposable supplies such as intravenous fluids and equipment, syringes and needles, airway equipment, and first aid supplies.

Emergency plans specific to both minor and major medical incidents are required (see Table 28-1). Minor medical events are not life or limb threatening and can be initially managed within the facility but they may be referred to a medical resource. Major medical emergencies that occur in the non-medical setting require an initial response by the staff followed by immediate transport to a medical facility. Emergency plans vary according to the type and size of facility, staff, location (hospital, physician's office, or fitness center) and local emergency response system. Because a medical emergency may arise at any time and any location, all employees, including secretarial, janitorial, and child care staff, should be certified in CPR and first aid (see Table 28-4 and 28-6).

In clinical and hospital-based programs, standing orders for a variety of emergencies such as hypotension, hypoglycemia, ventricular ectopy, angina, and cardiac arrest should be included in the policies and procedures manual. Many disciplines are involved in the execution of an emergency plan in the clinical setting; each staff member has a specific role to perform during emergency situations. All nursing staff and licensed physical therapists trained in advanced cardiac life support (ACLS) may perform defibrillation/cardioversion (per ACLS protocol and licensing practice acts). The clinical staff, including nurses, exercise physiologists, and physical therapists, should be trained in ACLS (see Table 28-7). There should be at least one (preferably two) licensed and trained ACLS personnel and a physician immediately available when high-risk patients are exercising or participating in graded exercise tests. After an emergency, an accident report should be completed and filed with the appropriate department for review and evaluation. Figures 49-1 and 49-2 provide sample emergency protocols for life-threatening and non–life-threatening emergencies and standing orders for the management of ventricular ectopy, respectively, in a cardiac rehabilitation setting.

Nonclinical settings, such as recreational and fitness facilities without access to a CPR code team, need a set of emergency procedures to manage life-threatening and non–life-threatening events until an emergency team arrives. In this setting, it is important to provide the 911 operator with a brief description of the problem as an advanced life support unit is dispatched in the event of a cardiac event or respiratory arrest. However, in non–life-threatening situations, such as seizures or bodily injury, a basic life support unit is often dispatched. In addition, the facility should have a signed medical release that provides authorization to release the victim's medical history and emergency contacts in the event that the emergency renders the victim unresponsive. Medical histories and other health care information should be kept in a locked file that is accessible to appropriate staff in the event of an emergency. When possible, a senior staff member should assume control of the emergency response, complete an accident report after the emergency, and file the report with the facility's director. The director or senior staff member should follow up with the victim or the victim's family regarding the victim's medical status as permitted by law and as the victim and family are willing to disclose information. Any information provided should be documented in the victim's personal file. Examples of non–life-threatening and life-threatening emergency procedures for a health and fitness facility are presented in Figure 49-3. Additional information about emergency policies and procedures is provided in Chapter 28 and in Appendix B of GETP7.

Given the availability and benefits of AEDs, a more detailed discussion of their role in the chain of survival during sudden cardiac arrest and recommendations regarding their location and utilization is warranted.

Ventricular Ectopy			
Symptomatic?			
Yes	No		
	Drop in blood pressure?		
	Yes	No	
1. Stop activity 2. Sit patient down 3. Check vitals 4. Document signs/symptoms 5. Document rhythm 6. Notify physician 7. Transfer to Emergency Room if not resolved 8. If patient remains symptomatic or becomes unconscious, initiate ACLS emergency procedure as needed for tachycardia and pulseless ventricular tachycardia	Treat as symptomatic		1. Notify physician if new ventricular ectopy 2. Observe closely

FIGURE 49-1. Standing orders for managing ventricular ectopy.

First Staff Member/Responder	Identify self as CPR and/or first-aid certified Determine if the emergency life-threatening or non life-threatening	
	Non life-threatening emergency	**Life-threatening emergency**
Nurse	1. Instruct victim to stop activity 2. Evaluate the victim's status (heart rate, blood pressure, or bodily injury) and determine appropriate emergency response 3. Ask exercise physiologist to get first-aid kit if warranted 4. Remain with victim monitoring heart rate and blood pressure 5. Administer first-aid as needed 6. Complete accident report and follow-up with patient	1. Determine if the victim is responsive 2. Ask a second staff member to call CPR Code and get crash cart 3. Evaluate airway, breathing and circulation 4. If victim has a pulse but not breathing, begin rescue breathing 5. If no pulse, begin CPR until AED/defibrillator arrives 6. If responsive, remain with victim, monitoring regularity, intensity and rate of pulse, blood pressure and signs and symptoms 7. If seizure, clear area of harmful objects and place mat or towel beneath head 8. Monitor heart rhythm and administer defibrillation/cardioversion per ACLS 9. Begin IV line and administer drugs per ACLS 10. Complete accident report and follow-up with patient
Exercise Physiologist	1. Call appropriate emergency number providing information about the patient 2. Retrieve first-aid kit 3. Assist with first-aid as needed 4. Clear the area around the victim, ensure there is a large open pathway for monitoring and EMT if activated.	1. Call CPR Code 2. Retrieve crash cart/AED 3. Get necessary drugs/supplies out of cart 4. Assist with 2-person CPR if required and monitoring of vital signs
Secretary	1. Call security 2. Call patient's family 3. Collect patient's belongings 4. Crowd control	1. Call security 2. Call patient's family 3. Collect patient's belongings 4. Crowd control

FIGURE 49-2. Example emergency plan for hospital-based cardiac rehabilitation program. The exercise physiologist, if trained and appropriately certified, can perform many of the procedures listed as the responsibility of the nurse.

Sudden cardiac arrest, which is caused by factors such as heart disease, rhythm disturbances, and congenital abnormalities, results in 335,000 deaths annually[9]. It is usually caused by an abnormal heart rhythm called ventricular fibrillation and causes the heart to beat in an uncoordinated fashion. Because blood is not effectively being pumped, the pulse and subsequently the breathing stop. If the heart is electrically shocked soon thereafter, normal rhythm may be restored. CPR alone can add only a few minutes to the time available for defibrillation. However, when immediate CPR is provided and defibrillation is performed during the first 3 to 5 minutes, survival rates can be as high as 48% to 70%. For every minute that defibrillation is delayed, there is a 7% to 10% reduction in the chance of survival[9].

An AED is a portable device that identifies heart rhythms amenable to defibrillation, uses audiovisual prompts to direct the correct response, and delivers the appropriate shock. Even children can be trained to operate AEDs safely and effectively[10]. Courses that incorporate AED training into traditional CPR training are available to the public. The Cardiac Arrest Survival Act extends Good Samaritan protection to AED users. The limited number of trial court verdicts on AEDs suggest that organizations adopting AED programs have a lower risk of liability than those who do not. The ACSM and the

AHA's joint position statement on automated external defibrillators in health and fitness facilities makes recommendations for the use and purchase of AEDs in the fitness setting[8]. The position statement recommends that AEDs be placed in health and fitness facilities with more than 2500 members, facilities that offer programs for clinical or elderly populations, and those with an anticipated response time (from cardiac arrest to delivery of the first shock) greater than 5 minutes. In addition, unsupervised facilities are encouraged to purchase AEDs as part of their emergency plans. AEDs should be placed in well-marked, easily accessible locations near telephones. It should take no more than 3 minutes for a responder to retrieve the AED and reach the victim[11]. This guideline and the expense associated with AED purchase will dictate the number of AEDs that should be placed in a facility. AEDs are not recommended for use in children under age 8 years. As more data become available, recommendations for the use of AEDs will be updated, necessitating the revision of policies and procedures for emergencies.

INFORMATION MANAGEMENT

This section of the policies and procedures manuals describes how to manage the storage, transmission, use,

First Staff Member/Responder	Identify self as CPR and/or first-aid certified	
	Determine if the emergency is life-threatening or non life-threatening	
	Non life-threatening emergency	**Life threatening emergency**
First Staff Member/Responder	1. Instruct victim to stop activity 2. Ask permission to assist 3. If given, evaluate the victim's status (heart rate, blood pressure, or bodily injury) and determine if an EMT response is warranted. 4. If EMT response is required, order second staff member to call 911 stating nature of emergency (injury to specific body part, seizure, etc.) and get the first-aid kit 5. Remain with victim monitoring rate, regularity and intensity of heart beat and blood pressure, clear area around victim and administer first-aid as needed 6. Complete accident report and file with senior staff member.	1. Determine if the victim is responsive 2. Ask permission to assist if responsive 3. Order a second staff member to call 911 for EMT giving reason and get the AED 4. Evaluate airway, breathing and circulation 5. If victim has a pulse but not breathing, begin rescue breathing 6. If no pulse, begin CPR until AED arrives 7. If responsive, remain with victim, monitoring regularity, intensity and rate of pulse, blood pressure and signs and symptoms 8. If seizure, clear area of harmful objects and place mat or towel beneath head 9. File report with senior staff member
Second Staff Member/Rescuer	1. Call 911 if needed with following information: phone number of facility, address/location, specific entrance instructions, brief description of type of emergency 2. Retrieve first-aid kit 3. Assist with first-aid as needed 4. Clear the area around the victim, ensure there is a large open pathway for monitoring and EMT if activated	1. Call 911 with the following information: phone number of facility, address/location, specific entrance instructions, brief description of problem – nonresponsive victim, person with chest pain, etc. 2. Retrieve AED 3. Attach pads, clear victim and analyze rhythm to determine if rhythm is shockable and proceed as instructed 4. Assist with 2-person CPR if required
Third Staff Member/Front Desk Person	1. Put elevator on hold (if applicable) 2. Wait at entrance and direct emergency team to victim if summoned 3. Direct crowds away from victim and emergency pathway 4. Retrieve medical information for emergency team or senior staff member if victim is unable to provide (Name, age, medications, medical conditions, and emergency contact numbers (if signed medical release) 5. Secure victim's belongings	1. Put elevator on hold (if applicable) 2. Wait at entrance and direct emergency team to victim 3. Clear area and direct crowds away from pathway to victim 4. Retrieve medical information for emergency team if victim is unconscious (Name, age, medications, medical conditions, and emergency contact numbers (if signed medical release) 5. Secure victim's belongings

FIGURE 49-3. An example emergency plan for a health and fitness facility.

and tracking of information related to operation. Included are policies and procedures with regard to the components listed in Box 49-4.

Policies for information management are usually determined by the parent organization. The **Health Insurance Portability and Accountability Act (HIPAA)** mandated that the Department of Health and Human Services (DHHS) develop high-level security and privacy guidelines and simplify billing procedures for the health care industry[12]. Each hospital organization is required by law to maintain the privacy of patient health information and provide a description of its privacy practices. HIPAA guidelines specific to information management are discussed in more detail in Chapter 50. The information services

department coordinates tracking programs, billing, membership and registration processes, and client records and is responsible for developing organization-wide policies related to client records, data collection, clinical outcomes, and reporting channels while maintaining client confidentiality. Individual services, such as cardiac rehabilitation and preventive services, may write program-specific guidelines unique to the application of those services and consistent with policies of the parent organization.

PERFORMANCE EVALUATION

Program evaluation is crucial to program success in both the clinical and preventive settings. This involves continual

- Clients' records, clients' privacy and confidentiality, storage, and outcome data
- Financial records, analysis, budget allocation, and capital and operational expenses
- Billing for insurance, memberships and value-added services, precertification, and reimbursement
- Provision of charity and scaled remunerative services
- Client registration and procedure scheduling
- Membership and guest enrollment procedures
- Protocol for member pre-activity screening and assessment
- Program outcomes and ongoing progress toward program goals
- Theft report forms

analysis and evaluation of performance within the context of scientific knowledge. In the clinical setting, documentation of patient outcomes is required by accrediting organizations. However, because accreditation is not required for health and fitness programs, outcome evaluation is often undervalued and underutilized in these settings. In addition, program evaluation in the form of direct and indirect monetary (revenue, program referrals, and reductions in employee health care costs) and nonmonetary (participation rates, improvements in employee health) program contributions, especially in the corporate and hospital fitness and wellness settings, can be used to justify continued funding during budget cutbacks. A facility cannot continue to grow, recruit new participants, offer cutting-edge programs, ensure the safety and efficacy of its services, and rise to meet developing market changes without regular objective program evaluation at all levels. Program evaluation should involve both process (determine if the implementation tasks assigned to staff were accomplished) and outcome (program objectives) evaluations and include the items listed in Box 49-5.

BOX 49-5 **Important Issues to Consider in Program Evaluation**

- Evaluation of performance dimensions (e.g., timeliness, effectiveness, continuity, safety, and efficiency)
- Evaluation of clients' satisfaction
- Continued scrutiny of national, regional, and local programs for benchmarking outcomes
- Demonstration of continuing evaluation of performance, outcomes, and processes, both as a whole facility and in individual departments
- Regular review of policies and procedures manuals to ensure comprehensiveness and accuracy

CLIENTS' RIGHTS AND ORGANIZATIONAL ETHICS

Preventive, rehabilitative, and exercise testing programs survive by the volume of clients they serve, either temporarily or through continuing membership. Maintaining client loyalty and satisfaction is an optimum requirement. Every hospital organization should post "The Patient Bill of Rights" within the facility and are required to provide patients with copies of the document. Clients have rights that must be posted within the facility. Clients have the right to:

- Considerate care that safeguards personal dignity
- Respect for cultural, psychosocial, and spiritual values
- Knowledge of the personal responsibility in the care process
- Information about their care plan and the health care professionals delivering those services

Equally important, clients have certain responsibilities and need to assume an active role in their care or wellness programs. Each facility should have a policy outlining which patients are appropriate for which programs. For example, participants may be excluded from a cardiac rehabilitation or fitness or wellness program if any of the following criteria are met:

- Their behavior is inappropriate to the point that it interferes with other participants.
- Personal hygiene is so poor that it affects other program participants and the individual fails to make changes after a one-on-one counseling.
- Physical limitations are present that do not allow the participant to safely participate in appropriate prescribed activity.
- The participant is noncompliant with program rules and guidelines for participant and staff safety.

A staff member should warn a participant that exceeds his or her target heart rate zone or participates in activities that are contraindicated based on his or her medical history. A staff member should review the exercise prescription with the noncompliant participant to ensure he or she understands the prescription. In addition, specific reasons for the warning and possible adverse outcomes should be presented. Finally, if the patient does not comply, he or she should no longer be allowed to participate in the program. In the health and fitness setting, a facility may also exclude an individual from participation to the extent permitted by law if the individual refuses to obtain a recommended medical evaluation or physician recommendation before participation[7]. The facility may instead require the noncompliant member to sign an assumption of risk document. A more detailed discussion of assumption of risk is presented in Chapter 50.

- Cognitive deficits exist that make it impossible for the participant to safely participate in the program.
- A participant falls under the guidelines of clinical contraindications for exercise programming.
- The medical director deems a participant inappropriate for program participation because of health risks or other reasons.

To further assist clients in taking responsibility in their medical care, advanced directives (ADs) should be discussed during clients' orientation sessions. An AD is a document that provides a client the opportunity to give directions about future medical care. There are two types of ADs, Durable Power of Attorney for Health Care and a "living will." A Durable Power of Attorney for Health Care allows persons to name an individual to make health care decisions when they are not able to do so. It is legal in all states but not in Washington, DC. A "living will" is a document that takes effect while the individual is alive and allows the client to state his or her wishes in writing but does not name a patient advocate. This document comes into effect if the client becomes incapacitated. Another type of directive called a Do Not Resuscitate (DNR) order tells hospital personnel that a patient does not wish for any lifesaving resuscitative actions (e.g. defibrillation or ventilator) to save his or her life. DNR orders should be specific, signed by the physician, and reviewed frequently. The medical director and legal department should be consulted regarding the implementation of and adherence to policies and procedures related to clients' rights and confidentiality.

CONFIDENTIALITY OF CLIENTS' RECORDS

In addition to clients' rights, policies and procedures should establish guidelines that ensure the confidentiality and privacy of client records. Record keeping includes informing clients of risks and processes in the provision of evaluation, exercise prescription, and rehabilitation services and receiving informed consent to provide these services. Forms for client consent, assumption of risk, physician's clearance, emergency medical authorization, and release of information should be placed in this section of the policies and procedures manuals, as well as HIPPA patient privacy guidelines. Although HIPAA regulations do not apply to most preventive programs offered by health and fitness facilities, some states have or are con-sidering similar or more stringent regulations than outlined in HIPAA, which may apply to health and fitness programs; thus, state and local legislation regarding confidentiality of client records should also be reviewed and placed in the policies and procedures manuals to ensure compliance at all government levels.

CLIENT ASSESSMENT AND PROVISION OF CARE AND EXERCISE PRESCRIPTION

The standard care plan includes three components of rehabilitation: medical, education, and exercise. The care plan should be individualized to meet the specific needs and goals of each patient as established by the patient or family, the referring physician, and therapists. Figure 49-4 depicts a sample care plan for a cardiac rehabilitation setting. The treatment plan should be discussed with the patient, and he or she should be informed of any treatment not covered by the insurance provider. Provision of comprehensive medical and rehabilitative services to the client occurs only when initial and ongoing assessments are the basis for determining and addressing specific care needs. Client assessment involves the collection of data such as physical and psychosocial status, health history, medications, physical needs, level of independence, diet, occupational activities, activities of daily living, and client goals and preferences. In the health and fitness setting, health history, appropriate pre-activity screening[7], and fitness assessment forms should be included in this section of the policies and procedures manuals.

After completion of the initial client assessment or screening, a rehabilitative care plan or exercise prescription is designed. The objective is to establish a protocol in which the client achieves optimal functioning, self-care and responsibility, independence, and an acceptable quality of life. It is also important to recognize that projected clinical outcomes are based on national norms and scientific data with the objective of reducing future clinical events and minimizing development or exacerbation of chronic illness[5,6]. These protocols are goal based with a maximum length of stay established for each program. However, discharge from the program is necessary after the patient's goals are met. Goals are reviewed every 30 days with the patient, and a progress note should be sent to the referring physician. In addition, a discharge note should be sent to the referring physician upon completion of the program. A rehabilitative care plan and exercise prescription should involve continued reassessment of the client and modification of the exercise program and include the components listed in Box 49-6.

With regard to the health and fitness setting, each client should have documentation of a fitness evaluation (if conducted), an equipment orientation session, and exercise prescription, as outlined above. In addition, confidential records of exercise progression, including any abnormal or unusual responses, should be documented for all personal training clients. All physician referrals and communication with clients' physicians or therapists should also be documented.

CLIENT AND FAMILY EDUCATION

Because education promotes healthy behavior, educational programs are a key function of any wellness, rehabilitative, or preventive center. It is important to establish policies regarding development of and referral to educational programs dealing with risk factors that are common across the chronic and acute disease spectrum,

CARDIAC REHABILITATION
PLAN OF CARE

PATIENT INFORMATION:

Name: _____ Age: _____ DOB: _____ Gender: _____

MD: _____ Phone/Fax #: _____

Surgeon: _____ Phone/Fax #: _____

Patient Phone #: _____

Emergency Contact: _____ Phone #: _____

Start date: _____ Visits approved: _____ Completion date: _____

DIAGNOSIS: (PROCEDURE / DATE)

_____
_____

Date referral received: _____

RISK STRATIFICATION:

__Low __Intermediate __High Explain: _____ Date/initials: _____

Patient presented to Medical Director: Risk level: _____ Date/initials: _____

CARDIAC CATHETERIZATION REPORT: Date: _____

Coronary Arteries of the Heart

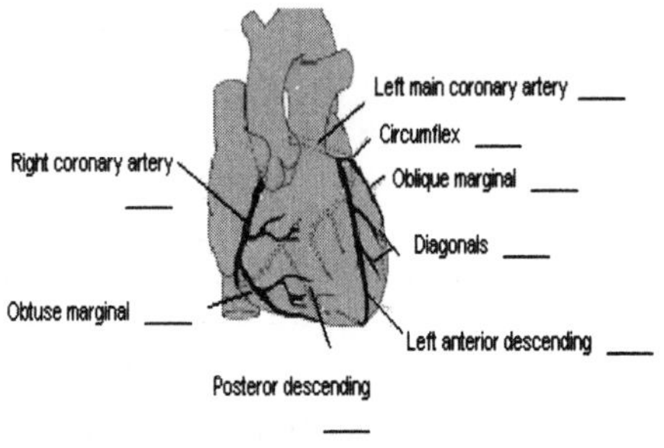

Left main coronary artery ____
Circumflex ____
Oblique marginal ____
Right coronary artery
____
Diagonals ____
Obtuse marginal ____
Left anterior descending ____
Posteror descending
____

CURRENT CARDIOVASCULAR HX
AND PREVIOUS MEDICAL HX:

_____
_____
_____
_____
_____
_____
_____
_____
_____
_____
_____
_____
_____
_____

Ejection fraction:_____

Target heart rate: _____per _____protocol. Date/initials: _____

Other: _____ per _____ Date/initials: _____

Age predicted THR: _____ Date/initials: _____

FIGURE 49-4. Sample plan of care.

CARDIAC RISK FACTORS:

__Age __HTN
__Gender __Smoking
__Family Hx __Sedentary Lifesyle
__DM Type:____ __Obesity
__High Chol/Triglycerides __Stress

NURSING ASSESSMENT:

Heart sounds:
__WNL (S1, S2, no S3, S4, no friction, rub or murmur)
__Other, explain: _____

Lung sounds:
__WNL
__Other, explain: _____

Pedal Edema:
__Yes __No
__Left __Right __Bilaterally
  Pitting? __Yes __No
__1+ __2+ __3+ __4+ Other: _____

Pain assessment (non-anginal):
__No __Yes, related to:_____Pain rated (1-10)_____
Pain education provided: __No __Yes

Incision:
__Yes __No
If yes, explain: _____
_____
_____

Goal: __No pain __Pain managed adequately with medications

RN signature: _____Date: _____

FUNCTIONAL ASSESSMENT / SEDENTARY LIFESTYLE   __N/A

Mobility limitations? __Yes   __No   If yes , explain: _____
Assistive device?   __Yes   __No   If yes, list: _____
Present level of exercise: _____
Occupation: _____
Recreational Activities/Household Chores: _____

Does patient have cardiac / orthopedic or other complications that would contraindicate
resistance training?   __Yes __No

If yes, list: _____

Goal: Patient will exercise within THR for 35 minutes and will have an increase in muscular
strength by 9th to 12th session. Patient will also achieve _____METS (metabolic
equivalent) by end of the program.

ANGINA   __NA

Did patient have angina prior to event? __Yes   __No
If yes, frequency and description of s/s: _____
Does patient have angina currently?   __Yes   __No

Goal: __No s/s of angina   __No s/s of angina with ADL's
    __No s/s of angina with moderate workload (5-7 mets)   __No s/s of angina with heavy
    workload (7-9 mets).
Goal will be achieved throughout program.

FIGURE 49-4. *Continued.*

HYPERTENSION   __N/A

# of yrs DX with hypertension: _____
Average blood pressure reported by patient: _____/_____ mm/Hg   __Does not monitor

Entry Blood Pressures:

Left sitting: _____/_____ mm/Hg Right sitting: _____/_____ mm/Hg

Left standing: _____/_____ mm/Hg Right standing: _____/_____ mm/Hg

Goal: Patient's blood pressure will be WNL at rest and will have a normal blood pressure response during exercise and after exercise. Goal will be achieved throughout program.

HYPERCHOLESTEROLEMIA / ELEVATED TRYGLYCERIDES   __N/A

# of yrs. DX with hyperlipidemia _____
TC: _____   LDL: _____   HDL: _____   TG: _____   Date of test: _____

Goal: Patient will implement a heart healthy diet in order to bring cholesterol levels WNL. Goal will be achieved by end of program.

DIABETES   __NA

# of yrs DX with type ___ diabetes: _____   Is patient currently on insulin? __Yes __No
Does patient monitor blood glucose? __Yes __No If yes, frequency: _____
Average fasting blood glucose: _____mg·dL^{-1}
Average blood glucose throughout day: _____mg·dL^{-1}
Hypoglycemic at BS < _____mg·dL^{-1}, s/s: _____

Goal: Patient's blood glucose will be WNL by 6th to 12th session, will have a normal response after exercise and will exhibit no s/s of hypoglycemia throughout program.

WEIGHT MANAGEMENT / BODY COMPOSITION   __N/A

Current weight: _____lbs.

BMI: _____kg·m^{-2} Waist Circumference: _____cm

Goal: Patient will maintain weight or have a goal body weight of _____lbs.

TOBACCO USE   __N/A

# of years patient has smoked or used tobacco: _____
Amount: _____
Has patient attempted to quit in the past? __Yes __No
Reason unsuccessful: _____
Goal: Patient will have no tobacco use by end of program.

FIGURE 49-4. Continued.

__Single __Married __Divorced __Widowed

Does patient have HX of alcohol/drug abuse __Yes __No

Psychosocial needs identified: _____

Goal: Patient will return to full pre-event family and social roles by end of program.

Level of stress: __Little __Moderate __High
Related to: _____

Does patient practice stress management / relaxation? __Yes __No

Goal: Patient will recognize s/s of stress and modify / reduce stress through stress management techniques. Goal will be accomplished by end of program.

CONGESTIVE HEART FAILURE   __N/A

# of yrs DX: _____

Symptoms: _____

See RN assessment for heart/lung sounds

Goal: Patient will have a decrease in s/s of CHF throughout program.

PRE- HEART TRANSPLANT / POST HEART TRANSPLANT   __N/A

__PRE

Symptoms: _____

Is patient currently on Transplant List? _____ Date: _____

Goal: Patient will have a decrease in s/s throughout program.

__POST

Has patient experienced any s/s of rejection since receiving transplant?   __Yes __ No
If yes, explain_____

Adjusting to transplant? _____ If no, explain: _____

Goal: Patient will be monitored closely for s/s of rejection throughout program and MD will be notified appropriately. Patient will also be able to recognize the s/s of rejection (such as fever, flu-like s/s, sudden change in pulse rate or rhythm, fluid retention, sudden increase in BP, and SOB).

CLAUDICATION__N/A

# of yrs DX: _____

Distance and pace patient able to walk before onset of s/s: _____
Symptoms relieved by: _____

Goal: Patient will be able to progress activity throughout program with no increase in s/s.

FIGURE 49-4. *Continued.*

```
┌─────────────────────────────────────────────────────────────────────────┐
│  KNOWLEDGE DEFICIT ASSESSMENT        __N/A                               │
│                                                                          │
│  Staff assessment of knowledge level:  __Good  __Fair  __Poor           │
│  Barriers to learning: _____ │
│                                                                          │
│  Goal: Patient will attend all appropriate lectures. Knowledge level     │
│  will increase in all pertinent topics.  Goal will be achieved           │
│  throughout program.                                                     │
│                                                                          │
│                                                                          │
│  PATIENT OVERALL GOALS FOR REHAB: _____   │
│  _____  │
│  _____  │
│                                                                          │
│  REHAB PLAN: _____   │
│  _____  │
│  _____  │
│  _____  │
│  _____  │
│  _____  │
│                                                                          │
│  Staff Signature/title: _____ Date: _____    │
└─────────────────────────────────────────────────────────────────────────┘
```

FIGURE 49-4. *Continued.*

such as smoking cessation; stress management; control of hypertension; management of pulmonary disease; relaxation and behavior management; and dietary programs for diabetes, cholesterol, weight loss, and sports nutrition. The goals of the educational programs are listed in Box 49-7.

Policies and procedures establish protocols for the client to become self-directed, participate in the decision-making process, and use experience and problem-solving skills as learning resources. The educational policies should be based on principles of adult education, evaluation of readiness to learn, and principles of lapse and relapse prevention. The intent of educational programs is to improve health outcomes by promoting healthy behavior, involve clients in their care and life decisions, and encourage acceptance of personal responsibility for self-teaching. The educational program should provide materials and knowledge that clients are unable to obtain themselves.

CONTINUUM OF CARE AND SERVICES

Policies describing the integration of all phases of the rehabilitative and preventive care continuum from entry through discharge should be in place. The needs of clients should be matched with appropriate services, appraisals, and programs, including referral to other disciplines as needed. This section should establish the process by which the client is able to move within the rehabilitative or health and fitness system and facility from parking through registration with a minimum of difficulty or excessive time and with a clear understanding of the process. Protocols and forms for ensuring that members

---

BOX 49-6 | Important Considerations Related to Exercise Prescription

- A description of the risk stratification process and assignment of risk status
- A decision concerning monitoring and supervision in light of risk status (e.g., continuous or intermittent electrocardiography, blood pressure, heart rate, signs and symptoms, rating of perceived exertion)
- Exercise prescription methodology, including mode, time, intensity, frequency, and progression
- Risk factor evaluation, goal setting, and expected outcomes
- Vocational retraining
- Discharge planning and follow-up

BOX 49-7 | Goals of Educational Programs

- Change lifestyle to bring about a positive health status.
- Exchange negative for positive health behaviors.
- Reduce risk of chronic and acute disease.
- Develop and use skills for coping with chronic disease.
- Help participants acquire physical skills.
- Optimize health status.
- Optimally function in vocational and recreational activities.

receive services included in their membership such as risk factor modification and fitness assessments, should be delineated in this section of the policies and procedures manuals. In addition, a plan to provide feedback to referring professionals and agencies should be outlined in the policies and procedures manual.

Summary

First and foremost, every clinical, fitness, and recreational facility should have a thorough set of policies and procedures in place to ensure adherence to national standards and guidelines, satisfy accrediting organizations, and provide a safe and effective exercise environment for all participants. Policies and procedures should be reviewed and revised on a regular basis. Employee training and practice of procedures for managing both major and minor medical events should be conducted at orientation and on a regular schedule thereafter to maintain optimal skill levels. An information management plan that ensures client or patient confidentiality, meets HIPAA guidelines, and integrates the required continuum of health care providers and services is crucial. Finally, policies and procedures detailing client or patient rights and responsibilities are necessary to produce optimal treatment and wellness outcomes.

Acknowledgments

The authors would like to acknowledge the contribution of Linda K. Hall, author of Chapter 78 in the previous edition of ACSM's Resource Manual for Guidelines for Exercise Testing and Prescription. Also, the authors would like to thank Jason Dudley for his review and contributions to this chapter and Medical City Hospital, Cardiac Rehabilitation, Dallas, Texas, for the care plan.

SELECTED REFERENCES FOR FURTHER READING

Heggestad J: Cardiac Health and Rehabilitation and Graded Exercise Testing Policies and Procedures Guidelines, 3rd ed. Academy Medical Systems; 2002.

National Strength and Conditioning Association Strength and Conditioning Professional Standards and Guidelines http://www.nsca-lift.org/publication/standards.shtml

Patton RW, Grantham WC, Gerson RF, Gettman LR: Developing and Managing Health/Fitness Facilities. Champaign, IL: Human Kinetics; 1989.

REFERENCES

1. Franklin BA: Exercise and cardiovascular events: A double-edged sword? J Sports Sci 17, 437–442, 1999.
2. Joint Commission on Accreditation of Healthcare Organizations, 1996: Comprehensive Accreditation Manual for Hospitals. Oakbrook Terrace, IL: Joint Commission on Accreditation of Healthcare Organizations; 1995.
3. Herbert DL, Herbert WG: Legal considerations. In Pollock ML, Schmidt DH, eds. Heart Disease and Rehabilitation. Champaign, IL: Human Kinetics; 1995.
4. American College of Sports Medicine: ACSM's Health/Fitness Facility Standards and Guidelines, 2nd ed. Champaign, IL: Human Kinetics; 1997.
5. American Association of Cardiovascular and Pulmonary Rehabilitation: Guidelines for Cardiac Rehabilitation and Secondary Prevention Programs, 4th ed. Champaign, IL: Human Kinetics; 2004.
6. American Association of Cardiovascular and Pulmonary Rehabilitation: Guidelines for Pulmonary Rehabilitation Programs, 3rd ed. Champaign, IL: Human Kinetics, 2004.
7. American College of Sports Medicine and American Heart Association: Joint statement: Recommendations for cardiovascular screening, staffing, and emergency policies at health/fitness facilities. Med Sci Sport Exerc 30:6, 1009–1018, 1998.
8. American College of Sports Medicine and American Heart Association: Automated external defibrillators in health/fitness facilities. Med Sci Sport Exerc 34:561–564, 2002.
9. American Heart Association: Heart disease and stroke statistics—2005 update. Dallas: American Heart Association; 2005.
10. Gundry JW, Comess KA, DeRook FA, et al: Comparison of naïve sixth-grade children with trained professionals in the use of an automated external defibrillator. Circulation 100:1703–1707, 1999.
11. National Center for Early Defibrillation. Available at: http://www.early-defib.org/03_deployment.html
12. U.S. Department of Health & Human Services: Health Insurance Portability and Accountability Act of 1996 (HIPAA) Available at: http://www.hhs.gov/ocr/hipaa

INTERNET RESOURCES

American Association of Cardiovascular and Pulmonary Rehabilitation: http://www.aacvpr.org

American Heart Association: http://www.americanheart.org

Americans with Disabilities Act: http://www.usdoj.gov/crt/ada/adahom1. htm

National Guideline Clearinghouse http://www.guideline.gov

National Strength and Conditioning Association http://www.nsca-lift.org

United States Department of Health & Human Services: Office for Civil Rights—HIPPA: http://www.hhs.gov/ocr/hipaa

50

Legal Considerations

DAVID L. HERBERT AND WILLIAM G. HERBERT

This chapter addresses KSAs from the following content areas:

1 Exercise Physiology and Related Exercise Science
2 Pathophysiology and Risk Factors
3 Health Appraisal, Fitness, and Clinical Exercise Testing
4 Electrocardiography and Diagnostic Techniques
5 Patient Management and Medications
6 Medical and Surgical Management
7 Exercise Prescription and Programming
8 Nutrition and Weight Management
9 Human Behavior and Counseling
10 Safety, Injury Prevention, and Emergency Procedures
11 Program Administration, Quality Assurance, and Outcome Assessment

---

Legal considerations constitute an important matter for those administering fitness evaluations and exercise tests, engaging in physical activity counseling, providing exercise recommendations, and directing fitness programs for apparently healthy adults or individuals with stable chronic diseases. One area of critical concern to exercise leaders, fitness instructors, rehabilitation specialists, and program administrators is the professional–client relationship and the activities performed within the confines of that relationship. Other considerations with special significance when evaluated from a legal perspective include the physical setting and areas in which program activities are conducted, the specific purpose for which exercise services are performed, the equipment used, and the techniques used with the program clients.

The law influences exercise professionals in each of these domains, as well as in others. Furthermore, expectations are substantially affected by the exercise environment—recreational, commercial, or clinical—and by the type of clientele being served. Regardless of the situation, sensitivity to issues of law, adherence to current professional guidelines, and the rigorous application of **risk management** principles may enhance the quality of service and client satisfaction. Moreover, practicing with a risk management perspective may reduce service-related injuries, the likelihood of personal injury litigation, and the extent of damage to the provider in the event of claim and lawsuit.

Laws that affect these matters vary considerably from state to state. Nonetheless, certain legal principles have broad application to pre-exercise screening, exercise testing, exercise program planning, activity supervision, and emergency response considerations. All exercise program personnel should know these principles and endeavor to develop practices aimed at reducing the risks of claims and lawsuits.

In carefully screened and supervised adult populations, the risks of serious cardiovascular accidents in exercise programs are very low. Even for those with some signs of disease who undergo clinical tests, the cardiovascular complication rate appears to be no greater than seven in 10,000 participants, and for aerobic exercise performed by cardiac patients, these rates are less than one in 20,000[1,2]. Recent survey findings indicate that facility readiness, staff training, and practice for serious adverse events in the health and fitness industry are abysmal despite the fact that more and more such facilities accept older clients and those with controlled chronic diseases[3–6]. More than 75% of these facilities reported that they had summoned emergency medical services at least once in 5 years. This suggests a high potential for personal injury lawsuits[3–6]. Until the 1990s, only a small fraction of all personal injury cases resulted in claims against exercise professionals. In recent years, however, there has been a definite increase in exercise-related claims processed through the legal system, especially claims against health and fitness facilities[7,8]. Those dealing with emergency response deficiencies in the industry also appear to be on the increase[9]. Although tort reform proposals may help stem this trend, the future portends an ever-increasing risk of claims and lawsuits for health care professionals generally; exercise professionals are not likely to escape the same problem.

Terminology and Concepts

Generally, legal claims against exercise professionals center on alleged violations of either contract or tort law.

KEY TERMS

Assumption of risk (waiver): An agreement by a client before beginning participation, to give up, relinquish, or waive the participant's rights to legal remedy (damages) in the event of injury, even when such injury arises as a result of provider negligence

Informed consent: A process that entails conveying complete understanding to a client or patient about their option to choose to participate in a procedure, test, service, or program

Negligence: A failure to conform one's conduct to a generally accepted standard or duty

Risk management: A process whereby a service or program is delivered in a manner to fully conform to the most relevant standards of practice and that uses operational strategies to ensure day-to-day fulfillment, optimum achievement of desired client outcomes, and minimize risk of harm or dissatisfaction with clients

These two broad concepts, along with written and statutory laws, define and govern most legal relationships between individuals, including the interrelationship of exercise professionals with clients.

CONTRACT LAW

The law of contracts defines undertakings that may be specified among individuals. A contract is simply a promise or performance bargained for and given in exchange for another promise or performance, all of which is supported by adequate consideration (i.e., something of value).

In examining exercise testing procedures and recommendations for structured physical activity provided to clients, it is important for professionals to understand how the law of contracts affects their relationships with clients. Examples are numerous and include clients receiving physical fitness information; recommendations given on intensity, duration, and modalities for exercise training; or even instructions on techniques for exercise participation. Likewise, the professional may perform exercise testing in exchange for payment or some other consideration of value. This contract relationship also encompasses any related activities that occur before and after exercise testing, such as health screening before testing, as well as first aid and emergency care that arises from or out of provider services. If expectations during this relationship are not fulfilled, a lawsuit for breach of contract may be instituted. Such potential suits allege nonfulfillment of certain promises or a breach of alleged warranties that the law sometimes imposes on many contractual relationships. Apart from the professional–client relationships, contract law also has implications for interprofessional relations, such as those with equipment companies, independent service contractors, and employees.

INFORMED CONSENT

Aside from breach of contract claims arising from a lack of promise fulfillment, claims against exercise professionals can be based on a type of breach of contract for failure to obtain adequate **informed consent** from exercise participants. Although claims based on lack of informed consent, founded upon contract principles, are somewhat archaic today, suits based on such failures are still put forth in some jurisdictions. More frequently today, however, such claims are brought forth in connection with negligence actions rather than breach of contract suits. Before an exercise professional administers a specific exercise procedure with a client, the individual must give informed consent to the procedure. Informed consent is intended to ensure that the client entered into the procedure with full knowledge of the relevant material risks, any alternative procedures that might satisfy certain of the objectives, and the benefits associated with that activity. This consent can be express (written) or implied by law simply as a function of how the two parties to the procedure conducted themselves. To give valid consent to a procedure, the person must be of legal age, not be mentally incapacitated, know and fully understand the importance and relevance of the material risks and benefits, and give consent voluntarily and not under any mistake of fact or duress[10]. Written consent is certainly preferable to any oral or implied form of consent; and of great importance, it expressly demonstrates the process if questions arise later as to whether that was the case.

In many states, adequate information must be provided to ensure that the participant knows and understands the risks and circumstances associated with a procedure before informed consent can be given. In such states, a so-called subjective test is used to determine whether that person understood and comprehended the risks and procedures associated with the matter at hand. Other states have adopted a less rigid rule and provide an objective test to determine consent to a procedure or treatment. Under this test, the determination centers on whether the participant, as a reasonable and ordinary person, understood the facts and circumstances associated with the procedure so as to give voluntary consent. Although some states do not require the use of informed consent for nonsurgical procedures or when a test is performed for non–health care–related purposes, adherence to the process is a desired approach. Examples of informed consent documents for exercise testing and training programs are available elsewhere[10–13].

In lawsuits arising out of the informed consent process, an injured party commonly claims that a professional was negligent in the explanation of the procedure, including the risks, and that the participant would not, if not for the negligence of the professional, have undergone the procedure. These cases are often decided upon the testimony of expert witnesses who determine whether the professional engaged in substandard conduct in securing the informed consent. These cases can involve claims related to contract law, warranties, negligence, and malpractice. Lawsuits arising from alleged deficiencies in the informed consent process related to testing, exercise prescription, or physical activity supervision have become more commonplace. The law is moving toward a broadening requirement for disclosure of risk to participants. Some courts have even gone so far as to require the disclosure of all possible risks, as opposed to those that are simply material[14]. Such a requirement imposes unusual burdens on programs and raises substantial medicolegal concerns[15]. These concerns require individual analysis and response.

One element of the informed consent process relates to confidentiality and disclosure of personal and sensitive information that may be gathered from the client in the course of evaluating his or her health status or delivering services. Provision should be made in the informed consent or other documentation to secure the written authorization to disclose specific test results, exercise progress reports, and so on, to health care professionals who have a need to know, such as a primary care physician. Written authorization may also be secured from clients if there is intent to use data in reporting group statistics for program evaluation or research purposes, even when such information is only to be presented in ways not identifiable with the client. Many states and the federal government have promulgated privacy statutes that may affect the release of personally identifiable material regarding a program participant that requires the creation and adoption of privacy policies as well as consents or authorizations for the disclosure of information.

The new federal privacy law, the Health Information Portability and Accountability Act (HIPAA) became effective in early 2003. The HIPAA law was enacted for several purposes, including the promotion of access for consumers to health insurance, protecting the privacy of health care data, and to standardize and promote efficiency of billing and insurance claims processing in the health care industry. Its provisions for protecting the rights of individual consumers define what providers and others must do to safeguard patients' personal medical and health information. The rule assures patients access to their own health information and, at the same time,

eliminates inappropriate uses. It applies to health care providers, medical claims clearinghouses, and health insurance carriers. Health and fitness and rehabilitative exercise professionals who interact with physicians, nurses, medical technicians, and billing clerks and who access a client's medical records in conjunction with delivery of their services are affected by the HIPAA rule. Just a few of the several important provisions include (a) individual patients or clients must be provided with copies of the HIPAA privacy rule, (b) patients' prior written authorization must be obtained before information disclosure or use by any third party, and (c) the purposes for which the information is to be used and the time limits of the authorization must be provided to the patient or client.

Most states have enacted laws to clarify and complement the HIPAA provisions, and these vary among jurisdictions. There are many examples of information routinely collected and maintained by health and fitness and exercise rehabilitation professionals, the uses and disclosure of which are affected by the HIPAA rule. These include not only data collected in the exercise service setting, such as clinical exercise test results, blood pressure and electrocardiographic records, but also untoward outcome events. With equal certainty, the rule affects the release of information to an exercise professional by health care professionals when the former seeks data needed for safeguarding clients in the process of delivering exercise services (e.g., medical history and laboratory data for preexercise screening or results of clinical exercise tests). The extent to which the HIPAA provisions apply to exercise professionals should be determined through consultation with risk managers and local legal counsel. Nonetheless, all should review and understand the rule, the content of which may be accessed on the Internet at the Health Resources and Services Administration's (USDHHS) website. The HIPAA provisions may be subject to revision or updating, as may the target website reference for related U.S. government information. At the time of this writing, the website containing this information may be found at: http://www.hhs.gov/ocr/hipaa/guidelines/guidanceallsections.pdf. The application of these laws to a program and rights to release information depends on a variety of factors that only individual counsel can properly address.

TORT LAW

A tort is simply a civil wrong. Most tort claims affecting exercise professionals are based on allegations of negligence or malpractice causing personal injury or death.

Negligence

Although **negligence** has no precise definition in law, it is regarded as failure to conform one's conduct to a generally accepted standard or duty. A legal cause of action based on claims of negligence may be established given proof of certain facts, specifically, that one person failed to provide due care to protect another to whom the former owed some duty or responsibility and that such failure proximately caused some injury to the latter person[10]. Thus, the validity of negligence claims is typically established through a specific process that examines certain facts and establishes whether:

- A defendant owed a particular duty or had specific responsibilities to some person who has asserted a claim of negligence
- One or more failures (breaches) occurred in the performance of that duty compared with a particular set of behaviors that were expected (due care, standard of care)
- The injury or damage in question was attributable to an established act or a failure to perform (i.e., a negligent act or omission was the proximate cause of the injury or damage)
- When negligence claims are asserted, the critical question centers on whether an exercise professional provided service in accordance with the so-called standard of care. After a duty is established, the nature and scope of expected performance are usually determined by one or more expert witness' references to published standards and guidelines from peer professional associations. Although standards of care are discussed in a different section of this chapter, ultimately, the most effective shield against claims of negligence may be the daily pattern of delivering services to clients and documenting fulfillment so as to show compliance with the most rigorous published guidelines that are relevant to the established activity.

Malpractice

Malpractice is a specific type of negligence action involving claims against defined professionals. Malpractice actions generally involve claims against professionals who have been provided with the public authority to practice (arising from specific state statutes) for alleged breaches of professional duties and responsibilities toward patients or other persons to whom they owed a particular standard of care or duty[10]. Historically, malpractice claims have been confined to actions against physicians and lawyers. By statute or case law, however, some states have expanded this group to include nurses, physical therapists, dentists, psychologists, and other health professionals. In 1995, Louisiana became the first state to pass legislation to license and regulate exercise practitioners who work under the authority of physicians with patients in cardiopulmonary rehabilitation treatment programs[16,17]. The Louisiana State Board of Medical Examiners now provides regulatory management for this practitioner group. Other states in recent years, such as Maryland, Massachusetts, and California, have also examined legislative proposals with various provisions to publicly regulate health and fitness and clinical exercise professionals, but no statutes have yet been enacted in jurisdictions

beyond Louisiana. To date, no published reports have addressed the effect of this relatively new public regulation on cardiac rehabilitation professionals in Louisiana. The more obvious possibilities of the effect include the level of autonomy in practice, changes in provisions of liability insurance, costs of such insurance, and exposure to claims of malpractice. The advantages and disadvantages of licensure for exercise practitioners have been debated for many years. The issues are complex and involve divergent perspectives from different stakeholders (e.g., those who have the goal of improving quality of service and safety for clients). Imposing added regulatory costs in an era of scarce public resources, intensifying competition with established licensed professions, raising the costs of credentialing and liability insurance for practitioners, and increasing negligence-type claims and suits are byproducts of licensure, and are not in the best interests of the profession. It remains to be seen whether the advent of licensure for exercise physiologists in Louisiana has generally succeeded in areas originally of greatest concern to the advocates.

Defenses to Negligence or Malpractice Actions

The proper conduct of the informed consent process can sometimes be used as defense against legal claims based on either tort or contract principles. In such cases, defense counsel may seek to characterize consent as an **assumption of risks** by the plaintiff. Assumption of risks to a procedure, however, is often difficult to establish without an explicit written statement or clear conduct that demonstrates such an assumption. In addition, an assumption of risks never relieves the exercise professional of the duty to perform in a competent and professional manner. Even when a valid informed consent with assumption of risks is obtained from a client, a spouse, children, or heirs can sometimes independently file suits against the exercise professional for loss of consortium-type claims, even when the participant could not have asserted these claims because of his or her own assumption of risks[18]. In some jurisdictions, it may be advisable or even necessary to obtain consent from a participant, a spouse, and perhaps, in a limited number of states, to make it binding on any children or the executor, administrators, and heirs to an estate. Certainly, such consents should be binding on estates if certain of these negligence and malpractice claims from some such parties are to be successfully avoided[19,20]. Thus, exercise professionals need to secure individual advice from legal counsel and, if applicable, their institutional risk managers to determine the legally sufficient elements of informed consent that must be presented to clients or patients in their settings and the extent to which "loss of consortium" issues should be addressed.

Informed consent often is confused with so-called releases. Releases are statements sometimes written into consent-type documents that contain exculpatory language—that is, wording that relieves the provider of legal responsibility in the event of an injury or death caused by any error, omission, or even negligence. Release documents, sometimes called prospective waivers of responsibility, are disfavored in some states. Moreover, in a medical setting, the use of such releases, with certain limited exceptions, has been declared invalid and against public policy. In non-medical settings, however, particularly with certain ultra-hazardous activities, such as auto racing, skydiving, and even exercise-related activities, the use of such releases may be valid in some jurisdictions, under certain circumstances, if they are properly drafted and used. In fact, when they are well defined and properly written, such documents may have substantial benefit to programs. In recent years, there has been a definite trend toward the increased use of waivers in health and fitness and recreational exercise settings to reduce providers' exposure to damage and loss arising from negligence actions. Improperly developed waivers can fail to protect providers. Consequently, a qualified attorney with a license in the jurisdiction should be consulted to determine their applicability and to prepare these documents. Materials are available to assist in the drafting and application of waivers[21].

Several other defenses to claims of negligence or malpractice are also available. In some states, for example, proof of negligence committed by the participant, referred to in law as contributory negligence, can preclude any recovery of damages from a defendant. In many states, however, this rule has been modified by adoption of a so-called system of comparative negligence. Under this rule, negligence of the injured party is compared with negligence of all defendants in the case. Then, if the negligence of the injured party is found to be less than that of all defendants in the case (or in some states, of any defendant in the case), the plaintiff is allowed to recover, albeit in an amount reduced by the contribution of negligence by the injured party[10].

Liability insurance is an effective mechanism to protect against financial loss in the event of claims and lawsuits. Such insurance policies pay for defense of any covered claims and lawsuits and provide indemnification from any judgment or settlement that is not excluded from the terms of coverage, up to the limits of coverage defined by the provisions of the policy. Proper professional liability insurance, which covers the activities and personnel in question, is readily available through individual purchase or many professional associations as a fee-based option for qualified members[22]. In some cases, these liability policies may include special categories, provisions, and pricing for members who hold special credentials (e.g., certification). The extent of liability policy coverage considered sufficient for a given exercise professional depends on individual judgment, exposure incurred in the delivery of service, and the advice of insurance professionals. This decision on purchase of insurance also should

be affected by whether the professional is self-employed, employed by an organization that extends coverage to the professionals who engage only in services on behalf of the organization, or function in both contexts at the same time.

Standards of Practice

Standards of practice (or care) express how contemporary services should be delivered to give reasonable assurance that desired outcomes will be achieved in a safe manner. In most professions, such standards are developed and periodically revised by consensus among professionals or national associations of providers. Standards documents address what are considered to be benchmark methods, procedures, processes, and protocols that are applied in almost all settings regardless of location, resources, or training of the provider.

In reality, the national standard of practice at any time typically is influenced by a variety of sources, including published statements from professional associations, government policies, state and national government regulations, litigation, and other factors. In recent years, the promulgation of standards for fitness and health care has increased dramatically. These circumstances mandate that professionals stay abreast of new pronouncements and regulations. Without knowledge of the most relevant and current standards and incorporation of these tenets into the operating protocols and records of service fulfillment, individual practitioners become vulnerable to damage and loss in the event of legal challenges arising from personal injury or wrongful death lawsuits.

Consider that in law, proof of negligence consequent to injury of a client (plaintiff) often depends on whether it can be established that there was a clear causal connection between the injury to the client and what the professional did (commission) or failed to do (omission). To establish what should or should not have been done in a given case, courts rely heavily on interpretations of standards from expert witnesses. The use of these standards in certain cases dealing with exercise testing and exercise leadership has already occurred[7].

In recent years, there has been a tendency for certain health care and fitness-related professionals to favor couching their pronouncements on how care should be delivered in the framework of "guidelines," as opposed to "standards" documents. The latter term implies an immutable requirement for practice and implies no flexibility or exceptions in individual applications. A "guideline" should be interpreted to mean a highly recommended method, procedure, or way of providing service that is advocated by leaders of the field or their consensus. The motivation for the "guidelines" approach is that, although it may have clarity and specificity, it is also written to express the importance of individual practitioners' being able to apply sound judgment in how they implement practice parameters for a particular situation or client without incurring increased risk of claim and lawsuit in the event of an untoward outcome. Although a profession-wide shift toward practice parameters that are defined as guidelines or recommendations rather than standards may have a solid rationale from a professional perspective, the extent to which this may add a margin of provider protection in the event of negligence-type lawsuits is difficult to predict. In the past, absence of definitive standards of practice has sometimes increased legal vulnerability for defendants. This has been because of the fact that, in the absence of clear and uniform standards from the profession, the opinions of individual expert witnesses brought by the plaintiff can have increased sway in the legal determination of what care was expected for a particular client who suffered an personal injury in given situation.

Many organizations have published documents that influence the legal standard of care in the health, fitness, exercise, and rehabilitation fields. Some of the most important are those of the American College of Sports Medicine[12,26] (ACSM) [GETP7], American Heart Association (AHA)[23-26], American Association of Cardiovascular and Pulmonary Rehabilitation (AACVPR)[11,13,27], Agency for Health Care Policy and Research, American College of Cardiology, American Medical Association, International Health Racquet & Sportsclub Association, Aerobics and Fitness Association of America, and National Strength and Conditioning Association[28] (also see Internet Resources). Documents from these organizations vary in their scope and applicability. Professionals should carefully examine the services, uses of technologies and procedures, and clientele before deciding which standards and guidelines are most applicable to their own programs or situations.

Published guidelines may be incomplete or not entirely uniform. In the event of injury or death of a participant, such deficits may create confusion rather than define the professional behavior expected in a specific setting. In the area of exercise testing, standards of the ACSM, AACVPR, and AHA are inconsistent with regard to the need for significant involvement of a physician during graded exercise testing[11-13,23-25].

On the matter of exercise prescription, one AHA publication[23] explicitly identifies a nurse as an individual who may "assess physical activity habits, prescribe exercise, and monitor responses in healthy persons and cardiac patients." Another contemporary AHA source[24] acknowledges that exercise by cardiac patients may be appropriately supervised by physicians, nurses, or exercise physiologists, as long as supervisors are trained and their duties are consistent with state statutes governing the practice of medicine and certain other allied health care professions. If deficiencies or disparities in the published guidelines have implications for safety and legal exposure in a particular situation, the development of low-risk protocols and procedures may be a matter of critical importance that requires the advice of local counsel.

Health care professions are in the midst of a movement that will eventually see written standards and guidelines covering nearly every major dimension of care. Fitness and rehabilitation professionals are in similar circumstances and must keep up to date with consensus publications that affect services. To reduce medicolegal risks, it is prudent to adopt the most stringent standards possible. Fulfillment is equally important: practitioners should not only update program operating manuals to verify adoption of current standards but also document day-to-day client records of service delivery to show what was done and how it was done.

In fact, documentation is vital to many aspects of risk management, not just verification of adherence to standards (see Chapter 49). Documentation should include contemporaneous recording of critical response levels that arise in exercise testing or training (e.g., important symptoms, estimations of effort, and activity demand, along with signs suggesting myocardial ischemia or poor ventricular response) and annotations about how these occurrences are referred to appropriate health care providers in a timely way. It also encompasses notations on program incidents, especially care delivered in emergencies (perhaps the most important setting in which to demonstrate, after the fact, what and when the essential steps were performed). Follow-up should always be performed and program records maintained to verify the outcome of the situation whenever emergency and non-emergency incidents occur.

Very recently, the AHA and ACSM released a joint position statement recommending certain basic policies and procedures for pre-exercise screening and emergency readiness in all health and fitness facilities, even in hotels offering only unsupervised access[26]. Every health club and recreational fitness center should evaluate the key features of their organizations and clientele, finding how best to structure written policies, procedures, and fulfillment relative to these important safety functions so as to adhere to this new recommendation[26]. From a risk management point of view, the adequacy of any policy or procedure is a function of its being committed to written form, kept up to date relative to changing professional guidelines, and linked to ongoing evidence of fulfillment[29]. With regard to emergency readiness, fulfillment may be partially shown by keeping dated records of regular emergency drills. Another dimension of documenting fulfillment may be achieved by maintaining records that show the names of staff members who practiced in emergency drills and notations on staff performance and any improvements made in the emergency drills. These formal drills prepare staff members for rapid and effective response when a genuine emergency arises. If a legal challenge should ever occur, this record of fulfillment may be quite helpful in establishing that a particular standard of care was adopted and routinely followed[30].

Forms may also be developed for staff members to use routinely in ensuring standardization in operational areas in which injury or legal risks are considered significant. Examples of these situations include forms for pre-exercise screening and consultation, instruction of new clients in exercise routines, specific cautions for avoidance of injury to clients, and staff inspection of equipment and facilities. Effective forms demonstrate how a facility has linked an important standard to a critical area of service. Use of such forms along with routine annotation of client records shows consistency of fulfillment.

Unauthorized Practice of Medicine and Allied Health Professional Statutes

In recent years, the growing prominence of exercise testing and other health and fitness services increasingly places exercise professionals in collaborative roles with licensed health care providers. This evolution has stimulated a variety of initiatives to clarify roles and responsibilities, promote professionalism, and increase professional opportunities. Competency credentials of the ACSM (e.g., ACSM Exercise Specialist, ACSM Health/Fitness Instructor, and ACSM Registered Clinical Exercise Physiologist) [see Appendix B], the AACVPR's core competency position statement for cardiac rehabilitation specialists, and efforts to establish licensure are illustrations of initiatives that affect the positioning of specialists and greater role delineation[17,27].

Providing exercise services with some degree of independence in collaboration with licensed providers can create legally precarious circumstances for exercise professionals. A prime example of confusion in this area is reflected in questions that often arise about the competency and legal authority needed to provide emergency cardiac care in community- or clinic-based settings for exercising cardiac patients. The standard for emergency response in this situation is clear and universal. It calls for a defibrillator; a crash cart with artificial airways, suction pump, and emergency drugs; and the competency of an onsite provider who can administer the AHA's advanced cardiac life support (ACLS) skills when needed[11,13,25]. This provider, however, must understand that he or she cannot assume such duties unless the physician in charge has given written standing orders to that effect or the individual also has legal authorization under state statutes to accept such standing orders or to otherwise carry out the activity. This is almost never the case for unlicensed exercise professionals who provide exercise services within the health care setting, such as a hospital-based exercise testing or cardiac rehabilitation program, with or without current ACLS training. Thus, there is no legal authority for an exercise professional to evaluate the need for or perform defibrillation on a patient in these circumstances, *unless* he or she has independently completed training and licensure requirements to perform these procedures in the

jurisdiction. Very recent advances in technology and new state and federal statutes are changing public expectations regarding use of automated external defibrillation (AEDs). This evolution may soon alter the standard of care for emergency service in the health and fitness setting[29]. It is expected, because of the ongoing development of published statements from professional organizations[31] and continuing litigation as to AED issues[32], that the use of AEDs is fast reaching the point that it will become the standard of care owed by health and fitness facilities toward their patrons. This time may already have come for facilities with moderate or large memberships that include marketing to older individuals, especially those with significant health risks.

The continuing evolution of health care reform further confuses the roles of health care providers. This may often be problematic for exercise professionals working in diagnostic exercise laboratories or rehabilitation centers. A significant part of this evolution has been aimed at reducing costs by using paraprofessionals in increasingly important clinical roles. In fact, various states have undertaken efforts to expand nursing practice and other provider practice laws beyond mere observation, reporting, and recording of a patient's signs and symptoms. Various physician assistant and similar paraprofessional practice laws provide expanded treatment authority to nonphysicians.

Until health care reform is complete, however, some nonphysicians will continue to be engaged in certain practices that might be characterized as the practice of medicine or some other statutorily defined and controlled allied health profession. In such situations, the unlicensed provider runs the risk of engaging in unauthorized practices that could lead to both criminal and civil sanctions. Many states have defined the practice of medicine broadly so that persons engaged in exercise testing and prescription activities could, under some circumstances, fall within the range of such statutes.

As previously indicated in this chapter, published standards are not always definitive in expressing the roles and responsibilities for exercise professionals, particularly with regard to the delivery of services for clients with documented diseases or even those with no outward signs of disease (e.g., silent myocardial ischemia). Thus, without the presence or assistance of a licensed physician or other allied health professional for certain aspects of the provision of exercise services, claims as to the unauthorized practice of medicine or some other provider practice could be put forth. Under some of these state statutes, such practices are often classified as crimes, usually misdemeanors, punishable by imprisonment for less than 1 year, a fine, or both. In some jurisdictions, felony classification for such offenses has been established with greater potential punishment.

In addition, a person found to have engaged in the unauthorized practice of medicine or some other allied health profession faces (after the fact) the legal expectation that he or she should have provided an elevated standard of care in the event of injury to or death of a participant. Under this rule, the actions of an exercise professional would be compared with the presumed standard of care of a physician or other allied health professional acting under the same or similar circumstances. In the event that the actions do not meet this standard (which the nonphysician or allied health professional cannot meet because of inadequacies of knowledge, skill, authorization, and experience), liability may result.

Tips for Exercise Professionals

Some tips for exercise professionals regarding legal matters include:

1. Know and apply in practice the most rigorous and current peer-developed guidelines applicable to your services, clients, and organization or environment.
2. Maintain credentials relevant to your service (e.g., personal certification or public licensure) and professional liability insurance coverage.
3. Use appropriate informed consent for all services in which such consent is relevant (consult with qualified attorney and risk manager).
4. Instruct clients in techniques of participation and limitations relevant to their health and physical capabilities, observe their related participation, correct problems, and follow up to verify that they manage their own participation safely and effectively.
5. Document fulfillment of your service in a manner consistent with standard of care and your written program policies and procedures.
6. Communicate critical information in a timely way to authorized parties.
7. Rehearse for emergencies.
8. Report incidents and follow up in order to continuously improve emergency readiness and performance.
9. Maintain equipment and inspect facilities on a frequent and regular basis.

Summary

More and more individuals are becoming exposed to organized exercise programs. Exercise professionals and fitness facility operators should note that middle-aged and older adults represent one of the fastest growing segments of their membership. These individuals tend to have more chronic disease risk factors, medical considerations affecting exercise participation, and likely a higher occurrence of undiagnosed diseases than any other group that might enter their programs. Therefore, the actual number of untoward events in exercise programs,

avoidable or otherwise, will inevitably increase. Increased numbers of these occurrences will result in negligence claims that will ultimately find resolution in court. The probabilities of such traumatic actions are low, particularly for individuals and organizations that operate programs in a manner commensurate with accepted professional standards. Awareness of the areas of special legal vulnerability and adoption of legally sensitive practices, however, will keep the risks of litigation low and lead to safer and more efficacious programs. Professionals are advised to keep current concerning developments in this ever-changing medicolegal field[10]. The reference list below includes key resources that may be consulted for further study on this topic[10-12,22].

REFERENCES

1. Rochmis P, Blackburn H: Exercise tests: A survey of procedures, safety and litigation experience in approximately 170,000 tests. JAMA 217:1061, 1971.
2. Foster C, Porcari JP:. The risks of exercise training. J Cardiopulm Rehab 21:347–352, 2001.
3. McInnis KJ, Herbert W, Herbert D, et al: Fitness clubs fail to adhere to AHA emergency standards. Circulation 102(suppl II):394, 2000.
4. McInnis KJ, Hayakawa S, Balady GJ: Cardiovascular screening and emergency procedures at health clubs and fitness centers. Am J Cardiol 80:380, 1997.
5. Herbert DL: Health clubs may not be meeting standards of care. Exerc Stand Malpract Rep 15:12, 2002.
6. American Heart Association: Health clubs not fit for cardiac emergencies [news release]. November 13, 2000.
7. Mathis v. New York Health Club, Inc. 690 N.Y.S.2d 433; 1999.
8. Mandel v. Canyon Ranch, Inc., et al: Superior Court of the State of Arizona, Puma County, Case No.3122777; 1998.
9. Herbert DL: Working out the risks: Inadequate response to emergencies by fitness center employees has led to lawsuits. Widespread use of defibrillators could avert tragedies and reduce claims Best's Review 99, May 2000.
10. Herbert DL, Herbert WG: Legal Aspects of Preventive, Rehabilitative and Recreational Exercise Programs, 4th ed. Canton, OH: PRC Publishing; 2002.
11. American Association for Cardiovascular and Pulmonary Rehabilitation: Guidelines for Pulmonary Rehabilitation Programs, 3rd ed. Champaign, IL: Human Kinetics, 2004.
12. American College of Sports Medicine: ACSM's Health/Fitness Facility Standards & Guidelines, 2nd ed. Champaign, IL: Human Kinetics; 1997.
13. American Association for Cardiovascular and Pulmonary Rehabilitation: Guidelines for Cardiac Rehabilitation and Secondary Prevention Programs, 4th ed. Champaign, IL: Human Kinetics; 2004.
14. Hedgecorth v. United States. 618 F. Supp.627 (E.D. Mo, 1985).
15. Herbert DL: Informed consent documents for stress testing to comport with Hedgecorth v. United States. Exerc Stand Malpract Rep 1:81, 1987.
16. Louisiana licenses clinical exercise physiologists [editorial]! Exerc Stand Malpract Rep 9:56, 1995.
17. Herbert WG: Licensure of clinical exercise physiologists: Impressions concerning the new law in Louisiana. Exerc Stand Malpract Rep 9:65, 1995.
18. Child sues for "loss of consortium." Lawyers Alert 3:249, 1984.
19. Herbert WG, Herbert DL: Exercise testing in adults: Legal and procedural considerations for the physical educator and exercise professionals. JOHPER 46:17, 1975.

20. Koeberle BE: Legal Aspects of Personal Fitness Training. Canton, OH: Professional Reports; 1990:35–38.
21. Cotten D, Cotten MB: Legal Aspects of Waivers in Sport, Recreation, and Fitness Activities. Canton, OH: PRC Publishing; 1997.
22. Eickhoff-Shemek J: Distinguishing "general" and "professional" liability insurance. CSM's Health & Fitness Journal 7:28, 2003.
23. American Heart Association: The AHA medical/scientific statement on exercise. Circulation 86:340, 1992.
24. American Heart Association: The AHA medical/scientific statement on cardiac rehabilitation programs. Circulation 90:1602, 1994.
25. American Heart Association: Guidelines for cardiopulmonary resuscitation and emergency cardiac care. JAMA 268:2171, 1992.
26. Balady GJ, Chaitman B, Driscoll D, et al: American College of Sports Medicine and American Heart Association joint position statement: Recommendations for cardiovascular screening, staffing, and emergency policies at health/fitness facilities. Circulation 97:2283, 1998.
27. American Association for Cardiovascular and Pulmonary Rehabilitation: Core competencies for cardiac rehabilitation specialists. J Cardiopulm Rehabil 14:87, 1994.
28. National Strength and Conditioning Association: Strength and Conditioning Professional Standards and Guidelines; May 2002. Available at: http://www.nsca-lift.org/Publications/Standards.shtml
29. Herbert DL: Standards of care for health and fitness facilities are ever evolving. ACSM's Health and Fitness Journal 4:18, 2000.
30. Herbert DL: Plan to save lives: Create and rehearse an emergency response plan. ACSM's Health and Fitness Journal 1:34, 1997.
31. YMCA of the USA: Automated external defibrillator (AED's). In YMCA's: A technical assistance paper; November 2001 [unpublished document].
32. Herbert DL: Lives, liabilities and lawsuits on the rise: Defibrillators are becoming part of the "standard of care" for recreation facilities. Recreation management 10:January/February, 2003.

SELECTED REFERENCES FOR FURTHER READING

Koeberle BE: Legal Aspects of Personal Fitness Training, 2nd ed. Canton, OH: Professional Reports; 1998.
Herbert DL, Herbert WG: Legal Aspects of Preventative, Rehabilitative, and Recreational Exercise Programs, 4th ed. Canton, OH: PRC Publishing; 2002.

INTERNET RESOURCES

Aerobics and Fitness Association
http://www.afaa.com

Agency for Health Care Policy Research
http://www.ahrq.gov

American Association of Cardiovascular and Pulmonary Rehabilitation
http://www.aacupr.org

American College of Cardiology
http://www.acc.org

American Heart Association
http://www.americanheart.org

American Medical Association
http://www.ama-assn.org

International Health, Racquet and Sportsclub Association
http://www.ihrsa.org

National Strength and Conditioning Association
http://www.nsca-lift.org

Compendium of Physical Activities: An Update of Activity Codes and MET Intensities

BARBARA E. AINSWORTH, WILLIAM L. HASKELL, MELICIA C. WHITT, MELINDA L. IRWIN,
ANN M. SWARTZ, SCOTT J. STRATH, WILLIAM L. O'BRIEN, DAVID R. BASSETT, JR.,
KATHRYN H. SCHMITZ, PATRICIA O. EMPLAINCOURT, DAVID R. JACOBS, JR., and ARTHUR S. LEON

Department of Epidemiology and Biostatistics, Department of Exercise Science, School of Public Health, University of South Carolina, Columbia, SC 29208; Stanford Center for Research in Disease Prevention, School of Medicine, Stanford University, Palo Alto, CA 94304; Division of Kinesiology, School of Kinesiology and Leisure Studies, University of Minnesota, Minneapolis, MN 55454; Division of Epidemiology, School of Public Health, University of Minnesota, Minneapolis, MN 55455; Department of Exercise Science and Sport Management, University of Tennessee, Knoxville, TN 37996; Department of Human Performance, University of Alabama, Tuscaloosa, AL 35487

ABSTRACT

AINSWORTH, B. E,., W. L. HASKELL, M. C. WHITT, M. L. IRWIN, A. M. SWARTZ, S .J. STRATH, W. L. O'BRIEN, D. R. BASSETT, JR., K. H. SCHMITZ, P. O EMPLAINCOURT, D. R. JACOBS, JR., and A. S. LEON. Compendium of physical activities: an update of activity codes and MET intensities. *Med. Sci. Sports Exerc.*, Vol. 32, No. 9, Suppl., pp. S498–S516, 2000. We provide an updated version of the Compendium of Physical Activities, a coding scheme that classifies specific physical activity (PA) by rate of energy expenditure. It was developed to enhance the comparability of results across studies using self-reports of PA. The Compendium coding scheme links a five-digit code that describes physical activities by major headings (e.g., occupation, transportation, etc.) and specific activities within each major heading with its intensity, defined as the ratio of work metabolic rate to a standard resting metabolic rate (MET). Energy expenditure in MET-minutes, MET-hours, kcal, or kcal per kilogram body weight can be estimated for specific activities by type or MET intensity. Additions to the Compendium were obtained from studies describing daily PA patterns of adults and studies measuring the energy cost of specific physical activities in field settings. The updated version includes two new major headings of volunteer and religious activities, extends the number of specific activities from 477 to 605, and provides updated MET intensity levels for selected activities. **Key Words:** EXERCISE, EXERTION, ENERGY EXPENDITURE

The Compendium of Physical Activities was developed to facilitate the coding of physical activities (PAs) obtained from PA records, logs, and surveys and to promote comparison of coded physical activity intensity levels across observational studies (1). The Compendium provides a coding scheme that links a five-digit code, representing the specific activities performed in various settings, with their respective metabolic equivalent (MET) intensity levels. Using the definition for a

MET as the ratio of work metabolic rate to a standard resting metabolic rate of 1.0 $(4.184 \text{ kJ}) \cdot \text{kg}^{-1} \cdot \text{h}^{-1}$, 1 MET is considered a resting metabolic rate obtained during quiet sitting. Activities are listed in the Compendium as multiples of the resting MET level and range from 0.9 (sleeping) to 18 METs (running at 10.9 mph).

We provide an update of the initial Compendium of Physical Activities, developed in 1989 and published in 1993. The updated Compendium reflects additional activities identified by researchers in the past 10 years and presents measured MET intensities for some activities in which METs were estimated from similar activities. The updated Compendium also reflects public

0195-9131/00/3209-0498/0
MEDICINE & SCIENCE IN SPORTS & EXERCISE® Copyright ©
2000 by the International Life Sciences Institute

health interests in evaluating the contributions of various types of physical activity to daily energy expenditure by providing additional categories for activities done during the day.

The initial Compendium has received widespread acceptance among PA specialists in the exercise science and public health fields. For example, in the United States, the coding scheme has been used to identify MET intensities for PAs in the third National Health and Nutrition Examination Survey (6), the 1991 National Health Interview Survey (11), the Paffenbarger College Alumni Study (15), and to evaluate the accuracy of the Minnesota Leisure Time Physical Activity Questionnaire (MN-LTPA) (26). Internationally, the Compendium has been used to identify MET intensities for activities listed in the MONICA Optional Survey of Physical Activity (MOSPA) (12). The coding scheme and MET intensities for activities listed in the Compendium of Physical Activities also have been published as an appendix or abstracted as a chart in several books (18–20,34).

In their landmark 1995 paper that presents the recommendation of the Centers for Disease Control and Prevention (CDC) and the American College of Sports Medicine (ACSM) for adults to accumulate at least 30 min of regular, moderate-intensity physical activity on most days of the week, Pate et al.(23) cite the Compendium as a reference that researchers, clinicians, and practitioners can use to identify examples of moderate intensity physical activities.

The updated Compendium includes two additional major headings and 129 new specific activities. It also provides modifications of 94 codes in the 1993 Compendium, adding or deleting specific activities or providing updated MET levels. The new major headings and most of the specific activities were identified from studies using PA records to identify daily PA habits among adults (2,3) and from personal communications from other investigators who reported activities omitted from the initial Compendium. Updated MET levels were obtained from laboratory and field studies designed to measure the energy cost for specific PAs (4,7–9,16,17,21, 22,24,27–30,32,35,37). We have also clarified the meaning of the letter T followed by three numbers (i.e., T010) as activities and their associated MET levels defined by Dr. Henry Taylor for the MN-LTPA (31). The letter T is now replaced by the words Taylor Code and followed by the MN-LTPA survey item number (e.g., Taylor Code 010). In this paper we present the updated Compendium of Physical Activities (Appendix 1) and recommendations for its implementation to identify PA habits using PA records.

CODING SCHEME

Activity coding. The reader is referred to the 1993 published version of the Compendium (1) for a detailed description of the coding scheme, organization, and methods used to calculate the energy cost of PAs. Briefly, the Compendium is organized to maximize flexibility in coding, data entry, and interpretation of energy cost for each class and type of PA. The coding scheme employs a five-digit code to categorize activities by their major purpose or heading (first two digits), specific activity (last three digits), and intensity (separate two- or three-digit column). For example, the five-digit code, 06100, is defined as follows:

Major Heading	Specific Activity	MET intensity
06	100	5.0
Home Repair	Cleaning Gutters	

Based on the model proposed by Pate et al. (23) for classifying the MET intensity of PAs (light, < 3 METs; moderate, 3–6 METs; vigorous, > 6 METs), the activity code 06100 is classified as moderate intensity.

Major headings. Two additional major headings were added to the updated Compendium of Physical Activities for a total of 21 major types of PAs (Table 1).

The two new categories, religious activities and volunteer activities, were identified from the use of PA records in the Cross-Cultural Activity Participation Study (CAPS) (2). CAPS was an observational study of PA habits among African American, Native American, and Caucasian women, ages 40 yr and older. The new categories include 43 specific activities that are culturally and socially relevant among ethnic minorities and/or older adults. Religious and ceremonial activities play a central role in the lives of many older adults, especially among ethnic minority groups (5). Among retired people and others not employed in occupational settings, volunteer activities also commonly represent an important contribution to daily energy expenditure.

Specific activities. The updated Compendium contains 605 specific activities, including 129 new activities added to the 1993 Compendium. Modifications were also made to 94 PAs listed in the 1993 Compendium, which involved adding or deleting specific activities associated with each code. For example, for the code 08030, lawn and garden activities, the phrase "wheelbarrow chores"

TABLE 1. Major Types of Activities in Version 2 of the Compendium of Physical Activities; New Major Headings are Italicized.

01–Bicycling	07–Inactivity	14–Sexual Activity
02–Conditioning Exercises	08–Lawn and Garden	15–Sports
	09–Miscellaneous	16–Transportation
03–Dancing	10–Music Playing	17–Walking
04–Fishing and Hunting	11–Occupation	18–Water Activities
	12–Running	19–Winter Activities
05–Home Activities	13–Self Care	20–Religious Activities
06–Home Repair		21–Volunteer Activities

Code	METS	Specific Activity	Examples
01009	8.5	bicycling	bicycling, BMX or mountain
01010	4.0	bicycling	bicycling, < 10 mph, leisure, to work or for pleasure (Taylor Code 115)
01015	8.0	bicycling	bicycling, general
01020	6.0	bicycling	bicycling, 10–11.9 mph, leisure, slow, light effort
01030	8.0	bicycling	bicycling, 12–13.9 mph, leisure, moderate effort
01040	10.0	bicycling	bicycling, 14–15.9 mph, racing or leisure, fast, vigorous effort
01050	12.0	bicycling	bicycling, 16–19 mph, racing/not drafting or > 19 mph drafting, very fast, racing general
01060	16.0	bicycling	bicycling, > 20 mph, racing, not drafting
01070	5.0	bicycling	unicycling
02010	7.0	conditioning exercise	bicycling, stationary, general
02011	3.0	conditioning exercise	bicycling, stationary, 50 watts, very light effort
02012	5.5	conditioning exercise	bicycling, stationary, 100 watts, light effort
02013	7.0	conditioning exercise	bicycling, stationary, 150 watts, moderate effort
02014	10.5	conditioning exercise	bicycling, stationary, 200 watts, vigorous effort
02015	12.5	conditioning exercise	bicycling, stationary, 250 watts, very vigorous effort
02020	8.0	conditioning exercise	calisthenics (e.g. pushups, situps, pullups, jumping jacks), heavy, vigorous effort
02030	3.5	conditioning exercise	calisthenics, home exercise, light or moderate effort, general (example: back exercises), going up & down from floor (Taylor Code 150)
02040	8.0	conditioning exercise	circuit training, including some aerobic movement with minimal rest, general
02050	6.0	conditioning exercise	weight lifting (free weight, nautilus or universal-type), power lifting or body building, vigorous effort (Taylor Code 210)
02060	5.5	conditioning exercise	health club exercise, general (Taylor Code 160)
02065	9.0	conditioning exercise	stair-treadmill ergometer, general
02070	7.0	conditioning exercise	rowing, stationary ergometer, general
02071	3.5	conditioning exercise	rowing, stationary, 50 watts, light effort
02072	7.0	conditioning exercise	rowing, stationary, 100 watts, moderate effort
02073	8.5	conditioning exercise	rowing, stationary, 150 watts, vigorous effort
02074	12.0	conditioning exercise	rowing, stationary, 200 watts, very vigorous effort
02080	7.0	conditioning exercise	ski machine, general
02090	6.0	conditioning exercise	slimnastics, jazzercise
02100	2.5	conditioning exercise	stretching, hatha yoga
02101	2.5	conditioning exercise	mild stretching
02110	6.0	conditioning exercise	teaching aerobic exercise class
02120	4.0	conditioning exercise	water aerobics, water calisthenics
02130	3.0	conditioning exercise	weight lifting (free, nautilus or universal-type), light or moderate effort, light workout, general
02135	1.0	conditioning exercise	whirlpool, sitting
03010	4.8	dancing	ballet or modern, twist, jazz, tap, jitterbug
03015	6.5	dancing	aerobic, general
03016	8.5	dancing	aerobic, step, with 6–8 inch step
03017	10.0	dancing	aerobic, step, with 10–12 inch step
03020	5.0	dancing	aerobic, low impact
03021	7.0	dancing	aerobic, high impact
03025	4.5	dancing	general, Greek, Middle Eastern, hula, flamenco, belly, and swing dancing
03030	5.5	dancing	ballroom, dancing fast (Taylor Code 125)
03031	4.5	dancing	ballroom, fast (disco, folk, square), line dancing, Irish step dancing, polka, contra, country
03040	3.0	dancing	ballroom, slow (e.g. waltz, foxtrot, slow dancing), samba, tango, 19th C, mambo, chacha
03050	5.5	dancing	Anishinaabe Jingle Dancing or other traditional American Indian dancing
04001	3.0	fishing and hunting	fishing, general
04010	4.0	fishing and hunting	digging worms, with shovel
04020	4.0	fishing and hunting	fishing from river bank and walking
04030	2.5	fishing and hunting	fishing from boat, sitting
04040	3.5	fishing and hunting	fishing from river bank, standing (Taylor Code 660)
04050	6.0	fishing and hunting	fishing in stream, in waders (Taylor Code 670)
04060	2.0	fishing and hunting	fishing, ice, sitting
04070	2.5	fishing and hunting	hunting, bow and arrow or crossbow
04080	6.0	fishing and hunting	hunting, deer, elk, large game (Taylor Code 170)
04090	2.5	fishing and hunting	hunting, duck, wading
04100	5.0	fishing and hunting	hunting, general
04110	6.0	fishing and hunting	hunting, pheasants or grouse (Taylor Code 680)
04120	5.0	fishing and hunting	hunting, rabbit, squirrel, prairie chick, raccoon, small game (Taylor Code 690)
04130	2.5	fishing and hunting	pistol shooting or trap shooting, standing

Figure A-1. Updated Compendium of Physical Activities.

Code	METS	Specific Activity	Examples
05010	3.3	home activities	carpet sweeping, sweeping floors
05020	3.0	home activities	cleaning, heavy or major (e.g. wash car, wash windows, clean garage), vigorous effort
05021	3.5	home activities	mopping
05025	2.5	home activities	multiple household tasks all at once, light effort
05026	3.5	home activities	multiple household tasks all at once, moderate effort
05027	4.0	home activities	multiple household tasks all at once, vigorous effort
05030	3.0	home activities	cleaning, house or cabin, general
05040	2.5	home activities	cleaning, light (dusting, straightening up, changing linen, carrying out trash)
05041	2.3	home activities	wash dishes - standing or in general (not broken into stand/walk components)
05042	2.5	home activities	wash dishes; clearing dishes from table—walking
05043	3.5	home activities	vacuuming
05045	6.0	home activities	butchering animals
05050	2.0	home activities	cooking or food preparation—standing or sitting or in general (not broken into stand/walk components),manual appliances
05051	2.5	home activities	serving food, setting table—implied walking or standing
05052	2.5	home activities	cooking or food preparation—walking
05053	2.5	home activities	feeding animals
05055	2.5	home activities	putting away groceries (e.g. carrying groceries, shopping without a grocery cart), carrying packages
05056	7.5	home activities	carrying groceries upstairs
05057	3.0	home activities	cooking Indian bread on an outside stove
05060	2.3	home activities	food shopping with or without a grocery cart, standing or walking
05065	2.3	home activities	non-food shopping, standing or walking
05070	2.3	home activities	ironing
05080	1.5	home activities	sitting—knitting, sewing, lt. wrapping (presents)
05090	2.0	home activities	implied standing—laundry, fold or hang clothes, put clothes in washer or dryer, packing suitcase
05095	2.3	home activities	implied walking—putting away clothes, gathering clothes to pack, putting away laundry
05100	2.0	home activities	making bed
05110	5.0	home activities	maple syruping/sugar bushing (including carrying buckets, carrying wood)
05120	6.0	home activities	moving furniture, household items, carrying boxes
05130	3.8	home activities	scrubbing floors, on hands and knees, scrubbing bathroom, bathtub
05140	4.0	home activities	sweeping garage, sidewalk or outside of house
05146	3.5	home activities	standing—packing/unpacking boxes, occasional lifting of household items light—moderate effort
05147	3.0	home activities	implied walking—putting away household items—moderate effort
05148	2.5	home activities	watering plants
05149	2.5	home activities	building a fire inside
05150	9.0	home activities	moving household items upstairs, carrying boxes or furniture
05160	2.0	home activities	standing—light (pump gas, change light bulb, etc.)
05165	3.0	home activities	walking—light, non-cleaning (readying to leave, shut/lock doors, close windows, etc.)
05170	2.5	home activities	sitting—playing with child(ren)–light, only active periods
05171	2.8	home activities	standing—playing with child(ren)–light, only active periods
05175	4.0	home activities	walk/run—playing with child(ren)–moderate, only active periods
05180	5.0	home activities	walk/run—playing with child(ren)–vigorous, only active periods
05181	3.0	home activities	carrying small children
05185	2.5	home activities	child care: sitting/kneeling—dressing, bathing, grooming, feeding, occasional lifting of child-light effort, general
05186	3.0	home activities	child care: standing—dressing, bathing, grooming, feeding, occasional lifting of child-light effort
05187	4.0	home activities	elder care, disabled adult, only active periods
05188	1.5	home activities	reclining with baby
05190	2.5	home activities	sit, playing with animals, light, only active periods
05191	2.8	home activities	stand, playing with animals, light, only active periods
05192	2.8	home activities	walk/run, playing with animals, light, only active periods
05193	4.0	home activities	walk/run, playing with animals, moderate, only active periods
05194	5.0	home activities	walk/run, playing with animals, vigorous, only active periods
05195	3.5	home activities	standing—bathing dog
06010	3.0	home repair	airplane repair
06020	4.0	home repair	automobile body work
06030	3.0	home repair	automobile repair
06040	3.0	home repair	carpentry, general, workshop (Taylor Code 620)
06050	6.0	home repair	carpentry, outside house, installing rain gutters, building a fence, (Taylor Code 640)
06060	4.5	home repair	carpentry, finishing or refinishing cabinets or furniture
06070	7.5	home repair	carpentry, sawing hardwood
06080	5.0	home repair	caulking, chinking log cabin
06090	4.5	home repair	caulking, except log cabin
06100	5.0	home repair	cleaning gutters

Figure A-1. *Continued.*

Code	METS	Specific Activity	Examples
06110	5.0	home repair	excavating garage
06120	5.0	home repair	hanging storm windows
06130	4.5	home repair	laying or removing carpet
06140	4.5	home repair	laying tile or linoleum, repairing appliances
06150	5.0	home repair	painting, outside home (Taylor Code 650)
06160	3.0	home repair	painting, papering, plastering, scraping, inside house, hanging sheet rock, remodeling
06165	4.5	home repair	painting, (Taylor Code 630)
06170	3.0	home repair	put on and removal of tarp - sailboat
06180	6.0	home repair	roofing
06190	4.5	home repair	sanding floors with a power sander
06200	4.5	home repair	scraping and painting sailboat or powerboat
06210	5.0	home repair	spreading dirt with a shovel
06220	4.5	home repair	washing and waxing hull of sailboat, car, powerboat, airplane
06230	4.5	home repair	washing fence, painting fence
06240	3.0	home repair	wiring, plumbing
07010	1.0	inactivity quiet	lying quietly, watching television
07011	1.0	inactivity quiet	lying quietly, doing nothing, lying in bed awake, listening to music (not talking or reading)
07020	1.0	inactivity quiet	sitting quietly and watching television
07021	1.0	inactivity quiet	sitting quietly, sitting smoking, listening to music (not talking or reading), watching a movie in a theater
07030	0.9	inactivity quiet	sleeping
07040	1.2	inactivity quiet	standing quietly (standing in a line)
07050	1.0	inactivity light	reclining—writing
07060	1.0	inactivity light	reclining—talking or talking on phone
07070	1.0	inactivity light	reclining—reading
07075	1.0	inactivity light	meditating
08010	5.0	lawn and garden	carrying, loading or stacking wood, loading/unloading or carrying lumber
08020	6.0	lawn and garden	chopping wood, splitting logs
08030	5.0	lawn and garden	clearing land, hauling branches, wheelbarrow chores
08040	5.0	lawn and garden	digging sandbox
08050	5.0	lawn and garden	digging, spading, filling garden, composting, (Taylor Code 590)
08060	6.0	lawn and garden	gardening with heavy power tools, tilling a garden, chain saw
08080	5.0	lawn and garden	laying crushed rock
08090	5.0	lawn and garden	laying sod
08095	5.5	lawn and garden	mowing lawn, general
08100	2.5	lawn and garden	mowing lawn, riding mower (Taylor Code 550)
08110	6.0	lawn and garden	mowing lawn, walk, hand mower (Taylor Code 570)
08120	5.5	lawn and garden	mowing lawn, walk, power mower
08125	4.5	lawn and garden	mowing lawn, power mower (Taylor Code 590)
08130	4.5	lawn and garden	operating snow blower, walking
08140	4.5	lawn and garden	planting seedlings, shrubs
08150	4.5	lawn and garden	planting trees
08160	4.3	lawn and garden	raking lawn
08165	4.0	lawn and garden	raking lawn (Taylor Code 600)
08170	4.0	lawn and garden	raking roof with snow rake
08180	3.0	lawn and garden	riding snow blower
08190	4.0	lawn and garden	sacking grass, leaves
08200	6.0	lawn and garden	shoveling snow, by hand (Taylor Code 610)
08210	4.5	lawn and garden	trimming shrubs or trees, manual cutter
08215	3.5	lawn and garden	trimming shrubs or trees, power cutter, using leaf blower, edger
08220	2.5	lawn and garden	walking, applying fertilizer or seeding a lawn
08230	1.5	lawn and garden	watering lawn or garden, standing or walking
08240	4.5	lawn and garden	weeding, cultivating garden (Taylor Code 580)
08245	4.0	lawn and garden	gardening, general
08246	3.0	lawn and garden	picking fruit off trees, picking fruits/vegetables, moderate effort
08250	3.0	lawn and garden	implied walking/standing—picking up yard, light, picking flowers or vegetables
08251	3.0	lawn and garden	walking, gathering gardening tools
09010	1.5	miscellaneous	sitting—card playing, playing board games
09020	2.3	miscellaneous	standing—drawing (writing), casino gambling, duplicating machine
09030	1.3	miscellaneous	sitting—reading, book, newspaper, etc.
09040	1.8	miscellaneous	sitting—writing, desk work, typing
09050	1.8	miscellaneous	standing—talking or talking on the phone
09055	1.5	miscellaneous	sitting—talking or talking on the phone
09060	1.8	miscellaneous	sitting—studying, general, including reading and/or writing

Figure A-1. *Continued.*

Code	METS	Specific Activity	Examples
09065	1.8	miscellaneous	sitting—in class, general, including note-taking or class discussion
09070	1.8	miscellaneous	standing—reading
09071	2.0	miscellaneous	standing—miscellaneous
09075	1.5	miscellaneous	sitting—arts and crafts, light effort
09080	2.0	miscellaneous	sitting—arts and crafts, moderate effort
09085	1.8	miscellaneous	standing—arts and crafts, light effort
09090	3.0	miscellaneous	standing—arts and crafts, moderate effort
09095	3.5	miscellaneous	standing—arts and crafts, vigorous effort
09100	1.5	miscellaneous	retreat/family reunion activities involving sitting, relaxing, talking, eating
09105	2.0	miscellaneous	touring/traveling/vacation involving walking and riding
09110	2.5	miscellaneous	camping involving standing, walking, sitting, light-to-moderate effort
09115	1.5	miscellaneous	sitting at a sporting event, spectator
10010	1.8	music playing	accordion
10020	2.0	music playing	cello
10030	2.5	music playing	conducting
10040	4.0	music playing	drums
10050	2.0	music playing	flute (sitting)
10060	2.0	music playing	horn
10070	2.5	music playing	piano or organ
10080	3.5	music playing	trombone
10090	2.5	music playing	trumpet
10100	2.5	music playing	violin
10110	2.0	music playing	woodwind
10120	2.0	music playing	guitar, classical, folk (sitting)
10125	3.0	music playing	guitar, rock and roll band (standing)
10130	4.0	music playing	marching band, playing an instrument, baton twirling (walking)
10135	3.5	music playing	marching band, drum major (walking)
11010	4.0	occupation	bakery, general, moderate effort
11015	2.5	occupation	bakery, light effort
11020	2.3	occupation	bookbinding
11030	6.0	occupation	building road (including hauling debris, driving heavy machinery)
11035	2.0	occupation	building road, directing traffic (standing)
11040	3.5	occupation	carpentry, general
11050	8.0	occupation	carrying heavy loads, such as bricks
11060	8.0	occupation	carrying moderate loads up stairs, moving boxes (16–40 pounds)
11070	2.5	occupation	chambermaid, making bed (nursing)
11080	6.5	occupation	coal mining, drilling coal, rock
11090	6.5	occupation	coal mining, erecting supports
11100	6.0	occupation	coal mining, general
11110	7.0	occupation	coal mining, shoveling coal
11120	5.5	occupation	construction, outside, remodeling
11121	3.0	occupation	custodial work—buffing the floor with electric buffer
11122	2.5	occupation	custodial work—cleaning sink and toilet, light effort
11123	2.5	occupation	custodial work—dusting, light effort
11124	4.0	occupation	custodial work—feathering arena floor, moderate effort
11125	3.5	occupation	custodial work—general cleaning, moderate effort
11126	3.5	occupation	custodial work—mopping, moderate effort
11127	3.0	occupation	custodial work—take out trash, moderate effort
11128	2.5	occupation	custodial work—vacuuming, light effort
11129	3.0	occupation	custodial work—vacuuming, moderate effort
11130	3.5	occupation	electrical work, plumbing
11140	8.0	occupation	farming, baling hay, cleaning barn, poultry work, vigorous effort
11150	3.5	occupation	farming, chasing cattle, non-strenuous (walking), moderate effort
11151	4.0	occupation	farming, chasing cattle or other livestock on horseback, moderate effort
11152	2.0	occupation	farming, chasing cattle or other livestock, driving, light effort
11160	2.5	occupation	farming, driving harvester, cutting hay, irrigation work
11170	2.5	occupation	farming, driving tractor
11180	4.0	occupation	farming, feeding small animals
11190	4.5	occupation	farming, feeding cattle, horses
11191	4.5	occupation	farming, hauling water for animals, general hauling water
11192	6.0	occupation	farming, taking care of animals (grooming, brushing, shearing sheep, assisting with birthing, medical care, branding)
11200	8.0	occupation	farming, forking straw bales, cleaning corral or barn, vigorous effort
11210	3.0	occupation	farming, milking by hand, moderate effort

Figure A-1. *Continued.*

Code	METS	Specific Activity	Examples
11220	1.5	occupation	farming, milking by machine, light effort
11230	5.5	occupation	farming, shoveling grain, moderate effort
11240	12.0	occupation	fire fighter, general
11245	11.0	occupation	fire fighter, climbing ladder with full gear
11246	8.0	occupation	fire fighter, hauling hoses on ground
11250	17.0	occupation	forestry, ax chopping, fast
11260	5.0	occupation	forestry, ax chopping, slow
11270	7.0	occupation	forestry, barking trees
11280	11.0	occupation	forestry, carrying logs
11290	8.0	occupation	forestry, felling trees
11300	8.0	occupation	forestry, general
11310	5.0	occupation	forestry, hoeing
11320	6.0	occupation	forestry, planting by hand
11330	7.0	occupation	forestry, sawing by hand
11340	4.5	occupation	forestry, sawing, power
11350	9.0	occupation	forestry, trimming trees
11360	4.0	occupation	forestry, weeding
11370	4.5	occupation	furriery
11380	6.0	occupation	horse grooming
11390	8.0	occupation	horse racing, galloping
11400	6.5	occupation	horse racing, trotting
11410	2.6	occupation	horse racing, walking
11420	3.5	occupation	locksmith
11430	2.5	occupation	machine tooling, machining, working sheet metal
11440	3.0	occupation	machine tooling, operating lathe
11450	5.0	occupation	machine tooling, operating punch press
11460	4.0	occupation	machine tooling, tapping and drilling
11470	3.0	occupation	machine tooling, welding
11480	7.0	occupation	masonry, concrete
11485	4.0	occupation	masseur, masseuse (standing)
11490	7.5	occupation	moving, pushing heavy objects, 75 lbs or more (desks, moving van work)
11495	12.0	occupation	skindiving or SCUBA diving as a frogman (Navy Seal)
11500	2.5	occupation	operating heavy duty equipment/automated, not driving
11510	4.5	occupation	orange grove work
11520	2.3	occupation	printing (standing)
11525	2.5	occupation	police, directing traffic (standing)
11526	2.0	occupation	police, driving a squad car (sitting)
11527	1.3	occupation	police, riding in a squad car (sitting)
11528	4.0	occupation	police, making an arrest (standing)
11530	2.5	occupation	shoe repair, general
11540	8.5	occupation	shoveling, digging ditches
11550	9.0	occupation	shoveling, heavy (more than 16 pounds/minute)
11560	6.0	occupation	shoveling, light (less than 10 pounds/minute)
11570	7.0	occupation	shoveling, moderate (10 to 15 pounds/minute)
11580	1.5	occupation	sitting—light office work, general (chemistry lab work, light use of hand tools, watch repair or micro-assembly, light assembly/repair), sitting, reading, driving at work
11585	1.5	occupation	sitting meetings, general, and/or with talking involved, eatting at a business meeting
11590	2.5	occupation	sitting; moderate (heavy levers, riding mower/forklift, crane operation), teaching stretching or yoga
11600	2.3	occupation	standing; light (bartending, store clerk, assembling, filing, duplicating, putting up a Christmas tree), standing and talking at work, changing clothes when teaching physical education
11610	3.0	occupation	standing; light/moderate (assemble/repair heavy parts, welding, stocking, auto repair, pack boxes for moving, etc.), patient care (as in nursing)
11615	4.0	occupation	lifting items continuously, 10–20 lbs, with limited walking or resting
11620	3.5	occupation	standing; moderate (assembling at fast rate, intermittent, lifting 50 lbs, hitch/twisting ropes)
11630	4.0	occupation	standing; moderate/heavy (lifting more than 50 lbs, masonry, painting, paper hanging)
11640	5.0	occupation	steel mill, fettling
11650	5.5	occupation	steel mill, forging
11660	8.0	occupation	steel mill, hand rolling
11670	8.0	occupation	steel mill, merchant mill rolling
11680	11.0	occupation	steel mill, removing slag
11690	7.5	occupation	steel mill, tending furnace
11700	5.5	occupation	steel mill, tipping molds
11710	8.0	occupation	steel mill, working in general
11720	2.5	occupation	tailoring, cutting

Figure A-1. *Continued.*

Code	METS	Specific Activity	Examples
11730	2.5	occupation	tailoring, general
11740	2.0	occupation	tailoring, hand sewing
11750	2.5	occupation	tailoring, machine sewing
11760	4.0	occupation	tailoring, pressing
11765	3.5	occupation	tailoring, weaving
11766	6.5	occupation	truck driving, loading and unloading truck (standing)
11770	1.5	occupation	typing, electric, manual or computer
11780	6.0	occupation	using heavy power tools such as pneumatic tools (jackhammers, drills, etc.)
11790	8.0	occupation	using heavy tools (not power) such as shovel, pick, tunnel bar, spade
11791	2.0	occupation	walking on job, less than 2.0 mph (in office or lab area), very slow
11792	3.3	occupation	walking on job, 3.0 mph, in office, moderate speed, not carrying anything
11793	3.8	occupation	walking on job, 3.5 mph, in office, brisk speed, not carrying anything
11795	3.0	occupation	walking, 2.5 mph, slowly and carrying light objects less than 25 pounds
11796	3.0	occupation	walking, gathering things at work, ready to leave
11800	4.0	occupation	walking, 3.0 mph, moderately and carrying light objects less than 25 lbs
11805	4.0	occupation	walking, pushing a wheelchair
11810	4.5	occupation	walking, 3.5 mph, briskly and carrying objects less than 25 pounds
11820	5.0	occupation	walking or walk downstairs or standing, carrying objects about 25 to 49 pounds
11830	6.5	occupation	walking or walk downstairs or standing, carrying objects about 50 to 74 pounds
11840	7.5	occupation	walking or walk downstairs or standing, carrying objects about 75 to 99 pounds
11850	8.5	occupation	walking or walk downstairs or standing, carrying objects about 100 pounds or over
11870	3.0	occupation	working in scene shop, theater actor, backstage employee
11875	4.0	occupation	teach physical education, exercise, sports classes (non-sport play)
11876	6.5	occupation	teach physical education, exercise, sports classes (participate in the class)
12010	6.0	running	jog/walk combination (jogging component of less than 10 minutes) (Taylor Code 180)
12020	7.0	running	jogging, general
12025	8.0	running	jogging, in place
12027	4.5	running	jogging on a mini-tramp
12030	8.0	running	running, 5 mph (12 min/mile)
12040	9.0	running	running, 5.2 mph (11.5 min/mile)
12050	10.0	running	running, 6 mph (10 min/mile)
12060	11.0	running	running, 6.7 mph (9 min/mile)
12070	11.5	running	running, 7 mph (8.5 min/mile)
12080	12.5	running	running, 7.5 mph (8 min/mile)
12090	13.5	running	running, 8 mph (7.5 min/mile)
12100	14.0	running	running, 8.6 mph (7 min/mile)
12110	15.0	running	running, 9 mph (6.5 min/mile)
12120	16.0	running	running, 10 mph (6 min/mile)
12130	18.0	running	running, 10.9 mph (5.5 min/mile)
12140	9.0	running	running, cross country
12150	8.0	running	running (Taylor Code 200)
12170	15.0	running	running, stairs, up
12180	10.0	running	running, on a track, team practice
12190	8.0	running	running, training, pushing a wheelchair
13000	2.0	self care	standing—getting ready for bed, in general
13009	1.0	self care	sitting on toilet
13010	1.5	self care	bathing (sitting)
13020	2.0	self care	dressing, undressing (standing or sitting)
13030	1.5	self care	eating (sitting)
13035	2.0	self care	talking and eating or eating only (standing)
13036	1.0	self care	taking medication, sitting or standing
13040	2.0	self care	grooming (washing, shaving, brushing teeth, urinating, washing hands, putting on make-up), sitting or standing
13045	2.5	self care	hairstyling
13046	1.0	self care	having hair or nails done by someone else, sitting
13050	2.0	self care	showering, toweling off (standing)
14010	1.5	sexual activity	active, vigorous effort
14020	1.3	sexual activity	general, moderate effort
14030	1.0	sexual activity	passive, light effort, kissing, hugging
15010	3.5	sports	archery (non-hunting)
15020	7.0	sports	badminton, competitive (Taylor Code 450)
15030	4.5	sports	badminton, social singles and doubles, general
15040	8.0	sports	basketball, game (Taylor Code 490)
15050	6.0	sports	basketball, non-game, general (Taylor Code 480)

Figure A-1. *Continued.*

Code	METS	Specific Activity	Examples
15060	7.0	sports	basketball, officiating (Taylor Code 500)
15070	4.5	sports	basketball, shooting baskets
15075	6.5	sports	basketball, wheelchair
15080	2.5	sports	billiards
15090	3.0	sports	bowling (Taylor Code 390)
15100	12.0	sports	boxing, in ring, general
15110	6.0	sports	boxing, punching bag
15120	9.0	sports	boxing, sparring
15130	7.0	sports	broomball
15135	5.0	sports	children's games (hopscotch, 4-square, dodge ball, playground apparatus, t-ball, tetherball, marbles, jacks, acrace games)
15140	4.0	sports	coaching: football, soccer, basketball, baseball, swimming, etc.
15150	5.0	sports	cricket (batting, bowling)
15160	2.5	sports	croquet
15170	4.0	sports	curling
15180	2.5	sports	darts, wall or lawn
15190	6.0	sports	drag racing, pushing or driving a car
15200	6.0	sports	fencing
15210	9.0	sports	football, competitive
15230	8.0	sports	football, touch, flag, general (Taylor Code 510)
15235	2.5	sports	football or baseball, playing catch
15240	3.0	sports	frisbee playing, general
15250	8.0	sports	frisbee, ultimate
15255	4.5	sports	golf, general
15265	4.5	sports	golf, walking and carrying clubs (See footnote at end of the Compendium)
15270	3.0	sports	golf, miniature, driving range
15285	4.3	sports	golf, walking and pulling clubs (See footnote at end of the Compendium)
15290	3.5	sports	golf, using power cart (Taylor Code 070)
15300	4.0	sports	gymnastics, general
15310	4.0	sports	hacky sack
15320	12.0	sports	handball, general (Taylor Code 520)
15330	8.0	sports	handball, team
15340	3.5	sports	hand gliding
15350	8.0	sports	hockey, field
15360	8.0	sports	hockey, ice
15370	4.0	sports	horseback riding, general
15380	3.5	sports	horseback riding, saddling horse, grooming horse
15390	6.5	sports	horseback riding, trotting
15400	2.5	sports	horseback riding, walking
15410	3.0	sports	horseshoe pitching, quoits
15420	12.0	sports	jai alai
15430	10.0	sports	judo, jujitsu, karate, kick boxing, tae kwan do
15440	4.0	sports	juggling
15450	7.0	sports	kickball
15460	8.0	sports	lacrosse
15470	4.0	sports	motor-cross
15480	9.0	sports	orienteering
15490	10.0	sports	paddleball, competitive
15500	6.0	sports	paddleball, casual, general (Taylor Code 460)
15510	8.0	sports	polo
15520	10.0	sports	racquetball, competitive
15530	7.0	sports	racquetball, casual, general (Taylor Code 470)
15535	11.0	sports	rock climbing, ascending rock
15540	8.0	sports	rock climbing, rappelling
15550	12.0	sports	rope jumping, fast
15551	10.0	sports	rope jumping, moderate, general
15552	8.0	sports	rope jumping, slow
15560	10.0	sports	rugby
15570	3.0	sports	shuffleboard, lawn bowling
15580	5.0	sports	skateboarding
15590	7.0	sports	skating, roller (Taylor Code 360)
15591	12.0	sports	roller blading (in-line skating)
15600	3.5	sports	sky diving
15605	10.0	sports	soccer, competitive

Figure A-1. *Continued.*

Code	METS	Specific Activity	Examples
15610	7.0	sports	soccer, casual, general (Taylor Code 540)
15620	5.0	sports	softball or baseball, fast or slow pitch, general (Taylor Code 440)
15630	4.0	sports	softball, officiating
15640	6.0	sports	softball, pitching
15650	12.0	sports	squash (Taylor Code 530)
15660	4.0	sports	table tennis, ping pong (Taylor Code 410)
15670	4.0	sports	tai chi
15675	7.0	sports	tennis, general
15680	6.0	sports	tennis, doubles (Taylor Code 430)
15685	5.0	sports	tennis, doubles
15690	8.0	sports	tennis, singles (Taylor Code 420)
15700	3.5	sports	trampoline
15710	4.0	sports	volleyball (Taylor Code 400)
15711	8.0	sports	volleyball, competitive, in gymnasium
15720	3.0	sports	volleyball, non-competitive, 6–9 member team, general
15725	8.0	sports	volleyball, beach
15730	6.0	sports	wrestling (one match = 5 minutes)
15731	7.0	sports	wallyball, general
15732	4.0	sports	track and field (shot, discus, hammer throw)
15733	6.0	sports	track and field (high jump, long jump, triple jump, javelin, pole vault)
15734	10.0	sports	track and field (steeplechase, hurdles)
16010	2.0	transportation	automobile or light truck (not a semi) driving
16015	1.0	transportation	riding in a car or truck
16016	1.0	transportation	riding in a bus
16020	2.0	transportation	flying airplane
16030	2.5	transportation	motor scooter, motorcycle
16040	6.0	transportation	pushing plane in and out of hangar
16050	3.0	transportation	driving heavy truck, tractor, bus
17010	7.0	walking	backpacking (Taylor Code 050)
17020	3.5	walking	carrying infant or 15 pound load (e.g. suitcase), level ground or downstairs
17025	9.0	walking	carrying load upstairs, general
17026	5.0	walking	carrying 1 to 15 lb load, upstairs
17027	6.0	walking	carrying 16 to 24 lb load, upstairs
17028	8.0	walking	carrying 25 to 49 lb load, upstairs
17029	10.0	walking	carrying 50 to 74 lb load, upstairs
17030	12.0	walking	carrying 74+ lb load, upstairs
17031	3.0	walking	loading/unloading a car
17035	7.0	walking	climbing hills with 0 to 9 pound load
17040	7.5	walking	climbing hills with 10 to 20 pound load
17050	8.0	walking	climbing hills with 21 to 42 pound load
17060	9.0	walking	climbing hills with 42+ pound load
17070	3.0	walking	downstairs
17080	6.0	walking	hiking, cross country (Taylor Code 040)
17085	2.5	walking	bird watching
17090	6.5	walking	marching, rapidly, military
17100	2.5	walking	pushing or pulling stroller with child or walking with children
17105	4.0	walking	pushing a wheelchair, non-occupational setting
17110	6.5	walking	race walking
17120	8.0	walking	rock or mountain climbing (Taylor Code 060)
17130	8.0	walking	up stairs, using or climbing up ladder (Taylor Code 030)
17140	5.0	walking	using crutches
17150	2.0	walking	walking, household walking
17151	2.0	walking	walking, less than 2.0 mph, level ground, strolling, very slow
17152	2.5	walking	walking, 2.0 mph, level, slow pace, firm surface
17160	3.5	walking	walking for pleasure (Taylor Code 010)
17161	2.5	walking	walking from house to car or bus, from car or bus to go places, from car or bus to and from the worksite
17162	2.5	walking	walking to neighbor's house or family's house for social reasons
17165	3.0	walking	walking the dog
17170	3.0	walking	walking, 2.5 mph, firm surface
17180	2.8	walking	walking, 2.5 mph, downhill
17190	3.3	walking	walking, 3.0 mph, level, moderate pace, firm surface
17200	3.8	walking	walking, 3.5 mph, level, brisk, firm surface, walking for exercise
17210	6.0	walking	walking, 3.5 mph, uphill

Figure A-1. *Continued.*

Code	METS	Specific Activity	Examples
17220	5.0	walking	walking, 4.0 mph, level, firm surface, very brisk pace
17230	6.3	walking	walking, 4.5 mph, level, firm surface, very, very brisk
17231	8.0	walking	walking, 5.0 mph
17250	3.5	walking	walking, for pleasure, work break
117260	5.0	walking	walking, grass track
17270	4.0	walking	walking, to work or class (Taylor Code 015)
17280	2.5	walking	walking to and from an outhouse
18010	2.5	water activities	boating, power
18020	4.0	water activities	canoeing, on camping trip (Taylor Code 270)
18025	3.3	water activities	canoeing, harvesting wild rice, knocking rice off the stalks
18030	7.0	water activities	canoeing, portaging
18040	3.0	water activities	canoeing, rowing, 2.0–3.9 mph, light effort
18050	7.0	water activities	canoeing, rowing, 4.0–5.9 mph, moderate effort
18060	12.0	water activities	canoeing, rowing, > 6 mph, vigorous effort
18070	3.5	water activities	canoeing, rowing, for pleasure, general (Taylor Code 250)
18080	12.0	water activities	canoeing, rowing, in competition, or crew or sculling (Taylor Code 260)
18090	3.0	water activities	diving, springboard or platform
18100	5.0	water activities	kayaking
18110	4.0	water activities	paddle boat
18120	3.0	water activities	sailing, boat and board sailing, windsurfing, ice sailing, general (Taylor Code 235)
18130	5.0	water activities	sailing, in competition
18140	3.0	water activities	sailing, Sunfish/Laser/Hobby Cat, Keel boats, ocean sailing, yachting
18150	6.0	water activities	skiing, water (Taylor Code 220)
18160	7.0	water activities	skimobiling
18180	16.0	water activities	skindiving, fast
18190	12.5	water activities	skindiving, moderate
18200	7.0	water activities	skindiving, scuba diving, general (Taylor Code 310)
18210	5.0	water activities	snorkeling (Taylor Code 320)
18220	3.0	water activities	surfing, body or board
18230	10.0	water activities	swimming laps, freestyle, fast, vigorous effort
18240	7.0	water activities	swimming laps, freestyle, slow, moderate or light effort
18250	7.0	water activities	swimming, backstroke, general
18260	10.0	water activities	swimming, breaststroke, general
18270	11.0	water activities	swimming, butterfly, general
18280	11.0	water activities	swimming, crawl, fast (75 yards/minute), vigorous effort
18290	8.0	water activities	swimming, crawl, slow (50 yards/minute), moderate or light effort
18300	6.0	water activities	swimming, lake, ocean, river (Taylor Codes 280, 295)
18310	6.0	water activities	swimming, leisurely, not lap swimming, general
18320	8.0	water activities	swimming, sidestroke, general
18330	8.0	water activities	swimming, synchronized
18340	10.0	water activities	swimming, treading water, fast vigorous effort
18350	4.0	water activities	swimming, treading water, moderate effort, general
18355	4.0	water activities	water aerobics, water calisthenics
18360	10.0	water activities	water polo
18365	3.0	water activities	water volleyball
18366	8.0	water activities	water jogging
18370	5.0	water activities	whitewater rafting, kayaking, or canoeing
19010	6.0	winter activities	moving ice house (set up/drill holes, etc.)
19020	5.5	winter activities	skating, ice, 9 mph or less
19030	7.0	winter activities	skating, ice, general (Taylor Code 360)
19040	9.0	winter activities	skating, ice, rapidly, more than 9 mph
19050	15.0	winter activities	skating, speed, competitive
19060	7.0	winter activities	ski jumping (climb up carrying skis)
19075	7.0	winter activities	skiing, general
19080	7.0	winter activities	skiing, cross country, 2.5 mph, slow or light effort, ski walking
19090	8.0	winter activities	skiing, cross country, 4.0–4.9 mph, moderate speed and effort, general
19100	9.0	winter activities	skiing, cross country, 5.0–7.9 mph, brisk speed, vigorous effort
19110	14.0	winter activities	skiing, cross country, > 8.0 mph, racing
19130	16.5	winter activities	skiing, cross country, hard snow, uphill, maximum, snow mountaineering
19150	5.0	winter activities	skiing, downhill, light effort
19160	6.0	winter activities	skiing, downhill, moderate effort, general
19170	8.0	winter activities	skiing, downhill, vigorous effort, racing
19180	7.0	winter activities	sledding, tobogganing, bobsledding, luge (Taylor Code 370)

Figure A-1. *Continued.*

Code	METS	Specific Activity	Examples
19190	8.0	winter activities	snow shoeing
19200	3.5	winter activities	snowmobiling
20000	1.0	religious activities	sitting in church, in service, attending a ceremony, sitting quietly
20001	2.5	religious activities	sitting, playing an instrument at church
20005	1.5	religious activities	sitting in church, talking or singing, attending a ceremony, sitting, active participation
20010	1.3	religious activities	sitting, reading religious materials at home
20015	1.2	religious activities	standing in church (quietly), attending a ceremony, standing quietly
20020	2.0	religious activities	standing, singing in church, attending a ceremony, standing, active participation
20025	1.0	religious activities	kneeling in church/at home (praying)
20030	1.8	religious activities	standing, talking in church
20035	2.0	religious activities	walking in church
20036	2.0	religious activities	walking, less than 2.0 mph - very slow
20037	3.3	religious activities	walking, 3.0 mph, moderate speed, not carrying anything
20038	3.8	religious activities	walking, 3.5 mph, brisk speed, not carrying anything
20039	2.0	religious activities	walk/stand combination for religious purposes, usher
20040	5.0	religious activities	praise with dance or run, spiritual dancing in church
20045	2.5	religious activities	serving food at church
20046	2.0	religious activities	preparing food at church
20047	2.3	religious activities	washing dishes/cleaning kitchen at church
20050	1.5	religious activities	eating at church
20055	2.0	religious activities	eating/talking at church or standing eating, American Indian Feast days
20060	3.0	religious activities	cleaning church
20061	5.0	religious activities	general yard work at church
20065	2.5	religious activities	standing—moderate (lifting 50 lbs., assembling at fast rate)
20095	4.0	religious activities	standing—moderate/heavy work
20100	1.5	religious activities	typing, electric, manual, or computer
21000	1.5	volunteer activities	sitting—meeting, general, and/or with talking involved
21005	1.5	volunteer activities	sitting—light office work, in general
21010	2.5	volunteer activities	sitting—moderate work
21015	2.3	volunteer activities	standing—light work (filing, talking, assembling)
21016	2.5	volunteer activities	sitting, child care, only active periods
21017	3.0	volunteer activities	standing, child care, only active periods
21018	4.0	volunteer activities	walk/run play with children, moderate, only active periods
21019	5.0	volunteer activities	walk/run play with children, vigorous, only active periods
21020	3.0	volunteer activities	standing—light/moderate work (pack boxes, assemble/repair, set up chairs/furniture)
21025	3.5	volunteer activities	standing—moderate (lifting 50 lbs., assembling at fast rate)
21030	4.0	volunteer activities	standing—moderate/heavy work
21035	1.5	volunteer activities	typing, electric, manual, or computer
21040	2.0	volunteer activities	walking, less than 2.0 mph, very slow
21045	3.3	volunteer activities	walking, 3.0 mph, moderate speed, not carrying anything
21050	3.8	volunteer activities	walking, 3.5 mph, brisk speed, not carrying anything
21055	3.0	volunteer activities	walking, 2.5 mph slowly and carrying objects less than 25 pounds
21060	4.0	volunteer activities	walking, 3.0 mph moderately and carrying objects less than 25 pounds, pushing something
21065	4.5	volunteer activities	walking, 3.5 mph, briskly and carrying objects less than 25 pounds
21070	3.0	volunteer activities	walk/stand combination, for volunteer purposes

METS for certain golfing activities were revised downward from 1993 estimates based on measurement of the activity using indirect calorimetry.

Figure A-1. *Continued.*

was added to the 1993 Compendium's specifications of clearing land and hauling branches. In other cases, activities were removed from existing codes and new codes were developed if the removed activities had a different MET level or were qualitatively different from other specific activities listed for the code. For example, the 1993 Compendium listed mopping as a specific activity in code 05020, home activities. However, Emplaincourt (7) measured the MET intensity for mopping as 3.5 METs and the MET intensity for the other activities in the code was listed as 3.0 METs. Thus, mopping was deleted from code 05020 and a new code, 05021, was created. Another example is watching television. In 1993, watching television was coded as 07010 (reclining) or 07020 (sitting) and was grouped with other specific activities that involved sitting quietly (i.e., riding in a car, listening to a lecture or to music) or reclining and doing nothing. Because watching television is a sedentary but modifiable leisure time activity that may be related to the increased prevalence of physical inactivity (36), over-weight, and obesity in the United States (13,14), the authors felt that watching television should have a separate code to monitor time spent in this activity. In the updated Compendium, the codes 07010 and 07020 refer to watching television only. New codes have been added for the remaining inactive reclining (07011) and sitting (07021) activities. Table 2 presents

TABLE 2. New Codes in Version 2 of the Compendium of Physical Activities.

Major Heading	Code Number	METs	Example
Bicycling	01015	8.0	Bicycling, general
Conditioning Exercises	02101	2.5	Mild stretching
Dancing	03016	8.5	Aerobic, step, with 6–8 inch step
	03017	10.0	Aerobic, step, with 10–12 inch step
	03031	4.5	Disco, folk, square, line dancing, Irish step dancing, polka, contra, and country dancing.
	03050	5.5	Anishinaabe Jingle Dancing or other traditional American Indian dancing
Home Activities	05021	3.5	Mopping
	05025	2.5	Multiple household tasks all at once, light effort
	05026	3.5	Multiple household tasks all at once, moderate effort
	05027	4.0	Multiple household tasks all at once, vigorous effort
	05043	3.5	Vacuuming
	05045	6.0	Butchering animals
	05053	2.5	Feeding animals
	05148	2.5	Watering plants
	05149	2.5	Building a fire inside
	05181	3.0	Carrying small children
	05187	4.0	Elder care, disabled adults, only active periods
	05188	1.5	Reclining with baby
	05190	2.5	Sitting, playing with animals, light, only active periods
	05191	2.8	Standing, playing with animals, light, only active periods
	05192	2.8	Walk/run, playing with animals, light, only active periods
	05193	4.0	Walk/run, playing with animals, moderate, only active periods
	05194	5.0	Walk/run, playing with animals, vigorous, only active periods
	05195	3.5	Standing–bathing dog
Lawn and Garden	06165	4.5	Painting (Taylor Code 630)
Inactivity	07011	1.0	Lying quietly, done nothing, lying in bed awake, listening to music (not talking or reading)
	07021	1.0	Sitting quietly, sitting smoking, listening to music (not talking or reading), watching a movie in a theater
Lawn and Garden	08125	4.5	Mowing lawn, power mower (Taylor Code 590)
	08165	4.0	Raking lawn (Taylor Code 600)
	04246	3.0	Picking fruit off trees, picking fruits/vegetables, moderate effort
Miscellaneous	09071	2.0	Standing–miscellaneous
	09075	1.5	Sitting—arts and crafts, light effort
	09080	2.0	Sitting—arts and crafts, moderate effort
	09085	1.8	Standing—arts and crafts, light effort
	09090	3.0	Standing—arts and crafts, moderate effort
	09095	3.5	Standing—arts and crafts, vigorous effort
	09100	1.5	Retreat/family reunion activities involving sitting, relaxing, talking, eating
	09105	2.0	Touring/traveling/vacation involving walking and riding
	09110	2.5	Camping involving standing, walking, sitting, light-to-moderate effort
	09115	1.5	Sitting at a sporting event, spectator
Occupation	11015	2.5	Bakery, light effort
	11121	3.0	Custodial, buffing the floor with an electric buffer
	11122	2.5	Custodial, cleaning sink and toilet, light effort
	11123	2.5	Custodial, dusting, light effort
	11124	4.0	Custodial, feathering arena floor, moderate effort
	11125	3.5	Custodial, general cleaning, moderate effort
	11126	3.5	Custodial, mopping, moderate effort
	11127	3.0	Custodial, take out trash, moderate effort
	11128	2.5	Custodial, vacuuming, light effort
	11129	3.0	Custodial, vacuuming, moderate effort
	11151	4.0	Farming, chasing cattle or other livestock on horseback, moderate effort
	11152	2.0	Farming, chasing cattle or other livestock, driving, light effort
	11191	6.0	Farming, taking care of animals (grooming, brushing, shearing sheep, assisting with birthing, medical care, branding)
	11495	12.0	Skin diving or SCUBA diving as a frogman (Navy Seal)
	11615	4.0	Lifting items continuously, 10–20 lbs, with limited walking or resting
	11765	3.5	Tailoring, weaving
	11796	3.0	Walking, gathering things at work, ready to leave
	11805	4.0	Walking, pushing a wheelchair

TABLE 2. New Codes in Version 2 of the Compendium of Physical Activities. *(continued)*

Major Heading	Code Number	METs	Example
Running	12027	4.5	Jogging on a mini-trampoline
Self Care	13036	1.0	Taking medication, sitting or standing
	13045	2.5	Hairstyling
	13046	1.0	Having hair or nails done by someone else, sitting
Sports	15265	4.5	Golf, walking and carrying clubs
	15285	4.3	Golf, walking and pulling clubs
	15591	12.5	Roller blading (in-line skating)
	15685	5.0	Tennis, doubles play
	15711	8.0	Volleyball, competitive play in a gymnasium
	15732	4.0	Track and field (shot, discus, hammer throw)
	15733	6.0	Track and field (high jump, long jump, triple jump, javelin, pole vault)
	15734	10.0	Track and field (steeplechase, hurdles)
Transportation	16015	1.0	Riding in a car or truck
	16016	1.0	Riding in a bus
Walking	17031	3.0	Loading/unloading a car
	17085	2.5	Bird watching
	17105	4.0	Pushing a wheelchair, non occupational setting
	17151	2.0	Walking, less than 2.0 mph, level ground, strolling, very slow
	17152	2.5	Walking, 2.0 mph, level, slow pace, firm surface
	17161	2.5	Walking from house to car or bus, from car or bus to go places, from car or bus to and from the work site
	17162	2.5	Walking to neighbor's house or family's house for social reasons
	17165	3.0	Walking the dog
	17231	8.0	Walking, 5.0 mph
	17280	2.5	Walking to and from an outhouse
Water Activities	18025	3.3	Canoeing, harvesting wild rice, knocking rice off the stalks
	18355	4.0	Water aerobics, water calisthenics
	18366	8.0	Water jogging
Religious Activities	20000–20100		Addition of 24 new codes and description of activities
Volunteer Activities	21000–21070		Addition of 19 new codes and description of activities

the new five-digit codes, and Table 3 presents the modifications for existing codes as incorporated in the updated Compendium.

Intensity of activities. All activities are assigned an intensity level based on the rate of energy expenditure expressed as METs. Intensity of activities in the Compendium is classified as multiples of 1 MET or as the ratio of the associated metabolic rate for the specific activity divided by a standard RMR. In the 1993 Compendium, MET values were assigned to each activity based on the "best representation" of an intensity level from published lists and selected unpublished data (1). For activities not in original lists or in other unpublished reports of the energy cost of physical activities, data were obtained from published literature and assigned a measured MET value or was estimated from similar activities with a known MET value (1).

MET levels for 42 activities in the updated Compendium were changed based on published and unpublished studies that measured the energy cost of PAs (4,7–9,16,17, 21,22,24,27–30,32,35,37). Since the publication of the 1995 Pate et al. (23) moderate activity recommendation, there has been widespread interest among health educators, clinicians, public health specialists, and fitness professionals to recommend types of activities that

are classified as moderate intensity. There was some concern, however, that the MET levels for many household, lawn and garden, walking, and some occupational activities frequently performed by older adults, people of color, and women of all ages had not been objectively measured, but had been assigned estimated MET intensities. Thus, in 1997–1998, a series of studies were funded by the International Life Sciences Institute Research Foundation to measure the energy cost of selected household, lawn and garden, walking, recreational, and occupational activities using indirect calorimetry methods in laboratory and field settings (4,9,29,30,35). Doctoral dissertations and other research studies have also focused on measuring the MET intensities of household, lawn and garden, cultural, and custodial activities (8,9,27,28).

Because changes in MET intensities for selected activities may change the energy cost of PA, investigators using the 1993 Compendium in cohort studies may wish to continue using the 1993 Compendium to compute the energy cost of activities. However, for newer activities, codes in the 2000 Compendium are appropriate for use.

As in the 1993 Compendium of Physical Activities, the updated Compendium provides data for adults without handicaps or other conditions that would significantly alter their mechanical or metabolic efficiency. Also, a study is

TABLE 3. Modified Codes in Version 2 of the Compendium of Physical Activities.

Major Heading	Code Number	Modification Made
Bicycling	01010	Removed word "general" from the description of activities
Conditioning Exercises	02010	Changed MET level from 5.0 to 7.0
	02020	Added "jumping jacks" to the description of activities
	02030	Changed MET level from 4.5 to 3.5
	02040	Added "including some aerobic movement with minimal rest" to the description of activities
	02065	Changed MET level from 6.0 to 9.0
	02070	Changed MET level form 9.5 to 7.0
	02080	Changed MET level from 9.5 to 7.0
	02090	Added "jazzercise" to the description of activities
	02100	Changed MET level from 4.0 to 2.5
Dancing	03010	Changed MET level from 6.0 to 4.8; Added "jazz, tap, jitterbug" to the description of activites
	03015	Changed MET level from 6.0 to 6.5
	03025	Added "Greek, Middle Eastern, hula, flamenco, belly, and swing dancing" to the description of activities
	03030	Changed description of activities to "ballroom dancing fast (Taylor Code 125)"
	03040	Added "samba, tango, 19th Century, mambo, chacha" to the description of activities
Fishing and Hunting	04001	Changed MET level from 4.0 to 3.0
	04020	Changed MET level from 5.0 to 4.0
Home Activities	05010	Changed MET level from 2.5 to 3.3
	05020	Changed MET level from 4.5 to 3.0; Removed "mopping" from the description of activities
	05030	Changed MET level from 3.5 to 3.0
	05040	Removed "vacuuming" and "moderate effort" from the description of activities
	05042	Changed MET level from 2.3 to 2.5
	05050	Changed MET level from 2.5 to 2.0; Added "manual appliances" to the description of activities
	05055	Added "carrying groceries" to the description of activities
	05056	Changed MET level from 8.0 to 7.5
	05060	Changed MET level from 3.5 to 2.3; Changed description of activities to "food shopping with or without a grocery cart, standing or walking"
	05066	Deleted this category for "Walking-shopping (non-grocery) shopping
	05120	Added, "carrying boxes"
	05130	Changed MET level from 5.5 to 3.8; Added activities "scrubbing bathroom, bathtub" to description of activities
	05145	Deleted this category for "moving household items, carrying boxes"
	05160	Changed MET level from 2.5 to 2.0
	05170	Added "only active periods" to the description of activities
	05171	Added "only active periods" to the description of activities
	05175	Added "only active periods" to the description of activities
	05180	Added "only active periods" to the description of activities
	05185	Changed MET level from 3.0 to 2.5; Added "general" to the description of activities
	05186	Changed MET level from 3.5 to 3.0
Home Repair	06020	Changed MET level from 4.5 to 4.0
	06050	Added "building a fence" to the description of activities
	06140	Added "repairing appliances" to the description of activities
	06230	Added "painting fence" to the description of activities
Inactivity	07010	Changed MET level from 0.9 to 1.0; Change description of activities to "lying quietly, watching television"
	07020	Changed description of activities to "Sitting quietly and watching television"
Lawn and Garden	08030	Added "wheelbarrow chores" to the description of activities
	08050	Added "composting" to the description of activities
	08060	Removed "(see occupation, shoveling)" and added "chain saw"
	08120	Changed MET level from 4.5 to 5.5; Removed "(Taylor Code 610)"
	08140	Changed MET level from 4.0 to 4.5
	08160	Changed MET level from 4.0 to 4.3; Removed "(Taylor Code 600)"
	08215	Added "Using leaf blower, edger" to description of activities
	08245	Changed MET level from 5.0 to 4.0
	08250	Added "picking flowers or vegetables" to description of activities
Miscellaneous	09020	Change MET level from 2.0 to 2.3; Add "duplicating machine" to description of activities
	09040	Added "typing" to description of activities
Occupation	11010	Added "moderate effort" to the description of activities
	11070	Added "making bed (nursing)" to the description of activities
	11140	Added "vigorous effort" to the description of activities
	11150	Added "(walking), moderate effort" to the description of activities
	11160	Added "cutting hay, irrigation work" to the description of activities
	11190	Added "horses" to the description of activities

TABLE 3. Modified Codes in Version 2 of the Compendium of Physical Activities. *(continued)*

Major Heading	Code Number	Modification Made
	11200	Added "cleaning corral or barn, vigorous effort" to the description of activities
	11220	Added "light effort" to the description of activities
	11230	Added "moderate effort" to the description of activities
	11528	Changed MET level from 8.0 to 4.0
	11580	Added "sitting, reading, driving at work" to the description of activities
	11585	Added "eating at a business meeting" to the description of activities
	11590	Added "teaching stretching or yoga"
	11600	Changed MET level from 2.5 to 2.3; Changed the description of activities to read "standing, light (bartending, store clerk, assembling, filing, duplicating, putting up a Christmas tree), standing and talking at work, changing clothes when teaching physical education"
	11620	Added "intermittent" to the description of activities
Running	12160	Replaced "running" with "jogging"; Changed to code 12025
	12190	Removed "wheelchair wheeling"
Self Care	13050	Changed MET level from 4.0 to 2.0
Sports	15250	Changed MET level from 3.5 to 8.0
	15260	Deleted this code for the Taylor Code 090 for "golf, carrying clubs"
	15280	Deleted this code for the Taylor Code 080 for "golf, pulling clubs"
	15380	Added "grooming horse" to the description of activities
	15680	Represents Taylor Code 430 intensity level for doubles tennis
	15710	Represents Taylor Code 400 intensity level for competitive volleyball
Walking	17010	Removed "general" from the description of activities
	17100	Added "or walk with children" to the description of activities
	17140	Changed the MET level from 4.0 to 5.0
	17150	Changed description of activities to "household walking"
	17160	Changed the MET level from 2.5 to 3.5 and changed description of activities to "walking for pleasure (Taylor Code 010)"
	17180	Changed the MET level from 3.0 to 2.8
	17190	Changed the MET level from 3.5 to 3.3
	17200	Changed the MET level from 4.0 to 3.8; Added "walking for exercise" to the description of activities
	17220	Changed MET level from 4.0 to 5.0
	17230	Changed MET level from 4.5 to 6.3
	17250	Removed "walking the dog" from the description of activities
Water Activities	18170	Changed code number to Occupational, 11495
	18240	Changed MET level from 8.0 to 7.0
	18250	Changed MET level from 8.0 to 7.0

underway at the University of North Carolina at Chapel Hill to measure the energy cost of individual and group PAs among youth, ages 8–18 yr (J. A. Harrell, School of Nursing, University of North Carolina at Chapel Hill, 1999). Another study is underway at the Edward Hines Jr. VA Hospital to measure the energy costs of physical activities in adults with spinal cord injuries (W. E. Langbein and E. Collins, Hine Hospital, Maywood, IL, 1999). When completed, the projects will provide compendiums of the PAs measured in the studies.

Calculation of energy cost. Methods used to calculate the energy cost of activities in the 1993 Compendium were explained in detail by Ainsworth et al. (1). There has been concern that the absolute MET intensities presented in the Compendium may be inaccurate for people of different body mass and body fat percentage (10,27). For weight-bearing activities, Schmitz et al. (27) and Howell et al. (10) showed that the energy cost of activity was higher among heavier individuals than indicated by the Compendium's MET intensities. For these individu-

als, use of the MET intensities in the Compendium would underestimate the actual energy cost of weight bearing activity. The opposite pattern would be observed for non–weight-bearing activities. Schmitz (27) discusses these concerns in relation to energy expended during household chores among obese and lean women. Similar observations may apply to individuals who differ in age, cardiorespiratory fitness levels, and mechanical efficiency and when activities are performed in varied geographic and environmental conditions (33). It should be emphasized that the Compendium was developed to facilitate the coding of PAs and to compare coding across studies. It does not take into account individual differences that may alter the energy cost of movement. Thus, a correction factor may be needed to adjust for individual differences when estimating the energy cost of PA in individuals; but no such general correction is available at this time.

Use of the Compendium in PA validation studies. The Compendium facilitates the use of PA records to record the type, intensity, and duration of activities in a systematic manner. PA records and the Compendium have been used to validate PA surveys commonly used in observational and clinical studies (25). In 1993, we presented a sample PA record for use with the Compendium (1). We have since developed an updated PA record that is easy to use and code and provides a detailed explanation for the use of PA records and the Compendium in PA validation studies.

DISCUSSION AND LIMITATIONS

The value and limitations of using the Compendium of Physical Activities to determine the energy cost of PA in adults was previously discussed in the 1993 publication (1). Because the MET levels presented in the Compendium are based on the energy cost of actual movement, investigators should remind participants to recall only the time spent in movement when using the Compendium to estimate the energy cost of activities. It should also be stressed that the Compendium was not developed to determine the precise energy cost of PA within individuals, but instead to provide an activity classification system that standardizes the MET intensities of PAs used in survey research. This limits the use of the Compendium in estimating the energy cost of PA in individuals in ways that account for differences in body mass, adiposity, age, sex, efficiency of movement, geographic and environmental conditions in which the activities are performed. Thus, individual differences in energy expenditure for the same activity can be large and the true energy cost for a person may or may not be close to the stated mean MET level as presented in the Compendium.

As was true with the original Compendium, the updated version contains specific activities in which the MET values were not derived from indirect calorimetry; however, many codes have been updated using measured MET values. The updated Compendium still has some codes in which MET values were estimated from activities having similar movement patterns. Therefore, these estimates may have ill-defined confidence limits around the mean MET values.

SUMMARY

The updated version of the 1993 Compendium of Physical Activities includes new major headings for religious and volunteer activities, new five-digit codes for 129 specific activities, and modifications to codes for 94 specific activities. Despite its known limitations, the Compendium has proven useful in coding physical activity surveys or records and in providing examples of activities within broad intensity ranges for use for PA counseling in research, education, and clinic settings. However, additional methods are needed to account for differences in individual characteristics that may alter the energy costs of physical activities.

NOTES

An unpublished edition of the Compendium was developed in 2000 to track changes from the first edition and to explore possible changes in future editions. The unpublished edition includes a two-digit number that identifies the version of the Compendium. The version number should make it simple to make corrections and additions to activity codes and their intensities while retaining the ability to code questionnaires consistently with questionnaires collected earlier on the same person. A copy of the unpublished tracking version of the Compendium may be obtained from Dr. Barbara Ainsworth.

Many people participated in the identification of specific activities and the modification of existing codes for the updated Compendium of Physical Activities. Although the individuals involved are too numerous to mention, we wish to thank a few colleagues and graduate students (listed by their institutional affiliation) for their valuable contributions to the updated Compendium of Physical Activities. The individuals are listed by their institutional affiliation: Jennifer Hootman and Angela Morgan (University of South Carolina), Mark Richardson (University of Alabama), Devra Hendelman and Patty Freedson (University of Massachusetts), Gregory Welk (Iowa State University), Steven Blair (Cooper Institute for Aerobics Research), Vivian Heyward, Lisa Stolarczyk, and Julia Orri (University of New Mexico), and Ava Walker (University of Minnesota).

This work was supported in part by the International Life Sciences Institute Center for Health Promotion (ILSI CHP). The use of trade names and commercial sources in this document is for purposes of identification only and does not imply endorsement by ILSI CHP. In addition, the views expressed herein are those of the individual authors and/or their organizations and do not necessarily reflect those of ILSI CHP.

Dr. Leon is supported in part by the Henry L. Taylor Professorship in Exercise Science and Health Enhancement. Dr. Ainsworth is supported in part by the NIH Women's Health Initiative SIP 22W-U48/CCU 409554−03. Support for the development of the initial Compendium of Physical Activities was provided by grants from the National Heart, Lung, and Blood Institute to Drs. Leon and Jacobs (RFA-86−37561), to Dr. Haskell (HL-362−72),to Dr. Montoye (5-R01- HL-37561), and to Dr. James Sallis (RFA-86-HL-9-P).

Address for correspondence: Barbara E. Ainsworth, Ph.D., MPH, FACSM, Department of Epidemiology and Biostatistics, University of South Carolina, Columbia, SC 29208; E-mail: bainsworth@sph.sc.edu.

REFERENCES

1. Ainsworth, B. E., W. L. Haskell, A.S.Leon, et al. Compendium of physical activities: energy costs of human movement. *Med. Sci. Sports Exerc.* 25:71–80, 1993.

2. Ainsworth, B. E., M. L. Irwin, C.L.Addy, M.C.Whitt, and L. M. Stolarczyk. Moderate physical activity patterns among minority women: the Cross-Cultural Activity Participation Study. *J. Women's Health* 8:805–813, 1999.

3. Ainsworth, B. E., B. Sternfeld, M.T.Richardson, and K. Jackson. Evaluation of the Kaiser Physical Activity Survey in Women. *Med. Sci. Sports Exerc.* 32(Suppl.), 2000.

4. Bassett,D.R.Jr., B. E. Ainsworth, A.M.Swartz, S.J.Strath, W. L. O'Brien, and G. A. King. Validity of four motion sensors in measuring moderate intensity physical activity. *Med. Sci. Sports Exerc.* 32(Suppl.):S471–S480, 2000.

5. Bayne-Smith,M. *Race, Gender, and Health.* Thousand Oaks, CA: Sage Publications, 1996, p. 134.

6. Crespo, C. J., S. J. Keteyian, G.W.Heath, and C. T. Sempos. Leisure-time physical activity among US adults: results from the Third National Health and Nutrition Examination Survey. *Arch. Intern. Med.* 156:93–98, 1996.

7. Emplaincourt, P.O. *Inter-individual Variability in the Energy Cost of Several Habitual Physical Activities.* Unpublished Ph. D. Dissertation, University of Alabama, Tuscaloosa, AL, 1999.

8. Gilman, M. B., H. Houle, L.Firzell, K.Headbird, J.L.Durstine, and B. E. Ainsworth. Metabolic cost of traditional American Indian activities in women over 40 years of age (Abstract). *Med. Sci. Sports Exerc.* 32:S53, 2000.

9. Hendelman, D., K. Miller, C.Bagget, E.Debold, and P. Freedson. Validity of accelerometry for the assessment of moderate intensity physical activity in the field. *Med. Sci. Sports Exerc.* 32(Suppl.): S442–S449, 2000.

10. Howell, W., C. Earthman, P.Reid, J.Delaney, and L. Houtkooper. Doubly labeled water validation of the Compendium of Physical Activities in lean and obese college women (Abstract). *Med. Sci. Sports Exerc.* 31:S142, 1999.

11. Jones, D. A., B. E. Ainsworth, J.B.Croft, J.R.Livengood, E. Lloyd, and H. R. Yusuf. Prevalences of moderate physical activity recommended by the Surgeon General's Report in U.S. adults: National Health Interview Survey, 1990. *Arch. Family Med.* 7:285–289, 1998.

12. Jones, D. A., C. D. Kimsey, C.Amacera, and C. M. Fuchs. Characteristics of physical activity among employed adults in selected WHO MONICA sites (Abstract). *Med. Sci. Sports Exerc.* 32:S187, 2000.

13. Kuczmarski, R. J., M. D. Carroll, K.M.Flegal, and R. P. Troiano. Varying body mass index cutoff points to describe over-weight prevalence among U.S. adults: NHANES III (1988–1994). *Obes. Res.* 5:542–548, 1997.

14. Kuczmarski, R. J., K. M. Flegal, S.M.Campbell, and C. L. Johnson. Increasing prevalence of overweight among U.S. adults: the National Health and Nutrition Examination Surveys 1960–1991. *JAMA* 272:205–211, 1994.

15. Lee, I-M., C-C. Hsieh, and R. S. Paffenbarger,Jr. Exercise intensity and longevity in men. *JAMA* 273:1179–1184, 1995.

16. Margaria, R., P. Cerretelli, P.Aghemo, and G. Sassi. Energy cost of running. *J. Appl. Physiol.* 18:367–370, 1963.

17. Melanson, E. L., P. S. Freedson, R.Webb, S.Jungbluth, and N. Kozlowski. Exercise responses to running and in-line skating at self-selected paces. *Med. Sci. Sports Exerc.* 28:247–250, 1996.

18. Montoye, H. J. The energy cost of exercise and competitive sport. In: *Nutrition in Sport: Olympic Encyclopaedia of Sports Medicine, Vol. VII,* R. J. Maughan (Ed.). Maldea, MA: Blackwell Science Inc., 2000, pp. 53–72.

19. Montoye, H. J., H. C. G. Kemper, W.H.M.Saris, and R. A. Washburn. *Measuring Physical Activity and Energy Expenditure.* Champaign, IL: Human Kinetics Publishers, 1996, pp. 34–41.

20. Nieman,D.C. *Fitness and Sports Medicine,* 2nd Ed. Palo Alto: Bull Publishing Co., 1995, pp. 685–691.

21. Noble R. M., and E. T. Howley. The energy requirement of selected tap dance routines. *Res. Q.* 50:438–442, 1979.

22. Olson M. S., H. N. Williford, D.L.Blessing, and R. Greathouse. The cardiovascular and metabolic effect of bench stepping exercise stepping in females. *Med. Sci. Sports Exerc.* 23:1311–1318, 1991.

23. Pate, R. R., M. Pratt, S.N.Blair, et al. Physical activity and public health: a recommendation from the Centers for Disease Control and Prevention and the American College of Sports Medicine. *JAMA* 273:402–407, 1995.

24. Patterson R., and S. V. Fisher. Cardiovascular stress of crutch walking. *Arch. Phys. Med. Rehabil.* 62:257–260, 1981.

25. Pereira, M. A., S. J. Fitzgerald, E. W., and Gregg, et al. A collection of physical activity questionnaires for health related research. *Med. Sci. Sports Exerc.* 29:S1–S205, 1997.

26. Richardson, M. T., A. S. Leon, D.R.Jacobs,Jr., B. E. Ainsworth, and R. C. Serfass. Comprehensive evaluation of the Minnesota Leisure Time Physical Activity Questionnaire. *J. Clin. Epidemiol.* 47:271–281, 1994.

27. Schmitz, M.K.H. *The Interactive and Independent Associations of Physical Activity, Body Weight, and Blood Lipid Levels.* Unpublished Ph. D. Dissertation, University of Minnesota, Minneapolis, MN, 1998.

28. Smith J. F. Energy cost of specific custodial work tasks. *Unpublished Doctoral Dissertation, University of Tennessee* 1975:.

29. Strath S. J., A. M. Swartz, D.R.Bassett,Jr., W. L. O'Brien, G. A. King, and B. E. Ainsworth. Evaluation of heart rate as a method for estimating moderate intensity physical activity. *Med. Sci. Sports Exerc.* 32(Suppl.):S471–S480, 2000.

30. Swartz, A. M., S. J. Strath, D.R.Bassett,Jr., W. L. O'Brien, G. A. King, and B. E. Ainsworth. Estimation of energy expenditure using CSA, Inc. accelerometer hip and wrist sites. *Med. Sci. Sports Exerc.* 32(Suppl.):S450–S456, 2000.

31. Taylor H. L., D. R. Jacobs Jr., B. Schuker, J.Knudsen,A.S. Leon, and G. Debacker. A questionnaire for the assessment of leisure time physical activities. *J. Chronic Dis.* 31:741–755, 1978.

32. Town G. P., N. Sol, and W. Sinning. The effect of rope skipping rate on energy expenditure of males and females. *Med. Sci. Sports Exerc.* 12:295–298, 1980.

33. U. S. Department of Health and Human Services. *Physical Activity and Health: A Report of the Surgeon General.* Atlanta, GA: U.S. Department of Health and Human Services, Centers for Disease Control and Prevention, National Center for Chronic Disease Prevention and Health Promotion, 1996, pp. 29–37.

34. U. S. Department of Health and Human Services,Public Health Service,Centers for Disease Control and Prevention,National Center for Chronic Disease Prevention and Human Promotion, Division of Nutrition and Physical Activity. *Promoting Physical Activity: A Guide for Community Action.* Champaign, IL: Human Kinetics, 1999.

35. Welk, G. J., S. N. Blair, K.Wood, S.Jones, and R. W. Thompson. A comparative evaluation of three accelerometry-based physical activity monitors. *Med. Sci. Sports Exerc.* 32(Suppl.):S489–S497, 2000.

36. Williams, C. D., J. F. Sallis, K.J.Calfas, and R. Burke. Psychosocial and demographic correlates of television viewing. *Am. J. Health Promot.* 13:207–214, 1999.

37. Zeni A. I., M. D. Hoffman, and P. S. Clifford. Energy expenditure with indoor exercise machines. *JAMA* 275:1424–1427, 1996.

The Compendium of Physical Activities Tracking Guide
(See "Notes" section of the preceding article for explanation)

KEY

Blue text = new activity was added to the descripton of that specific compendium code

If compcode and METS columns are blank under 1993 this means that the 2000 compcode and METS was **added** to the new addition to the compendium

If compcode and METS columns are blank under 2000 this means that the 1993 compcode and METS was **removed** from the new addition of the compendium

1993 compcode	1993 METS	2000 compcode	2000 METS	heading	description
01009	8.5	01009	8.5	bicycling	bicycling, BMX or mountain
01010	4.0	01010	4.0	bicycling	bicycling, < 10 mph, leisure, to work or for pleasure (Taylor Code 115)
		01015	8.0	bicycling	bicycling, general
01020	6.0	01020	6.0	bicycling	bicycling, 10–11.9 mph, leisure, slow, light effort
01030	8.0	01030	8.0	bicycling	bicycling, 12–13.9 mph, leisure, moderate effort
01040	10.0	01040	10.0	bicycling	bicycling, 14–15.9 mph, racing or leisure, fast, vigorous effort
01050	12.0	01050	12.0	bicycling	bicycling, 16–19 mph, racing/not drafting or > 19 mph drafting, very fast, racing general
01060	16.0	01060	16.0	bicycling	bicycling, > 20 mph, racing, not drafting
01070	5.0	01070	5.0	bicycling	unicycling
02010	5.0	02010	7.0	conditioning exercise	bicycling, stationary, general
02011	3.0	02011	3.0	conditioning exercise	bicycling, stationary, 50 watts, very light effort
02012	5.5	02012	5.5	conditioning exercise	bicycling, stationary, 100 watts, light effort
02013	7.0	02013	7.0	conditioning exercise	bicycling, stationary, 150 watts, moderate effort
02014	10.5	02014	10.5	conditioning exercise	bicycling, stationary, 200 watts, vigorous effort
02015	12.5	02015	12.5	conditioning exercise	bicycling, stationary, 250 watts, very vigorous effort
02020	8.0	02020	8.0	conditioning exercise	calisthenics (e.g. pushups, situps, pullups, jumping jacks), heavy, vigorous effort
02030	4.5	02030	3.5	conditioning exercise	calisthenics, home exercise, light or moderate effort, general (example: back exercises), going up & down floor (Taylor Code 150)
02040	8.0	02040	8.0	conditioning exercise	circuit training, including some aerobic movement with minimal rest, general
02050	6.0	02050	6.0	conditioning exercise	weight lifting (free weight, nautilus or universal-type), power lifting or body building, vigorous effort (Taylor Code 210)
02060	5.5	02060	5.5	conditioning exercise	health club exercise, general (Taylor Code 160)
02065	6.0	02065	9.0	conditioning exercise	stair-treadmill ergometer, general
02070	9.5	02070	7.0	conditioning exercise	rowing, stationary ergometer, general
02071	3.5	02071	3.5	conditioning exercise	rowing, stationary, 50 watts, light effort
02072	7.0	02072	7.0	conditioning exercise	rowing, stationary, 100 watts, moderate effort
02073	8.5	02073	8.5	conditioning exercise	rowing, stationary, 150 watts, vigorous effort
02074	12.0	02074	12.0	conditioning exercise	rowing, stationary, 200 watts, very vigorous effort
02080	9.5	02080	7.0	conditioning exercise	ski machine, general
02090	6.0	02090	6.0	conditioning exercise	slimnastics, jazzercise
02100	4.0	02100	2.5	conditioning exercise	stretching, hatha yoga
		02101	2.5	conditioning exercise	mild stretching
02110	6.0	02110	6.0	conditioning exercise	teaching aerobic exercise class
02120	4.0	02120	4.0	conditioning exercise	water aerobics, water calisthenics
02130	3.0	02130	3.0	conditioning exercise	weight lifting (free, nautilus or universal-type), light or moderate effort, light workout, general
02135	1.0	02135	1.0	conditioning exercise	whirlpool, sitting
03010	6.0	03010	4.8	dancing	ballet or modern, twist, jazz, tap, jitterbug

1993 compcode	METS	2000 compcode	METS	heading	description
03015	6.0	03015	6.5	dancing	aerobic, general
		03016	8.5	dancing	aerobic, step, with 6–8 inch step
		03017	10.0	dancing	aerobic, step, with 10–12 inch step
03020	5.0	03020	5.0	dancing	aerobic, low impact
03021	7.0	03021	7.0	dancing	aerobic, high impact
03025	4.5	03025	4.5	dancing	general, Greek, Middle Eastern, hula, flamenco, belly, and swing dancing
03030	5.5	03030	5.5	dancing	ballroom, dancing fast (Taylor Code 125)
		03031	4.5	dancing	ballroom, fast (disco, folk, square), line dancing, Irish step dancing, polka, contra, country
03040	3.0	03040	3.0	dancing	ballroom, slow (e.g. waltz, foxtrot, slow dancing), samba, tango, 19th C, mambo, chacha
		03050	5.5	dancing	Anishinaabe Jingle Dancing or other traditional American Indian dancing
04001	4.0	04001	3.0	fishing and hunting	fishing, general
04010	4.0	04010	4.0	fishing and hunting	digging worms, with shovel
04020	5.0	04020	4.0	fishing and hunting	fishing from river bank and walking
04030	2.5	04030	2.5	fishing and hunting	fishing from boat, sitting
04040	3.5	04040	3.5	fishing and hunting	fishing from river bank, standing (Taylor Code 660)
04050	6.0	04050	6.0	fishing and hunting	fishing in stream, in waders (Taylor Code 670)
04060	2.0	04060	2.0	fishing and hunting	fishing, ice, sitting
04070	2.5	04070	2.5	fishing and hunting	hunting, bow and arrow or crossbow
04080	6.0	04080	6.0	fishing and hunting	hunting, deer, elk, large game (Taylor Code 170)
04090	2.5	04090	2.5	fishing and hunting	hunting, duck, wading
04100	5.0	04100	5.0	fishing and hunting	hunting, general
04110	6.0	04110	6.0	fishing and hunting	hunting, pheasants or grouse (Taylor Code 680)
04120	5.0	04120	5.0	fishing and hunting	hunting, rabbit, squirrel, prairie chick, raccoon, small game (Taylor Code 690)
04130	2.5	04130	2.5	fishing and hunting	pistol shooting or trap shooting, standing
05010	2.5	05010	3.3	home activities	carpet sweeping, sweeping floors
05020	4.5	05020	3.0	home activities	cleaning, heavy or major (e.g. wash car, wash windows, clean garage), vigorous effort
		05021	3.5	home activities	mopping
		05025	2.5	home activities	multiple household tasks all at once, light effort
		05026	3.5	home activities	multiple household tasks all at once, moderate effort
		05027	4.0	home activities	multiple household tasks all at once, vigorous effort
05030	3.5	05030	3.0	home activities	cleaning, house or cabin, general
05040	2.5	05040	2.5	home activities	cleaning, light (dusting, straightening up, changing linen, carrying out trash)
05041	2.3	05041	2.3	home activities	wash dishes—standing or in general (not broken into stand/walk components)
05042	2.3	05042	2.5	home activities	wash dishes; clearing dishes from table—walking
		05043	3.5	home activities	vacuuming
		05045	6.0	home activities	butchering animals
05050	2.5	05050	2.0	home activities	cooking or food preparation—standing or sitting or in general (not broken into stand/walk components), manual appliances
05051	2.5	05051	2.5	home activities	serving food, setting table—implied walking or standing
05052	2.5	05052	2.5	home activities	cooking or food preparation—walking
		05053	2.5	home activities	feeding animals
05055	2.5	05055	2.5	home activities	putting away groceries (e.g. carrying groceries, shopping without a grocery cart), carrying packages
05056	8.0	05056	7.5	home activities	carrying groceries upstairs
		05057	3.0	home activities	cooking Indian bread on an outside stove
05060	3.5	05060	2.3	home activities	food shopping with or without a grocery cart, standing or walking
05065	2.0	05065	2.3	home activities	non-food shopping, standing or walking

Code	METs	Major Heading	Specific Activity
05066	2.3	home activities	walking shopping (non-grocery shopping)
05070	2.3	home activities	ironing
05080	1.5	home activities	sitting—knitting, sewing, lt. wrapping (presents)
05090	2.0	home activities	implied standing—laundry, fold or hang clothes, put clothes in washer or dryer, packing suitcase
05095	2.3	home activities	implied walking—putting away clothes, gathering clothes to pack, putting away laundry
05100	2.0	home activities	making bed
05110	5.0	home activities	maple syruping/sugar bushing (including carrying buckets, carrying wood)
05120	6.0	home activities	moving furniture, household items, carrying boxes
05130	3.8	home activities	scrubbing floors, on hands and knees, scrubbing bathroom, bathtub
05140	4.0	home activities	sweeping garage, sidewalk or outside of house
05145	7.0	home activities	moving household items, carrying boxes
05146	3.5	home activities	standing—packing/unpacking boxes, occasional lifting of household items light—moderate effort
05147	3.0	home activities	implied walking—putting away household items—moderate effort
05148	2.5	home activities	watering plants
05149	2.5	home activities	building a fire inside
05150	9.0	home activities	moving household items upstairs, carrying boxes or furniture
05160	2.5	home activities	standing—light (pump gas, change light bulb, etc.)
05165	3.0	home activities	walking—light, non-cleaning (readying to leave, shut/lock doors, close windows, etc.)
05170	2.5	home activities	sitting—playing with child(ren)—light, only active periods
05171	2.8	home activities	standing—playing with child(ren)—light, only active periods
05175	4.0	home activities	walk/run—playing with child(ren)—moderate, only active periods
05180	5.0	home activities	walk/run—playing with child(ren)—vigorous, only active periods
05181	3.0	home activities	carrying small children
05185	2.5	home activities	child care: sitting/kneeling—dressing, bathing, grooming, feeding, occasional lifting of child-light effort, general
05186	3.0	home activities	child care: standing—dressing, bathing, grooming, feeding, occasional lifting of child-light effort
05187	4.0	home activities	elder care, disabled adult, only active periods
05188	1.5	home activities	reclining with baby
05190	2.5	home activities	sit, play ing with animals, light, only active periods
05191	2.8	home activities	stand, playing with animals, light, only active periods
05192	2.8	home activities	walk/run, playing with animals, light, only active periods
05193	4.0	home activities	walk/run, playing with animals, moderate, only active periods
05194	5.0	home activities	walk/run, playing with animals, vigorous, only active periods
05195	3.5	home activities	standing—bathing dog
06010	3.0	home repair	airplane repair
06020	4.5	home repair	automobile body work
06030	3.0	home repair	automobile repair
06040	3.0	home repair	carpentry, general, workshop (Taylor Code 620)
06050	6.0	home repair	carpentry, outside house, installing rain gutters, building a fence, (Taylor Code 640)
06060	4.5	home repair	carpentry, finishing or refinishing cabinets or furniture
06070	7.5	home repair	carpentry, sawing hardwood
06080	5.0	home repair	caulking, chinking log cabin
06090	4.5	home repair	caulking, except log cabin
06100	5.0	home repair	cleaning gutters
06110	5.0	home repair	excavating garage
06120	5.0	home repair	hanging storm windows
06130	4.5	home repair	laying or removing carpet
06140	4.5	home repair	laying tile or linoleum, repairing appliances
06150	5.0	home repair	painting, outside home (Taylor Code 650)

1993 compcode	METS	2000 compcode	METS	heading	description
06160	4.5	06160	3.0	home repair	painting, papering, plastering, scraping, inside house, hanging sheet rock, remodeling
		06165	4.5	home repair	painting, (Taylor Code 630)
06170	3.0	06170	3.0	home repair	put on and removal of tarp - sailboat
06180	6.0	06180	6.0	home repair	roofing
06190	4.5	06190	4.5	home repair	sanding floors with a power sander
06200	4.5	06200	4.5	home repair	scraping and painting sailboat or powerboat
06210	5.0	06210	5.0	home repair	spreading dirt with a shovel
06220	4.5	06220	4.5	home repair	washing and waxing hull of sailboat, car, powerboat, airplane
06230	4.5	06230	4.5	home repair	washing fence, painting fence
06240	3.0	06240	3.0	home repair	wiring, plumbing
07010	0.9	07011	1.0	inactivity quiet	lying quietly, watching television
		07020	1.0	inactivity quiet	lying quietly, doing nothing, lying in bed awake, listening to music (not talking or reading)
07020	1.0	07021	1.0	inactivity quiet	sitting quietly and watching television
			1.0	inactivity quiet	sitting quietly, sitting smoking, listening to music (not talking or reading), watching a movie in a theater
07030	0.9	07030	0.9	inactivity quiet	sleeping
07040	1.2	07040	1.2	inactivity quiet	standing quietly (standing in a line)
07050	1.0	07050	1.0	inactivity light	reclining—writing
07060	1.0	07060	1.0	inactivity light	reclining—talking or talking on phone
07070	1.0	07070	1.0	inactivity light	reclining—reading
		07075	1.0	inactivity light	meditating
08010	5.0	08010	5.0	lawn and garden	carrying, loading or stacking wood, loading/unloading or carrying lumber
08020	6.0	08020	6.0	lawn and garden	chopping wood, splitting logs
08030	5.0	08030	5.0	lawn and garden	clearing land, hauling branches, wheelbarrow chores
08040	5.0	08040	5.0	lawn and garden	digging sandbox
08050	5.0	08050	5.0	lawn and garden	digging, spading, filling garden, composting, (Taylor Code 590)
08060	6.0	08060	6.0	lawn and garden	gardening with heavy power tools, tilling a garden, chain saw
08080	5.0	08080	5.0	lawn and garden	laying crushed rock
08090	5.0	08090	5.0	lawn and garden	laying sod
08095	5.5	08095	5.5	lawn and garden	mowing lawn, general
08100	2.5	08100	2.5	lawn and garden	mowing lawn, riding mower (Taylor Code 550)
08110	6.0	08110	6.0	lawn and garden	mowing lawn, walk, hand mower (Taylor Code 570)
08120	4.5	08120	5.5	lawn and garden	mowing lawn, walk, power mower
		08125	4.5	lawn and garden	mowing lawn, power mower (Taylor Code 590)
08130	4.5	08130	4.5	lawn and garden	operating snow blower, walking
08140	4.0	08140	4.5	lawn and garden	planting seedlings, shrubs
08150	4.5	08150	4.5	lawn and garden	planting trees
08160	4.0	08160	4.3	lawn and garden	raking lawn
		08165	4.0	lawn and garden	raking lawn (Taylor Code 600)
08170	4.0	08170	4.0	lawn and garden	raking roof with snow rake
08180	3.0	08180	3.0	lawn and garden	riding snow blower
08190	4.0	08190	4.0	lawn and garden	sacking grass, leaves
08200	6.0	08200	6.0	lawn and garden	shoveling snow, by hand (Taylor Code 610)
08210	4.5	08210	4.5	lawn and garden	trimming shrubs or trees, manual cutter
08215	3.5	08215	3.5	lawn and garden	trimming shrubs or trees, power cutter, using leaf blower, edger
08220	2.5	08220	2.5	lawn and garden	walking, applying fertilizer or seeding a lawn

Code	METs	Major Heading	Specific Activity
08230	1.5	lawn and garden	watering lawn or garden, standing or walking
08240	4.5	lawn and garden	weeding, cultivating garden (Taylor Code 580)
08245	4.0	lawn and garden	gardening, general
08246	3.0	lawn and garden	picking fruit off trees, picking fruits/vegetables, moderate effort
08250	3.0	lawn and garden	implied walking/standing—picking up yard, light, picking flowers or vegetables
08251	3.0	lawn and garden	walking, gathering gardening tools
09010	1.5	miscellaneous	sitting—card playing, playing board games
09020	2.3	miscellaneous	standing—drawing (writing), casino gambling, duplicating machine
09030	1.3	miscellaneous	sitting—reading, book, newspaper, etc.
09040	1.8	miscellaneous	sitting—writing, desk work, typing
09050	1.8	miscellaneous	standing—talking or talking on the phone
09055	1.5	miscellaneous	sitting—talking or talking on the phone
09060	1.8	miscellaneous	sitting—studying, general, including reading and/or writing
09065	1.8	miscellaneous	sitting—in class, general, including note-taking or class discussion
09070	1.8	miscellaneous	standing—reading
09071	2.0	miscellaneous	standing—miscellaneous
09075	1.5	miscellaneous	sitting—arts and crafts, light effort
09080	2.0	miscellaneous	sitting—arts and crafts, moderate effort
09085	1.8	miscellaneous	standing—arts and crafts, light effort
09090	3.0	miscellaneous	standing—arts and crafts, moderate effort
09095	3.5	miscellaneous	standing—arts and crafts, vigorous effort
09100	1.5	miscellaneous	retreat/family reunion activities involving sitting, relaxing, talking, eating
09105	2.0	miscellaneous	touring/traveling/vacation involving walking and riding
09110	2.5	miscellaneous	camping involving standing, walking, sitting, light-to-moderate effort
09115	1.5	miscellaneous	sitting at a sporting event, spectator
10010	1.8	music playing	accordion
10020	2.0	music playing	cello
10030	2.5	music playing	conducting
10040	4.0	music playing	drums
10050	2.0	music playing	flute (sitting)
10060	2.0	music playing	horn
10070	2.5	music playing	piano or organ
10080	3.5	music playing	trombone
10090	2.5	music playing	trumpet
10100	2.5	music playing	violin
10110	2.0	music playing	woodwind
10120	2.0	music playing	guitar, classical, folk (sitting)
10125	3.0	music playing	guitar, rock and roll band (standing)
10130	4.0	music playing	marching band, playing an instrument, baton twirling (walking)
10135	3.5	music playing	marching band, drum major (walking)
11010	4.0	occupation	bakery, general, moderate effort
11015	2.5	occupation	bakery, light effort
11020	2.3	occupation	bookbinding
11030	6.0	occupation	building road (including hauling debris, driving heavy machinery)
11035	2.0	occupation	building road, directing traffic (standing)
11040	3.5	occupation	carpentry, general
11050	8.0	occupation	carrying heavy loads, such as bricks
11060	8.0	occupation	carrying moderate loads up stairs, moving boxes (16–40 pounds)
11070	2.5	occupation	chambermaid, making bed (nursing)

1993 compcode	1993 METS	2000 compcode	METS	heading	description
11080	6.5	11080	6.5	occupation	coal mining, drilling coal, rock
11090	6.5	11090	6.5	occupation	coal mining, erecting supports
11100	6.0	11100	6.0	occupation	coal mining, general
11110	7.0	11110	7.0	occupation	coal mining, shoveling coal
11120	5.5	11120	5.5	occupation	construction, outside, remodeling
		11121	3.0	occupation	custodial work—buffing the floor with electric buffer
		11122	2.5	occupation	custodial work—cleaning sink and toilet, light effort
		11123	2.5	occupation	custodial work—dusting, light effort
		11124	4.0	occupation	custodial work—feathering arena floor, moderate effort
		11125	3.5	occupation	custodial work—general cleaning, moderate effort
		11126	3.5	occupation	custodial work—mopping, moderate effort
		11127	3.0	occupation	custodial work—take out trash, moderate effort
		11128	2.5	occupation	custodial work—vacuuming, light effort
		11129	3.0	occupation	custodial work—vacuuming, moderate effort
11130	3.5	11130	3.5	occupation	electrical work, plumbing
11140	8.0	11140	8.0	occupation	farming, baling hay, cleaning barn, poultry work, vigorous effort
11150	3.5	11150	3.5	occupation	farming, chasing cattle, non-strenuous (walking), moderate effort
		11151	4.0	occupation	farming, chasing cattle or other livestock on horseback, moderate effort
		11152	2.0	occupation	farming, chasing cattle or other livestock, driving, light effort
11160	2.5	11160	2.5	occupation	farming, driving harvester, cutting hay, irrigation work
11170	2.5	11170	2.5	occupation	farming, driving tractor
11180	4.0	11180	4.0	occupation	farming, feeding small animals
11190	4.5	11190	4.5	occupation	farming, feeding cattle, horses
		11191	4.5	occupation	farming, hauling water for animals, general hauling water
		11192	6.0	occupation	farming, taking care of animals (grooming, brushing, shearing sheep, assisting with birthing, medical care, branding)
11200	8.0	11200	8.0	occupation	farming, forking straw bales, cleaning corral or barn, vigorous effort
11210	3.0	11210	3.0	occupation	farming, milking by hand, moderate effort
11220	1.5	11220	1.5	occupation	farming, milking by machine, light effort
11230	5.5	11230	5.5	occupation	farming, shoveling grain, moderate effort
11240	12.0	11240	12.0	occupation	fire fighter, general
11245	11.0	11245	11.0	occupation	fire fighter, climbing ladder with full gear
11246	8.0	11246	8.0	occupation	fire fighter, hauling hoses on ground
11250	17.0	11250	17.0	occupation	forestry, ax chopping, fast
11260	5.0	11260	5.0	occupation	forestry, ax chopping, slow
11270	7.0	11270	7.0	occupation	forestry, barking trees
11280	11.0	11280	11.0	occupation	forestry, carrying logs
11290	8.0	11290	8.0	occupation	forestry, felling trees
11300	8.0	11300	8.0	occupation	forestry, general
11310	5.0	11310	5.0	occupation	forestry, hoeing
11320	6.0	11320	6.0	occupation	forestry, planting by hand
11330	7.0	11330	7.0	occupation	forestry, sawing by hand
11340	4.5	11340	4.5	occupation	forestry, sawing, power
11350	9.0	11350	9.0	occupation	forestry, trimming trees
11360	4.0	11360	4.0	occupation	forestry, weeding
11370	4.5	11370	4.5	occupation	furriery

Code	METS	Type	Description
11380	6.0	occupation	horse grooming
11390	8.0	occupation	horse racing, galloping
11400	6.5	occupation	horse racing, trotting
11410	2.6	occupation	horse racing, walking
11420	3.5	occupation	locksmith
11430	2.5	occupation	machine tooling, machining, working sheet metal
11440	3.0	occupation	machine tooling, operating lathe
11450	5.0	occupation	machine tooling, operating punch press
11460	4.0	occupation	machine tooling, tapping and drilling
11470	3.0	occupation	machine tooling, welding
11480	7.0	occupation	masonry, concrete
11485	4.0	occupation	masseur, masseuse (standing)
11490	7.5	occupation	moving, pushing heavy objects, 75 lbs or more (desks, moving van work)
11495	12.0	occupation	skindiving or SCUBA diving as a frogman (Navy Seal)
11500	2.5	occupation	operating heavy duty equipment/automated, not driving
11510	4.5	occupation	orange grove work
11520	2.3	occupation	printing (standing)
11525	2.5	occupation	police, directing traffic (standing)
11526	2.0	occupation	police, driving a squad car (sitting)
11527	1.3	occupation	police, riding in a squad car (sitting)
11528	4.0	occupation	police, making an arrest (standing)
11530	2.5	occupation	shoe repair, general
11540	8.5	occupation	shoveling, digging ditches
11550	9.0	occupation	shoveling, heavy (more than 16 pounds/minute)
11560	6.0	occupation	shoveling, light (less than 10 pounds/minute)
11570	7.0	occupation	shoveling, moderate (10 to 15 pounds/minute)
11580	1.5	occupation	sitting—light office work, general (chemistry lab work, light use of hand tools, watch repair or micro-assembly, light assembly/repair), sitting, reading, driving at work
11585	1.5	occupation	sitting meetings, general, and/or with talking involved, eatting at a business meeting
11590	2.5	occupation	sitting; moderate (heavy levers, riding mower/forklift, crane operation), teaching stretching or yoga
11600	2.3	occupation	standing; light (bartending, store clerk, assembling, filing, duplicating, putting up a Christmas tree), standing and talking at work, changing clothes when teaching physical/education
11610	3.0	occupation	standing; light/moderate (assemble/repair heavy parts, welding, stocking, auto repair, pack boxes for moving, etc.), patient care (as in nursing)
11615	4.0	occupation	lifting items continuously, 10–20 lbs, with limited walking or resting
11620	3.5	occupation	standing; moderate (assembling at fast rate, intermittent, lifting 50 lbs, hitch/twisting ropes)
11630	4.0	occupation	standing; moderate/heavy (lifting more than 50 lbs, masonry, painting, paper hanging)
11640	5.0	occupation	steel mill, fettling
11650	5.5	occupation	steel mill, forging
11660	8.0	occupation	steel mill, hand rolling
11670	8.0	occupation	steel mill, merchant mill rolling
11680	11.0	occupation	steel mill, removing slag
11690	7.5	occupation	steel mill, tending furnace
11700	5.5	occupation	steel mill, tipping molds
11710	8.0	occupation	steel mill, working in general
11720	2.5	occupation	tailoring, cutting
11730	2.5	occupation	tailoring, general
11740	2.0	occupation	tailoring, hand sewing
11750	2.5	occupation	tailoring, machine sewing

1993 compcode	1993 METS	2000 compcode	2000 METS	heading	description
11760	4.0	11760	4.0	occupation	tailoring, pressing
		11765	3.5	occupation	tailoring, weaving
11766	6.5	11766	6.5	occupation	truck driving, loading and unloading truck (standing)
11770	1.5	11770	1.5	occupation	typing, electric, manual or computer
11780	6.0	11780	6.0	occupation	using heavy power tools such as pneumatic tools (jackhammers, drills, etc.)
11790	8.0	11790	8.0	occupation	using heavy tools (not power) such as shovel, pick, tunnel bar, spade
11791	2.0	11791	2.0	occupation	walking on job, less than 2.0 mph (in office or lab area), very slow
11792	3.5	11792	3.3	occupation	walking on job, 3.0 mph, in office, moderate speed, not carrying anything
11793	4.0	11793	3.8	occupation	walking on job, 3.5 mph, in office, brisk speed, not carrying anything
11795	3.0	11795	3.0	occupation	walking, 2.5 mph, slowly and carrying light objects less than 25 pounds
		11796	3.0	occupation	walking, gathering things at work, ready to leave
11800	4.0	11800	4.0	occupation	walking, 3.0 mph, moderately and carrying light objects less than 25 lbs
		11805	4.0	occupation	walking, pushing a wheelchair
11810	4.5	11810	4.5	occupation	walking, 3.5 mph, briskly and carrying objects less than 25 pounds
11820	5.0	11820	5.0	occupation	walking or walk downstairs or standing, carrying objects about 25 to 49 pounds
11830	6.5	11830	6.5	occupation	walking or walk downstairs or standing, carrying objects about 50 to 74 pounds
11840	7.5	11840	7.5	occupation	walking or walk downstairs or standing, carrying objects about 75 to 99 pounds
11850	8.5	11850	8.5	occupation	walking or walk downstairs or standing, carrying objects about 100 pounds or over
11870	3.0	11870	3.0	occupation	working in scene shop, theater actor, backstage employee
		11875	4.0	occupation	teach physical education, exercise, sports classes (non-sport play)
		11876	6.5	occupation	teach physical education, exercise, sports classes (participate in the class)
12010	6.0	12010	6.0	running	jog/walk combination (jogging component of less than 10 minutes) (Taylor Code 180)
12020	7.0	12020	7.0	running	jogging, general
		12025	8.0	running	jogging, in place
		12027	4.5	running	jogging on a mini-tramp
12030	8.0	12030	8.0	running	running, 5 mph (12 min/mile)
12040	9.0	12040	9.0	running	running, 5.2 mph (11.5 min/mile)
12050	10.0	12050	10.0	running	running, 6 mph (10 min/mile)
12060	11.0	12060	11.0	running	running, 6.7 mph (9 min/mile)
12070	11.5	12070	11.5	running	running, 7 mph (8.5 min/mile)
12080	12.5	12080	12.5	running	running, 7.5 mph (8 min/mile)
12090	13.5	12090	13.5	running	running, 8 mph (7.5 min/mile)
12100	14.0	12100	14.0	running	running, 8.6 mph (7 min/mile)
12110	15.0	12110	15.0	running	running, 9 mph (6.5 min/mile)
12120	16.0	12120	16.0	running	running, 10 mph (6 min/mile)
12130	18.0	12130	18.0	running	running, 10.9 mph (5.5 min/mile)
12140	9.0	12140	9.0	running	running, cross country
12150	8.0	12150	8.0	running	running (Taylor Code 200)
12160	8.0			running	running, in place
12170	15.0	12170	15.0	running	running, stairs, up
12180	10.0	12180	10.0	running	running, on a track, team practice
12190	8.0	12190	8.0	running	running, training, pushing a wheelchair
12195	3.0			running	running, wheeling, general
13000	2.5	13000	2.0	self care	standing—getting ready for bed, in general
13009	1.0	13009	1.0	self care	sitting on toilet
13010	2.0	13010	1.5	self care	bathing (sitting)

Code	METs	Heading	Specific Activity
13020	2.0	self care	dressing, undressing (standing or sitting)
13030	1.5	self care	eating (sitting)
13035	2.0	self care	talking and eating or eating only (standing)
13036	1.0	self care	taking medication, sitting or standing
13040	2.0	self care	grooming (washing, shaving, brushing teeth, urinating, washing hands, putting on make-up), sitting or standing
13045	2.5	self care	hairstyling
13046	1.0	self care	having hair or nails done by someone else, sitting
13050	2.0	self care	showering, toweling off (standing)
14010	1.5	sexual activity	active, vigorous effort
14020	1.3	sexual activity	general, moderate effort
14030	1.0	sexual activity	passive, light effort, kissing, hugging
15010	3.5	sports	archery (non-hunting)
15020	7.0	sports	badminton, competitive (Taylor Code 450)
15030	4.5	sports	badminton, social singles and doubles, general
15040	8.0	sports	basketball, game (Taylor Code 490)
15050	6.0	sports	basketball, non-game, general (Taylor Code 480)
15060	7.0	sports	basketball, officiating (Taylor Code 500)
15070	4.5	sports	basketball, shooting baskets
15075	6.5	sports	basketball, wheelchair
15080	2.5	sports	billiards
15090	3.0	sports	bowling (Taylor Code 390)
15100	12.0	sports	boxing, in ring, general
15110	6.0	sports	boxing, punching bag
15120	9.0	sports	boxing, sparring
15130	7.0	sports	broomball
15135	5.0	sports	children's games (hopscotch, 4-square, dodge ball, playground apparatus, t-ball, tetherball, marbles, jacks, acrace games)
15140	4.0	sports	coaching: football, soccer, basketball, baseball, swimming, etc.
15150	5.0	sports	cricket (batting, bowling)
15160	2.5	sports	croquet
15170	4.0	sports	curling
15180	2.5	sports	darts, wall or lawn
15190	6.0	sports	drag racing, pushing or driving a car
15200	6.0	sports	fencing
15210	9.0	sports	football, competitive
15230	8.0	sports	football, touch, flag, general (Taylor Code 510)
15235	2.5	sports	football or baseball, playing catch
15240	3.0	sports	frisbee playing, general
15250	8.0	sports	frisbee, ultimate
15255	4.5	sports	golf, general
15260	5.5	sports	golf carrying clubs
15265	4.5	sports	golf, walking and carrying clubs (See footnote at end of the Compendium)
15270	3.0	sports	golf, miniature, driving range
15280	5.0	sports	golf, pulling clubs
15285	4.3	sports	golf, walking and pulling clubs (See footnote at end of the Compendium)
15290	3.5	sports	golf, using power cart (Taylor Code 070)
15300	4.0	sports	gymnastics, general
15310	4.0	sports	hacky sack

1993 compcode	METS	2000 compcode	METS	heading	description
15320	12.0	15320	12.0	sports	handball, general (Taylor Code 520)
15330	8.0	15330	8.0	sports	handball, team
15340	3.5	15340	3.5	sports	hand gliding
15350	8.0	15350	8.0	sports	hockey, field
15360	8.0	15360	8.0	sports	hockey, ice
15370	4.0	15370	4.0	sports	horseback riding, general
15380	3.5	15380	3.5	sports	horseback riding, saddling horse, grooming horse
15390	6.5	15390	6.5	sports	horseback riding, trotting
15400	2.5	15400	2.5	sports	horseback riding, walking
15410	3.0	15410	3.0	sports	horseshoe pitching, quoits
15420	12.0	15420	12.0	sports	jai alai
15430	10.0	15430	10.0	sports	judo, jujitsu, karate, kick boxing, tae kwan do
15440	4.0	15440	4.0	sports	juggling
15450	7.0	15450	7.0	sports	kickball
15460	8.0	15460	8.0	sports	lacrosse
15470	4.0	15470	4.0	sports	motor-cross
15480	9.0	15480	9.0	sports	orienteering
15490	10.0	15490	10.0	sports	paddleball, competitive
15500	6.0	15500	6.0	sports	paddleball, casual, general (Taylor Code 460)
15510	8.0	15510	8.0	sports	polo
15520	10.0	15520	10.0	sports	racquetball, competitive
15530	7.0	15530	7.0	sports	racquetball, casual, general (Taylor Code 470)
15535	11.0	15535	11.0	sports	rock climbing, ascending rock
15540	8.0	15540	8.0	sports	rock climbing, rappelling
15550	12.0	15550	12.0	sports	rope jumping, fast
15551	10.0	15551	10.0	sports	rope jumping, moderate, general
15552	8.0	15552	8.0	sports	rope jumping, slow
15560	10.0	15560	10.0	sports	rugby
15570	3.0	15570	3.0	sports	shuffleboard, lawn bowling
15580	5.0	15580	5.0	sports	skateboarding
15590	7.0	15590	7.0	sports	skating, roller (Taylor Code 360)
		15591	12.0	sports	roller blading (in-line skating)
15600	3.5	15600	3.5	sports	sky diving
15605	10.0	15605	10.0	sports	soccer, competitive
15610	7.0	15610	7.0	sports	soccer, casual, general (Taylor Code 540)
15620	5.0	15620	5.0	sports	softball or baseball, fast or slow pitch, general (Taylor Code 440)
15630	4.0	15630	4.0	sports	softball, officiating
15640	6.0	15640	6.0	sports	softball, pitching
15650	12.0	15650	12.0	sports	squash (Taylor Code 530)
15660	4.0	15660	4.0	sports	table tennis, ping pong (Taylor Code 410)
15670	4.0	15670	4.0	sports	tai chi
15675	7.0	15675	7.0	sports	tennis, general
15680	6.0	15680	6.0	sports	tennis, doubles (Taylor Code 430)
		15685	5.0	sports	tennis, doubles
15690	8.0	15690	8.0	sports	tennis, singles (Taylor Code 420)
15700	3.5	15700	3.5	sports	trampoline

Code	METs	Category	Specific Activity
15710	4.0	sports	volleyball (Taylor Code 400)
15711	8.0	sports	volleyball, competitive, in gymnasium
15720	3.0	sports	volleyball, non-competitive, 6–9 member team, general
15725	8.0	sports	volleyball, beach
15730	6.0	sports	wrestling (one match = 5 minutes)
15731	7.0	sports	wallyball, general
15732	4.0	sports	track and field (shot, discus, hammer throw)
15733	6.0	sports	track and field (high jump, long jump, triple jump, javelin, pole vault)
15734	10.0	sports	track and field (steeplechase, hurdles)
16010	2.0	transportation	automobile or light truck (not a semi) driving
16015	1.0	transportation	riding in a car or truck
16016	1.0	transportation	riding in a bus
16020	2.0	transportation	flying airplane
16030	2.5	transportation	motor scooter, motorcycle
16040	6.0	transportation	pushing plane in and out of hangar
16050	3.0	transportation	driving heavy truck, tractor, bus
17010	7.0	walking	backpacking (Taylor Code 050)
17020	3.5	walking	carrying infant or 15 pound load (e.g. suitcase), level ground or downstairs
17025	9.0	walking	carrying load upstairs, general
17026	5.0	walking	carrying 1 to 15 lb load, upstairs
17027	6.0	walking	carrying 16 to 24 lb load, upstairs
17028	8.0	walking	carrying 25 to 49 lb load, upstairs
17029	10.0	walking	carrying 50 to 74 lb load, upstairs
17030	12.0	walking	carrying 74+ lb load, upstairs
17031	3.0	walking	loading /unloading a car
17035	7.0	walking	climbing hills with 0 to 9 pound load
17040	7.5	walking	climbing hills with 10 to 20 pound load
17050	8.0	walking	climbing hills with 21 to 42 pound load
17060	9.0	walking	climbing hills with 42+ pound load
17070	3.0	walking	downstairs
17080	6.0	walking	hiking, cross country (Taylor Code 040)
17085	2.5	walking	bird watching
17090	6.5	walking	marching, rapidly, military
17100	2.5	walking	pushing or pulling stroller with child or walking with children
17105	4.0	walking	pushing a wheelchair, non-occupational setting
17110	6.5	walking	race walking
17120	8.0	walking	rock or mountain climbing (Taylor Code 060)
17130	8.0	walking	up stairs, using or climbing up ladder (Taylor Code 030)
17140	5.0	walking	using crutches
17150	2.0	walking	walking, household walking
17151	2.0	walking	walking, less than 2.0 mph, level ground, strolling, very slow
17152	2.5	walking	walking, 2.0 mph, level, slow pace, firm surface
17160	3.5	walking	walking for pleasure (Taylor Code 010)
17161	2.5	walking	walking from house to car or bus, from car or bus to go places, from car or bus to and from the worksite
17162	2.5	walking	walking to neighbor's house or family's house for social reasons
17165	3.0	walking	walking the dog
17170	3.0	walking	walking, 2.5 mph, firm surface
17180	2.8	walking	walking, 2.5 mph, downhill

Code	METs
15710	4.0
15720	3.0
15725	8.0
15730	6.0
15731	7.0
16010	2.0
16020	2.0
16030	2.5
16040	6.0
16050	3.0
17010	7.0
17020	3.5
17025	9.0
17026	5.0
17027	6.0
17028	8.0
17029	10.0
17030	12.0
17035	7.0
17040	7.5
17050	8.0
17060	9.0
17070	3.0
17080	6.0
17090	6.5
17100	2.5
17105	4.0
17110	6.5
17120	8.0
17130	8.0
17140	4.0
17150	2.0
17160	2.5
17170	3.0
17180	3.0

1993 compcode	METS	2000 compcode	METS	heading	description
17190	3.5	17190	3.3	walking	walking, 3.0 mph, level, moderate pace, firm surface
17200	4.0	17200	3.8	walking	walking, 3.5 mph, level, brisk, firm surface, walking for exercise
17210	6.0	17210	6.0	walking	walking, 3.5 mph, uphill
17220	4.0	17220	5.0	walking	walking, 4.0 mph, level, firm surface, very brisk pace
17230	4.5	17230	6.3	walking	walking, 4.5 mph, level, firm surface, very, very brisk
		17231	8.0	walking	walking, 5.0 mph
17250	3.5	17250	3.5	walking	walking, for pleasure, work break
17260	5.0	17260	5.0	walking	walking, grass track
17270	4.0	17270	4.0	walking	walking, to work or class (Taylor Code 015)
		17280	2.5	walking	walking to and from an outhouse
18010	2.5	18010	2.5	water activities	boating, power
18020	4.0	18020	4.0	water activities	canoeing, on camping trip (Taylor Code 270)
		18025	3.3	water activities	canoeing, harvesting wild rice, knocking rice off the stalks
18030	7.0	18030	7.0	water activities	canoeing, portaging
18040	3.0	18040	3.0	water activities	canoeing, rowing, 2.0–3.9 mph, light effort
18050	7.0	18050	7.0	water activities	canoeing, rowing, 4.0–5.9 mph, moderate effort
18060	12.0	18060	12.0	water activities	canoeing, rowing, > 6 mph, vigorous effort
18070	3.5	18070	3.5	water activities	canoeing, rowing, for pleasure, general (Taylor Code 250)
18080	12.0	18080	12.0	water activities	canoeing, rowing, in competition, or crew or sculling (Taylor Code 260)
18090	3.0	18090	3.0	water activities	diving, springboard or platform
18100	5.0	18100	5.0	water activities	kayaking
18110	4.0	18110	4.0	water activities	paddle boat
18120	3.0	18120	3.0	water activities	sailing, boat and board sailing, windsurfing, ice sailing, general (Taylor Code 235)
18130	5.0	18130	5.0	water activities	sailing, in competition
18140	3.0	18140	3.0	water activities	sailing, Sunfish/Laser/Hobby Cat, Keel boats, ocean sailing, yachting
18150	6.0	18150	6.0	water activities	skiing, water (Taylor Code 220)
18160	7.0	18160	7.0	water activities	skimobiling
18170	12.0				
18180	16.0	18180	16.0	water activities	skindiving, fast
18190	12.5	18190	12.5	water activities	skindiving, moderate
18200	7.0	18200	7.0	water activities	skindiving, scuba diving, general (Taylor Code 310)
18210	5.0	18210	5.0	water activities	snorkeling (Taylor Code 320)
18220	3.0	18220	3.0	water activities	surfing, body or board
18230	10.0	18230	10.0	water activities	swimming laps, freestyle, fast, vigorous effort
18240	8.0	18240	7.0	water activities	swimming laps, freestyle, slow, moderate or light effort
18250	8.0	18250	7.0	water activities	swimming, backstroke, general
18260	10.0	18260	10.0	water activities	swimming, breaststroke, general
18270	11.0	18270	11.0	water activities	swimming, butterfly, general
18280	11.0	18280	11.0	water activities	swimming, crawl, fast (75 yards/minute), vigorous effort
18290	8.0	18290	8.0	water activities	swimming, crawl, slow (50 yards/minute), moderate or light effort
18300	6.0	18300	6.0	water activities	swimming, lake, ocean, river (Taylor Codes 280, 295)
18310	6.0	18310	6.0	water activities	swimming, leisurely, not lap swimming, general
18320	8.0	18320	8.0	water activities	swimming, sidestroke, general
18330	8.0	18330	8.0	water activities	swimming, synchronized
18340	10.0	18340	10.0	water activities	swimming, treading water, fast vigorous effort
18350	4.0	18350	4.0	water activities	swimming, treading water, moderate effort, general

Code	Category	METs	Description
18355	water activities	4.0	water aerobics, water calisthenics
18360	water activities	10.0	water polo
18365	water activities	3.0	water volleyball
18366	water activities	8.0	water jogging
18370	water activities	5.0	whitewater rafting, kayaking, or canoeing
19010	winter activities	6.0	moving ice house (set up/drill holes, etc.)
19020	winter activities	5.5	skating, ice, 9 mph or less
19030	winter activities	7.0	skating, ice, general (Taylor Code 360)
19040	winter activities	9.0	skating, ice, rapidly, more than 9 mph
19050	winter activities	15.0	skating, speed, competitive
19060	winter activities	7.0	ski jumping (climb up carrying skis)
19075	winter activities	7.0	skiing, general
19080	winter activities	7.0	skiing, cross country, 2.5 mph, slow or light effort, ski walking
19090	winter activities	8.0	skiing, cross country, 4.0–4.9 mph, moderate speed and effort, general
19100	winter activities	9.0	skiing, cross country, 5.0–7.9 mph, brisk speed, vigorous effort
19110	winter activities	14.0	skiing, cross country, > 8.0 mph, racing
19130	winter activities	16.5	skiing, cross country, hard snow, uphill, maximum, snow mountaineering
19150	winter activities	5.0	skiing, downhill, light effort
19160	winter activities	6.0	skiing, downhill, moderate effort, general
19170	winter activities	8.0	skiing, downhill, vigorous effort, racing
19180	winter activities	7.0	sledding, tobogganing, bobsledding, luge (Taylor Code 370)
19190	winter activities	8.0	snow shoeing
19200	winter activities	3.5	snowmobiling
20000	religious activities	1.0	sitting in church, in service, attending a ceremony, sitting quietly
20001	religious activities	2.5	sitting, playing an instrument at church
20005	religious activities	1.5	sitting in church, talking or singing, attending a ceremony, sitting, active participation
20010	religious activities	1.3	sitting, reading religious materials at home
20015	religious activities	1.2	standing in church (quietly), attending a ceremony, standing quietly
20020	religious activities	2.0	standing, singing in church, attending a ceremony, standing, active participation
20025	religious activities	1.0	kneeling in church/at home (praying)
20030	religious activities	1.8	standing, talking in church
20035	religious activities	2.0	walking in church
20036	religious activities	2.0	walking, less than 2.0 mph—very slow
20037	religious activities	3.3	walking, 3.0 mph, moderate speed, not carrying anything
20038	religious activities	3.8	walking, 3.5 mph, brisk speed, not carrying anything
20039	religious activities	2.0	walk/stand combination for religious purposes, usher
20040	religious activities	5.0	praise with dance or run, spiritual dancing in church
20045	religious activities	2.5	serving food at church
20046	religious activities	2.0	preparing food at church
20047	religious activities	2.3	washing dishes/cleaning kitchen at church
20050	religious activities	1.5	eating at church
20055	religious activities	2.0	eating/talking at church or standing eating, American Indian Feast days
20060	religious activities	3.0	cleaning church
20061	religious activities	5.0	general yard work at church
20065	religious activities	2.5	standing—moderate (lifting 50 lbs., assembling at fast rate)
20095	religious activities	4.0	standing—moderate/heavy work
20100	religious activities	1.5	typing, electric, manual, or computer
21000	volunteer activities	1.5	sitting—meeting, general, and/or with talking involved
21005	volunteer activities	1.5	sitting—light office work, in general

1993 compcode	1993 METS	2000 compcode	METS	heading	description
		21010	2.5	volunteer activities	sitting—moderate work
		21015	2.3	volunteer activities	standing—light work (filing, talking, assembling)
		21016	2.5	volunteer activities	sitting, child care, only active periods
		21017	3.0	volunteer activities	standing, child care, only active periods
		21018	4.0	volunteer activities	walk/run play with children, moderate, only active periods
		21019	5.0	volunteer activities	walk/run play with children, vigorous, only active periods
		21020	3.0	volunteer activities	standing—light/moderate work (pack boxes, assemble/repair, set up chairs/furniture)
		21025	3.5	volunteer activities	standing—moderate (lifting 50 lbs., assembling at fast rate)
		21030	4.0	volunteer activities	standing—moderate/heavy work
		21035	1.5	volunteer activities	typing, electric, manual, or computer
		21040	2.0	volunteer activities	walking, less than 2.0 mph, very slow
		21045	3.3	volunteer activities	walking, 3.0 mph, moderate speed, not carrying anything
		21050	3.8	volunteer activities	walking, 3.5 mph, brisk speed, not carrying anything
		21055	3.0	volunteer activities	walking, 2.5 mph slowly and carrying objects less than 25 pounds
		21060	4.0	volunteer activities	walking, 3.0 mph moderately and carrying objects less than 25 pounds, pushing something
		21065	4.5	volunteer activities	walking, 3.5 mph, briskly and carrying objects less than 25 pounds
		21070	3.0	volunteer activities	walk/stand combination, for volunteer purposes

METS for certain golfing activities were revised downward from 1993 estimates based on measurement of the activity using indirect calorimetry.

American College of Sports Medicine Certifications

This appendix details information about American College of Sports Medicine (ACSM) Certification and Registry Programs, as well as a complete listing of the current knowledge, skills, and abilities (KSAs) that comprise the foundations of these certification and registry examinations. The mission of the ACSM Committee on Certification and Registry Boards is to develop and provide high quality, accessible and affordable credentials and continuing education programs for health and exercise professionals who are responsible for preventive and rehabilitative programs that influence the health and well-being of all individuals.

ACSM Certifications and The Public

The first of the ACSM clinical certifications was initiated nearly 30 years ago in conjunction with publication of the first edition of the Guidelines for Exercise Testing and Prescription. That era was marked by rapid development of exercise programs for patients with stable coronary artery disease (CAD). ACSM sought a means to disseminate accurate information on this health care initiative through expression of consensus from its members in basic science, clinical practice, and education. Thus, these early clinical certifications were viewed as an aid to the establishment of safe and scientifically based exercise services within the framework of cardiac rehabilitation.

Over the past 30 years, exercise has gained widespread favor as an important component in programs of rehabilitative care or health maintenance for an expanding list of chronic diseases and disabling conditions. The growth of public interest in the role of exercise in health promotion has been equally impressive. In addition, federal government policy makers have revisited questions of medical efficacy and financing for exercise services in rehabilitative care of selected patients. Over the past several years, recommendations from the U.S. Public Health Service and the U.S. Surgeon General have acknowledged the central role for regular physical activity in the prevention of disease and promotion of health.

The development of the health/fitness certifications in the 1980s reflected ACSM's intent to increase the availability of qualified professionals to provide scientifically sound advice and supervision regarding appropriate physical activities for health maintenance in the apparently healthy adult population. Since 1975, more than 30,000 certificates have been awarded. With this consistent growth, ACSM has taken steps to ensure that its competency-based certifications will continue to be regarded as the premier program in the exercise field. For example, since 2002 ACSM has provided guidelines to assist colleges and universities with establishing standardized curricula that are focused on the knowledge, skills, and abilities (KSAs) requisite in the examinations for the ACSM Health/Fitness Instructor®, ACSM Exercise Specialist® and ACSM Registered Clinical Exercise Physiologist®.

Additionally, the ACSM University Connection Endorsement Program is designed to recognize institutions with educational programs that meet all of the KSAs specified by the ACSM Committee on Certification and Registry Boards (CCRB). Other examples include publishing a periodical addressing professional practice issues targeted to those who are certified, ACSM's Certified News, and oversight of continuing education requirements for maintenance of certification is another. Continuing education credits can be accrued through ACSM-sponsored educational programs such as ACSM workshops (Health/Fitness Instructor® and Exercise Specialist®), regional chapter and annual meetings, and other educational programs approved by the ACSM Professional Education Committee. These enhancements are intended to support the continued professional growth of those who have made a commitment to service in this rapidly growing health and fitness field.

Recently, ACSM, as a founder member of the multiorganizational Committee on Accreditation for the Exercise Sciences (CoAES), assisted with the development of Standards and Guidelines for educational programs seeking accreditation under the auspices of the Commission on Accreditation of Allied Health Education Programs (CAAHEP). Additional information on outcomes-based, programmatic accreditation can be obtained by visiting www.caahep.org, and specific information regarding the standards and guidelines can be obtained by visiting www.coaes.org. Because the standards and guidelines refer to the KSAs that follow, reference to specific KSAs as they relate to given sets of standards and guidelines will be noted when appropriate.

ACSM also acknowledges the expectation from successful candidates that the public will be informed of the high standards, values, and professionalism implicit in meeting these certification requirements. The College has formally organized its volunteer committee structure and national office staff to give added emphasis to informing the public, professionals, and government agencies about issues of critical importance to ACSM. Informing these constituencies about the meaning and value of ACSM certification is one important priority that will be given attention in this initiative.

ACSM Certification Programs

The ACSM certified Personal Trainer™ is a fitness professional involved in developing and implementing an individualized approach to exercise leadership in healthy populations and/or those individuals with medical clearance to exercise. Using a variety of teaching techniques, the Personal Trainer is proficient in leading and demonstrating safe and effective methods of exercise by applying the fundamental principles of exercise science. The ACSM certified Personal Trainer™ is familiar with forms of exercise used to improve, maintain, and/or optimize health-related components of physical fitness and performance. The ACSM certified Personal Trainer™ is proficient in writing appropriate exercise recommendations, leading and demonstrating safe and effective methods of exercise, and motivating individuals to begin and to continue with their healthy behaviors.

The ACSM Health/Fitness Instructor® (HFI) is a professional qualified to assess, design, and implement individual and group exercise and fitness programs for low risk individuals and individuals with controlled disease. The HFI is skilled in evaluating health behaviors and risk factors, conducting fitness assessments, writing appropriate exercise prescriptions, and motivating individuals to modify negative health habits and maintain positive lifestyle behaviors for health promotion.

The ACSM Exercise Specialist® (ES) is a is a healthcare professional certified by ACSM to deliver a variety of exercise assessment, training, rehabilitation, risk factor identification and lifestyle management services to individuals with or at risk for cardiovascular, pulmonary, and metabolic disease(s). These services are typically delivered in cardiovascular/pulmonary rehabilitation programs, physicians' offices or medical fitness centers. The ACSM Exercise Specialist® is also competent to provide exercise-related consulting for research, public health, and other clinical and non-clinical services and programs.

The ACSM Registered Clinical Exercise Physiologist® (RCEP) is an allied health professional who works with persons with chronic diseases and conditions in which exercise has been shown to be beneficial. The RCEP performs health, physical activity, and fitness assess-

ments, and prescribes exercise and physical activity primarily in hospitals or other health provider settings.

Certification at a given level requires the candidate to have a knowledge and skills base commensurate with that specific level of certification. In addition, the HFI level of certification incorporates the KSAs associated with the ACSM certified Personal Trainer™ certification, and the ES level of certification incorporates the KSAs associated with the HFI certification, as illustrated in Figure F-1. In addition, each level of certification has minimum requirements for experience, level of education, or other certifications.

How to Obtain Information and Application Materials

The certification programs of ACSM are subject to continuous review and revision. Content development is entrusted to a diverse committee of professional volunteers with expertise in exercise science, medicine, and program management. Expertise in design and procedures for competency assessment is also represented on this committee. Administration of certification is the responsibility of the ACSM National Center. Inquiries concerning certifications, application requirements, fees, and examination test sites and dates may be made to

ACSM Certification Resource Center
1-800-486-5643
Website: www.lww.com/acsmcrc
E-mail: certification@acsm.org

Knowledge, Skills, and Abilities (KSAs) Underlining ACSM Certifications

Minimal competencies for each certification level are outlined below. Certification examinations are constructed based upon these KSAs. Two companion ACSM publications, *ACSM's Resource Manual for Guidelines for Exercise Testing and Prescription, fifth edition,* and *ACSM's Certification Review Book, second edition,* may also be used to gain further insight pertaining to the topics identified here. However, neither the Guidelines for Exercise Testing and Prescription nor either of the above mentioned Resource Manuals provides all of the information upon which the ACSM Certification examinations are based. Each may prove to be beneficial as a review of specific topics and as a general outline of many of the integral concepts to be mastered by those seeking certification.

CLASSIFICATION/NUMBERING SYSTEM FOR KNOWLEDGE, SKILLS, AND ABILITIES (KSAS)

The system for classifying and numbering KSAs has been changed. It is designed to be easier to use for certification candidates, where all the KSAs for a given certification/

FIGURE F-1:

Level	Requirements	Recommended Competencies
ACSM certified Personal Trainer™	*18 years of age or older *High school diploma or equivalent (GED) *Possess current Adult CPR certification that has a practical skills examination component (*such as the American Heart Association or the American Red Cross*).	*Demonstrate competence in the KSAs required of the ACSM certified Personal Trainer™ as listed in the current edition of the *ACSM's Guidelines for Exercise Testing and Prescription* *Adequate knowledge of and skill in risk factor and health status identification, fitness appraisal and exercise prescription *Demonstrate ability to incorporate suitable and innovative activities that will improve an individual's functional capacity Demonstrate the ability to effectively educate and/or communicate with individuals regarding lifestyle modification
ACSM Health/Fitness Instructor®	*An Associate's Degree or a Bachelor's degree in a health-related field from a regionally accredited college/university (one is eligible to sit for the exam if the candidate is in the last term of their degree program), AND *Possess current Adult CPR certification that has a practical skills examination component (*such as the American Heart Association or the American Red Cross*).	*Demonstrate competence in the KSAs required of the ACSM Health/Fitness Instructor® as listed in the current edition of the *ACSM's Guidelines for Exercise Testing and Prescription* *Work-related experience within the health and fitness field *Adequate knowledge of, and skill in, risk factor and health status identification, fitness appraisal, and exercise prescription *Demonstrate ability to incorporate suitable and innovative activities that will improve an individual's functional capacity *Demonstrate the ability to effectively educate and/or counsel individuals regarding lifestyle modification *Knowledge of exercise science including kinesiology, functional anatomy, exercise physiology, nutrition, program administration, psychology, and injury prevention
ACSM Exercise Specialist®	*A Bachelor's Degree in an allied health field from a regionally accredited college of university (one is eligible to sit for the exam if the candidate is in the last term of their degree program); AND *Minimum of 600 hours of practical experience in a clinical exercise program (e.g. cardiac/pulmonary rehabilitation programs, exercise testing, exercise prescription, electrocardiography, patient education and counseling, disease management of cardiac, pulmonary, and metabolic diseases, and emergency management); AND *Current certification as a Basic Life Support Provider or CPR for the Professional Rescuer (*available through the American Heart Association or the American Red Cross*).	*Demonstrate competence in the KSAs required of the ACSM Exercise Specialist®, Health/Fitness Instructor®, as listed in the current edition of *ACSM's Guidelines for Exercise Testing and Prescription*. *Ability to demonstrate extensive knowledge of functional anatomy, exercise physiology, pathophysiology, electrocardiography, human behavior/psychology, gerontology, graded exercise testing for healthy and diseased populations, exercise supervision/leadership, patient counseling, and emergency procedures related to exercise testing and training situations.

Level	Requirements	Scope of Practice
ACSM Registered Clinical Exercise Physiologist®	*Master's Degree in exercise science, exercise physiology or kinesiology from a regionally accredited college or university *Current certification as a Basic Life Support Provider or CPR for the Professional Rescuer (*available through the American Heart Association or the American Red Cross*). *Minimum of 600 clinical hours are required with hours in each of the clinical practice areas, which may be completed as part of a formal degree program in exercise physiology. cardiovascular-200; pulmonary-100 ; metabolic-120; orthopedic/musculoskeletal-100; neuromuscular-40; immunological/hematological-40; These hours may be obtained with patients with co-morbid conditions. For example, time spent working with a patient who has Coronary Heart Disease and Parkinson's Disease may be counted in two practice areas IF you were providing exercise evaluation or programming specific to each of the conditions.	The RCEP is an allied health professional who uses exercise and physical activity to assess and treat patients at risk of or with chronic diseases or conditions where exercise has been shown to provide therapeutic and/or functional benefit. Patients for whom RCEP services are appropriate may include, but are not limited to, persons with cardiovascular, pulmonary, metabolic, cancerous, immunologic, inflammatory, orthopedic, musculoskeletal, neuromuscular, gynecological, and obstetrical diseases and conditions. The RCEP provides scientific, evidence-based primary and secondary preventive and rehabilitative exercise and physical activity services to populations ranging from children to older adults. The RCEP performs exercise screening, exercise testing, exercise prescription, exercise and physical activity counseling, exercise supervision, exercise and health education/promotion, and evaluation of exercise and physical activity outcome measures. The RCEP works individually and as part of an interdisciplinary team in clinical, community, and public health settings. The practice and supervision of the RCEP is guided by published professional guidelines, standards, and applicable state and federal regulations. The practice of clinical exercise physiology is restricted to patients who are referred by and are under the care of a licensed physician.

credential are listed in their entirety across a given Practice area and/or Content Matter area for each level of certification. Within each certification's/credential's KSA set, the numbering of individual KSAs uses a three-part number as follows:

First number–denotes Practice Area (1.x.x)

Second number–denotes Content Area (x.1.x)

Third number–denotes the sequential number of each KSA (x.x.1), within each Content Area

The Practice Areas (the first number) are numbered as follows:

1.x.x   General Population/Core
2.x.x   Cardiovascular
3.x.x   Pulmonary
4.x.x   Metabolic
5.x.x   Orthopedic/Musculoskeletal
6.x.x   Neuromuscular
7.x.x   Immunologic

The Content Matter Areas (the second number) are numbered as follows:

x.1.x   Exercise Physiology and related Exercise Science
x.2.x   Pathophysiology and Risk Factors
x.3.x   Health Appraisal, Fitness and Clinical Exercise Testing
x.4.x   Electrocardiography and Diagnostic Techniques
x.5.x   Patient Management and Medications
x.6.x   Medical and Surgical Management
x.7.x   Exercise Prescription and Programming
x.8.x   Nutrition and Weight Management
x.9.x   Human Behavior and Counseling
x.10.x Safety, Injury Prevention, and Emergency Procedures

x.11.x Program Administration, Quality Assurance, and Outcome Assessment
x.12.x Clinical and Medical Considerations (ACSM certified Personal Trainer™ only)

EXAMPLES by Level of Certification/Credential:

ACSM certified Personal Trainer™ KSAs:

0.1.10   Knowledge to describe the normal acute responses to cardiovascular exercise.

In this example, the **practice** area is General Population/Core; the **content matter** area is Exercise Physiology and Related Exercise Science; and this KSA is the **tenth** KSA within this content matter area.

ACSM Health/Fitness Instructor® KSAs:

0.3.8   Skill in accurately measuring heart rate, blood pressure, and obtaining rating of perceived exertion (RPE) at rest and during exercise according to established guidelines.

In this example, the **practice** area is General Population/Core; the **content** matter area is Health Appraisal, Fitness and Clinical Exercise Testing; and this KSA is the **eighth** KSA within this content matter area.

ACSM Exercise Specialist® KSAs°:

1.7.17   **Design a strength and flexibility programs for individuals with cardiovascular, pulmonary and/or metabolic diseases, elderly, and children.**

In this example, the **practice** area is General Population/Core; the **content** matter area is Exercise Prescription and Programming; and this KSA is the **seventeenth**

KSA within this content matter area. Furthermore, because this specific KSA appears in **bold**, it covers multiple practice areas and content areas.

°A special note about ACSM Exercise Specialist® KSAs:

Like the other certifications presented thus far, the ACSM Exercise Specialist® KSAs are categorized by content area. However, some ES KSAs cover multiple practices areas within each area of content. For example, a number of them describe a specific topic with respect to both exercise testing and training, which are two distinct content areas. Rather than write out each separately (which would have greatly expanded the KSA list length) they have been listed under a single content area. When reviewing these KSAs, please note that KSAs in **bold text** cover multiple content areas. Also, where appropriate, some KSAs mention specific patient populations (i.e., practice area). If a specific practice area is not mentioned within a given KSA, then it applies equally to each of the general population, cardiovascular, pulmonary and metabolic practice areas. Note that "metabolic patients" are defined as those with at least one of the following: overweight or obese, diabetes (type I or II), metabolic syndrome. Each KSA describes either a single or multiple knowledge (K), skill (S), or ability (A), or a combination of K, S or A, that an individual should have mastery of to be considered a competent ACSM Exercise Specialist®. Finally, as stated previously, the ACSM Exercise Specialist® candidate is also responsible for the mastery of both the ACSM Health/Fitness Instructor® and the ACSM certified Personal Trainer™ KSAs.

ACSM Registered Clinical Exercise Specialist® KSAs:

7.6.1 "List the drug classifications commonly used in the treatment of patients with a National Institutes of Health (NIH) disease, name common generic and brand names drugs within each class, and explain the purposes, indications, major side effects, and the effects, if any, on the exercising individual."

The **practice** area is Immunologic; the **content matter** area is Medical and Surgical Management; and this KSA is the **second** KSA within this content matter area.

ACSM certified Personal Trainer™ Knowledge, Skills, and Abilities (KSAs):

EXERCISE PHYSIOLOGY AND RELATED EXERCISE SCIENCE

1.1.1   Knowledge of the basic structures of bone, skeletal muscle, and connective tissues.

1.1.2   Knowledge of the basic anatomy of the cardiovascular system and respiratory system.

1.1.3   Knowledge of the definition of the following terms: inferior, superior, medial, lateral, supination, pronation, flexion, extension, adduction, abduction, hyperextension, rotation, circumduction, agonist, antagonist, and stabilizer.

1.1.4   Knowledge of the plane in which each muscle action occurs.

1.1.5   Knowledge of the interrelationships among center of gravity, base of support, balance, stability, and proper spinal alignment.

1.1.6   Knowledge of the following curvatures of the spine: lordosis, scoliosis, and kyphosis.

1.1.7   Knowledge to describe the myotatic stretch reflex.

1.1.8   Knowledge of the biomechanical principles for the performance of the following activities: walking, jogging, running, swimming, cycling, weight lifting, and carrying or moving objects.

1.1.9   Ability to define aerobic and anaerobic metabolism.

1.1.10   Knowledge to describe the normal acute responses to cardiovascular exercise.

1.1.11   Knowledge to describe the normal acute responses to resistance training.

1.1.12   Knowledge of the normal chronic physiological adaptations associated with cardiovascular exercise.

1.1.13   Knowledge of the normal chronic physiological adaptations associated with resistance training.

1.1.14   Knowledge of the physiological principles related to warm-up and cool-down.

1.1.15   Knowledge of the common theories of muscle fatigue and delayed onset muscle soreness (DOMS).

1.1.16   Knowledge of the physiological adaptations that occur at rest and during submaximal and maximal exercise following chronic aerobic and anaerobic exercise training.

1.1.17   Knowledge of the physiological principles involved in promoting gains in muscular strength and endurance.

1.1.18   Knowledge of blood pressure responses associated with acute exercise, including changes in body position.

1.1.19   Knowledge of how the principle of specificity relates to the components of fitness.

1.1.20   Knowledge of the concept of detraining or reversibility of conditioning and its implications in fitness programs.

1.1.21   Knowledge of the physical and psychological signs of overtraining and to provide recommendations for these problems.

1.1.22   Knowledge of the following terms: progressive resistance, isotonic/isometric, concentric, eccentric, atrophy, hypertrophy, sets, repetitions, plyometrics, Valsalva maneuver.

1.1.23 Ability to identify the major bones and muscles. Major muscles include, but are not limited to, the following: trapezius, pectoralis major, latissimus dorsi, biceps, triceps, rectus abdominis, internal and external obliques, erector spinae, gluteus maximus, quadriceps, hamstrings, adductors, abductors, and gastrocnemius.

1.1.24 Ability to identify the major bones. Major bones include, but are not limited to the clavicle, scapula, strernum, humerus, carpals, ulna, radius, femur, fibia, tibia, and tarsals.

1.1.25 Ability to identify the joints of the body.

1.1.26 Knowledge of the primary action and joint range of motion for each major muscle group.

1.1.27 Ability to locate the anatomic landmarks for palpation of peripheral pulses.

HEALTH APPRAISAL, FITNESS AND CLINICAL EXERCISE TESTING

1.3.1 Knowledge of and ability to discuss the physiological basis of the major components of physical fitness: flexibility, cardiovascular fitness, muscular strength, muscular endurance, and body composition.

1.3.2 Knowledge of the importance of a health/medical history.

1.3.3 Knowledge of the value of a medical clearance prior to exercise participation.

1.3.4 Knowledge of the categories of participants who should receive medical clearance prior to administration of an exercise test or participation in an exercise program.

1.3.5 Knowledge of relative and absolute contraindications to exercise testing or participation.

1.3.6 Knowledge of the limitations of informed consent and medical clearance prior to exercise testing.

1.3.7 Knowledge of the advantages/disadvantages and limitations of the various body composition techniques including, but not limited to: air displacement, plethysmography, hydrostatic weighing, Bod Pod, bioelectrical impedence.

1.3.8 Skill in accurately measuring heart rate, and obtaining rating of perceived exertion (RPE) at rest and during exercise according to established guidelines.

1.3.9 Ability to locate common sites for measurement of skinfold thicknesses and circumferences (for determination of body composition and waist-hip ratio).

1.3.10 Ability to obtain a basic health history and risk appraisal and to stratify risk in accordance with ACSM Guidelines.

1.3.11 Ability to explain and obtain informed consent.

1.3.12 Ability to instruct participants in the use of equipment and test procedures.

1.3.13 Knowledge of the purpose and implementation of pre-activity fitness testing, including assessments of cardiovascular fitness, muscular strength, muscular endurance, and flexibility, and body composition.

1.3.14 Ability to identify appropriate criteria for terminating a fitness evaluation and demonstrate proper procedures to be followed after discontinuing such a test.

EXERCISE PRESCRIPTION AND PROGRAMMING

1.7.1 Knowledge of the benefits and risks associated with exercise training in prepubescent and postpubescent youth.

1.7.2 Knowledge of the benefits and precautions associated with resistance and endurance training in older adults.

1.7.3 Knowledge of specific leadership techniques appropriate for working with participants of all ages.

1.7.4 Knowledge of how to modify cardiovascular and resistance exercises based on age and physical condition.

1.7.5 Knowledge of and ability to describe the unique adaptations to exercise training with regard to strength, functional capacity, and motor skills.

1.7.6 Knowledge of common orthopedic and cardiovascular considerations for older participants and the ability to describe modifications in exercise prescription that are indicated.

1.7.7 Knowledge of selecting appropriate testing and training modalities according to the age and functional capacity of the individual.

1.7.8 Knowledge of the recommended intensity, duration, frequency, and type of physical activity necessary for development of cardiorespiratory fitness in an apparently healthy population.

1.7.9 Knowledge to describe, and the ability to demonstrate (such as technique and breathing), exercises designed to enhance muscular strength and/or endurance of specific major muscle groups.

1.7.10 Knowledge of the principles of overload, specificity, and progression and how they relate to exercise programming.

1.7.11 Knowledge of the components incorporated into an exercise session and the proper sequence (i.e., preexercise evaluation, warm-up, aerobic stimulus phase, cool-down, muscular strength and/or endurance, and flexibility).

1.7.12 Knowledge of special precautions and modifications of exercise programming for participation at altitude, different ambient temperatures, humidity, and environmental pollution.

1.7.13 Knowledge of the importance and ability to record exercise sessions and performing periodic evaluations to assess changes in fitness status.

1.7.14 Knowledge of the advantages and disadvantages of implementation of interval, continuous, and circuit training programs.

1.7.15 Knowledge of the concept of "Activities of Daily Living" (ADLs) and its importance in the overall health of the individual.

1.7.16 Knowledge of Progressive Adaptation in resistance training and it's implications on program design and periodization

1.7.17 Understanding of personal training client's "personal space" and how it plays into a trainer's interaction with their client.

1.7.18 Skill to teach and demonstrate the components of an exercise session (i.e., warm-up, aerobic stimulus phase, cool-down, muscular strength/endurance, flexibility).

1.7.19 Skill to teach and demonstrate appropriate modifications in specific exercises for the following groups: older adults, pregnant and postnatal women, obese persons, and persons with low back pain.

1.7.20 Skill to teach and demonstrate appropriate exercises for improving range of motion of all major joints.

1.7.21 Skill in the use of various methods for establishing and monitoring levels of exercise intensity, including heart rate, RPE, and METs.

1.7.22 Knowledge of and ability to apply methods used to monitor exercise intensity, including heart rate and rating of perceived exertion.

1.7.23 Ability to describe modifications in exercise prescriptions for individuals with functional disabilities and musculoskeletal injuries

1.7.24 Ability to differentiate between the amount of physical activity required for health benefits and the amount of exercise required for fitness development.

1.7.25 Ability to determine training heart rates using two methods: percent of age-predicted maximum heart rate and heart rate reserve (Karvonen).

1.7.26 Ability to identify proper and improper technique in the use of resistive equipment such as stability balls, weights, bands, resistance bars, and water exercise equipment.

1.7.27 Ability to identify proper and improper technique in the use of cardiovascular conditioning equipment (e.g., stairclimbers, stationary cycles, treadmills, elliptical trainers).

1.7.28 Ability to teach a progression of exercises for all major muscle groups to improve muscular strength and endurance.

1.7.29 Ability to modify exercises based on age and physical condition.

1.7.30 Ability to explain and implement exercise prescription guidelines for apparently healthy clients or those who have medical clearance to exercise

1.7.31 Ability to adapt frequency, intensity, duration, mode, progression, level of supervision, and monitoring techniques in exercise programs for apparently healthy clients or those who have medical clearance to exercise

1.7.32 Ability to design resistive exercise programs to increase or maintain muscular strength and/or endurance.

1.7.33 Ability to periodize a resistance training program for continued muscular strength development

1.7.34 Ability to evaluate, prescribe, and demonstrate appropriate flexibility exercises for all major muscle groups.

1.7.35 Ability to design training programs using interval, continuous, and circuit training programs.

1.7.36 Ability to describe the advantages and disadvantages of various commercial exercise equipment in developing cardiorespiratory fitness, muscular strength, and muscular endurance.

NUTRITION AND WEIGHT MANAGEMENT

1.8.1 Knowledge of the role of carbohydrates, fats, and proteins as fuels for aerobic and anaerobic metabolism.

1.8.2 Knowledge to define the following terms: obesity, overweight, percent fat, Body Mass Index, lean body mass, anorexia nervosa, bulimia nervosa, and body fat distribution.

1.8.3 Knowledge of the relationship between body composition and health.

1.8.4 Knowledge of the effects of diet plus exercise, diet alone, and exercise alone as methods for modifying body composition.

1.8.5 Knowledge of the importance of an adequate daily energy intake for healthy weight management.

1.8.6   Knowledge of the importance of maintaining normal hydration before, during, and after exercise.

1.8.7   Knowledge of the USDA Food Pyramid.

1.8.8   Knowledge of the female athlete triad

1.8.9   Knowledge of the myths and consequences associated with inappropriate weight loss methods (e.g., saunas, vibrating belts, body wraps, electric simulators, sweat suits, fad diets).

1.8.10   Knowledge of the number of kilocalories in one gram of carbohydrate, fat, protein, and alcohol.

1.8.11   Knowledge of the number of kilocalories equivalent to losing 1 pound of body fat.

1.8.12   Knowledge of the guidelines for caloric intake for an individual desiring to lose or gain weight.

1.8.13   Knowledge of common nutritional ergogenic aids, the purported mechanism of action, and any risk and/or benefits (e.g., carbohydrates, protein/amino acids, vitamins, minerals, sodium bicarbonate, creatine, bee pollen, etc.)

1.8.14   Ability to describe the health implications of variation in body fat distribution patterns and the significance of the waist to hip ratio.

HUMAN BEHAVIOR AND COUNSELING

1.9.1   Knowledge of at least five behavioral strategies to enhance exercise and health behavior change (e.g., reinforcement, goal setting, social support).

1.9.2   Knowledge of the stages of motivational readiness.

1.9.3   Knowledge of the 3 stages of learning: Cognitive, Associative, Autonomous

1.9.4   Knowledge of specific techniques to enhance motivation (e.g., posters, recognition, bulletin boards, games, competitions). Define extrinsic and intrinsic reinforcement and give examples of each.

1.9.5   Knowledge of the different types of learners (Auditory, Visual, Kinesthetic) and how to apply teaching and training techniques to optimize a client's training session

1.9.6   Knowledge of the types of feedback and ability to use communication skills to optimize a client's training session.

SAFETY, INJURY PREVENTION, AND EMERGENCY PROCEDURES

1.10.1   Knowledge of and skill in obtaining basic life support and cardiopulmonary resuscitation certification.

1.10.2   Knowledge of appropriate emergency procedures (i.e., telephone procedures, written emergency procedures, personnel responsibilities) in a health and fitness setting.

1.10.3   Knowledge of basic first aid procedures for exercise-related injuries, such as bleeding, strains/sprains, fractures, and exercise intolerance (dizziness, syncope, heat injury).

1.10.4   Knowledge of basic precautions taken in an exercise setting to ensure participant safety.

1.10.5   Knowledge of the physical and physiological signs and symptoms of overtraining.

1.10.6   Knowledge of the effects of temperature, humidity, altitude, and pollution on the physiological response to exercise.

1.10.7   Knowledge of the following terms: shin splints, sprain, strain, tennis elbow, bursitis, stress fracture, tendonitis, patello-femoral pain syndrome, low back pain, plantar fasciitis, and rotator cuff tendonitis.

1.10.8   Knowledge of hypothetical concerns and potential risks that may be associated with the use of exercises such as straight leg sit-ups, double leg raises, full squats, hurdlers stretch, yoga plough, forceful back hyperextension, and standing bent-over toe touch.

1.10.9   Knowledge of safety plans, emergency procedures, and first aid techniques needed during fitness evaluations, exercise testing, and exercise training.

1.10.10   Knowledge of the cPT's responsibilities, limitations, and the legal implications of carrying out emergency procedures.

1.10.11   Knowledge of potential musculoskeletal injuries (e.g., contusions, sprains, strains, fractures), cardiovascular/pulmonary complications (e.g., tachycardia, bradycardia, hypotension/hypertension, tachypnea) and metabolic abnormalities (e.g., fainting/syncope, hypoglycemia/hyperglycemia, hypothermia/hyperthermia).

1.10.12   Knowledge of the initial management and first aid techniques associated with open wounds, musculoskeletal injuries, cardiovascular/pulmonary complications, and metabolic disorders.

1.10.13   Knowledge of the components of an equipment maintenance/repair program and how it may be used to evaluate the condition of exercise equipment to reduce the potential risk of injury.

1.10.14   Knowledge of the legal implications of documented safety procedures, the use of incident documents, and ongoing safety training.

1.10.15   Skill in demonstrating appropriate emergency procedures during exercise testing and/or training.

1.10.16 Ability to identify the components that contribute to the maintenance of a safe environment.

1.10.17 Ability to assist or "spot" a client in a safe and effective manner during resistance exercise

PROGRAM ADMINISTRATION, QUALITY ASSURANCE, AND OUTCOME ASSESSMENT

1.11.1 Knowledge of the cPT's role in administration and program management within a health/fitness facility.

1.11.2 Knowledge of and the ability to use the documentation required when a client shows abnormal signs or symptoms during an exercise session and should be referred to a physician.

1.11.3 Knowledge of professional liability and most common types of negligence seen in training environments

1.11.4 Understand the practical and legal ramifications of the employee vs. independent contractor classifications as they relate to personal trainers

1.11.5 Knowledge of appropriate professional conduct, practice standards, and ethics in relationships dealing with clients, employers, and other allied health/medical/fitness professionals.

1.11.6 Knowledge of the types of exercise programs available in the community and how these programs are appropriate for various populations.

1.11.7 knowledge of and ability to implement effective, professional business practices and ethical promotion of personal training services

CLINICAL AND MEDICAL CONSIDERATIONS

1.12.1 Knowledge of cardiovascular, respiratory, metabolic, and musculoskeletal risk factors that may require further evaluation by medical or allied health professionals before participation in physical activity.

1.12.2 Knowledge of risk factors that may be favorably modified by physical activity habits.

1.12.3 Knowledge of the risk factor concept of Coronary Artery Disease (CAD) and the influence of heredity and lifestyle on the development of CAD.

1.12.4 Knowledge of how lifestyle factors, including nutrition, physical activity, and heredity, influence blood lipid and lipoprotein (i.e., cholesterol: high-density lipoprotein and low-density lipoprotein) profiles.

1.12.5 Knowledge of cardiovascular risk factors or conditions that may require consultation with medical personnel before testing or training, including inappropriate changes of resting or exercise heart rate and blood pressure, new onset discomfort in chest, neck, shoulder, or arm, changes in the pattern of discomfort during rest or exercise, fainting or dizzy spells, and claudication.

1.12.6 Knowledge of respiratory risk factors or conditions that may require consultation with medical personnel before testing or training, including asthma, exercise-induced bronchospasm, extreme breathlessness at rest or during exercise, bronchitis, and emphysema.

1.12.7 Knowledge of metabolic risk factors or conditions that may require consultation with medical personnel before testing or training, including body weight more than 20% above optimal, BMI > 30, thyroid disease, diabetes or glucose intolerance, and hypoglycemia.

1.12.8 Knowledge of musculoskeletal risk factors or conditions that may require consultation with medical personnel before testing or training, including acute or chronic back pain, osteoarthritis, rheumatoid arthritis, osteoporosis, tendonitis, and low back pain.

1.12.9 Knowledge of the basic principles of electrical conduction of the heart, it's phases of contraction, and it's implications.

1.12.10 Knowledge of common drugs from each of the following classes of medications and describe their effects on exercise: antianginals; antihypertensives; antiarrhythmics; bronchodilators; hypoglycemics; psychotropics; and vasodilators.

1.12.11 Knowledge of the effects of the following substances on exercise: antihistamines, tranquilizers, alcohol, diet pills, cold tablets, caffeine, and nicotine.

ACSM Health/Fitness Instructor® Knowledge, Skills, and Abilities (KSAs):

GENERAL POPULATION/CORE: EXERCISE PHYSIOLOGY AND RELATED EXERCISE SCIENCE

1.1.1 Knowledge of the basic structures of bone, skeletal muscle, and connective tissues.

1.1.2 Knowledge of the basic anatomy of the cardiovascular system and respiratory system.

1.1.3 Knowledge of the definition of the following terms: inferior, superior, medial, lateral, supination, pronation, flexion, extension, adduction, abduction, hyperextension, rotation, circumduction, agonist, antagonist, and stabilizer.

1.1.4 Knowledge of the plane in which each muscle action occurs.

1.1.5 Knowledge of the interrelationships among center of gravity, base of support, balance, stability, and proper spinal alignment.

1.1.6 Knowledge of the following curvatures of the spine: lordosis, scoliosis, and kyphosis.

1.1.7 Knowledge to describe the myotatic stretch reflex.

1.1.8 Knowledge of fundamental biomechanical principles that underlie performance of the following activities: walking, jogging, running, swimming, cycling, weight lifting, and carrying or moving objects.

1.1.9 Ability to define aerobic and anaerobic metabolism.

1.1.10 Knowledge of the role of aerobic and anaerobic energy systems in the performance of various activities.

1.1.11 Knowledge of the following terms: ischemia, angina pectoris, tachycardia, bradycardia, arrhythmia, myocardial infarction, cardiac output, stroke volume, lactic acid, oxygen consumption, hyperventilation, systolic blood pressure, diastolic blood pressure, and anaerobic threshold.

1.1.12 Knowledge to describe normal cardiorespiratory responses to static and dynamic exercise in terms of heart rate, blood pressure, and oxygen consumption.

1.1.13 Knowledge of how heart rate, blood pressure, and oxygen consumption responses change with adaptation to chronic exercise training.

1.1.14 Knowledge of the physiological adaptations associated with strength training.

1.1.15 Knowledge of the physiological principles related to warm-up and cool-down.

1.1.16 Knowledge of the common theories of muscle fatigue and delayed onset muscle soreness (DOMS).

1.1.17 Knowledge of the physiological adaptations that occur at rest and during submaximal and maximal exercise following chronic aerobic and anaerobic exercise training.

1.1.18 Knowledge of the differences in cardiorespiratory response to acute graded exercise between conditioned and unconditioned individuals.

1.1.19 Knowledge of the structure of the skeletal muscle fiber and the basic mechanism of contraction.

1.1.20 Knowledge of the characteristics of fast and slow twitch fibers.

1.1.21 Knowledge of the sliding filament theory of muscle contraction.

1.1.22 Knowledge of twitch, summation, and tetanus with respect to muscle contraction.

1.1.23 Knowledge of the physiological principles involved in promoting gains in muscular strength and endurance.

1.1.24 Knowledge of muscle fatigue as it relates to mode, intensity, duration, and the accumulative effects of exercise.

1.1.25 Knowledge of the basic properties of cardiac muscle and the normal pathways of conduction in the heart.

1.1.26 Knowledge of the response of the following variables to acute static and dynamic exercise: heart rate, stroke volume, cardiac output, pulmonary ventilation, tidal volume, respiratory rate, and arteriovenous oxygen difference.

1.1.27 Knowledge of blood pressure responses associated with acute exercise, including changes in body position.

1.1.28 Knowledge of and ability to describe the implications of ventilatory threshold (anaerobic threshold) as it relates to exercise training and cardiorespiratory assessment.

1.1.29 Knowledge of and ability to describe the physiological adaptations of the respiratory system that occur at rest and during submaximal and maximal exercise following chronic aerobic and anaerobic training.

1.1.30 Knowledge of how each of the following differs from the normal condition: dyspnea, hypoxia, and hypoventilation.

1.1.31 Knowledge of how the principle of specificity relates to the components of fitness.

1.1.32 Knowledge of the concept of detraining or reversibility of conditioning and its implications in fitness programs.

1.1.33 Knowledge of the physical and psychological signs of overtraining and to provide recommendations for these problems.

1.1.34 Knowledge of and ability to describe the changes that occur in maturation from childhood to adulthood for the following: skeletal muscle, bone structure, reaction time, coordination, heat and cold tolerance, maximal oxygen consumption, strength, flexibility, body composition, resting and maximal heart rate, and resting and maximal blood pressure.

1.1.35 Knowledge of the effect of the aging process on the musculoskeletal and cardiovascular structure and function at rest, during exercise, and during recovery.

1.1.36 Knowledge of the following terms: progressive resistance, isotonic/isometric, concentric, eccentric, atrophy, hypertrophy, sets, repetitions, plyometrics, Valsalva maneuver.

1.1.37 Knowledge of and skill to demonstrate exercises designed to enhance muscular strength and/or endurance of specific major muscle groups.

1.1.38 Knowledge of and skill to demonstrate exercises for enhancing musculoskeletal flexibility.

1.1.39 Ability to identify the major bones and muscles. Major muscles include, but are not limited to, the following: trapezius, pectoralis major, latissimus dorsi, biceps, triceps, rectus abdominis, internal and external obliques, erector spinae, gluteus maximus, quadriceps, hamstrings, adductors, abductors, and gastrocnemius.

1.1.40 Ability to identify the major bones. Major bones include, but are not limited to the clavicle, scapula, strernum, humerus, carpals, ulna, radius, femur, fibia, tibia, and tarsals.

1.1.41 Ability to identify the joints of the body.

1.1.42 Knowledge of the primary action and joint range of motion for each major muscle group.

1.1.43 Ability to locate the anatomic landmarks for palpation of peripheral pulses.

PATHOPHYSIOLOGY AND RISK FACTORS

1.2.1 Knowledge of the physiological and metabolic responses to exercise associated with chronic disease (heart disease, hypertension, diabetes mellitus, and pulmonary disease).

1.2.2 Knowledge of cardiovascular, respiratory, metabolic, and musculoskeletal risk factors that may require further evaluation by medical or allied health professionals before participation in physical activity.

1.2.3 Knowledge of risk factors that may be favorably modified by physical activity habits.

1.2.4 Knowledge to define the following terms: total cholesterol (TC), high-density lipoprotein cholesterol (HDL-C), TC/HDL-C ratio, low-density lipoprotein cholesterol (LDL-C), triglycerides, hypertension, and atherosclerosis.

1.2.5 Knowledge of plasma cholesterol levels for adults as recommended by the National Cholesterol Education Program.

1.2.6 Knowledge of the risk factor concept of CAD and the influence of heredity and lifestyle on the development of CAD.

1.2.7 Knowledge of the atherosclerotic process, the factors involved in its genesis and progression, and the potential role of exercise in treatment.

1.2.8 Knowledge of how lifestyle factors, including nutrition, physical activity, and heredity, influence lipid and lipoprotein profiles.

HEALTH APPRAISAL, FITNESS AND CLINICAL EXERCISE TESTING

1.3.1 Knowledge of and ability to discuss the physiological basis of the major components of

physical fitness: flexibility, cardiovascular fitness, muscular strength, muscular endurance, and body composition.

1.3.2 Knowledge of the importance of a health/medical history.

1.3.3 Knowledge of the value of a medical clearance prior to exercise participation.

1.3.4 Knowledge of the categories of participants who should receive medical clearance prior to administration of an exercise test or participation in an exercise program.

1.3.5 Knowledge of relative and absolute contraindications to exercise testing or participation.

1.3.6 Knowledge of the limitations of informed consent and medical clearance prior to exercise testing.

1.3.7 Knowledge of the advantages/disadvantages and limitations of the various body composition techniques including air displacement, plethysmography, hydrostatic weighing, skinfolds and bioelectrical impedence.

1.3.8 Skill in accurately measuring heart rate, blood pressure, and obtaining rating of perceived exertion (RPE) at rest and during exercise according to established guidelines.

1.3.9 Skill in measuring skinfold sites, skeletal diameters, and girth measurements used for estimating body composition.

1.3.10 Skill in techniques for calibration of a cycle ergometer and a motor-driven treadmill.

1.3.11 Ability to locate the brachial artery and correctly place the cuff and stethoscope in position for blood pressure measurement.

1.3.12 Ability to locate common sites for measurement of skinfold thicknesses and circumferences (for determination of body composition and waist-hip ratio).

1.3.13 Ability to obtain a health history and risk appraisal that includes past and current medical history, family history of cardiac disease, orthopedic limitations, prescribed medications, activity patterns, nutritional habits, stress and anxiety levels, and smoking and alcohol use.

1.3.14 Ability to obtain informed consent.

1.3.15 Ability to explain the purpose and procedures for monitoring clients prior to, during, and after cardiorespiratory fitness testing.

1.3.16 Ability to instruct participants in the use of equipment and test procedures.

1.3.17 Ability to describe the purpose of testing, determine an appropriate submaximal or maximal protocol, and perform an assessment of cardiovascular fitness on the cycle ergometer or the treadmill.

1.3.18 Ability to describe the purpose of testing, determine appropriate protocols, and perform assessments of muscular strength, muscular endurance, and flexibility.

1.3.19 Ability to perform various techniques of assessing body composition, including the use of skinfold calipers.

1.3.20 Ability to analyze and interpret information obtained from the cardiorespiratory fitness test and the muscular strength and endurance, flexibility, and body composition assessments for apparently healthy individuals and those with stable disease.

1.3.21 Ability to identify appropriate criteria for terminating a fitness evaluation and demonstrate proper procedures to be followed after discontinuing such a test.

1.3.22 Ability to modify protocols and procedures for cardiorespiratory fitness tests in children, adolescents, and older adults.

1.3.23 Ability to identify individuals for whom physician supervision is recommended during maximal and submaximal exercise testing.

ELECTROCARDIOGRAPHY AND DIAGNOSTIC TECHNIQUES

1.4.1 Knowledge of how each of the following differs from the normal condition: premature atrial contractions and premature ventricular contractions.

1.4.2 Ability to locate the appropriate sites for the limb and chest leads for resting, standard, and exercise (Mason Likar) electrocardiograms (ECGs), as well as commonly used bipolar systems (e.g., CM-5).

PATIENT MANAGEMENT AND MEDICATIONS

1.5.1 Knowledge of common drugs from each of the following classes of medications and describe the principal action and the effects on exercise testing and prescription: antianginals; antihypertensives; antiarrhythmics; bronchodilators; hypoglycemics; psychotropics; and vasodilators.

1.5.2 Knowledge of the effects of the following substances on exercise response: antihistamines, tranquilizers, alcohol, diet pills, cold tablets, caffeine, and nicotine.

EXERCISE PRESCRIPTION AND PROGRAMMING

1.7.1 Knowledge of the relationship between the number of repetitions, intensity, number of sets, and rest with regard to strength training.

1.7.2 Knowledge of the benefits and risks associated with exercise training in prepubescent and postpubescent youth.

1.7.3 Knowledge of the benefits and precautions associated with resistance and endurance training in older adults.

1.7.4 Knowledge of specific leadership techniques appropriate for working with participants of all ages.

1.7.5 Knowledge of how to modify cardiovascular and resistance exercises based on age and physical condition.

1.7.6 Knowledge of the differences in the development of an exercise prescription for children, adolescents, and older participants.

1.7.7 Knowledge of and ability to describe the unique adaptations to exercise training in children, adolescents, and older participants with regard to strength, functional capacity, and motor skills.

1.7.8 Knowledge of common orthopedic and cardiovascular considerations for older participants and the ability to describe modifications in exercise prescription that are indicated.

1.7.9 Knowledge of selecting appropriate testing and training modalities according to the age and functional capacity of the individual.

1.7.10 Knowledge of the recommended intensity, duration, frequency, and type of physical activity necessary for development of cardiorespiratory fitness in an apparently healthy population.

1.7.11 Knowledge of and the ability to describe exercises designed to enhance muscular strength and/or endurance of specific major muscle groups.

1.7.12 Knowledge of the principles of overload, specificity, and progression and how they relate to exercise programming.

1.7.13 Knowledge of the various types of interval, continuous, and circuit training programs.

1.7.14 Knowledge of approximate METs for various sport, recreational, and work tasks.

1.7.15 Knowledge of the components incorporated into an exercise session and the proper sequence (i.e., preexercise evaluation, warm-up, aerobic stimulus phase, cool-down, muscular strength and/or endurance, and flexibility).

1.7.16 Knowledge of special precautions and modifications of exercise programming for participation at altitude, different ambient temperatures, humidity, and environmental pollution.

1.7.17 Knowledge of the importance of recording exercise sessions and performing periodic evaluations to assess changes in fitness status.

1.7.18 Knowledge of the advantages and disadvantages of implementation of interval, continuous, and circuit training programs.

1.7.19   Knowledge of the types of exercise programs available in the community and how these programs are appropriate for various populations.

1.7.20   Knowledge of the concept of "Activities of Daily Living" (ADLs) and its importance in the overall health of the individual.

1.7.21   Skill to teach and demonstrate the components of an exercise session (i.e., warm-up, aerobic stimulus phase, cool-down, muscular strength/endurance, flexibility).

1.7.22   Skill to teach and demonstrate appropriate modifications in specific exercises for the following groups: older adults, pregnant and postnatal women, obese persons, and persons with low back pain.

1.7.23   Skill to teach and demonstrate appropriate exercises for improving range of motion of all major joints.

1.7.24   Skill in the use of various methods for establishing and monitoring levels of exercise intensity, including heart rate, RPE, and METs.

1.7.25   Ability to identify and apply methods used to monitor exercise intensity, including heart rate and rating of perceived exertion.

1.7.26   Ability to describe modifications in exercise prescriptions for individuals with functional disabilities and musculoskeletal injuries

1.7.27   Ability to differentiate between the amount of physical activity required for health benefits and the amount of exercise required for fitness development.

1.7.28   Ability to determine training heart rates using two methods: percent of age-predicted maximum heart rate and heart rate reserve (Karvonen).

1.7.29   Ability to identify proper and improper technique in the use of resistive equipment such as stability balls, weights, bands, resistance bars, and water exercise equipment.

1.7.30   Ability to identify proper and improper technique in the use of cardiovascular conditioning equipment (e.g., stairclimbers, stationary cycles, treadmills, elliptical trainers).

1.7.31   Ability to teach a progression of exercises for all major muscle groups to improve muscular strength and endurance.

1.7.32   Ability to communicate effectively with exercise participants.

1.7.33   Ability to design, implement, and evaluate individualized and group exercise programs based on health history and physical fitness assessments.

1.7.34   Ability to modify exercises based on age and physical condition.

1.7.35   Knowledge and ability to determine energy cost, $\dot{V}O_2$, METs, and target heart rates and apply the information to an exercise prescription.

1.7.36   Ability to convert weights from pounds (lb) to kilograms (kg) and speed from miles per hour (mph) to meters per minute ($m.min^{-1}$).

1.7.37   Ability to convert METs to $\dot{V}O_2$ expressed as $mL.kg^{-1}.min^{-1}$, $L.min^{-1}$, and/or $mL.kg$ $FFW^{-1}.min^{-1}$.

1.7.38   Ability to determine the energy cost in METs and kilocalories for given exercise intensities in stepping exercise, cycle ergometry, and during horizontal and graded walking and running.

1.7.39   Ability to prescribe exercise intensity based on $\dot{V}O_2$ data for different modes of exercise, including graded and horizontal running and walking, cycling, and stepping exercise.

1.7.40   Ability to explain and implement exercise prescription guidelines for apparently healthy clients, increased risk clients, and clients with controlled disease.

1.7.41   Ability to adapt frequency, intensity, duration, mode, progression, level of supervision, and monitoring techniques in exercise programs for patients with controlled chronic disease (e.g., heart disease, diabetes mellitus, obesity, hypertension), musculoskeletal problems, pregnancy and/or postpartum, and exercise-induced asthma.

1.7.42   Ability to design resistive exercise programs to increase or maintain muscular strength and/or endurance.

1.7.43   Ability to evaluate flexibility and prescribe appropriate flexibility exercises for all major muscle groups.

1.7.44   Ability to design training programs using interval, continuous, and circuit training programs.

1.7.45   Ability to describe the advantages and disadvantages of various commercial exercise equipment in developing cardiorespiratory fitness, muscular strength, and muscular endurance.

1.7.46   Ability to modify exercise programs based on age, physical condition, and current health status.

NUTRITION AND WEIGHT MANAGEMENT

1.8.1   Knowledge of the role of carbohydrates, fats, and proteins as fuels for aerobic and anaerobic metabolism.

1.8.2   Knowledge to define the following terms: obesity, overweight, percent fat, lean body mass, anorexia nervosa, bulimia, and body fat distribution.

1.8.3   Knowledge of the relationship between body composition and health.

1.8.4   Knowledge of the effects of diet plus exercise, diet alone, and exercise alone as methods for modifying body composition.

1.8.5   Knowledge of the importance of an adequate daily energy intake for healthy weight management.

1.8.6   Knowledge of the difference between fat-soluble and water-soluble vitamins.

1.8.7   Knowledge of the importance of maintaining normal hydration before, during, and after exercise.

1.8.8   Knowledge of the USDA Food Pyramid.

1.8.9   Knowledge of the importance of calcium and iron in women's health.

1.8.10   Knowledge of the myths and consequences associated with inappropriate weight loss methods (e.g., saunas, vibrating belts, body wraps, electric simulators, sweat suits, fad diets).

1.8.11   Knowledge of the number of kilocalories in one gram of carbohydrate, fat, protein, and alcohol.

1.8.12   Knowledge of the number of kilocalories equivalent to losing 1 pound of body fat.

1.8.13   Knowledge of the guidelines for caloric intake for an individual desiring to lose or gain weight.

1.8.14   Knowledge of common nutritional ergogenic aids, the purported mechanism of action, and any risk and/or benefits (e.g., carbohydrates, protein/amino acids, vitamins, minerals, sodium bicarbonate, creatine, bee pollen).

1.8.15   Knowledge of nutritional factors related to the female athlete triad syndrome (i.e., eating disorders, menstrual cycle abnormalities, and osteoporosis).

1.8.16   Knowledge of the NIH Consensus statement regarding health risks of obesity, Nutrition for Physical Fitness Position Paper of the American Dietetic Association, and the ACSM Position Stand on proper and improper weight loss programs.

1.8.17   Ability to describe the health implications of variation in body fat distribution patterns and the significance of the waist to hip ratio.

HUMAN BEHAVIOR AND COUNSELING

1.9.1   Knowledge of at least five behavioral strategies to enhance exercise and health behavior change (e.g., reinforcement, goal setting, social support).

1.9.2   Knowledge of the five important elements that should be included in each counseling session.

1.9.3   Knowledge of specific techniques to enhance motivation (e.g., posters, recognition, bulletin boards, games, competitions). Define extrinsic and intrinsic reinforcement and give examples of each.

1.9.4   Knowledge of extrinsic and intrinsic reinforcement and give examples of each.

1.9.5   Knowledge of the stages of motivational readiness.

1.9.6   Knowledge of three counseling approaches that may assist less motivated clients to increase their physical activity.

1.9.7   Knowledge of symptoms of anxiety and depression that may necessitate referral to a medical or mental health professional.

1.9.8   Knowledge of the potential symptoms and causal factors of test anxiety (i.e., performance, appraisal threat during exercise testing) and how it may affect physiological responses to testing.

SAFETY, INJURY PREVENTION, AND EMERGENCY PROCEDURES

1.10.1   Knowledge of and skill in obtaining basic life support and cardiopulmonary resuscitation certification.

1.10.2   Knowledge of appropriate emergency procedures (i.e., telephone procedures, written emergency procedures, personnel responsibilities) in a health and fitness setting.

1.10.3   Knowledge of basic first aid procedures for exercise-related injuries, such as bleeding, strains/sprains, fractures, and exercise intolerance (dizziness, syncope, heat injury).

1.10.4   Knowledge of basic precautions taken in an exercise setting to ensure participant safety.

1.10.5   Knowledge of the physical and physiological signs and symptoms of overtraining.

1.10.6   Knowledge of the effects of temperature, humidity, altitude, and pollution on the physiological response to exercise.

1.10.7   Knowledge of the following terms: shin splints, sprain, strain, tennis elbow, bursitis, stress fracture, tendonitis, patellar femoral pain syndrome, low back pain, plantar fasciitis, and rotator cuff tendonitis.

1.10.8   Knowledge of hypothetical concerns and potential risks that may be associated with the use of exercises such as straight leg sit-ups, double leg raises, full squats, hurdlers stretch, yoga plough, forceful back hyperextension, and standing bent-over toe touch.

1.10.9   Knowledge of safety plans, emergency procedures, and first aid techniques needed during fitness evaluations, exercise testing, and exercise training.

1.10.10 Knowledge of the health/fitness instructor's responsibilities, limitations, and the legal implications of carrying out emergency procedures.

1.10.11 Knowledge of potential musculoskeletal injuries (e.g., contusions, sprains, strains, fractures), cardiovascular/pulmonary complications (e.g., tachycardia, bradycardia, hypotension/hypertension, tachypnea) and metabolic abnormalities (e.g., fainting/syncope, hypoglycemia/hyperglycemia, hypothermia/hyperthermia).

1.10.12 Knowledge of the initial management and first aid techniques associated with open wounds, musculoskeletal injuries, cardiovascular/pulmonary complications, and metabolic disorders.

1.10.13 Knowledge of the components of an equipment maintenance/repair program and how it may be used to evaluate the condition of exercise equipment to reduce the potential risk of injury.

1.10.14 Knowledge of the legal implications of documented safety procedures, the use of incident documents, and ongoing safety training.

1.10.15 Skill to demonstrate exercises used for people with low back pain.

1.10.16 Skill in demonstrating appropriate emergency procedures during exercise testing and/or training.

1.10.17 Ability to identify the components that contribute to the maintenance of a safe environment.

PROGRAM ADMINISTRATION, QUALITY ASSURANCE, AND OUTCOME ASSESSMENT

1.11.1 Knowledge of the health/fitness instructor's role in administration and program management within a health/fitness facility.

1.11.2 Knowledge of and the ability to use the documentation required when a client shows signs or symptoms during an exercise session and should be referred to a physician.

1.11.3 Knowledge of how to manage of a fitness department (e.g., working within a budget, training exercise leaders, scheduling, running staff meetings).

1.11.4 Knowledge of the importance of tracking and evaluating member retention.

1.11.5

1.11.6 Ability to administer fitness-related programs within established budgetary guidelines.

1.11.7 Ability to develop marketing materials for the purpose of promoting fitness-related programs.

1.11.8 Ability to create and maintain records pertaining to participant exercise adherence, retention, and goal setting.

1.11.9 Ability to develop and administer educational programs (e.g., lectures, workshops) and educational materials.

CARDIOVASCULAR: PATHOPHYSIOLOGY AND RISK FACTORS

2.2.1 Knowledge of cardiovascular risk factors or conditions that may require consultation with medical personnel before testing or training, including inappropriate changes of resting or exercise heart rate and blood pressure, new onset discomfort in chest, neck, shoulder, or arm, changes in the pattern of discomfort during rest or exercise, fainting or dizzy spells, and claudication.

2.2.2 Knowledge of the causes of myocardial ischemia and infarction.

2.2.3 Knowledge the pathophysiology of hypertension, obesity, hyperlipidemia, diabetes, chronic obstructive pulmonary diseases, arthritis, osteoporosis, chronic diseases, and immunosuppressive disease.

2.2.4 Knowledge the effects of the above diseases and conditions on cardiorespiratory and metabolic function at rest and during exercise.

PULMONARY: PATHOPHYSIOLOGY AND RISK FACTORS

3.2.1 Knowledge of respiratory risk factors or conditions that may require consultation with medical personnel before testing or training, including asthma, exercise-induced bronchospasm, extreme breathlessness at rest or during exercise, bronchitis, and emphysema.

METABOLIC: PATHOPHYSIOLOGY AND RISK FACTORS

4.2.1 Knowledge of metabolic risk factors or conditions that may require consultation with medical personnel before testing or training, including body weight more than 20% above optimal, BMI > 30, thyroid disease, diabetes or glucose intolerance, and hypoglycemia.

ORTHOPEDIC/MUSCULOSKELETAL: PATHOPHYSIOLOGY AND RISK FACTORS

5.2.1 Knowledge of musculoskeletal risk factors or conditions that may require consultation with medical personnel before testing or training, including acute or chronic back pain, osteoarthritis, rheumatoid arthritis, osteoporosis, tendonitis, and low back pain.

NOTE: The KSAs listed above for the ACSM Health/Fitness Instructor® are the same KSAs for educational programs seeking undergraduate (bachelor's degree) academic accreditation through the CoAES. Specifically, these programs are typically Exercise Science, Kinesiology, and/or Physical Education departments with professional development tracks for those students interested in careers in the fitness industry. For more information, please visit www.coaes.org.

ACSM Exercise Specialist® Knowledge, Skills, and Abilities (KSAs):

EXERCISE PHYSIOLOGY AND RELATED EXERCISE SCIENCE

1.1.1   Describe coronary anatomy.

1.1.2   Describe the physiological effects of bed rest and discuss the appropriate physical activities that might be used to counteract these changes.

1.1.3   Identify the cardiorespiratory responses associated with postural changes.

1.1.4   Describe activities that are primarily aerobic and anaerobic.

1.1.5   Identify the metabolic equivalent (MET) requirements of various occupational, household, sport/exercise, and leisure time activities.

1.1.6   Knowledge of the unique hemodynamic responses of arm versus leg exercise and of static versus dynamic exercise.

1.1.7   Define the determinants of myocardial oxygen consumption and the effects of exercise training on those determinants.

1.1.8   Determine maximal oxygen (O_2) consumption and describe the methodology for measuring it.

1.1.9   Plot the normal resting and exercise values associated with increasing exercise intensity (and how they may differ for diseased populations) for the following: heart rate, stroke volume, cardiac output, double product, arteriovenous O_2 difference, O_2 consumption, systolic and diastolic blood pressure, minute ventilation, tidal volume, breathing frequency, Vd/Vt, $\dot{V}_E/\dot{V}O_2$, and $\dot{V}_E/\dot{V}CO_2$.

1.1.10   Discuss the effects of isometric exercise in individuals with cardiovascular, pulmonary, and/or metabolic diseases or with low functional capacity.

1.1.11   Knowledge of acute and chronic adaptations to exercise for apparently healthy individuals (low risk) and for those with cardiovascular, pulmonary, and metabolic diseases.

1.1.12   Describe the effects of variation in environmental factors (e.g. temperature, humidity, altitude) for normal individuals and those with cardiovascular, pulmonary, and metabolic diseases.

PATHOPHYSIOLOGY AND RISK FACTORS

1.2.1   Summarize the atherosclerotic process, including current hypotheses regarding onset and rate of progression and/or regression.

1.2.2   Compare and contrast the differences between typical, atypical, and vasospastic angina.

1.2.3   Describe the pathophysiology of the healing myocardium and the potential complications after acute myocardial infarction (MI) (extension, expansion, rupture)

1.2.4   Describe silent ischemia and its implications for exercise testing and training.

1.2.5   Examine the role of diet on cardiovascular risk factors such as hypertension, blood lipids and body weight.

1.2.6   Describe the lipoprotein classifications and define their relationship to atherosclerosis or other diseases.

1.2.7   Describe the cardiorespiratory and metabolic responses that accompany or result from pulmonary diseases at rest and during exercise.

1.2.8   Describe the influence of exercise on cardiovascular risk factors.

1.2.9   Describe the normal and abnormal cardiorespiratory responses at rest and exercise.

1.2.10   Identify the mechanisms by which functional capacity and cardiovascular, pulmonary, metabolic, and neuromuscular adaptations occur in response to exercise testing and training in healthy and disease states.

1.2.11   Describe the cardiorespiratory and metabolic responses in myocardial dysfunction and ischemia at rest and during exercise.

HEALTH APPRAISAL, FITNESS AND CLINICAL EXERCISE TESTING

1.3.1   Describe common procedures and apply knowledge of results from radionuclide imaging (e.g., thallium, technetium, sestamibi, single photon emission computed tomography (SPECT)).

1.3.2   Knowledge of exercise testing procedures for various clinical populations including those individuals with cardiovascular, pulmonary, and metabolic diseases in terms of exercise modality, protocol, physiological measurements, and expected outcomes.

1.3.3   Describe anatomical landmarks as they relate to exercise testing and programming.

1.3.4   Locate and palpate anatomic landmarks of radial, brachial, carotid, femoral, popliteal, and tibialis arteries.

1.3.5 Select an appropriate test protocol according to the age and functional capacity of the individual.

1.3.6 Identify individuals for whom physician supervision is recommended during maximal and submaximal exercise testing.

1.3.7 Conduct pre-exercise test procedures.

1.3.8 Describe basic equipment and facility requirements for exercise testing.

1.3.9 Instruct the test participant in the use of the RPE scale and other appropriate subjective rating scales, such as the dyspnea and angina scales.

1.3.10 Obtain informed consent and describe its purpose.

1.3.11 Describe the importance of accurate and calibrated testing equipment (e.g., treadmill, ergometers, electrocardiograph, and sphygmomanometers).

1.3.12 Measure physiological and subjective responses (e.g., symptoms, ECG, blood pressure, heart rate, RPE and other scales, oxygen saturation, and oxygen consumption) at appropriate intervals during the test.

1.3.13 Describe the effects of age, weight, level of fitness, and health status on the selection of an exercise test protocol.

1.3.14 Ability to measure oxygen consumption during an exercise test.

1.3.15 Ability to provide testing procedures and protocol for children and the elderly with or without various clinical conditions.

1.3.16 Obtain and interpret medical history and physical examination findings as they relate to health appraisal and exercise testing.

1.3.17 Accurately record and interpret right and left arm pre-exercise blood pressures in the supine and upright positions.

1.3.18 Describe and analyze the importance of the absolute and relative contraindications of an exercise test.

1.3.19 Select and perform appropriate procedures and protocols for the exercise test, including modes of exercise, starting levels, increments of work, ramping versus incremental protocols, length of stages, and frequency of data collection.

1.3.20 Describe and conduct immediate postexercise procedures and various approaches to cool-down.

1.3.21 Record, organize, perform, and interpret necessary calculations of test data.

1.3.22 Describe the differences in the physiological responses to various modes of ergometry (e.g., treadmill, cycle and arm ergometers) as they relate to exercise testing and training.

1.3.23 Describe normal and abnormal chronotropic and inotropic responses to exercise testing and training.

1.3.24 Describe and apply Baye's theorem as it relates to pretest likelihood of CAD and the predictive value of positive or negative diagnostic exercise ECG results.

1.3.25 Compare and contrast obstructive and restrictive lung diseases and their effect on exercise testing and training.

1.3.26 Identify orthopedic limitations (e.g., gout, foot drop, specific joint problems) as they relate to modifications of exercise testing and programming.

1.3.27 Identify neuromuscular disorders (e.g., Parkinson's disease, multiple sclerosis) as they relate to modifications of exercise testing and programming.

1.3.28 Describe the aerobic and anaerobic metabolic demands of exercise testing and training in individuals with cardiovascular, pulmonary, and/or metabolic diseases undergoing exercise testing or training.

1.3.29 Identify the variables measured during cardiopulmonary exercise testing (e.g., heart rate, blood pressure, rate of perceived exertion, ventilation, oxygen consumption, ventilatory threshold, pulmonary circulation) and their potential relationship to cardiovascular, pulmonary, and metabolic disease.

1.3.30 Discuss the appropriate use of static and dynamic exercise for individuals with cardiovascular, pulmonary, and metabolic disease.

ELECTROCARDIOGRAPHY AND DIAGNOSTIC TECHNIQUES

1.4.1 Summarize the purpose of coronary angiography.

1.4.2 Describe myocardial ischemia and identify ischemic indicators of various cardiovascular diagnostic tests.

1.4.3 Describe the differences between Q-wave and non-Q-wave infarction.

1.4.4 Identify the ECG patterns at rest and responses to exercise in patients with pacemakers and ICDs.

1.4.5 Identify resting and exercise ECG changes associated with the following abnormalities: bundle branch blocks and bifascicular blocks; atrioventricular blocks; sinus bradycardia and tachycardia; sinus arrest; supraventricular premature contractions and tachycardia; ventricular premature contractions (including frequency, form, couplets, salvos, tachycardia); atrial flutter and fibrillation; ventricular fibrillation; myocardial ischemia, injury, and infarction.

1.4.6 Define the ECG criteria for initiating and/or terminating exercise testing or training.

1.4.7 Identify ECG changes that correspond to ischemia in various myocardial regions.

1.4.8 Describe potential causes of various cardiac arrhythmias.

1.4.9 Identify potentially hazardous arrhythmias or conduction defects observed on the ECG at rest, during exercise, and recovery.

1.4.10 Describe the diagnostic and prognostic significance of ischemic ECG responses and arrhythmias at rest, during exercise, or recovery.

1.4.11 Identify resting and exercise ECG changes associated with cardiovascular disease, hypertensive heart disease, cardiac chamber enlargement, pericarditis, pulmonary disease, and metabolic disorders.

1.4.12 Administer and interpret basic resting spirometric tests and measures including FEV1.0, FVC, and MVV.

1.4.13 Locate the appropriate sites for the limb and chest leads for resting, standard, and exercise (Mason Likar) electrocardiograms (ECGs), as well as commonly used bipolar systems (e.g., CM-5).

1.4.14 Obtain and interpret a pre-exercise standard and modified (Mason-Likar) 12-lead ECG on a participant in the supine and upright position.

1.4.15 Ability to minimize ECG artifact.

1.4.16 Describe the diagnostic and prognostic implications of the exercise test ECG and hemodynamic responses.

1.4.17 Identify ECG changes that typically occur due to hyperventilation, electrolyte abnormalities, and drug therapy.

1.4.18 Identify the causes of false positive and false negative exercise ECG responses and methods for optimizing sensitivity and specificity.

1.4.19 Identify and describe the significance of ECG abnormalities in designing the exercise prescription and in making activity recommendations.

1.4.20 Explain indications and procedures for combining exercise testing with radionuclide or echocardiographic imaging.

PATIENT MANAGEMENT AND MEDICATIONS

1.5.1 List indications for use of streptokinase, tissue plasminogen activase, and other thrombolytic agents.

1.5.2 Describe mechanisms and actions of medications that may affect exercise testing and prescription.

1.5.3 Recognize medications associated in the clinical setting, their indications for care, and their effects at rest and during exercise (e.g., antianginals, antihypertensives, antiarrythmics, bronchodilators, hypoglycemics, psychotropics, vasodilators, anticoagulant and antiplatelet drugs, and lipid-lowering agents).

MEDICAL AND SURGICAL MANAGEMENT

1.6.1 Describe percutaneous coronary and peripheral interventions (e.g., PTCA, stent) as an alternative to medical management or bypass surgery.

1.6.2 Describe indications and limitations for medical management and interventional techniques in different subsets of individuals with CAD and PAD.

EXERCISE PRESCRIPTION AND PROGRAMMING

1.7.1 Describe basic joint movements, muscle actions, and points of insertions as it relates to exercise programming.

1.7.2 Compare and contrast benefits and risks of exercise for individuals with CAD risk factors and for individuals with cardiovascular, pulmonary, and/or metabolic diseases.

1.7.3 Design appropriate exercise prescription in environmental extremes for normal individuals and those with cardiovascular, pulmonary, and metabolic diseases.

1.7.4 Design, implement and supervise individualized exercise prescriptions for people with chronic disease and disabling conditions.

1.7.5 Design a supervised exercise program beginning at hospital discharge and continuing for up to six months for the following conditions: MI; angina: LVAD; congestive heart failure; PCI; CABG; medical management of CAD; chronic pulmonary disease; weight management; diabetes; and cardiac transplants.

1.7.6 Knowledge of the concept of "Activities of Daily Living" (ADLs) and its importance in the overall rehabilitation of the individual.

1.7.7 Prescribe exercise using nontraditional modalities (e.g., bench stepping, elastic bands, isodynamic exercise, water aerobics) for individuals with cardiovascular, pulmonary, or metabolic diseases.

1.7.8 Discuss equipment adaptations necessary for different age groups.

1.7.9 Identify individuals who require exercise testing prior to exercise training.

1.7.10   Organize GXT and clinical data and counsel patients regarding issues such as ADL, return to work and physical activity.

1.7.11   Describe relative and absolute contraindications to exercise training.

1.7.12   Identify characteristics that correlate or predict poor compliance to exercise programs, and strategies to increase exercise adherence.

1.7.13   Describe the importance of warm-up and cool-down sessions with specific reference to angina and ischemic ECG changes, and for overal patient safety.

1.7.14   Identify and explain the mechanisms by which exercise may contribute to preventing or rehabilitating individuals with cardiovascular, pulmonary, and metabolic diseases.

1.7.15   Describe common gait abnormalities as they relate to exercise testing and programming.

1.7.16   Describe the principle of specificity of training as it relates to the mode of exercise testing and training.

1.7.17   Design a strength and flexibility programs for individuals with cardiovascular, pulmonary and/or metabolic diseases, elderly, and children.

1.7.18   Determine appropriate testing and training modalities according to the age and functional capacity of the individual.

1.7.19   Describe the indications and methods for ECG monitoring during exercise testing and training.

1.7.20   Describe the importance of and appropriate methods for resistance training in older individuals.

1.7.21   Ability to modify exercise testing and training to the limitations of peripheral arterial disease (PAD).

NUTRITION AND WEIGHT MANAGEMENT

1.8.1   Describe and discuss dietary considerations for cardiovascular and pulmonary diseases, chronic heart failure, and diabetes that are recommended to minimize disease progression and optimize disease management.

1.8.2   Compare and contrast dietary practices used for weight reduction and address the benefits, risks, and scientific support for each practice. Examples of dietary practices are high protein/low carbohydrate diets, Mediterranean diet, and low fat diets such as the American Heart Association recommended diet.

1.8.3   Calculate the effect of caloric intake and energy expenditure on weight management.

HUMAN BEHAVIOR AND COUNSELING

1.9.1   List and apply five behavioral strategies as they apply to lifestyle modifications, such as exercise, diet, stress, and medication management.

1.9.2   Describe signs and symptoms of maladjustment and/or failure to cope during an illness crisis and/or personal adjustment crisis (e.g., job loss) that might prompt a psychological consult or referral to other professional services.

1.9.3   Describe the general principles of crisis management and factors influencing coping and learning in illness states.

1.9.4   Identify the psychological stages involved with the acceptance of death and dying and ability to recognize when it is necessary for a psychological consult or referral to a professional resource.

1.9.5   Recognize observable signs and symptoms of anxiety or depressive symptoms and the need for a psychiatric referral.

1.9.6   Describe the psychological issues to be confronted by the patient and by family members of patients who have cardiovascular disease and/or who have had an acute MI or cardiac surgery.

1.9.7   Identify the psychological issues associated with an acute cardiac event versus those associated with chronic cardiac conditions.

SAFETY, INJURY PREVENTION, AND EMERGENCY PROCEDURES

1.10.1   Respond appropriately to emergency situations (e.g. cardiac arrest, hypoglecemia and hyperglycemia; bronchospasm; sudden onset hypotension; serious cardiac arrhythmias; implantable cardiac defibrillator (ICD) discharge; transient ischemic attack (TIA) or stroke; MI) which might arise before, during, and after administration of an exercise test and/or exercise session.

1.10.2   List medications that should be available for emergency situations in exercise testing and training sessions

1.10.3   Describe the emergency equipment and personnel that should be present in an exercise testing laboratory and rehabilitative exercise training setting.

1.10.4   Describe the appropriate procedures for maintaining emergency equipment and supplies.

1.10.5   Describe the effects of cardiovascular, pulmonary, and metabolic diseases on performance and safety during exercise testing and training.

1.10.6 Risk stratify individuals with cardiovascular, pulmonary, and metabolic diseases, using appropriate materials and understanding the prognostic indicators for high-risk individuals.

PROGRAM ADMINISTRATION, QUALITY ASSURANCE, AND OUTCOME ASSESSMENT

1.11.1 Discuss the role of outcome measures in chronic disease management programs such as cardiovascular and pulmonary rehabilitation programs.

1.11.2 Identify and discuss various outcome measurements that could be used in a cardiac or pulmonary rehabilitation program.

1.11.3 Identify and discuss specific outcome collection instruments that could be used to collect outcome data in a cardiac or pulmonary rehabilitation program.

ACSM Registered Clinical Exercise Physiologist® Knowledge, Skills, and Abilities (KSAs):

KSA # GENERAL POPULATION/CORE: EXERCISE PHYSIOLOGY AND RELATED EXERCISE SCIENCE

1.1.1 Describe the acute responses to aerobic and resistance exercise training on the function of the cardiovascular, respiratory, musculoskeletal, neuromuscular, metabolic, endocrine, and immune systems.

1.1.2 Describe the chronic effects of aerobic, resistance, and flexibility exercise training on the structure and function of the cardiovascular, respiratory, musculoskeletal, neuromuscular, metabolic, endocrine, and immune systems.

1.1.3 List typical values in sedentary and trained persons for oxygen uptake, heart rate, mean arterial pressure, systolic and diastolic blood pressure, cardiac output, stroke volume, minute ventilation, respiratory rate, and tidal volume at rest and during submaximal and maximal exercise.

1.1.4 Describe the physiological determinants of VO2, MVO2, and mean arterial pressure and explain how these determinants may be altered with aerobic and resistance exercise training.

1.1.5 Explain how environmental factors may affect the physiological responses to exercise, including ambient temperature, humidity, air quality (e.g. CO, ozone, air pollution) and altitude, and describe appropriate alterations in exercise recommendations due to environmental conditions and patient health status.

1.1.6 Explain the health benefits of a physically active lifestyle, the hazards of sedentary behavior and summarize key recommendations of US national reports of physical activity (e.g. US Surgeon General, Institute of Medicine, ACSM, AHA)

1.1.7 Explain the physiological adaptations to exercise training that may result in improvement in or maintenance of health, including metabolic (i.e., Metabolic syndrome, glucose and lipid metabolism), cardiovascular (i.e., atherosclerosis), musculoskeletal (i.e. bone density), neuromuscular, pulmonary (i.e. lung function), and immune system (i.e. colds, acute illness) health.

1.1.8 Explain the mechanisms underlying the physiological adaptations to aerobic and resistance exercise training including those resulting in changes in or maintenance of maximal and submaximal oxygen consumption, lactate and ventilatory (anaerobic) threshold, myocardial oxygen consumption, heart rate, blood pressure, ventilation (including ventilatory (anaerobic) threshold), muscle structure, bioenergetics (e.g., substrate utilization), and immune function.

1.1.9 Explain the physiological effects of physical inactivity, including bed rest, and methods that may counteract these effects.

1.1.10 Recognize and respond to abnormal signs and symptoms during exercise.

GENERAL POPULATION/CORE: HEALTH APPRAISAL, FITNESS AND CLINICAL EXERCISE TESTING

1.3.1 Conduct pre-test procedures including explaining test procedures to the patient and obtaining informed consent, obtaining a focused medical history and results of prior tests and physical exam, disease-specific risk factor assessment (i.e., CVD, Metabolic, Pulmonary diseases), presenting concise information to other health care providers and third party payers.

1.3.2 Conduct a brief physical examination including evaluation of peripheral edema, measuring blood pressure, peripheral pulses, respiratory rate, and ausculating heart and lung sounds.

1.3.3 Calibrate lab equipment used frequently in the practice of clinical exercise physiology (e.g. motorized/computerized treadmill, mechanical cycle ergometer and arm ergometer, electrocardiograph, spirometer, respiratory gas analyzer (Metabolic cart)).

1.3.4   Administer exercise tests consistent with US nationally accepted standards for testing (I.e., ACSM, AHA).

1.3.5   Identify contraindications to an exercise session

1.3.6   Appropriately select and administer functional tests to measure patient outcomes and functional status including the 6 minute walk, Get Up and Go, Berg Balance Scale, Physical Performance Test.

1.3.7   Evaluate patient outcomes from serial outcome data collected before, during and after exercise interventions.

1.3.8   Interpret the variables that may be assessed during clinical exercise testing including maximal oxygen consumption, resting Metabolic rate, ventilatory volumes and capacities, respiratory exchange ratio, ratings of perceived exertion and discomfort (chest pain, dyspnea, claudication), ECG, heart rate, blood pressure, rate pressure product, ventilatory (anaerobic) threshold, oxygen saturation, breathing reserve, muscular strength, and muscular endurance and other common measures employed for diagnosis and prognosis of disease.

1.3.9   Determine atrial and ventricular rate from rhythm strip and 12-lead ECG and explain the clinical significance of abnormal atrial or ventricular rate (e.g.. tachycardia, bradycardia).

1.3.10   Identify ECG changes associated with drug therapy, electrolyte abnormalities, subendocardial and transmural ischemia, myocardial injury, and infarction and explain the clinical significance of each.

1.3.11   Identify SA, AV, and bundle branch blocks from a rhythm strip & 12-lead ECG, and explain the clinical significance of each.

1.3.12   Identify sinus, atrial, functional, and ventricular dysrhythmias from a rhythm strip & 12-lead ECG, and explain the clinical significance of each.

1.3.13   Identify contraindications to exercise testing.

1.3.14   Determine an individual's pre-test and post-test probability of CHD, identify factors associated with test complications, and apply appropriate precautions to reduce risks to the patient.

1.3.15   Extract and interpret clinical information needed for safe exercise management of individuals with chronic disease.

1.3.16   Identify probable disease-specific endpoints for testing in a patient with chronic disease or disability.

1.3.17   Select and employ appropriate techniques for preparation and measurement of ECG, heart rate, blood pressure, oxygen saturation, RPE, symptoms (e.g., angina, dyspnea, claudication), expired gases, and other measures as needed before, during and following exercise, pharmacologic, echocardiography, and radionuclide tests.

1.3.18   Select and administer appropriate exercise tests to evaluate functional capacity, strength, and flexibility in patients with chronic disease.

1.3.19   Discuss strengths and limitations of various methods of measures and indices of body composition.

1.3.20   Appropriately select, apply, and interpret body composition tests and indices.

GENERAL POPULATION/CORE: EXERCISE PRESCRIPTION AND PROGRAMMING

1.7.1   Adapt Exercise Prescriptions for patients with comorbid conditions and disease complications.

1.7.2   Design and supervise comprehensive exercise programs for outpatients with chronic disease

1.7.3   Determine the appropriate level of supervision and monitoring recommended for individuals with known disease based on chronic disease risk stratification (e.g., cardiovascular, metabolic, musculoskeletal, etc), and current health status.

1.7.4   Develop and supervise an appropriate Exercise Prescription (e.g., aerobic, strength and flexibility training) for individuals with comorbid disease.

1.7.5   Implement appropriate precautions prior to, during, and following exercise in patients with chronic disease according to health status, medical treatment, environmental conditions, and other relevant factors.

1.7.6   Instruct individuals with chronic disease in techniques for performing physical activities safely and effectively in an unsupervised exercise setting.

1.7.7   Modify the Exercise Prescription or discontinue exercise based upon patient symptoms, current health status, musculoskeletal limitations, and environmental considerations.

GENERAL POPULATION/CORE: HUMAN BEHAVIOR AND COUNSELING

1.9.1   Summarize contemporary theories of health behavior change including social cognitive theory, theory of reasoned action, theory of planned behavior, Transtheoretical model, health belief model and apply techniques to promote healthy behaviors including physical activity .

1.9.2   Describe characteristics associated with poor adherence to exercise programs.

1.9.3   Describe the psychological issues associated with acute and chronic illness such as depression, social isolation, hostility, aggression, and suicidal ideation.

1.9.4   Counsel patients with chronic diseases and conditions on topics such as disease processes, treatments, diagnostic techniques, and lifestyle management.

1.9.5   Select and apply behavioral techniques such as goal setting, relapse prevention, and social support, which enhance adoption of and adherence to healthy behaviors including exercise.

1.9.6   Explain factors that may increase anxiety prior to or during exercise testing and describe methods to reduce anxiety.

1.9.7   Recognize signs and symptoms of failure to cope during personal crises such as job loss, bereavement, and illness.

GENERAL POPULATION/CORE: SAFETY, INJURY PREVENTION, AND EMERGENCY PROCEDURES

1.10.1   List routine emergency equipment, drugs, and supplies present in an exercise testing laboratory and therapeutic exercise session area.

1.10.2   Provide immediate responses to emergencies (I.e., first responder) including basic cardiac life support, AED, joint immobilization, activation of EMS.

1.10.3   Verify operating status of emergency equipment including defibrillator, laryngoscope, oxygen, etc.

1.10.4   Explain Universal Precautions procedures and apply as appropriate.

1.10.5   Develop and implement a plan for responding to emergencies.

GENERAL POPULATION/CORE: PROGRAM ADMINISTRATION, QUALITY ASSURANCE AND OUTCOME ASSESSMENT

1.11.1   Describe appropriate staffing for exercise programs and exercise testing laboratories based on factors such as patient health status, facilities, and program goals.

1.11.2   List necessary equipment and supplies for exercise programs and exercise testing laboratories.

1.11.3   Select, document and report treatment outcomes using patient-relevant results of tests (e.g., exercise tests, physical work simulations, biomarkers, and other laboratory tests) and surveys (e.g., physical functioning and health-related quality of life).

1.11.4   Explain legal issues pertinent to health care delivery by licensed and non-licensed health care professionals providing rehabilitative services and exercise testing (e.g., torts, contracts, informed consent, negligence, malpractice, liability, standards of care) and legal risk management techniques .

1.11.5   Identify patients requiring referral to a physician or allied health services such as physical therapy, dietary counseling, stress management, weight management, psychosocial and social services.

1.11.6   Develop a plan for patient discharge from therapeutic exercise program, including community referrals.

CARDIOVASCULAR: EXERCISE PHYSIOLOGY AND RELATED EXERCISE SCIENCE

2.1.1   Describe the indications for, physiologic responses to, and potential complications of pharmacological and pacing stress testing in individuals with cardiovascular diseases.

2.1.2   Describe the potential benefits and hazards of aerobic, resistance, and flexibility exercise in individuals with cardiovascular diseases.

2.1.3   Explain how cardiovascular diseases may affect the physiological responses to exercise training on the ischemic cascade and the components of the Fick equation.

CARDIOVASCULAR: PATHOPHYSIOLOGY AND RISK FACTORS

2.2.1   Explain current hypotheses regarding the pathophysiology of atherosclerosis, including the etiology and rate of progression of disease.

2.2.2   Describe the epidemiology, pathophysiology, risk factors, and key clinical findings of cardiovascular diseases

2.2.3   Explain the ischemic cascade and its effect on myocardial function.

CARDIOVASCULAR: HEALTH APPRAISAL, FITNESS AND CLINICAL EXERCISE TESTING

2.3.1   Describe common techniques used to diagnose cardiovascular disease, including echocardiography, radionuclide imaging, angiography, pharmacologic testing, and biomarkers (e.g., Troponin, CK, etc) and explain the indications, limitations, risks and normal and abnormal results for each.

2.3.2   Explain how cardiovascular disease may affect physical examination findings

2.3.3   List the key clinical findings during a physical exam of a patient with cardiovascular diseases.

2.3.4   Recognize and respond to abnormal signs and symptoms in individuals with cardiovascular diseases such as pain, peripheral edema, dyspnea, fatigue.

CARDIOVASCULAR: MEDICAL AND SURGICAL MANAGEMENT

2.6.1   Describe the epidemiology, pathophysiology, risk factors, and key clinical findings of cardiovascular diseases.

2.6.2   Explain the common medical and surgical treatments of cardiovascular diseases including pharmacologic therapy, revascularization procedures, ICD, pacemakers, and transplant.

2.6.3   Summarize key recommendations current U.S. clinical practice guidelines for the prevention, treatment and management of cardiovascular diseases (e.g., AHA, ACC, NHLBI)

2.6.4   List the drug classifications commonly used in the treatment of individuals with cardiovascular diseases, name common generic and brand names drugs within each class, and explain the purposes, indications, major side effects, and the effects, if any, on the exercising individual.

2.6.5   Explain how treatments for cardiovascular disease, including preventive care, may affect the rate of progression of disease.

2.6.6   Apply current U.S. national guidelines for primary and secondary prevention of heart disease (e.g., lipoproteins, obesity, pharmacologic, behavioral) to identify and manage cardiovascular risk.

CARDIOVASCULAR: EXERCISE PRESCRIPTION AND PROGRAMMING

2.7.1   Develop an appropriate Exercise Prescription (e.g., aerobic, strength and flexibility training) for individuals with cardiovascular disease.

2.7.2   Design & adapt Exercise Prescriptions for individuals with cardiovascular disease to accomodate physical disabilities and complications due to cardiovascular diseases

2.7.3   Design and supervise comprehensive outpatient exercise programs for individuals with cardiovascular disorders.

2.7.4   Instruct an individual with cardiovascular diseases and disabilities in techniques for performing physical activities safely and effectively in an unsupervised exercise setting.

PULMONARY: EXERCISE PHYSIOLOGY AND RELATED EXERCISE SCIENCE

3.1.1   Describe the potential benefits and hazards of aerobic, resistance, and flexibility exercise in individuals with Pulmonary diseases.

3.1.2   Explain how Pulmonary diseases may affect the physiologic responses to aerobic, resistance, and flexibility exercise.

3.1.3   Explain how scheduling of exercise relative to meals can affect dyspnea.

3.1.4   Explain how Pulmonary diseases may affect range of motion, muscular strength and endurance.

PULMONARY: PATHOPHYSIOLOGY AND RISK FACTORS

3.2.1   Describe the epidemiology, pathophysiology, risk factors, and key clinical findings of Pulmonary diseases

3.2.2   Explain the common medical and surgical treatments of Pulmonary diseases including pharmacologic therapy, surgery, and transplant.

PULMONARY: HEALTH APPRAISAL, FITNESS AND CLINICAL EXERCISE TESTING

3.3.1   Explain how Pulmonary disease may affect physical examination findings

3.3.2   List the key clinical findings during a physical exam of a patient with Pulmonary disease

3.3.3   Have knowledge of lung volumes and capacities (e.g., tidal volume, residual volume, inspiratory volume, expiratory volume, total lung capacity, vital capacity, functional residual capacity, peak flow rate) and how they may differ between normals and patients with Pulmonary disease.

3.3.4   Recognize and respond to abnormal signs and symptoms in individuals with Pulmonary diseases such as wheezing, cough, sputum, edema, dyspnea, fatigue.

PULMONARY: MEDICAL AND SURGICAL MANAGEMENT

3.6.1   Describe the epidemiology, pathophysiology, risk factors, and key clinical findings of Pulmonary diseases

3.6.2   List the drug classifications commonly used in the treatment of individuals with Pulmonary diseases and disabilities, name common generic and brand names drugs within each class, and explain the purposes, indications, major side effects, and the effects, if any, on the exercising individual.

3.6.3 Explain how treatments for Pulmonary disease, including preventive care, may affect the rate of progression of disease.

3.6.4 List the risk factors for Pulmonary disease and explain methods of reducing risk.

PULMONARY: EXERCISE PRESCRIPTION AND PROGRAMMING

3.7.1 Develop an appropriate Exercise Prescription (e.g., aerobic, strength, flexibility training) for individuals with chronic Pulmonary diseases.

3.7.2 Design & adapt Exercise Prescriptions for individuals with chronic Pulmonary diseases to accommodate physical disabilities and complications due to Pulmonary diseases

3.7.3 Design and supervise comprehensive outpatient exercise programs for individuals with chronic Pulmonary disease.

3.7.4 Instruct an individual with Pulmonary diseases in proper breathing techniques and exercises and methods for performing physical activities safely and effectively in an unsupervised exercise setting.

METABOLIC: PATHOPHYSIOLOGY AND RISK FACTORS

4.2.1 Describe the epidemiology, pathophysiology, risk factors, and key clinical findings of Metabolic diseases (e.g. Renal Failure, Diabetes, Hyperlipidemia, Obesity, Frailty)

4.2.2 Explain current hypotheses regarding the pathophysiology of Metabolic diseases, including the etiology and rate of progression of disease.

4.2.3 Describe the potential benefits and hazards of aerobic, resistance, and flexibility exercise in individuals with Metabolic diseases.

4.2.4 Explain how Metabolic diseases may affect the physiologic responses to aerobic, resistance, and flexibility exercise.

4.2.5 Describe the probable effects of dialysis treatment on exercise performance, functional capacity, and safety, and explain methods for preventing adverse effects

4.2.6 Describe the probable effects of hypo/hyperglycemia on exercise performance, functional capacity, and safety, and explain methods for preventing adverse effect

METABOLIC: HEALTH APPRAISAL, FITNESS AND CLINICAL EXERCISE TESTING

4.3.1 Describe common techniques used to diagnose Metabolic diseases including biomarkers, glucose tolerance testing, GFR, and explain the indications, limitations, risks and normal and abnormal results for each.

4.3.2 List the key clinical findings during a physical exam of a patient with Metabolic disease(s).

4.3.3 Explain appropriate techniques for monitoring blood glucose before, during, and after an exercise session.

4.3.4 Recognize and respond to abnormal signs and symptoms in individuals with Metabolic diseases such as hypo/ hyperglycemia, peripheral neuropathies, fluid overload, loss of appetite, low hematocrit, and hypotension, and orthopedic problems.

METABOLIC: MEDICAL AND SURGICAL MANAGEMENT

4.6.1 Describe the epidemiology, pathophysiology, risk factors, and key clinical findings of Metabolic diseases (e.g. Renal Failure, Diabetes, Hyperlipidemia, Obesity, Frailty).

4.6.2 Summarize key recommendations of current U.S. clinical practice guidelines (e.g. ADA, NIH, NHLBI) for the prevention, treatment and management of Metabolic diseases (e.g. Renal Failure, Diabetes, Hyperlipidemia, Obesity, Frailty)

4.6.3 Explain the common medical and surgical treatments of Metabolic diseases including pharmacologic therapy, surgery, and transplant.

4.6.4 List the drug classifications commonly used in the treatment of patients with Metabolic disease, name common generic and brand names drugs within each class, and explain the purposes, indications, major side effects, and the effects, if any, on the exercising individual.

4.6.5 Explain how treatments for Metabolic diseases, including preventive care, may affect the rate of progression of disease.

4.6.6 Apply current U.S. national guidelines for prevention of Metabolic diseases to identify and manage disease complications and reduce cardiovascular risk (i.e. ADA).

4.6.7 Apply current U.S. national guidelines for primary prevention of heart disease (e.g., lipoproteins, obesity, pharmacologic, behavioral) to identify and manage cardiovascular risk.

METABOLIC: EXERCISE PRESCRIPTION AND PROGRAMMING

4.7.1 Develop an appropriate Exercise Prescription (e.g., aerobic, strength, flexibility training) for individuals with Metabolic disease.

4.7.2   Design, adapt, and supervise an Exercise Prescription for patients with complications due to Metabolic diseases (e.g., amputations, retinopathy, autonomic neuropathies, vision impairment, hypotension, hypertension and during hemodialysis treatments)

4.7.3   Design and supervise comprehensive outpatient exercise programs for individuals with Metabolic diseases.

4.7.4   Instruct individuals with Metabolic diseases in techniques for performing physical activities safely and effectively in an unsupervised exercise setting.

ORTHOPEDIC/MUSCULOSKELETAL: EXERCISE PHYSIOLOGY AND RELATED EXERCISE SCIENCE

5.1.1   Describe the potential benefits and hazards of aerobic, resistance, and flexibility exercise in individuals with musculoskeletal diseases and disabilities (e.g., low back pain, arthritis, osteoporosis/fibromyalgia, and tendinitis/impingement syndrome, amputation).

5.1.2   Explain how musculoskeletal diseases may affect the physiologic responses to aerobic, resistance, and flexibility exercise.

5.1.3   Describe the appropriate use of rest, spinal extension-flexion exercises vs. lumbar stabilization, and the appropriate dose of avoidance of physical activity in patients with back pain.

5.1.4   Explain how musculoskeletal diseases and disabilities may affect functional capacity, range of motion, balance, agility, muscular strength and endurance.

ORTHOPEDIC/MUSCULOSKELETAL: PATHOPHYSIOLOGY AND RISK FACTORS

5.2.1   Describe the epidemiology, pathophysiology, risk factors, and key clinical findings of orthopedic/musculoskeletal diseases & disabilities (e.g., low back pain, arthritis, osteoporosis, tendonitis/impingement syndrome, and amputation)

ORTHOPEDIC/MUSCULOSKELETAL: HEALTH APPRAISAL, FITNESS AND CLINICAL EXERCISE TESTING

5.3.1   Recognize and respond to abnormal signs and symptoms in individuals with musculoskeletal diseases and disabilities such as pain, muscle weakness.

ORTHOPEDIC/MUSCULOSKELETAL: MEDICAL AND SURGICAL MANAGEMENT

5.6.1   List the drug classifications commonly used in the treatment of patients with musculoskeletal diseases and disabilities, name common generic and brand names drugs within each class, and explain the purposes, indications, major side effects, and the effects, if any, on the exercising individual.

5.6.2   Explain how treatments for musculoskeletal disease, including preventive care, may affect the rate of progression of disease.

ORTHOPEDIC/MUSCULOSKELETAL: EXERCISE PRESCRIPTION AND PROGRAMMING

5.7.1   Explain exercise training concepts specific to industrial or occupational rehabilitation, which includes work hardening, work conditioning, work fitness, and job coaching.

5.7.2   Design, adapt, and supervise an Exercise Prescription (aerobic, strength, and flexibility training) to accommodate patients with complications due to musculoskeletal diseases & disabilities (e.g., low back pain, arthritis, osteoporosis, tendonitis/impingement syndrome and amputation)

5.7.3   Instruct an individual with musculoskeletal diseases and disabilities in techniques for performing physical activities safely and effectively in an unsupervised exercise setting.

NEUROMUSCULAR: EXERCISE PHYSIOLOGY AND RELATED EXERCISE SCIENCE

6.1.1   Describe the potential benefits and hazards of aerobic, resistance, and flexibility exercise in individuals with Neuromuscular diseases & disabilities (e.g., Multiple Sclerosis, Muscular Dystrophy, Parkinson's Disease, Polio and Post Polio Syndrome, Stroke and Head Injury, Cerebral Palsy, Amyotrophic Lateral Sclerosis, Peripheral Neuropathy, Spinal cord injury, Epilepsy)

6.1.2   Explain how Neuromuscular diseases may affect the physiologic responses to aerobic, resistance, and flexibility exercise.

6.1.3   Describe the effects of nonmotor complications, such as fatigue, on exercise performance in patients with Neuromuscular diseases and disabilities.

6.1.4   Explain how Neuromuscular diseases and disabilities may affect range of motion, balance, agility, muscular strength and endurance.

NEUROMUSCULAR: HEALTH APPRAISAL, FITNESS AND CLINICAL EXERCISE TESTING

6.3.1 Recognize and respond to abnormal signs and symptoms in individuals with Neuromuscular diseases and disabilities such as muscle weakness, cognitive deficit, fatigue.

NEUROMUSCULAR: EXERCISE PRESCRIPTION AND PROGRAMMING

6.7.1 Adapt the Exercise Prescription based on the functional limits and benefits of assistive devices (e.g. wheelchairs, crutches, and canes).

6.7.2 Develop an appropriate Exercise Prescription (e.g. aerobic, strength, flexibility training) for individuals with Neuromuscular diseases and disabilities including those treated with surgery.

6.7.3 Design, Adapt, and Supervise aerobic, strength training and flexibility exercise routines to accommodate patients with complications due to Neuromuscular diseases and disabilities (e.g., Multiple Sclerosis, Muscular Dystrophy, Parkinson's Disease, Polio and Post Polio Syndrome, Stroke and Head Injury, Cerebral Palsy, Amyotrophic Lateral Sclerosis, Peripheral Neuropathy, Spinal cord injury, Epilepsy)

6.7.4 Instruct an individual with Neuromuscular diseases and disabilities in techniques for performing physical activities safely and effectively in an unsupervised exercise setting.

IMMUNOLOGIC: EXERCISE PHYSIOLOGY AND RELATED EXERCISE SCIENCE

7.1.1 Describe the immediate and long-term influence of medical therapies for NIH on Cardiopulmonary and musculoskeletal responses to exercise training.

7.1.2 Describe the potential benefits and hazards of aerobic, resistance, and flexibility exercise in individuals with NIH disease (e.g. cancer, anemia, bleeding disorders, AIDS, organ transplant, Chronic Fatigue Syndrome)

7.1.3 Explain how NIH diseases may affect the physiologic responses to aerobic, resistance, and flexibility exercise.

7.1.4 Explain how cancer therapy (e.g., surgery, radiation, and chemotherapy) may affect functional capacity, range of motion, and the physiological responses to exercise.

7.1.5 Apply current U.S. national guidelines for primary and secondary prevention of NIH disease (e.g. ACS, NIH).

IMMUNOLOGIC: PATHOPHYSIOLOGY AND RISK FACTORS

7.2.1 Describe the epidemiology, pathophysiology, risk factors, and key clinical findings of NIH diseases (e.g. cancer, anemia, bleeding disorders, AIDS, organ transplant, Chronic Fatigue Syndrome)

IMMUNOLOGIC: HEALTH APPRAISAL, FITNESS AND CLINICAL EXERCISE TESTING

7.3.1 Recognize and respond to abnormal signs and symptoms in individuals with NIH diseases such as fatigue, dyspnea, tachycardia.

IMMUNOLOGIC: MEDICAL AND SURGICAL MANAGEMENT

7.6.1 List the drug classifications commonly used in the treatment of patients with NIH disease, name common generic and brand names drugs within each class, and explain the purposes, indications, major side effects, and the effects, if any, on the exercising individual.

7.6.2 Summarize key recommendations of current U.S. clinical practice guidelines (e.g. ACS, NIH) for the prevention, treatment and management of NIH diseases (e.g. cancer, anemia, bleeding disorders, AIDS, organ transplant, Chronic Fatigue Syndrome)

7.6.3 Explain the common medical and surgical treatments of NIH diseases including pharmacologic therapy, and surgery.

IMMUNOLOGIC: EXERCISE PRESCRIPTION AND PROGRAMMING

7.7.1 Develop an appropriate Exercise Prescription (e.g. aerobic, strength, flexibility training) for individuals with NIH disorders (e.g. cancer, anemia, bleeding disorders, AIDS, organ transplant, Chronic Fatigue Syndrome)

7.7.2 Design, adapt, and supervise the Exercise Prescription to accommodate patients with physical disabilities and complications due to NIH diseases

7.7.3 Design and supervise comprehensive outpatient exercise programs for individuals with immunologic/hematological disorders (e.g. cancer, anemia, bleeding disorders, AIDS, organ transplant, Chronic Fatigue Syndrome)

7.7.4 Instruct an individual with immunologic/hematological diseases and disabilities in techniques for performing physical activities safely and effectively in an unsupervised exercise setting.

NOTE: The KSAs listed above for the ACSM Registered Clinical Exercise Specialist® are the same KSAs for educational programs in Clinical Exercise Physiology seeking graduate (master's degree) academic accreditation through the CoAES . For more information, please visit www.coaes.org.

Additional KSAs required (in addition to the ACSM Health/Fitness Instructor® KSAs) for programs seeking academic accreditation in Applied Exercise Physiology

The KSAs that follow, IN ADDITION TO the ACSM Health/Fitness Instructor® KSAs above, represent the KSAs for educational programs in Applied Exercise Physiology seeking graduate (master's degree) academic accreditation through the CoAES. For more information, please visit www.coaes.org.

KSA # GENERAL POPULATION/CORE: EXERCISE PHYSIOLOGY AND RELATED EXERCISE SCIENCE

1.1.1   Ability to describe modifications in exercise prescription for individuals with functional disabilities and musculoskeletal injuries.

1.1.2   Ability to describe the relationship between biomechanical efficiency, oxygen cost of activity (economy), and performance of physical activity.

1.1.3   Knowledge of the muscular, cardiorespiratory, and metabolic responses to decreased exercise intensity.

GENERAL POPULATION/CORE: PATHOPHYSIOLOGY AND RISK FACTORS

1.2.1   Ability to define atherosclerosis, the factors causing it, and the interventions that may potentially delay or reverse the atherosclerotic process.

1.2.2   Ability to describe the causes of myocardial ischemia and infarction.

1.2.3   Ability to describe the pathophysiology of hypertension, obesity, hyperlipidemia, diabetes, chronic obstructive pulmonary diseases, arthritis, osteoporosis, chronic diseases, and immunosuppressive disease.

1.2.4   Ability to describe the effects of the above diseases and conditions on cardiorespiratory and metabolic function at rest and during exercise.

GENERAL POPULATION/CORE: HEALTH APPRAISAL, FITNESS AND CLINICAL EXERCISE TESTING

1.3.1   Knowledge of the selection of an appropriate behavioral goal and the suggested method to evaluate goal achievement for each stage of change.

1.3.2   Knowledge of the use and value of the results of the fitness evaluation and exercise test for various populations.

1.3.3   Ability to design and implement a fitness testing/health appraisal program that includes, but is not limited to, staffing needs, physician interaction, documentation, equipment, marketing, and program evaluation.

1.3.4   Ability to recruit, train, and evaluate appropriate staff personnel for performing exercise tests, fitness evaluations, and health appraisals.

GENERAL POPULATION/CORE: MEDICAL AND SURGICAL MANAGEMENT

1.5.1   Ability to identify and describe the principal action, mechanisms of action, and major side effects from each of the following classes of medications: Antianginals, Antihypertensives, Antiarrhythmics, Bronchodilators, Hypoglycemics, Psychotropics, and Vasodilators.

GENERAL POPULATION/CORE: HUMAN BEHAVIOR AND COUNSELING

1.9.1   Knowledge of and ability to apply basic cognitive-behavioral intervention such as shaping, goal setting, motivation, cueing, problem solving, reinforcement strategies, and self-monitoring.

1.9.2   Knowledge of the selection of an appropriate behavioral goal and the suggested method to evaluate goal achievement for each stage of change.

GENERAL POPULATION/CORE: SAFETY, INJURY PREVENTION, AND EMERGENCY PROCEDURES

1.10.1   Ability to identify the process to train the exercise staff in cardiopulmonary resuscitation.

1.10.2   Ability to design and evaluate emergency procedures for a preventive exercise program and an exercise testing facility.

1.10.3   Ability to train staff in safety procedures, risk reduction strategies, and injury care techniques.

1.10.4 Knowledge of the legal implications of documented safety procedures, the use of incident documents, and ongoing safety training.

GENERAL POPULATION/CORE: PROGRAM ADMINISTRATION, QUALITY ASSURANCE AND OUTCOME ASSESSMENT

1.11.1 Ability to manage personnel effectively.

1.11.2 Ability to describe a management plan for the development of staff, continuing education, marketing and promotion, documentation, billing, facility management, and financial planning.

1.11.3 Ability to describe the decision-making process related to budgets, market analysis, program evaluation, facility management, staff allocation, and community development.

1.11.4 Ability to describe the development, evaluation, and revision of policies and procedures for programming and facility management.

1.11.5 Ability to describe how the computer can assist in data analysis, spreadsheet report development, and daily tracking of customer utilization.

1.11.6 Ability to define and describe the total quality management (TQM) and continuous quality improvement (CQI) approaches to management.

1.11.7 Ability to interpret applied research in the areas of exercise testing, exercise programming, and educational programs to maintain a comprehensive and current state-of-the-art program.

1.11.8 Ability to develop a risk factor screening program, including procedures, staff training, feedback, and follow-up.

1.11.9 Knowledge of administration, management and supervision of personnel.

1.11.10 Ability to describe effective interviewing, hiring, and employee termination procedures.

1.11.11 Ability to describe and diagram an organizational chart and show the relationships between a health/fitness director, owner, medical advisor, and staff.

1.11.12 Knowledge of and ability to describe various staff training techniques.

1.11.13 Knowledge of and ability to describe performance reviews and their roll in evaluating staff.

1.11.14 Knowledge of the legal obligations and problems involved in personnel management.

1.11.15 Knowledge of compensation, including wages, bonuses, incentive programs, and benefits.

1.11.16 Knowledge of methods for implementing a sales commission system.

1.11.17 Ability to describe the significance of a benefits program for staff and demonstrate an understanding in researching and selecting benefits.

1.11.18 Ability to write and implement thorough and legal job descriptions.

1.11.19 Knowledge of personnel time management techniques.

1.11.20 Knowledge of administration, management, and development of a budget and of the financial aspects of a fitness center.

1.11.21 Knowledge of the principles of financial management.

1.11.22 Knowledge of basic accounting principles such as accounts payable, accounts receivable, accrual, cash flow, assets, liabilities, and return on investment.

1.11.23 Ability to identify the various forms of a business enterprise such as sole proprietorship, partnership, corporation, and S-corporation.

1.11.24 Knowledge of the procedures involved with developing, evaluating, revising, and updating capital and operating budgets.

1.11.25 Ability to manage expenses with the objective of maintaining a positive cash flow.

1.11.26 Ability to understand and analyze financial statements, including income statements, balance sheets, cash flows, budgets, and pro forma projections.

1.11.27 Knowledge of program-related break-even and cost/benefit analysis.

1.11.28 Knowledge of the importance of short-term and long-term planning.

1.11.29 Knowledge of the principles of marketing and sales.

1.11.30 Ability to identify the steps in the development, implementation, and evaluation of a marketing plan.

1.11.31 Knowledge of the components of a needs assessment/market analysis.

1.11.32 Knowledge of various sales techniques for prospective members.

1.11.33 Knowledge of techniques for advertising, marketing, promotion, and public relations.

1.11.34 Ability to describe the principles of developing and evaluating product and services, and establishing pricing.

1.11.35 Knowledge of the principles of day-to-day operation of a fitness center.

1.11.36 Knowledge of the principles of pricing and purchasing equipment and supplies.

1.11.37 Knowledge of facility layout and design.

1.11.38 Ability to establish and evaluate an equipment preventive maintenance and repair program.

1.11.39 Ability to describe a plan for implementing a housekeeping program.

1.11.40   Ability to identify and explain the operating policies for preventive exercise programs, including data analysis and reporting, confidentiality of records, relationships with health care providers, accident and injury reporting, and continuing education of participants.

1.11.41   Knowledge of the legal concepts of tort, negligence, liability, indemnification, standards of care, health regulations, consent, contract, confidentiality, malpractice, and the legal concerns regarding emergency procedures and informed consent.

1.11.42   Ability to implement capital improvements with minimal disruption of client or business needs.

1.11.43   Ability to coordinate the operations of various departments, including, but not limited to, the front desk, fitness, rehabilitation, maintenance and repair, day care, housekeeping, pool, and management.

1.11.44   Knowledge of management and principles of member service and communication.

1.11.45   Skills in effective techniques for communicating with staff, management, members, health care providers, potential customers, and vendors.

1.11.46   Knowledge of and ability to provide strong customer service.

1.11.47   Ability to develop and implement customer surveys.

1.11.48   Knowledge of the strategies for management conflict.

1.11.49   Knowledge of the principles of health promotion and ability to administer health promotion programs.

1.11.50   Knowledge of health promotion programs (e.g., nutrition and weight management, smoking cessation, stress management, back care, body mechanics, and substance abuse).

1.11.51   Knowledge of the specific and appropriate content and methods for creating a health promotion program.

1.11.52   Knowledge of and ability to access resources for various programs and delivery systems.

1.11.53   Knowledge of the concepts of cost-effectiveness and cost-benefit as they relate to the evaluation of health promotion programming.

1.11.54   Ability to describe the means and amounts by which health promotion programs might increase productivity, reduce employee loss time, reduce health care costs, and improve profitability in the workplace.

Index

Page numbers in *italics* denote figures; those followed by t denote tables, those followed by b denote boxes

A

A band, 25–26
AACVPR, (*See* American Association of Cardiovascular and Pulmonary Rehabilitation)
ABCDE treatment, of angina pectoris, 433
Abdomen, acute and chronic musculoskeletal injuries of, 396t
ABI, (*See* Ankle-brachial index)
Acarbose (Precose), 474
ACC, (*See* American College of Cardiology)
Accelerometer(s), 136, 137, 139, 140–141
Accommodating resistance, 352
Acquired immune deficiency syndrome (AIDS), 529
Acquired immunity, 529
ACS, (*See* Acute coronary syndromes)
ACSM, (*See* American College of Sports Medicine)
ACSM certified Personal Trainer™, 700
knowledge, skills, abilities required for, 703–707
requirements for, *701*
ACSM Exercise Specialist®, 700
knowledge, skills, abilities required for, 714–718
requirements for, *701*
ACSM Health/Fitness Instructor®, 700
knowledge, skills, abilities required for, 707–714
requirements for, *701*
ACSM Registered Clinical Exercise Physiologist®, 700
requirements for, *702*
knowledge, skills, abilities required for, 718–725
Actin, 25–26
Active listening, 589–590
Active range of motion (AROM), 21
Active stretching, 217
ACTIVITYGRAM, 137
Acute coronary syndromes (ACS), 412
diagnosis of, 432–433
pathophysiology of, 418–419 (*See also* Acute myocardial infarction; Angina pectoris; Sudden cardiac arrest)
treatment of, 430t, 432–433
Acute mountain sickness (AMS), 46, 71–72
Acute myocardial infarction, 303, 412, 418
classification of, 419
complications of, 420b
diagnosis of, 418–419
electrocardiographic interpretation in, 305–309, 419
pathological Q wave differentiation, 307
pathological Q waves, 305–306, 420t
ST segment changes, 305–309

leads and injured regions in, 306–307
pathophysiology of, 416–418, *418–419*
symptoms of, 418
treatment of, post infarction, 432–433
triggers of, 418, 419b
Acute pericarditis, 304
ST segment changes in, 307–308, *308*
ADA, (*See* Americans with Disabilities Act)
Adaptation, principle of, 336
Adaptive immunity, 529
Adenosine triphosphate (ATP)
in bioenergetic pathways, 52–53
and creatine phosphate system, 46
glycolysis in formation of, 47
hydrolysis of, 46
mechanisms of formation of, 47t
oxidative phosphorylation of, 47–48
Adherence, to regular physical activity, 565–580, (*See also* Exercise compliance)
behavioral factors influencing, 567–568 (*See also* Health behavior change)
decisional balance in, 548, 593–594
demographics of, 566
enhancing, 577–580
factors influencing, 565
environmental, 568–569, 573–577
personal, 566–567, 572–573
program related, 568–569, 573–577
in specific populations, 569
goal setting in, 574–576, 594, 596
Internet resources on, 571, 580
problem solving in, 594, 595b
references on, 570–571, 580
relapse prevention in, 555–556, 596
self-efficacy in, 549, 573, 596
stages of change access in, 590–591, 591b (*See also* Health behavior change)
tracking client activity in, 591–593
Adipocyte, 367
Administration, of exercise programs and facilities, (*See* Exercise program facilities)
Adolescents, resistance training programs for, 360–361
Advanced directives, 651
Advocacy, 559, 563
AED, (*See* Automated external defibrillator)
Aerobic energy sources, 46–49, *49*
Aerobic exercise, mixed impact, 380–381
Aerobic fitness, 313–314, 336, 337, 376, 602, (*See also* Cardiopulmonary adaptation)
Aerobic kickboxing, 382
Aerobics and Fitness Association of America, standards of practice of, 663
Agency for Health Care Policy and Research, standards of practice of, 663
Aging, and older adults, 79–83
cardiovascular system in, 79–81
fluid regulation in, 82–83

immune system in, 82
Internet resources on, 92
muscle strength assessment in, 214–215
musculoskeletal system in, 81–82
nervous system in, 82
neuromuscular adaptation in, to resistance training, 334
neuromuscular changes in, 333, 333b
preparticipation health screening in, 118
pulmonary system in, 81
references on, 89–92
renal function in, 82–83
resistance training programs for, 361
stages of, 80t
system changes in, 83t
thermoregulation in, 82–83
Agonist muscles, 4, 32
of lower extremities, 24t
of upper extremities, 23t
AHA, (*See* American Heart Association)
AHA/ACSM Health/Fitness Facility Preparticipation Screening Questionnaire, 116–117, 391, *391*
AIDS, (*See* HIV (human immunodeficiency virus) infection)
Air displacement, in body composition analysis, 202
Air pollutants
avoiding, 73
and effect on exercise physiology, 72–74, 274, 406
and National Ambient Air Quality Standards, 73t
outdoor, 72–73
primary and secondary, 72
and short term health effects, 74t
Air quality index (AQI), 388, 405t
Akinesis, in echocardiographic interpretation, 278, 283
Alcohol abuse, 586
Alcohol consumption, dietary, 154
Alendronate, 493
Allosterism, 52
Alpha-glucosidase inhibitors, 474
Altitude, and effect on exercise physiology, 70–72, 274, 406
Altitude sickness, preventing, 72
Alveolar-capillary membrane, 15
Alveoli, 15
major cells of, *15*, 15–16
Amantadine (Symmetrel), 517t, 522t
Ambulatory payment classification (APC) system, 634–635
AMDRs (Acceptable Macronutrient Distribution Ranges), 172
American Association of Cardiovascular and Pulmonary Rehabilitation (AACVPR)